Language Intervention Strategies in Aphasia and Related Neurogenic Communication Disorders

FOURTH EDITION

Language Intervention Strategies in Aphasia and Related Neurogenic Communication Disorders

FOURTH EDITION

Editor

Roberta Chapey, Ed.D.

Professor
Department of Speech Communication Arts and Sciences
Brooklyn College
The City University of New York
Brooklyn, New York

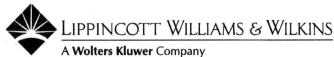

LIPPINCOTT WILLIAMS & WILKINS
A **Wolters Kluwer** Company
Philadelphia • Baltimore • New York • London
Buenos Aires • Hong Kong • Sydney • Tokyo

Editor: John Butler
Managing Editor: Linda S. Napora
Marketing Manager: Christen DeMarco
Production Manager: Susan Rockwell
Compositor: PRD Group
Printer: Courier

The publisher is not responsible (as a matter of product liability, negligence or
otherwise) for any injury resulting from any material contained herein. This
publication contains information relating to general principles of medical care, which
should not be construed as specific instructions for individual patients.
Manufacturers' product information and package inserts should be reviewed for
current information, including contraindications, dosages and precautions.

Printed in the United States of America

First Edition, 1981
Second Edition, 1986
Third Edition, 1994

Library of Congress Cataloging-in-Publication Data is available

*The publishers have made every effort to trace the copyright holders for borrowed material. If they have inadvertently
overlooked any, they will be pleased to make the necessary arrangements at the first opportunity.*

To purchase additional copies of this book, call our customer service department at **(800) 638-3030** or fax
orders to **(301) 824-7390**. International customers should call **(301) 714-2324**.

1   2   3   4   5   6   7   8   9   10   01   02   03   04   05

To the memory of my dad,
Robert (Bob) Chapey,
for his boundless generosity, kindness, love,
understanding, tolerance, support, humanness,
and humor—and for his truly brilliant strategies
for living. He was a super parent.
    R.C.

Preface

Welcome to the first edition of *Language Intervention Strategies in Aphasia and Related Neurogenic Communication Disorders* for the 21st century. The first edition of the book was published in 1981, the second in 1986, and the third in 1994. All three editions of *Language Intervention Strategies in Adult Aphasia* (the original title) grew out of the realization that the discussion of aphasia therapy had become a major theme in clinical aphasiology literature but that the specification of numerous types or strategies of intervention was of fairly recent origin. All four texts grew out of the belief that there continues to be a substantial number of approaches applicable to the remediation of language-disordered adults that should be brought together and shared. The four texts are also grounded in the realization that a variety of different therapeutic principles and approaches need to be articulated, assembled, applied, and critiqued in order to strengthen the quality of future work in our field.

The major purpose of the *Fourth Edition* is to bring together significant thoughts on intervention and to stimulate further developments in the remediation of adult aphasic patients. It is noted, however, that some of the models presented in this text still need to be supported by controlled studies and long-term clinical application.

Each of the editions of the text increasingly moves away from a "container view" of language and communication and is informed by the observation that language is idea-oriented, not word-oriented; that it is socially constructed by participants communicating with someone, about something, for some reason; and that judgments of competence/incompetence involve evaluations about issues such as role, context, content, intent, timing, volume, movements, intonation, gender, age, taste, group membership, etc. (Bloom and Lahey, 1988; Kovarsky, Duchan and Maxwell, 1999). In addition, the **dual goals** of communication—that of **transaction** or the exchange of information and that of **interaction** or the fulfillment of social needs (such as affiliation with other people, assertion of individuality, demonstration of competence, gaining and maintaining membership in social circles, etc.) (Simmons-Mackie, 2001) are increasingly reflected in the texts.

Further, the texts increasingly reflect the fact that we have a responsibility to individuals with aphasia and their significant others to foster their membership in a communicating society and their participation in personally relevant activities (Simmons-Mackie, 2001). Toward that end, there is a growing emphasis on the importance of our role as clinicians, educators, counselors, and advocates for individuals dealing with aphasia, and the importance that support organizations such as the National Aphasia Association (naa@aphasia.org, 800-92204622) and the Well Spouse Foundation (wellspouse@aol.com, www.wellspouse.org, 800-838-0879) can have in their lives. This emphasis also reflects the belief that two of the most important factors in positive human health for all individuals are living a life of purpose and quality connection to others.

Another current theme that affects our practice is a shift away from management by evaluation, control, and bureaucracy to leadership that brings out the best in others. Specifically, leadership by authoritarian, evaluative, military models is no longer seen as preferable since such bullies are seen to have low self-esteem, unresolved anger, and jealousy. Leadership that brings out the best in others (clinicians, clients, significant others, etc.) fosters personal growth and development through inspiration, empowerment, flexibility, creativity, encouragement, caring, support, sensitivity to market and clinical trends, and the provision of appropriate resources.

In addition, the Internet continues to have a major impact on our clinical practice—acting as a bridge to connect us to ideas and resources that add richness and depth to our assessment, intervention, research, advocacy, and counseling techniques. Research into each of these areas continues to expand and inform our clinical practice and leadership styles.

The *Fourth Edition* contains 36 chapters organized in five sections. Section I covers basic considerations such as the incidence of stroke and aphasia, the role of the aphasiologist, the neural basis of language, medical aspects of language assessment and intervention, and the assessment of language and communication. Section II presents five chapters on principles of language intervention such as research methods appropriate to our field, treatment recovery, prognosis, and clinical effectiveness, teams and partnerships in clinical practice, as well as special considerations for the treatment of bilingual and culturally diverse patients. A number of issues related to service delivery are discussed.

Section III contains five chapters on psychosocial and functional approaches to intervention—models that focus on improving ability to perform communication activities of daily living. Such approaches consider the impact of aphasia on the well-being of the individual, their family, and environment. Section IV, the largest section, covers 'Traditional Approaches to Language Intervention.' It is divided into four units containing seven stimulation approaches, four cognitive neuropsychological and three neurolinguistic approaches, and five 'specialized' interventions. Section V provides suggestions for remediation of disorders that frequently accompany aphasia or are related to or confused with aphasia; namely, traumatic brain injury, right hemisphere damage, dementia, apraxia, and dysarthria.

The 36 chapters can be read in any order. In addition, all the chapters do not need to be read at one time. For example, when I teach our graduate course in adult aphasia, I use 12 to 15 chapters as a core, and then refer to other chapters as they come up in class discussions, presentations or term papers, and/or when students ask questions about a specific individual with aphasia that they are observing or working with in clinical practicum. I use the remaining chapters to give additional options, depth, and resources for actual work with individuals affected by aphasia.

Language Intervention Strategies in Aphasia and Related Neurogenic Communication Disorders—Fourth Edition can be used in classes for advanced undergraduate and graduate students in speech language pathology. Clinical aphasiologists who are no longer formal students, but who desire to keep abreast of new ideas in their field will also find the material of interest. Further, the material will be valuable to students and professionals in nursing, medicine, and other health-related disciplines.

Roberta Chapey

References

Bloom, L., and Lahey, M. (1988). *Language Disorders and Language Development*. New York: Macmillan

Kovarsky, D., Duchan, J. F., and Maxwell, M. (1999). Constructing (In) Competence. *Disabling Evaluations in Clinical and Social Interactions*. Mahwah, NJ: Lawrence Erlbaum.

Simmons-Mackie-N. (2001). Social approaches to aphasia intervention. In R. Chapey (Ed.), *Language Intervention Strategies in Aphasia and Related Neurogenic Communication Disorders*—Fourth Ed. Baltimore, MD: Lippincott Williams & Wilkins.

Acknowledgments

To those who have contributed to my personal life and professional career, past and present, I express my deep appreciation. I am also grateful to the authors and publishers who granted me permission to quote from their works.

Many concerned and dedicated people have helped bring this textbook to fruition. Sincere appreciation is extended to each. Special thanks are extended to Bob Marshall for his invaluable suggestions for the organization of the table of contents, to Argye E. (Beth) Hillis for her professionalism and enthusiasm in organizing the section on cognitive neuropsychology, and to Nina Simmons-Mackie, Linda Garcia, Karen Riedel, and Brooke Hallowell for their insightful comments and help. As editor, I would especially like to thank each contributor for helping to make this text a kaleidoscope of enriching and rewarding experiences for me as well as for each of our patients. I am deeply appreciative of their caring and support and for many "one and only moments" of connection.

I am also thankful to the staff of Lippincott Williams & Wilkins for their dedication to making this a first rate text and for facilitating so many relentless details of this project. For the tireless support and help, I thank John Butler, Senior Acquisitions Editor; Linda Napora, Managing Editor; Susan Katz, Vice President, Medical Education and Health Professions; and Tim Satterfield, CEO, Medical Education and Health Professions.

In gratitude for friendship and support, I extend special thanks to my family: my mother, Geraldine, and her significant other, John Dolan; my sister, Geraldine, and my brother in-law, Eugene Pasternack; my ex-husband, Kris Thiruvillakkat, Sr., and my stepsons Kris, Michael, and David Thiruvillakkat; and my cousins Irene, John, and T.J. Hughes; Gerry and Gerry Keck; Michael, Maura, Michael, Brenden, and Liz Chapey, Paul R. Mcrowski, the Murphys, the Chapeys, and to Honore and Peter Beletti, Pat Bombicino, Gerry Cammarata, Meg Cowles, Sr. William Daley, Pummy Dhody, Brian Dumon and Amy Marks, Dottie and Dan Fortini, Lynn Fox, Debra La Perch, Linda and Jim Gardner, Debra Hayden, Ann Jablon, Bette Lane, Barbara Levine, Patty Mattone, Joan and Bob McDougall, Sandy and Jessica Milton, Pat O'Brien, Connie O'Donnel, Helene Pelowitz, Belinda Pennington, Guillermo Pieras, Donna and Frank Prete, Karen Riedel, Karen Roulston, Regina and Irving Schild, Linda Sharlin and Michael Vitale, Diane Solomon and Barry Jarrett, Barbara and Wayne Stonell, Paula Square, Patricia Sweeting, Katherine M. Twyford, Randi Thompson and Jonah Finkelstein, Mary Lu Verderame.

To the faculty and staff of Marymount Manhattan College, for giving me an absolutely outstanding undergraduate education, for their continued support and caring, and for the fun I've had as President of the alumni association, I extend special thanks.

I also extend special thanks to the speech pathology faculty at Columbia University and thank them for their financial and emotional support during my doctoral studies. I mourn the passing of Dr. Edward Mysak, Dr. Eleanor Morrison, Dr. Joan Baken, and Cynthia Contreras. With their passing I have lost special colleagues and friends who were very supportive of my academic career and of me, and the world has lost very unique people.

In addition, I thank the Board and the many members of the NYC Speech Language Hearing Association for their help and support during my tenure as Vice President and then President of the association. I am very grateful for their warmth, enthusiasm, help, and laughter.

And last, but never least, special thanks to all who made Chapey Therapy Consultants, Inc. and Chapey Health Link, Inc. enriching and rewarding personal and professional experiences.

I feel very blessed.

Roberta Chapey

Contributors

Donna L. Bandur, MCISC, CCC-SLP
Professional Practice Leader
Speech-Language Pathology
London Health Sciences Centre
London, Ontario, Canada

Kathryn A. Bayles, PhD, CCC-SLP
Professor and Head
Department of Speech and Hearing Sciences
Associate Director
The National Center for Neurogenic Communication
  Disorders
The University of Arizona
Tucson, Arizona

Pelagie M. Beeson, PhD, CCC-SLP
Assistant Research Scientist
National Center for Neurogenic Communication
  Disorders
Department of Speech and Hearing Sciences
The University of Arizona
Tucson, Arizona

Rita Sloan Berndt, PhD
Department of Neurology
University of Maryland School of Medicine
Baltimore, Maryland

David R. Beukelman, PhD
Professor
Special Education and Communication Disorders
University of Nebraska, Lincoln
Lincoln, Nebraska
University of Nebraska Medical Center
Director of Education and Research
Speech Language Pathology Division
Munroel/Meyer Institute for Genetics and Rehabilitation
Omaha, Nebraska

Arpita Bose, MSc
Doctoral Student
Department of Speech-Language Pathology
Faculty of Medicine
University of Toronto
Toronto, Ontario, Canada

Roberta Chapey, EdD
Professor
Department of Speech Communication Arts and
  Sciences
Brooklyn College
City University of New York
Brooklyn, New York

Leora R. Cherney, PhD, BC-NCD
Associate Professor
Physical Medicine and Rehabilitation
Northwestern University Medical School
Chicago, Illinois
Clinical Educator/Researcher
Communicative Disorders
Rehabilitation Institute of Chicago
Chicago, Illinois

Carl A. Coelho, PhD
Associate Professor
Communication Sciences
University of Connecticut
Storrs, Connecticut
Consultant
Speech Pathology
Rehabilitation Medicine
Hospital for Special Care
New Britain, Connecticut

Hanna Damasio, MD
Professor and Director
Human Neuroanatomy & Neuroimaging
  Laboratory
Department of Neurology
Division of Behavioral Neurology and Cognitive
  Neuroscience
University of Iowa College of Medicine
Iowa City, Iowa

Judith F. Duchan, PhD, CCC
Professor
Department of Communicative Disorders and
  Sciences
State University of New York at Buffalo
Buffalo, New York

Joseph R. Duffy, PhD, CCC, BC-NCD
Professor
Head
Division of Speech Pathology
Department of Neurology
Mayo Clinic
Rochester, MN

Roberta J. Elman, PhD, CCC-SLP, BC-NCD
President/Founder
Aphasia Center of California
Oakland, California

Timothy Feeney
The Wildwood Institute
Schenectady, New York

Linda J. Garcia, PhD, S-LP (C), CCC-SLP
Audiology and Speech-Language Pathology Program
University of Ottawa and SCO Health Service
Ottawa, Ontario, Canada

Lee Ann C. Golper, PhD, BC-NCD
Director
Vanderbilt Bill Wilkerson Center
Nashville, Tennessee

Brooke Hallowell, PhD
Associate Professor
School of Hearing and Speech Sciences
Ohio University
Athens, Ohio

Argye Elizabeth Hillis, MD, MA
Assistant Professor of Neurology
Department of Neurology
Divisions of Cognitive Neurology and Stroke
Johns Hopkins University School of Medicine
Baltimore, Maryland

Tammy Hopper, PhD, CCC-SLP
Department of Speech and Hearing Sciences
The National Center for Neurogenic Communication
  Disorders
The University of Arizona
Tucson, Arizona

Karen Hux, PhD
Associate Professor
Barkley Memorial Center for Special Education
  and Communication Disorders
University of Nebraska at Lincoln
Lincoln, Nebraska

Aura Kagan
Program, Research, and Education Director
The Aphasia Institute
Toronto, Ontario, Canada

Richard C. Katz, PhD, CCC SLP, BC-NCD
Chair
Audiology and Speech Pathology Department
Carl T. Hayden VA Medical Center
Phoenix, Arizona
Adjunct Professor
Department of Speech and Hearing Science
Arizona State University
Tempe, Arizona

Kevin P. Kearns, PhD, CCC
Professor and Director
Communication Sciences and Disorders
Massachusetts General Hospital Institute of Health
  Professions
Boston, Massachusetts

Rosemary Lubinski, EdD, CCC
Professor
Department of Communication Disorders and
  Sciences
University of Buffalo
Amherst, New York

Amy P. Lustig, MEd, MA, CCC-SLP
Communications Sciences and Disorders
University Center for Social and Urban Research
University of Pittsburgh
Pittsburgh, Pennsylvania

Jon G. Lyon, PhD, CCC-SLP
Director
Living with Aphasia, Inc
Mazomanie, Wisconsin

Nancy J. Manasse, M.A., CCC-SLP
University of Nebraska
Lincoln, Nebraska

Robert C. Marshall, PhD, BC-NCD
Professor
Department of Communicative Disorders
University of Rhode Island
Kingston, Rhode Island

Ruth E. Martin, PhD
Assistant Professor
School of Communication Sciences and Disorders
Faculty of Health Sciences
University of Western Ontario
London, Ontario, Canada

Malcolm R. McNeil, PhD
Professor and Chair
Department of Communication Science and
    Disorders
Adjunct Professor
Department of Otolaryngology
University of Pittsburgh
Co-Director
Pittsburgh Aphasia Treatment, Research and
    Education Center
Pittsburgh, Pennsylvania

E. Jeffrey Metter, MD
National Institute on Aging
Gerontology Research Center
Baltimore, Maryland

Charlotte C. Mitchum, MS, CCC (SLP)
Department of Neurology
University of Maryland School of Medicine
Baltimore, Maryland

Anthony G. Mlcoch, PhD
Speech-Language Pathologist
Audiology and Speech Pathology Service
Hines Veterans Affairs Hospital
Hines, Illinois

Shirley Morganstein, MA
Director
Speech and Audiology
Kessler Institute for Rehabilitation
West Orange, New Jersey

Laura L. Murray, PhD, CCC-SLP, SLP (C)
Assistant Professor
Speech and Hearing Sciences
Indiana University
Bloomington, Indiana

Penelope S. Myers, PhD, CCC-SLP
Research Associate
Division of Speech Pathology
Department of Neurology
Mayo Clinic
Rochester, Minnesota

Stephen E. Nadeau, MD
Professor of Neurology
University of Florida College of Medicine
Staff Neurologist
Malcolm Randall Veterans AdministrationVA
    Medical Center
Gainesville, Florida

Richard K. Peach, PhD
Professor
Otolaryngology and Bronchoesophagology and
    Neurological Sciences
Rush Medical College
Chicago, Illinois
Professor
Communication Disorders and Sciences
College of Health Sciences
Rush University
Chicago, Illinois

Bruce E. Porch, PhD
Professor Emeritus
Communicative Disorders/Neurology
University of New Mexico
Albuquerque, New Mexico

Paul R. Rao, PhD
Vice President
Clinical Services
National Rehabilitation Hospital
Washington, District of Columbia
Visiting Professor
Audiology and Speech Language Pathology
Gallaudet University
Washington, District of Columbia
and Visiting Professor
Speech Language Pathology
Loyola College
Baltimore, Maryland

Anastasia M. Raymer, PhD
Assistant Professor
Department of Early Childhood
Speech-Language Pathology and Special Education
Old Dominion University
Norfolk, Virginia

Patricia M. Roberts, PhD, CCC-SLP, SLP(C)
Audiology and Speech Language Pathology Program
University of Ottawa
Ottawa, Ontario, Canada

Randall R. Robey, PhD
Director
Communication Disorders Program
University of Virginia
Charlottesville, Virginia

Leslie J. Gonzalez Rothi, PhD, CCC
Professor of Neurology
Department of Neurology
University of Florida
Gainesville, Florida
Program Director
Neurology Service
Veterans Affairs Medical Center
Gainesville, Florida

Barbara B. Shadden, PhD, CCC-SLP, BC-NCD
Professor and Director
Program in Communication Disorders
University of Arkansas–Fayetteville
Fayetteville, Arkansas

Cynthia M. Shewan, PhD, CCC
Director, Research and Scientific Affairs Department
American Academy of Orthopaedic Surgeons
Rosemont, Illinois

Nina Simmons-Mackie, PhD, BC-NCD
Professor
Department of Communication Sciences and
    Disorders
Southeastern Louisiana University
Hammond, Louisiana

Marilyn Certner Smith, MA
Director of Rehabilitation Sciences, East Facility
Kessler Institute for Rehabilitation
East Orange, New Jersey

Robert W. Sparks, MSc
Chief, Speech Pathology/Audiology (retired)
Veterans Affairs Medical Center
Boston, Massachusetts

Paula A. Square, PhD
Professor and Chair
Department of Speech-Language Pathology
Faculty of Medicine
University of Toronto
Toronto, Ontario, Canada

Shirley F. Szekeres, PhD
Associate Professor
Nazareth College of Rochester
Rochester, New York

Cynthia K. Thompson, PhD
Professor
Department of Communication Sciences and
    Disorders, and Department of Neurology
Northwestern University
Evanston, Illinois

Connie A. Tompkins, PhD, CCC-SLP, BC-NCD
Professor
Department of Communication Science and
    Disorders
University of Pittsburgh
Pittsburgh, Pennsylvania

Amy C. Weiss, MS, CCC-SLP
University of Nebraska-Lincoln
Lincoln, Nebraska

Mark Ylvisaker, PhD
Associate Professor
Department of Communication Disorders
College of Saint Rose
Albany, New York

Contents

Section I

Basic Considerations

Chapter 1

Introduction to Language Intervention Strategies in Adult Aphasia

Roberta Chapey and Brooke Hallowell

OBJECTIVES

The objectives of this chapter are to present both a concise and comprehensive definition of aphasia; present theoretical frameworks for conceptualizing aphasia; review key etiologic factors related to aphasia; highlight the interdisciplinary nature of aphasiology; consider appropriate ways to refer to individuals with aphasia; present a rationale for language intervention for adults with neurogenic communication disorders; and address future trends in aphasiology.

INTRODUCTION

The present text grew out of a desire to bring researchers and practitioners in adult neurogenic communication disorders together to present an accurate and coherent picture of current language practice in assessment and intervention and to make it available in useful form. Foremost is the desire to bring together significant thoughts on language intervention, while stimulating further study concerning the effectiveness of the approaches presented.

Before proceeding with the discussion of specific intervention strategies, we will consider several general issues that are relevant to clinical aphasiology. In this chapter we consider: a brief definition of aphasia; frameworks for conceptualizing aphasia; etiology and epidemiology; the interdisciplinary nature of aphasia; a rationale for intervention; and future trends in aphasiology.

APHASIA BRIEFLY DEFINED

The study of aphasia is complex because of the variable manifestations of aphasia, the heterogeneity of its underlying neurological substrates, and the sophistication required to understand the mechanisms behind its associated symptomatology. Therefore, there are many ways of conceptualizing it. However, students and professionals interested in exploring the world of neurogenic communication disorders often need to be able to articulate a clear and concise definition of aphasia. Such a definition might be **"aphasia" is an acquired communication disorder caused by brain damage, characterized by an impairment of language modalities: speaking, listening, reading and writing;** it is not the result of a sensory deficit, a general intellectual deficit, or a psychiatric disorder (e.g., Brookshire, 1992; Goodglass, 1993).

What is critical to an adequate definition is the mention of four primary facts: it is neurogenic; it is acquired; it affects language; and it excludes general sensory and mental deficits.

1. **Aphasia is neurogenic.** Aphasia always results from some form of damage to the brain. The specific structures affected vary across cases, as do the means by which the damage may occur. Still, the underlying cause of aphasia is always neurological. Aphasia is most often caused by stroke, but may also arise from head trauma, surgical removal of brain tissue, growth of brain tumors, or infections.

2. **Aphasia is acquired.** Aphasia is not characterized as a developmental disorder; an individual is not born with it. Rather, it is characterized by the partial or complete loss of language function in a person who had previously developed some language ability. The term "childhood aphasia" refers to an acquired language problem in children; it is not, by definition, applicable to children who never had language abilities to lose. (Childhood aphasia is not discussed in this text.) It should be noted, though, that children who have suffered neurological incidents such as gunshot wounds, surgical removal of tumors, or even stroke, may develop a true form of "aphasia" if those incidents cause them to lose communication abilities they had already gained earlier in life.

3. **Aphasia involves language problems.** In defining aphasia it is important to recognize that any or all

modalities of symbolic communication may be affected: speaking, listening, reading and writing. Most cases involve some impairments in all four language modalities.

4. **Aphasia is not a problem of sensation or intellect.** Aphasia excludes general sensory and mental deficits. By definition, aphasia does not involve a problem of sight, touch, smell, hearing, or taste. Although aphasia may be *accompanied* by any number of other deficits in perceptual acuity, its definition excludes such deficits. Further, aphasia is not a result of general intellectual deterioration, mental slowing, or psychiatric disturbance. The exclusionary characteristics of the definition of aphasia are especially critical in the differential diagnosis of a wide array of neurogenic communication, cognitive, and perceptual disorders.

CONCEPTUAL FRAMEWORKS OF APHASIA

Although it is simple to define the term "aphasia," there are a number of in-depth definitions or frameworks for studying the nature of aphasia. An understanding of basic differences among ways of conceptualizing aphasia is essential to developing a solid theoretical framework of one's own.

Propositional Language Framework

According to Hughling Jackson, aphasia is an impairment in one's ability to make propositions, or to convey the intent of an utterance (Jackson, 1878). In referring to the "propositional" aspects of language, Jackson emphasizes the intellectual, volitional, and rational aspects of language that involve the use of linguistic symbols for the communication of highly specific and appropriate ideas and relationships. In a proposition, both the words and the manner in which they are related to one another are important. Jackson contrasts propositional aspects of language with subpropositional aspects, which he characterizes as inferior, automatic, highly learned responses (Goodglass & Wingfield, 1977; Head, 1915; Jackson, 1878).

Within this framework, a person with aphasia is seen as having difficulty communicating specific meaning and integrating words into particular contexts to express specific ideas and relationships. Patients may know words, but may habitually use them incorrectly, and often fail at embedding words in a variety of sentence forms. Jackson noted that even when propositional language is impaired, many patients retain automatic language. For example, even with severe propositional deficits, an individual may be able to name the days of the week, complete sentences such as "The grass is____," or produce highly learned responses such as "Hi. How are you?"

According to proponents of the framework, an individual with aphasia has an impairment in the use of spontaneous language to communicate *specific meaning*. The more propositional language required in a particular communication context, the more the patient is impaired. Assessment involves an analysis of the patient's ability to use spontaneous speech to express specific ideas. Intervention focuses on stimulation of the patient's ability to use propositional language.

Concrete-Abstract Framework

Goldstein and Scheerer (1948) observed that having an "abstract attitude" implies an ability to react to things in a conceptual manner. This attitude is necessary to isolate properties that are common to several objects, and for the formulation of concepts as opposed to sensory impressions of individual objects. It is also used to comprehend relationships between objects and events in the world. An abstract attitude gives the individual the power to inhibit actions or reactions and to use past experiences. These experiences help the individual organize perceptual rules and therefore to create and continue interactions with other people. Language that reflects an abstract attitude is propositional language. In contrast, the individual in the concrete attitude passively responds to reality and is bound to the immediate experience of objects and situations. Concrete language consists of speech automations, emotional utterances, sounds, words, and series of words (Goldstein & Scheerer, 1948) (see Table 1–1).

In general, impairment in abstract attitude is reflected in propositional language. If one cannot abstract, one cannot symbolize or embed symbols in appropriate contexts. An individual who is impaired in abstract attitude, then, is unable to consider things that are possibilities rather than actualities, to keep in mind simultaneously various aspects of a situation, to react to two stimuli that do not belong intrinsically together, to inhibit reactions, and to ideationally isolate parts of a whole (see Table 1–1).

Goldstein and Scheerer (1948) developed a number of tests of ability to assume the abstract attitude. The tests include object sorting tasks involving form, color, and combined color and form sorting. When observing sorting test results, one may ask: Is the sort concrete (perceptual) or abstract (conceptual)? Can the individual verbally account for a sort presented by the examiner (abstract)? The intervention implications of this framework would be to stimulate the patient to comprehend and produce language that is increasingly more abstract.

Thought Process Framework

Wepman (1972a) suggested that aphasia may be a thought process disorder in which impairment of semantic expression is the result of an impairment of thought processes that "serve as the catalyst for verbal expression" (p. 207). He noted that patients with aphasia frequently substitute words that are associated with words they are attempting to produce, and that the remainder of the individual's communicative effort appears to relate to the approximated rather than the intended word. An inaccurate verbal formulation may lead

TABLE 1–1

The Abstract-Concrete Model of Aphasia[a]

Abstract	Concrete
• Adaptive behavior	• Adaptive behavior
• Propositional	• Nonpropositional (automatic, serial content, social gesture)
• Assumes a mental set voluntarily and volitionally, and a conceptual framework	• Unable to assume a mental set . . . interruption disrupts behavior
• Takes initiative (begins performance)	• Unreflexive, passive
• Actions determined by the way the individual thinks about them	• Actions determined by objects
• Shifts voluntarily from one aspect of a situation to another, making a choice	• Reactive, unable to shift to a new situation, perseverates (no rule to change)
• Keeps various aspects of a situation in mind simultaneously	• Impressed by one property exclusively—experiences only this one and reacts to it
• Reacts to two stimuli that do not belong intrinsically together	• Cannot react to two stimuli that do not belong intrinsically together
• Conscious, aware, volitional, rational, reasoning	
• Grasps essential of given whole	• Cannot grasp essential of given whole
• Permits use of past experience to form rules and to continue	• Reacts to "here and now" only
• Breaks whole into parts, isolating them voluntarily and combining them to wholes	• Cannot grasp essentials of a given whole
• Abstracts common properties, transcends the immediate	• Deals with "here and now"; deals with the specific or immediate sense impressions
• Plans ahead ideationally	• Deals with the "here and now"; no rule to change
• Assumes an attitude toward the merely possible	• Thinking and acting are determined by the immediate claims made by the particular aspect of an object or situation
• Able to account to oneself, to verbally account for what one does	
• Thinks and performs symbolically	
• Detaches ego from the outer world and inner experience	• Cannot detach ego from inner experience; reacts to "here and now"—immediate sense impressions
• Permits inhibition	• Reacts to "here and now"

[a]From Goldstein, K. (1948). *Language and language disturbances.* New York: Grune & Stratton.

to interference with thought processes, as there is a drive to establish consonance between the thought process and the actual utterance. For example, if a patient is trying to say "circle" and instead utters "square," the concept of circle may be modified to be consistent with the utterance, and the patient may begin to think of a circle as a square.

Individuals who cannot retrieve the most appropriate lexical symbol for a context are impaired in their ability to communicate a number and variety of specific propositional ideas. When the continued efforts relate to the approximated rather than the intended word, spontaneous language becomes even more impaired.

Within a framework in which aphasia is seen primarily as a disorder of thought process, assessment involves determining if individuals can follow a train of thought in their communication or spontaneous language, and if they can expand on topics and ideas. For Wepman (1972b, 1976), the first stage of therapy is thought-centered or content-centered discussion

in which patients are stimulated to attend to their thoughts and remain on topic. During the second stage of therapy, patients are encouraged to elaborate on various topics.

Unidimensional Framework

A unidimensional view of aphasia relates language behaviors to a single common denominator. The expressive and receptive, as well as the semantic and syntactic components of language are considered to be inseparable. This view suggests that damage to the language mechanism results in general language impairment in which there is an effect on all aspects of language. Aphasiologists who subscribe to this framework **do not** promote the use of Broca's-Wernicke's, fluent-nonfluent, sensory-motor, receptive-expressive, or input-output dichotomies in aphasia.

One of the most popular and in-depth unidimensional theories, that proposed by Schuell and her colleagues (Schuell et al., 1964), regards aphasia as a general language impairment that crosses all language modalities: speaking, listening, reading, and writing. These authors noted that the behaviors impaired in aphasia involve integrations that cannot be attributed merely to organization of motor responses or to events in outgoing pathways; rather, they involve use of an ability that is dependent on higher-level integrations.

According to proponents of this framework, aphasia is not modality specific. Rather, it involves the inability to access or retrieve words and rules of an acquired language for communication (Schuell et al., 1964). The person with aphasia has lost functional spontaneous language, or the ability to use connected language units to communicate according to the established conventions of the language. Schuell's concept of the cause of this general language breakdown reflects a broad and dynamic view of the language process.

The assessment implications of the unidimensional framework involve an analysis of the patient's ability to comprehend and produce language within all four modalities, and in contexts ranging from single words to spontaneous discourse. Schuell's test, the Minnesota Test for Differential Diagnosis of Aphasia (MTDDA) (Schuell, 1973) is based on this model (see Chapters 4 and 17).

The intervention applications are similarly unidimensional and multimodal. Treatment focus is on stimulation, the use of strong, controlled, and intensive auditory activation of the impaired symbol system in order to maximize patient reorganization of language. The clinician manipulates and controls specific dimensions of stimuli in order to make complex events happen in the brain, thus aiding the patient in making maximal responses (see Chapter 17).

Microgenetic View

Brown (1972, 1977, 1979) and Brown and Perecman (1986) challenge the notion that language production can be explained by an array of cortical speech centers and connecting pathways that convey memories and images from one processing center to another. These authors propose an alternative conceptual framework in which language processing is conceived as an event that emerges over different levels of the brain corresponding to different levels of evolutionary development, not across specific cortical areas. Phylogenetically older limbic mechanisms are thought to mediate early stages in cognition and linguistic representation, while the more recently evolved left lateralized neocortex (encompassing Broca's and Wernicke's areas) mediates the final stages in cognition and linguistic processing. Having evolved from common limbic structures, the anterior and posterior language zones are considered to be fundamentally united. **Language is considered to be processed simultaneously by complementary systems in the anterior and posterior part of the brain, rather than sequentially from one component to the next.** The function of cerebral pathways is

considered to be the coordination of different regions of the brain rather than the mere conveyance of information between regions.

According to this view, varying forms of aphasia correspond to lesions of brain structures that have emerged at varying stages of evolution. A lesion in one of the language areas of the brain gives rise to the relative prominence of an earlier stage of language processing. Thus, the symptoms of aphasia serve to magnify the processing events that, in normal language, would be mediated by the lesioned area. According to Brown and Perecman (1986), treatment focuses on facilitation of the transition from one stage to the next in the microgenetic sequence.

Multidimensional Frameworks

Proponents of a multidimensional framework conceptualize aphasia as having multiple forms, each corresponding to a different underlying site of lesion and having a characteristic list of hallmark features. For individuals who hold a multidimensional view of aphasia, assessment involves determining what symptomatology is present and subsequently classifying a patient in one category or another. Some conceptualize aphasia dichotomously, for example, as Broca's versus Wernicke's, fluent versus nonfluent, semantic versus syntactic, or anterior versus posterior. Usually, such dichotomies are associated with the cerebral localization of the lesions that result in aphasia. The Boston Diagnostic Aphasia Examination (BDAE) (Goodglass & Kaplan, 1983), the Western Aphasia Battery (Kertesz, 1982; Kertesz & Poole, 1974), and the Language Modalities Test for Aphasia (Wepman & Jones, 1961) reflect such classification systems. Intervention, according to this framework, is oriented toward specific deficits. That is, the clinician attempts to rehabilitate a specific language modality (such as speaking) or behavior (such as confrontation naming or phonemic production) that is found to be impaired (c.f., Cubelli et al., 1988).

Classification of Multidimensional Types of Aphasia

For the sake of simplicity and presentation of basic terminology, one may consider the basic subtypes of aphasia across different multidimensional classification schemes to fall into the categories of "fluent," "nonfluent," and "other" aphasias. The reader should be aware, though, that the terms fluent and nonfluent are not highly descriptive terms in and of themselves. It is important to specify what is meant by the use of these terms when describing the language of any individual patient. An individual may appear to be nonfluent for any of a variety of reasons, or according to any of a large array of measures. Generally, persons with aphasia are considered fluent if they are able to speak in spontaneous conversation without abnormal pauses, abundant nonmeaningful filler phrases, or long periods of silence. Nonfluent patients tend to have a reduced rate of speech and to express less communicative content per unit of time than normal speakers do. Of course, patients who are completely nonverbal are nonfluent. Damasio (1998) presents an excellent synopsis of the various categorical terms used throughout the history of the study of aphasia. A more thorough discussion of the classification of aphasia according to neuroanatomical substrates is presented by Hannah Damasio in the next chapter.

Fluent Aphasias

There are three basic types of fluent aphasia: conduction aphasia, Wernicke's aphasia, and transcortical sensory aphasia.

Wernicke's Aphasia. The critical features of Wernicke's aphasia are impaired auditory and reading comprehension and fluently articulated but paraphasic speech (Goodglass & Kaplan, 1983) in which syntactic structure is relatively preserved. In many cases, patients with Wernicke's aphasia present with logorrhea, or press of speech, characterized by excessive verbal production. Paraphasias are most often in the form of sound transpositions and word substitutions (Goodglass et al., 1964). Patients with Wernicke's aphasia experience naming difficulty that is severe in relation to their fluent spontaneous speech (Goodglass et al. 1964). Neologisms are frequent. Those who produce frequent neologistic expressions are often unintelligible and are sometimes referred to as having "jargon aphasia" (Wepman & Jones, 1961). Patients with Wernicke's aphasia also have difficulty reading, writing, and repeating words (Damasio, 1998). They often demonstrate a lack of awareness of their deficits, especially compared to patients with other types of aphasia. Some authors and many clinicians use the term "receptive aphasia" to refer to the disability of patients with Wernicke's aphasia because of their primary deficit in the area of linguistic comprehension. Likewise, because lesions that lead to this form of aphasia tend to be located in the temporal lobe, Wernicke's aphasia represents a classic form of "posterior" aphasia.

Conduction Aphasia. The speech of persons with conduction aphasia is fluent, although generally less abundant than the speech of those with Wernicke's aphasia (Damasio, 1998). A hallmark feature is impaired repetition of words and sentences relative to fluency in spontaneous speech, which is often normal or near normal. Auditory comprehension is also relatively spared (Goodglass & Kaplan, 1983). Most patients "repeat words with phonemic paraphasias, but often they will omit or substitute words, and they may fail to repeat anything at all if function words rather than nouns are requested" (Damasio, 1998, p. 35). Literal paraphasias repeatedly interfere with speech.

Transcortical Sensory Aphasia (TSA). Individuals with TSA have fluent, well-articulated speech with frequent paraphasias and neologisms (Goodglass & Kaplan, 1983). Global paraphasias occur more frequently than phonemic paraphasias (Damasio, 1998). A key feature that differentiates TSA from conduction aphasia is intact repetition ability. Auditory comprehension is generally poor. Confrontation naming is impaired, and the patient may offer an irrelevant response or echo the words of the examiner (Goodglass & Kaplan, 1983).

Nonfluent Aphasias

There are three basic types of nonfluent aphasia: Broca's, transcortical motor, and global aphasia.

Broca's Aphasia. Broca's aphasia is the most classic form of nonfluent aphasia. It is often considered the "opposite" of Wernicke's aphasia (Damasio, 1998, p. 35). The essential characteristics of Broca's aphasia include awkward articulation, restricted vocabulary, agrammatism, and relatively intact auditory and reading comprehension (Goodglass & Kaplan, 1983). Typically, writing is at least as severely impaired as speech. Persons with Broca's aphasia are usually aware of their communicative deficits, and are more prone to depression and sometimes catastrophic reactions than are patients with other forms of aphasia. Some authors and clinicians use the term "expressive aphasia" to refer to the disability of patients with Broca's aphasia because of their primary deficit in the area of language formulation and production. Likewise, because lesions that lead to this form of aphasia tend to be located in the frontal lobe, Broca's aphasia represents a classic form of "anterior" aphasia.

Transcortical Motor Aphasia (TMA). In patients with TMA, repetition is intact relative to "otherwise limited speech" (Goodglass & Kaplan, 1983). Such patients exhibit phonemic and global paraphasias, syntactic errors, perseveration, and difficulty imitating and organizing responses in conversation (Damasio, 1998; Goodglass & Kaplan, 1983). Confrontation naming is usually preserved, but auditory comprehension is impaired.

Global Aphasia. Global aphasia is a disorder of language characterized by impaired linguistic comprehension and expression. It is often considered a combination of both Wernicke's and Broca's aphasia. Patients with global aphasia tend to produce few utterances and have a highly restricted lexicon. They have little or no understanding in any modality and little or no ability to communicate (Wepman & Jones, 1961).

Other Forms of Aphasia

Anomic Aphasia. Anomic aphasia is a form of aphasia characterized primarily by significant word retrieval problems (Damasio, 1998; Goodglass, 1993; Goodglass & Wingfield,

1997). It is differentiated from the symptom of anomia, or dysnomia, which is typical in most forms of aphasia. Speech is generally fluent except for the hesitancies and pauses associated with word finding deficits. Grammar is generally intact.

Primary Progressive Aphasia. Primary progressive aphasia is a type of aphasia that has an insidious rather than an acute onset. The term "primary" refers to the fact that deficits in language are the primary symptoms noted, with cognitive skills remaining intact relative to linguistic skills. The term "progressive" refers to the fact that the condition is degenerative, with communication skills worsening over time. The underlying etiology for progressive aphasia may be any of a number of degenerative diseases affecting the brain. Many patients with this form of aphasia eventually present with significant cognitive deficits as part of a syndrome of dementia (Ceccaldi et al., 1996; Damasio, 1998).

Alexia and Agraphia. Alexia, a deficit in reading ability, occurs in most forms of aphasia, especially in those involving significant auditory comprehension deficits, such as Wernicke's aphasia or TSA. Consequently, it is very infrequently considered a form of aphasia in and of itself. There are some rare patients, though, who present with deficits in reading that are markedly more severe than other communicative deficits, such as auditory comprehension and speech. Such forms of alexia may occur with or without agraphia, a deficit in writing ability. Forms of aphasia involving alexia with and without agraphia are described in formidable detail by Damasio and Damasio (1983), Goodglass (1993), and Geschwind (1965).

Exceptions to Multidimensional Aphasia Subtypes

Numerous systems for the multidimensional categorization of aphasia have been proposed. Further, most textbooks addressing aphasia offer creative means of categorizing the various subtypes of aphasia based on derivations of previous authors' suggestions. Acknowledging the diversity in diagnostic criteria and nomenclature used throughout the history of the study of aphasia, A. Damasio (1998) refers to the task of classifying the subtypes of aphasia as a "necessary evil" (p. 32). Most aphasiologists might agree with Damasio that "attempting to review the classification systems of aphasia is probably foolhardy" (p. 32). Most clinical aphasiologists attest to the fact that it is common to meet patients with forms of aphasia that do not fit neatly into any one category described according to a known multidimensional classification scheme (c.f., Caplan & Chertkow, 1989). Even those with a form of aphasia that fits a particular classification at one point in time may demonstrate a different form of aphasia as their condition evolves. Patients with right or bilateral cerebral

dominance for language functions, subcortical lesions, degenerative conditions, traumatic brain injury, and multiple or unknown sites of lesion often present further challenges to the classification of aphasia subtypes, as explored in other chapters of this book. Still, it is essential that those studying aphasia and working with people who have aphasia understand traditional multidimensional models of classification. Such an understanding helps ensure improved communication among clinicians and researchers, improve the validity and reliability of diagnostic reporting, clarify theoretical differences in how experts differ in their ways of conceptualizing aphasia, and highlight the similarities and distinctions between one's idealized concept of any subtype of aphasia as compared to the actual manifestations of aphasia in an individual patient.

Psycholinguistic/Problem Solving/Information Processing Framework

Psycholinguistic approaches to language recognize its three integrated and interrelated components: cognition, language and communication (Muma, 1978) and the integration of language content, form, and use (Bloom & Lahey, 1978). **Content** involves meaning. Language refers to the structures of language or the rule-based systems of phonology, morphology, syntax, and semantics. **Communication** involves the use, purpose, or function that a particular utterance or gesture serves at any one time and its contextual realization. **Cognition** involves the acquisition of knowledge of the world, and the continued processing of this knowledge. It refers to all of the mental processes by which information is transformed, reduced, elaborated, stored, recovered and used (Neisser, 1997). According to Chapey (1994) cognition can be operationally defined as the mental operations in the Guilford (1967) Structure-of-Intellect Model, namely, recognition/understanding, memory, and convergent, divergent and evaluative thinking (see Chapter 17).

According to Chapey (1986; 1994), a psycholinguistic view of aphasia may be defined as an acquired impairment in language content, form and use and the cognitive processes that underlie language, such as memory and thinking (convergent, divergent, and evaluative thinking). The impairment may be manifested in listening, speaking, reading, and writing, although not necessarily to the same degree in each.

Chapey (1994) also suggests that aphasia is an impairment in problem solving and information processing. Problem solving and information processing both involve the use of all five cognitive operations (recognition/understanding, memory, and convergent, divergent and evaluative thinking), the four types of content [figural, symbolic, semantic (content, form and use) and behavioral (use/pragmatics)] and five products or associations (units, classes, relations, systems, and transformations) of the Guilford (1967) model (see Chapter 17). The specific components that are used depend upon the problem presented and/or the information being processed.

Within this model, assessment of individuals with aphasia centers on an analysis of the cognitive, linguistic, and communicative strengths and weaknesses (Chapey, 1986; 1994) of each individual. Intervention focuses on the stimulation of these abilities, but especially the stimulation of the cognitive processes underlying language comprehension and production (see Chapter 17).

Body Structure and Function, Activity, and Participation Framework

The World Health Organization (WHO) has launched a worldwide effort to re-define functioning and disability in an effort to heighten awareness of its holistic components and the very complex interaction of conditions within the individual and in the environment that affect functioning. The three levels proposed for this International Classification of Functioning and Disability (ICIDH-2, 1999) are body structure and function, activity, and participation.

Such terminology represents a move away from the classic biomedical model and takes into consideration both the organic and the complex functional consequences of disease. It enables us "to deconstruct the social exclusion creation process" and prevents us from saying "that persons are responsible for the social consequences of their disease" (Fougeyrollas et al., 1997, p. 15). Fougeyrollas et al.'s (1997) system, based on the WHO ICIDH-2, shows the dynamic interaction of important variables such as risk factors/causes, personal factors such as organic systems and capabilities, environmental factors, and life habits of social participation in the "Handicap Creation Process" (Fougeyrollas et al., 1997). For example, a consistent and dependable support system will likely decrease the impact of impairment; a depressed, uninvolved spouse may increase it. Therefore, all individuals in the environment and the environment itself impact functioning and participation in life (see Chapter 10).

This literature also focuses on the fact that the core features of positive human health or well-being involve leading a life of purpose, quality connection to others (and zest for life comes from such connections), positive self-regard, and mastery (Kahneman et al., 1999; Ryff & Singer, 1998). Unfortunately, subsequent to the loss of language due to stroke, all of these areas are affected not only for the individual with aphasia but for significant individuals in their environment. This, in turn, impacts their health, well-being, and quality of life.

For individuals with aphasia, **body structure and function** refers to impairments of brain and brain functions. **Activity limitations** primarily involve the four language modalities: speaking, listening, reading and writing (see also Chapter 4) as well as tasks necessary for daily living such as conversing with the nurse or family member, writing a check, making a phone call, reading a paper or menu, and so forth. These modalities have been the traditional focus of assessment and intervention in aphasia. During the last ten years, such functional tasks have increasingly been the focus of care. Current thinking also includes **participation** in daily life and realizing immediate and long-term real life goals (LPAA, 2000) (see Chapter 10). This might include playing golf, shopping for clothes, getting a job, going on vacation, participating in clubs and organizations, and so forth. How aphasia might affect these activities is the concern of such classifications as the ICIDH-2 and the Handicap Creation Process. Communication is seen as an integral part of the execution/involvement of life participation events. Therefore, the National Joint Committee for the Communicative Needs of Persons with Severe Disabilities defines communication as "a basic need and basic right of all human beings" (National Joint Committee, 1992, p. 2) (see Chapter 10).

Within this framework, assessment and treatment target all three areas from day one. Without a cause to communicate, there is no practical need for communication. Therefore, assessment and treatment focus on a reason to communicate as much as on communication repair. In addition, as a result of these classifications, there is an increased interest in focusing on the social and physical environmental factors which might contribute to full participation.

This approach to intervention also encourages us to advocate for our clients "to seek modifications in the socioeconomic organization, to act on attitudes and social representations, and to make resources and compensatory and adaptive services" available for functional and life participation differences (Fougeyrollas et al., 1997, p. 15).

ETIOLOGY AND EPIDEMIOLOGY OF STROKE AND APHASIA OF STROKE

Stroke

Stroke, or cerebrovascular accident (CVA), is the most prevalent cause of aphasia. A stroke occurs when blood flow to an area of the brain is interrupted by the blockage of a blood vessel or artery, or by the rupturing of an artery. Blood carries essential nutrients, especially glucose and oxygen, to brain cells. Since brain cells do not have the capacity to store these nutrients, they are in need of constant blood supply. Even brief periods of interruption in blood supply to the brain can have lasting devastating effects on brain tissue (see Chapters 2 and 3).

Stroke is the third leading cause of death in the United States and the most common cause of adult disability (Centers for Disease Control, 1999; Zivin & Choi, 1991). Zivin and Choi (1991) note that in the United States "of approximately 500,000 new victims each year, roughly 30 percent die, and 20 to 30 percent become severely and permanently disabled" (p. 56). Thus, for at least 40 percent of those who survive, stroke is a seriously crippling disease. Many survivors have lasting problems with movement and motor control of the body, perceptual deficits, cognitive problems, and swallowing disorders, as well as problems of speech and language.

There are several types of stroke. Chapters 2 & 3 contain a discussion of the most common forms of stroke leading to aphasia, namely thrombotic, embolic, and hemorrhagic strokes.

Incidence of Aphasia

Statistics regarding the incidence of aphasia and of the various subtypes of aphasia are variable, due to subject sampling and description methods (c.f., Scarpa et al., 1987). Marquardsen (1969) estimates that approximately one-third of patients who survive the first week of stroke have aphasia. Pedersen et al., (1995) demonstrate incidences as high as 40 percent in patients evaluated within the first three days of stroke. Scarpa et al. (1987) estimate that about 55 percent of patients with strokes affecting the left hemisphere have aphasia when examined 15 to 30 days after a stroke. Approximately 80,000 Americans develop aphasia each year, leaving more than a million Americans with this seriously handicapping condition (Brody, 1992; National Institute for Deafness and Other Communication Disorders, 1999). According to the National Institute for Deafness and Other Communication Disorders (1999), about one million people in the United States currently have aphasia.

Risk Factors for Stroke and Aphasia

Although some studies have reported gender differences in the incidence of aphasia and in the location of associated lesions (Kimura, 1980; McGlone, 1980), other researchers have discounted such findings (Hier et al., 1994; Pedersen et al., 1995; Scarpa et al., 1987). Likewise, handedness does not appear to have a significant effect on stroke incidence or severity (Pedersen et al., 1995). Diagnoses of hypertension, diabetes, and high cholesterol are factors that increase an individual's likelihood of experiencing stroke and aphasia, as are lifestyle factors of smoking, stress, inactivity, excessive consumption of alcohol, and dietary intake high in cholesterol, fat and sodium (Centers for Disease Control, 1999; Flack & Yunis, 1997; Kuller, 1995; Yusuf et al., 1998). Additionally, access to health care is a critical factor in prevention, as well as in recovery through medical and rehabilitative treatment following stroke.

While advancing age is consistently associated with stroke (Stegmayr et al., 1994), reports of the influence of age on the incidence of aphasia within stroke patient populations have not been substantiated in studies employing controlled sampling and subject description methods (Habib et al., 1987; Miceli et al., 1981).

Data from the 42-year-long Framingham Study conducted by the National Institutes of Health (Willich, 1987) suggest that strokes are twice as likely to occur between 6 A.M. and noon than at any other time of the day and that more than half (especially hemorrhagic strokes) occur on Mondays. Other studies have confirmed this finding, attributing it to the fact that those times correspond to periods when the body's supply and demand for oxygen is at its greatest level of imbalance, that is, when there is an increase in oxygen requirements simultaneous with reduced levels of blood flow (Flack & Yunis, 1997).

Racial, Ethnic, and Cultural Factors Influencing Incidence of Stroke and Aphasia

Many researchers report an influence of racial and ethnic origins on the incidence of stroke and aphasia. Stroke mortality is generally reported to be substantially higher in African American and Hispanic populations than in Caucasians (Gaines, 1997; Sacco et al., 1998). Discrepancies among reports on the relationship of race and ethnicity to stroke and aphasia may be attributable to sampling methods and to the sophistication and accuracy of diagnostic methods (c.f., Gillum, 1994; 1995). Most of the racial differences in the incidence of stroke and aphasia may be accounted for by differences in cultural influences on such lifestyle factors as diet, exercise, smoking, and access to health care services (Kuller, 1995). Persons of lower socioeconomic status also have higher risk factors for stroke, further influencing epidemiological studies of stroke and aphasia (Centers for Disease Control, 1999). The role of race, ethnicity, socioeconomic status, and culture have important implications not only for the incidence of aphasia, but also for its diagnosis and treatment. It is for this reason that an entire chapter of this book and several components of other chapters are devoted to multicultural issues pertinent to intervention in adult aphasia.

Geographic location appears to play an important role in the prevalence and incidence rates of stroke and aphasia. For example, the southeastern region of the United States has been labeled by many as the "Stroke Belt" because of higher stroke mortality rates than other geographic areas, even when researchers account for age, gender, and race. Regional differences appear to be primarily influenced by the levels of risk factors such as high blood pressure, obesity, poor diet, and smoking, not on the physical properties of the areas involved (Casper et al., 1995; Centers for Disease Control, 1999; Gaines, 1997).

Etiologies Other Than Stroke

Much of the empirical literature on aphasia is based on the study of patients who acquired aphasia because of a cerebrovascular accident. There are two good reasons for this. First, the majority of patients who have a clear and definite diagnosis of aphasia have had a stroke. Second, because stroke patients tend to have well-defined, localizable focal lesions, the etiologies associated with their manifestations of aphasia can be documented in research reports and controlled for in experimental paradigms, making such patients attractive research participants. Still, it is important to acknowledge that there are many other etiologies that may be associated with aphasia. For example, patients who have experienced traumatic brain injury, neoplasm, degenerative conditions, or exposure to neurotoxic agents often present with aphasia. The diffuse brain damage and frequently ill-defined sites of lesion associated with such etiologies preclude a large volume of controlled research pertaining specifically to aphasia in these complex populations. It is nonetheless important to recognize and treat patients who have aphasia regardless of the underlying cause.

While the nature of aphasia is not always best studied with non-stroke populations, there is a growing body of treatment research pertaining to such populations. This book includes several chapters that address issues especially relevant to intervention with patients with traumatic brain injury and dementing illness. Additionally, much of what has been learned about the treatment of aphasia in stroke patients may be applied to the treatment of acquired neurogenic communication problems in other patient populations.

Other Acquired Neurogenic Disorders

The study of aphasia is vitally related to the study of other acquired neurogenic disorders. Clinical aphasiologists are ideally trained in the diagnosis and treatment of a host of neurogenic conditions and have a solid understanding of their underlying neuropathologies. Academic knowledge and clinical expertise in the areas of dementia and other cognitive disorders, right brain damage, traumatic brain injury, motor speech disorders, confusional states, and normal aging are essential to excellence in clinical aphasiology. Also of increasing importance is competence in the area of dysphagia because of the critical relationships among the acquired neurogenic disorders that each of these areas have to one another. Each of these are addressed in the current text.

Prevention

Data pertaining to risk factors enable researchers, clinicians, and laypersons to better reduce the likelihood of any individual experiencing the life-altering consequences of stroke and aphasia. Recognizing the tremendous cost-saving advantages of preventing stroke, many health insurance companies have launched programs to promote wellness and help reduce consumers' risk of stroke (Thomas, 1997). Key lifestyle changes to reduce the risk of stroke and aphasia include dietary modification (e.g., reduced cholesterol and sodium intake, increased dietary fiber, vitamin therapy, moderation of consumption of caffeine and alcohol, and weight reduction

in overweight patients), increased physical activity, smoking cessation, and stress reduction (He & Whelton, 1997; Khaw, 1996; Shinton, 1997). Numerous pharmacological treatments reduce the risk of stroke by helping to control hypertension and blood lipids (Centers for Disease Control, 1999). In light of the increased risk of stroke in the early morning hours and on Mondays, scheduling of stressful tasks at times other than these is advised, as is the careful timing of the daily administration of anti-hypertensive medications (Flack & Yunis, 1997).

Many preventive health programs also target factors such as those discussed in an article entitled "The Contours of Positive Human Health" by Ryff and Singer (1998). These authors focus on the core features of positive human health, well-being and quality of life, namely, leading a life of purpose (life participation), quality connection to others (zest for life comes from such connections), positive self-regard, and mastery (see also Kahneman et al., 1999). Active intervention programs focusing on these factors is especially important for patients and their significant others in order to prevent further illness such as additional strokes in individuals with aphasia (see section "Impairment, Activities, Participation In Life") and disease in their significant others.

Aging and Communication

The past three decades have brought an increasing interest in age-related changes in adults. Toward this end, numerous professionals have measured cognition, perception, sensation, mobility, communication, and other neurological and psychological systems in an attempt to identify key variables that may or may not change with age. Although an increase in incidence with age is reported for many diseases and other problems affecting the cardiovascular, pulmonary, gastrointestinal, genitourinary, hematological, musculoskeletal, metabolic, and endocrine systems (Abrams & Berko, 1990), some research has focused on positive changes and functioning in the elderly. The "myth... that to be old is to be sick, sexless and senile" (Frady et al., 1985) is being countered by many vigorous and independent aging adults. In fact, there has been gradual improvement in the overall health of the elderly (Manton et al., 1998). The majority of those who are over 85 are continuing to care for themselves (Elias, 1992).

Studies suggesting relationships between age and health or cognitive factors are often confounded by concomitant problems faced by elderly individuals. For example, those who perform poorly on mental ability tests may have other problems, such as depression, amnesia, dementia, vitamin deficiencies, or alcoholism. Additionally, they may be hindered by medications, including sedatives and/or nonsteroidal anti-inflammatory drugs, or by environmental insults such as pollution and stress (Allison, 1991).

Evidence of neurobiological changes that may come with age can be derived from animal research, which suggests that elderly animals are as capable of growing new connections between brain cells as are younger animals (Wu et al., 1999). This also appears to be true in humans (Saurwein-Teissl et al., 1998). New neuroimaging and behavioral methods, as well as evolving technology for the molecular study of the nervous system, have allowed researchers to conclude that, despite the loss of neurons with aging, the brain undergoes continuous adaptation as it ages. Some authors (e.g., Eriksson et al., 1998) have recently presented claims that support the possibility of regenerating nerve cells in the hippocampi of older adults. One type of neuron in the brain replete with the enzyme acetylcholinesterase (necessary for communication among cells) "actually becomes more abundant during adulthood, and is preserved in healthy older people" (Allison, 1991, p. 7). Mesulam (as cited in Allison, 1991) claims that such age-related changes may underlie "wisdom," suggesting that "programmed neuronal death and the growth of new connections could be the brain's way of sculpting new and better pathways" (p. 8).

INTERDISCIPLINARY APPROACHES TO APHASIOLOGY

The study of aphasia and related neurogenic communication disorders is inherently interdisciplinary (see Chapter 8). Although clinical practice in intervention for patients with aphasia requires specific training, certification and/or licensure in much of the world, the study of aphasia does not fall within the bounds of any single discipline. The disciplines that help understand the nature of neurogenic communication disorders and provide the most effective intervention include speech-language pathology, audiology, neuroscience, cognitive science, biology, engineering, physics, psychology, pharmacology, linguistics, communication, social work, counseling, anthropology, sociology, multiculturalism, mathematics, rehabilitation, physiatry, neurology, gerontology, physical therapy, occupational therapy, music therapy, and health care administration. This list is far from exhaustive. It is interesting to note that many of the disciplines just mentioned are also hybrid ones, drawing from basic science, theory, and practice in a variety of content areas. Thus, the student or professional who is truly committed to the study of aphasia must also be committed to life-long learning across disciplinary boundaries.

A NOTE ON REFERRING TO PERSONS WITH APHASIA

Before progressing with further study of aphasia and its management, it is important to note that the term "aphasic" is not a noun but an adjective, just as are most of the words we use to describe disabilities. While one might defend the stylistic use of the adjectival form as a label for a person who

has aphasia ("an aphasic"), such labeling may convey a lack of respect for, and sensitivity toward, individuals who have aphasia (Brookshire, 1992).

Indeed, the WHO has launched worldwide efforts to modify the ways in which we refer to persons with disabilities (see p. 9). The WHO classification emphasizes that disablement is not considered an attribute of an individual, but rather the complex interactions of conditions involving a person in the context of his or her social environment (World Health Organization, 1999). Health care professionals and researchers throughout the world are following suit by de-emphasizing the reference to individuals according to medically based diagnostic categories, focusing instead on their holistic functional concerns and what might be done to address them.

While, occasionally, the term "aphasic" may be used to refer to an "individual with aphasia" in the writings of the diverse authors in this book, there is a widespread movement among health care professionals to heighten sensitivity to individuals served by choosing terminology that does not objectify and label people primarily through their impairments or disabilities. Readers are encouraged to join this movement.

LIFE-CHANGING EFFECTS OF APHASIA

Within a matter of minutes, the lives of individuals who have aphasia change completely. They become prisoners in their own minds. Many, through the effects of neurological impairments, become prisoners in their own bodies as well. Some want to move and walk but cannot; some want to think and communicate but are significantly limited in their ability to do so. Persons with aphasia may be unable to maintain employment, leading not only to financial stress but also to feelings of isolation, frustration and worthlessness. Some people with aphasia are lonely and desperate. Some are even suicidal (Brody, 1992). Others tolerate the condition remarkably well.

Despite worldwide efforts to improve the ways that individuals with handicaps are treated and regarded, strong negative attitudes toward persons with communicative and physical handicaps remain. Individuals with stroke and aphasia face attitudinal barriers, marginal social status, suspicion, rejection, distrust, stigmatization and loss of esteem (Brody, 1992; Love, 1981; Post & Leith, 1983; Sahs & Hartman, 1976).

Patients' significant others are usually dramatically affected by the onset of aphasia in a friend, colleague or loved one. The onset of acquired aphasia, so life-changing in practically every dimension of daily living, inspires many to appreciate just how central communicative ability is to the human race (c.f., Parr et al., 1997).

Language: The Human Essence

The need for socialization is the core of human existence, and the ability to communicate with others is the essence of that socialization (Chapey, 1994). Language is basic to what Chomsky (1972) calls the "human essence." More than any other attribute, language distinguishes humans from other animals. It is the most basic characteristic of the intellect and the very means through which the mind matures and develops (Chapey, 1994). Language enables individuals to describe and clarify their thoughts for themselves and others (Fromkin & Rodman, 1974).

Human experience and interaction are welded to language (Chapey, 1994). According to Goodman (1971), the ability to share experience through language is a means of homeostasis that enables human beings to maintain and/or restore an equilibrium in which they can survive. Goodman also observes that language is the basis of personality, revealing our innate being and our psychic ties with the world.

Language is also the essence of maturity, which is defined as an ability to relate warmly to and intimately with others—with their goals, aspirations, and hopes. It involves a "fitting in," carrying one's share of personal and social responsibility, and conveying one's seasoned intelligence (Chapey, 1994). Thus, definitions of maturity involve and revolve around the ability to use language effectively (Chapey, 1994).

Insofar as persons with aphasia are impaired in their ability to use language, they are impaired in their human essence (Chapey, 1994). Part of the personality often appears lost, and the ability to maintain interpersonal relationships, to convey wants and needs, and to be a mature self-reliant, self-actualized person is impaired. Many individuals who lose language perceive that their equilibrium is devastated and that they are not fully functioning, mature adults (Chapey, 1994).

There is tremendous variability in how aphasia affects an individual's sense of self and social ability. The effects may be disproportionate to the degree of neurological impairment. Even mild deficits may be traumatizing to persons who identify closely with their active roles as communicators. Others with severe neurological impairments and language deficits tolerate the effects of their condition with remarkable serenity.

RATIONALE FOR LANGUAGE INTERVENTION IN APHASIA

A rationale for language intervention with persons who have aphasia is based on the belief that language constitutes what is considered the human essence and that treatment can effect a change in a patient's communicative performance (Chapey, 1994). Aphasia is not considered by most to be a disorder that can be cured. Still, skilled intervention enables many individuals to be able to comprehend and produce language and to communicate more effectively. Through intervention, aphasiologists attempt to heighten each patient's potential to function maximally within his or her environment,

to facilitate meaningful relationships, and to restore self-esteem, dignity, and independence (Chapey, 1994; Wepman, 1972a).

It is unfortunate that many post-trauma and post-stroke patients with good potential for rehabilitation are left untreated. Many individuals have the capacity to communicate more effectively and yet are not encouraged to do so (Chapey, 1994; Wepman, 1972a). Quality health care means going beyond the provision of basic physical care and meeting the holistic needs of patients with high standards and dignity. Individuals should be granted the right to be treated by qualified clinicians providing the best techniques known. Not to allow persons to communicate to the best of their ability is to deprive them of their own human essence (Chapey, 1994).

FUTURE TRENDS

The explosion of new knowledge and new technology is leading scientists to a progressively greater understanding of the brain's biology. Molecular answers are now increasingly available for questions we have addressed only indirectly. New and evolving imaging methods provide promise for richer information about the nature of neurogenic disorders in adults, and about their treatment. New approaches to pharmacological intervention are producing promising preliminary results related to facilitation of cerebrovascular recovery following stroke or brain injury, and cognitive improvement through neurotrophic factors.

Research in all of the areas related to the study of aphasia will continue to illuminate our understanding of neurogenic communication disorders. Many of these research areas are explored further in this book. It is important that aphasiologists continue to learn about how the brain organizes language and to reflect on how this kind of knowledge can affect the growth and development of new approaches to treatment. The more we know about how intervention changes brain function, the more effective we can make our intervention approaches.

Demographic characteristics of patient populations will continue to stimulate new development in adult language intervention. Increased life expectancies and the progressive aging of the world's population will continue to influence the nature of the patients served by the clinical aphasiologists, as will the growth of multilingual and multicultural populations. Other important influences will include the increased incidence of certain relevant etiological factors such as hepatitis, HIV, and AIDS (ASHA, 1989a; Larsen, 1998; Flower & Sooy, 1987).

RATIONALE FOR THIS TEXT

The primary purpose of the present text is the presentation of various models of intervention for adult aphasia patients and for patients with related disorders. Such models can provide a framework with which to focus therapy, to generate intervention tasks, and to analyze empirically the efficiency of rehabilitation efforts. Some of these strategies have appeared in part or in whole in previous literature; others have not. It should be recognized, however, that it is not the purpose of this text to assess any of the models or to resolve the inconsistencies in these approaches. These functions are better performed in appropriate professional journals or through further research.

It is hoped that this text will provoke theoretical speculation and that those chapters that are rich conceptually will prompt the collection of further data and generate the production of new approaches. The readings are organized into sections to help shape the reader's perspective on the field. However, the sections of the book—and its chapters—may be used in any order.

▶ *Acknowledgment*–This work was supported in part by grant DC00153-01A1 from the National Institute on Deafness and Other Communication Disorders. Thanks to Jessica DeSimone, Kirsten C. Carr and Jacquie Kurland for editorial assistance and to Linda Garcia for her insights regarding the WHO model.

KEY POINTS

1. There are four essential features to a definition of aphasia.
2. Varied theoretical frameworks influence the way one conceptualizes aphasia and therefore may influence the diagnosis and treatment of aphasia.
3. There are multiple etiological factors associated with aphasia, the most common of which is stroke.
4. Traditional classification schemes help to elucidate various manifestations of aphasia, but are often limited in terms of characterizing the conditions of individual patients.
5. The study of aphasia is interdisciplinary.
6. The term "aphasic" is an adjective, not a noun.
7. A solid rationale for language intervention in adult aphasia is based on the notion that language is essential to one's human essence and that treatment can effect a change in a patient's communicative competence.

Activities for Reflection and Discussion

1. Write your own definition of the term "aphasia," employing each of the four components mentioned for an ideal definition. Compare your definition with those of your colleagues. How might the way one conceptualizes aphasia influence one's choice of words in defining aphasia?

2. Make a list of risk factors for stroke and aphasia. What are some ways that you might serve as a role model to patients and their families in the ways you exhibit stroke prevention tactics in your own life?

3. A background in basic terminology used in the study of communication disorders is assumed by the authors of this book. Reviewing terminology as presented in other texts may be helpful. Define in your own words the following terms used to describe the symptoms associated with aphasia:
   - perseveration
   - catastrophic reaction
   - logorrhea
   - press of speech
   - paraphasia (including the terms literal, phonemic, semantic, verbal, and global paraphasia)
   - transposition
   - neologism
   - anomia
   - jargon
   - alexia
   - agraphia

   Note that some authors use the prefix *dys*- rather than *a*- for many of these terms, referring, for example, to dysnomia, dyslexia, dysgraphia, and even dysphasia rather than using the corresponding terms anomia, alexia, agraphia, and aphasia. What is the literal semantic distinction between terms beginning with *dys*- as compared to *a*-? The choice of prefixes in the usage of such terms among aphasiologists appears to be a function of stylistic convention more than a function of the literal significance of the prefixes in question.

4. Explain why many patients with "fluent" aphasia are also considered to have "receptive" aphasia.

5. Describe the hallmark features of each of the classic subtypes of aphasia described: Wernicke's aphasia, transcortical motor aphasia, conduction aphasia, Broca's aphasia, global aphasia, transcortical sensory aphasia, anomic aphasia, alexia, and primary progressive aphasia. As you read the upcoming chapter, it will be helpful to continue to reflect on how these hallmark symptoms are associated with the underlying neuropathologies of aphasia. As you consider diagnostic issues in aphasia as discussed further in this text, it will be helpful to further consider how the way in which one conceptualizes aphasia is relevant to the diagnostic process.

6. How might the way one conceptualizes the nature of aphasia, and classifies its subtypes, influence the process of assessing an individual with aphasia? How might it influence treatment?

References

Abrams, W., & Berko, R. (1990). *The Merck manual of geriatrics*. Rahway, NJ: Merck, Sharp & Dohme Research Laboratories.

Allison, M. (1991, October). Stopping the brain drain. *Harvard Health Letter, 16* (12), 6–8.

Basso, A., Capitani, M., Laiacona, M., & Luzzatti, C. (1980). Factors influencing type and severity of aphasia. *Cortex, 16,* 631–636.

Bloom, L. & Lahey, M. (1978). *Language development and language disorders*. New York: Wiley.

Brookshire, R.H. (1992). *An introduction to neurogenic communications disorders*. St. Louis: Mosby–Year Book.

Brody, J. (1992, June 10). When brain damage disrupts speech. *New York Times*, p. C13.

Brown, J.W. (1972). *Aphasia, apraxia and agnosia: Clinical and theoretical aspects*. Springfield, IL: Charles C. Thomas.

Brown, J.W. (1977). *Mind, brain and consciousness*. New York: Academic Press.

Brown, J.W. (1979). Language representation in the brain. In Steklis, H. & Raleigh, M. (eds.), *Neurobiology of social communication in primates*. New York: Academic Press.

Brown, J.W., & Grober, E. (1983). Age, sex, and aphasia type: Evidence for a regional cerebral growth process underlying localization. *The Journal of Nervous and Mental Disease, 171* (7), 431–434.

Brown, J.W., & Perecman, E. (1986). Neurological basis of language processing. In Chapey, R. (ed.), *Language intervention strategies in adult aphasia*. Baltimore MD: Williams & Wilkins.

Caplan, D. & Chertkow, H. (1989). Neurolinguistics. In Kuehn, D.P., Lemme, M.L., Baumgartner, J.M. (eds.). *Neural bases of speech, hearing, and language*. Austin, TX: Pro-Ed, 292–302.

Casper, M.L., Wing, S., Anda, R.F., et al. (1995). The shifting stroke belt: Changes in the geographic pattern of stroke mortality in the United States, 1962 to 1988. *Stroke, 26* (5), 755–760.

Ceccaldi, M., Soubrouillard, C., Poncet, M., & Lecours, A.R. (1996). A case reported by Serieux: The first description of a "primary progressive word deafness"? In Code, Wallesch, Jaonette, & Roch (eds.), *Classic cases in neuropsychology*. East Sussex, UK: Psychology Press, 45–52.

Centers for Disease Control (1999, August). Achievements in public health, 1900–1999. *Morbidity and Mortality Weekly Report, 48* (30).

Chapey, R. (1986). An introduction to language intervention strategies in adult aphasia. In Chapey, R. (ed.), *Language intervention strategies in adult aphasia*. Baltimore, MD: Williams & Wilkins.

Chapey, R. (1994). Introduction to language intervention strategies in adult aphasia. In Chapey, R. (ed.), *Language intervention strategies in adult aphasia*. Baltimore, MD: Williams & Wilkins, 3–26.

Chapey, R. (1994). Cognitive intervention: Stimulation of cognition, memory, convergent thinking, divergent thinking, and evaluative thinking. In Chapey, R. (ed.), *Language intervention strategies in adult aphasia*. Baltimore, MD: Williams & Wilkins.

Chomsky, N. (1972). *Language and mind*. New York: Harcourt, Brace & World.

Cubelli, R., Foresti, A., & Consolini, T. (1988). Reeducation strategies in conduction aphasia. *Journal of Communication Disorders, 21,* 239–249.

Damasio, A. (1998). Signs of aphasia. In Sarno, M.T. (ed.), *Acquired aphasia*. New York: Academic Press, 25–41.

Damasio, A., & Damasio, H. (1983). The anatomic basis of pure alexia. *Neurology, 33,* 1573–1583.

Damasio, A., & Damasio, H. (1992). Brain and language. *Scientific American, 267,* 89–95.

Damasio, A., & Damasio, H. (1994). Cortical systems for retrieval of concrete knowledge: The convergence zone framework. In Koch, C. (ed.), *Large-scale neuronal theories of the brain*. Cambridge, MA: MIT Press, 61–74.

DeRenzi, E., Faglioli, P., & Ferrari, P. (1980). The influence of sex and age on the incidence and type of aphasia. *Cortex, 16,* 627–630.

Elias, S. (1992). What is independence? *Generations, 16* (1), 49–52.

Eriksson, P.S., Perfilieva E., Bjork-Eriksson T., Alborn A.M., Nordborg C., Peterson D.A., & Gage F.H. (1998). Neurogenesis in the adult human hippocampus. *Nature Medicine, 4* (11), 1313–1317.

Flack, J.M., & Yunis, C. (1997). Therapeutic implications of the epidemiology and timing of myocardial infarction and other cardiovascular diseases. *Journal of Human Hypertension, 11,* 23–28.

Flower, W. & Sooy, D. (1987). AIDS: An introduction for speech-language pathologists and audiologists. *ASHA, 29,* 25–30.

Frady, M., Gerdau, R., Lennon, T., Sherman, W., & Singer, S. (1985, December 28). *Growing old in America*. ABC News Close-Up.

Fromkin, V., & Rodman, R. (1974). *An introduction to language*. New York: Holt, Rinehart & Winston.

Fougeyrollas, P., Cloutier, R., Bergeron, H., Cote, J., Cote, M., & St. Michel, G. (1997). *Revision of the Quebec Classification: Handicap creation process*. Lac St-Charles, Quebec: International Network on the Handicap Creation Process.

Gaines, K. (1997). Regional and ethnic differences in stroke in the southeastern United States Population. *Ethnicity and Disease, 7,* 150–264.

Geschwind, N. (1965). Disconnexion syndromes in animals and man. *Brain, 88,* 237–294, 585–644.

Gillum, R.F. (1994). Epidemiology of stroke in Native Americans. *Stroke, 26* (3), 514–521.

Gillum, R.F. (1995). Epidemiology of stroke in Hispanic Americans. *Stroke, 26* (9), 1707–1712.

Goldstein, K., & Scheerer, M. (1948). Abstract and concrete behavior in experimental study with special tests. *Psychological Monograph, 53,* 2.

Goodglass, H. (1993). *Understanding aphasia*. San Diego: Academic Press.

Goodglass, H., & Kaplan, E. (1983). *The assessment of aphasia and related disorders*. Philadelphia: Lea & Febiger.

Goodglass, H., Quadfasel, F., & Timberlake, W. (1964). Phrase length and type and severity of aphasia. *Cortex, 1,* 133–153.

Goodglass, H., & Wingfield, A. (1997). Anatomical and theoretical considerations in anomia. In Goodglass, H., & Wingfield, A. (eds.), *Anomia: Neuroanatomical and cognitive correlates*. San Diego: Academic Press, 20–29.

Goodman, P. (1971). *Speaking and language: Defense of poetry.* New York: Random House.

Habib, M., Ali-Cherif, A., Poncet, M., & Salamon, G. (1987). Age-related changes in aphasia type and stroke location. *Brain and Language, 31* (2), 245–251.

He, J., & Whelton, P.K. (1997). Epidemiology and prevention of hypertension. *Medical Clinics of North America, 81* (5), 1077–1097.

Head, H. (1915). Hughlings Jackson on aphasia and kindred affections of speech. *Brain, 38,* 1–27.

Hier, D.B., Yoon, W.B., Mohr, J.P., Price, T.R., & Wolf, P.A. (1994). Gender and aphasia in the Stroke Data Bank. *Brain and Language, 47,* 155–67.

ICIDH-2: International Classification of Functioning and Disability: Beta-2 draft, Full Version. (1999). Geneva, World Health Organization.

Jackson, H.H. (1878). On affectations of speech from disease of the brain. *Brain, 1,* 304–330.

Kahneman, D., Diener, E., & Schwarz, N. (1999). **Well-being**. New York: Russell Sage Foundation.

Kertesz, A., & Sheppard, A. (1981). The epidemiology of aphasic and cognitive impairment in stroke: Age, sex, aphasia type and laterality differences. *Brain 104,* 117–128.

Kertesz, A. (1982). *Western Aphasia Battery.* New York: Grune & Stratton.

Kertesz, A., & Poole, E. (1974). The aphasia quotient: The taxonomic approach to the measurement of aphasic disability. *Canadian Journal of Neurological Science, 1,* 7–16.

Khaw, K. (1996). Epidemiology of stroke. *Journal of Neurology, Neurosurgery, and Psychiatry, 61,* 333–338.

Kimura, D. (1980). Sex differences in intrahemispheric organization of speech. *Behavioral and Brain Sciences 3,* 240–241.

Kuller, L.H. (1995). Stroke and diabetes. In National Diabetes Data Group (eds.), Diabetes in America. 2nd Ed. Bethesda, MD: National Institutes of Health, 449–456.

Larsen, C. (1998). *HIV-1 and communication disorders: What speech and hearing professionals need to know.* San Diego: Singular Publishing Group, Inc.

Love, R.J. (1981). The forgotten minority: The communicatively disabled. *ASHA, 23,* 485–490.

LPAA Project Group (in alphabetical order: Roberta Chapey, Judith F. Duchan, Roberta J. Elman, Linda J. Garcia, Aura Kagan, Jon Lyon, & Nina Simmons Mackie) (February, 2000). Life Participation Approach to Aphasia: A Statement of Values for the Future. The *ASHA* Leader, Vol 5, 3.

Manton, K.G., Stallard, E., & Corder, L.S. (1998). The dynamics of dimensions of age-related disability 1982 to 1994 in the U.S. elderly population. *Journals of Gerontology: Series A: Biological Sciences & Medical Sciences, 53A* (1), B59–B70

Marquardsen, J. (1969). The natural history of acute cerebrovascular disease: A retrospective study of 769 patients. *Acta Neurologica Scandinavica, 45:* supplement 38.

McGlone, J. (1980). Sex difference in human brain asymmetry: A critical survey. *Behavioral and Brain Sciences, 3,* 215–263.

Miceli, G., Caltagirone, C., Gainotti, G., Masullo, C., Silveri, M.C., & Villa, G. (1981). Influence of age, sex, literacy and pathologic lesion on incidence, severity and type of aphasia. *Acta Neurologica Scandinavica, 64* (5), 370–382.

Muma, J. (1978). *Language handbook: Concepts, assessment and intervention.* Englewood Cliffs, NJ: Prentice-Hall.

National Institute for Deafness and Other Communication Disorders (1999). Health information: Voice, speech, and language. [on-line]. Available: http://www.nih.gov/nidcd/health/pubs_vsl/aphasia.htm

National Joint Committee for the Communicative Needs of Persons with Severe Disabilities. (1992). Guidelines for meeting the communication needs of persons with severe disabilities. *ASHA, 34* (March, Supp. 7), 1–8.

Neisser, U. (1967). *Cognitive psychology.* New York: Appleton-Century Crofts.

Parr, S., Byng, S., & Gilpin, S. (1997). *Talking about aphasia.* Buckingham, UK: Open University Press.

Pedersen, P.M., Jorgensen, H.S., Nakayama, H., Raaschou, H.O., & Olsen, T.S. (1995). Aphasia in acute stroke: Incidence, determinants, and recovery. *Annals of Neurology, 38* (4), 659–666.

Post, J., & Leith, W. (1983). I'd rather tell a story than be one. *ASHA 25,* 23–26.

Ryff, C., & Singer, B. (1998). The Contours of Positive Human Health. *Psychological Inquiry, 9,* 1, 1–28.

Sacco, R.L., Boden-Albala, B., Gan, R., Chen, X., Kargman., D.E., Shea, S., Paik, M.C., & Hauser, W.A. (1998, Feb). Stroke incidence among white, black, and Hispanic residents of an urban community: the Northern Manhattan Stroke Study. *American Journal of Epidemiology, 147* (3), 259–268.

Sahs, A.L., & Hartman, E.C. (1976). *Fundamentals of stroke care.* Washington, DC: U.S. Department of Health, Education and Welfare.

Saurwein-Teissl, M., Schonitzer, D., & Grubeck-Loebenstein, B. (1998). Dendritic cell responsiveness to stimulation with influenza vaccine is unimpaired in old age. *Experimental Gerontology, 33* (6), 625–631.

Scarpa, M., Colombo, P., Sorgato, P., & DeRenzi, E. (1987). The incidence of aphasia and global aphasia in left brain-damaged patients. *Cortex, 23,* 331–336.

Schuell, H. (revised by J. Sefer) (1973). *Differential diagnosis of aphasia with the Minnesota test.* Minneapolis, MN: University of Minnesota Press.

Schuell, H., Jenkins, J.J., & Jiminez-Pabon, E. (1964). *Aphasia in adults.* New York: Harper Medical Division.

Shinton, R. (1997). Lifelong exposures and the potential for stroke prevention: The contribution of cigarette smoking, exercise, and body fat. *Journal of Epidemiology and Community Health, 51* (2), 138–143.

Stegmayr, B., Asplund, K., & Wester, P.O. (1994). Trends in incidence, case-fatality rate, and severity of stroke in northern Sweden. *Stroke, 25* (9), 1738–45.

Thomas, T.N. (1997). The medical economics of stroke. *Drugs, 54* (3), 51–58.

Wepman, J. (1972a). Aphasia therapy: A new look. *Journal of Speech and Hearing Disorders, 37,* 203–214.

Wepman, J. (1972b). Aphasia therapy: Some relative comments and some purely personal prejudices. In Sarno, M. (ed.), *Aphasia: Selected readings.* New York: Appleton-Century-Crofts.

Wepman, J. (1976). Aphasia: Language without thought or thought without language. *ASHA, 18,* 131–136.

Wepman, J., & Jones, L. (1961). *Studies in aphasia: An approach to testing: The Language Modalities Test for Aphasia*. Chicago: Education-Industry Service.

Willich, S.N., Levy, D., Rocco M.B., Tofler, G.H., Stone, P.H., & Muller, J.E. (1987, Oct). Circadian variation in the incidence of sudden cardiac death in the Framingham Heart Study population. *American Journal of Cardiology, 60* (10), 801–806.

World Health Organization (1999). ICIDH-2: International Classification of Impairments, Activities and Participation: A manual of dimensions of disablement and health [on-line]. Available: http://www.who.int/msa/mnh/ems/icidh/introduction.htm

Wu, G.Y., Zou, D.J., Rajan, I., & Cline, H. (1999). Dendritic dynamics in vivo change during neuronal maturation. *Journal of Neuroscience, 19* (11), 4472–4483.

Yusuf, H.R., Giles, W.H, Croft, J.B., Anda, R.F., & Casper, M.L. (1998). Impact of risk factor profiles on determining cardiovascular disease risk. *Preventive Medicine, 27* (1), 1–9.

Zivin, J., & Choi, D. (1991, July). Stroke therapy. *Scientific American, 265* (1), 56–63.

Chapter 2

Neural Basis of Language Disorders

Hanna Damasio

OBJECTIVES AND INTRODUCTION

Based on what has been learned from pathologic alterations in patients with aphasia due to focal brain damage, human neuroanatomy related to language processing is discussed in this chapter. Aphasia refers to a compromise in the process of comprehending language, formulating language, or both, which occurs in a language-competent and intellectually competent individual. Aphasia is a breakdown in the two-way translation process that establishes the relation between thought and language. As a consequence, people with aphasia have an inability to translate, with reasonable fidelity, a nonverbal set of images (thoughts) into linguistic symbols and grammatical relationships (or the inverse problem – translating a received language message into thought).

Aphasia is a defect in linguistic processing and not a defective process of perception or movement or thought. As discussed in other chapters of this volume, aphasia can affect varied aspects of language processing (e.g., syntax, the lexicon, the phonemic and morphemic morphology of a word). In each individual patient several or even all of these aspects can be compromised, but the emphasis of the defect can also befall one particular aspect only. Deafness, even when due to central processes, precludes comprehension of language through the auditory channel but not through the visual channel. Incoordination of speech movements causes dysarthria but not a linguistic breakdown of speech output. A thought disorder such as schizophrenia does not cause aphasia but rather produces a correct linguistic translation of a deranged thought process.

Aphasia is not the exclusive province of auditory-based languages. Languages based on visuomotor communication, such as American Sign Language (ASL), can also be compromised following focal brain damage, along similar symptom clusters (Bellugi et al., 1983).

Most often aphasia is the result of cerebrovascular disease leading to stroke but it can also appear following head injury, cerebral tumors, and degenerative diseases such as Alzheimer's or Pick's. The constellation of defects does not really depend on the underlying pathological process but rather on the specific brain region that becomes affected. The differences one might witness between aphasias caused by some of these pathological processes, or others, have more to do with the way the process affects the underlying brain tissue than with a specific effect on the language dysfunction. (For example, see Anderson et al., 1988 and 1990; Damasio, 1987a).

Most aphasic syndromes are seen in disease processes affecting the left hemisphere given that the vast majority of individuals share a left-hemisphere language dominance, even when they are left-handed. However, in some instances, some left-handers develop aphasia after lesions of the right hemisphere (or may fail to show aphasia after lesions in language areas of the left hemisphere) possibly because both hemispheres are more involved in language processing than is standard. Even more rarely, we can witness either the presence of aphasia with a right-hemisphere lesion in a right-handed person, or conversely, the absence of aphasia with a typical left-hemisphere insult also in a right-handed subject. These cases are known as "crossed aphasia" and "crossed non-aphasia," respectively.

HISTORICAL OVERVIEW

The history of aphasia and the history of neuroscience share the same starting point: neuroscience began with the description, in 1861, of a patient who had lost the ability to communicate through the spoken word because of damage to the left frontal operculum. The original description was outlined by Paul Broca (1861), and it formed the basis for what was later coined Broca Aphasia, a severe disruption of language output which far exceeded a difficulty in language comprehension. About a decade later Carl Wernicke was to describe another seminal patient with aphasia (Wernicke, 1874 and 1886). The cause was another lesion of the left hemisphere but this time in the posterior temporal region rather than in the frontal lobe. So began what was later termed Wernicke Aphasia in which the deficit in language comprehension far exceeded the disruption of language output. It did not take long to transform these observations of specific language deficits, which occurred after circumscribed areas of left-hemisphere damage, into generalizations about the neural basis of language. The idea that the left hemisphere was the site of human spoken language became accepted. With it came the idea that there were brain "centers" responsible for this function – an anterior center responsible for the production of language located in the frontal operculum or Broca's Area and a posterior center responsible for language comprehension, located in the posterior half of the superior temporal gyrus or Wernicke's Area. Further studies of patients with differently placed lesions and slight variations of the presenting deficits helped cement the traditional view, which mapped language-related brain areas to Broca and Wernicke areas, and their anatomical connection through a unidirectional fiber tract, the arcuate fasciculus, which carried speech signals from Wernicke's area to Broca's area. This cartoon of the key set of structures necessary to receive and produce language still pervades most textbooks and monographs on the subject, and even some modern texts on cognitive science and linguistics continue to use this phrenologic picture of the language brain despite their otherwise non-phrenologic models of the processes of thought and language. In the meantime, however, much has occurred in the history of aphasia. This includes a major backlash against localizationism that occurred along with the advent of behaviorisms in psychology, an approach that led to the opposite point of view, namely that nothing but the whole brain was responsible for cognition. During the heyday of this approach, virtually all and any part of the brain was seen as equipotential, and language processes were no longer localized. The other initial historical development occurred when Norman Geschwind, working in the mid-1960s, struck a healthy balance between the excesses of phrenology and those of behavioristic theories. With his landmark articles on disconnection syndromes (Geschwind, 1965) he placed the classical observations on the anatomy of aphasia in a new functional perspective. He also went further in the anatomical explanations he provided for some of the previously described aphasic syndromes and enlarged the original set of language-related areas to include the left supramarginal gyrus and the left angular gyrus, both located in the inferior sector of the parietal lobe (see also Geschwind, 1971). At about the same time, detailed evaluation of aphasic patients was beginning to be performed with measurement tools which considered the linguistic and cognitive aspects of language processing. Modern test batteries and classifications of the aphasias started in earnest in the 1960s.

Over the years numerous other aphasia classifications have appeared, all having their origin in the difficulties encountered by previous classifications in the accommodation to the unavoidable variability in the presentation of aphasic patients. I will not discuss the several available classification systems of aphasia, or their respective advantages and disadvantages. This topic is covered in other chapters in this book. In general, I will follow the separation of aphasic syndromes associated with the Boston and Iowa schools (Benton & Hamsher, 1978; Goodglass & Kaplan, 1983).

The availability of MR imaging and more recently 3-D reconstruction of the human brain has empowered the human lesion method and made way for a new wave of cognitive experiments. (For more on the lesion method see Damasio, 2000, and Damasio & Damasio, 1989.) The results of these studies have shown that language processing is not "centered" on Broca and Wernicke's areas, but rather on systems composed of many neural sites working in close cooperation. Some of these sites include Broca and Wernicke's areas. Language processing will, for instance, engage several regions of left temporal and prefrontal/premotor cortices in the left hemisphere which lie outside the classical language areas (Damasio, 1990; Damasio et al., 1990; Damasio & Tranel, 1993; Goodglass et al., 1986). It has also been shown that structures in the left basal ganglia, thalamus, and supplementary motor areas are engaged in language production (Damasio et al., 1982; Graff-Radford et al., 1985a and b; Naeser et al., 1982). The advent of functional neuroimaging has also helped reveal important related facts.

For instance, in normal subjects, visual word processing activates left occipital and temporal cortices other than the traditional Wernicke's area (Frith et al., 1991; Habib et al., 1996; Myerson & Goodglass, 1972; Wise et al., 1991); and areas in left temporal pole, left infero-temporal cortices, and left prefrontal cortices are active when normal subjects attempt successfully to retrieve words denoting objects belonging to different conceptual categories (Damasio et al., 1996; Martin et al., 1996; Mazoyer et al., 1993).

Further support of the view that brain structures engaged in language processing are not confined to the classical language areas has come from electrophysiological studies in patients undergoing surgery for the treatment of epilepsy. Here again, cerebral cortex outside the traditional language areas has been shown to be engaged in a whole host of language processes (Lesser & Gordon, 1994; Luders et al., 1991; Nobre et al., 1994; Ojemann, 1983 and 1991).

ANATOMICAL OVERVIEW

Sulci, Gyri and Cytoarchitectonic Fields

To understand the neural underpinnings of the aphasias, we must begin with an understanding of normal brain anatomy. Knowledge of neuroanatomy has been gathered over the years mostly through the study of brains at the autopsy table, although today it is possible to study macroscopic anatomy at the computer screen, thanks to the technique of magnetic resonance (MR) and to programs that manipulate MR information and allow for 3-dimensional (3-D) reconstruction of brain tissue viewed on the computer screen. The brain anatomy reviewed in this chapter is based on normal brains, i.e., brains of normal individuals without any neurological or psychiatric disease. The brains I use have been reconstructed in 3-D from thin MR slices (1.5 mm thick). The slices are contiguous, T1 weighted, and obtained in the coronal direction. A collection of about 124 such coronal slices is stripped of scalp, meninges, blood vessels, cerebellum and brainstem, and reconstructed in 3-D on the computer screen of a silicon graphics workstation, using Brainvox (Damasio & Frank, 1992; Frank et al., 1997). Brainvox is a family of programs developed to analyze normal and lesioned brains at the computer screen. It allows us to identify and color code sulci, gyri, lesions, or any structure on the 3-D rendered volume, on the original coronal slices, or on any slice obtained by slicing through the 3-D volume. Any such markings are immediately available on any 2-D view intersecting the marked structure and on the 3-D reconstructed brain. The 3-D reconstructed brain can be viewed in any direction, can be split into smaller regions, and can be measured volumetrically. Surface and linear measurements can also be obtained.

Figure 2–1 A and B shows the two hemispheres of such a reconstructed normal brain seen from the lateral and mesial views. Some major sulci that divide the hemispheres into their basic constituents, the lobes and the gyri, are marked. (See also Damasio, 1995; Duvernoy, 1991; Ono, 1990; among others for more anatomical information.) On the lateral surface the most prominent sulcus is the Sylvian Fissure (SF), a mostly horizontal sulcus running anteroposteriorly. The SF separates the temporal lobe, below, from the frontal and parietal lobes, above. The posterior end of the Sylvian Fissure usually shows an asymmetric course when the right and left hemispheres are compared, as is the case in the example at hand. It tends to be longer and lower on the left, and shorter and turning upward on the right. The other prominent sulcus, usually continuous, on the lateral surface of the hemispheres is the central sulcus (CS). It runs from the interhemispheric fissure (the separation between the two hemispheres) above, toward the Sylvian Fissure, below, taking a posteroanterior course. It may or may not reach the Sylvian Fissure proper. This sulcus separates the frontal lobe, in front, from the parietal lobe (behind). Parallel to the central sulcus there are two other sulci, which are more often than not subdivided into more than one segment. They are, anteriorly, the pre-central sulcus (preCS), and posteriorly, the post-central sulcus (postCS). Together with the central sulcus they define the pre-central and post-central gyri (preCG, postCG), respectively, the most posterior sector of the frontal lobe, often designated as motor cortex (where the primary motor cortex or Brodmann's area 4 can be found), and the most anterior sector of the parietal lobe, the sensory cortex (where primary sensory cortices or Brodmann's areas 3, 1 and 2 are seen). Very often we speak of these two gyri as the sensorimotor cortices. There are two other prominent sulci to consider in the dorso-lateral surface of the frontal lobe, namely the superior frontal sulcus (SFS) and the inferior frontal

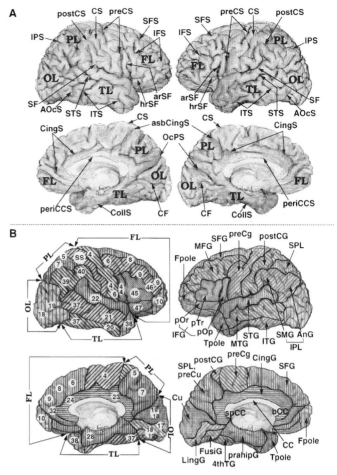

Figure 2–1. A. Lateral and mesial views of the two hemispheres with the identification of major sulci. Abbreviations as mentioned in the text. (Left hemisphere on the right and right hemisphere on the left.) B. The same lateral and mesial views of two hemispheres, with different shadings for the different gyri. The left hemisphere shows the name of the gyri (abbreviations as mentioned in the text) and the right hemisphere contains the numbers for Brodmann's cytoarchitectonic areas. SS corresponds to primary somatosensory regions (Brodmann's areas 3, 1, and 2).

sulcus (IFS). Both run anteroposteriorly from the pre-central sulcus toward the polar region of the frontal lobe, usually stopping before reaching the pole. In relation to language, the inferior frontal sulcus is probably the more important of the two, given that it forms the superior limit of the inferior frontal gyrus (IFG) in which we find the frontal operculum (FOp), traditionally called Broca's area when the left hemisphere is considered. The frontal operculum is divided into three subregions by two small sulci called the anterior terminal branches of the Sylvian Fissure. The more posterior of these sulci, the ascending ramus of the Sylvian Fissure (arSF), forms the anterior limit of the pars opercularis (or Brodmann's area 44). The posterior limit of this sector is formed by the lower segment of the pre-central sulcus. The more anterior of the sulci, the horizontal ramus of the Sylvian Fissure (hrSF) serves as the anteroinferior limit of the pars triangularis (or Brodmann's area 45) and the superior limit of the pars orbitalis (or Brodmann's area 47). Between the inferior frontal sulcus and the superior frontal sulcus lies the middle frontal gyrus (MFG) occupied by Brodmann's areas 46, 9, 8 and 6. The superior frontal sulcus constitutes the lateral and inferior limit of the superior frontal gyrus (SFG), which continues into the mesial surface of the hemisphere. On this dorsolateral aspect of the gyrus we find Brodmann's areas 9, 8 and 6. The most anterior sector of the frontal lobe, the polar region just in front of the three horizontal frontal gyri just described, is occupied by Brodmann's area 10.

In the temporal lobe there is one consistent sulcus, more or less parallel to the Sylvian Fissure, the superior temporal sulcus (STS). Together with the Sylvian Fissure it delineates the superior temporal gyrus (STG), which corresponds to Brodmann's area 22. Another sulcus, also parallel, can be seen on the lateral surface, the inferior temporal sulcus (ITS). This sulcus is constituted, more often than not, by several small segments and can be difficult to recognize. It creates the separation between the middle temporal gyrus (MTG) containing Brodmann's area 21, above, and the inferior temporal gyrus (ITG) containing Brodmann's area 20, below. The posterior sector of both these gyri contain Brodmann's area 37, which continues into the infero-mesial surface of the temporal lobe.

The parietal lobe is also subdivided by a prominent anteroposteriorly running sulcus, the intraparietal sulcus (IPS), starting at the post-central sulcus and going in the direction of the occipital lobe. This sulcus separates the inferior parietal lobule (IPL), containing Brodmann's areas 40 and 39, from the superior parietal lobule (SPL), containing Brodmann's areas 5 and 7. The inferior parietal lobule is itself subdivided into two major gyri, namely the supramarginal gyrus (SMG), anteriorly (Brodmann's area 40) sitting on top of the Sylvian Fissure and around its posterior end, and the angular gyrus (AnG) or Brodmann's area 39 sitting behind the former, around the posterior end of the superior temporal sulcus.

There is no clear demarcation between the parietal, temporal, and occipital lobes on the lateral surface of the hemispheres. The anterior occipital sulcus (AOcS), when it exists, is a sulcus that runs more or less vertically from the lower edge of the hemisphere upward, and can be considered the dividing line between temporal and occipital lobes. In relation to the parietal lobe, the posteroinferior edge of the angular gyrus is considered the separation between occipital and parietal regions.

On the mesial surface of the hemispheres, there are several major sulci to be considered. One is the cingulate sulcus (CingS), continuous or subdivided into several segments, more or less parallel to the contour of the corpus callosum (CC). The corpus callosum is the midline white matter structure containing the fibers connecting the cortices of the two hemispheres. Together with the pericallosal sulcus

(periCCS), directly around the corpus callosum, it creates the limit of the cingulate gyrus (CingG), containing prominently Brodmann's areas 23, 24, and 32, plus several other regions buried within the sulcus itself. At its posterior end, the cingulate sulcus turns upward in what is known as the ascending branch of the cingulate sulcus (asbCingS). The identification of this terminal segment is important because it serves as an indicator for the position of the mesial termination of the central sulcus, a small anteroposteriorly oriented sulcus that is just in front of the ascending ramus of the cingulate sulcus. The termination of the pre-central sulcus is immediately in front. The termination of the post-central sulcus is usually behind the ascending branch of the cingulate sulcus. It is not rare to find a double cingulate sulcus, particularly in its anterior sector.

In the mesial aspect of the temporal lobe there is one consistent sulcus, parallel to the long axis of the temporal lobe, the collateral sulcus (CollS), which separates the fifth or parahippocampal gyrus (parahipG), containing Brodmann's areas 28, 36, and 35, from the inferotemporal region (ITr), the name often given to the temporal cortices between the collateral sulcus and the superior temporal sulcus described earlier (see also **Fig. 2–2A** for a better view of this sulcus). This inferotemporal region includes the middle temporal gyrus (already mentioned), the inferior temporal gyrus (ITG), and the fourth temporal gyrus (4thTG), containing both Brodmann's areas 20 and 37. The inferior temporal gyrus is separated from the fourth temporal gyrus by a very inconsistent and variable sulcus, the temporo-occipital sulcus (TOS).

Mesially, the parietal lobe, the sector behind the ascending branch of the cingulate sulcus, is clearly separated from the occipital lobe by a sulcus running superoinferiorly and slightly posteroanteriorly, the occipito-parietal sulcus (OPS). The parietal region in front of this sulcus is also known as the pre-cuneus (preCu) or Brodmann's area 7.

There is no distinct sulcus separating the occipital from the temporal lobe. However, in the mesial aspect of the occipital lobe itself there is a distinct and consistent sulcus, running anteroposteriorly, the calcarine fissure (CF), whose two lips contain the primary visual cortex or Brodmann's area 17. The calcarine fissure separates the mesial aspect of the occipital lobe into two sectors: the supracalcarine region (sCR), or cuneus (CU), containing Brodmann's areas 18 and 19, and the infracalcarine region (iCR), also containing Brodmann's areas 18 and 19. The infracalcarine sector is subdivided into two parallel gyri, the lingual gyrus (LingG) superiorly and the fusiform gyrus (FusiG) inferiorly, by the continuation of the collateral sulcus. The lingual gyrus is the continuation of the parahippocampal gyrus and the fusiform gyrus the continuation of the fourth temporal gyrus. This is probably the reason why we may find the designation of fusiform gyrus applied to the fourth temporal gyrus. However, in order to maintain a separation between the nomenclature applied to the occipital and temporal regions, we should refer to the temporal fusiform gyrus when referring to the fourth temporal gyrus as fusiform gyrus.

Typically, the occipito-parietal sulcus and the calcarine sulcus join just behind the posterior end of the corpus callosum, which is also known as splenium. The cortex between the splenium and the juncture of the occipito-parietal and calcarine sulci is usually referred to as the retrosplenial area, which contains several different cytoarchitectonic areas.

Let us consider now the inferior surface of the hemispheres (Fig. 2–2A, B). This is a very wide surface, particularly when the temporal and frontal lobes are concerned, something that is difficult to appreciate if we only look at the lateral and mesial views of the brain. Looking at the temporal lobe from below, we realize the enormous expanse of

the inferior and fourth temporal gyri. This is also the view in which we can more easily see the temporo-occipital sulcus when it exists.

The inferior surface of the frontal lobe, or orbital surface, has one anteroposterior sulcus, positioned medially, the medial orbital sulcus (MOS), which separates the gyrus rectus (GR), or primary olfactory cortex, from the rest of the orbital surface. There is also an array of lateral-orbital sulci (LOS), often designated as the H-shaped orbital sulci. The major cytoarchitectonic fields in this region are Brodmann's area 12, mesially, areas 11 and 13 lateral to the former, and area 10 at the pole.

Most of the cerebral cortex is actually not readily visible in any of the views we have been dealing with but rather hidden within the hemispheric sulci, something that can be more easily appreciated if we look at coronal cuts throughout the hemispheres (see Fig. 2–3). Furthermore, there are

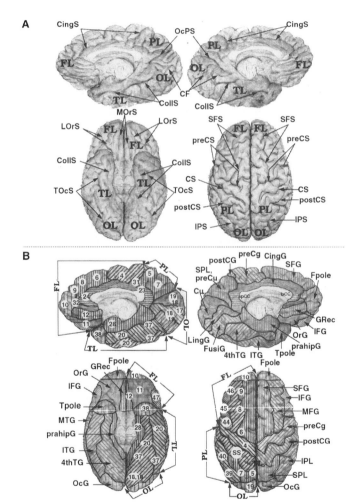

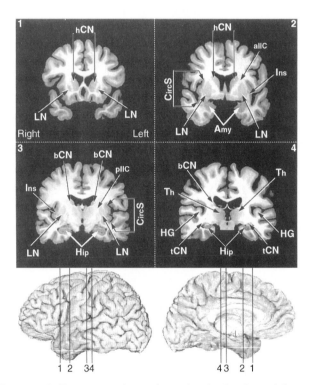

Figure 2–3. Four coronal cuts through a brain whose left hemisphere is depicted in the bottom tier. The lines on the 3-D hemisphere represent the placement of the cuts above. Note that most of the cortical rim is actually not on the visible surface of the hemisphere but rather buried within the sulci. The ventricles appear as clearly delineated black structures. The subcortical gray areas, as well as the insula, can easily be identified in these cuts. Abbreviations are those used in the text. (The coronal slices are presented according to the radiological convention with the right hemisphere on the left and the left hemisphere on the right. This convention is respected in all illustrations. Brain slices are always presented from anterior to posterior or from the most inferior view to the most superior view.).

Figure 2–2. A. The upper tier shows the tilted mesial view of the two hemispheres so as to reveal the collateral sulcus (CollS); the lower tier shows the ventral view of the brain on the left, and the dorsal view on the right. Sulci are marked with the abbreviations mentioned in the text. B. Same views as in A. Gyri are shaded and named on the mesial view of the left hemisphere and on the ventral and dorsal view of the right hemisphere. Brodmann's cytoarchitectonic numbers are on the opposite hemisphere.

also two surfaces of cortex that are completely hidden from view when we look only at lateral, mesial, inferior, or superior views. These are the insula (In) and Heschl's gyrus (HG), the latter also known as primary auditory cortex containing Brodmann's areas 41 and 42 (Fig. 2–4). Heschl's gyrus occupies the superior surface of the superior temporal gyrus and is limited posteriorly by the transverse temporal sulcus

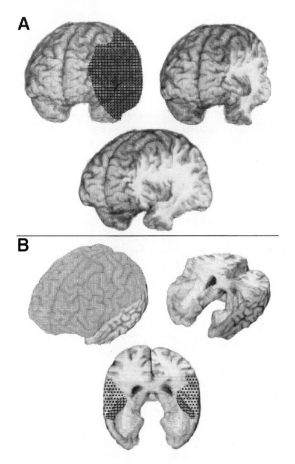

Figure 2–4. A. 3-D reconstructed brain is seen from the front and left. The cross-hatched area in the left image shows the region of the brain that was removed so as to allow the viewing of the insula, on the right. Below is the same brain but rotated more to a left lateral view. The insula cortex can readily be recognized as an island of gray matter in the midst of the white matter. B. 3-D reconstructed brain seen from above and the left, with a cross-hatched region corresponding to the frontal and the parietal lobes and superior sector of the occipital lobe (on the left). On the right, the same view after the cross-hatched structures were removed. In the left temporal lobe the superior surface of the superior temporal gyrus is now visible. Two transverse sulci are visible. The bottom image shows the cut brain seen from above with the occipital pole pointing up. In this view the transverse gyri of Heschl are clearly seen (cross-hatched area) and behind them the posterior surface of the superior temporal gyri, the plana temporale (dotted areas). Note that in this case the planum on the left is larger than on the right (the common left/right asymmetry seen in right-handed subjects).

(TTS), which has a posteromesial-to-anterolateral course. This structure divides the superior temporal gyrus into two distinct segments, one anterior and one posterior to it, both containing Brodmann's area 22. The posterior sector is also known as the planum temporale (PlT), which typically shows a marked asymmetry between the right and the left hemispheres, being usually larger on the left where it constitutes the major portion of the classical Wernicke's area.

The insula is also completely hidden. It can be found by opening up the Sylvian Fissure, separating the temporal lobe from the fronto-parietal operculum. In Figure 2–4, after removal of part or most of the lateral sector of the hemisphere, a region of cortex is shown, completely encircled by a sulcus, the circular sulcus (CircS) that delineates an island of cortex, or the insula. In the insula several gyri can be identified, more or less parallel to each other, and with a lateromesial course. These gyri are known as the short insular gyri—those located more anteriorly, and the long insular gyri—those located posteriorly.

We should also refer briefly to some of the more important subcortical gray matter structures (see Fig. 2–3). Within the temporal lobe, in the depth of the parahippocampal gyrus we find the hippocampus proper (Hip) and the amygdala (Amy). Within the frontal lobe we find the basal ganglia (BG) with its separate constituents, the caudate nucleus (CN) and the lenticular nucleus (LN), which can be further subdivided into the putamen (Pu) laterally and the pallidum (Pa) mesially. In the caudate nucleus we consider the head (hCN), the more voluminous anterior sector, the body (bCN), and the tail (tCN), these latter two in the depth of the parietal lobe. Posterior and inferior to the basal ganglia sits the thalamus (Th), mostly in the depth of the parietal lobe. The thalamus is separated from the basal ganglia by a white matter structure known as the posterior limb (pl) of the internal capsule. Between the caudate and the putamen we can find the anterior limb (al) of the internal capsule. The internal capsule is a white matter structure containing the ascending and descending fibers of the post- and precentral gyri. Lateral to the lateral limit of the putamen, under the insula, is another gray matter structure, the claustrum (Clau), which is separated from the putamen and the insular cortex by the external capsule and the extreme capsule, respectively.

All these gray matter structures, cortical and subcortical, are highly linked by reciprocal connections. These are massive and multiple, and connect most of these regions to each other, but not in an indiscriminate way. The connections are highly patterned and specific. However, it is beyond the scope of this chapter to go into details of these connections. A lot is known about them, and a lot is still to be learned. For interested readers, I recommend a text by Jones and Peters (1986). Here I just emphasize a few general principles that are useful in our further discussion.

The first principle is that the primary sensory cortices, e.g., visual, auditory, olfactory, and somatosensory, receive connections from the sensory organs in the body's periphery, usually through intermediary stages, at subcortical levels, and project "forward" or "downstream" to early association cortices, in a divergent fashion. Downstream from these early association cortices, pathways project systematically to higher- and higher-order association cortices in convergent fashion. At each station, the forward-directed projections are accompanied by back-projecting projections that are often just as numerous as those projecting forward. This is to say that from primary sensory regions there is a massive forward, mostly convergent system, going to higher-order association cortices, and that this system is accompanied by a back-projecting system that is mostly divergent. The areas in which these "feedforward" and "feedback" systems pivot have been designated as convergence zones (Damasio, 1989). It is the coordinated functioning of this convergent/divergent system that allows, among others, for the translation of nonverbal thought processes into linguistic processes that constitute the basis for our language-based communication, be it spoken, written, or signed.

Vascular Supply of the Cerebral Hemispheres

Before we begin our discussion about the neurological underpinnings of the aphasias, we need one more aside, namely, a very brief overview of the brain's vascular supply (Fig. 2–5). This is important since the most common cause of aphasia is vascular lesions, and because the vascular lesions causing aphasia have allowed us to use the lesion method efficiently to find the neural underpinnings of language disorders.

The brain's vascular supply comes from the internal carotid artery (the external carotid giving blood supply to the extracranial tissues). (See also Lazorthes, 1976; Waddington, 1974; Szikla et al., 1977; Day, 1987; and Damasio, 1987b, for more detail of the vascular supply of the brain.) We should consider five distinct vascular territories: the territory of the anterior cerebral arteries (ACA), (one on the left, and one on the right); the territory of the middle cerebral arteries (MCA), again, one left and one right; and the territory of the posterior cerebral artery (PCA), one for the two hemispheres. These different territories are connected through the circle of Willis. The circle of Willis is formed by the anterior communicating artery (AcomA), which links the two anterior cerebral arteries; the initial segments of the two anterior cerebral arteries, which arise, together with the middle cerebral artery, from the internal carotid artery; and the two posterior communicating arteries (PComA) (right and left), which link the internal carotid artery to the posterior cerebral artery and the basilar artery. This basic pattern is variable and one or several of the linking segments may be missing.

The anterior cerebral artery supplies the territory of the inferior and mesial aspect of the frontal lobe, the mesial parietal lobe, and the cingulate gyrus. It can be divided into several subsegments as seen in Figure 2–5.

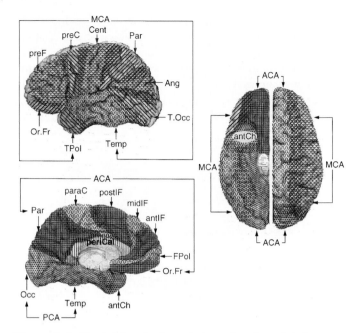

Figure 2–5. The left hemisphere, in lateral and mesial views, and the right hemisphere, in ventral and dorsal views. The main subdivisions of each of the three cerebral arteries are marked on the left hemisphere images. Note that the cross-hatched markings of each artery overlap with its neighbor. On the ventral and dorsal views of the right hemisphere the three main arteries are marked. The double cross-hatched area corresponds to the watershed area. ACA = anterior cerebral artery; MCA = middle cerebral artery; PCA = posterior cerebral artery; antCh = anterior choroidal artery. Under MCA: Orb.Fr = orbito-frontal artery; preF = pre-frontal artery; preC = pre-central artery; Cent = central artery; Par = parietal arteries (includes anterior parietal and posterior parietal); Ang = angular artery; T.Occ = temporo-occipital artery; Temp = temporal arteries (includes anterior, middle, and posterior branches); TPol = temporo-polar arteries. Under ACA: Or.Fr = orbito-frontal artery; FPol = fronto-polar artery; antIF = anterior-internal-frontal artery; midIF = middle-internal-frontal artery; postIF = posterior-internal-frontal artery; paraC = paracentral artery; Par = parietal artery; periCal = pericallosal artery. Under PCA: Occ = occipital branches; Temp = temporal branches.

The middle cerebral artery supplies the territory of most of the lateral surface of the hemispheres. The main subdivisions to be considered are those of the anterior or frontal branches, the posterior or parieto-occipital branches, and the temporal branches. In each of them independent arteries can be considered as shown in Figure 2–5.

The posterior cerebral artery supplies the territory of the occipital pole and the mesial surface of the occipital and temporal lobes. Again, different branches can be considered with their distinct territory as Figure 2–5 shows. The mesial aspect of the most anterior sector of the temporal lobe gets its blood supply from the anterior choroidal artery (antChA), a branch of the internal carotid artery before the internal carotid subdivides into middle and anterior cerebral arteries.

The area at the edges of each of the three main territories mentioned above receives capillaries from the two arterial territories as they meet. This "horseshoe" region occupies a sector on the superior frontal gyrus, the superior parietal lobule and the angular gyrus and the postero-lateral aspect of the occipital lobe, continuing on the inferior surface of the temporal lobe toward the temporal pole. It is normally designated as the watershed area. It is important to have an idea about this region for two specific reasons. First, because of its dual blood supply, this region is more resistant to infarction. Second, because its supply is achieved by terminal, thinner vessels, the region is more vulnerable to severe decreases in arterial pressure. In such events, this is one of the regions that suffers the most intense deprivation of oxygen. For instance, in a stroke consequent to cardiac arrest and a severe and sustained drop in blood pressure, these areas are compromised in the left hemisphere and may cause aphasias of the transcortical type.

There is another region that is supplied by terminal arteries, but does not have dual blood supply: the region of the basal ganglia. This region gets its blood supply from multiple, thin and fragile perforating vessels that leave the stem of the middle cerebral artery at almost right angles. This configuration makes them very vulnerable to sudden decreases in blood pressure in the main supplying vessel as well as to arterial blockage by emboli.

Because the blood supply to the brain is carried out by small vessels that penetrate the hemispheres through the cortex in the direction of the underlying white matter, an obstruction of any of the major supply vessels tends to create an area of infarct that is broader on the surface than in the depth. It is the reason for the well-known and traditional description of the image of a stroke as a wedge-shaped form with the base turned towards the cortex.

NEUROANATOMICAL CORRELATES OF THE APHASIAS

Classic Aphasias

Broca Aphasia

Broca's description of the language impairment seen in his patient Leborgne suggests that the condition was worse than that we associate today with a typical Broca aphasia. The speech output was so sparse that it was largely confined to the word "tant" and comprehension of spoken language was also severely compromised (Broca, 1861). In modern terms, the case that began the history of aphasiology and whose lesion became associated with Broca aphasia, would probably be described as a global aphasia.

It was precisely the severity of this presentation that gave rise to one of the famous debates in the history of aphasia and of neuroscience, that between Déjérine and Pierre Marie at the Paris Society of Medicine in 1908 (Déjérine & Marie, 1908). Because of the severity of lack of speech output and comprehension deficits, Pierre Marie defended the notion that not only Broca's area would have been damaged in this patient, but that the lesion would also have included the basal ganglia and the posterior temporal structures of Wernicke's area. On the other hand, Déjérine defended the notion that damage would have been limited to the frontal lobe and would not extend into posterior temporal areas. The controversy was only put to rest in 1980 when researchers at the Salpetrière Hospital decided to obtain a CT scan of the brain of Mr. Tant (the name by which the patient is generally known), a brain that had been preserved uncut, and continues to be so preserved, for over a century (Castaigne et al., 1980). The scan clearly showed damage to Broca's area, to the underlying basal ganglia, and to the insula, but not to Wernicke's area or to surrounding areas, which were intact.

Even today, there is still some controversy about the anatomical underpinnings of Broca's aphasia. For instance, in 1978 Mohr and collaborators pointed out that infarctions confined to the inferior frontal gyrus cause only a brief period of mutism which resolves into effortful speech but generally does not cause significant linguistic deficits (Mohr et al., 1978). They claimed that such lesions do not cause a Broca aphasia in the proper sense. The same investigators suggested that the lesion necessary to produce the more severe language disturbance usually classified as Broca aphasia is far larger, requiring the involvement of all of the frontal operculum and of the insula. In our experience, chronic and long-lasting language deficits conforming to the characteristics of a Broca aphasia in the chronic epoch do indeed require damage of a sizable area of the frontal operculum and surrounding tissue. However, in the acute epoch of the condition, a small and circumscribed infarct of the frontal operculum can also produce a nonfluent language deficit with all the characteristics of a typical Broca aphasia (Fig. 2–6). Similar findings have been described by Tonkonogy and Goodglass (1981). These authors pointed out that a small lesion involving the frontal operculum had caused linguistic deficits in the acute epoch, although the deficits were not long lasting. In the same study, the authors showed that an equally small lesion placed in an immediately posterior position, in the rolandic operculum, did not cause any phonemic, lexical, or syntactical processing difficulties, but rather dysarthric and dysprosodic speech output (see also Schiff et al., 1983).

When language deficits are classified as a Broca aphasia in the acute phase and when they persist for months, it is usually the case that damage in a large sector of the inferior frontal gyrus is found, as seen in Figure 2–7, for example. (See also Alexander et al., 1990, and Naeser & Hayward, 1978.)

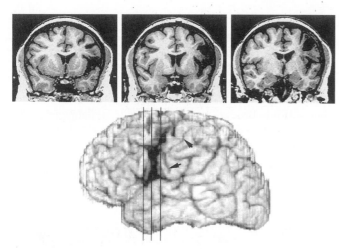

Figure 2–6. 3-D reconstruction of the brain of a patient. Acutely she had Broca aphasia and mild right-arm and face paresis as a result of an infarction in the territory of the pre-central artery. Recovery was fairly quick. In the chronic epoch she had no motor defects and her language had improved remarkably. The lesion occupies the anterior half (lower two-thirds) of the pre-central gyrus not damaging the motor cortex in the central sulcus (arrow) in the left hemisphere. The lesion also damages the pars opercularis of the frontal operculum. It does not damage insula or basal ganglia, which can be seen to be intact in the coronal slices. In summary, it is a lesion that partially damages premotor cortices 6 and 44.

In other cases, the infarct may be in the territory of most of the anterior branches of the MCA and will have damaged not just the cortex of the frontal operculum (Brodmann's areas 44 and 45), but also have extended into the underlying white matter and involve the insula and the basal ganglia, as well as the inferior sector of the pre-central gyrus. Other such chronic Broca aphasias will have started as a global aphasia in the acute period. (See also Global Aphasia and Fig. 2–11.)

Wernicke Aphasia

There has never been the same degree of controversy in relation to the symptom complex or to the anatomical correlate of the prototypical fluent aphasia: Wernicke aphasia. Wernicke's original description of the language impairment and of its underlying brain damage (Wernicke, 1886) is consonant with contemporary investigations (Damasio, 1981 and 1987a; Kertesz, 1979; Kertesz et al., 1979 and 1993; Knopman et al., 1984; Mazzocchi & Vignolo, 1979; Naeser & Hayward, 1978; and Selnes et al., 1983, 1984, 1985; among others). A typical case of Wernicke's aphasia due to an infarct of the temporal arteries is depicted in Figure 2–8. The lesion is seen in the posterior sector of the superior temporal gyrus (Brodmann's area 22). This region is the core of Wernicke's area. The lesion also extends into the posterior region of

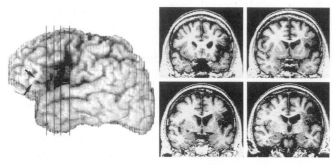

Figure 2–7. 3-D reconstruction of the brain of a patient. Acutely he had Broca aphasia and face and arm paresis as a result of an infarction in the territories of the pre-frontal and pre-central arteries. He also recovered but was left with mild weakness in his right arm and with language deficits that were still classified as a mild Broca aphasia. In this case the lesion occupies the inferior third of the entire pre-central gyrus involving the central sulcus region in the left hemisphere. It also involves the entire frontal operculum including pars opercularis and triangularis and even part of pars orbitalis. It is only the outer rim of the inferior frontal gyrus that is spared. There is damage to pre-motor regions 6 and 44 as well as motor region 4 and pre-frontal regions 45 and 47. The lesion also extends further into the underlying white matter than in the previous case (Fig. 2–6). It damages insula but does not damage the basal ganglia.

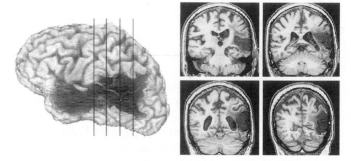

Figure 2–8. 3-D reconstruction of the brain of a patient. Acutely she presented with Wernicke aphasia and right hemianopsia as a result of an infarction in the territory of the temporal branches of the MCA. The visual field persisted in the chronic epoch as did the aphasia. The lesion involves most of the dorsolateral aspect of the left temporal lobe. The superior and middle temporal gyri are completely occupied by damaged tissue, as well as the inferior sector of the supramarginal gyrus, and the anterior sector of the angular gyrus. The damage extends deep into the underlying white matter, destroying the posterior segment of the insula and reaching the ventricle at the level of the trigone. Cortical areas that are destroyed beyond the insula include the primary auditory cortices (Brodmann's areas 41 and 42 in the transverse gyrus of Heschl), all of surrounding area 22 (including the posterior portion or Wernicke's area), all of area 21, the superior sector of area 37, the inferior sector of area 40, and the anterior sector of area 39.

the middle and inferior temporal gyri (part of Brodmann's areas 37, 20 and 21), and into part of the inferior parietal lobule, destroying the lower sector of the supramarginal and the angular gyri (Brodmann's areas 40 and 39). In such cases, recovery is limited and a severe fluent aphasia may persist for months. A noticeable aphasia may persist for years.

Conduction Aphasia

When damage is limited to the supramarginal gyrus (Brodmann's area 40) the result is a fluent aphasia, distinct from Wernicke's aphasia, known as conduction aphasia. The fundamental clinical characteristic of conduction aphasia is a severe inability to repeat a heard sentence verbatim. In severe cases, even single words are not repeated. This repetition deficit is disproportionately severe in comparison to the ability to produce spontaneous speech or understand speech (see Benson et al., 1973; Geschwind, 1965; Konorski et al., 1961; Liepmann & Pappenheim, 1914, for the early descriptions of the syndrome and its underlying brain damage, and Damasio & Damasio, 1980; Kertesz et al., 1979; Naeser & Hayward, 1978; Rubens & Selnes, 1986, among others for later descriptions).

Typical cases of conduction aphasia are often caused by damage to the supramarginal gyrus (see Figure 2–9 for an example). This is the case of a patient who, at age 33, suffered an intracerebral hemorrhage to the left parietal lobe which led to the diagnosis of an intracerebral arteriovenous (AV) malformation. In order to excise the entire AV malformation, the neurosurgeon had to remove the entire supramarginal gyrus, while being able to spare the entire superior temporal gyrus. After surgery this patient presented with a typical conduction aphasia. She was unable to repeat even short sentences, e.g., "Take this home." As is typical of conduction aphasia, comprehension of the sentences to be repeated was preserved. For example, asked to repeat "The orchestra played and the audience applauded," verbatim, the patient failed entirely. Yet, when asked about the meaning of the sentence she paraphrased it as "There was music and they liked it, they clapped." Even today, almost 20 years after the onset of her aphasia, this patient has difficulty in repeating sentences longer than 3 or 4 words, although her other acute deficits, for instance, her naming impairment, have improved remarkably.

Damage to the cortex of the supramarginal gyrus and to its underlying white matter compromises the arcuate fasciculus, the pathway which connects posterior and anterior language areas as first described by Déjérine (1901 and 1906). Geschwind proposed (1965) that the inability to repeat was a result of damage to the pathway and although the essence of this explanation may well be correct for some cases of conduction aphasia, it may not be adequate for all. It is certainly the case that conduction aphasia can result from somewhat different lesion patterns. In 1980 we described patients with

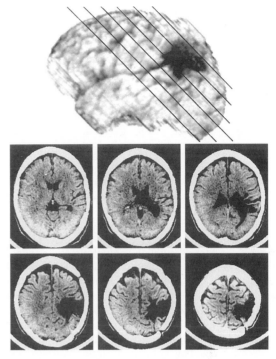

Figure 2–9. 3-D reconstruction (in this instance from a thin-cut CT scan) of the brain of a patient with conduction aphasia resulting from an arteriovenous malformation that ruptured and bled. The condition required the subsequent surgical removal of most of the supramarginal gyrus. In the chronic epoch this patient continues to display a mild conduction aphasia. The lesion involves the supramarginal gyrus (Brodmann's area 40). Wernicke's area is mostly intact.

lesions in left auditory cortex and insula, without involvement of supramarginal gyrus, who presented with a typical conduction aphasia (Damasio & Damasio, 1980). Rubens and Selnes also described a similar presentation with exclusively left insular damage (Rubens & Selnes, 1986). Interestingly, the arcuate fasciculus seems not to course exclusively in the depth of the supramarginal gyrus as described by Déjérine but may instead be a large sheath of white matter whose lower segment courses under the insula (Galaburda & Pandya, 1983).

Global Aphasia

While occlusion of some of the anterior branches of the middle cerebral artery causes a nonfluent Broca type of aphasia, and occlusion of posterior temporal and parietal branches causes a fluent, Wernicke type of aphasia, occlusion of the middle cerebral artery itself, prior to its branching, causes extensive damage to frontal, parietal, and temporal regions, and results in a more severe language deficit known as global aphasia. As the description indicates, the ensuing deficits involve both production and comprehension of language and patients may be left with little speech other than for stereotyped and automated words and stock sentences. This

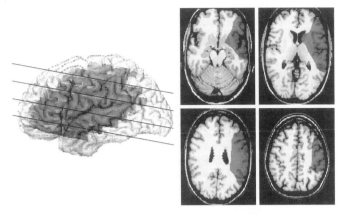

Figure 2–10. MAP-3 of the brain of a patient with a large left MCA infarct resulting in severe global aphasia and right hemiparesis. [MAP-3 is a technique that allows the 3-D visualization of lesions of individual subjects in a common normal target brain. For details about the technique see Damasio, 2000 and Frank et al., 1997.]. The lesion involves most of the frontal lobe structure in the territory of the anterior branches of the MCA, including Broca's area, most of the sensorimotor cortices, and the supramarginal gyrus, as well as all of the superior temporal gyrus, including Wernicke's area. The insula and the basal ganglia, as well as the white matter in the frontal and parietal lobes are also damaged.

sort of stroke also causes a severe restriction of movement in the right side of the body, a right hemiplegia. A typical image of the brain lesion of such a patient is shown in Figure 2–10.

The signs of global aphasia, namely, little language output, severe comprehension deficits in both oral and written form, inability to repeat, and inability to write, may appear in association with more restricted lesions. A large left frontal lobe lesion, involving not only Broca's area but extending into other frontal gyri, the pre- and post-central gyri, the supramarginal gyrus, the insula, and the basal ganglia, sparing the temporal lobe altogether, may present as a severe global aphasia. Such an "acute" global aphasia may resolve into a less severe albeit remarkable language deficit and be eventually classified as a severe Broca aphasia (see Fig. 2–11 for example).

One other anatomical presentation of global aphasia deserves mention. The severe and pervasive linguistic deficit of global aphasia which is usually accompanied by a right hemiplegia, may, on occasion, present without any motor deficits (see Legatt et al., 1987, and Tranel et al., 1987). Such a presentation is the consequence of two separate lesions due, for instance, to multiple emboli causing infarctions in both anterior and posterior branches of the middle cerebral artery. In other words, instead of a blockage of the main trunk of the artery, at the level of the stem, resulting in one large lesion, there are more peripheral blockages and thus more than one lesion. As described in Tranel et al. (1987), there may be an area of infarct in the left prefrontal/premotor cortices, and then another in the left posterior-tempora parietal region,

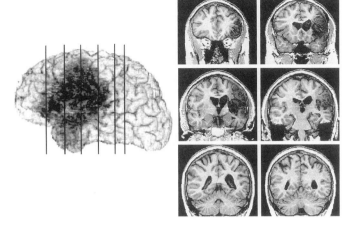

Figure 2–11. 3-D reconstruction of the brain of a patient with a large infarct in the territory of the anterior branches of the left MCA, the temporal-polar branch and the anterior-temporal branches. This patient presented acutely with a right hemiparesis and global aphasia. In the chronic epoch, however, his language had improved enough to have his aphasia reclassified as a severe Broca aphasia. The infarct involves prefrontal cortices in both the inferior and part of the middle-frontal gyri (Brodmann's areas 45, 47, and part of 46 and 9), premotor regions in the same gyri (Brodmann's areas 44 and 6), sensorimotor regions in the pre- and post-central gyri (Brodmann's areas 4, 3, 1, and 2), the anterior sector of the superior temporal gyrus (Brodmann's area 22), and the dorsolateral sector of the temporal pole (Brodmann's area 38). The insula is equally damaged and the infarct extends deep into the subcortical structures damaging the caudate and putamen, therefore damaging also the claustrum and the extreme and external capsules. The internal capsule is also damaged. What is important to note is that the primary auditory cortex (Brodmann's areas 41, 42) in Heschl's gyrus is only partially damaged (see cut 4) and that both Wernicke's area (posterior Brodmann's area 22) and the supramarginal gyrus (Brodmann's area 40) are spared, as can be seen in the two posterior cuts.

sparing the sensorimotor cortices in between (see Fig. 2–12). As is to be expected from the lesion placement, patients with this form of global aphasia recover faster and better than do those with classic global aphasia.

Transcortical Aphasias

The transcortical aphasias are characterized by normal word and sentence repetition. Transcortical sensory aphasia is diagnosed when a patient presents with fluent paraphasic speech and with poor auditory comprehension but with intact word and sentence repetition. There is a practical value in recognizing this type of aphasia as separate from Wernicke aphasia because it indicates to the clinician that both the primary auditory cortices (Brodmann's areas 41 and 42 in the transverse gyrus of Heschl) and the posterior sector of the superior temporal gyrus (Wernicke's area proper) are spared.

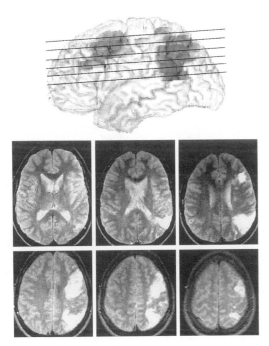

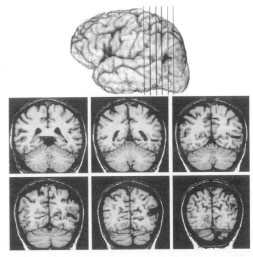

Figure 2–12. T2-weighted MR image and MAP-3 of the brain of a patient who acutely presented with global aphasia without a hemiparesis. This patient improved rapidly and was eventually left with only a mild language deficit. Note the two separate areas of infarction in the left hemisphere: one in the pre-central artery territory damaging the superior sector of the frontal operculum and the posterior region of the middle frontal gyrus, and the other in the territory of the parietal artery damaging the supramarginal gyrus and possibly part of the posterior sector of the superior temporal gyrus. The sensorimotor cortices, the insula and the basal ganglia are intact, as is most of the frontal operculum and most of Wernicke's area.

In transcortical sensory aphasia, the damage is posterior and inferior to the above-mentioned regions. It may involve the angular gyrus (Brodmann's area 39) and the posterior sector of the middle temporal gyrus (Brodmann's area 37).

On occasion the lesions may extend into the lateral aspect of the occipital lobe (Brodmann's areas 19 and 18) or into more anterior sectors of the middle temporal gyrus (Brodmann's area 21) (see Alexander et al., 1989b; Damasio, 1981 and 1987a; Freedman et al., 1984; and Kertesz et al., 1979, among others). In some instances, this same type of aphasia can be detected with exclusively subcortical lesions underlying the cortical regions mentioned above, as described in Damasio (1987a). See Figure 2–13 for an example of a transcortical sensory aphasia.

When patients present with a nonfluent language deficit and preserved repetition, we talk about a transcortical motor aphasia. The location of the lesions responsible for this type of aphasia is less consistent than for the transcortical sensory type. We may find transcortical motor aphasia in patients with small subcortical lesions located immediately anterior to the frontal horn of the left lateral ventricle, a part of the

Figure 2–13. 3-D reconstruction of the brain of a patient who presented with a fluent aphasia but intact repetition, a typical transcortical sensory aphasia. The cause of the syndrome was an acute intracerebral hemorrhage in the left hemisphere. In the chronic epoch, after resolution of the hemorrhage, we see an area of encephalomalacia in the left angular gyrus (Brodmann's area 39) and underlying white matter.

so-called anterior watershed area (Fig. 2–14). We also may find transcortical motor aphasia with lesions in the left frontal lobe involving prefrontal and premotor cortices (Brodmann's areas 10, 9, 46, 8, and 6, respectively).

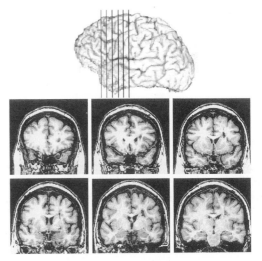

Figure 2–14. 3-D reconstruction of the brain of a patient who suffered a relatively small infarct in the left hemisphere, in the region of the anterior watershed territory. The external surface of the brain is intact, including all of the cortical mantle in Broca's and Wernicke's areas. The area of damage can only be seen in the coronal slices as an area of decreased signal in the white matter just anterior to the frontal horn of the left ventricle (see the first coronal cut). It extends posteriorly lateral to the lateral ventricle. It does not damage the caudate nucleus nor the insula.

Isolation of the Speech Areas

The combinations of the lesion described for transcortical motor aphasia, with those responsible for transcortical sensory aphasia, may result in an extensive lesion which isolates the "speech area." Patients with such lesions have a severe dual deficit in language comprehension and intentional language formulation, associated with a remarkably preserved capacity for aural repetition of even long sentences, devoid of any proper comprehension of sentence meaning. The repetition is achieved with so much ease that it is best described as echolalia, the immediate and rather accurate repetition of any verbal material received auditorially. When asked a question the patient may actually repeat the question verbatim instead of providing an answer. Geschwind described one of these rare cases, which was due to severe carbon monoxide poisoning (Geschwind et al., 1968). The underlying pathology was a watershed infarction nearly occupying the totality of the watershed region between the anterior and middle cerebral arteries and the posterior and middle cerebral arteries.

Crossed Aphasia

As mentioned earlier, the diagnosis of crossed aphasia applies when a fully right-handed subject has a lesion in the right hemisphere and becomes aphasic as a consequence of that lesion (Fig. 2–15). The incidence of such cases is low (Alexander et al., 1989a; Castro-Caldas et al., 1987). The same sort of individuals may fail to develop aphasia following lesions located in "language-related" areas of the left hemisphere, a situation known as "crossed non-aphasia" (Fig. 2–16).

Atypical Aphasias

With the advent of the modern neuroimaging techniques, beginning with early CT scans in 1972 and then with MR scans since the early 1980s, it became possible to identify the neural underpinnings of some aphasic presentations that were classified as "atypical." The atypicality was usually the result of a mixture of features of nonfluent and fluent aphasias that produced a blend quite distinctive from the severe and all-encompassing deficits of a global aphasia.

In the early 1980s several authors provided anatomical evidence for the connection between such a mixture of symptoms and infarcts in the basal ganglia. More specifically, the infarcts were located in the left hemisphere, in the head of the caudate nucleus and in the putamen (Aran et al., 1983; Brunner et al., 1982; Damasio et al., 1982; Damasio et al., 1984; Fromm et al., 1985; and Naeser et al., 1982). No aphasia at all is seen when the damage occurs in the right hemisphere. The vascular territory affected here was that of the striate arteries, a set of small terminal arteries arising from the stem of the middle cerebral artery. When infarcts are placed more laterally involving only the lateral aspect of the putamen and

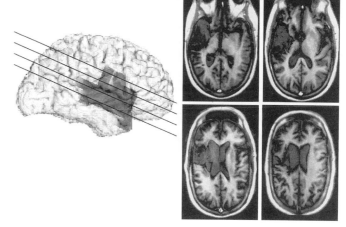

Figure 2–15. T1-weighted MR image and MAP-3 of a right-handed patient with infarct in the territory of the right anterior branches of the MCA (pre-frontal, pre-central, and central) and the territory of the anterior and middle temporal arteries. He presented with a left hemiparetic visual neglect, anosognosia, visuospatial deficits, and severe atypical aphasia. A typical presentation for a crossed aphasia. There is damage to the frontal operculum (Brodmann's areas 44 and 45 as well as 47), to sensorimotor cortices (in the lower tier of both the pre- and post-central gyri, involving Brodmann's areas 6, 4, 3, 1, and 2), to the inferior sector of the supramarginal gyrus (Brodmann's area 40), most of the anterior sectors of the superior temporal gyrus (Brodmann's areas 22, 41, and 42), as well as extension into insula and deep structures such as the caudate, the putamen, and internal capsule.

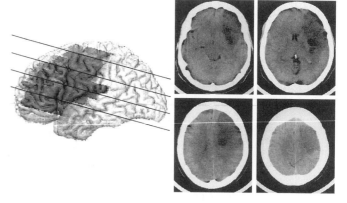

Figure 2–16. CT scan and MAP-3 of the brain of a right-handed patient with a very large left MCA infarct followed by a partial fronto-temporal brain resection. Neither the infarct nor the subsequent surgery resulted in aphasia; there was only mild dysarthria. The patient, however, did present severe impairment of visual memory, visuoconstructional abilities, and some degree of anosognosia. These symptoms are suggestive of a lesion in the nondominant hemisphere, suggesting reversed language dominance in this right-handed subject. We would talk about a "crossed non-aphasia."

the external and extreme capsules, and even the anterior insula, no aphasia is observed although the patient may show dysarthria and dysprosodia.

The early reports, based on relatively low-resolution scans of the 1970s, raised the possibility that there might be undetected damage in cortical regions. In a post-mortem study, however, Barat demonstrated that there was no damage outside the basal ganglia (Barat et al., 1981). Under the microscope, no area of abnormality could be seen in the cortical language areas. Modern, high-resolution MR scans confirm that this syndrome does occur as a result of damage to the left basal ganglia without involvement of the cortical language regions (Fig. 2–17).

The occurrence of aphasia with damage in the left thalamus has been noted with vascular lesions (Alexander & Loverme, 1980; Cappa & Vignolo, 1979; McFarling et al., 1982; Mohr et al., 1975), and with thalamic tumors (Arseni, 1958; Cheek & Taveras, 1966). The modern neuroimaging techniques have helped establish a precise anatomical basis for these aphasias (Archer et al., 1981; Cohen et al., 1980; Graff-Radford & Damasio, 1984; Graff-Radford et al., 1985a,b). Lesions in the anterior nuclei of the left thalamus, involving mostly the latero-ventral and antero-ventral nuclei were related to aphasias of the transcortical type

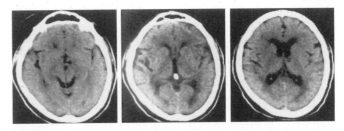

Figure 2–18. CT scan of a patient who presented acutely with an atypical aphasia due to an infarct of the anterior thalamic arteries. There is a low density lesion in the anteromesial region of the left thalamus.

(see Fig. 2–18). Lesions of the left thalamus which spare the anterior nuclei, and lesions of the right thalamus, result in sensory and motor deficits but not in aphasia.

Anomic Aphasia

Difficulty in producing the words that denote concrete entities presented visually, the most typical situation of "confrontation naming," is often present in most types of aphasia. On occasion, however, such a deficit is disproportionate in relation to other language deficits, or can even occur in isolation, something that was noted as early as 1898 by Pitres (Pitres, 1898). In such situations, it may be reasonable to use the label "anomic aphasia" or "amnesic aphasia."

In 1986 Goodglass called attention to the fact that a dissociation between the production of words denoting actions and those denoting concrete entities could be found in nonfluent and fluent aphasics, respectively (Goodglass et al., 1986; see also Daniele et al., 1994) and in 1984 Warrington and Shallice had called attention to the presentation of different patients with category-specific semantic impairments (Hart et al., 1985; Hillis & Caramazza, 1991; Semenza & Zettin, 1989; Silveri & Gainotti, 1988; Warrington & McCarthy, 1994; Warrington & Shallice, 1984).

The possible anatomical underpinnings for such category-specific word retrieval deficits only began to be elucidated over the past decade. Today there is ample evidence that the inferotemporal cortex of the left cerebral hemisphere can be segregated into distinct areas whose damage causes category-specific word retrieval defects for visually presented concrete entities (Caramazza & Hillis, 1991; Damasio et al., 1990; Damasio & Tranel, 1993; Damasio et al., 1996; Hillis & Caramazza, 1991; Miozzo et al., 1994; Perani et al., 1995; Tranel et al., 1997a and 1997b). Convergent findings have come through functional studies of non-lesioned brains (Buchel et al., 1998; Bunn et al., 1998; Damasio et al., 1996; Frith et al., 1991; Martin et al., 1996; Mazoyer et al., 1993; Nobre et al., 1994; Ojemann, 1983 and 1991; Petersen et al., 1988; Schlaghecken, 1998).

Work from our laboratory has shown that lesions located exclusively in the left temporal pole can cause deficits in the

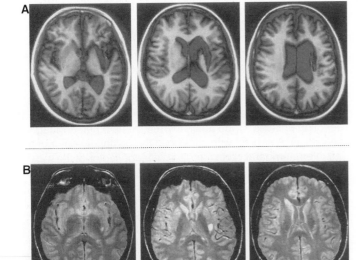

Figure 2–17. A. T1-weighted MR image of a patient who presented acutely with a left basal ganglionic hemorrhage and an atypical aphasia. This scan, obtained in the chronic epoch, shows a lesion in the head of the caudate nucleus and the putamen, as well as the internal capsule. However, there is no damage to cortical regions in the frontal operculum nor to posterior temporal cortices. B. T2-weighted MR image of a patient who presented acutely with dysarthria, but no aphasia, as a result of a ventriculostriatal infarct affecting the posterior sector of the putamen. Most of the putamen is, however, spared, as is the caudate nucleus.

retrieval of proper names for unique persons, in the presence of normal recognition of those persons (Damasio et al., 1996). Such deficits are not seen with lesions in the temporal pole of the nondominant hemisphere although damage to the right temporal pole may result in a deficient recognition of unique persons (Tranel et al., 1997b). [See Damasio et al., 1996, and Tranel et al., 1997b, for details of the testing procedures required to separate the processes of recognition and name retrieval.] When the lesion extends into the left anterior sector of IT in addition to damaging the temporal pole, the deficit encompasses not only the retrieval of words denoting unique persons but also that of nonunique animals. If the lesion spares the temporal pole but damages the anterior sector of IT, the deficit may be limited to the retrieval of words denoting animals alone. Again, recognition is not affected (in order for recognition of animals to be affected, the lesions must involve the mesial occipito-temporal cortices, especially those in the right hemisphere). When the retrieval of words denoting nonunique manipulable tools is the predominant feature of a naming deficit, the lesion usually involves the left posterior IT region at the level of the lateral occipito-temporal junction. Normal individuals tested in a PET study with the same stimuli used for the brain-damaged patient population show maximal activation in the temporal pole, anterior IT and posterior IT, respectively, for the retrieval of words denoting unique persons, nonunique animals, and nonunique manipulable tools (Damasio et al., 1996). See Figure 2–19 for a summary of lesions producing category-specific deficits.

We should consider here another group of patients who often present with pure naming deficits in the early stages of disease, the so-called "progressive aphasias." The term refers to subjects who show a progressive impairment in language performance, usually starting with a deficit in unique name retrieval, later proceeding to encompass deficits in the retrieval of words denoting nonunique entities, and finally encompassing more typical features of aphasia. The underlying damage is usually found in the left temporal lobe in the form of atrophy. The atrophy usually starts in the polar region and gradually comes to involve more of the temporal region, especially in IT regions. Many of these patients have a progressive degenerative disease, for example, a variant of Pick's disease. On occasion, the disease may affect first the frontal lobe with particular atrophy in the inferior frontal gyrus. In such cases, the presenting signs are those of difficulty retrieving words denoting actions and words denoting relationship of entities.

Mutism

Mutism is a condition that is not strictly an aphasia but is often taken as such. For instance, patients with akinetic mutism do not have abnormal language: they simply do not communicate in any form or fashion. They do not speak

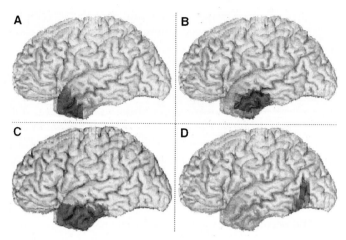

Figure 2–19. MAP-3 of the brains of four different patients with anomia. A. A subject with left temporal lobectomy who after surgery was left with severe impairment of naming of unique persons whom he could, however, recognize. The excised area was limited to the temporo-polar region (Brodmann's area 38). B. A subject with a resection of an arteriovenous malformation in the anterior sector of the left temporal lobe. After surgery there was a lesion in the anterior sector of the middle and inferior temporal lobes (Brodmann's areas 21 and 20) without extensive damage to the temporal pole. This subject showed deficit in retrieval of words denoting living entities such as animals, which he could, however, recognize. There were no other aphasic symptoms nor were there deficits in the retrieval of unique names. C. A subject with left temporal lobectomy, more extensive than the one depicted in (A). In this case the excision included the temporo-polar region (Brodmann's area 38) as well as the most anterior sector of the infero-temporal region (Brodmann's areas 21 and 20). This subject not only showed impairment in retrieving the name of unique persons he still recognized, but also showed deficits in retrieving words denoting animals. Once again there were no other language deficits. D. A subject with a lesion in the posterior sector of the left infero-temporal cortex and the anterior sector of the occipital cortices (Brodmann's areas 37 and 19). This subject showed deficits in the retrieval of words denoting manipulable tools, in the setting of some further cognitive deficits that would characterize her as having a transcortical sensory aphasia.

spontaneously; they do not speak when spoken to; and they fail to show any intention to communicate with the interlocutor. The attitude is in sharp contrast with that of the patients discussed so far. A hallmark of aphasic patients is the intent to communicate albeit with incorrectly found language. Akinetic mute patients are usually immobile, in body and speech. Akinetic mutism occurs with lesions of the anterior cingulate gyrus, either bilateral or unilateral, usually as a result of infarcts of the anterior branches of the anterior cerebral artery. Rupture of an anterior communicating aneurysm can produce vascular spasm in both anterior cerebral arteries and also cause such infarcts. The patients may remain akinetic and mute for weeks or months and eventually recover

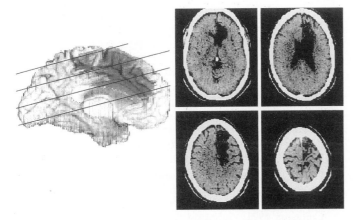

Figure 2–20. CT scan and MAP-3 of a patient who suffered the rupture of an anterior communicating aneurysm and had, as a result, an infarct in the territory of the internal-frontal and paracentral arteries. The patient presented suddenly with what was thought to be right hemiplegia and mutism. The infarcted region occupies the anterior cingulate (Brodmann's area 24 and part of area 23) and the mesial surface of the superior frontal gyrus, including the supplementary motor area (Brodmann's area 6) and part of the mesial motor region (Brodmann's area 4). It was soon recognized that in fact there were some motor deficits in the right leg but that there were no motor deficits in the right arm. The patient was simply akinetic. The patient improved over a period of a few weeks and began using sparse language which in time became completely normal.

without language deficits. Predictably, the recovery is speedier with unilateral infarcts. See Figure 2–20 for an example of such a lesion. When the lesion occurs only in the supplementary motor area (mesial section of Brodmann's area 6), the condition is restricted to mutism, with only minor akinesia. During the recovery of the latter sort of patient, the condition may resemble a transcortical motor aphasia.

▶ *Acknowledgment*–This work was supported by NIH Program Project Grant P01NS19632, and NIH Program Project Grant 1P50DCO3189-01A1. I thank Donna Wenell and Carol Devore for their help in the preparation of this manuscript.

KEY POINTS

1. The anatomical descriptions of classic Broca and Wernicke aphasias have stood the test of time. The location of the lesions that can produce those aphasias is, in essence, the same that was proposed originally.
2. The notion of "language centers" derived from those early anatomical studies did not prevail. All aspects of language performance depend on the concerted functioning of multi-component systems. The deficits caused by a lesion in a specific location correspond to the removal of the contribution of a particular anatomical component toward the overall function of the system.
3. The traditional Broca and Wernicke "language areas" are not sufficient to explain all that goes on in language production and comprehension. Many other areas must be added to the list if we are to explain normal language processing and account for the language deficits due to focal brain lesions.

References

Alexander, M.P., Fischette, M.R., & Fischer, R.S.: Crossed aphasia can be mirror image or anomalous. *Brain, 112,* 953–973, 1989a.

Alexander, M.P., Hiltbronner, B., & Fischer, R.: The distributed anatomy of transcortical sensory aphasia. *Arch. Neurol., 46,* 885–892, 1989b.

Alexander, M.P. & Loverme, S.R. Jr.: Aphasia after left hemispheric intracerebral hemorrhage. *Neurology, 30,* 1193–1202, 1980.

Alexander, M.P., Naeser, M.A., & Palumbo, C.: Broca's area aphasia. *Neurology, 40,* 353–362, 1990.

Anderson, S.W., Damasio, H., & Tranel, D.: The use of tumor and stroke patients in neuropsychological research: A methodological critique. *J. Clin. Exp. Neurpsychol., 10,* 32, 1988.

Anderson, S.W., Damasio, H., & Tranel, D.: Neuropsychological impairments associated with lesions caused by tumor or stroke. *Arch. Neurol., 47,* 397–405, 1990.

Aran, D.M., Rose, D.F., Rekate, H.L., & Whiteaker, H.A.: Acquired capsular/striatal aphasia in childhood. *Arch. Neurol., 40,* 614–617, 1983.

Archer, C.R., Ilinsky, I.A., Goldfader, P.R., & Smith, K.R.: Aphasia in thalamic stroke: CT stereotactic localization. *J. Comput. Assist. Tomogr., 5,* 427–432, 1981.

Arseni, C.: Tumors of the basal ganglia. *AMA Arch. Neurol. Psychiatry, 80,* 18–26, 1958.

Barat, M., Mazaux, J.M., Bioulac, B., Giroire, J.M., Vital, C., & Arne, L.: Troubles du langage de type aphasique et lesions putamino-caudees. *Rev. Neurol. (Paris), 137,* 343–356, 1981.

Bellugi, V., Poizner, H., & Klima, E.S.: Sign language aphasia. *Human Neurobiol., 2,* 155–170, 1983.

Benson, D.F., Sheremata, W.A., Bouchard, R., Segarra, J.M., Price, D.L., & Geschwind, N.: Conduction aphasia: a clinicopathological study. *Arch. Neurol. (Chicago), 28,* 339–346, 1973.

Benton, A.L. & Hamsher, K.: *Multilingual aphasia examination.* Iowa City: Benton Laboratory of Neuropsychology.

Broca, P.: Remarques sur le siège de la faculté de langage articulé, suivie d'une observation d'aphémie (perte de la parole). *Bull. Soc. Anat., 36,* 330–357, 1861.

Brunner, R.J., Kornhuber, H.H., Seemuller, E., Suger, G., & Wallesch, C.W.: Basal ganglia participation in language pathology. *Brain Lang., 16,* 281–299, 1982.

Buchel, C., Price, C., & Friston, K.: A multimodal language region in the ventral visual pathway. *Nature, 394,* 272–277, 1998.

Bunn, E.M., Tyler, L.K., & Moss, H.E.: Category-specific semantic deficits: The role of familiarity and property type reexamined. *Neuropsychology, 12,* 367–379, 1998.

Cappa, S.F. & Vignolo, L.A.: "Transcortical" features of aphasia following left thalamic hemorrhage. *Cortex, 15,* 121–130, 1979.

Caramazza, A. & Hillis, A.: Lexical organization of nouns and verbs in the brain. *Nature, 349,* 788–790, 1991.

Castaigne, P., Lhermitte, F., Signoret, J.L., & Abelante, R.: Description et étude scannographique du cerveau de Leborgne (la découverte de Broca). *Rev. Neurol. (Paris), 136,* 563–583, 1980.

Castro-Caldas, A., Confraria, A., & Poppe, P.: Nonverbal disturbances in crossed aphasia. *Aphasiology, 1,* 403–413, 1987.

Cheek, W.R. & Taveras, J.: Thalamic tumors. *J. Neurosurg., 24,* 505–513, 1966.

Cohen, J.A., Gelfer, C.E., & Sweet, R.D.: Thalamic infarction producing aphasia. *Mt. Sinai J. Med. (NY), 47,* 398–404, 1980.

Damasio, A.R.: The brain binds entities and events by multiregional activation from convergence zones. *Neural Computa., 1,* 123–132, 1989.

Damasio, A.R.: Category-related recognition defects as a clue to the neural substrates of knowledge. *Trends Neurosci., 13,* 95–98, 1990.

Damasio, A.R. & Tranel, D.: Nouns and verbs are retrieved with differently distributed neural systems. *Proc. Natl. Acad. Sci. USA, 90,* 4957–4960, 1993.

Damasio, A.R., Damasio, H., Tranel, D., & Brandt, J.P.: Neural regionalization of knowledge access. *Symposia on Quantitative Biology, Vol. 55,* New York: Cold Spring Harbor Laboratory Press, 1990, pp. 1039–1947.

Damasio, A., Damasio, H., Rizzo, M., Varney, N., & Gersh, F.: Aphasia with nonhemorrhagic lesions in the basal ganglia and internal capsule. *Arch. Neurol., 39,* 15–20, 1982.

Damasio, H.: Cerebral localization of the aphasias. In M.T. Sarno (ed.). *Acquired Aphasia.* New York: Academic Press, 1981.

Damasio, H.: Anatomical and neuroimaging contributions to the study of aphasia. In H. Goodglass (ed.). *Handbook of Neuropsychology, Vol. I, Language.* Amsterdam: Elsevier Publishers, 1987a.

Damasio, H.: The lesion method in cognitive neuroscience. In J. Grafman (ed.). *Handbook of Neuropsychology, Vol. 1.* Amsterdam: Elsevier Publishers, 2000.

Damasio, H.: Vascular territories defined by computer tomography. In J.H. Wood (ed.). *Cerebral Blood Flow: Physiologic and Clinical Aspects.* New York: McGraw-Hill Book Company, 1987b, pp. 324–332.

Damasio, H.: *Human Brain Anatomy in Computerized Images.* New York: Oxford University Press, 1995.

Damasio, H. & Damasio, A.R.: The anatomical basis of conduction aphasia. *Brain, 103,* 337–350, 1980.

Damasio, H. & Damasio, A.: *Lesion Analysis in Neuropsychology.* New York: Oxford University Press, 1989.

Damasio, H. & Frank, R.: Three-dimensional in vivo mapping of brain lesions in humans. *Arch. Neurol., 49,* 137–143, 1992.

Damasio, H., Eslinger, P., & Adams, H.P.: Aphasia following basal ganglia lesions: New evidence. *Semin. Neurol., 4,* 151–161, 1984.

Damasio, H., Grabowski, T.J., Tranel, D., Hichwa, R.D., & Damasio, A.R.: A neural basis for lexical retrieval. *Nature: 380,* 499–505, 1996.

Daniele, A., Giustolisi, L., Silveri, M.C., Colosimo, C., & Gainotti, G.: Evidence for a possible neuroanatomical basis for lexical processing of nouns and verbs. *Neuropsychologia, 32,* 1325–1341, 1994.

Day, A.L.: Arterial Distributions and Variants. In Wood, J.H. (ed.). *Cerebral Blood Flow: Physiologic and Clinical Aspects.* New York: McGraw-Hill Book Company, 1987, pp. 19–36.

Déjérine, J.: Anatomie des Centres Nerveux. Paris: Reuff, 1901.

Déjérine, J.: L'aphasie sensorielle et l'aphasie motrice. *Presse Medicale, 14,* 437–439, 453–457, 1906.

Déjérine, J., Marie, P.: Society of Neurology of Paris, Meeting of June 11, 1908. Discussion on Aphasia. Revue Neurologique: 16, 1–611. In M. F. Cole & M. Cole. *Pierre Marie's Papers on Speech Disorders.* New York: Hafner Publishing Company, 1971.

Duvernoy, H.: *The Human Brain: Surface, Three-Dimensional Sectional Anatomy and MRI.* Vienna: Springer-Verlag, 1991.

Frank, R.J., Damasio, H., & Grabowski, T.J.: Brainvox: an interactive, multimodal, visualization and analysis system for neuroanatomical imaging. *NeuroImage, 5,* 13–30, 1997.

Freedman, M., Alexander, M.P., & Naeser, M.A.: Anatomic basis of transcortical motor aphasia. *Neurology, 34,* 409–417, 1984.

Frith, C.D., Friston, K.J., Liddle, P.F., & Frackowiak, R.S.J.: A PET study of word finding. *Neuropsychologia, 29,* 1137–1148, 1991.

Fromm, D., Holland, A.L., Swindell, C.S., & Reinmuth, O.M.: Various consequences of subcortical stroke. *Arch. Neurol., 42,* 943–950, 1985.

Galaburda, A.M. & Pandya, D.N.: The intrinsic architectonic and connectional organization of the superior temporal region of the rhesus monkey. *J. Comp. Neurol., 221,* 169–184, 1983.

Geschwind, N.: Disconnexion syndromes in animals and man. *Brain, 88,* 237–294, 1965.

Geschwind, N.: Aphasia. *N. Engl. J. Med., 284,* 654–656, 1971.

Geschwind, N., Quadfaset, F.A., & Segarra, J.M.: Isolation of the speech area. *Neuropsychologia, 6,* 327–340, 1968.

Goodglass, H. & Kaplan, E.: *The Assessment of Aphasia and Related Disorders.* Philadelphia: Lea & Febiger, 1982.

Goodglass, H., Wingfield, A., Hyde, M.R., & Theurkauf, J.: Category specific dissociations in naming and recognition by aphasic patients. *Cortex, 22,* 87–102, 1986.

Graff-Radford, N. & Damasio, A.: Disturbances of speech and language associated with thalamic dysfunction. *Semin. Neurol., 4,* 162–168, 1984.

Graff-Radford, N., Schelper, R.L., Ilinsky, I., & Damasio, H.: Computed tomography and post mortem study of a nonhemorrhagic thalamic infarction. *Arch. Neurol. (Chicago), 42,* 761–763, 1985a.

Graff-Radford, N., Damasio, H., Yamada, T., Eslinger, P., & Damasio, A.: Nonhemorrhagic thalamic infarctions: Clinical, neurophysiological and electrophysiological findings in four anatomical groups defined by CT. *Brain, 108,* 485–516, 1985b.

Habib, M., DéMonet, J-F., & Frackowiak, R.: Neuroanatomic cognitive du langage: Contribution de l'imagerie fonctionnelle cérébrale. *Rev. Neurol. (Paris), 152,* 249–260, 1996.

Hart, J., Berndt, R.S., & Caramazza, A.: Category-specific naming deficit following cerebral infarction. *Nature, 316,* 439–440, 1985.

Hillis, A.E. & Caramazza, A.: Category-specific naming and comprehension impairment: A double dissociation. *Brain, 114,* 2081–2094, 1991.

Jones, E.G. & Peters, A. (eds.): *Cerebral Cortex, Vol. 5, Sensory-Motor Areas and Aspects of Cortical Connectivity.* New York: Plenum Press, 1986.

Kertesz, A.: *Aphasia and Associated Disorders.* New York: Grune & Stratton, 1979.

Kertesz, A., Harlock, W., & Coates, R.: Computer tomographic localization, lesion size, and prognosia in aphasia and nonverbal impairment. *Brain Lang., 8,* 34–50, 1979.

Kertesz, A., Lau, W.K., & Polk, M.: The structural determinants of recovery in Wernicke's aphasia. *Brain Lang., 44,* 153–164, 1993.

Knopman, D.S., Selnes, O.A., Niccum, N., & Rubens, A.B.: Recovery of naming in aphasia: Relationship to fluency, comprehension and CT findings. *Neurology, 34,* 1461–1470, 1984.

Konorski, J., Kozniewska, H., & Stepien, L.: Analysis of symptoms and cerebral localization of audio-verbal aphasia. *Proc. VII Int. Congr. Neurol., 2,* 234–235, 1961.

Lazorthes, G., Gouaze, A., & Salamon, G.: *Vascularisation et Circulation de l'Encephale.* Paris: Masson, 1976.

Legatt, A.D., Rubin, A.J., Kaplan, L.R., Healton, E.B., & Brust, J.C.: Global aphasia without hemiparesis. *Neurology, 37,* 201–205, 1987.

Lesser, R. & Gordon, B.: Electrical stimulation and language. *J. Clin. Neuropsychol., 11,* 191–204, 1994.

Liepmann, H., & Pappenheim, M.: Über einem Fall von sogenannter Leitungsaphasie mit anatomischem Befund. *Z. Neurot. Psychiatr., 27,* 1–41, 1914.

Luders, H., Lesser, R.P., Hahn, J., Dinner, D.S., Morris, H.H., Wyllie, E., & Godoy, J.: Basal temporal language area. *Brain, 114,* 743–754, 1991.

Martin, A., Wiggs, C.L., Ungerleider, L.G., & Haxby, J.V.: Neural correlates of category-specific knowledge. *Nature, 379,* 649–652, 1996.

Mazoyer, B.M., Tzourio, N., Frak, V., Syrota, A., Murayama, N., Levrier, O., Salamon, G., Dehaene, S., Cohen, L., & Mehler, J.: The cortical representation of speech. *J. Cog. Neurosci., 5,* 467–479, 1993.

Mazzocchi, F., & Vignolo, L.A.: Localization of lesions of aphasia: Clinical CT scan correlations in stroke patients. *Cortex, 15,* 627–654, 1979.

McFarling, D., Rothi, L.J., & Heilman, K.M.: Transcortical aphasia from ischemic infarcts of the thalamus. *J. Neurol. Neurosurg. Psychiatry, 45,* 107–112, 1982.

Miozzo, A., Soardi, S., & Cappa, S.F.: Pure anomia with spared action naming due to a left temporal lesion. *Neuropsychologia, 32,* 1101–1109, 1994.

Mohr, J.P., Watters, W.C., & Duncan, G.W.: Thalamic hemorrhage and aphasia. *Brain Lang., 2,* 3–17, 1975.

Mohr, J.P., Pessin, M.S., Finkelstein, S., Funkenstein, H.H., Duncan, G.W., & Davis, K.R.: Broca's aphasia: Pathologic and clinical. *Neurology, 28,* 311–324, 1978.

Myerson, R. & Goodglass, H.: Transformational grammars of three agrammatic patients. *Lang. Speech, 15,* 40–50, 1972.

Naeser, M.A., Alexander, M.P., Helm-Estabrooks, N., Levine, H.L., Laughlin, S.A., & Geschwind, N.: Aphasia with predominantly subcortical lesion sites. *Arch. Neurol., 39,* 2–14, 1982.

Naeser, M.A. & Hayward, R.W.: Lesion localization in aphasia with cranial computed tomography and the Boston Diagnostic Aphasia Exam. *Neurology, 28,* 545–551, 1978.

Nobre, A.C., Allison, T., & McCarthy, G.: Word recognition in the human inferior temporal lobe. *Nature, 372,* 260–263, 1994.

Ojemann, G.A.: Brain organization for language from the perspective of electrical stimulation mapping. *Behav. Brain Sci., 189,* 230, 1983.

Ojemann, G.A.: Cortical organization of language. *J. Neurosci., 11,* 2281–2287, 1991.

Ono, M., Kubik, S., & Abernathey, C.D.: *Atlas of the cerebral sulci.* Stuttgart: George Thieme Verlag, 1990.

Perani, D., Cappa, S.F., Bettinardi, V., Bressi, S., Gorno-Tempini, M., Matarrese, M., & Fazio, F.: Different neural systems for the recognition of animals and man-made tools. *NeuroReport, 6,* 1637–1641, 1995.

Petersen, S.E., Fox, P.T., Posner, M.I., Mintun, M., & Raichle, M.E.: Positron emission tomographic studies of the cortical anatomy of single-word processing. *Nature, 331,* 585–589, 1988.

Pitres, A.: L'aphasic amnesique et ses variétés cliniques. *Prog. Med., 28,* 17–23, 1898.

Rubens, A. & Selnes, O.: Aphasia with insular cortex infarction. *Proceedings of the Academy of Aphasia Meeting,* Nashville, TN, 1986.

Schiff, H.B., Alexander, M.P., Naeser, M.A., & Galaburda, A.M.: Aphemia: Clinical-anatomic correlations. *Arch. Neurol., 40,* 720–727, 1983.

Schlaghecken, F.: On processing BEASTS and BIRDS: An event-related potential study on the representation of taxonomic structure. *Brain Lang., 64,* 53–82, 1998.

Selnes, O.A., Knopman, D.S., Niccum, N., & Rubens, A.B.: The critical role of Wernicke's area in sentence repetition. *Arch. Neurol., 17,* 549–557, 1985.

Selnes, O.A., Niccum, N., Knopman, D.S., & Rubens, A.B.: Recovery of single word comprehension: CT scan correlates. *Brain Lang., 21,* 72–84, 1984.

Selnes, O.A., Knopman, D.S., Niccum, N., Rubens, A.B., & Larson, D.: Computed tomographic scan correlates of auditory comprehension deficits in aphasia: A prospective recovery study. *Arch. Neurol., 13,* 558–566, 1983.

Semenza, C. & Zettin, M.: Evidence from aphasia for the role of proper names as pure referring expressions. *Nature, 342,* 678–679, 1989.

Silveri, M.C. & Gainotti, G.B.: Interaction between vision and language in category specific semantic access impairment. *Cogn. Neuropsychol, 5,* 677–709, 1988.

Szikla, G., Bouvier, G., Hori, T., & Petrov, V.: *Angiography of the Human Brain Cortex.* Berlin: Springer-Verlag, 1977.

Tonkonogy, J. & Goodglass, H.: Language function, foot of the third frontal gyrus, and rolandic operculum. *Arch. Neurol, 38,* 486–490, 1981.

Tranel, D., Damasio, D., & Damasio, A.R.: On the neurology of naming. In H. Goodglass & A. Wingfield (eds.). *Anomia: Neuroanatomical and Cognitive Correlates.* New York: Academic Press, 1997a, pp. 67–92.

Tranel, D., Logan, C.G., Frank, R.J., & Damasio, A.R.: Explaining category-related effects in the retrieval of conceptual and lexical knowledge for concrete entities: Operationalization and analysis of factors. *Neuropsychologia, 35,* 1329–1339, 1997b.

Tranel, D., Biller, J., Damasio, H., Adams, H., & Cornell, S.: Global aphasia without hemiparesis. *Arch. Neurol., 44,* 304–308, 1987.

Waddington, M.M.: *Atlas of Cerebral Angiography with Anatomic Correlation.* Boston: Little, Brown & Co., 1974.

Warrington, E.K. & McCarthy, R.A.: Multiple meaning systems in the brain: A case for visual semantics. *Neuropsychologia, 32,* 1465–1473, 1994.

Warrington, E.K. & Shallice, T.: Category specific semantic impairments. *Brain, 107,* 829–853, 1984.

Wernicke, C.: *Der aphasische Symptomen-Komplex.* Breslau: Cohn & Weigert, 1874.

Wernicke, C.: Einige neuere Arbeiten über Aphasie. *Fortschr Med., 4,* 377–463, 1886.

Wise, R., Chollet, F., Hadar, U., Friston, K., Hoffner, E., & Frackowiak, R.: Distribution of cortical neural networks involved in word comprehension and word retrieval. *Brain, 114,* 1803–1817, 1991.

Chapter 3

Medical Aspects of Stroke Rehabilitation

Anthony G. Mlcoch and E. Jeffrey Metter

INTRODUCTION AND OBJECTIVES

Stroke is the leading cause of death and disability. Each year, it is estimated that nearly 731,000 individuals will suffer from the sequelae of stroke including death, paralysis, sensory loss, mental status changes, and speech and language disturbances (Broderick et al., 1998). By definition it is a "...sudden and severe attack..." implying that the signs of stroke occur abruptly with little warning and are usually persistent (Dorland's Illustrated Medical Dictionary, 1994). The etiology of stroke is vascular in origin and is due to an interruption of blood flow to various brain regions or to bleeding within the brain or spinal cord. The term *cerebral vascular accident* (CVA) is used synonymously with the term *stroke* to denote this vascular etiology. Keeping in mind the sudden onset, the persistent nature, and the vascular origins, the World Health Organization (1989) defines stroke as a series of "...rapidly developing clinical signs of focal (or global) disturbance of cerebral function, with symptoms lasting 24 hours or longer or leading to death with no apparent cause other than of vascular origin."

It is important for the healthcare professional to know the warning signs of stroke and how strokes are manifested, diagnosed, and treated for several reasons. First, the nurse, physical therapist, occupational therapist or speech pathologist may be the first to recognize that a stroke is occurring. As will be reviewed later in this chapter, early detection of the signs of stroke is critically important since acute treatment may minimize the effects that a stroke will have on the individual. Second, these professionals will be working with others or within a dedicated team of stroke professionals. A command of the stroke vernacular is necessary to effectively communicate with these professionals and to develop and participate in a plan-of-treatment for the stroke victim. Lastly, the healthcare professional will be responsible for counseling the patient and his/her family, providing information pertaining to the prognosis, treatment and outcome of stroke. An understanding of the pathogenesis, diagnostic procedures and the purpose of various treatments is obviously needed.

The purpose of this chapter is to provide the information outlined above. It will review the risk factors (epidemiology), etiology and diagnosis of stroke, including the major neuroimaging procedures and the current acute and chronic stroke treatments. In addition, pharmaceuticals and their effect on stroke recovery will be reviewed.

EPIDEMIOLOGY

Stroke ranks third behind heart disease and cancer as an underlying cause of death in the United States. The current death rate from stroke is approximately 1 person per 1000 population per year and accounts for 10–12% of all deaths (Bonita, 1992). The annual incidence is between 1 and 2 per 1000, while the prevalence rates are between 4 and 6 per 1000 (Kurtzke, 1980). These numbers imply that approximately 1 million individuals at a given time will be living after suffering from a stroke, while 250,000 to 500,000 will suffer from a stroke annually, and half this number will die related to the stroke. The cost of stroke in lost wages is estimated at 20 billion dollars (American Heart Association, 1992) with overall costs being much higher.

The incidence of stroke increases geometrically with age and is primarily a disorder of aging. Thus, for individuals under age 50, the incidence is less than 1 per 1000 annually, while by age 70 it approaches 10 per 1000 and by age 80 is about 20 per 1000 (Kurtzke, 1980). About 1 in 4 men and 1 in 5 women aged 45 will have a stroke if they live to an age of 85 (Bonita, 1992).

Epidemiological studies (see Whisnant, 1983) demonstrated that the annual incidence of strokes declined from the 1950s through the 1970s. However, from 1980, the rates have been increasing. For example, in Rochester, Minnesota, the incidence of stroke increased from 1980–1984 (Broderick et al., 1989) and from 1985–1989 (Brown et al., 1996). The increases are likely due to improved diagnostic methods caused by the introduction of CT scanning and better identification of hemorrhagic strokes (Mayo et al., 1991).

Preventive measures may contribute to lowering the incidence of major disability and mortality. Table 3–1 lists factors that have been associated with increased risk for stroke. Many of these factors can be altered by life style changes, proper

TABLE 3–1

Risk Factors Associated with Ischemic and Hemorrhagic Stroke

Hypertension
Hypercholesterolemia
Cigarette smoking
Cardiac disease
Diabetes mellitus
Alcohol
Obesity
Homocystinemia
Sickle cell disease
Male sex
African-American race
Hyperviscosity
Lack of physical activity
Transient ischemic attacks

counseling, and earlier recognition of changes in patient health status. Improved recognition and treatment of such factors have helped to reduce the incidence of stroke. As an example, the improved treatment of hypertension by lowering blood pressure has been shown to decrease the incidence of stroke and myocardial infarctions (Veteran's Administration Cooperative Study Group on Antihypertensive Agents, 1970; SHEP Cooperative Research Group, 1991). Likewise, the use of antiplatelet and anticoagulant agents in patients with atrial fibrillation have been shown to effectively reduce the incidence of stroke (Ezekowitz & Levine, 1999). Lastly, the recognition of transient ischemic attacks (described below) can also forewarn of impending disaster, and appropriate referral becomes critical. Improved recognition and treatment of such factors have helped to reduce the incidence of stroke.

Stroke-related mortality results from the stroke itself and from other vascular diseases, particularly coronary artery disease and associated heart attacks. Early mortality varies between 17 and 34% during the first month post stroke (Bonita, 1992). The most significant factors associated with early mortality have been alteration in consciousness, which implies a greater and more extensive stroke, and increasing age (Truscott et al., 1974). Myocardial infarction, congestive heart failure, and hypertension have been correlated with early mortality in some studies (Ford & Katz, 1966). Late mortality occurs after the initial hospitalization and is much higher than for the general age-adjusted population. Terent (1989) noted a 1-year fatality rate of 33%.

The scope of the problem becomes clearer when examining what becomes of stroke survivors. Marquardsen (1969) in an extensive review of the literature noted that of unselected stroke survivors 1–25% were able to return to work,

50–75% were able to walk unaided and were discharged home, and 20–30% required continued institutionalization. Thorngren and Westling (1990) found a similar rate of survivors living at home 1 year post-onset of stroke. Held (1975) notes "the percentage of patients who can resume their capability to earn wages is lower than in virtually all other handicaps, physical or intellectual." From these observations it is apparent that stroke will have a devastating effect on the patient and the entire family.

STROKE ETIOLOGY

The most common cause of stroke-like illnesses is related to vascular disease. A partial differential diagnosis for stroke is shown in Table 3–2. The two main mechanisms are related to either loss of blood circulation to parts of the brain through thrombosis with infarction or to hemorrhage of blood into or surrounding the brain. Both mechanisms result in rapid disruption of the ability of brain neurons to function properly, and if severe and persistent, to the death of neuronal tissue. Resulting symptoms depend on the area of the brain damaged and the effect that the damaged region has on the remainder of the brain.

The circulation to the brain arises from two pairs of arteries: the internal carotids and vertebrals. The carotid arteries course in the anterior aspects of the neck and divide into an external and internal branch. The internal carotid artery proceeds to enter the cranium and supply much of the forebrain. The internal carotid artery bifurcates into the anterior and middle cerebral arteries, which supply the cerebral hemispheres over the anterior and much of the lateral surfaces of the cerebral hemisphere (Williams, 1995; Parent, 1996).

The vertebral artery is the first branch of the subclavian artery and proceeds into the cranium through the foramen magnum. The two vertebral arteries unite to form the basilar artery. The basilar artery continues along the midline of the pons. At the upward end of the pons, the artery divides into two posterior cerebral arteries which proceed posteriorly to the inferior medial surfaces of the hemispheres to the occipital lobes. The artery supplies blood to those regions by which it passes, including the brain stem, inferior and medial aspects of the hemispheres, and the occipital area.

At the base of the brain, interconnections occur between the carotid and vertebral arteries, forming a circular passage that allows for mixing of blood from the anterior and posterior circulations. This interconnection is called the circle of Willis. Collateral circulation, which refers to the ability of blood from separate brain arteries to redistribute to other brain areas, is extensive, including the circle of Willis and connections between the external and internal carotids, the left and right anterior cerebral arteries via the anterior communicating artery, and the three cerebral artery systems. Collateral circulation is particularly important when the

TABLE 3–2

Partial Differential Diagnosis for Stroke

Vascular Pathology
  Hemorrhage
    Intracranial hemorrhage
    Subarachnoid hemorrhage
      Aneurysm
        Arteriovenous malformation
    Subdural hematoma
    Epidural hematoma
  Infarction
    Thrombotic
    Embolism
Etiology
  Hypertension
  Atherosclerosis
  Heart disease
    Rheumatic valvular disease
    Atrial fibrillation
    Prosthetic valve
    Infectious endocarditis
  Infectious
  Trauma
  Drugs
    Anticoagulants
    Antiplatelets
    Heparin
  Arterial dissection
  Cocaine
  Congenital absence or atresia of artery
  Radiation fibrosis
  Trauma
  Vasculitis
  HIV
  Fibromuscular hyperplasia
  Moyamoya disease
  Hypertensive encephalopathy
  Sickle cell disease

principal artery to a region becomes compromised. If collateral circulation is adequate, no brain damage may occur. This is accounted for by the ability of collateral arteries to take over and supply an adequate blood supply to the affected internal carotid (Gillilan, 1980).

Ischemic Strokes

Ischemic strokes occur with the complete or partial occlusion of arteries. When blood flow to a region falls below a critical level needed to maintain cellular function and to remove accumulating toxic waste, (e.g., lactic acid) cells begin to die and an infarct develops with necrosis and loss of tissue bulk (Plum & Posner, 1980; Raichle, 1983). Typically,

in ischemic regions, there will be an inner zone of infarction with a surrounding zone of ischemia. Most research on treatment attempts to protect the ischemic zone to prevent the extension of the inner zone of infarction and thus limit functional disability.

The most common cause of ischemic strokes is thrombotic and/or embolic occlusion of the artery related to atherosclerosis. Atherosclerosis is a proliferation of the smooth muscle cells in the intima of the arterial wall with an expansion and deposition of lipid within the associated connective tissue (Ross & Glomset, 1973; Ross, 1980). Atheroma deposition within the arterial wall results in narrowing or stenosis of the artery. If the stenosis reaches a critical level, usually considered greater than about 70%, changes occur in distal blood flow. As stenosis increases and flow becomes stagnate, the likelihood of thrombosis within the artery increases. A second change results from injury to the friable and easily damaged atherosclerotic lesion with the development of an ulcer. The blood system responds to the ulcer as it would to any other injury within the arterial wall with the laying down of fibrin material, platelet adhesion, and trapping of blood cells. This deposition is called a thrombus. It can either occlude the blood vessel, called a thrombosis, or break apart and be released into the blood stream as an embolus, which can occlude a distal artery. Embolism can result from thrombus formed for any reason, not just from an ulcerated arterial lesion. Another site of embolic material is the left ventricle of the heart when the chamber has been significantly damaged by a myocardial infarction. These two mechanisms—thrombosis and embolus—are the principal causes of ischemic strokes. The clinical picture with ischemic stroke as with any neurologic disorder depends on the regions of the brain damaged and the involved artery (Table 3–3).

Hemorrhagic Strokes

A hemorrhagic stroke results from the rupture of a blood vessel within the intracranium. The hemorrhage can occur within three different spaces: the parenchyma of the brain, or the subarachnoid, or subdural spaces. The most frequent type of hemorrhage which would result in consultation with a speech-language pathologist would be an intraparenchymal hemorrhage. Such hemorrhages occur secondary to rupturing of a small artery within the brain, or occasionally by bleeding from a complex of abnormally formed blood vessels called an arteriovenous malformation. Intracerebral hemorrhage causes symptomatology by mass displacement of brain tissue, increased pressure in adjacent and distal brain regions, and tissue destruction at the site of bleeding. With the advent of x-ray computed tomography (CT), small hemorrhages are now being identified which have a good prognosis.

Clinical features are relatively distinct depending on type and location of the hemorrhage. The onset frequently occurs

---

TABLE 3–3

Focal Neurological Findings in Stroke

Middle cerebral artery distribution
    Hemiplegia/hemiparesis
    Hemisensory loss
    Homonymous hemianopsia
    Perceptual dysfunction
    Aphasia
Anterior cerebral artery distribution
    Hemiparesis, legs more than arms
    Hemisensory loss, legs more than arms
    Mute
    Decreased spontaneity
    Bradyphrenia (extreme fatigability)
    Apraxia
    Abulia (lack of will)
    Akinetic mutism
Posterior cerebral artery distribution
    Coma
    Hemiplegia
    Ataxia
    Tremor
    Hemiballismus (motor restlessness)
    Sensory loss
    Intractable pain
    Vision loss (uni or bilateral hemianopsia)
    Prosopagnosia (inability to recognize familiar faces)
Vertebral-basilar artery distribution
    Paresis
    Sensory loss
    Cranial nerve
    Ataxia
    Diplopia (double vision)
    Dysarthria
    Vertigo
    Coma

during activity or exertion. The patient has the sudden onset of a severe headache, with rapid development of alteration of consciousness. Neurologic symptoms are similar to those experienced in corresponding strokes resulting from infarctions (Table 3–3).

Transient Ischemic Attacks

Transient ischemic attacks (TIAs) are particularly important for the speech-language pathologist to understand because an individual who has such an attack is at a high risk of having a stroke. In fact, there is a 10 to 20% chance of having a stroke within 1 year, and a 30 to 60% of having one in 5 years. Great variability has been found in the incidence of stroke in TIA patients, as found by a number of investigators (see Brust, 1977). Part of the difference is related to the definitions used for accepting a patient as having a TIA. For such reasons, when reading papers on TIA, it is extremely important to read clinical criteria carefully, and to understand the group of patients actually being studied. A TIA is a brief focal cerebral event where the symptoms develop rapidly. The duration of an attack ranges from 2 to 30 minutes, to as long as 24 hours, while most are less than 23 hours in duration. The patient may have two or more such attacks over a variable period of time (The Joint Committee for Stroke Facilities, 1974). During a TIA, part of the brain has temporarily become ischemic, resulting in the clinical symptoms. With resolution of the ischemia, the symptoms disappear.

Carotid territory TIAs show one or more of the following (Joint Committee, 1974): 1) hemiparesis—muscular weakness or clumsiness of an arm and/or leg on one side of the body; 2) hemisensory changes; 3) transient aphasia; 4) amaurosis fugax—transient loss of vision in one eye; and/or 5) homonymous hemianopsia—transient loss of vision with an inability to see one side of the visual field.

Vertebral-basilar TIAs show a different combination of symptoms determined by the structures that receive their blood flow from this arterial complex. Symptoms include one or more of the following: 1) Motor dysfunction involving one or more extremities; 2) Sensory changes involving one or more extremities usually including the face; 3) Visual loss—both total or partial loss of vision; 4) Gait or posture instability with ataxia, imbalance, or unsteadiness, but not vertigo; and/or 5) Double vision (diplopia), swallowing problems (dysphagia), dysarthria or vertigo occurring in combination with the above.

The following are not considered symptoms of TIA since each of these are common and are not associated with stroke: 1) Altered conscious or faints; 2) Dizziness; 3) Amnesia alone; 4) Confusion alone; 5) Seizure activity; 6) March (progression) of motor or sensory symptoms; 7) Vertigo alone; 8) Diplopia alone; 9) Dysphagia alone; 10) Dysarthria alone; or 11) Symptoms associated with migraine (e.g., scintillating scotomata—a transient blind gap in a visual field) (Joint Committee, 1974).

TIAs are important because they suggest the patient is at a higher risk of having a stroke compared with age-matched population. In fact, there is a 10–20% chance of having a stroke within 1 year, and a 30–60% chance of having one in 5 years.

Treatment for TIA is successful at decreasing the risk of impending strokes. It attempts to prevent the formation of thrombus and the release of emboli. Two major approaches are being used. The surgical approach is to remove the atheromatous material from within the carotid artery, i.e., endarterectomy. Recent cooperative studies have shown that carotid endarterectomies are beneficial to patients with recent hemispheric or retinal transient ischemic attacks (Barnett et al., 1991; Mayberg et al., 1991; European Carotid Trialists' Collaborative Group, 1991). Patients with stenosis >70% of the vessel lumen to their symptomatic carotid artery were less likely to incur a stroke after undergoing an endarterectomy than if they had received only antiplatelet treatment (e.g., aspirin). Patients with stenosis in the 50–69% range showed less consistent benefits (Henry et al., 1998). However, there is a risk from the angiogram required to define the anatomy of the blood vessels, and from the surgical procedure itself (Whisnant et al., 1983). Endarterectomy seems warranted only when overall morbidity and mortality from the angiogram and surgical procedure are less than 5% (Sundt et al., 1975).

The second treatment approach is medical and consists of preventing thrombus formation. Immediately following a first TIA, a patient may be treated with heparin and then placed on an anticoagulant for a variable period of time (Sandok et al., 1978). Anticoagulants prevent the formation of the thrombus, thus preventing the release of emboli. The risk of anticoagulants is bleeding, and this can be a high risk. In using these medications, bleeding parameters of the blood, primarily the prothrombin time (measure of the blood's ability to coagulate), need to be carefully followed and adjusted. In general, the physician attempts to keep the value at 1.5 to 2.0 times normal, which minimizes the bleeding risk. Because of the high risk of bleeding, anticoagulants are typically used for periods of 3 to 6 months. The second medical treatment has been antiplatelet agents such as aspirin. Aspirin decreases the stickiness of platelets so that they will not adhere to the atheromatous lesions. Several studies have shown that the use of aspirin lowers the risk of subsequent TIA, strokes and death, particularly in males (Fields et al., 1977; Canadian Cooperative Study Group, 1978; Antiplatelet Trialists Collaboration, 1994). At present, one aspirin or less a day seems to be an appropriate dose. However, no dose has been shown to definitely be most efficacious. The low risk of complications other than gastrointestinal make this an appealing treatment.

Other Causes

A large number of other disorders can result in stroke-like syndromes (Table 3–2). Such illnesses include brain tumors, chronic subdural hematoma (Moster et al., 1983), infections of the brain, multiple sclerosis, residual head trauma, etc. At times there are clinical clues suggesting that what appears to be a stroke may be something else. Recognition of such differences in the clinical course suggest that something is occurring other than a "simple stroke." The key is that over time the patient is not showing normal recovery, but rather is becoming worse. This can appear as slowly increasing weakness, seizures, increasing confusion, or aphasia, or the development of new signs or symptoms that were not noted previously.

DIAGNOSIS

A diagnosis is made based on a history, physical examination, and diagnostic studies. The history is the most important part of the evaluation. Without adequate information, the physician typically does not know what to look for. The purpose of the physical examination is to confirm the history.

In making a neurologic diagnosis, answers are needed to several key questions. The first question is whether the problem is based on a nervous system dysfunction. For example, a patient being seen because of a sudden episode of loss of consciousness lasting 2 to 3 minutes could have had a seizure, which is of neurologic origin, or a syncopal episode (faint), which is usually not neurologic but more likely of cardiovascular origin. The second question asks where in the nervous system does the dysfunction occur. Can the clinical picture be explained by a single or multiple lesions? The third question concerns the etiology of the lesion. The answers to these three questions dictate the nature and extent of intervention.

Laboratory Evaluation

A variety of nonatherosclerotic causes of stroke syndromes can occur (Table 3–2). Routine tests are usually done to define hematologic, connective tissue, and inflammatory disorders. Typically, blood studies include counts of the red and white blood cells. A screening panel is done which examines blood electrolytes (sodium, potassium, chloride, bicarbonate, calcium), glucose and liver and kidney function. Other blood tests include syphilis serology, as well as screening tests for connective tissue diseases. Routine studies also include an electrocardiogram to evaluate the heart. Additional cardiac studies are frequently done including 24-hour ambulatory monitoring of the heart and transthoracic or transesophageal echocardiography. These tests are done because of their low cost, safety and high return of information, which may not be available from other sources.

Noninvasive Carotid Studies

Since carotid endarterectomy has become an appropriate therapy for nonhemorrhagic strokes related to atherosclerotic disease, techniques are needed to evaluate the extent of disease at the carotid bifurcation. The ideal would be to have a procedure that would be 100% accurate in detecting the extent of disease, and would carry no risk. The accepted procedure to evaluate this area is cerebral angiography, but this carries a definite risk. Other tests have been developed which can evaluate the carotid bifurcation and intracranial arterial structure with 80–90% accuracy and far less risk, with 35% false positives in experienced laboratories.

Ultrasound approaches are used to study the carotid bifurcation. The first is based on the Doppler effect, i.e., a sound source which moves toward you has a higher pitch than if it is standing still, and a lower pitch if it is moving away from you (Evans et al., 1989). Doppler imaging registers echoes of ultrasound waves in relation to the velocity of blood flow. It presents an image of the vessel lumen and in particular the blood column. The second approach uses B-scan mode ultrasonography, which registers echoes related to variations in the acoustical carrying properties of tissues. It images the vessel wall instantaneously as a real-time image.

Doppler techniques have been applied to the study of intracranial arteries. The procedures allow for the estimation of whether intracranial arterial stenosis, aneurysm, or arteriovenous malformations are present. The procedure is valuable in assisting the physician in understanding the blood flow dynamics in patients with complex cerebrovascular problems (Asslid, 1992).

Cerebral Angiography

Cerebral angiography represents the "gold standard" for determining the nature and extent of the vascular abnormality in cerebral blood vessels. Angiography is particularly necessary when considerations are being made to do a surgical procedure, or where clinical diagnosis is uncertain. Typically, the procedure is carried out by placing a small-bore tubing into the femoral artery in the groin and passing it up the artery to the aortic arch and into the appropriate arteries, including both carotid arteries and a vertebral artery. When in place, contrast medium is forced through the tubing and into the arterial circulation while x-ray pictures are taken in rapid sequence over a 10 to 20 second period. Pictures are taken in several planes, resulting in three-dimensional reconstruction of the arteries. In the hands of a good angiographer, the risk is typically less than 1% morbidity and mortality, the major risk being the development of a stroke during or shortly after the procedure.

Magnetic resonance angiography has been developed which takes advantage of the power of magnetic resonance imaging (see below). This technique offers the advantage of imaging carotid and intracerebral circulation without the use of injected contrast media (Ruggieri et al., 1991). Because this method is noninvasive, it is becoming a screening tool for studying extracranial and intracranial vascular disease.

Brain Imaging

The techniques examined so far have studied what occurs within the blood vessel. An important issue for the physician is the type and nature of the damage to the brain, which can be studied by several imaging technologies. Using these technologies, two types of neuroimaging methods that enable the physician to obtain three-dimensional images of the central nervous system have emerged: those that measure the transmission of energy through tissue such as computed transmission tomography; and those that produce images from natural or introduced energy sources, which include magnetic resonance imaging, positron emission tomography, and single photon emission tomography (Fig. 3–1).

Transmission tomography examines differential tissue absorption of externally administered energy and includes

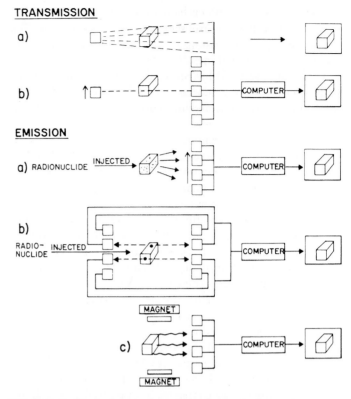

Figure 3–1. Illustrations representing transmission and emission methods. Transmission: a) standard planar radiography; b) computed transaxial tomography. Emission: a) single photon emission computed tomography; b) positron emission tomography; and c) magnetic resonance imaging. (From Metter & Hanson, 1985).

standard radiography and computed tomography (CT). In standard radiography, the brain is irradiated by x-ray. The x-rays that are unabsorbed or transmitted through the brain are recorded by sensitive film or a video image device (fluoroscopy). This provides a planar or two-dimensional image which has excellent spacial but poor contrast resolution (i.e., the ability to distinguish white matter from grey matter). CT obtains three-dimensional images of the brain by measuring the amount of transmitted radiation using multiple detectors placed around the head. The amount of transmitted radiation at each integral point (pixel) is then calculated using a dedicated computer. A three-dimensional image of the brain is constructed using this information.

CT studies brain structure, pathology, and anatomy. Contrast between structures depends on the amount of x-ray absorbed, and the thickness, density, and atomic number of the structures. For example, bone, which contains a high concentration of calcium, absorbs x-ray much more readily than other tissues, and is clearly delineated by both conventional radiography and CT. Distinctive structures within the brain are more difficult to see because specific gravity differences between adjacent structures are small. CT is capable of differentiating tissues with small absorption differences. With standard x-ray, resolution is basically continuous, while with CT it is dependent on pixel size, since each pixel represents an average value of transmitted radiation within its borders. (Oldendorf, 1981; Ketonen, 1997).

Emission tomography produces images utilizing data from internal energy sources. Such sources include magnetic radionuclides injected intravenously, intra-arterially, or by inhalation, and the electrophysiological characteristics of the brain. Emission techniques include magnetic resonance imaging (MRI), positron emission tomography (PET), and single photon emission computed tomography (SPECT).

Magnetic resonance imaging (MRI) is the most recent development in brain imaging. It does not utilize radioactive substances but examines the response of selected elements in response to a large magnetic field. Current techniques are primarily concerned with the study of proton distribution, i.e., water. The resolution of MRI is on the order of CT, but has better contrast in distinguishing grey from white matter. The technique is particularly useful in studying the posterior fossa, where CT has difficulty.

MRI utilizes a very different set of physical properties, taking advantage of the behavior of nuclei as small dipoles or very weak magnets. Under normal circumstances, the axes of the nuclei point in random directions. In a strong magnetic field, the nuclei line up so that their dipoles are either parallel or antiparallel with the field. The nuclei can flip back and forth between the parallel and antiparallel positions, which requires energy absorption and the emission of a radiowave. MRI uses this property by applying a radiofrequency wave to the fixed magnetic field, encouraging nuclei to flip back and forth (resonate) between parallel and antiparallel positions, and measuring the radiowaves emitted in the process. (Bradley, 1982; Crooks et al., 1981).

Each element in a magnetic field resonates at specific frequencies, making the physical properties of the fields specific to a given element. Hydrogen is most commonly scanned because of its excellent resonating ability and abundance in tissue as a component of water and all organic molecules. Two measures usually studied are magnetic relaxation times "T1" and "T2", which are dependent on nuclear density and environment. T1 is the "thermal relation", or "spin-lattice" reaction time and represents the time for the nuclei to become aligned and magnetized when placed in a magnetic field. T1 depends on the physical properties of the sample, e.g., liquids are held together by looser forces than are solids, will become magnetized more quickly than solids, and will have a shorter T1.

T2 is the "spin-spin" or "transverse" relaxation time. Nuclei tend to spin much as a top would. As a top spins it points perpendicular to the ground when under stable conditions. If a second energy source is applied (as by touching it with a finger), it begins to wobble. The wobble represents a torque which describes a second axis of rotation for the top. Nuclei in a strong magnetic field when pulsed by a radiofrequency wave behave in a similar manner. T2 is a measure of how well and how long this wobble is maintained following the radiofrequency pulse. For solids, T2 is very short, because of the fixed rigid structure of the molecules; it is long for liquids (Bradley, 1982).

Contrast has been striking with MRI. Principal advantages include improved contrast between grey and white matter, and the ability to examine the posterior fossa. The contrast is on the order of 10 times better than that found with CT (Crooks et al., 1981). In stroke, MRI demonstrates infarction and edema as early as 90 minutes after occlusion (Spetzler et al., 1983). Furthermore, MRI can be used to study blood flow. Such applications are being used to study how the brain responds to specific tasks. Also, diffusion weighted and perfusion imaging are being used more frequently, as they are sensitive to the early changes that occur with cerebral infarction (Fisher & Albers, 1999; Ay et al., 1999).

PET and SPECT are two tomographic techniques based on the technology of detecting gamma ray emissions from intravenously injected radioisotopes. PET and SPECT are designed to measure functional changes such as regional cerebral blood flow (rCBF), metabolism and neurotransmitters. These methods are distinguished by the type of radiopharmaceuticals and equipment each employs. PET uses isotopes with short half-lives, necessitating the availability of a cyclotron, which adds considerable expense to the procedure. These isotopes are unique since the annihilation of their electrons produces two gamma photons which discharge at 180 degrees from each other. Detection of both photons is made by a gamma camera with a series of parallel gamma ray detectors. Using a dedicated computer, the site at which the dual photons were emitted are located with excellent accuracy.

SPECT also uses isotopes injected intravenously. At present there are only three SPECT radioisotopes approved by the Federal Drug Administration for clinical use; N-isopropyl-p-iodoamphetamine (IMP), 99mTc-hexamethylpropylene amine oxide (HMPAO) and technetium-99m-ethyl cysteinate dimer (ECD). These radiotracers have relatively long half-lives and do not require an on site cyclotron. They are either made from kits or are shipped directly from the manufacturer. They also differ from those isotopes used by PET in that they emit one gamma photon. The site at which the photon was emitted is located by using a collimator, which is a lead shield with a series of holes cut into it. The collimator is mounted on the head of the gamma camera. Spacial resolution is less than with the other imaging methods.

SPECT has not been used extensively in the diagnosis of stroke. The reason for this is that while SPECT detects focal and diffuse changes of cerebral blood flow (CBF), it is insensitive to specific etiologies, such as discerning whether the observed behavioral changes are ischemic, neoplastic, or metabolic. At best the physician requests a SPECT scan in those cases where the CT and MRI are negative and the patient exhibits mental status changes which are stroke-like. In these cases SPECT might be helpful in determining whether these changes are secondary to a progressive dementia or neuropsychiatric disease (Talbot et al., 1998).

Brain Imaging in the Study of Aphasia

X-ray Computed Tomography

CT has been a powerful tool in correlating brain structural abnormalities with speech and language pathology. More recently, MRI is serving the same role. Studies have described the relationship between lesion site and type of aphasia (Hayward et al., 1977; Naeser & Hayward, 1978; Kertesz et al., 1979; Mazzocchi & Vignolo, 1979; Noel et al., 1980). Specific lesions have resulted in specific aphasia syndromes in a manner consistent with classical descriptions. The pre-rolandic/post rolandic separation of nonfluent and fluent aphasias seems well supported by CT (Naeser & Hayward, 1978; Kertesz et al., 1979). A number of cases do not fit within the model (Mazzocchi & Vignolo, 1979; Metter et al., 1981). It has been demonstrated that the location of brain lesions can be predicted from aphasia type with reasonable accuracy; however, the reverse does not appear to be true (Noel et al., 1980). In general, larger lesions result in poorer outcome and more severe aphasia than do small single lesions (Kertesz et al., 1979; Yarnell et al., 1976). Lesion localization independent of size may also be critical for recovery, as noted by the poor prognosis of lesions involving the posterior superior temporal and infrasylvian supramarginal regions, which are associated with poor comprehension (Selnes et al., 1983). Some large lesions are less devastating than very critically placed smaller lesions. The value of knowing the site of brain lesions in predicting the recovery potential of aphasia patients has been demonstrated (Selnes et al., 1983). Such information may be of value in planning language therapy for aphasic patients. This includes identifying patients with Wernicke's or global aphasia who might benefit from intensive auditory comprehension therapy as well as those who might benefit from treatment specifically designed to increase their spontaneous speech (Naeser et al., 1990; Naeser & Helm-Esterbrooks, 1985; Naeser et al., 1987; Naeser et al., 1989).

CT has been particularly valuable in the identification of subcortical lesions and their correlation to language disturbance. Subcortical infarctions of the dominant hemisphere with basal ganglia involvement have resulted in aphasia that is characterized by word finding difficulties, phonemic paraphasias, intact repetition and rapid recovery (Brunner et al., 1982). More severe and long-lasting aphasic symptoms were observed when subcortical lesions appeared in combination with cortical lesions. Nonhemorrhagic infarctions of the anterior limb of the internal capsule and of the striatum in the dominant hemisphere have produced aphasia syndromes that do not correspond to the classic descriptions of cortical aphasia (Damasio et al., 1982). Recovery of aphasic symptoms tended to occur rapidly with these lesions. A specific type of "thalamic speech" has also been recognized with paucity of spontaneous speech, hypophonia, anomia, perseveration, and neologisms with intact comprehension and word repetition characteristic of the aphasia associated with thalamic CT lesions (Alexander & LoVerme, 1980). Patients with capsular/putaminal lesion sites with anterior superior white matter lesion extension had a different syndrome with good comprehension; slow, dysarthric speech and lasting right hemiplegia (Naeser et al., 1982). On the other hand, patients with capsular/putaminal lesion sites with posterior white matter lesion extension had poor comprehension and fluent Wernicke's-type speech. It is the hope of investigators that identification of specific syndromes may lead to specific and improved treatments.

Positron Emission Computed Tomography

Fluorodeoxyglucose (FDG) PET studies have demonstrated that cerebral glucose metabolism in stroke patients extends beyond the zone of infarction as determined by CT (Kuhl et al., 1980; Metter et al., 1981). Figure 3–2 shows an example of the distant effects that may be seen with cerebral infarction (Metter & Hanson, 1985). In this case, the CT study, 1 month post event and 1 week before his death, shows several lacunar infarcts in the left and right internal capsule/basal ganglia regions. The same lesions can be seen on the gross section of the brain. The FDG scan shows similar but subtler changes in the regions. In addition, there is prominent metabolic depression in the left frontal region where there is no evidence of structural changes on CT or the gross brain specimen. The case seems to demonstrate a disconnection syndrome where the left frontal region has been disconnected from its input and output which runs through the internal capsule. The left internal capsule has been destroyed by the lacunar infarct in the internal capsule. Similar remote changes have been found in many stroke cases (Kuhl et al., 1980; Metter et al., 1981; Lenzi et al., 1981; Baron et al., 1981; Martin & Raichle, 1983; Metter et al., 1987). The presence of distant regions with hypometabolism suggests that function in undamaged tissue may be aberrant and might account for some aspects of the aphasic language disturbance and in the recovery process (Metter et al., 1992). Furthermore, functional activation studies in aphasia have shown changing brain organization with increasing activity in the right hemisphere (Muller et al., 1999; Heiss et al., 1999; Cappa & Vallar, 1992).

Studies that examine brain blood flow and metabolism demonstrate that focal brain regions have clear effects on other parts of the brain. Such observations appear to allow for more unifying concepts regarding the development of aphasia following stroke. For example, it has been found that

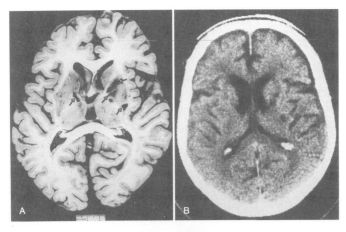

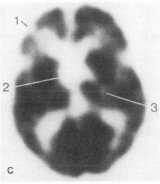

Figure 3–2. Comparison of imaging techniques in a patient with multiple brain infarctions. The three sections are taken from the same level of the brain. A. Gross brain section. Arrows have been added to point out four regions of lacunar infarction. Note that the overlying cortex in this brain section appears to be normal. B. CT scan of the same section. Note that each area of lacunar infarction found on the brain section can be seen in this scan. The scan and brain agree closely in anatomy. C. FDG PET scan of the same section. Arrows 2 and 3 point out the areas of lacunar infarction noted in (A) and (B). In addition, an abnormality can be seen in the left frontal region (arrow 1). This metabolic abnormality does not correspond to any structural abnormality demonstrated in the gross brain section (A) or CT scan (B). The metabolic abnormality at 1 represents the effect of disconnecting the left frontal region from its input and output caused by the lesion in the left internal capsule (the arrow on the left in A). The PET scan gives physiologic information that allows for the understanding of the effects of structural lesions, which can be demonstrated using CT.

essentially all aphasic patients studied by FDG PET demonstrated metabolic abnormalities in the left temporoparietal regions independent of where the structural lesion causing the aphasia was located (Metter et al., 1990). Furthermore, differences between Wernicke's, Broca's, and conduction aphasias were found to differ on the extent of metabolic abnormalities in prefrontal cortex, a part of the brain not felt to be directly responsible for most aphasias (Metter et al., 1989). The data also suggested that language function may

not be attributable only to the structural lesion, but rather to what occurs in other brain areas when the perisylvian region (which functions as a unit involved with language function) is structurally damaged.

Studying brain metabolism has also demonstrated aspects of the role of subcortical brain structures in aphasia (Metter, 1992). Differences in the location of subcortical structural damage are associated with differences in the location changes in overlying cortex. As shown in Figure 3–2, lesions of the anterior internal capsule result in frontal lobe hypometabolism. For most middle cerebral artery distribution strokes, the presence of subcortical extension of the infarct will be associated with frontal lobe hypometabolism. These metabolic and the associated subcortical structural changes are associated with the expressive aspects of the aphasia (Metter et al., 1988).

Single Photon Emission Computed Tomography

The future role of SPECT might lie in its ability to predict recovery. Like PET, SPECT often detects areas of reduced Cerebral Blood Flow (CBF) larger than and remote from the ischemic lesion identified on CT and MRI. These include subcortical infarcts resulting in cortical hypoperfusion and cortical frontoparietal infarcts resulting in contralateral cerebellar diaschisis (Bogousslavsky et al., 1988; Vallar et al., 1988; Megans et al., 1992; Okuda et al., 1994; Halka et al., 1997; Abe et al., 1997). The behavior associated with this phenomenon (i.e., ataxia and aphasia) often resolves as blood flow returns to the remote region (Vallar et al., 1988; Megens et al., 1992). In addition to the "distant effects" associated with cerebral infarction, the size of the CBF defect is inversely correlated with stroke recovery (Lee et al., 1984; Defer et al., 1987; Bushnell et al., 1989; Giulibei et al., 1990; Limburg et al., 1991; Gupta et al., 1991). That is, the larger the defect, the less likely the patient will exhibit good recovery.

The utility of SPECT to predict aphasia recovery has been studied. Investigations have demonstrated that increases of CBF to the dominant left and non-dominant right cerebral hemispheres may be associated with good recovery from aphasia. Using SPECT, Yamaguchi et al. (1980) showed that poor aphasia recovery was associated with failure of increased CBF in the fronto-temporal regions in both cerebral hemispheres in response to counting, conversational speech, and listening to music. Similarly in two investigations by Knopman et al. (1983) and Cardebat et al. (1994), good aphasia recovery was associated with increases of CBF in the right inferior frontal region and the right middle temporal cortex respectively, in response to a listening task. Other studies have shown that good language recovery was related to whether the cortical language region was perfused. Good recovery was associated with reduced but not absent CBF activity in the language region in the left cerebral hemisphere, whereas this region was hypoperfused in patients with poor language recovery (Tikofsky et al., 1985; Mlcoch et al., 1994).

The time at which a SPECT scan is made is important in the study of aphasia recovery (Mimura et al., 1998). The mean right and left hemispheric CBFs measured at or before 9 months post-onset were not predictive of long-term language recovery, while right hemispheric CBFs measured at 7 years post-onset were significantly higher for those patients demonstrating good language recovery. This finding along with those of the previously reviewed studies tend to support the notion that early recovery from aphasia is likely influenced by increased CBF to areas adjacent to damaged regions in the dominant left cerebral hemisphere, whereas long-term language recovery may be related to the compensatory functions of the non-dominant right cerebral hemisphere.

TREATMENT

The treatment of a patient who has developed a stroke can be divided into two parts. The initial, or acute, therapy is directed to the preservation of life, and to preventing expansion of the disability associated with stroke. The second part, or chronic therapy, is directed towards rehabilitation with the reestablishment of as normal a lifestyle as possible.

Acute Therapy

With ischemic strokes there is a region of infarction surrounded by a zone whose tissue can either recover or progress to infarction. This zone is called the *ischemic penubra* and extensive efforts have been made to develop methods to protect and improve blood flow to this region during the early stages of stroke. These include the use of vasodilators to increase cerebral blood flow and to increase arterial pressure in an attempt to force blood into the zone, and the use of corticosteroids, drugs aimed at reducing the swelling of the brain associated with the acute stage of stroke. Unfortunately, none of these neuroprotective methods have proved to be beneficial and until recently the medical treatment of acute ischemic stroke has been limited to the preservation of life.

In 1995 the National Institute of Neurological Disorders and Stroke (NINDS) reported a double-blind study to determine the efficacy of recombinant tissue plasminogen activator (t-PA) for the treatment of acute ischemic stroke. t-PA is a drug delivered intravenously and is essentially a "clot buster" in that it breaks the embolism apart allowing blood flow to return to the deprived region of the brain. The NINDS found that patients who had received t-PA within 3 hours of onset of stroke symptoms demonstrated significantly better recovery at 3 months post-onset. As compared with a placebo control group, patients treated with t-PA were at least 30%

more likely to have minimal or no disability at 3 months post stroke onset. The one negative result was that at 36 hours after onset there was a higher incidence of symptomatic intracerebral hemorrhage in the t-PA group (6.4 vs. 0.6%). However, mortality was lower for the t-PA group at 3 months (17 vs. 21%).

Based on the findings of the NINDS study, t-PA received formal Food and Drug Administration approval in 1996 for the treatment of patients with acute ischemic stroke. To be eligible for this drug, the patient must have had an ischemic stroke within 3 hours of taking the drug; had a CT scan showing no evidence of intracranial hemorrhage; had not had another stroke or serious head trauma within the preceding 3 months; had not undergone major surgery within 14 days; had no history of subarachnoid or intracranial hemorrhage; showed no evidence of significant hypertension; did not have a history of gastrointestinal or urinary tract hemorrhage within 21 days; and was not taking anticoagulants. Since approval, t-PA has been shown to be an effective treatment for ischemic stroke in community hospitals as well as in large medical centers (Chui et al.,1998; Grand et al., 1998).

For those patients who do not meet these stringent criteria and cannot take t-PA, treatment is dependent on identifying the etiology or where the stroke-producing emboli are formed: the internal carotid artery or the heart. Treatment of the former is by either removing the thrombus from the artery by a surgical procedure called a *carotid endarterectomy* (CEA) or by providing antiplatelets such as aspirin. CEA has been shown to significantly reduce the chances of having a second stroke (North American Symptomatic Carotid Endarterectomy Trial Collaborators, 1991a, 1991b; Mayberg et al., 1991; Haynes et al., 1994; Gasecki et al., 1994; Moore et al., 1995). The relative risk of having a second symptomatic stroke within 3 years is reduced by as much as 50% after undergoing a CEA when compared with medically treated patients (ECSTC, 1991). On the other hand, if the etiology is cardiogenic, anticoagulants such as heparin and warfarin (Coumadin) are given to prevent further embolization. Evidence suggests that such treatment reduces overall morbidity and mortality (Easton & Sherman, 1980; Ezekowitz & Levine, 1999).

Chronic Therapy

Chronic therapy begins as soon as the patient is medically stable. The goals of treatment are rehabilitative at this stage and are generally aimed at teaching or providing the means whereby the patient can walk, communicate and carry out activities of daily living (ADL). Initially, this might be as simple as preventing contractures and decubiti (breakdowns and ulcerations of the skin) from forming, especially in seriously disabled patients. This entails passive ranging of a hemiparetic arm and/or leg and rotating the patient in his/her bed routinely. Another goal is to provide stimulation by either talking to the patient or having him/her actively participate in ADL and gradually getting the patient into a lounge chair or wheelchair for progressively longer periods each day. Early mobilization is advocated whenever possible (U.S. Department of Health & Human Services, 1995). This will help the patient actively participate in a rehabilitative program by preventing him/her from becoming deconditioned.

Formal rehabilitation entails the disciplines of physiatry, nursing, social services, psychology and physical, occupational, speech-language, and vocational therapy. Rehabilitation programs can be conducted in a number of settings. There is modest evidence that patients do better in a dedicated stroke unit. Stroke care can be provided in a rehabilitation unit, nursing facility, outpatient clinic or in the home. At present, recommendations are that rehabilitation units should be used for patients with multiple disabilities and who can tolerate at least 3 hours of physical activity each day (U.S. Department of Health & Human Services, 1995).

The goals and techniques used by each type of therapy are beyond the scope of this chapter. The optimal extent and intensity of rehabilitation is still unclear (Kwakkel et al., 1997). Furthermore, the time course of recovery is variable. For example, continued improvement in language performance can be observed for many years following the onset of aphasia (Hanson et al., 1989).

An American Heart Association panel has stated that there are 6 major areas of focus in stroke rehabilitation: 1) dealing with comorbid illnesses and complications; 2) maximizing independence; 3) maximizing psychosocial coping for patient and family; 4) promotion of societal reintegration; 5) improving quality of life; and 6) preventing recurrent vascular events (Gresham et al., 1997; U.S. Department of Health & Human Services, 1995). However, note those factors that affect overall stroke rehabilitation or outcome.

The severity of the neurological impairment has been shown to have the most effect on the outcome of stroke recovery (Lorenze et al., 1958; Gersten et al., 1970). Patients demonstrating severe to profound neurological impairment and/or hemiplegia (vs. hemiparesis) tend to stay longer in the hospital and become less functional (Harvey et al., 1998). Degree of communication deficit also plays a role in the stroke recovery. Patients with global aphasia or hemineglect tend to respond poorly to rehabilitative efforts aimed at teaching ADL and improving mobility (Paolucci et al., 1998). Patients with these deficits are likely to be less independent than those with other types of aphasia (with better comprehension of spoken language) or without sensory neglect (the ability to attend to events in the left or right hemispace) (Paolucci et al., 1996). Lastly, the effects of psychiatric disorders such as depression and apathy may also have a negative effect on stroke recovery. Surprisingly, poststroke depression has not been found to be consistently correlated with outcome or length of stay on a rehabilitative unit (Eastwood et al., 1989; Sinyor et al., 1986). Stroke patients with depression are not less

functionally competent but tend to have less active lifestyles than patients without depression (Clark & Smith, 1998). In contrast, patients demonstrating *apathy syndrome or negative symptom complex* tend to stay longer in rehabilitation and are less functionally competent and independent at the end of treatment (Galynker et al., 1997; Clark & Smith, 1998). This type of patient is indifferent to his/her environment. He/she expresses no concerns about the effect his/her stroke has on others, often explaining his/her lack of motivation as being tired. He/she shows little or no ambition and makes feeble efforts at achieving independence. These patients respond poorly to rehabilitation regardless of their degree of physical disability (Dombovy et al., 1986; Schmel'kov, 1982). However, the clinician should not assume that this behavior is purposeful. It is often the sequela of brain damage such as *abulia* (lack of willfulness) associated with frontal lobe disease or *anosognosia* (lack of awareness of disability) resulting from right cerebral hemisphere or left temporal lobe damage.

PHARMACOLOGICAL EFFECTS AND TREATMENT

The stroke patient often presents with complications which may compromise his/her health and overall recovery. These include seizures, hyperanxiety, depression, and hypertension. Drugs are frequently prescribed by the physician to treat these disorders. While many of these drugs have been shown to impede recovery in laboratory animals, few studies have investigated their effects on humans (Table 3–4) (also see Goldstein, 1997, 1998 for a review).

In a retrospective study, the motor recovery of stroke patients who had received drugs detrimental to recovery in laboratory animals was investigated (Goldstein et al., 1990). These were commonly prescribed drugs and included the antihypertensives, clonidine and prazosin, dopamine receptor antagonists, anxiolytics, and the antiseizure agent, phenytoin. When compared with a group of patients who were not taking these drugs, the drug group demonstrated significantly poorer motor recovery. In another retrospective investigation the detrimental effects of these commonly prescribed drugs were also found (Goldstein, 1995). Irrespective of other factors such as the degree of initial motor impairment, the drug group showed less recovery of motor function and were less independent in ADL. However, the major drawback to both these retrospective studies is that it is difficult to determine whether the negative effect was due to the drugs or the disorders treated by the drugs (i.e., depression, anxiety, etc.). A double-blind prospective investigation of a specific drug or class of drugs is needed to determine its effect on stroke recovery.

Pharmacological agents that act on the central nervous system can be classified according to whether they increase production or retard metabolism (agonists) or impede

TABLE 3–4

Common Drugs and Their Effect on Stroke Recovery in Laboratory Animals and Humans

Neurotransmitter Action	Clinical Use	Effect	
		Animal	Human
Norepinephrine Agonists			
Amphetamine	Stimulant	+	+
Methylphenidate (Ritalin)	Stimulant	+	+
Norepinephrine Antagonists			
Prazosin	Antihypertensive	–	ID
Clonidine	Antihypertensive	–	ID
Propranolol	Antihypertensive	NE	NE
Dopamine Agonists			
Bromocriptine	Stimulant	ND	ID
Apomorphine	Stimulant	+	ND
Dopamine Antagonists			
Halperidol (Haldol)	Tranquilizer	–	ID
Spiroperidol	Tranquilizer	–	ND
GABA Agonists			
Diazepam	Anxiolytic	–	ID
Phenytoin (Dilantin)	Anti-seizure	–	ID
Phenobarbital	Anti-seizure	–	ID
Carbamazepine (Tegretol)	Anti-seizure	NE	ID
Seratonin (5-HT) Agonists			
Trazodone	Antidepressant	–	+
Desipramine	Antidepressant	+	ND
Fluoxetine	Antidepressant	NE	+
Amitriptyline (Elavil)	Antidepressant	NE	NE
Nortriptyline (Pamelor)	Antidepressant	ND	NE

+ – positive effect
– – negative effect
NE – no effect
ID – insufficient data
ND – no data

production or enhance the metabolism (antagonists) of specific neurotransmitters such as norepinephrine (NE), gamma-aminobutyric-acid (GABA), serotonin (5-HT), and dopamine (DA). Of these only the effects of NE and DA agonists have been extensively studied in both animals and humans after brain injury.

NE is produced within the pons and the lateral tegmental areas of the midbrain and is projected to all areas of the cerebral cortex, as well as specific thalamic and subthalamic nuclei. NE acts on the sympathetic nervous system in that it prepares the brain to cope with stressful situations and is associated with wakefulness and alertness. A reduction of NE has been found in rat and cat brainstems after cerebral infarction (Cohen et al., 1975). Based on the assumption that motor deficits secondary to cerebral injury might be reversed by increasing the production of NE, several investigations have looked at the effect that amphetamine, a powerful NE agonist, has on the motor recovery in laboratory animals (Feeney et al., 1982; Boyeson & Feeney, 1984; Hovda & Feeney, 1984). The common finding of these studies is that amphetamine tends to expedite motor recovery in rats and cats after cerebral injury is induced and the improvement is enduring. In addition, this improvement only occurred when amphetamine was given in conjunction with motor training. Amphetamine treatment alone did not accelerate recovery, indicating that this psychostimulant is a *performance-enhancing* drug.

Similar findings have been found in humans. Cristostomo et al. (1988) showed that stroke patients who took amphetamine with physical therapy demonstrated a rate of improvement 40% greater than patients who received physical therapy and a placebo. Walker-Batson et al. (1995) also showed that this accelerated recovery continues after the patient stops taking amphetamine and well past the period of spontaneous recovery. Hemiplegic patients who received 10 mg of amphetamine every fourth day for 10 sessions paired with physical therapy demonstrated continued accelerated motor recovery up to 12 months post stroke onset. Methylphenidate (ritalin), another NE agonist, has been also shown to have a positive effect on stroke recovery (Grade et al., 1998). Acute stroke patients receiving this drug exhibited significant improvements in mood, ability to carry out ADL, and motor functioning.

Walker-Batson and her colleagues (1991; 1992) also have studied the effects of amphetamine in a small group of patients with aphasia. Using an experimental paradigm similar to that employed in the animal and human studies, six patients, within 30 days of their strokes, were given 10 to 15 mg of amphetamine followed by a 1 hour session of intensive speech and language therapy every fourth day for 10 sessions. The Porch Index of Communicative Ability (PICA) was administered 3 days prior to initiation of treatment, 1 week after the treatment was terminated, then again at 3 months post stroke onset. Comparisons of their 3-month PICA overall scores and their 6-month predicted overall PICA scores were made. Of the six patients, four had achieved over 94% of their projected 6-month score at the end of their 10 weeks of amphetamine and language therapy sessions. At 3 months post onset, five of the six aphasic patients demonstrated over 100% of their 6-month predicted score. While these results are preliminary at best, they indicate that amphetamine might increase the rate of language recovery in aphasia. Whether this agent enhances the overall extent of aphasia recovery is not known. A double-blind, placebo-controlled study is needed.

The neurotransmitter, dopamine (DA), is produced in the substantia nigra and the ventral tegmental regions and projected to the caudate nucleus, putamen, globus pallidus and mesial frontal cortex. DA agonists such as Sinemet and bromocriptine have been used for many years to improve the initiation and ease of movement of patients with Parkinson's disease. Other uses include the treatment of akinetic mutism (Echiverri et al., 1988) and apathy due to bilateral thalamic strokes (Catsman-Berrevoets & Hartskamp, 1988).

The effect of bromocriptine on stroke recovery from aphasia has been studied. Early studies were promising, indicating that this drug may improve the speech fluency of patients with nonfluent aphasia secondary to stroke (Albert et al., 1988; Bachman & Morgan, 1988; Gupta & Mlcoch, 1992; MacLennan et al., 1991; Sabe et al., 1992). However, the data from these studies were generally episodal, employing a single subject test-retest design without adequate experimental controls such as including a placebo condition and blinding the patient and the examiner as to what the patient was taking.

Only two double-blind, placebo-controlled group investigations have been undertaken (Gupta et al., 1995; Sabe et al., 1995). Both studies used patients who were at least 1 year post-stroke and who exhibited a nonfluent aphasia. Each patient in each study took a specified daily dose (15 mg and 60 mg, respectively) of bromocriptine and after a wash-out period, was placed on placebo tablets. Language skills were measured before and after each phase (drug and placebo trials). Regardless of the dosage given in each study, bromocriptine had no effect on the patient's ability to speak fluently, name objects, to write, and to understand spoken and printed language when compared with the placebo condition. Bromocriptine did not prove to be an effective treatment of chronic nonfluent aphasia.

Interestingly, the question of whether bromocriptine (or DA agonists in general) is a performance-enhancing drug, like amphetamine, was not tested. Both studies used patients with chronic nonfluent aphasia and drug administration was not tightly coupled with language therapy. In fact, the Gupta et al. study (1995) did not provide language treatment to their patients during the study. To date there has not been an investigation of whether bromocriptine is a performance-enhancing drug in either laboratory animals or humans. Obviously a study of this type is needed.

FUTURE TRENDS

Since the third edition of this book was printed in 1994, some things have changed but much is unchanged in the diagnosis and treatment of stroke. For the most part, stroke remains a neurological disease of prevention. The physician's responsibility is to identify those risk factors associated with stroke and to eliminate or minimize their potential effect by encouraging implementation of lifestyle changes or by treating the patient surgically (i.e., carotid endarterectomy) and/or pharmaceutically (i.e., antiplatelet, antihypertensive, and anticoagulation therapy).

In the past 5 years much effort has been directed at reducing the extent of functional brain damage resulting from stroke. In an attempt to save the tissue surrounding the infarct (i.e., ischemic penumbra) many neuroprotective agents have been studied. Unfortunately, except for t-PA, none have been found to be effective in stopping the cascade of events resulting in brain cell death. As reviewed, t-PA has the potential of reducing the degree of brain damage by quickly returning blood flow to the affected region. This will hopefully enhance the stroke patient's overall recovery.

The future of stroke treatment lies in how we view the brain. In the past we considered the brain as a *static organ*, one that is "hard wired" and changes little after puberty. We now understand that the brain is a *dynamic structure*, one that is constantly changing as the environment requires and is continually adding new cells which may have the power to enhance the cognitive skills of the individual. It is this view that has led researchers to the implantation of fetal stem brain cells into the brains of patients with Parkinson's disease as well as adult brain cells created by specialized tumors into the brains of stroke victims. While the preliminary (and unpublished) results from this research are mixed and in their infancy, the research may potentially lead to an effective treatment of brain disorders including stroke within the near future.

References

Abe, K., Ukita, N., Yorifuji, S., & Yanagihara, T. (1997). Crossed cerebellar diaschisis in chronic Broca's aphasia. *Neuroradiology*, *39*, 624–626.

Albert, M.L., Bachman, D.L., Morgan, A., & Helm-Estabrook, N. (1988). Pharmacotherapy for aphasia. *Neurology*, *38*, 877–879.

Alexander, M. & LoVerme, S.R. (1980). Aphasia after left hemispheric intracerebral hemorrhage. *Neurology*, *30*, 1193–1202.

American Heart Association (1992). Heart and Stroke Facts. Dallas, American Heart Association.

Antiplatelet Trialists Collaboration (1994). Collaborative overview of randomized trials of antiplatelet therapy. Prevention of death, myocardial infarction and stroke by prolonged antiplatelet therapy in various categories of patients. *British Medical Journal*, *308*, 81–106.

Asslid, R. (1992). *Transcranial Doppler Sonography*. New York, Springer-Verlag.

Ay, H., Buonanno, F.S., Rordorf, G., Schaefer, P.W., Schwamm, L.H., Wu, O., Gonzalez, R.G., Yamada, K., Sorensen, G.A., & Koroshetz, W.J. (1999). Normal diffusion-weighted MRI during stroke-like deficits. *Neurology*, *52*, 1784–1791.

Bachman, D.L. & Morgan, A. (1988). The role of pharmacotherapy in the treatment of aphasia: preliminary results. *Aphasiology*, *2*, 225–228.

Barnett, H.J.M., Taylor, D.W., Haynes, R.B., Sackett, D.L., Peerless, S.J., & Ferguson, G.G. (1991). Beneficial effect of carotid endartectomy in symptomatic patients with high-grade carotid stenosis. *N. Engl. J. Med.*, *325*, 445–453.

Baron, J.C., Bousser, M.G., Comar, D., Duquesnoy, N., Sastre, J., & Castaigne, P. (1981). Crossed cerebellar diaschisis: A remote functional depression secondary to supratentorial infarction in man. *J. Cereb. Blood Flow Metabol.*, *1* (Suppl. 1), S500–S501.

Bogousslavsky, J., Miklossy, J., & Regli, F. (1988). Subcortical neglect: Neuropsychological correlations with anterior choroidal artery territory infarction. *Ann. Neurol.*, *23*, 448–452.

Bonita, R. (1992). Epidemiology of stroke. *Lancet*, *339*, 342–344.

Boyeson, M.G. & Feeney, D. (1984). The role of norepinephrine in recovery from brain injury. *Soc. Neurosci. Abstr.*, *10*, 638.

Bradley, W.G. (1982). NMR tomography. Diasonic Interactive Education Program. Diasonics Inc, Militas, CA.

Broderick, J., Brott, T., Kathari, R., Miller, R., Khoury, J., Pancoli, A., Gebel, J., Mills, D., Minneci, L., & Shukla, R. (1998). The Greater Cincinnati/Northern Kentucky Stroke Study: Preliminary first-ever and total incidence rates of strokes among blacks. *Stroke*, *29*, 415–421.

Broderick, J.P., Phillips, S.J., Whisnant, J.P., O'Fallon, W.M., & Bergstralh, E.J. (1989). Incidence rates of stroke in the eighties: the end of the decline in stroke. *Stroke*, *20*, 577–582.

Brown, R.D., Whisnant, J.P., Sicks, J.D., O'Fallon, W.M., & Wiebers, D.O. (1996). Stroke incidence, prevalence, and survival secular trends in Rochester, Minnesota, through 1989. *Stroke*, *27*, 373–380.

Brunner, R.J., Kornhuber, H.H., Seemuller, E., Suger, G., & Wallesch, C.W. (1982). Basal ganglia participation in language pathology. *Brain Lang.*, *16*, 281–299.

Brust, J.C.M. (1977). Transient ischemic attacks: Natural history and anticoagulation. *Neurology*, *27*, 701–707.

Bushnell, D.L., Gupta, S., Mlcoch, A.G., & Barnes, E. (1989) Prediction of language and neurologic recovery after cerebral infarction with SPECT imaging using N-isopropyl-p-(I123) iodoamphetamine. *Arch. Neurol.*, *46*, 665–669.

Canadian Cooperative Study Group. (1978). A randomized trial of asp sulfinpyrazone in threatened stroke. *N. Engl. J. Med.*, *299*, 53–59.

Cappa, S.F. & Vallar, G. (1992). The role of the left and right hemispheres in recovery from aphasia. *Aphasiology*, *6*, 359–372.

Cardebat, D., Demonet, J.F., Celsis, P., Puel, M., Vaillord, G., & Marc-Vergnes, J.P. (1994). Right temporal compensatory mechanism in a deep dysphasic patient: A case report with activation study by SPECT. *Neuropsychologia*, *32*, 97–103.

Catsman-Berrevoets, C.E. & Harkskamp, F.V. (1988). Compulsive presleep behavior and apathy due to bilateral thalamic stroke. *Neurology*, *38*, 647–649.

Chui, D., Krieger, D., Villar-Cordova, C., Kasner, S.E., Morgenstern, L.B., Brantina, P.L., Yatsu, F.M., & Grotta, J.C. (1998).

Intravenous tissue plasminogen activator for acute ischemic stroke: Feasibility, safety, and efficacy in the first year of clinical practice. *Stroke, 29,* 18–22.

Clark, M.S. & Smith, D.S. (1998). The effects of depression and abnormal illness behavior on outcome following rehabilitation from stroke. *Clin. Rehab., 12,* 73–80.

Cohen, M.P., Waltz, A.G., & Jacobson, R.L. (1975). Catecholamine content of cerebral tissue after occlusion or manipulation of the middle cerebral artery in cats. *J. Neurosurg., 43,* 32–36.

Crisostomo, E.A., Duncan, P.W., Propst, M.A., Dawson, D.V., & Davis, J.N. (1988). Evidence that amphetamine with physical therapy promotes recovery of motor function in stroke patients. *Ann. Neurol., 23,* 94–97.

Crooks, L., Herfkens, R., & Kaufman, L. (1981). Nuclear magnetic resonance imaging. *Prog. Nucl. Med., 7,* 149–163.

Damasio, A.R., Damasio, H., Rizzo, M., Varney, N., & Gersch, F. (1982). Aphasia with nonhemorrhagic lesions in the basal ganglia and internal capsule. *Arch. Neurol., 39,* 15–20.

Defer, G., Moretti, J.L., & Cesaro, P. (1987). Early and delayed SPECT using N-isopropyl-p-iodoamphetamine iodine 123 in cerebral ischemia: A prognostic index for clinical recovery. *Arch. Neurol., 44,* 715–718.

Dorland's Illustrated Medical Dictionary, 26th Edition. Philadelphia, Saunders, 1994.

Dumbovy, M.L., Sandok, B.A., & Basford, J.R. (1986). Rehabilitation for stroke: A review. *Stroke, 17,* 363–369.

Easton, J.D. & Sherman, D.G. (1980). Management of cerebral embolism of cardiac origin. *Stroke, 11,* 433–442.

Eastwood, M.R., Rifat, S.L., Nobbs, H., & Ruderman, J. (1989). Mood disorders following CVA. *Br. J. Psych., 154,* 195–200.

Echiverri, H.C., Tatum, W.O., Merens, T.A., & Coker, S.B. (1988). Akinetic mutism: Pharmacologic probe of dopminergic mesencephalofrontal activating system. *Pediatric Neurol., 4,* 228–230.

ECSTC (1991). MRC European carotid surgery trial: Interim results for symptomatic patients with severe (70–90%) or with (0–29%) carotid stenosis. *Lancet, 337,* 1235–1243.

European Carotid Trialists' Collaborative Group MRC/European Carotid Surgery Trial. (1991). Interim results for symptomatic patients with severe (70–99%) or with mild (0–29%) carotid stenosis. *Lancet, 1,* 1235–1245.

Evans, D.H., McDicken, W.N., Skidmore, R., & Woodcock, J.P. (1989). Doppler ultrasound physics, instrumentation, and clinical applications. Chichester, England, John Wiley & Sons.

Ezekowitz, M.D. & Levine, J.A. (1999). Preventing strokes in patients with atrial fibrillation. *JAMA, 281,* 1830–1835.

Feeney, D., Gonzales, J., & Law, W. (1982). Amphetamine, haloperidol and experience interact to affect rate of recovery after motor cortex injury. *Science, 217,* 855–857.

Fields, W.S., Lemak, N.A., Frankoski, R.F., & Hardy, R.J. (1977). Controlled trial of aspirin in cerebral ischemia. *Stroke, 8,* 301–315.

Fisher, M. & Albers, G.W. (1999). Applications of diffusion-perfusion magnetic imaging in acute ischemic stroke. *Neurology, 52,* 1750–1756.

Ford, A.B. & Katz, S. (1966). Prognosis after strokes. *Medicine, 45,* 223–246.

Galynker, I., Prikhojan, A., Phllips, E., Facsenseanu, M., Ieronimo, C., & Rosenthal, R. (1997). Negative symptoms of stroke patients and length of hospital stay. *J. Nervous Mental Dis., 185,* 616–621.

Gasecki, A.P., Ferguson, G.G., Eliasziw, M., Cagett, G.P., Fox, A.J., Hachinski, V., & Barnett, H.J. (1994). Early endarterectomy for severe carotid artery stenosis after a nondisabling stroke: Results from the North American Symptomatic Carotid Endarterectomy Trial. *J. Vasc. Surg.,* 288–295.

Gersten, J.W., Ager, C., Anderson, K., & Cenkovich, F. (1970). Relation of muscle strength and range of motion to activities of daily living. *Arch. Phys. Med. Rehab., 51,* 137–142.

Gillilan, L.A. (1980). Anatomy of the blood supply to the brain and spinal cord. *In Cerebrovascular Survey Report for Joint Council Subcommittee on Cerebrovascular Disease, National Institute of Neurological and Communicative Disorders, and Stroke and National Heart and Lung Institute.* Bethesda, MD.

Giubilei, F., Lenzi, G.L., & Dipiero, V. (1990). Predictive value of brain perfusion single photon emission computed tomography in acute ischemic stroke. *Stroke, 21,* 895–900.

Goldstein, L.B. (1997). Influence of common drugs and related factors on stroke outcome. *Curr. Opin. Neurol., 10,* 52–57.

Goldstein, L.B. (1995). Common drugs may influence motor recovery after stroke. *Neurology, 45,* 865–871.

Goldstein, L.B. (1998). Potential effects of common drugs on stroke recovery. *Arch. Neurol., 55,* 454–456.

Goldstein, L.B., Matchar, D.B., Morganlander, J.C., & Davis, J.N. (1990). The influence of drugs on the recovery of sensorimotor function after stroke. *J. Neurol. Rehab., 4,* 137–144.

Grade, C., Redford, B., Chrotowski, J., Toussaint, L., & Blackwell, B. (1998). Methylphenidate in early poststroke recovery: A double-blind placebo controlled study. *Arch. Phys. Med. Rehab., 79,* 1047–1050.

Grand, M., Stenzel, C., Schmullins, S., Rudolf, J., Neveling, M., Lechleuthner, Schneweiss, S., & Heiss, W.D. (1998). Early intravenous thrombolysis for acute stroke in a community-based approach. *Stroke, 29,* 1544–1549.

Gresham, G.E., Alexander, D., Bishop, D.S., Giuliani, C., Goldberg, G., Holland, A., Kelly-Hayes, M., Linn, R.T., Roth, E.J., Stason, W.B., & Trombly, C.A. (1997). Rehabilitation. *Stroke, 28,* 1522–1526.

Gupta, S., Bushnell, D., Mlcoch, A.G., Eastman, G., Barnes, W.E., & Fisher, S.G. (1991). Utility of late N-isopropyl-p-(I 123)-iodoamphetamine brain distribution in the predictive recovery/outcome following cerebral infarction. *Stroke, 22,* 1512–1518.

Gupta, S.R. & Mlcoch, A.G. (1992). Bromocriptine treatment of nonfluent aphasia. *Arch. Phys. Med. Rehab., 73,* 373–376.

Gupta, S.R., Mlcoch, A.G., Scolaro, C., & Moritz, T. (1995). Bromocriptine treatment of nonfluent aphasia. *Neurology, 45,* 2170–2173.

Halkar, R.K., Sisterhen, C., Ammons, J., Galt, J.R., & Alazraki, N.P. (1997). Tc-99m ECD SPECT imaging in aphasia caused by cortical infarct. *Clin. Nucl. Med., 22,* 850–851.

Hanson, W.R., Metter, E.J., & Riege, W.H. (1989). The course of chronic aphasia. *Aphasiology, 3,* 1929.

Harvey, R.L., Roth, E.J., Heinemann, A.W., Lovell, L.L., McGuire, J.R., & Diaz, S. (1998). Stroke rehabilitation: Clinical predictors of resource utilization. *Arch. Phys. Med. Rehab., 79,* 1349–1355.

Haynes, R.B., Taylor, D.W., Sackett, D.L., Thorpe, K., Ferguson, G.G., & Barnett, H.J. (1994). Prenetion of functional impairment by endarterectomy for symptomatic high-grade carotid stenosis. *JAMA, 271,* 1256–1259.

Hayward, R.W., Naeser, M.A., & Zatz, L.M. (1977). Cranial computed tomography in aphasia. *Radiology, 123,* 653–660.

Heiss, W.D., Kessler, J., Thiel, A., Ghaemi, M., & Karbe, H. (1999). Differential capacity of left and right hemispheric areas for compensation of poststroke aphasia. *Ann. Neurol., 45,* 430–438.

Held, J.P. (1975). The natural history of stroke. In S. Licht (ed.), *Stroke and its Rehabilitation.* Baltimore, Waverly Press.

Henry, J.M., Barnett, D., Wayne Taylor, Michael Eliasziw, Allan, J., Fox, Gary, G., Ferguson, R., Brian Haynes, Richard, N., Rankin, G., Patrick Clagett, Vladimir, C., Hachinski, David, L., Sackett, Kevin, E., Thorpe, Heather, E., Meldrum, & David Spence, J. for the North American Symptomatic Carotid Endarterectomy Trial Collaborators (1998). Benefit of Carotid Endarterectomy in Patients with Symptomatic Moderate or Severe Stenosis. *N. Engl. J. Med., 339:*1415–1425.

Hovda, D.A. & Feeney, D. (1984). Amphetamine and experience promotes recovery of locomotor function after unilateral frontal cortex injury in the cat. *Brain Res., 298,* 358–361.

Joint Committee for Stroke Facilities. (1974). XI. Transient focal cerebral ischemia: Epidemiological and clinical aspects. *Stroke, 5,* 276–287.

Kertesz, A., Harlock, W., & Coates, R. (1979). Computer tomographic localization, lesion size and prognosis in aphasia and nonverbal impairment. *Brain Lang., 8,* 34–50.

Ketonen, L. (1997). Computerized tomography in clinical neurology. In R.J. Joynt & R.C. Griggs (eds.). *Clinical Neurology.* Philadelphia, Lippincott Williams & Wilkins.

Knopman, D.S., Rubens, A.B., & Selnes, O. (1983). Right hemisphere participation in recovery from aphasia: Evidence from xenon133 inhalation rCBF studies. *J. Cerebral Blood Flow Metab, 3* (Suppl. 1), S250–S251.

Kuhl, D.E., Phelps, M.E., Kowell, A.P., Metter, E.J., Selin, C., & Winter, J. (1980). Effect of stroke on local cerebral metabolism and perfusion: Mapping by emission computed tomography of 18FDG and 13NH3. *Ann. Neurol., 8,* 47–60.

Kurtzke, J. (1980). Epidemiology of cerebrovascular disease. In *Cerebrovascular Survey Report for Joint Council Subcommittee on Cerebrovascular Disease.* NINCDS. Bethesda, MD.

Kwakkei, G., Wagenaar, R.C., Koelman, T.W., Lankhorst, G.J., & Koetsier, J.C. (1997). Effects of intensity of rehabilitation after stroke: A research synthesis. *Stroke, 28,* 1550–1556.

Lee, R.G., Hillman, T.C., & Holman, B.L. (1984). Predictive value of perfusion defect size using N-isopropyl-(I-123)-p-iodoamphetamine emission tomography in acute stroke. *J. Neurosurg., 61,* 449–452.

Lenzi, G.L., Frackowiak, R.S., & Jones, T. (1981). Regional cerebral blood flow (rCBF), oxygen utilization (CMRO2) and oxygen extraction ratio (OER) in acute hemispheric stroke. *J. Cerebral Blood Flow Metab, 1* (Suppl. 1), S504–S505.

Levine, J. & Swanson, P.D. (1969). Nonatherosclerotic causes of stroke. *Ann. Intern. Med., 70,* 807–816.

Limburg, M., Royen, E.A., Hijdra, A., & Verbeeten, B. (1991). RCBF-SPECT in brain infarction: When does it predict outcome? *J. Nucl. Med., 32,* 382–387.

Lorenze, E.J., DeRosa, A.J., & Keenan, E.L. (1958) Ambulation problems in hemiplegia. *Arch. Phys. Med. Rehab., 39,* 366–370.

MacLennan, D.L., Nicholas, L.E., Morley, G.K., & Brookshire, R.H. (1991). The effects of bromocriptine on speech and language function in a with transcortical motor aphasia. In T.E. Prescott (ed.). *Clinical Aphasiology:* Vol. 20 (pp. 145–156). Boston, College Hill.

Marquardsen, J. (1969). The natural history of acute cerebrovascular disease. *Acta Neurol. Scand.,* (Suppl. 38). *45,* 11–92.

Martin, W.R.W. & Raichle, M.E. (1983). Cerebellar blood flow and metabolism in cerebral hemisphere infarction. *Ann. Neurol., 14,* 168–176.

Mayberg, M.R., Wilson, S.E., Yatsu, F., Weiss, D.G., Messina, L., & Colling, C. (1991). Carotid endarterectomy and prevention of cerebral ischemia in symptomatic carotid stenosis. *JAMA, 266,* 3289–3294.

Mayo, N.E., Goldberg, M.S., Leve, A.R., Danys, I., & Korner-Bitensky, N. (1991). Changing rates of stroke in the province of Quebec, Canada. *Stroke, 22,* 590–595.

Mazzocchi, F. & Vignolo, L.A. (1979). Localization of lesions in aphasia: Clinical CT scan correlation in stroke patients. *Cortex, 15,* 627–653.

Megens, J., van Loon, J., Goffin, J., & Gybels, J. (1992). Subcortical aphasia from a thalamic abscess. *J. Neurol. Neurosurg., 55,* 319–321.

Metter, E.J. (1992). Role of subcortical structures in aphasia: Evidence from resting cerebral glucose metabolism. In G. Vallar, S.F. Cappa, & C.W. Walesch (eds.). *Neuropsychological Disorders Associated with Subcortical Lesions* (pp. 478–500). New York, Oxford University Press.

Metter, E.J. & Hanson, W.R. (1985). Brain imaging as related to speech and language. In J. Darby (ed.). *Speech Evaluation in Neurology* (pp. 123–160). New York, Grune and Stratton.

Metter, E.J., Hanson, W.R., Jackson, C.A., Kempler, D., Van Lancker, D., & Mazziotta, J.C. (1990). Temporoparietal cortex in aphasia, evidence from positron emission tomography. *Arch. Neurol., 47,* 1235–1238.

Metter, E.J., Kempler, D., Jackson, C., Hanson, W.R., Mazziotta, J.C., & Phelps, M.E. (1989). Cerebral glucose metabolism in Wernicke's, Broca's, and conduction aphasias. *Arch. Neurol., 46,* 27–34.

Metter, E.J., Kempler, D., Jackson, C.A., Hanson, W.R., Riege, W.H., & Camras, L.R. (1987). Cerebral glucose metabolism in chronic aphasia. *Neurology, 37,* 1599–1606.

Metter, E.J., Mazziotta, J.C., Itabashi, H.H., Mankovich, N.J., Phelps, M.E., & Kuhl, D.E. (1985). Comparison of x-ray CT, glucose metabolism and postmortem data in a patient with multiple infarctions. *Neurology, 35,* 1695–1701.

Metter, E.J., Riege, W.H., Hanson, W.R., Phelps, M.E., & Kuhl, D.E. (1988). Evidence for a caudate role in aphasia from FDG positron computed tomography. *Aphasiology, 2,* 33–43.

Metter, E.J., Wasterlain, C.G., Kuhl, D.E., Hanson, W.R., & Phelps, M.E. (1981). 18FDG positron emission computed tomography in a study of aphasia. *Ann. Neurol., 10,* 173–183.

Metter, E.J., Jackson, C.A., Kempler, D., & Hanson, W.R. (1992). Temporoparietal cortex and the recovery of language comprehension in aphasia. *Aphasiology, 6,* 349–358.

Mimura, M., Kato, M., Sano, Y., Kojima, T., Naeser, M., & Kashima, H. (1998). Prospective and retrospective studies of recovery in aphasia. Changes in cerebral blood flow and language functions. *Brain, 121,* 2083–2094.

Mlcoch, A.G., Bushnell, D.L., Gupta, S., & Milo, T.J. (1994). Speech fluency in aphasia: Regional cerebral blood flow correlates of recovery using single photon emission computed tomography. *J. Neuroimaging, 4,* 6–10.

Moore, W.S., Barnett, H.J., Beebe, H.G., Bernstein, E.F., Brener, B.J., Brott, T., Caplan, L.R., Day, A., Goldstone, J., & Hobson, R.W. (1995). A multidiscipline consensus statement for the ad hoc committee, American Heart Association. *Stroke, 26,* 188–201.

Moster, M.L., Johnston, D.E., & Reinmuth, O.M. (1983). Chronic subdural hematoma with transient neurological deficits: A review of 15 cases. *Ann. Neurol., 14,* 539–542.

Muller, R.A., Tothermel, R.D., Behen, M.E., Muzik, O., Chakraborty, P.K., & Chugani, H.T. (1999). Language organization in patients with early and late left-hemispheric lesion: A PET study. *Neuropsychologia, 37,* 545–557.

Naeser, M.A., Alexander, M.P., HelmEstabrooks, N., Levine, H.L., Laughlin, S.A., & Geschwind, N. (1982). Aphasia with predominantly subcortical lesion sites. *Arch. Neurol., 39,* 214.

Naeser, M.A., Gaddie, A., Palumbo, C.L., & Staissny-Eder, D. (1990). Late recovery of auditory comprehension in global aphasia: Improved recovery observed with subcortical isthmus lesion versus Wernicke's cortical area lesion. *Arch. Neurol., 47,* 425–432.

Naeser, M.A. & Hayward, R.W. (1978). Lesion localization in aphasia with cranial computed tomography and the Boston Diagnostic Aphasia Exam. *Neurology, 28,* 545–551.

Naeser, M.A. & Helm-Esterbrooks, N. (1985). CT scan lesion localization and response to melodic intonation therapy with nonfluent aphasia cases. *Cortex, 21,* 203–223.

Naeser, M.A., Helm-Esterbrooks, N., Hass, G., Auerbach, S., & Srinivasan, M. (1987). Relationship between lesion extent in Wernicke's area on CT scan and predicting recovery of comprehension in Wernicke's aphasia. *Arch. Neurol., 44,* 73–82.

Naeser, M.A., Palumbo, C.L., Helm-Esterbrooks, N., Stiassny-Eder, D. & Albert, M.L. (1989). Role of medial subcallosal fasciculus plus other white matter pathways in recovery of spontaneous speech. *Brain, 112,* 1–38.

National Institute of Neurological Disorders and Stroke Study Group (1995). Tissue plasminogen activator for the acute ischemic stroke. *N. Engl. J. Med., 333,* 1581–1587.

Noel, G., Bain, H., Collard, M., & Huvelle, R. (1980). Clinicopathological correlations in aphasiology by means of computerized axial tomography: Interest of using printout and prospective considerations. *Neuropsychobiology, 6,* 190–200.

North American Symptomatic Carotid Endarterectomy Trial Collaborators. (1991a). Beneficial effect of carotid endarterectomy in symptomatic patients with high-grade carotid stenosis. *N. Engl. J. Med., 325,* 445–453.

North American Symptomatic Carotid Endarterectomy Trial Collaborators. (1991b). North American Symptomatic Carotid Endarterectomy Trial: Methods, patient characteristics, and progress. *Stroke, 22,* 11–20.

Okuda, B., Tanaka, H., Tachibana, H., Kawabata, K., & Sugita, M. (1994). Cerebral blood flow in subcortical global aphasia. Perisylvian cortical hypoperfusion as a crucial role. *Stroke, 25,* 1495–1499.

Oldendorf, W.H. (1981). Nuclear medicine in clinical neurology: An update. *Ann. Neurol., 10,* 207–213.

Paolucci, S., Antonucci, G., Gialloret, L.E., Traballes, M., Lubich, S., Pratesi, L., & Palombi, L. (1996). Predicting stroke inpatient rehabilitation outcome: The prominent role of neuropsychological disorders. *Euro. Neurol., 36,* 385–390.

Paolucci, S., Antonucci, G., Pratesi, L., Traballesi, M., Lubich, S., & Grasso, M.G. (1998). Functional outcome in stroke inpatient rehabilitation: Predicting no, low, and high response patients. *Cerebrovascular Diseases, 8,* 228–234.

Parent, A. (1996). Carpenter's Human Neuroanatomy, Ninth Edition. Baltimore, Williams & Williams.

Plum, F. & Posner, J.B. (1980). The Diagnosis of Stupor and Coma. Edition 3. Philadelphia, Davis.

Raichle, M.E. (1983). The pathophysiology of brain ischemia. *Ann. Neurol., 13,* 210.

Ross, R. (1980). Atherosclerosis. *In Cerebrovascular Survey Report for Joint Council Subcommittee on Cerebrovascular Disease, National Institute of Neurological and Communicative Disorders and Stroke, and National Heart and Lung Institute.* Bethesda, MD.

Ross, R. & Glomset, J.A. (1973). Atherosclerosis and the arterial smooth muscle cell. *Science, 180,* 1332–1339.

Ruggieri, P.M., Masayk, T.J., & Ross, J.S. (1991). Magnetic resonance angiography: Cerebrovascular applications. *Curr. Concepts Cerebrovascular Dis. Stroke., 26,* 29–36.

Sabe, L., Leiguarda, R., & Starkstein, S.E. (1992). An open-label trial of bromocriptine in nonfluent aphasia. *Neurology, 42,* 1637–1638.

Sabe, L., Salverezza, F., Cuerva, A.G., Leiguarda, R., & Starkstein, S. (1995). A randomized double-blind, placebo-controlled study of bromocriptine in nonfluent aphasia. *Neurology, 45,* 2272–2274.

Sandok, B.A., Furlan, A.J., Whisnant, J.P., & Sundt, T.M. (1978). Guidelines for management of transient ischemic attacks. *Mayo Clin. Proc., 53,* 665–674.

Schmel'kov, V.N. (1982). Restoration of motor function in stroke patients: Peculiarities relating to damage of the right or left hemisphere. *Neurosci. Behav. Psychol., 12,* 96–100.

Selnes, O.A., Knopman, D.S., Niccums, N., Rubens, A.B., & Larson, D. (1983). Computed tomographic scan correlates of auditory comprehension deficits in aphasia: A prospective recovery study. *Ann. Neurol., 5,* 558–566.

SHEP Cooperative Research Group (1991). Prevention of stroke by antihypertensive drug treatment in older persons with isolated systolic hypertension: Final results of the systolic hypertension in the elderly program (SHEP). *JAMA, 265,* 3255–3264.

Sinyor, D., Amato, P., Kaloupek, D.G., Becker, R., Goldenberg, M., & Coopersmith, H. (1986). Post-stroke depression: Relationship to functional impairment, coping strategies, and rehabilitative outcome. *Stroke, 17,* 1102–1107.

Spetzler, R.F., Zabramski, J.M., Kaufman , B., & Yeung, H. (1983). NMR imaging: Preliminary laboratory and clinical evaluation of focal cerebral ischemia. *J Cerebral Blood Flow Metab, 3* (Suppl. 1), S87–S88.

Sundt, T.M., Sandok, B.A., & Whisnant, J.P. (1975). Carotid endarterectomy: Complications and preoperative assessment of risk. *Mayo Clin. Proc., 50*, 301–306.

Terent, A. (1989). Survival after stroke and transient ischemic attacks during the 1970s and 1980s. *Stroke, 20*, 1320–1326.

Thorngren, M. & Westling, B. (1990). Rehabilitation and achieved health quality after stroke: A population-based study of 258 hospitalized cases followed for one year. *Acta Neurol. Scand., 82*, 374–380.

Talbot, P.R., Lloyd, J.J., Snowden, J.S., Neary, D., & Testa, H.J. (1998). A clinical role for 99m Tc-HMPAO SPECT in the investigation of dementia?. *J. Neurosurg. Psych., 64*, 306–313.

Tikofsky, R.S., Collier, B.D., Hellman, R.S., Sapena, V.K., Zielonka, J.S., Krohn, L., & Gresch, A. (1985). Cerebral blood flow patterns determined by SPECT I-123 iodoamphetamine (IMP) imaging and WAB AQs in chronic aphasia: A preliminary report. Poster presented at the Academy of Aphasia, Nashville, Tennessee.

Truscott, B.L., Kretschmann, C.M., Toole, J.F., & Pajak, T.F. (1974). Early rehabilitative care in community hospitals: Effect on quality of survivorship following a stroke. *Stroke, 5*, 623–629.

U.S. Department of Health & Human Services (1995). Clinical Practice Guidelines, Number 16, Post-stroke Rehabilitation. Rockville, Maryland, Public Health Service, AHCPR Publication 950662.

Vallar, G., Perani, D., Cappa, S., Messa, C., Lenzi, G.L., & Fazio, F. (1988). Recovery from aphasia and neglect after subcortical stroke: Neuropsychological and cerebral perfusion study. *J. Neurol. Neurosurg. Psych., 51*, 1269–1276.

Veteran's Administration Cooperative Study Group on Antihypertensive Agents. (1970). Effect of treatment on morbidity in hypertension. II. Results in patients with diastolic blood pressure averaging 90 through 114 mm. hg. *JAMA, 213*, 1143–1152.

Walker-Batson, D., Devous, M.D., Curtis, S.S., Unwin, H., & Greenlee, R.G. (1991). Response to amphetamine to facilitate recovery from aphasia subsequent to stroke. In T.E. Prescott (ed.). *Clinical Aphasiology:* Vol. 20. Boston, College Hill.

Walker-Batson, D., Smith, P., Curtis, S., Unwin, H., & Greenlee, R. (1995). Amphetamine paired with physical therapy accelerates motor recovery after stroke: Further evidence. *Stroke, 26*, 2254–2259.

Walker-Batson, D., Unwin, H., Curtis, S., Allen, E., Wood, M., & Smith, P. (1992). Use of amphetamine in the treatment of aphasia. *Restorative Neurology and Neurosciences, 4*, 47–50.

Whisnant, J.P. (1983). The role of the neurologist in the decline of stroke. *Ann. Neurol., 14*, 17.

Whisnant, J.P., Sandok, B.A., & Sundt, T.M. (1983). Carotid endarterectomy for unilateral carotid system transient cerebral ischemia. *Mayo Clin. Proc., 58*, 171–175.

Williams, P.L. (ed.) (1995). Gray's Anatomy. Edinburgh, Churchill Livingstone.

World Health Organization (1989). Stroke 1989: Recommendations on stroke prevention, diagnosis, and therapy: Report of the WHO task force and other cerebrovascular disorders. *Stroke, 20*, 1407–1431.

Yamaguchi, F., Meyer, J.S., Sakai, F., & Yamamoto, M. (1980). Case reports of three dysphasic patients to illustrate rCBF responses during behavioral activation. *Brain Lang., 9*, 145–148.

Yarnell, P., Monroe, P., & Sobel, L. (1976). Aphasic outcome in stroke: A clinical neuroradiological correlation. *Stroke, 7*, 516–522.

Chapter 4

Assessment of Language Disorders in Adults

Laura L. Murray and Roberta Chapey

OBJECTIVES

The focus of this chapter is on the assessment of the language impairment in aphasia in relation to the three interrelated and integrated components of language and the three components of the World Health Organization definition of functioning and disability. We emphasize the importance of accurate analysis of spontaneous language production and comprehension skills as well as informed presentation of standard tests of aphasia. Specifically, the objectives of this chapter are as follows: (a) to list general and specific goals of assessment as well as the hallmark characteristics of a quality assessment; (b) to provide detailed descriptions of the general components germane to the assessment process; and, (c) to review specific procedures for each of the goals of language assessment.

INTRODUCTION

Language has three highly interrelated and integrated components: cognitive, linguistic, and pragmatic (Muma, 1978) (Fig. 4–1). **Cognitive** refers to the manner in which individuals acquire knowledge about the world and in which they continue to process this knowledge. It refers to all of the processes by which sensory input is transformed, reduced, elaborated, stored, recovered, and used (Neisser, 1967). Through cognitive processes, we achieve knowledge and command of our world; that is, we process information. According to Chapey (1986; 1992; 1994), these processes can be operationally defined as the five mental operations in the Guilford (1967) Structure-of-Intellect (SOI) model: recognition/understanding (attention/perception), memory, convergent thinking, divergent thinking, and evaluative thinking (see Chapter 17). In addition, the term executive function is identified as a component of our cognitive system (Johnson, 1997; Ylvisaker & Feeney, 1998).

Linguistic refers to language content, form, and use. Language **content**, or semantics, is the meaning, topic, or subject matter involved in an utterance (Owens, 1984; Wiig & Semel, 1984). Language **form** consists of a system of rules for communicating meaning and includes three rule systems: phonology, morphology, and syntax. **Pragmatic** refers to a system of rules and knowledge that guides how we use language in social settings (Bates, 1976). It includes a knowledge of how to converse with and what to say to different partners and in different contexts, and how to initiate, maintain, and terminate discourse and conversation (Craig, 1983). It also refers to the use, purpose, or function that a particular utterance serves. For example, the same content and form "Where are my keys?" can be used to question a statement, request information, indirectly request an action, and so on.

Within this context, **adult aphasia** is defined as an acquired impairment in language production and comprehension and in other cognitive processes that underlie language. Aphasia is secondary to brain-damage, and is most frequently caused by stroke. It is characterized by reduction in or an impaired ability to access language content or meaning, language form or structure, language use or function, and the cognitive processes that underlie and interact with language, such as attention, memory, and thinking (Chapey, 1994). Aphasia is considered a multimodality disorder since it may affect listening, speaking, reading, writing, and gesturing abilities, although not necessarily to the same degree in each modality (see Chapter 15).

Aphasia does not refer to single modality deficits including perceptual impairments such as agnosia or motor impairments such as apraxia of speech or dysarthria. **Agnosia** refers to an inability to imitate, copy, or recognize the significance of incoming sensory information in the absence of perceptual deficits in the affected sensory modality (Stringer, 1996). That is, in visual agnosia, the patient might be unable to recognize a circle even though the visual sensation is intact. **Apraxia of speech** is a motoric impairment that disrupts central motor planning, and consequently, voluntary positioning of the speech musculature and sequencing of muscle movements in the absence of an impairment in muscular control (Darley et al., 1975; Square-Storer & Roy, 1989) (see Chapter 36). When a motor speech deficit is caused by

COGNITIVE	LINGUISTIC
Recognition/Understanding	
Attention	Content
Perception	Semantics
Comprehension	
	Form/Structure
Memory	Phonology
Working memory	Morphology
Long-term memory	Syntax
Executive Functions	
Self-Awareness	
Inhibition	
Problem Solving/Abstract Reasoning	
Recognition/Comprehension	
Memory	
Convergent Thinking	
Divergent Thinking	
Evaluative Thinking	

PRAGMATICS

Figure 4–1. Three interrelated and integrated components of language (modified from Chapey, 1994; Lahey, 1988; Muma, 1978).

impaired strength, speed, or coordination of the speech musculature, it is diagnosed as **dysarthria** (Darley et al., 1975). However, because aphasia, agnosia, apraxia, and dysarthria can co-occur in a patient, an important aspect of assessment involves determining which, if any, of these disorders exist, and subsequently defining the nature and extent of each particular disorder (see also Chapter 36).

Body Structure and Function, Activities, and Participation in Life

Aphasia can also be defined within the context of The World Health Organization's (WHO) International Classification of Impairments, Disabilities and Handicaps (ICIDH) (WHO, 1980). This classification system proposes three levels, namely, Body Structure and Function, Activities, and Participation (ICIDH-2) (WHO, 1998) in order to heighten our awareness of the holistic components of functioning and disability and the very complex interaction of conditions within the individual and the environment that affect functioning. That is, it takes into consideration both the organic and the complex functional consequences of disease. Fougeyrollas et al. (1997) expands on this definition and attempts to show the dynamic interaction of important variables such as risk factors/causes, personal factors such as organic systems and capabilities, environmental factors, and life habits of social participation on functioning in the "Handicap Creation Process."

For individuals with aphasia, body structure and function refer to impairments of brain and brain functions. Activity

limitations primarily involve the four language modalities of speaking, listening, reading, and writing as well as tasks necessary for daily living such as conversing with the nurse or family member, writing a check, making a phone call, reading a paper or menu, and so forth. The four language modalities have been the traditional focus of assessment and intervention in aphasia. However, during the last ten years functional tasks have increasingly been the focus of care. More recently, thinking also includes participation in daily life and realizing immediate and long-term real life goals (Chapey et al., 2000) (see Chapter 10). This might include playing golf, shopping for clothes, getting a job, going on vacation, participating in clubs and organizations, and so forth. How aphasia might affect these activities is the concern of classifications such as the ICIDH-2 and the Handicap Creation Process (see also Chapter 10).

This literature also focuses on the fact that the core features of positive human health or well-being involve leading a life of purpose, quality connection to others (and zest for life comes from such connections), positive self-regard, and mastery (Kahneman et al., 1999; Ryff & Singer, 1998). Subsequent to the loss of language due to stroke, all of these areas are affected not only for the individual with aphasia but for significant individuals in their environment. This, in turn, impacts their health, well-being, and quality of life.

In addition, without a cause to communicate, there is no practical need for communication. Therefore, within this definition, assessment and treatment target all three areas from day one and focus on a reason to communicate as much as on communication repair (Chapey et al., 2000). As a result of these classifications, then, there is an increased focus on the social and physical environmental factors which might contribute to full participation in life (Chapey et al., 2000).

Assessment: Definition

Assessment is defined as an organized, goal-directed evaluation of the variety of cognitive, linguistic, and pragmatic components of language. Such an evaluation is carried out to determine each patient's language strengths and weaknesses and the degree to which language weaknesses can be modified (Chapey, 1986; 1994; Lahey, 1988). Ideally, it explores "the nature of the language impairment and indicate(s) what aspects of language performance are most appropriate for treatment" (Byng et al., 1990, p. 67). This type of in-depth assessment may seem contrary to current health care philosophy that underscores frugality and efficiency. However, it is essential that clinicians advocate for the best quality of services for their patients. This includes requesting sufficient time and funding to complete a sensitive and reliable assessment from which to develop the most appropriate treatment goals and procedures. Such a thorough, specific, and detailed assessment is essential if one is to see patterns of behavior,

---

Etiologic Goals

---

1. Determination of the presence or absence of aphasia
2. Identification and definition of complicating conditions that have precipitated or are maintaining the communication impairment to determine if they can be eliminated, reduced, or changed

Cognitive, Linguistic, and Pragmatic Goals

    (For each of the following goals, behaviors are analyzed to specify the nature and extent of the strengths and weaknesses in that particular behavior)
3. Analysis of cognitive abilities
4. Analysis of the ability to comprehend language content
5. Analysis of the ability to comprehend language form
6. Analysis of the ability to produce language content
7. Analysis of the ability to produce language form
8. Analysis of pragmatic abilities

Treatment Goals

---

9. Determination of candidacy for and prognosis in treatment
10. Specification and prioritization of treatment goals

Figure 4–2. Specific Goals of Assessment.

describe the complexity of the patient's language behavior, and develop a specific hierarchy of therapeutic goals that are appropriate to each patient (Chapey, 1986; 1994). That is, there should be a strong connection among one's definition of language, one's description of the patient's language, and the goals that are established for treatment (Chapey, 1986; 1994). Indeed, as Brookshire (1997) states, clinicians "must work to ensure that gains in economy and efficiency do not come at the expense of their understanding of their patients' impairments and do not compromise their ability to provide the most efficacious treatment for those impairments" (p. 206).

Assessment Goals

The purposes of assessment are to describe language behaviors in terms of both strengths and weaknesses, to identify existing problems, to determine intervention goals, and to define factors that facilitate the comprehension, production, and use of language (Chapey, 1994). Specific goals (Fig. 4–2) are divided into etiologic goals, cognitive/linguistic/pragmatic goals, and treatment goals (Chapey, 1994).

Hallmarks of a Quality Assessment

The nature of the language deficit in aphasia dictates the need to perform a high-quality and thorough assessment. Some of the characteristics that typify a quality evaluation include (a) a current knowledge of significant characteristics

and patterns of the language impairment in aphasia as well as restrictions to personal activities and participation in life based on both first-hand experiences with patients with aphasia as well as dedicated review of the aphasia language and disability literature; (b) a collection of comprehensive and detailed language samples of patients performing tasks at diverse levels of difficulty; (c) repeated observation, abstraction of behavior patterns, and formulation of hypotheses to account for the language impairment; (d) a quantitative and qualitative description of performance to generate information regarding the course, extent, and scope of treatment; and (e) respect for each and every individual patient, including that patient's past history and accomplishments as well as his or her future contributions.

THE ASSESSMENT PROCESS

Assessment in aphasia involves three interrelated components: data collection, hypothesis formation, and hypothesis testing (Chapey, 1994). Data collection is the process of obtaining information that is linked directly or indirectly to the language strengths and weaknesses of the patient (Lahey, 1988). Hypothesis formation involves categorizing the data or forming taxonomies based on regularities or similarities observed in the collected information; furthermore, it requires interpreting the data and making decisions regarding the presence of aphasia, candidacy for treatment, prognosis, and appropriate treatment goals (Lahey, 1988). The third component germane to the assessment process consists of hypothesis testing or the ongoing assessment and analysis of treatment goals, procedures, and patient progress (Lahey, 1988).

Data Collection

The data collected during the assessment process are based upon reported as well as direct observation of the patient's language abilities (Lahey, 1988).

Reported Observations

Reported observations consist of those data gathered from others who have assessed the patient or who are familiar with the patient's history. These observations may be collected via interviews and written correspondence, as well as review of the patient's pertinent medical records. For example, the clinician may interview professional workers or review the written reports of physicians, nurses, nursing assistants, occupational and physical therapists, neuropsychologists, and social workers who have already assessed or treated the patient. When possible, the patient's perceptions of his or her current language strengths and weakness is also explored. Likewise, family members, friends, and/or members of the community who live with or who have frequent contact with the patient can provide valuable information concerning the patient's current language skills, activities, and participation in life. These relatives and friends may be asked to keep a diary or complete checklists or rating scales that relate to their perception of the patient's language abilities, activities, and life participation. For example, the spouse might compile a diary of how her husband typically makes his needs and wants known in different contexts or with different communicative partners throughout the day.

One possible tool for gathering such information from caregivers is the Communicative Effectiveness Index (CETI; Lomas et al., 1989). This index requires caregivers to indicate "not at all able" and "as able as before the stroke" to rate their partner's current performance in specific particular daily communicative situations (Table 4–1).

Direct Observations

During direct observation, the clinician observes the behavior of the patient over several assessment sessions. Repeated

---

TABLE 4–1

The Sixteen Items of the Communicative Effectiveness Index (CETI)[a]

Please rate _____'s performance for that particular communication situation.
1. Getting somebody's attention.
2. Getting involved in group conversations that are about him/her.
3. Giving yes and no answers appropriately.
4. Communicating his/her emotions.
5. Indicating that he/she understands what is being said to him/her.
6. Having coffee-time visits and conversations with friends and neighbors (around the bedside or at home).
7. Having a one-to-one conversation with you.
8. Saying the name of someone whose face is in front of him/her.
9. Communicating physical problems such as aches and pains.
10. Having a spontaneous conversation (i.e., starting the conversation and/or changing the subject).
11. Responding to or communicating anything (including yes or no) without words.
12. Starting a conversation with people who are not close family.
13. Understanding writing.
14. Being part of a conversation when it is fast and there are a number of people involved.
15. Participating in a conversation with strangers.
16. Describing or discussing something in depth.

[a] From Lomas, J., Pickard, L., Bester, S., Elbard, H., Finlayson, A. and Zoghaib, C. (1989). The Communicative Effectiveness Index: Development and psychometric evaluation of a functional communication measure for adult aphasia. *Journal of Speech and Hearing Disorders*, 54, 113–124. Reprinted by permission. © 1989, the American Speech-Language-Hearing Association.

---

observations are necessary to maximize patient ability to respond and to minimize fatigue, stress, and possible failure. Multiple samples also are essential because qualitative and quantitative aspects of the language abilities of patients with aphasia vary across different communication contexts, contents, and tasks (Chapey, 1994; Glosser et al., 1988). In addition, an aphasic patient's performance of a certain language behavior may also vary despite identical communication conditions (Boyle et al., 1991; Freed et al., 1996), since "an inconsistent response is one of the most striking results produced by a lesion of the cerebral cortex" (Head, 1920, p. 89). Therefore, the clinician elicits language in several contexts, such as unstructured, moderately structured, and highly structured contexts, and appraises the effects of sampling methodology on the language elicited (Chapey, 1994; Lahey, 1988).

Unstructured Observations

In unstructured observation, the clinician describes the patient's cognitive, linguistic, and pragmatic behaviors in a natural setting when there is a minimum of control or interference. The setting should be familiar to the client and provide opportunity for the individual to interact verbally with others. For example, a clinician working in the home health setting may spend an initial session simply observing the spontaneous communicative interactions of both the patient and spouse during a meal time. During such a session, a clinician may be able to identify maladaptive strategies (e.g., a spouse who pretends to understand aphasic jargon) that lead to communication interference or breakdown, as well as positive strategies (e.g., an aphasic patient who requests repetitions, a spouse who accompanies his or her speech with gesture) that the patient or the spouse is now using to facilitate his or her communication interactions (Holland, 1991).

Moderately Structured Observations

At times, the clinician may take a moderately active role in structuring observations and use predetermined questions or tasks to elicit spontaneous language production and comprehension. For example, the client might be asked to retell a story, describe pictures, or answer direct questions or requests, such as: "How do you change a tire?" or "How do you make scrambled eggs?" The clinician and patient may also role play specific situations such as (a) ordering in a restaurant and paying the bill, (b) relating the date and time of a doctor's appointment, or (c) answering the phone and relaying a message (Chapey, 1994). When possible, descriptive, narrative, procedural, and conversational types of discourse are elicited since several studies have documented that type of discourse may significantly affect quantitative and qualitative aspects of aphasic patients' language (Li et al., 1996; Shadden, 1998; Shadden et al., 1991). The use of moderately structured observations permits the clinician to collect and

---

TABLE 4–2

Screening or Bedside Tests of Aphasia

Instrument	Source
Acute Aphasia Screening Protocol (AASP)	Crary et al. (1989)
Aphasia Language Performance Scales (ALPS)	Keenan & Brassell (1975)
Aphasia Screening Test	Reitan (1991)
Bedside Evaluation Screening Test, Second Edition (BEST-2)	Fitch-West & Sands (1998)
Frenchay Aphasia Screening Test	Enderby et al. (1987; Enderby & Crow, 1996)
Halstead-Wepman Aphasia Screening Test*	Sall & Wepman (1945)
Sheffield Screening Test for Acquired Language Disorders	Syder et al. (1993)
Sklar Aphasia Scale (SAS)	Sklar (1983)
The Aphasia Screening Test (AST)	Whurr (1996)
Quick Assessment for Aphasia	Tanner & Culbertson (1999)

*This aphasia screening instrument is no longer published.

observe a larger language sample and more language behaviors than might otherwise be possible and/or explore specific aspects of spontaneous language production and comprehension that had not emerged in a totally natural and unstructured context (Chapey, 1994; Lahey, 1988).

Highly Structured Observations

The language assessment also includes highly structured observations based upon the use of bedside and screening assessment tools, comprehensive aphasia batteries, and/or tests of specific language functions.

Bedside and Screening Tests. Screening tests provide an efficient means to determine the presence or absence of aphasia and to develop ideas for further assessment or initial treatment procedures (Al Khawaja et al., 1996). However, since they are short in length and sample a limited amount of language, they do not provide a detailed description of the patients' language ability. Screening tests may be useful, however, in the early post acute stages of recovery, when patients are too ill to complete a lengthy aphasia evaluation, in certain clinical settings where the length of stay in the facility is brief, or where cost containment necessitates fast clinical information without extensive testing. Although a clinician could develop a reliable bedside or screening evaluation using a small set of functional objects, published screening tests are more convenient and may also enhance measurement reliability (Davis, 1993).

There are several standardized and frequently used aphasia screening instruments (Table 4–2) such as the Aphasia Language Performance Scales (ALPS; Keenan & Brassell, 1975). This instrument consists of four scales (i.e., Listening, Talking, Reading, Writing), each of which has 10 items of increasing difficulty. The actual screening requires minimal administration and scoring time and is suitable for patients

regardless of aphasia severity or type. A Spanish version is also currently available.

Shortened versions of several comprehensive tests of aphasia are also available for screening purposes. These include the adaptation of the Minnesota Test for Differential Diagnosis of Aphasia by Powell et al. (1980) and the SPICA version of the Porch Index of Communicative Ability by Holtzapple et al. (1989).

Comprehensive Aphasia Tests. In many instances, clinicians rely upon comprehensive aphasia batteries to provide the major portion of their highly structured observations. These tests are designed to evaluate specific language functions along a continuum of complexity and to reduce the biasing effects of internal and external factors on language performance (e.g., education, socioeconomic status), and to independently assess each language modality (i.e., listening, speaking, reading, and writing) (Davis, 1993).

Many comprehensive aphasia batteries are available, each of which is associated with particular administration and interpretation strengths and weaknesses. Five tests that are commonly used in both clinical and research settings in the United States and Canada include the Minnesota Test for Differential Diagnosis of Aphasia (MTDDA; Schuell, 1965b), the Boston Diagnostic Aphasia Examination (BDAE; Goodglass & Kaplan, 1983), the Western Aphasia Battery (WAB; Kertesz, 1982), the Aphasia Diagnostic Profiles (ADP; Helm-Estabrooks, 1992), and the Porch Index of Communicative Ability (PICA; Porch, 1967, 1981).

One of the oldest and most comprehensive test batteries for aphasia is the MTDDA (Schuell, 1965b). It consists of 46 subtests that are designed to assess a patient's strengths and weaknesses in speaking, listening, reading, and writing language modalities. A plus/minus scoring is used for most subtests. In addition, a severity rating scale from 0 to 6 can be used to quantify performance in the four assessed language modalities. The test provides a classification system based on Schuell's view that aphasia is a unidimensional, multimodality impairment (see Chapter 15). This system categorizes according to whether the patient presents with aphasia alone or aphasia plus sensory and/or motor deficits (e.g., simple aphasia, aphasia with sensorimotor involvement, aphasia with visual impairment). The test manual provides guidelines for the prediction of recovery based on Schuell's extensive clinical experience.

The BDAE (Goodglass & Kaplan, 1983) provides a comprehensive exploration of a range of communicative abilities and is used to classify aphasic patients' language profiles into one of the localization-based classifications of Broca's, Wernicke's, anomic, conduction, transcortical motor, transcortical sensory, and global aphasia syndromes (see also Chapters 1, 2, and 3). It contains 27 subtests that assess conversational and narrative speech, auditory comprehension, oral expression, repetition, reading, and writing. Supplementary tests to examine additional verbal as well as nonverbal skills (e.g., passive subject-object discrimination and drawing to command, respectively) are also provided. Scoring of the conversational and narrative speech is accomplished with a seven-point aphasia severity rating scale and a profile of speech characteristics: melodic line, phrase length, articulatory agility, grammatical form, paraphasia in running speech, repetition, word-finding, and auditory comprehension. Scoring of the other sections varies from plus/minus scores, four-point scales, to counts of the number of paraphasias in the oral expression subtests. Raw scores can be related to percentiles and help determine aphasia classification. For ease of interpretation, performance patterns can be compared to example profiles provided in the manual.

An upcoming revision of the BDAE (Goodglass et al., 1998) will contain several new subtests targeting assessment of narrative speech, category-specific word comprehension, syntax comprehension, and specific reading disorders (e.g., surface and deep dyslexia). (NB: the revised version incorporates a cartoon strip story retelling task rather than the Cookie Theft picture.) This version will also include a shortened form of the BDAE.

Like the BDAE, the WAB (Kertesz, 1982) is designed to diagnose localization-based aphasic syndromes. However, unlike the BDAE, the WAB identifies syndromes on the basis of specific test scores and provides summary scores which allow documentation of progress. The oral language abilities portion of the WAB contains 10 subtests which assess spontaneous speech (i.e., content and fluency), auditory comprehension, repetition, and naming. The seven subtests of the visual language and the other subtests portion examine reading, writing, praxis, and construction abilities. Three summary scores can be calculated from WAB performances: (a) an Aphasia Quotient (AQ) is derived from performance of the oral language subtests, (b) a Language Quotient (LQ) is derived from performance of all language subtests (i.e., oral language abilities subtests as well as reading and writing

subtests) (Shewan & Kertesz, 1984), and (c) a Cortical Quotient (CQ) is derived from performance of all subtests. A Western Aphasia Battery Scoring Assistant (Kertesz, 1993) is also available to facilitate scoring and data reporting. However, clinicians will need to refer to Shewan and Kertesz (1984) for specific information concerning the calculation of LQ summary scores since the WAB manual and Scoring Assistant only describe AQ and CQ summary scores.

The ADP (Helm-Estabrooks, 1992) allows for documentation of the nature and severity of aphasia, recovery of impairment, and information concerning the general social-emotional status of each patient. The test consists of 10 subtests that assess speaking, listening, reading, writing, and gestural modalities (the reading and writing portions are short and therefore may require follow-up testing in some patients with aphasia). The scoring methods vary across subtests from a four-point scale and plus/minus scoring to calculation of the number of correct information units and phrase length for Verbal Fluency tasks. Subtest raw scores can be converted to standard scores and percentiles, as well as summed to determine overall Lexical Retrieval, Aphasia Severity, and Alternative Communication summary scores. Like the WAB, subtest and summary standard scores are used to determine aphasia type in terms of the Boston classifications of aphasia. In addition to these localization-based classifications, the ADP includes a borderline fluent aphasia type. Clinicians can also plot confidence ranges (i.e., standard error of measurement intervals) for each subtest and summary standard scores to determine patient progress over time.

The PICA (Porch, 1967, 1981) is a highly standardized test designed to provide a reliable measure of deficit severity and recovery prognosis (see Chapter 28). It contains 18 subtests that assess verbal, gestural, and graphic modalities through the use of 10 common objects. However, it does not contain any spontaneous discourse production tasks. Performance on each of these subtests is scored using an elaborate 16-point multidimensional scoring system that is intended to be sensitive to the completeness, accuracy, promptness, responsiveness, and efficacy of each response (Table 4–3). The number assigned to each response in a subtest can then be averaged to provide 18 subtest scores or scores for the language functions of pantomime, reading, auditory, visual, writing, and copying. In his 1981 revision of the PICA, Porch added diacritical markings to this scoring system to provide more specific and sensitive characterization of responses; for example, an intelligible response that received a score of 5 would be augmented by a diacritical "p" if it was a perseverative response. The PICA scoring system is highly informative. However, it requires a recommended 40 hours of formal training to be able to use it (Martin, 1977; McNeil et al., 1975).

The batteries described above are among those most frequently used by clinicians. In addition, several other comprehensive aphasia tests are available including the Neurosensory Center Comprehensive Examination for Aphasia

TABLE 4–3

Multidimensional Scoring System of the Porch Index of Communicative Ability[a]

Score	Level	Description
16	Complex	Accurate, responsive, complex, immediate, elaborative response to test item
15	Complete	Accurate, responsive, complete, immediate response to test item
14	Distorted	Accurate, responsive, complete response to test item, but with reduced facility of production
13	Complete-Delayed	Accurate, responsive, complete response to test item which is significantly slow or delayed
12	Incomplete	Accurate, responsive response to test item which is lacking in completeness
11	Incomplete-Delayed	Accurate, responsive, incomplete response to test item which is significantly slowed or delayed
10	Corrected	Accurate response to test item self-correcting a previous error without request or after a prolonged delay
9	Repetition	Accurate response to test item after a repetition of the instructions by request or after a prolonged delay
8	Cued	Accurate response to test item stimulated by a cue, additional information, or another test item
7	Related	Inaccurate response to test item which is clearly related to or suggestive of an accurate response
6	Error	Inaccurate response to test item
5	Intelligible	Intelligible response which is not associated with the test item; for example, perseverative or automatic responses or an expressed indication of inability to respond
4	Unintelligible	Unintelligible or incomprehensible response which can be differentiated from other responses
3	Minimal	Unintelligible response which cannot be differentiated from other responses
2	Attention	Patient attends to test item but gives no response
1	No Response	Patient exhibits no awareness of test item

[a] From Porch, B. (1971). Multidimensional scoring in aphasia testing. *Journal of Speech and Hearing Research*, 14, 776–792. Reprinted by permission. © 1971, The American Speech-Language-Hearing Association.

(Spreen & Benton, 1977), Examining for Aphasia (Eisenson, 1994), the Appraisal of Language Disturbances (Emerick, 1971), and the Burns Brief Inventory of Communication and Cognition (Burns, 1997).

For patients who do not speak English or who speak English as a second language, aphasia batteries are available in other languages (e.g., Aachen Aphasia Battery; Huber et al., 1983, 1984) and translated versions of many English aphasia tests (e.g., Hua et al., 1997; Mazaux & Orgozo, 1981) are available. In addition, a few aphasia batteries such as the Multilingual Aphasia Examination (Benton et al., 1994; Rey & Benton, 1991) and the Bilingual Aphasia Test (Paradis & Libben, 1987, 1993) assess various language abilities of bilingual and multilingual patients. These tests provide different language versions (e.g., Spanish, Arabic, French, Swedish) that appear functionally and culturally equivalent in content rather than simply direct translations of the stimulus items.

Two other comprehensive batteries, the Boston Assessment of Severe Aphasia (BASA; Helm-Estabrooks et al., 1989) and the Assessment of Communicative Effectiveness in Severe Aphasia (Cunningham et al., 1995), have been developed for patients with severe language impairments. Because these batteries are designed to measure the language abilities of severely aphasic patients, their test procedures differ slightly from those of traditional aphasia tests. For example, the BASA probes for spared language abilities across a variety of tasks and modalities including auditory, visual, and gestural expression and comprehension, as well as visual-spatial

and praxis tasks. The scoring system for this measure includes the identification of affect and perseveration, as well as partial verbal and gestural responses. Consequently, clinicians can acquire more explicit information regarding the communicative strengths and weaknesses of their severely aphasic patients than can be typically obtained using one of the more traditional aphasia batteries.

Tests of Specific Language Functions. Clinicians may need to supplement or substitute comprehensive aphasia batteries with tests of specific language functions to allow more in-depth quantification and/or qualification of abilities in specific language modality and/or to include a greater range of item difficulty. Such testing may be particularly important when an aphasic patient performs at either a basal (very low) or ceiling (very high) level on an aphasia battery and little information is obtained with respect to areas of relative strength or weakness for treatment planning. Therefore, Table 4–4 contains a list of some of the tests available for measuring auditory comprehension, verbal expression, reading comprehension, writing, and gestural abilities of patients with aphasia.

For many of these tests, normative data are provided in the test manual so that an aphasic patient's performance may be compared with those of brain-damaged or non-brain-damaged peers. For other tests, clinicians must look to the empirical literature to find the appropriate normative data. For example, several studies have been conducted to extend

TABLE 4–4

Tests of Specific Language Functions That May Be Used to Augment or Replace Comprehensive Aphasia Batteries

Language Function	Instrument	Source
Auditory Comprehension	Auditory Comprehension Test for Sentences	Shewan (1979)
	Functional Auditory Comprehension Task	LaPointe & Horner (1978)
	Discourse Comprehension Test	Brookshire & Nicholas (1997)
	Peabody Picture Vocabulary Test-3	Dunn & Dunn (1997)
	Psycholinguistic Assessments of Language Processing in Aphasia	Kay et al. (1997)
	Pyramids and Palm Trees	Howard & Patterson (1992)
	Revised Token Test	McNeil & Prescott (1978)
	Test for Reception of Grammar	Bishop (1983)
Verbal Expression Naming	Action Naming Test	Obler & Albert (1979)
	Boston Naming Test	Kaplan et al. (1983)
	Comprehensive Receptive and Expressive Vocabulary Test-Adult	Wallace & Hammill (1997)
	Controlled Oral Word Association Test	Benton et al. (1994)
	Object Naming Test	Newcombe et al. (1971)
	Psycholinguistic Assessments of Language Processing in Aphasia	Kay et al. (1997)
	Test of Adolescent and Adult Word-Finding	German (1990)
	The Naming Test	Williams (1996)
	The Word Test-Adolescent	Zachman et al. (1989)
Syntax	Northwestern Syntax Screening Test	Lee (1971)
	Shewan Spontaneous Language Analysis	Shewan (1988a, 1988b)
	The Reporter's Test	DeRenzi & Ferrari (1978)
Reading Comprehension	Gray Oral Reading Tests-3	Wiederholt & Bryant (1992)
	Johns Hopkins University Dyslexia Battery	Goodman & Caramazza (1986b)
	Peabody Individual Achievement Test-Revised	Markwardt (1998)
	Psycholinguistic Assessments of Language Processing in Aphasia	Kay et al. (1997)
	Nelson Reading Skills Test	Hanna et al. (1977)
	New Adult Reading Test	Nelson (1984)
	Reading Comprehension Battery for Aphasia-2	LaPointe & Horner (1998)
	Test of Reading Comprehension-3	Brown et al. (1995)
	Wide Range Achievement Test-3	Wilkinson (1994)
Writing	Johns Hopkins University Dysgraphia Battery	Goodman & Caramazza (1986a)
	Psycholinguistic Assessments of Language Processing in Aphasia	Kay et al. (1997)
	Test of Written Language-3	Hammill & Larson (1996)
	Thurstone Word Fluency Test	Thurstone & Thurstone (1962)
	Wide Range Achievement Test-3	Wilkinson (1993)
	Writing Process Test	Warden & Hutchinson (1993)
	Written Language Assessment	Grill & Kirwin (1989)
Gesture	Assessment of Nonverbal Communication	Duffy & Duffy (1984)
	Pantomime Recognition Test	Benton et al. (1993)
	Test of Oral and Limb Apraxia	Helm-Estabrooks (1991)

the normative sample of the Boston Naming Test (Kaplan et al., 1983) to individuals who (a) live in institutionalized or community settings (Neils et al., 1995), (b) represent a wide age range (Henderson et al., 1998; Tombaugh & Hubley, 1997; Welch et al., 1996), and (c) represent diverse educational, racial, and socioeconomic backgrounds (Henderson et al., 1998; Neils et al., 1995; Tombaugh & Hubley, 1997). Likewise, expanded normative data for verbal fluency tests such as the Controlled Oral Word Association Test (Benton et al., 1994) and the Thurstone Word Fluency Test (Thurstone & Thurstone, 1962) are also available in the research literature (Ivnik et al., 1996; Heaton et al.,1992; Kempler et al., 1998). Further expansion of the norms for many published language tests is needed since the demographic characteristics of the aphasic population in North America is slowly changing over time (Neils-Strunjas, 1998).

Nonstandard Observations

Nonstandardized observations are also used as data. Indeed, some tests of aphasia and some measures of specific language functions rely primarily upon nonstandard observations. These observations are moderately or highly structured observations that do not have published norms (Lahey, 1988). They are typically cited as tasks in empirical research studies and doctoral dissertations and can easily be adopted for assessment purposes. Such measures often yield valuable insights into the language, communication, or cognitive abilities and impairments of patients. For example, using divergent semantic tasks such as "Can you think of all of the objects that can be folded?" or "that will break if they are dropped," the clinician can score patient responses in terms of fluency (or the number of ideas produced), flexibility (or the variety of ideas produced), originality, and/or elaboration (Chapey, 1994). However, these tasks do not have published norms.

Psychometric Considerations

Clinicians should be knowledgeable about the basic psychometric properties of aphasia batteries or tests that they use. Specifically, clinicians should evaluate each test in terms of its validity, reliability, and standardization (Carmines & Zeller, 1979; Cronbach, 1990).

Validity

There are several types of validity that are important in language sciences: content, construct, and criterion-related validity. Determining the content validity of a test involves deciding if the instrument is measuring all of the behaviors that it should be measuring (Carmines & Zeller, 1979); that is, an aphasia test should examine the full domain of language behaviors that are perceived as being theoretically and functionally germane to successful communication. Construct validity refers to the extent to which a test relates to other measures of the same construct, in this case, aphasia or language abilities. Criterion-related or predictive validity concerns the accuracy to which a test predicts whether a patient is aphasic. Ideally, an aphasia test should be able to discriminate not only between aphasic and non-brain-damaged adults but also between aphasic and other brain-damaged populations (e.g., dementia, right hemisphere brain-damage) (Spreen & Risser, 1998).

Unfortunately, aphasia batteries have been questioned on the basis of all forms of validity. Spreen and Risser (1998) note that although an aphasia test may have strong criterion-related validity, analysis often does not indicate whether trivial test items are responsible for discriminating aphasic from non-brain-damaged adults. The content and construct validity of some aphasia tests are also suspect because they include no clear operational definition of what is being assessed and fail to stipulate the specific model of language upon which test construction was based (Chapey, 1986; 1994; Byng et al., 1990; David, 1990; Kay et al., 1990; Martin, 1977; Weniger, 1990). For example, the conceptual schemata underlying aphasia tests have often ignored the complexity factor in language (Chapey, 1986; 1994). Tests have not reflected the fact that the communication of meaning is the essence of language (Goodman, 1971), and results do not supply enough information about the content, context, intent, structure, relevance, and meaningfulness of utterances (Chapey, 1994). Furthermore, the majority of aphasia batteries do not provide a description of the patient's language impairment in relation to recently advanced cognitive neuropsychological models of language (e.g., Ellis & Young, 1988; Patterson et al., 1985), and consequently fail to yield information concerning the nature of the underlying disorder. As Byng et al. (1990) suggest, "most standardized tests neither clarify what is wrong with the patient, nor specify what treatment should be provided" (p. 67). Lastly, many tasks in aphasia batteries assess composite abilities or more than one linguistic and/or cognitive ability at a time. For example, instructing a patient to "Put the pen on top of the book, then give it to me" (WAB item) engages linguistic processing abilities as well as attention, memory, initiation, and limb praxis abilities. Because linguistic and cognitive skills are both composite abilities and because they are highly interrelated processes, testing one particular aspect of language (e.g., confrontation written naming) without directly or indirectly involving associated processes (e.g., visuoperception, graphomotor constructional abilities) involves sophisticated clinical skill and acumen.

Reliability

Test reliability reflects the extent to which similar results are obtained during repeated administrations of the test under similar testing conditions. The more consistent the repeated measurements are, the more reliable the test is (Carmines & Zeller, 1979; Cronbach, 1990). Although measuring any phenomenon is always associated with some degree of chance error, a test should contain detailed administration and scoring instructions and examples in order to minimize intra- and inter-examiner measurement error that can affect test reliability as well as validity.

Because of the extensive physiologic changes that typically occur during the early, acute phases of recovery, the reliability of aphasia tests can be poor. However, regardless of time post-onset, intra- and inter-examiner reliability should be satisfactory (i.e., reliability coefficient of at least .80). Clinicians should examine the reliability of overall test scores as well as individual subtests.

Standardization

Test administration procedures should be standardized (Cronbach, 1990; Spreen & Risser, 1998) in order to minimize measurement error and to allow valid comparison of patient performance to published norms. To establish such norms, standardized tests are administered to a large number of individuals who represent a cross-section of the population to whom the test will be administered in clinical practice. In addition, many test authors revise their tests in an attempt to improve their sampling procedures and to expand normative data to a greater variety of reference groups (e.g., increased age range, improved minority representation in the normative sample) (see Table 4–4).

Progress/Recovery and Ethnocultural Test Considerations

In addition to meeting psychometric criteria, tests designed for use with aphasic patients should allow for measurement of recovery or progress in treatment and be ethnoculturally sensitive.

Several researchers have noted that standardized tests are clearly unsuitable measures of language change or recovery (David, 1990; Kay et al., 1990; Weniger, 1990). For example, the subtests of most aphasia batteries include too few items to provide a sensitive and reliable measure of that particular language modality or function. Likewise, real change made by the patient in specific areas of language functioning may not be represented in the overall test score, and the effectiveness of specific treatments may not therefore be adequately measured.

Clinicians also examine whether or not the testing procedures are designed with respect to ethnocultural considerations. This applies not only to the aphasia and language tests used by the clinician, but also to those tests regularly administered by other team members (Garcia & Desrochers, 1997). For example, Lu (1996) studied the intercultural variations of specific aspects of language use during informal conversations or "small talk" for Chinese and for American-born English-speaking individuals. He found very specific

differences in discourse structure, content (topic), situations, communication styles, and self-presentation. Chapey and Lu (1998) suggest that such important differences in language and the value that a given culture places upon different aspects of language are important in selecting tasks and priorities for both assessment and intervention. In addition, variables such as the duration of residency in the United States, English proficiency, and the value that a given culture places upon different language and cognitive abilities, test stimuli, and tasks all influence an individual's performance (Ardila, 1995; Jacobs et al., 1997; Payne-Johnson, 1992). Consequently, clinicians must be aware of how salient and suitable stimuli and procedures are to particular cultural groups. Likewise, assessment findings will be more accurate and valid if the normative group for a given aphasia test is representative of an aphasic patient's corresponding cultural and language group.

Body Structure and Function, Activities, and Participation

The World Health Organization's (1998) model of body structure and function, activities, and participation (ICIDH-2) influences how aphasia is conceptualized and consequently assessed and treated. Within this model, a handicap is created not only by the degree and nature of impairments in bodily structure, bodily function, and language, but also by the limitations of personal activities and restrictions to participation in society. Therefore, the WHO model involves consideration of contextual factors, including social and physical environmental variables (e.g., social attitudes in the patient's community, architectural design of the patient's home) and personal variables (e.g., age, education, co-existing physical and mental health conditions), that may interact with impairment, activity, and participation and therefore influence the individual's functioning. Within the context of this model, clinicians appraise each of these areas of handicap creation since there is no one-to-one correspondence among these variables or levels (Frattali, 1998a; Fougeyrollas et al., 1997; Ross & Wertz, 1999); that is, it is difficult to estimate the nature and extent of activity and participation assets and limitations solely on the basis of bodily function and structure (see Chapters 10–14).

Body Function and Structure

An impairment of body structure and function refers to a loss or anomaly in anatomical, physiological, or psychological structure or function. Examples of conditions at this level include aphasia, hemiparesis, hemianopsia, and dysphagia.

Activities

Within the activity level of this framework, aphasia limitations involve the four language modalities of speaking, listening, reading, and writing, as well as tasks necessary for daily living (World Health Organization, 1998). Such limitations in language-related activities of daily living refer to any communication difficulties that arise in everyday contexts (e.g., trouble using the telephone, writing checks, reading the newspaper). Therefore, assessment at the limitation and activity level can involve use of aphasia tests and batteries or probes of specific language abilities (e.g., naming or productive syntax abilities) as well as functional status measures to assess the extent and type of language with which aphasic patients may present (Frattali, 1998b; Holland & Thompson, 1998). In addition, analyses of spontaneous language within the context of activities of daily living and other personally meaningful activities is seen as an essential component of assessment.

Because of this recent emphasis on function, many clinicians may be required to summarize patient data on rating scales such as the Functional Independence Measure (FIM; State University of New York at Buffalo, 1993). The FIM, part of the Uniform Data Set for medical rehabilitation, was developed in part as a means to set reimbursement rates in response to cost containment efforts by the government, and to document a patient's performance of a minimum set of skills at intake and discharge (Ottenbacher et al., 1996). However, the FIM includes a very, very limited number of items to summarize language abilities (Table 4–5). Consequently, the brevity of description alone on this rudimentary scale makes it an instrument of questionable reliability, validity, and sensitivity (Chapey, 1994; Gallagher, 1998; Odell & Flynn, 1998). In fact, Ottenbacher and colleagues (1996) found the poorest rating reliability for the comprehension item. Although other scales such as the Functional Assessment Measure (FAM; Hall et al., 1988), Frenchay Activities Index (Holbrook & Skilbeck, 1983), and the Functional Communication Measure (FCM; American-Speech-Language-Hearing Association, 1995) contain more communication-related information, they are similar to the FIM in terms of limited content, sensitivity, and/or validity (Golper, 1996; Odell et al., 1997).

Rather than rely on these scales to summarize communication-related activity limitations, clinicians may adopt other longer but more precise functional language inventories or scales such as the CETI (Lomas et al., 1989), the ASHA Functional Assessment of Communication Skills for Adults (ASHA FACS; Frattali et al., 1995), the Communicative Abilities in Daily Living-2 (Holland et al., 1999), or The Amsterdam-Nijmegen Everyday Language Test (ANELT; Blomert et al., 1994) (see Goal 8: Analysis of Pragmatic Ability, pp. 92–97).

Participation in Society

Sustained life participation in personally, culturally, and intrinsically valued tasks and goals enhances individual well-being for all human beings (Cantor & Sanderson, 1999). Such participation and concomitant well-being depend in part on social, personal, and tangible resources which increase or decrease an individual's likelihood of participating in various tasks (Cantor & Sanderson, 1999). These resources are assessed, and, when necessary, supported or added to facilitate and motivate "continued participation (even) in the face of threat or frustration" (Cantor & Sanderson, 1999, p. 230) in order to keep individuals "vigilant as they find new ways to participate in life" (p. 230) and thereby gain renewed health and well-being.

Participation restrictions refer to obstacles that limit or prevent the patient from fulfilling his or her social, occupational, or personal role or goals (World Health Organization, 1998). For example, aphasic patients may be unable to return to work, may become socially isolated, and may undergo role changes (e.g., from provider to dependent) because of their aphasia/functional communication problems and because of transportation barriers in the community. To assess deficits at the participation level, clinicians may use measures of psychosocial status such as the Visual Analog Mood Scales (VAMS; Stern, 1998), quality of life measures such as the Sickness Impact Profile (Bergner et al., 1981), and wellness measures such as the Duke-UNC Health Profile (Parkerson et al., 1981). With the exception of the VAMS, few of these measures are designed specifically for patients with language deficits; consequently, the results obtained from using such measures with aphasic patients may need to be interpreted cautiously in terms of reliability and validity (see also Chapter 10).

Hypothesis Formation

The information obtained during data collection needs to be organized, systematized, and condensed in a meaningful way (Chapey, 1994; Lahey, 1988). In this decision making component of assessment, the clinician sifts through all of the information obtained, delicately balancing and blending the data to arrive at a penetrating understanding of a patient's total behavior. Hypothesis formation, then, is a sophisticated clinical judgment applied to the information collected (Lahey, 1988). It is an evaluation of the type, frequency, and pattern of behaviors produced by the patient and an exploration of the interrelatedness of various behaviors (Lahey, 1988). A synthesis of the diagnostic findings will not only aid in determining the suitability of the patient for therapy, but will also indicate priorities and specific plans for a program of intervention.

Aphasia Classification

Many classification systems have been developed for adults with aphasia. Some clinicians use one of the dichotomous classifications (e.g., fluent vs. nonfluent aphasia; receptive vs. expressive aphasia) or one of the anatomically based classification systems (e.g., Broca's, Wernicke's, or conduction aphasia) available in the aphasia literature, while others use

TABLE 4–5

Functional Independence Measure (FIM)

	7	Complete Independence (Timely, Safely)	NO
	6	Modified Independence (Device)	
L		**Modified Dependence**	
E	5	Supervision	
V	4	Minimal Assist (Subject = 75%)	
E	3	Moderate Assist (Subject = 50%+)	HELPER
L		**Complete Dependence**	
S	2	Maximal Assist (Subject = 25%+)	
	1	Total Assist (Subject = 0%+)	

Self-Care   FOLLOW-UP
A. Eating
B. Grooming
C. Bathing
D. Dressing-Upper Body
E. Dressing-Lower Body
F. Toileting

Sphincter Control
G. Bladder Management
H. Bowel Management

Mobility Transfer
I. Bed, Chair, Wheelchair
J. Toilet
K. Tub, Shower

Locomotion
L. Walk/Wheelchair

M. Stairs

Communication
N. Comprehension

O. Expression

Social Cognition
P. Social Interaction
Q. Problem Solving
R. Memory   Total FIM:_____

NOTE: Leave no blanks; enter 1 if patient not testable due to risk.
From Research Foundation. (1990). Guide for use of the Uniform Data Set for Medical Rehabilitation.
Buffalo, NY: Research Foundation, State University of New York.

the system developed by Schuell and colleagues (1964) to categorize or label the results of their assessment. However, there is still no universally acceptable classification system (Holland et al., 1986; Kertesz, 1979). In addition, the validity of such classification systems has been called into question for several reasons (Byng et al., 1990; Caplan, 1993; Gordon, 1998; Wertz et al., 1984; Varney, 1998): (a) the language profile of many patients cannot be fitted into one of the categories (estimates range from 25% to as many as 70% of aphasic patients); (b) patients in these categories cannot be said to be homogeneously impaired; (c) certain aphasia classifications such as receptive/expressive or sensory/motor are misleading since most if not all aphasic patients display some degree of impairment in both language comprehension and production abilities; (d) a patient can evolve from one classification to another during the course of recovery; (e) the inclusionary criteria for the different aphasia types frequently overlap (e.g., all aphasia types include anomia as a symptom); (f) classification of aphasia type may vary as a function of the aphasia battery used (e.g., BDAE vs. WAB results); (g) discrepancies in interjudge reliability can possibly stem from a lack of agreement as to how to assign and weight specific responses; (h) categories convey little information concerning the nature of the underlying language impairment (e.g., which particular level [semantic vs. phonologic] of language processing is impaired); and (i) syndrome classification in itself does not provide the basis for any comprehensive treatment program. Despite these concerns, the use of aphasia classifications remains a common and often useful means of describing language deficits in both clinical and research settings. For example, for some patients, a particular aphasia type may succinctly describe their language profile, and consequently the label may, at times, be useful to include in a medical chart note, clinical report, or research paper.

Severity Classification

Determining the severity of an aphasic patient's language impairment may guide the clinician in choosing appropriate testing materials. For example, for patients with severe language impairments, clinicians may wish to avoid a frustrating assessment experience for themselves and their patients by selecting shorter tasks or tests for initial assessment. Severity ratings may also provide a useful guide for assigning patients to language treatment groups (Beeson & Holland, 1994). However, regardless of the measure used to determine or index a patient's overall aphasia severity (e.g., clinical judgment, severity rating scale, severity score), clinicians will want to determine whether or not it has been examined with respect to validity and reliability. For example, Lezak (1995) noted that the severity estimate derived from a standardized battery, even the CADL, may underestimate a patient's ability to communicate in everyday situations because contextual cues, routines, and familiarity with vocabulary are qualities of everyday communication that are difficult to replicate in a standardized examination.

Cognitive Neuropsychological, Psycholinguistic, and Information Processing Models

In addition, rather than summarize assessment results with two or three scores, clinicians may use cognitive neuropsychological, psycholinguistic, or information processing models to describe their clinical findings (Byng et al., 1990; Caplan, 1993; Kay et al., 1996; and see Davis, 1996, for a comparison of cognitive neuropsychology and psycholinguistics). In these models, a particular language behavior (e.g., picture naming) is visualized as a sequence of operations (e.g., visuo-perceptual analysis, accessing semantic stores, accessing phonological output lexicon) (Fig. 4–3). The clinician's task is to determine the integrity of each of these language operations or components within each language modality in order to localize the level or levels at which the language behavior is breaking down. Additionally, clinicians following this approach may assess the type(s) of errors made and the manner in which the patient goes about completing each

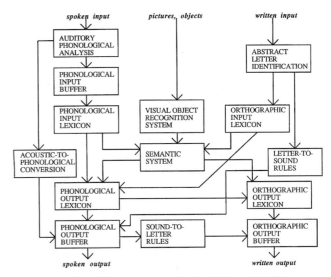

Figure 4–3. Cognitive neuropsychological model of the language processing system. Adapted from Kay, J., Lesser, R., & Coltheart, M. (1996). Psycholinguistic Assessments of Language Processing in Aphasia (PALPA): An introduction. *Aphasiology, 10,* 159–215.

language task. That is, according to information processing approaches, clinicians analyze what underlying mechanisms of processing impairment may be causing surface-level symptoms in order to understand the nature of the language deficit. This approach acknowledges that similar aphasic behaviors (e.g., anomia) may result from different underlying processing problems; for example, one patient may have difficulty with written naming because of a breakdown at the semantic level, whereas another patient may be unable to access information within the orthographic output lexicon.

Summary

In summary, this assessment approach and others support the need for clinicians to go beyond the administration of aphasia batteries and the labeling of aphasia type and severity, and describe and summarize the actual cognitive, linguistic (content and form), and pragmatic strengths and weaknesses of each aphasic patient (Chapey, 1981; 1986; 1994). This type of information is essential in clarifying and facilitating the choice of treatment goals and activities (Chapey, 1994). Such an approach to assessment can yield descriptive summaries that indicate the level at which language performance (a) is completely accurate, (b) begins to break down, and (c) breaks down completely (Chapey, 1994). Additionally, such summaries can identify factors that facilitate and retard the patient's language abilities and can help clinicians to determine initial goals of therapy and to aid in reassessing the patient to determine when goals have been reached. Thus, when descriptive language summaries are accurately written, well-organized, easy to understand, and free of professional jargon, slang, and vague terminology, they can clarify and facilitate the choice of treatment goals and strategies (Chapey, 1981; 1986; 1994).

Hypothesis Testing

The results of hypothesis formation, and specifically the treatment goals that are established, are considered tentative and flexible enough to change as new evidence emerges (Chapey, 1994; Lahey, 1988). Hypothesis testing, then, enables the clinician to continue to secure additional data about the language abilities and impairments of each patient in order to determine the validity, accuracy, and appropriateness of hypotheses that were formulated. Separation of assessment and intervention allow for the presentation of information in an organized manner. However, in practice, assessment should be an ongoing part of treatment and must occur at every phase of rehabilitation (Chapey, 1986; 1994).

Reporting Assessment Results

An important aspect of the assessment process involves sharing the results of the language assessment with other individuals and professionals on the team, as well as with the patient, family, and significant others. Assessment findings are usually shared when all of the data are assembled (e.g., unstructured and structured observations, case history, observations and reports from other team members) and have been collectively analyzed and interpreted. The findings, conclusions, and recommendations may be conveyed verbally at family and/or staff conferences, as well as in the form of a short and concise written report. Frequently, visual illustrations (e.g., a diagram of the brain to assist in describing anatomic areas that have been affected by the patient's stroke) help patients, caregivers, and other professionals comprehend the information provided (Shipley & McAfee, 1998). In addition, clinicians usually try to avoid overloading the patient and family with too much information at one time and are prepared to repeat information across several sessions in order to assure that the patient and his or her family understand the assessment results (Luterman, 1996).

A widely used written format for sharing assessment data is the SOAP note (Fig. 4–4). In this type of format, "S" stands for the clinician's subjective comments about the patient and the session or assessment, "O" for the objective findings obtained during the session or assessment, "A" for the clinician's assessment or interpretation of the patient's session or assessment performance, and "P" for the plan regarding further assessment or treatment. Such notes are usually as succinct as possible since, as Golper (1996) notes, "brief notes get read and long narratives do not" (p. 69).

World Health Organization Model

Clinicians are also increasingly summarizing assessment data with reference to the World Health Organization's (1998)

S (Subjective): Mr. O appeared motivated and cooperative throughout the session. He demonstrated and commented about frustration with his word-finding difficulties.

O (Objective): The Test of Adolescent/Adult Word Finding was administered. Mr. O achieved the following:

	Percent Correct
Picture Naming: Nouns	28%
Sentence Completion Naming	19%
Description Naming	8%
Picture Naming: Verbs	5%
Category Naming	19%
Total Naming	17%
Comprehension	90%
Average Item Response Time	12 s

A (Assessment): Mr. O presented with severe (below the 1st percentile rank) word-finding difficulties across a variety of word types (i.e., verbs and nouns) and a variety of word-finding tasks. Additionally, Mr. O required substantial time to produce the name of a given test item.

P (Plan): Biweekly, one hour therapy sessions will be arranged. The focus of therapy will be to increase the accuracy and speed of Mr. O's word-finding abilities at the isolated word level using a cuing hierarchy treatment approach.

Figure 4–4. Reporting assessment results: An example of a SOAP note.

---

model of body structure and function, activities, and life participation (see above and Chapters 1, 10–14). Such information can be particularly useful in prioritizing goals for intervention.

GOALS OF ASSESSMENT

Goal 1: Determination of the Presence of Aphasia

A frequent assessment goal is to determine whether the patient presents with aphasia or whether his or her language skills are within normal limits when with those compared his or her peers. Frequently, the presence or absence of aphasia can be determined during an initial observation or interaction with the patient. For example, when the language impairment is severe or moderate, the presence of aphasia is obvious and a diagnosis can be made within a brief period of time. The remainder of the assessment can then focus on specifying the nature and extent of the disorder. However, when symptoms are mild, it may be more difficult to confirm the presence of a language impairment. That is, language problems may not be apparent when conversation is limited and expected responses are highly convergent. In such cases, despite the presence of aphasia as identified by the family or the physician, persons with aphasia may be so mildly impaired that they achieve perfect or near perfect scores on traditional aphasia batteries. For some patients, difficulty in determining the presence of aphasia may be a result of the fact that test norms do not accurately reflect a given patient's peer group (Garcia & Desrochers, 1997; Neils-Strunjas, 1998) in terms of age, language, cultural, and/or educational background. Therefore, clinicians compare the demographic characteristics of a patient and normed population.

A limited range of tasks on some aphasia batteries may also make determining the presence of language impairments difficult. For example, using the Western Aphasia Battery, Wertz and colleagues (1984) found that 5 out of 45 patients were diagnosed with normal language skills; however, using the Boston Diagnostic Aphasia Examination, all of these patients were diagnosed with aphasia. Therefore, at times, the final decision regarding the presence of aphasia in mildly impaired patients may be tentative and must be based on carefully documented observation and clinical judgment (Chapey, 1986; 1994).

In addition to determining the presence of aphasia, it is frequently the responsibility of the clinician to differentiate between the language impairment in aphasia and a language impairment that results from a different etiology. Careful analysis of the case history is performed to confirm the fact that the language symptoms do not solely reflect right hemisphere damage, dementia, traumatic brain injury (see Chapters 33–36), or other neurological (e.g., schizophrenia), pharmacological, or emotional (e.g., clinical depression) disorders. The language disorders associated with these conditions not only have different underlying sources of disturbance, but also follow different clinical courses and consequently demand different treatment approaches. Likewise, it is important to note that having aphasia does not exempt a patient from also presenting with one or more of the above conditions.

Right Hemisphere Damage (RHD)

In most cases, the communication problems of patients with RHD are not purely language based (Brownell, 1988; Myers, 1999; Tompkins, 1995; Varley, 1995). That is, most RHD patients are capable of functioning adequately on superficial communicative levels but experience difficulty in more complex and sophisticated communicative situations (see Chapter 34). Communication difficulties following RHD may arise directly or indirectly from a variety of impairments including deficits of perception, affect and emotion, and cognitive and communicative skills. In addition, patients with RHD represent a very heterogeneous population in terms of the extent and types of cognitive and communicative disorders they present.

The perceptual deficits of RHD patients can include various visuospatial problems and visual agnosias (such as complex visual discrimination deficits; visual integration deficits; visual imagery deficits; topographical, geographic, and spatial disorientation; prosopagnosia/facial recognition deficits; object agnosia; achromatopsia/color perception deficits; and visuoconstruction deficits), despite adequate sensory abilities (Cummings & Burns, 1996; Tompkins, 1995). Similar perceptual problems may also be observed in the auditory modality (such as auditory agnosia, amusia, sound localization deficits, impaired discrimination of prosody, and music perception deficits). These perceptual problems are associated with difficulties in appreciating the external context in which the stimulus is embedded and with problems in integrating the stimulus with internal associations. Although many of these perceptual problems and agnosias are primarily associated with bilateral lesions, some of them may occur following unilateral right hemisphere brain-damage.

When affect is impaired, the patient with RHD may have difficulty in the discrimination and production of a normal range of facial expressions that convey various emotions (Myers, 1999; Tompkins, 1995). RHD patients may also display prosodic impairments in which they have a reduced ability to comprehend or use linguistic or emotional prosody. However, currently this research has produced mixed findings (Baum & Pell, 1997; Tompkins, 1995; Ryalls & Behrens, 1988) and some researchers suggest that emotional and prosodic comprehension problems may, at least in part, reflect lower level perceptual difficulties (Joanette et al., 1990; Tompkins & Flowers, 1985).

RHD patients may also present with a variety of cognitive impairments (Cherney & Halper, 1996; Cummings & Burns, 1996; Myers, 1999; Tompkins, 1995). In terms of attention, RHD patients may have difficulty orienting, sustaining, focusing, or dividing their attention. Neglect is also common following RHD and is frequently attributed to impaired attentional mechanisms. Memory impairments following RHD include working memory and long-term, visuospatial memory deficits. These patients, particularly those with frontal lobe involvement, may also display executive function problems such as anosognosia (i.e., a lack of awareness of one's deficits), perseveration, and planning, integrating, and problem solving deficits.

The communicative deficits that are common among RHD patients do not resemble those of aphasic patients, and become most apparent in prolonged conversation or other open-ended and more sophisticated communication tasks (Brownell et al., 1995; Myers, 1999; Tompkins, 1995). Similarly, as communication tasks or contexts become less concrete and more complex, RHD patients are more likely to manifest the following comprehension and production deficits: (a) difficulty in organizing and summarizing information in an efficient, meaningful way; (b) a tendency to produce impulsive answers that are tangential and/or provide unnecessary detail; (c) difficulty in distinguishing between information that is relevant and irrelevant; (d) problems in assimilating and using contextual cues; (e) difficulty in conveying information in a cohesive and coherent manner; (f) a tendency to overpersonalize external events; (g) a tendency to lend a literal or superficial interpretation to figurative language (e.g., idioms, metaphors, indirect requests); and (h) a reduced sensitivity to their communicative context and partners and to the pragmatic or extralinguistic aspects of communication (e.g., turn-taking, topic maintenance, topic shifting). Many researchers hypothesize that the variety of perceptual, affective, and/or cognitive deficits that many RHD patients have underlie or at least contribute to their higher level communication disorders (e.g., Tompkins et al., 1994; Myers, 1999).

Dementia

Dementia is a condition of acquired, progressive degeneration of intellectual abilities affecting several cognitive domains such as language, memory, visuospatial skills, emotion or personality, and executive functions such as reasoning or abstraction (Cummings & Benson, 1992; Grabowski & Damasio, 1997) (see Chapter 35). Symptomatology varies from subtle changes during the early stages of the dementing illness that may not be noticeable to profound changes during the later stages that may render the patient unable to function socially or occupationally. Dementia may result from a variety of reversible and irreversible disorders (Cummings, 1987; Kaufer & Cummings, 1997; Molloy & Lubinski, 1995) (Table 4–6). Cognitive symptoms associated with reversible dementias can be remediated by treating the underlying medical condition; in contrast, researchers have yet to identify treatments that will reduce or eliminate the cognitive symptoms associated with irreversible dementing diseases. Consequently, it is very important that reversible causes of dementia be ruled out prior to diagnosing a patient with irreversible dementia.

The various **types of dementia** may also be categorized on the basis of the neuroanatomic location of the causative neuropathology (Cummings, 1990; Ripich, 1995; Webster-Ross et al., 1990): (a) **cortical dementias** (e.g., Alzheimer's disease, Pick's disease), in which the pathology primarily affects cortical brain tissue; (b) **subcortical dementias** (e.g., Parkinson's disease, Huntington's disease), in which the pathology primarily affects subcortical structures such as the basal ganglia and thalamus; and (c) **mixed dementias** (e.g., multi-infarct dementia), in which both cortical and subcortical structures are affected by the disease process. There are some differences among the symptom profiles associated with each of these dementia classifications. For example, in terms of communication profiles, patients with cortical dementia have logorrhea, empty speech, verbal paraphasias, impaired comprehension, relatively preserved repetition, and topic digression; in contrast, patients with subcortical dementia tend to have decreased output on verbal fluency tests (divergent thinking), agraphia, and motor

TABLE 4–6

Examples of Reversible and Irreversible Causes of Dementia

Reversible Causes that can Resemble Dementia
  Depression (pseudodementia)
  Drug use (e.g., anticholinergic side effects)
  Infection (e.g., meningitis, encephalitis)
  Hearing loss
  Neoplasm
  Normal pressure hydrocephalus
  Mental and/or sensory deprivation
  Renal failure (dialysis dementia)
  Thyroid disease
  Toxin exposure (e.g., lead poisoning)
  Vitamin deficiency (e.g., pellagra, Wernicke-Korsakoff syndrome)
Irreversible Causes
  Alzheimer's disease
  Creutzfeld-Jakob disease
  Human immunodeficiency virus encephalopathy
  Huntington's disease
  Multi-infarct dementia
  Multiple sclerosis
  Parkinson's disease
  Pick's disease
  Progressive supranuclear palsy
  Traumatic brain injury (e.g., dementia pugilistica)

speech disturbances such as slow rate, hypophonia, and articulation and intonation difficulties.

Despite some differences in symptomatology among patients with varying dementia etiologies, there are also some similarities, particularly as the dementing disease progresses over time (Bayles & Kaszniak, 1987; Hart & Semple, 1990) (see also Chapter 35 by Bayles). Typically, in the **early stages** of dementia, patients are forgetful and disoriented for time but generally not for place or person, and both their short- and long-term memory abilities are already affected. In terms of language abilities, patients may still appear to be successful communicators, especially during casual conversations; however, they may sometimes digress from the topic and ramble at length during conversation. During these stages, dementia patients may also display periodic word-finding problems and difficulty in interpreting higher-level language forms such as humor or sarcasm.

During the **middle stages** of dementia, patients become further disoriented and have difficulty with both time and place information. Memory abilities become further impaired and patients can no longer manage personal finances, employment, or medication. Conversational problems are now prominent, with patients having difficulty adhering to conversational rules such as turn-taking, topic maintenance, and topic shifting. Language output becomes vague, empty, perseverative, and often irrelevant, and patients will frequently produce semantic paraphasias and may misuse syntactic forms that affect meaning. Auditory and reading comprehension problems also become prominent during this stage of dementia.

In the **later stages** of dementia, the patient becomes disoriented for time, place, and person, and is now dependent for most activities of daily living. Language output may be completely void of meaning, and many patients eventually become mute; language comprehension abilities are similarly devastated.

Review of the linguistic and cognitive changes that occur in dementia indicates that there are some similarities between patients with aphasia and those with dementia, particularly patients with anomic aphasia and patients in the early stages of dementia (Nicholas et al., 1985). However, there are several linguistic and cognitive **features** that may help **distinguish** aphasic from demented populations. For example, **errors in language form** (i.e., morphology and syntax) are less common in the language output of dementia patients, whereas **perseveration of ideas** is less common in the language output of aphasic patients (Bayles & Kaszniak, 1987). In terms of cognitive symptoms, Bayles et al. (1989) finds that patients with mild and moderate dementia perform significantly more poorly on delayed **recall** compared with their immediate recall performance; in contrast, there is no such disparity between the delayed and immediate recall performances of aphasic patients. Patients with dementia also display much greater difficulty on **memory** tests of delayed spatial and verbal recognition than do patients with aphasia.

Traumatic Brain Injury (TBI)

According to the National Head Injury Foundation (1989), TBI refers to any insult to the brain produced by an external force that may result in a variety of temporary or permanent physical, cognitive, and behavioral impairments. TBI may be caused by discrete and focal brain damage or may be the result of extensive and diffuse brain damage. Patients with discrete lesions may display language impairments that are similar to those incurred by stroke (i.e., aphasia). However, patients with diffuse lesions may display cognitive-communicative impairments associated with deficits of attention, memory, and executive functions such as problem solving, abstraction, conceptual organization, and self-monitoring (Adamovich & Henderson, 1985; American Speech-Language-Hearing Association, 1991; Chapman et al., 1995) (see TBI Chapter 33).

Generally, patients who survive their TBI are less likely to present with frank aphasia as opposed to cognitive-communicative problems which affect more subtle and higher level aspects of language and communication (Gil et al., 1996; Schwartz-Cowley & Stepanik, 1989). In contrast to the content and form difficulties of aphasic patients, TBI patients with cognitive-communicative impairments, or what

Darley (1982) termed "language of confusion," display difficulties primarily with the pragmatic aspects of language. Examples of pragmatic deficits include difficulties organizing verbal and written output so that it is coherent, cohesive, and concise, problems selecting and maintaining appropriate conversational topics, and the frequent production of irrelevant, tangential, or confabulatory verbal and written output (Chapman et al., 1995; Hartley, 1995; Hartley & Levin, 1990). Other higher level language difficulties of TBI patients such as problems attending to, comprehending, and retaining complex and abstract commands, stories, or other linguistic material are usually secondary to cognitive impairments of attention, memory, or executive functions. Although both aphasic and TBI patients may have word retrieval problems, there are often some qualitative differences between the types of errors produced by these two patient populations (Boles, 1997; Holland, 1982; Levin et al., 1981). Specifically, in addition to the circumlocutions, semantic paraphasias, and reduced word fluency that are typical of both groups, TBI patients may make naming errors that are related to their personal situation or to the nature of the stimulus, that are errors of confabulation, or that are a product of visual misperception.

Primary Progressive Aphasia

Primary progressive aphasia (PPA) is a clinical syndrome in which patients suffer progressive language deterioration despite unidentifiable stroke, tumor, infection, or metabolic disease and relative preservation of cognition and independence in activities of daily living (Mesulam & Weintraub, 1992; Weintraub et al., 1990) (see also Chapter 20). In addition, Weintraub and colleagues (1990) suggest that patients should present with at least a two-year history of isolated and progressive language impairment before being diagnosed with PPA. Currently, there is some debate about whether PPA is a separate clinical entity. That is, some researchers regard PPA as a precursor or variant of more generalized dementias such as Alzheimer's or Pick's disease (Green et al., 1990; Kertesz et al., 1994). Others believe that the clinical behavior and histopathological results of PPA are sufficiently different from these diseases (Duffy & Petersen 1992; Kirshner et al., 1987).

Although distinguishing PPA from the language impairments caused by progressive dementing diseases remains controversial, differentiating PPA from traditional aphasia can be made on the bases of etiology (i.e., unknown or diffuse versus focal brain-damage) and course (i.e., progressive versus relatively static presentation of symptoms). The language symptoms of patients with PPA may be quite variable and aphasia types such as anomic aphasia, Broca's aphasia, conduction aphasia, pure word deafness, nonfluent aphasia, mixed transcortical aphasia, and global aphasia are reported (Duffy & Petersen, 1992; Rogers & Alarcon, 1997;

Westbury & Bub, 1997). Despite this variability, the incidence of nonfluent PPA is reported more frequently in the literature. For these patients, specific language symptoms appear to be similar to those associated with traditional aphasia and most frequently include word finding deficits (the most common initial symptom as well), repetition difficulties, and auditory comprehension problems (Westbury & Bub, 1997). Interestingly, in their review of 112 published cases of PPA, Westbury and Bub note that both reading and writing modalities tend to remain relatively strong for years after the onset of the disorder.

Psychiatric Disorders

Of the several psychiatric disorders that can negatively affect an individual's communication abilities, schizophrenia generally receives the most attention in the speech-language pathology literature. Schizophrenia is a relatively common, chronic psychotic disorder that most frequently manifests in late adolescence or early adulthood. However, a form of schizophrenia with symptom onset in the second half of life is also reported (Jeste, 1993; Keefe & Harvey, 1994). This disorder is associated with both positive (i.e., the presence of abnormal behavior) and negative (i.e., the absence of normal behavior) symptoms. Positive symptoms include thought disorder, delusions, and hallucinations; negative symptoms include flat affect, apathy, and social withdrawal. Individuals with schizophrenia also present with a variety of neuropsychological problems including memory and attention deficits, and executive function impairments such as anosognosia (i.e., lack of awareness of deficits), perseveration, and difficulties with planning and problem solving (Elliott et al., 1998; Elliott & Shakian, 1995).

Communication impairment of individuals with schizophrenia may include word finding difficulties, language output characterized by reduced content, disturbed affective prosody, perseveration, irrelevance, and cohesion and organizational problems (DiSimoni et al., 1977; Docherty et al., 1996; Goren et al., 1996). Productive morphosyntactic abilities and basic auditory and reading comprehension abilities are typically spared. These communication difficulties and associated problems in social functioning are the result of the neuropsychological and negative symptoms described above (Dickerson et al., 1996). Although the communication problems of patients with aphasia are generally sufficiently different from those of patients with schizophrenia, difficulty distinguishing between the two may arise in some cases such as aphasic patients with premorbid psychotic disorders.

Goal 2: Identification of Complicating Conditions

The clinician aids in determining which factors precipitated and which are continuing to contribute to the language problem. The purpose of this part of the assessment is to determine what variables can be reduced, eliminated, or changed to facilitate the language comprehension and production abilities of the aphasic patient. To identify complicating conditions that affect language, clinicians compile a comprehensive case history and complete interviews of the patient, his or her caregivers and appropriate individuals in the community.

Case History and Interviews

To identify the precipitating and maintaining factors affecting language, the clinician completes a thorough and systematic review of a patient's demographic, medical, and behavioral information including educational, medical, family, mental health, and occupational history, as well as past, present, and future communication environments and goals. This information can be gathered by reviewing the patient's medical chart and by asking the patient, family, and significant others to complete pre-interviews or referral forms. The clinician obtains much of the information regarding the patient's history prior to the initial patient contact. This enables the clinician to formulate an opinion concerning the possible areas that need greater specificity during testing.

For example, use of forms such as those in Appendix 4-1 or published inventories (e.g., Caregiver Administered Communication Inventory; Tanner & Culberston, 1999) can often save time, provide a systematic method for obtaining information, and provide a focus and direction for subsequent interviews.

During subsequent interviews, specific areas that seem unclear or that need greater specificity are explored. Interviews provide an opportunity to verify and to clarify information obtained on the referral forms, and to pursue data that may be pertinent to the nature of the patient's communication problem but that are not included on the form. For example, the clinician may attempt to determine the degree to which the verbal and nonverbal behaviors of individuals in the patient's environment facilitate or impede language recovery. Other areas that may be described are the relationships between and among persons in the environment, the social role change of the client and family subsequent to aphasia, patient and family understanding of and attitudes toward aphasia, needs and expectations concerning treatment and treatment outcome, and the realistic or unrealistic nature of these expectations.

Further information can be gained by interviewing or reviewing the reports of other assessment and/or intervention team members who have evaluated some aspect of the patient's physical, psychological, emotional, social, or occupational functioning. Such a team may be composed of the attending physician and nursing staff, a neurologist, a physiatrist, a geriatrician, an occupational therapist, a physical therapist, a neuropsychologist, a social worker, a therapeutic recreational specialist, a dietician, a rehabilitation counselor, and family members (see also Chapter 8). It is crucial to have good communication among team members, particularly in those clinical settings in which others such as the neuropsychologist or occupational therapist may share the responsibility of determining the cognitive and linguistic abilities of patients with aphasia.

Complicating Conditions

During testing of the patient with aphasia, the clinician is alert for signs of dysfunction in areas that do not appear to be generally equivalent in severity with overall performance. This is done to determine if there are conditions that may interfere with recovery. More detailed assessment of these areas is subsequently made to determine the presence of complicating conditions, and is usually completed prior to the in-depth evaluation of language abilities. Testing included in this category would be procedures designed to discern auditory and visual sensitivity, auditory and visual agnosia, behaviors frequently associated with right hemisphere functions, motoric impairments, and post-stroke psychobehavioral disorders such as clinical depression.

Auditory and Visual Sensitivity

Assessment of auditory sensitivity should, at the very least, include a hearing screening. Preferably, the clinician has access to information concerning a patient's (a) threshold for the awareness of sound; (b) standard pure tone thresholds (i.e., both air and bone conduction); and (d) speech discrimination scores. Although aphasia is not a problem of auditory sensitivity, hearing loss can obviously negatively affect a patient's auditory comprehension abilities. The necessity of testing hearing sensitivity is made even more obvious by the fact that many aphasic patients are older and therefore at high risk for hearing disorders (Formby et al., 1987; Gates et al., 1990). However, testing the hearing acuity of some patients may be very difficult if they are severely language impaired and therefore unable to understand test instructions or to grasp the nature of the response requirements (Wilson et al., 1981). Accordingly, collaboration between the clinician and the audiologist is necessary to assure a valid assessment of hearing abilities. Additionally, for those aphasic patients who wear hearing aids or rely upon other assistive listening devices, it is important for the clinician to check whether these devices are in working order (e.g., buildup of cerumen, check for working batteries) prior to the language evaluation.

It is equally important to determine that the patient's visual acuity (e.g., cataracts, myopia) and visual fields (i.e., right homonymous hemianopia) are intact enough so that they will not significantly impede assessment and treatment procedures. Assuring adequate vision is particularly important for clinicians working with older aphasic patients since at least one-third of the elderly have some degree of vision loss (Atkins, 1998). When a visual defect is suspected, the patient is referred to an ophthalmologist for testing. For aphasic patients with identified visual acuity problems, clinicians should assure that any assistive devices (e.g., glasses, contacts lens, magnifying glass) are available and in appropriate condition (e.g., clean, most recent prescription) when completing the language assessment. For aphasic patients with identified visual field cuts, the clinician can arrange visual stimuli in a vertical presentation to avoid eliciting visual-versus language-based errors.

Auditory and Visual Agnosia

Occasionally, patients with aphasia, particularly those who have suffered bilateral brain damage, may present with auditory or visual agnosia. Patients with auditory agnosia have difficulties recognizing auditory stimuli even though they may recognize the same stimuli in other modalities and even though they have adequate hearing sensitivity (Bauer & Zawacki, 1997). Patients with aphasia may demonstrate one or more of the following types of auditory agnosia (Albert & Bear, 1974; Buchman et al., 1986; Gates & Bradshaw, 1977): (a) amusia, or the inability to recognize music rhythms or forms, (b) auditory sound agnosia, or the inability to recognize nonverbal sounds, and (c) pure word deafness, or the inability to recognize and repeat spoken language with a relatively preserved ability to recognize nonverbal sounds.

Visual agnosia refers to an impairment in the recognition of visual stimuli despite adequate visual sensitivity (Farah & Feinberg, 1997). Several types of visual agnosia can occur with aphasia (De Renzi, 1997a; Feinberg et al., 1986; Stringer, 1996): (a) prosopagnosia, or a difficulty in recognizing familiar faces, (b) autopagnosia, or a difficulty in recognizing body parts, or (c) visual object agnosia, or a difficulty in recognizing actual or pictured objects. In diagnosing auditory or visual agnosia, it is important to exclude (a) sensory deficits in the affected modality, (b) comprehension deficits, (c) expressive disturbances, and (d) unfamiliarity with the test stimuli (Stringer, 1996).

Right Hemisphere Functions

Aphasic patients may demonstrate nonverbal impairments that are more frequently associated with right hemisphere brain-damage and that may directly or indirectly interfere with the therapeutic process. For example, some aphasic patients present with constructional apraxia or difficulties copying or composing drawings of two- or three-dimensional figures (Arena & Gainotti, 1978; De Renzi, 1997b). Such patients might construct drawings that are oversimplified and reduced in size but that improve with repetition. Therefore, several aphasia batteries (e.g., WAB, PICA) include subtests that examine for the presence of constructional impairments.

Aphasic patients may also display inattention or neglect to the right side of space. Although neglect is more frequently associated with right hemisphere brain-damage, recent research indicates that it is also quite common following left hemisphere brain-damage (incidence rates of between 15 to 65%) (Pedersen et al., 1997; Stone et al., 1993). Therefore, during assessment, clinicians may use published tests such as the Behavioral Inattention Test (Wilson et al., 1987), or may develop cancellation, line bisection, copying, and other pencil-and-paper tasks to identify neglect in their aphasic patients. In addition, since neglect may affect any modality, testing is done in other modalities as well.

Motoric Impairments

It is not uncommon for patients with aphasia to present with a variety of motoric impairments that may directly or indirectly affect their functional communicative abilities. Specifically, motoric deficits may impair the speed and accuracy of a patient's motor speech, gestural, and graphomotor abilities. Three frequently co-occurring motoric impairments are apraxia, dysarthria, and hemiparesis.

Apraxia. Apraxia generally refers to an impairment in the capacity to position muscles and to plan and sequence muscle movements for volitional purposes (Darley, 1975). This motoric performance problem cannot be attributed to muscular weakness, slowness, or incoordination as these same muscles may be used without difficulty in reflexive or automatic motor acts. Likewise, patients who have difficulties performing skilled and purposeful motor acts because of cognitive or motivational problems would not be considered apraxic. Two common forms of apraxia that may co-occur with aphasia and that may negatively impact a patient's communication abilities are apraxia of speech and limb apraxia.

In patients with apraxia of speech, the apraxia involves the speech musculature, resulting in difficulty with the volitional production of phonemes and phoneme sequences (McNeil et al., 1997; Square-Storer & Roy, 1989; Yorkston et al., 1999). Consequently, these patients demonstrate articulatory breakdown in the form of variable and inconsistent articulatory substitutions, distortions, omissions, repetitions, or additions. These patients also present with prosodic alterations including abnormal stress patterns, slow speech rate, and pauses which are inappropriate or of increased duration. Some of the speech symptom variability in apraxia of speech is related to the context in which the utterance is produced, such as word or utterance length, word frequency, the phonetic complexity of the word or utterance, and the nature of the task being performed (e.g., repetition vs. spontaneous production). Since this disorder is frequently associated with damage to premotor cortex or insular regions of the left hemisphere (Dronkers, 1996; Duffy, 1995), it is commonly associated with aphasia.

Therefore, many aphasia batteries include subtests to examine for the presence of apraxia of speech (e.g., BDAE). In addition, clinicians may also choose to further examine the motor speech abilities of their aphasic patients using standardized tests such as the Apraxia Battery for Adults (Dabul, 1979) or the Comprehensive Apraxia Test (DiSimoni, 1989).

Limb apraxia refers to an inability to execute acquired and volitional movements of the fingers, wrist, elbow, or shoulder that is unrelated to motoric, sensory, or cognitive deficits (Heilman et al., 1997; Helm-Estabrooks & Albert, 1991). Limb apraxia is another frequent correlate of aphasia but may often remain undiagnosed, particularly in patients with hemiparesis who must attempt to perform skilled movements with their nondominant arm (i.e., their difficulty is attributed to using their nonpreferred arm versus an apraxic disorder). Generally, patients with limb apraxia have more difficulty performing distal versus proximal movements, and transitive (i.e., involving a tool or instrument) versus intransitive movements. Patients with this disorder may make the following types of errors (Rothi et al., 1988): (a) content errors, in which they perform the wrong movement or action (e.g., when asked to show how to brush their teeth, they show how to comb their hair), and (b) production errors, in which the spatial or temporal organization of the movement or action is incorrect (e.g., pantomiming brushing one's teeth by holding the toothbrush vertically versus horizontally).

The assessment of ideomotor praxis should occur prior to administering any language or cognitive tests (Helm-Estabrooks & Albert, 1991). Failure to do so may result in patients with limb apraxia being mistakenly diagnosed with comprehension or other neuropsychological deficits (e.g., memory, attention), because of their difficulties with completing commands that require purposeful movements, and possibly, because of problems providing a reliable pointing or yes/no head response. Clinicians may assess the presence or absence of limb apraxia by developing a battery of tasks that represent a range of difficulty and complexity (see Belanger et al., 1996 and Rothi et al., 1997) or by utilizing one of the commercially available apraxia tests such as the Test of Oral and Limb Apraxia (Helm-Estabrooks, 1991) or the Apraxia Battery for Adults (Dabul, 1979).

Dysarthria. Dysarthria refers to a group of neurologic motor speech disorders that result from impaired control or changes in the tone (i.e., weakness, slowness, imprecision, and/or incoordination) of the speech musculature (Darley et al., 1975; Yorkston et al., 1999). Patients with dysarthria have difficulty with one or more of the basic components of motor speech, including respiration, phonation, resonance, articulation, and prosody. Motor speech symptoms of the specific patient tend to be relatively consistent across speaking contexts. However, motor speech symptoms may vary considerably among patients with this disorder due to different etiologies and different muscular involvement. Persistent dysarthria is most likely to be present in aphasic patients who have suffered bilateral brain-damage since the speech musculature is innervated bilaterally (Duffy, 1995).

Clinicians may use a variety of published tools to quantify and qualify dysarthric speech disturbances including the

TABLE 4–7

Items of Paired-Word Intelligibility Test Listed by Phonetic Contrast

Category of Feature	Pair 1	Pair 2	Pair 3
Initial voicing	bee-pea	do-two	goo-coo
Final voicing	add-at	buzz-bus	need-neat
Vowel duration	eat-it	gas-guess	pop-pup
Stop vs. fricative	see-tea	sew-toe	do-zoo
Glottal vs. null	high-eye	hit-it	has-as
Fricative vs. affricate	shoe-chew	shop-chop	ship-chip
Stop vs. nasal	dough-no	bee-me	buy-my
Alveolar vs. palatal	see-she	sew-show	sip-ship
Tongue height	eat-at	soup-soap	eat-eight
Tongue advancement	hat-hot	tea-two	day-dough
Stop place	pan-can	dough-go	bow-go
Diphthong	buy-boy	high-how	aisle-oil
r/l	ray-lay	rip-lip	raw-law
w/r	way-ray	row-woe	won-run
Liquid vs. vowel	string-stirring	spring-spurring	bring-burring
Cluster with one intrusive vowel	blow-below	plight-polite	claps-collapse

From Kent, R., Weismer, B., Kent, J., and Rosenbek, J. (1989). Toward phonetic intelligibility testing in dysarthria. *Journal of Speech and Hearing Disorders, 54,* 493.

Assessment of Intelligibility of Dysarthric Speech (Yorkston et al., 1984), the Frenchay Dysarthria Assessment (Enderby, 1983), and the Dysarthria Examination Battery (Drummond, 1993). Another assessment option is the word intelligibility test developed by Kent et al. (1989). This test is "designed to examine 19 acoustic-phonetic contrasts that are likely to (a) be sensitive to dysarthric impairment, and (b) contribute significantly to speech intelligibility" (p. 482) (Table 4–7). Importantly, Kent and colleagues provide a discussion of the therapeutic implications of their test.

Hemiparesis. Many aphasic patients may present with hemiparesis or muscular weakness of the right side of their body. If the motoric impairment is so severe that the left side of the body is paralyzed, the term hemiplegia may be used. Such weakness of the right hand or a reliance on their nondominant, left hand may compromise the speed and precision of many aphasic patients' writing, typing, drawing, and/or gesturing.

Post-Stroke Psychobehavioral Disorders

Many patients suffer from post-stroke psychobehavioral disorders including depression, anxiety, catastrophic reaction, mania, psychosis, adjustment disorders, and behavioral problems such as aggressiveness and sexual inappropriateness (Bishop & Pet, 1995; Craig & Cummings, 1995). These psychobehavioral disorders may be the result of one or more of the following (Koenig, 1997): a premorbid mood disorder, medications (e.g., depression is a common side effect of certain antihypertensives), brain-damage, or a psychological reaction to the stress associated with acquiring communication as well as other possible cognitive and physical impairments. Such psychobehavioral problems are viewed as serious medical problems that can compromise the overall assessment and rehabilitative process, including speech-language evaluation and treatment (Swindell & Hammons, 1991; Teresi & Holmes, 1997).

Because it is the most commonly observed mood disorder subsequent to brain-damage, research has focused primarily on issues relating to depression in aphasia. Specifically, the relation between depression and several patient characteristics such as lesion location and time post-onset of aphasia has been examined. Although several studies report a greater incidence of depression among aphasic patients with frontal lesions (e.g., Robinson & Benson, 1981; Starkstein & Robinson, 1988), the reliability of this relation remains equivocal due to inadequate assessment procedures, excessive subject exclusionary criteria, or both (Spencer et al., 1997). With respect to time post-stroke, aphasic patients appear to be at greatest risk for depression beyond the acute stages of recovery. For example, Smollan and Penn (1997) found that patients who were at approximately 4 years post-onset reported higher levels of depression than patients who were at earlier or later stages of recovery. Although there are few data available concerning the effects of depression on recovery from aphasia, it has been shown that depression adversely affects recovery from general post-stroke impairments. That is, depressed stroke patients have been found to participate less actively in their rehabilitation programs and to show greater functional and cognitive impairments than nondepressed stroke patients (Robinson et al., 1986; Sinyor et al., 1986).

Because of the negative impact of depression on the therapeutic process, speech-language pathologists need to identify aphasic patients who might possibly be clinically depressed and make appropriate referrals for further psychological assessment and/or medical or psychological intervention. Unfortunately, many of the depression scales that are used to diagnose depression are inappropriate for the aphasic population because they place high demands upon the patients' linguistic, attention, and memory abilities (Black, 1995; Spencer et al., 1997). However, clinicians may now use some newly devised tests which attempt to minimize linguistic and cognitive requirements. For example, both the Stroke and Aphasia Depression Scale (SAD; Smollan & Penn, 1997) and the Visual Analog Mood Scales (VAMS; Stern, 1998) require patients to indicate their self-perceptions of their current emotional functioning on visual analog scales that are anchored by both picture and written stimuli; additionally, both scales evaluate a variety of moods and therefore provide information not only about depression, but other possible psychobehavioral disorders as well.

Goal 3: Analysis of Cognitive Abilities

Cognition is a generic term for any process whereby an organism becomes aware of or obtains knowledge of an object (English & English, 1958). It "refers to all the processes by which sensory input is transformed, reduced, elaborated, stored, recovered, and used" (Neisser, 1967, p. 4). It is a group of processes that we use in a coordinated and integrated manner in order to achieve knowledge and command of our world. That is, cognition is our means of processing and handling information.

Mental Operations

A multitude of specific processes contribute to our overall cognitive proficiency. According to Chapey (1983; 1994) these can be operationally defined as the five mental operations of the Guilford (1967) Structure-of-Intellect model, namely, recognition/understanding (including perception and attention), memory, and thinking (convergent, divergent, and evaluative) (see also Chapter 17).

Recognition/Understanding

Recognition/comprehension involves knowing, awareness, immediate discovery or rediscovery, recognition of information in various forms, perception, attention, and comprehension or understanding. Recognition involves acknowledgment that something has been seen or perceived previously (Guilford, 1967). There is a great deal of research in the area of comprehension (see goals 4 and 5). Less focus has been placed on areas such as attention. However, several attentional behaviors have been identified, including

(a) sustained attention, or the ability to maintain attention and therefore, consistent performance over a long period of time; (b) focused or selective attention, or the ability to focus on and prioritize part of our external or internal environment in the presence of competing stimuli; and (c) divided attention, or the ability to attend to and complete more than one task, or to attend and process multiple stimuli simultaneously.

Memory

Memory is the power, act, or process of fixing newly gained information in storage as well as retaining and retrieving this new information (Guilford, 1967; Squire, 1987). This refers to short-term or working memory or a capacity-limited arena (which is usually thought to hold seven items plus or minus two), in which information is processed and temporarily stored (Baddeley, 1986). It is hypothesized to contain buffers (e.g., phonological loop, visuospatial sketchpad) which briefly hold incoming information as well as an executive component that controls what information is processed and stored.

Impairments of both working memory and long-term memory have been observed in patients with aphasia. In fact, Allport (1986) proposes that "the dysphasias...are a class of memory disorder" (p. 32). Specifically, aphasic patients demonstrate working memory deficits when completing both verbal as well as visuospatial and other nonverbal memory tasks (Burgio & Basso, 1997; Tompkins et al., 1994). Additionally, there is some evidence to suggest that there is a relation between aphasic patients' working memory and language abilities (Caspari et al., 1998; Tompkins et al., 1994).

According to Chapey (1994), long-term memory contains Guilford's entire Structure-of-Intellect (SOI) cube: operations, contents, and products (see also Chapter 17). It is not a unitary storage system but rather information is hypothesized to be stored in different sites or in a different manner depending on the type of memory. Research identifies long-term memory deficits among aphasic patients for both verbal and nonverbal information (Beeson et al., 1993; Burgio & Basso, 1997; Ween et al., 1996). Although minimal research has been completed to examine the relation between long-term memory deficits and language abilities in aphasia, there is some evidence from other patient populations (e.g., temporal lobectomy patients) that impairments to certain long-term memory stores may negatively affect vocabulary acquisition skills as well as pragmatic language abilities (Gabrieli et al., 1988; Wilson & Wearing, 1995).

Thinking

There are three types of thinking: convergent thinking, divergent thinking, and evaluative thinking. **Convergent thinking** is the generation of logical conclusions from given information, where emphasis is on achieving the conventionally best outcomes. Usually, the information given fully determines the outcome (Guilford & Hoepfner, 1971).

Convergent production is in the area of logical deductions or compelling inferences. It involves the generation of logical necessities.

Divergent thinking involves the generation of logical alternatives from given information where emphasis is on variety, quantity, and relevance of output from the same source. It is concerned with the generation of logical possibilities, with the ready flow of ideas and with the readiness to change the direction of one's responses (Guilford, 1967). It involves providing ideas in situations where a proliferation of ideas on a specific topic is required. Such behavior necessitates the use of a broad search of memory storage, and the production of multiple possible solutions to a problem. It is the ability to extend previous experience and knowledge or to widen existing concepts (Cropley, 1967). Divergent behavior is directed toward new responses—new in the sense that the thinker was not aware of the response before beginning the particular line of thought (Gowan et al., 1967). Divergent questions are open ended and do not have a single correct answer. Responses are scored according to the number of ideas produced (fluency), and the variety of ideas suggested (flexibility). They can also be scored according to originality or the frequency or unusualness of the response and/or elaboration or the ability to specify numerous details in planning an event or making a decision (Guilford, 1967).

According to Guilford (1967), **evaluative thinking** or judgment involves the ability of the individual to use knowledge to make appraisals or comparisons or to formulate evaluations in terms of known specifications or criteria, such as correctness, completeness, identity, relevance, adequacy, utility, safety, consistency, logical feasibility, practical feasibility, or social custom.

Other Thinking and Executive Function Abilities

Various researchers use the term "executive functions" to refer to a collection of cognitive abilities (or composite abilities) that enable us to successfully complete independent, deliberate, and novel behaviors (Dugbarty et al., 1999; Ylvisaker & Feeney, 1998) that allow us to generate, choose, plan, and monitor responses that are goal directed and adaptive (Alexander et al., 1989; Borkowski & Burke, 1996; Denckla, 1996; Ylvisaker & Feeney, 1998). Such functions include (a) self-awareness of one's strengths and weaknesses and level of task difficulty (which involves recognition/understanding), (b) inhibition of incompatible responses, and (c) reasoning, problem solving, strategic thinking, and decision making. Within the Guilford model, problem solving, decision making, and learning are composite abilities that involve many or all of these executive functions. The specific aspects of functioning that are used depend on the problem presented, the decision to be made, the reasoning required, and/or the information to be learned (see also Chapter 17).

Individuals with aphasia may have executive function difficulties such as problem-solving/decision, making deficits

(Archibald et al., 1967; Chapey, 1994; Tatemichi et al., 1994; Vilkki, 1988) and preservation or failure to inhibit or shift a response (Albert & Sanderson, 1986; Glosser & Goodglass, 1990). Some aphasic individuals with left hemisphere brain damage also present with executive function difficulties thought to be characteristic of right hemisphere brain-damage such as lack of awareness or anosognosia (Cutting, 1978; LeBrun, 1987; Marshall et al., 1998; Stone et al., 1993). For example, they may demonstrate lack of awareness of their physical symptoms (e.g., right hemiparesis), language impairments, or both.

Contents of the Guilford SOI Model

According to Guilford (1967), there are four broad, substantive, basic kinds (or areas) of information or content that the organism discriminates: figural, symbolic, semantic, and behavioral. The two that are relevant to language are semantic and behavioral. Semantic content pertains "to information in the form of conceptions or mental constructs to which words are often applied." Therefore, it involves thinking and verbal communication. However, it need not necessarily be dependent on words (Guilford & Hoepfner, 1971). Behavioral content pertains to the psychological aspects of human interactions or to information that is essentially nonfigural and nonverbal, where the attitudes, needs, desires, moods, intentions, perceptions, and thoughts of others and of ourselves are involved. It involves some of the cues that the human organism obtains about the attention, perception, thinking, feeling, emotions, and intentions of others that come indirectly through nonverbal means.

Products of the Guilford SOI Model

There are six products in the Guilford model. Units enter into classes, which enter into relations, which enter into systems, which enter into transformations, which enter into implications. That is, at each level there are a larger and larger number of associations between and among items or concepts. Indeed, according to Guilford and Hoepfner (1971), products are the way in which things are associated in the mind. They may also form a continuum from simple to complex or concrete to abstract (Chapey, 1994).

Units are relatively "segregated or circumscribed items" or "chunks" of information having "thing" character (Guilford & Hoepfner, 1971). They are items to which nouns are often applied. Classes are "conceptions underlying sets of items of information grouped by virtue of their common properties" (Guilford & Hoepfner, 1971) and involve common properties within sets. Relations are meaningful connections "between items of information based upon variables or points of contact that apply to them" (Guilford & Hoepfner, 1971). Systems are organized patterns of information or "complexes of interrelated or interacting parts" (Guilford & Hoepfner, 1971). Transformations are changes of various kinds (such as redefinitions, shifts, transitions,

TABLE 4–8

Tests Available to Evaluate the Neuropsychological Abilities of Patients with Aphasia

Cognitive Function	Instrument	Source
Comprehensive	Burns Brief Inventory of Communication and Cognition	Burns (1997)
	Cognitive Linguistic Quick Test	Helm-Estabrooks (in press)
	Ross Information Processing Assessment-2	Ross-Swain (1996)
Attention	Behavioral Inattention Test	Wilson et al. (1987)
	Color Trails Test	D'Elia et al. (1996)
	Criterion-Oriented Test of Attention	Williams (1994)
	d2 Test	Brickencamp (1962)
	SCAN-A: A Test for Auditory Processing Disorders in Adolescents and Adults	Keith (1993)
	Symbol Search subtest of the WAIS-3	Wechsler (1997a)
	Test of Everyday Attention	Robertson et al. (1994)
	Vigil Continuous Performance Test	The Psychological Corporation (1996)
Memory	Benton Visual Retention Test	Sivan (1992)
	Continuous Visual Memory Test	Trahan & Larrabee (1988)
	Figural Memory subtest of the WMS-3	Wechsler (1997b)
	Rey Complex Figure Test and Recognition Trial	Meyers & Meyers (1995)
	Rivermead Behavioral Memory Test	Wilson et al. (1985)
	Spatial Span subtest of the WMS-3	Wechsler (1997b)
	Visual Memory Span subtest of the WMS-3	Wechsler (1997b)
	Visual Reproduction subtests of the WMS-3	Wechsler (1997b)
Executive Functions	Behavioral Assessment of the Dysexecutive Syndrome	Wilson et al. (1996)
	Coloured Progressive Matrices	Raven et al. (1984)
	Comprehensive Test of Nonverbal Intelligence	Hammill et al. (1996)
	Delis-Kaplan Executive Function System	Delis et al. (in press)
	Matrix Reasoning subtest of the WAIS-3	Wechsler (1997a)
	Picture Arrangement subtest of the WAIS-3	Wechsler (1997a)
	Porteus Maze Test	Porteus (1959)
	Purdue Pegboard Test	Purdue Research Foundation (1948)
	Test of Nonverbal Intelligence-3	Brown et al. (1997)
	Williams Inhibition Test	Williams (1994)
	Wisconsin Card Sorting Test	Grant & Berg (1993)

or modifications) in existing information. Implications are "circumstantial connections between items of information, as by virtue of contiguity, or any condition that promotes "belongingness" (Guilford & Hoepfner, 1971). Implications involve information expected, anticipated, suggested, or predicted by other information.

Assessment of Cognition

Since cognition is the way in which or the process by which language is learned and used, each of the cognitive processes is assessed. Specifically, ability to produce semantic and behavioral units, classes (concepts), systems, relations, transformations, and implications under all five mental operations are explored. The tests developed by Guilford and his colleagues can be used for this purpose (see Chapter 17). In addition, other tests that tap these abilities can be used. For example, recognition/understanding and

convergent thinking are assessed on many standard tests of aphasia.

Examples of specific areas that are assessed are described below.

Attention

The status of an aphasic patient's attention abilities are evaluated in both unstructured and structured contexts in an attempt to provide information about if and how such problems interfere with activities of daily living. In unstructured observations, the clinician determines if the individual appears alert and able to maintain attention over a specific length of time. Patient ability to resist distraction by either external or internal stimuli is also noted. These and other aspects of attention may also be assessed using published tests such as those listed in Table 4–8. For example, the Test of Everyday Attention (Robertson et al., 1994) contains real-

QUESTIONNAIRE

Therapist _____ Discipline _____ Date _____

Could you please answer the following questions about _____ by ticking the box which most nearly applies to his or her behaviour now:

Has _____ recently?	Not at all (0)	Occasionally (1)	Sometimes (2)	Almost always (3)	Always (4)
1. Seemed lethargic (i.e. lacking energy)					
2. Tired easily					
3. Been slow in movement					
4. Been slow to respond verbally					
5. Performed slowly on mental tasks					
6. Needed prompting to get on with things					
7. Stared into space for long periods					
8. Had difficulty concentrating					
9. Been easily distracted					
10. Been unable to pay attention to more than one thing at once					
11. Made mistakes because he/she wasn't paying attention properly					
12. Missed important details in what he/she was doing					
13. Been restless					
14. Been unable to stick at an activity for very long					

Total:

Score:

Figure 4–5. Rating Scale of Attentional Behavior. Reprinted with permission from Ponsford, J. & Kinsella, G. (1991). The use of a rating scale of attentional behavior. *Neuropsychological Rehabilitation, 1,* 241–257.

life materials and tasks that target a variety of attentional processes: sustained attention, focused attention, divided attention, and attentional switching skills. Clinicians may also use rating scales such as that developed by Ponsford and Kinsella (1991), which are completed by both the clinician and the patient (Fig. 4–5).

Memory

Unstructured observations may provide some information about patient memory abilities such as whether or not the individual is oriented to place, time, and person. For highly structured assessment, there are many commercially available tests of memory that are accessible. However, there are relatively few that are appropriate for aphasic patients since most rely heavily upon processing of linguistic stimuli, verbal responses, or both (Fig. 4–4 and Table 4–8). The Rivermead Behavioral Memory Test (RBMT; Wilson

et al., 1985) represents an exception and includes subtests such as remembering an appointment and a short route. Cockburn and colleagues (1990) demonstrate that most RBMT subtests can be validly administered to aphasic patients, since performance of only a few subtests are significantly affected by language impairment. Other appropriate structured evaluations include the Visual Memory Span subtest of the Wechsler Memory Scales-3 (Wechsler, 1997b) to assess working memory abilities (particularly the Backward Tapping portion), and the Rey Complex Figure Test (Meyers & Meyers, 1995) to examine long-term visuospatial recall. Although performance is usually quantified in terms of the number and length of items remembered or the length of time items can be retained, responses may also be analyzed to identify patterns of impairment (such as remembering only the beginning or end of the material or the production of random errors).

TABLE 4–9

Sentence Types that May Be Used to Probe Syntactic Comprehension[a]

Sentence Structure	Number of			Canonicity of Thematic Roles
	Words	Propositions	Thematic Roles	
Active The lion kicked the elephant (Foil: The elephant kicked the lion)	5	1	2	canonical
Active Conjoined Theme The pig chased the lion and the cow (Foil: The lion chased the pig and the cow)	8	1	2	canonical
Active with Adjunct The elephant pulled the dog to the horse (Foil: The dog pulled the elephant to the horse)	8	1	3	canonical
Passive with Adjunct The dog was pulled to the horse by the elephant (Foil:The horse pulled the dog to the elephant)	9	1	3	noncanonical
Truncated Passive (TP) The pig was touched (Foil: The animal that was depicted as touching the pig was touched)	4	1	2	noncanonical
Passive (P) The elephant was pushed by the cow (Foil: The cow pushed the elephant)	7	1	2	noncanonical
Cleft Object (CO) It was the dog that the horse passed (Foil: The dog passed the horse)	8	1	2	noncanonical
Conjoined (C) The elephant followed the lion and pulled the dog (Foil: The elephant followed the lion that pulled the dog)	9	2	4	canonical
Object Subject (OS) The horse kicked the elephant that touched the dog (Foil: The horse kicked the elephant and touched the dog)	9	2	4	canonical
Subject Object (SO) The dog that the pig followed touched the horse (Foil: The pig that followed the dog touched the horse)	9	2	4	noncanonical

[a] From Caplan, D., Waters, G.S., & Hildebrandt, N. (1997). Determinants of sentence comprehension in aphasic patients in sentence-picture matching tasks. *Journal of Speech, Language, and Hearing Research, 40,* 542–555. Reprinted by permission. © 1997, The American Speech-Language-Hearing Association.

Executive Functions

The assessment of executive functions also includes observations as well as the administration of psychometric tests (see Table 4–8). For example, The Torrance Test of Creative Thinking (Torrance, 1966) can be used to measure divergent thinking and The Test of Problem Solving (Zachman et al., 1983) may be used to explore processes such as explaining inferences, determining causes, answering negative questions, determining solutions, and avoiding problems. (In both tests norms are only provided for children.) Sohlberg's (1992) Profile of Executive Control System involves both observation

of the individual performing daily tasks as well as a patient interview. Structured tests may include the Test of Nonverbal Intelligence-3 (Brown et al., 1997) and the Williams Inhibition Test (Williams, 1994).

Goal 4: Analysis of Ability to Comprehend Language Content

Language content is the meaning, topic, or subject matter of individual words, individual utterances, and/or conversation (Lahey, 1988; Owens, 1984; Wiig & Semel, 1984). Content also refers to the characterization or conceptualization of topics according to how they relate or are similar to one another in different messages (Lahey, 1988). A topic is the particular idea expressed in a message, such as comments about a specific object (e.g., a pipe); a particular action (e.g., eating lunch); or a specific relation (e.g., the relation between Harry and his pipe or a patient and his shoes) (Lahey, 1988). It is important to note that the meaning of words and concepts may change over time and across cultures, and may depend on the social and experiential context in which they are used.

The ability to comprehend the content of language is always impaired in aphasia (e.g., Webb & Love, 1983). These deficiencies involve assigning meaning to incoming auditory or written messages and/or to understanding words as they relate to objects, persons, actions, ideas, and experiences. For many aphasic patients, this impairment is confounded by deficiencies in cognitive abilities such as perception (e.g., visual or auditory discrimination), memory, and thinking. Assessment, therefore, centers not only on analyzing the patient's comprehension of language content but also on perceptual and cognitive abilities. Content is assessed for both auditory and reading comprehension. Both assessments are necessary since there are many patients in whom auditory comprehension is better than reading comprehension as well as those who display better reading than auditory comprehension skills (see also Chapter 25 by Beeson/Hillis and Appendix 4-2).

Comprehension of Content in Isolated Words

Receptive vocabulary is assessed by asking aphasic patients to point to real or pictured objects, actions, attributes, and relationships, and categories of objects, actions, numbers, and letters (e.g., "Point to car," "Point to drinking," "Show me yellow."). Knowledge of language categories is assessed by requiring the patient to point to objects, pictures, or words that belong to a specific class or group of words (e.g., "Show me the words that are the names of fruit"), and to identify rhyme words, synonyms, and antonyms. Most aphasia batteries include subtests to examine word-level comprehension of objects, actions, and so forth. However, few of them include subtests to examine understanding of word relationships and categories. Therefore, clinicians must rely upon probe tasks to assess this aspect of word comprehension (see Appendix 4-2). Another option is to use tests such as the Pyramids and Palm Trees test (Howard & Patterson, 1992). During administration of this instrument, patients are asked to match on the basis of a semantic association (e.g., for the target "pyramid," the response choices are "palm tree" and "pine tree"). The six versions of this test available allow the clinician to determine if the patient has a general semantic deficit or modality-specific problems.

Generally, pointing tasks can be made more difficult by increasing the number of items or words from which the patient must select the target (e.g., increase from two to six distractor items), by increasing the similarity of the target and distractors items (e.g., for the target word "car," printed distractors could be changed from "lemon," "glass," and "toe," to "cab," "bus," and "bar"), or both. The influence of other variables such as word frequency or familiarity, length, and image ability on a patient's understanding is also examined.

Comprehension of Content in Connected Language

Comprehension of labels for objects, actions, attributes, and relationships and of categories of objects, actions, and relationships are also assessed in connected language at both the sentence and discourse levels. At the sentence level, the clinician evaluates patient ability to point to common objects by description (e.g., "Read this sentence and point to the object that it describes"), by function (e.g., "Point to something that cuts"), and/or the patient's ability to follow directions or commands (e.g., "Write your address and then underline the name of your street"). Testing also includes assessment of the ability to understand concrete and abstract sentences. For example, in evaluating concrete sentences, the clinician might ask, "Is this a cup?" Items that evaluate more abstract comprehension abilities typically assess the patient's understanding of complex relationships such as comparative (e.g., "Are grapefruits larger than lemons?"), spatial (e.g., "Is California west of Arizona?"), temporal (e.g., "Does November come before October?"), inferential (e.g., "The man cut the steak. Did the man use a knife?"), cause-effect ("Can smoke cause a fire?"), or synonym (e.g., "Does sob mean the same as cry?") relations (Wiig & Semel, 1984) (see also Appendix 4-2). In addition to manipulating vocabulary characteristics (e.g., word frequency or imageability), clinicians alter variables such as sentence length and/or relational complexity to increase or decrease the difficulty of sentence-level comprehension tasks.

During **highly structured** assessment of both language content and form, response requirements are carefully controlled to be sure that success or failure are dependent on the stimulus characteristics and not on an inability to respond. For example, requiring a patient to gesture a response (e.g., "Pretend to use a hammer") may be complicated by a co-existing limb apraxia. Therefore, patients are usually required to respond by pointing to a word or picture or by producing or pointing to a one-word answer such as yes/no, true/false, or right/wrong. Abilities and impairments can then be ascribed to the specific input parameter that is being systematically controlled.

Comprehension of **discourse-length** spoken or written material is also performed, since there may be a difference between sentence- and discourse-level comprehension abilities (Nicholas & Brookshire, 1986; Stachowiak et al., 1977). Most aphasia batteries include subtests designed to assess auditory and reading comprehension abilities at this level. However, research revealed that aphasic patients were able to answer more than half of the reading items from several popular aphasia batteries correctly (e.g., BDAE, WAB) at a significantly greater rate than by chance only (relatively low passage dependency) (Nicholas et al., 1986). Consequently, when clinicians use these materials they may be assessing reading comprehension at the sentence rather than discourse level. In comparison to the reading subtests of aphasia batteries, the NRST, the Nelson Reading Skills Test (NRST; Hanna et al., 1977), was found to have more acceptable passage dependency. That is, patients with aphasia and adults with no brain-damage had to read the paragraphs to answer the test questions correctly (Nicholas & Brookshire, 1987). Another assessment option, the Discourse Comprehension Test (DCT; Brookshire & Nicholas, 1997), is designed to examine understanding of information that varies in terms of salience (main ideas vs. detailed information), as well as directness (explicitly stated information vs. implied information). Therefore, it can be administered as either a test of listening or reading comprehension.

Lastly, the aphasic patient's ability to understand meaning in **unstructured, spontaneous language** is determined. This is done by noting the type and amount of content that appears to be understood, as demonstrated by appropriate response to conversation. For example, if a patient hears the statements "No, this belongs to the nurse. Is this hers?" and "This is mine. Please give it to me" and responds appropriately, the clinician may begin to hypothesize that the patient comprehends the relationship of possession. However, it is important to be cautious when basing judgements about discourse-level abilities on the basis of general conversational speech since aphasic patients frequently nod or gesture appropriately as a response to social or prosodic cues and may not be comprehending the language content.

Gesture

Clinicians also assess the ability to comprehend gestures or pantomime since, for some aphasic patients with severe aphasia, gestures may represent a patent modality for comprehension (Daniloff et al., 1982; Varney, 1982). In particular, aphasic patients with severe auditory comprehension impairments but relatively minimal or mild reading impairments have been found to display better gestural recognition abilities than those patients with severe auditory and reading comprehension impairments (Kirshner & Webb, 1981; Seron et al., 1979). This finding has led some researchers to suggest that reading comprehension abilities may be a

better indicator of the ability to communicate effectively via gestures than overall aphasia severity (Daniloff et al., 1982; Peterson & Kirshner, 1981). In contrast, other studies have found a relationship between praxis and pantomime recognition impairments (Bell, 1994; Wang & Goodglass, 1992). With respect to gestural codes, iconic gestures (e.g., pantomiming the function of objects), and AmerInd signs (i.e., a modification of American Indian hand talk) are easier to discern than American Sign Language (ASL) by naive viewers, and consequently may be more suitable for assessing and treating aphasia (Campbell & Jackson, 1995; Christopoulou & Bonvillian, 1985; Daniloff et al., 1986) (see Chapter 30).

Gestural recognition abilities are not typically tested as part of most aphasia batteries. Therefore, clinicians may use one of the few commercially available tests such as the Assessment of Nonverbal Communication (Duffy & Duffy, 1984), one of the nonstandardized tasks described in the literature (e.g., Bell, 1994; Daniloff et al., 1982; Rothi et al., 1997), or a probe task developed by themselves. Generally, gestural comprehension is assessed with videotaped or live presentation of gestures, and the patient points to the correct picture in a multiple-choice format. In addition to assessing gesture comprehension abilities in isolation, clinicians may also examine the effect of providing gestural information in concert with auditory information (Records, 1994). That is, clinicians can determine if gestural information aids auditory comprehension.

Influential Variables

A variety of variables may positively or negatively influence aphasic patients' abilities to comprehend language content as well as language form (see Goal 5 for further information about assessing comprehension of language form). Research indicates that comprehension of both content and form are inversely proportional to the level of intellectual complexity (Shewan & Canter, 1971; Siegel, 1959), length (Shewan & Canter, 1971; Weidner & Lasky, 1976), and degree of semantic similarity among response choices (Baker et al., 1981; Duffy & Watkins, 1984). In contrast, there is a positive relationship between comprehension abilities and other stimulus variables such as **word frequency** (Croskey & Adams, 1970; Schuell et al., 1961), **imageability** (Kay et al., 1990), **emotional content** (Boller et al., 1979), **salience** (i.e., main ideas vs. details), **directness** (i.e., stated vs. implied) (Ernest-Baron et al., 1987; Nicholas & Brookshire, 1986, 1995a), **sentence constraint** (Faust & Kravetz, 1998; Puskaric & Pierce, 1997), **redundancy** (Gardner et al., 1975; Stachowiak et al., 1977), **context** (Cannito et al., 1989; Hough et al., 1997), and **personal significance** of the material. Additionally, for some aphasic patients, the **grammatical class** or part of speech (e.g., verbs vs. nouns) can influence their comprehension abilities (Caramazza & Hillis,

TABLE 4–10

Concepts Elicited from Normal Speakers Describing the "Cookie Theft" Picture

Two	little	mother	in the kitchen (indoors)
children	girl	woman (lady)	general statement about
little	sister	children behind her	disaster
boy	standing	standing by sink	lawn
brother	by boy	washing (doing)	sidewalk
standing	reaching up	dishes	house next door
on stool	asking for	drying	open windows
wobbling (off balance)	cookie	faucet on	curtains
3-legged	has finger to mouth	full blast	
falling over	saying "shhh"	ignoring (daydreaming)	
on the floor	(keeping him quiet)	water	
hurt himself	trying to help (not	overflowing	
reaching up	trying to help)	onto floor	
taking (stealing)	laughing	feet getting wet	
cookies		dirty dishes left	
for himself		puddle	
for his sister			
from the jar			
on the high shelf			
in the cupboard			
with the open door			
handing to sister			

From Yorkston, K. & Beukelman, D. (1980). An analysis of connected speech samples of aphasic and normal speakers. *Journal of Speech and Hearing Disorders, 45,* 27–36. Reprinted by permission. © 1980, The American Speech-Language-Hearing Association.

1991; Daniloff et al., 1982). The influence of each of these variables and of rehearsal, repetition, modeling, and expansion are explored.

Several factors that are related to the presentation of the verbal stimuli also contribute to aphasic patients' success and failure in comprehension (Blumstein et al., 1985; Gardner et al., 1975; Hough et al., 1997; Kimelman & McNeil, 1989; Lasky et al., 1976; Murray et al., 1997; Records, 1994; Toppin & Brookshire, 1978). Consequently, the degree to which a patient's comprehension is facilitated or retarded by tone of voice, intensity, stress, attentional demands (e.g., focused vs. divided attention tasks), concomitant gestures or pictorial cues, presentation rate, pauses at intervals, prolongation of words, and imposed response delays can be determined.

Goal 5: Analysis of Ability to Comprehend Language Form

Language form includes **syntax,** a system of rules used to order words and relate them to one another in order to express ideas, and **morphology,** a system of rules used to construct words (Owens, 1984). In aphasia, impairments in the ability to understand syntax or grammatical morphology are common. Consequently, assessment involves an analysis of the

aphasic patient's ability to understand language form at both the word and sentence levels (see Appendix 4-3).

Comprehension of Form Words and Morphology

Form words can be of two types: **substantive or open class words** (e.g., verbs, nouns, adjectives, adverbs) and **relational or closed class** words (e.g., prepositions, conjunctions, and articles) (Saffran et al., 1989). Because most aphasia batteries focus primarily on examining comprehension of nouns, clinicians may devise tests of their own or borrow from nonstandardized measures to assess comprehension of form words. The ability to comprehend the meaning of both substantive and relational words can be assessed through the use of picture verification tasks in which the aphasic patient sees a picture, hears or reads a word or phrase, and points to the best picture for that word or phrase. For example, a picture verification task to evaluate comprehension of prepositions might include stimuli such as "Point to (a) The cup is on the table; (b) The cup is under the table; or (c) the cup is near the table." Because of interest in the patient's ability to comprehend prepositions, the clinician may first assure that the patient can accurately recognize the substantive words within the test stimuli (e.g., "cup," "table") (see Appendix 4-3). In each instance, responses are analyzed to determine the type and frequency of words the patient is able to understand, the length of stimulus that can be understood, and the latency or length of time needed to comprehend the material.

Morphology involves the rules used to form words into other words (Caplan, 1993). More specifically, in English, word formation is accomplished via affixing derivational or inflectional morphemes. Addition of a derivational morpheme changes a word into a different form word (e.g., "pain" into "painful") whereas addition of an inflectional morpheme signifies a certain syntactic relationship (e.g., subject-verb agreement of "read" for "She reads."). Deficits comprehending both types of morphology are observed in aphasic patients (Badecker & Caramazza, 1987; Tyler & Cobb, 1987). However, few assessment tools have been developed to examine such abilities. Two exceptions to this are the commercially available Psycholinguistic Assessments of Language Processing in Aphasia (PALPA; Kay et al., 1997) and in the research literature, a test developed by Caplan and Bub (1990). Caplan and Bub's test includes subtests to assess recognition and comprehension of morphologically complex words. The recognition subtest contains real, affixed words (e.g., "runs") and nonwords (e.g., "runned"), and aphasic patients make a lexical decision regarding whether the item heard or read was a real or made-up word. In the comprehension subtest, aphasic patients complete a word picture matching task and a similarity judgement task.

Comprehension of Syntactic Constructions

Processing syntactic structures involves the knowledge of how one orders words within an utterance and how to construct various sentence types such as active, passive, negative, and negative–passive. To comprehend syntactic information, aphasic patients need adequate knowledge of syntactic rules (i.e., the ability to parse the structures that organize phrase elements into hierarchically translatable constituents such as subject NP, or object NP). They also need to be able to quickly process a transient auditory signal (if it is a listening situation) and to retain a memory representation of the signal to assure that sentential elements are not missed or misinterpreted (Berndt, 1998; Caplan, 1993). Disruption to this temporal aspect of syntactic processing will likely result in slow, labored reading abilities although in reading there may be multiple opportunities to extract syntactic information from the written material.

Aphasic patients' difficulties comprehending the syntactic structure of spoken or written language range from minimal difficulty to very selective deficits (i.e., problems interpreting only certain sentence types such as cleft-object sentences), to profound impairments (i.e., patients must rely on semantic and pragmatic knowledge to comprehend sentences) (Caplan & Hildebrandt, 1988; Schwartz et al., 1980).

In terms of assessment, patient ability to comprehend basic sentence types is determined. However, aphasia batteries rarely include items that assess syntactic comprehension

abilities. Other tests, with the exception of the PALPA (Kay et al., 1997), have been criticized because they do not allow differentiation between disorders of syntactic comprehension or short-term or working memory limitations (Caplan, 1993). Therefore, clinicians also probe the syntactic processing abilities of their aphasic patients using commercially available tests such as the Revised Token Test (McNeil & Prescott, 1978), tests from the research literature (e.g., Caplan & Bub, 1990; Caplan et al., 1997), or probes they develop based on these test procedures.

Assessment often takes the form of a picture sentence verification task in which the patient decides if a spoken or written phrase or sentence is true or false or if it answers the question yes or no. For example, the patient might be presented with a picture of a boy pushing a girl. Subsequently, he would point to the printed word "true" or "false" after each of the following sentences: "The boy is pushing the girl"; "The girl is pushing the boy"; "The boy is being pushed by the girl," and so forth. Caplan and colleagues (1997) also have patients demonstrate or act out sentence stimuli using the objects provided. The stimuli are constructed so that sentences cannot be interpreted solely on the basis of semantic processing or word knowledge, and so that distractor items represent plausible sentence interpretations (Berndt, 1998). During analysis of responses, clinicians attend to accuracy of response and to error types.

In determining the complexity of structures that the patient can comprehend, clinicians attend to the following syntactic features of a sentence: (a) **canonicity of thematic role order** (e.g., canonical order refers to sentences with the structure of Subject-Verb-Object), (b) the **number of verbs** in a sentence, and (c) the **number of propositions or thematic roles** played by nouns around a given verb (Caplan et al., 1996). Table 4–9 contains a list of the sentence types (as well as possible foils) in an order of increasing complexity. That is, aphasic patients (Caplan et al., 1985, 1997) respond more accurately and more quickly to sentence types at the top versus the bottom of this table. Therefore, clinicians compare their patients' understanding of active versus truncated passive, active conjoined versus cleft object, active with adjunct versus passive with adjunct, object subject versus subject object, and conjoined versus subject object. This hierarchy of sentence types may serve as a possible framework to identify the approximate level at which she or he is functioning and to describe the syntactic features that the aphasic patient can comprehend.

Goal 6: Analysis of Ability to Produce Language Content

Impairments in the ability to produce language content are always part of aphasia (Benson, 1979; Henderson, 1995). Deficiencies are observed in the appropriate use of vocabulary words relating to objects, events, relationships, and content categories. The aphasic patient may have difficulty in word finding, labeling, and categorizing, and/or in the spontaneous selection or substitution of one appropriate word for another. Therefore, assessment involves an analysis of the ability to provide the spoken and written label or name of objects, actions, events, attributes, and relationships in response to highly structured tasks as well as during connected and spontaneous language. Importantly, clinicians should not assume that a given patient's writing deficits will parallel his or her spoken language deficits. Indeed, writing disturbances may differ both quantitatively as well as qualitatively from disturbances in their spoken language (Varney, 1998) (see also Chapters 22–25).

Production of Content in Highly Structured Tasks

An important component of content assessment involves determining the patient's ability to provide the verbal and written label of objects, actions, events, attributes, and relationships at various levels of task and stimulus difficulty. Several common structured word-finding tasks that vary in terms of difficulty include (a) defining referents, (b) superordinate or category naming, (c) verbal fluency, (d) confrontation naming, (e) automatic closure naming, (f) automatic serial naming, (g) recognition naming, and (h) repetition naming (Chapey, 1994). For each task, a variety of psycholinguistic variables such as word frequency, picturability, length, and concreteness can be varied to enable the clinician to specify the nature and extent of the word finding impairment (Deloche et al., 1996; Nickels, 1995; Nickels & Howard, 1995). Most aphasia batteries and tests of spoken or written naming, such as the Test of Adolescent and Adult Word Finding (German, 1990), include subtests which examine several if not all of these types of word finding abilities (see Table 4–4).

Defining Referents

A patient's ability to define words is assessed by asking the patient questions such as "What does anchor mean?" "What does robin mean?" Responses are analyzed to determine the type of explanation produced, such as definition by usage, by location, by classification, and so forth. The ability to name words that are defined can also be explored (e.g., "A person who rides horses in a horse race is called a _____.").

Category Naming

The ability to classify semantically related words and concepts is assessed in various word frequency categories. The patient's ability to categorize in his or her own language can be scored according to (a) perceptual categories: classifying on the basis of a relevant sensory quality of a stimulus such as shape, size, or color (e.g., banana, lemon, grapefruit are all yellow), (b) conceptual or semantic categories: classifying on the basis of a generalized idea of a class of objects

(e.g., banana, lemon, grapefruit are all fruit), and (c) functional categories: classifying on the basis of an action or function associated with a class of objects (e.g., banana, lemon, grapefruit are all for eating) (Goldstein, 1948). The clinician may also examine the degree of concreteness or abstractness of a patient's category responses. For example, grouping items on the basis of perceptual categories would be considered a more concrete response versus grouping on the basis of semantic or functional category.

To explore the ability to decipher categories, patients may be asked to (a) provide the verbal or written name of an object category (e.g., "Rose, tulip, and carnation are all a type of _____."), (b) name as many words as possible that belong to a certain category (e.g., "Write down the names of as many animals as you can.") (a divergent semantic task), (c) produce word associations (e.g., "What is the first word that you think of when I say school?"), and (d) sort objects into categories and explain the rationale for their sort (e.g., Goldstein's [1948] sort task).

Verbal Fluency

Verbal fluency tasks are divergent semantic tasks and require patients to name as many words as they can think of within a certain category (as described above) or starting with a particular letter such as P, R, F, or C. For the letter task, patients are instructed to not use proper nouns. A time limit of at least 60 seconds is typically imposed, and the patient is given more than one test trial. Normative data for these types of naming tasks are available in the research literature (Heaton et al., 1992; Spreen & Strauss, 1991).

Confrontation Naming

Verbal and written naming in response to visual presentation is assessed by presenting objects, actions, events, and relationships or pictures of these that vary in frequency and type of category. For example, naming of objects, geometric forms, letters, animals, colors, body parts, and actions is almost always evaluated. For patients with right hemiparesis or other motoric impairments that may affect legibility, it may also be beneficial to assess writing skills with block letters that can be ordered to spell words (e.g., for a picture of a circle, the clinician gives the patient blocks with the letters "I," "R," "C," "E," "C," and "L" and asks him or her to spell the name of this picture); to make this task more difficult, distractor letter blocks could be added.

Automatic Closure Naming

The capacity to complete an open-ended sentence or phrase stem such as "The sky is _____" is often a component of assessment. These sentence or phrase stems can be varied in terms of constraint or the degree to which a stem generates a particular response (Fischler & Bloom, 1979; Schwanenflugel &

Shoben, 1985). For example, the stimulus "It's raining cats and ____" would be considered highly constrained because only one response, "dogs," is appropriate. In contrast, the stimulus "He ate the ____" would be minimally constrained because there are numerous plausible responses. For both aphasic and non-brain-damaged adults, automatic closure naming is facilitated when the sentence or phrase stem is highly constrained or convergent and there are a limited number or closed set of response choices (Breen & Warrington, 1994; McCall et al., 1997; Treisman, 1965).

Automatic Serial Naming

The ability to produce rote or over learned material is also appraised. For example, the patient may be asked to count to 20, name the days of the week, write out the letters of the alphabet, and/or recite well-known prayers or nursery rhymes.

Recognition Naming

When patients are unable to name an item, the correct word can be offered to them to determine if they are capable of recognizing words they cannot name. For example, for the target stimulus "elephant," a patient may be required to indicate which of three verbal or written choices is the appropriate label (e.g., "giraffe," "elephant," or "telephone"). To increase the difficulty of this task, distractor items can be manipulated to be semantically (e.g., "giraffe") and/or phonologically/orthographically (e.g., "telephone") similar to the target.

Repetition Naming

Repetition or copying of words is assessed to determine if the patient can repeat or copy words that he or she cannot verbally name or write, respectively (e.g., the clinician says "Now repeat: elephant.").

Production of Content in Connected Language

The ability to retrieve precise words for objects, events, relationships, and so forth during unstructured, spontaneous language is important to the communication of meaning. In addition, an aphasic patient's ability to produce content during highly structured tasks may differ from his or her abilities during less structured communication activities that require greater amounts of verbal or written output and require more thinking. Therefore, clinicians analyze samples of their patients' spoken or written connected language to determine the accuracy, responsiveness, completeness, promptness, and efficiency of their content.

Picture description tasks are often used to elicit such spoken and written discourse. The data generated can provide a controlled source for analyzing parameters of language content, form, and use (Shadden, 1998a,b). Although several

aphasia test batteries include spoken and written picture description tasks, eliciting larger samples using other connected language tasks may improve the reliability and validity of assessment results. In addition, to assure adequate test-retest stability for measures of connected language, clinicians may wish to use at least four or five stimuli to collect language samples that are at least 300 to 400 words in length (Brookshire & Nicholas, 1994). These stimuli should include more than picture description tasks since they tend to elicit labeling behavior. Such naming responses may limit the number and variety of lexical and pragmatic behaviors produced as well as the complexity of morphosyntactic structures generated by patients (Li et al., 1996; Shadden et al., 1991; Shadden, 1998a,b). Other language tasks that may be used to elicit spoken or written language samples include conversational discourse, sequential events illustrated through multiple pictures, story-retelling, video-narration, or procedural description tasks (e.g., "How do you change a tire?") (Bracy & Drummond, 1993; Ulatowska et al., 1983a,b; Cherney, 1998; Shadden, 1998a,b).

Numerous methods are available to analyze content in connected language samples (Shadden, 1998a,b). For example, one popular scoring system, developed by Yorkston and Beukelman (1980), requires the clinician to determine the number of content units or "grouping of information that was always expressed as a unit" (p. 30), per unit time (see Table 4–10). These researchers provide a list of content units for the "cookie theft" picture description task of the BDAE. One limitation of this system, however, is that it only provides responses to this one picture. Consequently, Nicholas and Brookshire (1993) expanded on this idea and describe a scoring system to analyze content in language samples derived from a variety of stimuli. In their system, rules are provided to help the clinician determine the number of words and "correct information units" (CIUs), or words that are "accurate, relevant and informative relative to the eliciting stimulus" (p. 340). Nicholas and Brookshire recommend that clinicians calculate both words per minute and the percentage of CIUs (i.e., number of CIUs/number of words) to obtain the most information about both the content and efficiency of their aphasic patients' connected language. They also describe a rule-based system for scoring the presence, completeness, and accuracy of content pertaining to the main concepts or gist in the connected language of aphasic patients (Nicholas & Brookshire, 1995b). In addition, they list the main concepts consistently identified by non-brain-damaged adults in response to the "cookie theft" picture from the BDAE (Nicholas & Brookshire, 1995b) and to their stimulus 'the birthday party picture' (Nicholas & Brookshire, 1992). These content measures (developed by Nicholas & Brookshire, 1993; 1995b) are excellent predictors of how informative aphasic patients are perceived by unfamiliar listeners (Doyle et al., 1996). In addition, changes on these measures over time correlate positively with unfamiliar listeners' perceptions of socially relevant changes in the communicative ability of aphasic patients (Ross & Wertz, 1999).

Gesture

Although gestural abilities are often impaired in aphasia due to linguistic, cognitive, and/or apraxic deficits, many patients, even those with severe and global aphasia, have been able to acquire simple forms of gestural communication (Helm-Estabrooks et al., 1982; Skelly, 1979) (see Chapter 30). With respect to gestural codes, iconic (e.g., demonstrating how to use a toothbrush), symbolic (e.g., showing how to salute), and AmerInd gestures are often more suitable than ASL signs as assessment and treatment stimuli because they can be discerned more easily by unfamiliar viewers, and because they have been created or adapted for one-handed gesturing (Campbell & Jackson, 1995; Daniloff et al., 1986; Skelly, 1979).

Most aphasia batteries (e.g., ADP, PICA) include a subtest that examines ability to produce a limited number of iconic gestures, common symbolic gestures, or both. Commercially available tests such as the Assessment of Nonverbal Communication (Duffy & Duffy, 1984) can also be used to obtain a more in-depth evaluation of gestural production abilities. Another option is to assess the gestural production skills using one of the several nonstandardized procedures described in the research literature (e.g., Alexander & Loverso, 1993; Conlon & McNeil, 1989; Rothi et al., 1997).

Drawing

For some severely impaired patients with aphasia, it may be useful to examine their ability to reproduce or spontaneously produce drawings in order to communicate content (Lyon & Helm-Estabrooks, 1987; Ward-Lonergan & Nicholas, 1995). However, before communicative drawing is adapted as a viable option, Lyon and Helm-Estabrooks (1987) suggest that the following abilities be considered as prerequisites: (a) an intact visuosemantic system for the concepts to be drawn, (b) adequate access to the symbols within this visuosemantic system, (c) adequate motoric and praxic abilities to draw these symbols, and (d) the ability to manipulate or augment drawn output "in a communicatively interactive and problem-solving manner" (p. 62). Therefore, assessment may involve determining the integrity of the aphasic patient's abilities in each of these areas via probes such as copying and drawing from memory, and via an evaluation of hand and limb motoric and praxic skills. The Daily Mishaps Test, which requires the patient to draw enacted scenarios which contain one- to three-part scenes, may also be used to evaluate patients' drawing abilities (Helm-Estabrooks & Albert, 1991). Although no formal scoring procedures are provided, clinicians can develop their own or borrow

from scoring criteria described in the research literature (e.g., Murray, 1998).

Cognitive Neuropsychological and Neurolinguistic Approach

Clinicians who adhere to a neuropsychological/neurolinguistic approach to assessment attempt to determine the nature of their aphasic patients' language impairment with respect to models of language (Caplan, 1993; Kay et al., 1996; Mitchum, 1993). That is, the clinician attempts to localize which particular component(s) of the model are impaired (see Fig. 4–2) (see Chapters 22–25). In terms of word-finding abilities, for example, aphasic patients have been found to have breakdowns at the semantic and/or phonological/graphemic output lexicon level. These symptoms are most frequently characterized as impairments of access to or egress from memory, rather than loss of these respective linguistic representations (Beeson et al., 1995; Deloche et al., 1996; Robinson & Grossman, 1997; Saffran & Schwartz, 1994). Aphasic patients may also display difficulties at the articulatory/graphic planning stage or with the motor realization of that plan, but these difficulties are often viewed as a motoric (e.g., apraxia of speech, apractic agraphia), rather than a linguistic problem per se.

The research literature contains many articles that provide guidance for performing such a neuropsychological/neurolinguistic assessment. For example, Rothi and colleagues (1991) describe a model of the nature of word-retrieval impairments. Specifically, Rothi et al. recommend that the consistency of a patient's word-finding errors be examined across modalities, tasks, and sessions in order to distinguish impaired access/egress from degradation of linguistic knowledge; that is, access/egress deficits are associated with inconsistent errors, and knowledge impairments are associated with consistent errors. To discriminate the level or levels at which a patient's word-finding abilities are breaking down, Rothi et al. describe a number of naming and comprehension tasks that are helpful for such analysis. For example, failure on tasks such as sorting or matching stimuli according to semantic category or naming to definitions may indicate semantic level impairments, whereas failure on tasks such as matching rhyming pictures or printed words may indicate lexical level (phonologic or orthographic, respectively) impairments.

Currently, there are also two test batteries available, the Psycholinguistic Assessments of Language Processing in Aphasia (PALPA; Kay et al., 1997) and the Psycholinguistic Assessment of Aphasia (PAL; Caplan & Bub, 1990), which adopt a neuropsychological/neurolinguistic approach to the assessment of aphasia[1]. These batteries include a variety of tasks to help the clinician identify the locus or loci of impairments in producing spoken or written language content and form at the word level. However, only the PAL includes

TABLE 4–11

Categories of Performance Deviations That May Be Examined in Connected Language Samples

Category	Definition	Examples
Non-word		
Part-word or unintelligible production	Word fragments or productions that are intelligible in context	...on a *st..sk*...stool ...on a *frampi*
Non-word filler	Utterances such as "uh" or "um"	...on a..*um*..stool..*uh*...
Non-CIU		
Inaccurate	Not accurate with regard to the stimulus, and no attempt to correct	...on a *chair* (for stool)
False start	False start or abandoned utterance	...on a *chair*..no, a stool
Unnecessary exact	Exact repetition of words, unless used purposefully for emphasis or cohesion	...on a..*on a* stool
Nonspecific or vague	Nonspecific or vague words lacking an unambiguous referent	...on a *thing*
Filler	Empty words that do not communicate information about the stimulus	...on a ..*you know*..stool
And	All occurrences of the word *and*	...a boy *and* a stool
Off-task or irrelevant	Commentary on the task or the speaker's performance	*I've seen this one before.* *I can't say it.*

NOTE. In the examples, only nonwords and words printed in italics were scored as performance deviations. From Brookshire, R.H. & Nicholas, L.E. (1995). Performance deviations in the connected speech of adults with no brain damage and adults with aphasia. *American Journal of Speech-Language Pathology, 4*, 118–123. Reprinted by permission. © 1995, The American Speech-Language-Hearing Association.

subtests to determine language production skills at the sentence level; neither battery examines language skills at the discourse level. In addition, neither battery is standardized nor provides comprehensive normative data.

Analysis of Ability to Produce Language Content Responses

In addition to observing the accuracy and quantity of content in aphasic patients' verbal and written output, clinicians analyze the nature and pattern of errors made. In terms of types of paraphasias or naming errors, aphasic patients frequently produce one or more of the following: (a) **phonemic** or literal paraphasia: the response contains substitution, addition, omission, and/or rearrangement of the target word's phonemes (e.g., "skoon" for the target "spoon"), (b) **semantic** paraphasia: the substituted word is semantically related to the target word (e.g., "fork" for the target "spoon"), (c) **random paraphasia**: the substituted word has no apparent semantic relation to the target word (e.g., "tractor" for the target "spoon"), (d) **circumlocution**: the response is a description or definition of the target word (e.g., "it's metallic and is used to eat soup" for the target "spoon"), (e) **neologism**: the response is a nonsense word (e.g., "clumpter" for the target "spoon"), (f) **indefinite substitution**: the response is a nonspecific word or description (e.g., "a thing for doing stuff" for the target "spoon"), and (g) **no response**.

Several researchers have developed detailed coding systems to describe the word-finding errors of aphasic patients (e.g., Mitchum et al., 1990; Zingeser & Berndt, 1988). For example, Brookshire and Nicholas (1995) describe a set of categories to quantify and to qualify performance deviations in language output that could not be scored as real words or correct information units (Table 4–11) (see also Nicholas & Brookshire, 1993). These authors used this system to analyze the language of their aphasic patients and found that they produced a significantly greater proportion of inaccurate words, false starts, and part-words or unintelligible words in comparison with their non-brain-damaged peers.

Cohesion Analysis

Cohesion is defined as the relations of meaning that "tie" or "glue" linguistic items (such as one main clause and all subordinate clausal and nonclausal elements attached or embedded in it) together, thereby creating meaningful interdependencies among the words in a text or within a discourse sample. Cohesion is achieved linguistically through a variety of cohesive devices that contribute to the overall coherence of the verbal or written output. Various researchers recommend exploring semantic cohesion in the spontaneous connected speech of aphasic patients (Glosser & Deser, 1990; Lemme et al., 1984; Liles & Coelho, 1998).

Of the numerous **types of cohesive devices,** the following types are most frequently examined in the language of aphasic patients (Glosser & Deser, 1990; Lemme et al., 1984): (a) **reference:** reference items such as personal (e.g., "he," "us") and demonstrative (e.g., "these," "here") pronouns are used to refer to a previously stated or written, unambiguous antecedent; (b) **lexical ties:** vocabulary is selected to exemplify previously stated or written information (e.g., repetition of nouns, provision of a synonym or superordinate); (c) **conjunction:** conjunctive devices such as "and" and "then" are included; and (d) **ellipsis:** certain items are omitted because they can be presupposed from the previous stated or written text.

During assessment, we explore the relationship between the clarity of a message and the amount of cohesion it contains. Specifically, clinicians identify the occurrence of these cohesive devices in connected language to determine the degree and accuracy of their use, which may be either appropriate (Coelho et al., 1994) or inappropriate (Glosser & Deser, 1990; Uryase et al., 1991; Liles & Coelho, 1998), complete (i.e., the antecedent easily identified), incomplete (i.e., the antecedent was not provided), or inaccurate (i.e., an ambiguous antecedent) (Liles, 1985).

Influential Variables

During assessment we also determine the variables that facilitate or impede the production of language content in order to specify the nature and extent of the word-finding impairment. Such analyses give us very valuable information about the treatment activities and stimuli that we will use. For example, psycholinguistic variables such as the target words' frequency (Deloche et al., 1996), age of acquisition (Deloche et al., 1997), length (Nickels & Howard, 1995), concreteness (Nickels, 1995), semantic category (Goodglass et al., 1966), grammatical class (Zingeser & Berndt, 1988), degree of certainty (Mills et al., 1979), and operativity (Nickels & Howard, 1995) are examined. In addition, a variety of contextual and task factors that have been found to affect word retrieval in aphasia are explored. These include type of sensory input (Benton et al., 1972), stimulus novelty (Faber & Aten, 1979), length of trial and inter-trial time (Brookshire, 1971), type of naming task (Berndt et al., 1997; Williams & Canter, 1987), concomitant gesturing (Hanlon et al., 1990), verbal reinforcement (Stoicheff, 1960), attention condition (Murray, 1996), and word retrieval success rate (Brookshire, 1972). It is important to note that these variables may not only influence the content produced by aphasic patients during word-level or structured language, but also during connected language. Therefore, clinicians introduce conversational topics that vary in terms of abstraction, intellectual complexity, length, and frequency to examine which topics facilitate and which retard the amount of meaningful content, jargon, and/or

TABLE 4–12

An Example of a Cuing Hierarchy

1. The clinician imposes a delay or the patient requests additional time to produce the word
2. The clinician provides a semantically related word or the patient generates one or more words that are semantically related to the target (e.g., "sugar" or "tea" for the target "coffee")
3. The clinician provides a phonemic cue (e.g., /k/ for the target "coffee") or the patient produces one or more words that are phonetically similar to the target (e.g., "cost" or "caddy")
4. The clinician or the patient provides a description of the target word (e.g., "I drink this every morning." for the target "coffee").
5. The clinician provides a carrier phrase for the target word (e.g., "A cup of _____").

word-finding errors in their patients' spoken or written language.

Evaluation also includes an analysis of patient ability to use clinician-produced and/or self-generated cues. That is, clinicians explore what type of word-retrieval cues (e.g., phonemic cues) or self-correction strategies (e.g., delay) assist the patient's word-finding abilities. Cue hierarchies, such as that displayed in Table 4–12, can be explored to examine word-finding stimulability and to determine what type of self-correction strategies a patient uses.

Goal 7: Analysis of Ability to Produce Language Form

Linguistic form includes morphology, syntax, and phonology. Morphology refers to the set of rules that govern the structure of words and the construction of word forms from the basic elements of meaning (i.e., morphemes), syntax refers to our rule system for ordering words into sentences, and phonology refers to our sound system as well as the rules we use to combine those sounds (Owens, 1984). Aphasia may result in difficulties producing one or more aspects of form. Consequently, each should be assessed during an in-depth language evaluation.

Production of Form Words and Morphology

Morphologic and syntactic impairments in verbal production are common in patients with aphasia. Such deficiencies are observed in the use of relational words such as articles, prepositions, conjunctions, and personal pronouns (Goodglass et al., 1993; Hofstede & Kolk, 1994). In addition, morphological inflections such as the plural /-s/, possessive /-s/, or present progressive /-ing/ are frequently omitted or inappropriately used. In aphasia, the hierarchy of difficulty for producing these various morphemes has been found to be a function of grammatical rather than phonological complexity (Goodglass & Berko, 1960; Haarman & Kolk, 1992). Specifically, aphasic patients tend to display relatively greater difficulty as they shift from producing determiners to prepositions to pronouns to auxiliary verbs for form words, and as they shift from producing plural to adjective to verb inflections for grammatical morphemes.

Most traditional aphasia batteries do not assess this aspect of language. However, both the PALPA (Kay et al., 1997) and the PAL (Caplan & Bub, 1990) include subtests to assess production of morphology. For example, on the PAL, patients are given a word that they insert into a given sentence (e.g., "courage" must be affixed to fit into the sentence "If a man is brave, we say he is ____."). Goodglass and Berko's (1960) sentence completion test examines patient ability to affix several types of grammatical morphemes. For example, to examine the regular past tense/-ed/ morpheme, the clinician reads the stimuli aloud and the patient then supplies the final word/target morphological inflection: "He is using the fly swatter to swat flies. Yesterday, several flies were ____."

The above tests elicit form words and morphology via relatively structured or constrained, very highly structured tasks. In addition, there are also a number of scoring systems described in the aphasia literature that may be used to examine these syntactic features in connected language samples (Menn et al., 1994; Saffran et al., 1989; Thompson et al., 1995). For example, Menn and colleagues (1994) developed an Index of Grammatical Support to examine the average number of form words and grammatical morphemes that are correctly used in the spoken output of patients with aphasia.

Production of Syntactic Constructions

In terms of syntax, aphasic patients experience difficulty in combining words into both simple and complex constructions in order to express relationships. More specifically, patients demonstrate restricted use of syntactic forms and therefore produce incomplete syntactic structures, simple syntactic structures, or both (Bird & Franklin, 1995, 1996; Edwards, 1998; Goodglass et al., 1994). They may also produce few complex syntactic structures or sentence forms and commit more errors when attempting them.

In terms of assessment, the clinician determines the specific syntactic structures that are available to each aphasic patient. To examine the production of spoken and written sentences in highly structured contexts, clinicians may choose from one of the few structured tests (see Table 4–4) or subtests that are designed to elicit a variety of syntactic forms (e.g., passives, datives, relative clauses). For example, on the PAL (Caplan & Bub, 1990), patients are asked to describe a picture with the constraint that they must begin their description with a certain word such as "bicycle" (to elicit the passive sentence, "The bicycle is being pushed by the man.").

TABLE 4–13

The Types and Examples of Syntactic Constructions That May Be Analyzed

Construction	Examples
Noun Phrase	cookies; the boss
Verb	stealing; hurry up
Adjective	big; warm
Prepositional Phrase	in the basket
Expanded Noun Phrase	cookies in the jar
Expanded Verb	get up in the morning
Expanded Adjective	sick of the office
Expanded Prepositional Phrase	in bed in the morning
Subject+Auxiliary	so is the woman; aren't they? (tag question)
Subject Verb	the man's running
Subject+Predicate	he's the president
Verb Object	dry the dishes
Subject Object	the dog...chicken
Topic-Comment	boy...off stool; burglar...policeman
Expanded Subject Verb	the guy's running to work
Expanded Subject+ Predicate	the woman's angry with her husband
Expanded Verb Object	grab the chicken quickly/from the basket
Expanded Subject Object	dog...chicken in basket
Expanded Topic-Comment	burglar policeman outside
Subject Verb Object	the dog stole the chicken
Expanded Subject Verb Object	the mother's washing dishes in the kitchen
Complex	I hope he gets to work on time
Multicomplex	he picks the corn to see if it's ripe
Aborted Utterance	this boy has...
Abandoned Utterance	the sink is overflowing on to the ...

From Goodglass, H., Christiansen, J.A., & Gallagher, R. (1994). Syntactic constructions used by agrammatic speakers: Comparison with conduction aphasics and normals. *Neuropsychology, 8,* 598–613. Reprinted by permission. © 1994, The American Speech-Language-Hearing Association.

Another assessment option is to examine connected, spoken, or written language samples using one of the several syntactic scoring systems described in the aphasia literature (Edwards, 1995; Goodglass et al., 1994; Rochon et al., 1998; Saffran et al., 1989; Thompson et al., 1995) (Table 4–13). Although some of these analysis systems were developed to characterize agrammatic language output (e.g., Saffran et al., 1989), other systems are aimed at characterizing structural aspects of fluent or paragrammatic language output (e.g., Edwards, 1995). Most of these scoring systems provide detailed procedures for collecting language samples (typically using picture description or story retelling tasks), separating samples into utterances or T-units (i.e., an independent main clause and any dependent clauses modifying it; see also Cannito et al., 1988), and identifying a variety of syntactic forms (e.g., proportion of grammatical sentences, proportion of simple vs. complex grammatical sentences, number and type of sentential constituents). Because the procedures are so explicit, researchers report good inter-rater reliability.

Analysis of Responses

The type of form errors that are produced are determined. Specifically, this involves examining whether the morphologic or syntactic errors are a substitution or omission of target structures. Omission errors might, for example, involve production of verbs in their infinitive form (e.g., without person or number agreement or tense endings), or the omission of a whole group of words such as relational words or auxiliary verbs. Substitution errors might involve the interchangeability of constituents. For example, the patient might confuse nouns with verbs or affix the inappropriate morphological inflection. Substitutions may be further examined to determine whether errors are within- (e.g., "in" for "with") or across-category (e.g., "her" for "with") substitutions (Haarman & Kolk, 1992). Such error analysis also involves determining whether sentences are understandable in spite of omissions and substitutions. Interestingly, in English, word order violations are relatively uncommon among aphasic patients (Bates et al., 1988; Menn & Obler, 1990); therefore, identifying word order violations is not a major focus of error analysis.

The frequency and consistency of production of various syntactic structures is also evaluated to determine which structures are frequently, infrequently, or never used and which are consistently or inconsistently used correctly. For example, some patients with fluent types of aphasia may produce a variety of syntactic forms but produce these complex forms at a reduced frequency compared with their non-brain-damaged peers (Edwards, 1995, 1998). When aphasic patients demonstrate inconsistent use of form words, morphological inflections, or syntactic forms, the clinician tries to identify whether or not there are any influential linguistic or task variables. For example, for some aphasic patients, there is a relationship between the degree of structure or task constraint (e.g., sentence completion vs. conservational activities) and the number and type of grammatical errors produced (Hofstede & Kolk, 1994).

Phonology

Phonology refers to the set of sounds in one's language as well as the rules used to distribute and sequence those sounds into words (Owens, 1984). Basically, phonology has two components: a segmental part that consists of phonemes and syllables and a suprasegmental part that includes intonation, stress, and pauses.

Segmental Phonology

Aphasia is frequently accompanied by a segmental phonological disorder or an impairment in the ability to produce the distinctive sound elements of a word or syllable in the standard manner. In fact, Blumstein (1998) concludes that "nearly all aphasic patients produce phonological errors in their speech output" (p. 162). Often, segmental phonological disorders are associated with dysarthria or apraxia of speech and consequently with breakdown in terms of phonetic implementation. Both of these disorders are frequent accompaniments of aphasia and have been described above under Goal 2. When either or both of them are present, phonology is assessed in detail. The data collected include (a) phonemic errors produced during unstructured spontaneous language and the phonological context of those errors, (b) errors produced on a standard articulation test, (c) results of stimulability testing or the patient's ability to modify his or her production of error phonemes following auditory and visual stimulation, and (d) results of an evaluation of the patient's peripheral speech mechanism.

Suprasegmental Phonology

The production of suprasegmental components of phonology such as intonation and stress may also be problematic for some patients with aphasia.

Intonation. Intonation refers to modulations of the pitch or musical flow of an utterance and is primarily dependent upon laryngeal control (Blumstein, 1998). Ability to produce such normal melodic intonation or prosodic quality is assessed to determine if the patient has problems using pitch variations to indicate grammatical segmentation or complexity (Goodglass, 1968), such as at the end of a phrase or sentence. Difficulties in the production of intonation have been reported, particularly in patients with Broca's aphasia or anterior left hemisphere lesions (Cooper et al., 1984).

Stress. Stress refers to the force or accentuation of a particular sound or syllable (Blumstein, 1998). The clinician determines if the aphasic patient uses normal stress patterns or if he or she manifests incorrect stress placement and subsequent reduction or omission of vowels or morphemes that would normally have been stressed. Stress is assessed at both the phrase and sentence level (Goodglass, 1968).

Generally, the specific suprasegmental phonological variables that the aphasic patient can produce or that he or she can be stimulated to produce are determined. This can be accomplished during moderately structured observations or by administering certain aphasia batteries (e.g., WAB, BDAE) in which suprasegmental features of spoken output are examined, such as when rating the fluency of connected speech. Additionally, those suprasegmentals that can be used to facilitate or increase the intelligibility of spontaneous speech or the communicating of meaning are identified and incorporated when formulating therapeutic goals.

Goal 8: Analysis of Pragmatic Ability

Communication is a reciprocal act of sending and receiving information that is profoundly influenced by the context in which it is used and the partners involved. That is, both the communication environment and the partners are dynamic components of the communication itself. Therefore, language (including content and form) varies with each context and partner. Indeed, the language produced or comprehended by an individual at any point in time will be an interactive product of contextual variables and the individual's structural linguistic knowledge (Gallagher, 1983).

Pragmatics refers to the system of rules that regulate the use of language in context (Bates, 1976). It involves the interactional aspects of communication and the use of language for communication (Prutting & Kirchner, 1983). The emphasis is not on sentence structure but rather on how meaning is communicated—how units of language function in discourse. Pragmatics is a knowledge of who can say what to whom, in what way, where, when, and why, and by what means (Prutting, 1979). It is the knowledge of how to converse with different partners and in different contexts, as well as the knowledge of the rights, obligations, and expectations underlying the initiation, maintenance, and termination of discourse.

Pragmatic abilities include a communicator's proficiency in constantly adjusting the content, form, and acceptability of his or her message, in switching or shifting sets of reference as in topic changes, and in being sensitive to the influence of the communication partner's social status and communicative abilities and to the physical context in which communication occurs (Craig, 1983; Prutting & Kirchner, 1983). It also refers to the ability to use language for a variety of functions or intents such as requesting, greeting, warning, and protesting (Lucas, 1980).

In assessing pragmatics, there is a functional communication perspective in which the aphasic patient's ability to convey messages is examined, regardless of whether the patient uses deviant language content, form, or both to convey these messages. With respect to the WHO model, such assessment often focuses more on testing at the activity and participation levels rather than the impairment level (Holland & Thompson, 1998).

Generally, pragmatic aspects of language remain an area of relative strength for many aphasic patients. Indeed, most patients with aphasia can communicate better than they can speak (Holland, 1975). However, "pragmatic skills certainly can be affected by focal brain damage" (Holland, 1996, p. 162). Consequently, clinicians assess pragmatic skills to determine if these abilities are an area of strength that may be capitalized upon during treatment or whether they are

problematic and need to be remediated during treatment. Specifically, it is important to examine use and understanding of the various speech acts and intents and of the many discourse rules that govern conversational skills such as turn-taking and topic selection, maintenance, and code switching and to determine how they are influenced by various contexts and partners (Chapey, 1994).

Communication Environment

Various communication settings and activities may affect the length, morphosyntactic complexity (e.g., anaphoric pronouns), redundancy, fluency, responsiveness (e.g., elaborations of comments), semantic relatedness, and lexical selections (e.g., technical jargon) of the language that is produced or that is understood (Labov, 1970; Wiener et al., 1984). For example, clinicians frequently observe variations in production and comprehension of spoken and written language when comparing communicative performance in the therapy room to that observed in more naturalistic environments (Holland, 1975). Also, Glosser et al. (1988) found that verbal complexity and language errors vary significantly with different contents and contexts of communication. For example, in conditions that restrict visual contact between the speaker and listener (e.g., communicating over the telephone or through an opaque barrier), aphasic patients, like non-brain-damaged adults, produce fewer communicative gestures and more complex verbalizations. Hofstede and Kolk (1994) also have observed changes in the morphosyntactic output of aphasic patients across different speaking conditions (e.g., conversation, formal interview, picture description). Further, "aphasic patients show appropriate and predictable linguistic changes in response to nonlinguistic social contextual variables" (Glosser et al., 1988, p. 115). Therefore, assessment involves an analysis of whether or not the aphasic patient's linguistic behavior changes with various contexts, and if so, how specific contexts facilitate or hinder the number and variety of his or her communicative behaviors.

Communication Partners

Specific communicative partners may also affect the form, content, and intent of language that is produced or that is to be understood (Gallagher, 1983). Partner characteristics such as age, sex, familiarity, and authoritative status as well as internal variables such as world knowledge, values, previous experiences, and emotional status affect communication (Davis, 1993). Therefore, clinicians analyze such variability and note patterns of performance.

Part of successful communication involves having the opportunity to communicate highly personal thoughts and emotions to those who are judged to be important partners, as well as feeling the fulfillment associated with sending and receiving messages (Lubinski, 1995). That is, successful

TABLE 4–14

Family Interaction Analysis: Scoring Form[a,b]

Significant Other Behaviors	S	U	R
Nonfacilitative			
1. Inattentive posture	_____	_____	_____
2. Incongruent affect	_____	_____	_____
3. Lengthy response	_____	_____	_____
4. Self-focus	_____	_____	_____
5. Inappropriate topic change	_____	_____	_____
6. Advice giving	_____	_____	_____
7. Judgmental response	_____	_____	_____
8. Premature confrontation	_____	_____	_____
9. Interrupting	_____	_____	_____
10. Guessing	_____	_____	_____
11. Repeating	_____	_____	_____
12. Simple language	_____	_____	_____
13. Loud voice	_____	_____	_____
14. Abrupt topic change	_____	_____	_____
15. Speaking for patient	_____	_____	_____
Facilitative			
16. Closed question	_____	_____	_____
17. Verbal following	_____	_____	_____
18. Minimal encouragers	_____	_____	_____
19. Open question	_____	_____	_____
20. Paraphrasing content	_____	_____	_____
21. Reflecting feeling	_____	_____	_____
22. Summarizing content	_____	_____	_____
23. Summarizing feeling	_____	_____	_____
24. Sharing	_____	_____	_____
25. Confrontation	_____	_____	_____
26. Interpretation	_____	_____	_____
27. Verbal cueing	_____	_____	_____
28. Gesturing	_____	_____	_____
29. Instruction	_____	_____	_____
30. Labeling	_____	_____	_____
31. Modeling	_____	_____	_____
32. Physical cue	_____	_____	_____
33. Request for attention	_____	_____	_____

[a] From Florance, C. (1981). Methods of communication analysis used in family interaction therapy. *Clinical Aphasiology, 11*, 204–211.

[b] S = successful; U = unsuccessful; R = rejection.

communication gives the individual the feeling of social connectedness and quality connection to others. Unfortunately, some aphasic patients may have few opportunities for successful, meaningful communication due to a lack of sensitivity to the value of interpersonal communication, few reasons to talk, lack of privacy, excessive background noise, no viable communication partner, negative perceptions of their communicative competence, and/or lack of stimulation in general (Kagan, 1995; Lubinski, 1995; McCooey et al., in press). Therefore, the aphasia assessment includes an evaluation of the communication opportunities afforded the patient and the barriers to such communication using tools such as

the Profile of the Communication Environment of the Adult Aphasic (Lubinski, 1994). In addition, clinicians determine whether a particular patient has anyone with whom to talk, and/or who the frequent and infrequent communicative partners are and how they affect communicative behavior.

Other nonstandardized tools such as the Family Interaction Analysis (Florance, 1981) (Table 4–14) may also help the clinician identify the psychosocial factors that promote successful communication interaction and those that contribute to a communication-impaired environment. Completing these types of analyses may help provide information about the caregivers' and significant others' sensitivity to the aphasic patient's communication difficulties, as well as about their successful and unsuccessful strategies for communicating with the patient. Subsequently, the clinician can help the patient, significant communication partners, and specific individuals in the community to create a positive and rewarding communication environment that contains stimulating activities and a variety of interesting communication partners.

Speech Acts and Intents

Pragmatics involves the acquisition and use of conversational knowledge and of the semantic rules necessary to communicate a variety of intentions (Lucas, 1980). This semantic knowledge develops and is used within the context of a speech act, a theoretical unit of communication between a speaker and a hearer. According to Searle (1969), the speech act includes what the message-sender means, what the message (or other linguistic elements) means, what the message-sender intends, what the message-receiver intends, what the message-receiver understands, and what the rules governing the linguistic utterance are. In Searle's theory, the proposition is the words or sentences produced, and the illocutionary force of this proposition is the message-sender's intent in producing the utterance.

A number of taxonomies have been developed to describe the variety of intentions that we use in language (Dore, 1974; Searle, 1969; Tough, 1977). Frequently identified **intents** include (a) **response:** the intention to attend to and respond to another's utterance or question; (b) **request:** the intention to address another for help whether it be to solicit information, action, or perhaps acknowledgment; (c) **greeting:** the intention to convey a conventional greeting; (d) **protesting:** the intention to object to another person's behavior, or to reject or resist the action, statement, or command of another; (e) **description/comment:** the intention to give a mental image of something seen or heard; (f) **assertion:** the intention to point out to another that some statement or proposition is true; this intent includes a subset called affirmation, which includes instances in which the speaker is agreeing with or confirming a proposition; and (g) **informing:** the intention to report on present and past experiences.

Many of these intents are used in one or more of the following four communication categories proposed by Lomas et al. (1989) (see Table 4–1): (a) **basic need:** communication skills are needed to accomplish basic needs such as eating and daily hygiene; (b) **health threat:** communication skills are needed to maintain physical well-being or health (e.g., calling for assistance after falling, telephoning 911 for emergency help); (c) **life skill:** the ability to provide or understand information is needed to complete daily activities such as shopping, home maintenance, and driving; and (d) **social need:** communication skills are needed to participate in social activities such as playing cards, going to church, or writing a letter to a friend.

Intents may be communicated and comprehended through semantic-syntactic utterances and/or by previous or subsequent utterances. In addition, they may be expressed (and comprehended) through facial expression or accompanying actions, gestures, or tone of voice. What is not said may also communicate intent. We can also say one thing and mean another. That is, individuals frequently use their knowledge of the communication environment and their partners to help them decipher between what is said and what is meant.

Aphasic patients have a relatively preserved ability to interpret a variety of speech acts and intents, including the ability to respond correctly to indirect requests (Foldi, 1987; Wilcox et al., 1978). In terms of production, some patients maintain the ability to produce a variety of speech acts or intents including requests for clarification, responses to requests for clarification, and greetings (Apel et al., 1981; Newhoff et al., 1985; Prinz, 1980; Ulatowska et al., 1992). Despite these preserved pragmatic abilities, however, impairments in other aspects of pragmatics are reported. First, aphasic patients use a restricted range of speech acts and intents (Prutting & Kirchner, 1987; Wilcox & Davis, 1977). For example, Doyle et al. (1994) found that aphasic patients primarily produced responses (to direct requests). In contrast, assertions predominated the verbal output of non-brain-damaged adults. Secondly, different pragmatic impairments are observed among patients with different types of aphasia and different sites of brain-damage (Prutting & Kirchner, 1987; Murray & Holland, 1995). Because of these possible pragmatic limitations, examining patients' ability to communicate and comprehend various speech acts or intents is an important part of a comprehensive aphasia assessment.

Discourse Skills

The reciprocal nature of discourse involves the initiation of the speech act or the maintenance of that interaction via turn-taking, topic maintenance and shifts, and repair and/or revision strategies. Sufficient skill in these various behaviors is necessary to attain cooperative discourse participation. That is, Grice (1975) proposed that successful discourse is achieved when (a) the message-sender provides a sufficient amount of information (i.e., not too much and not too little); (b) the messages being shared are truthful; (c) the vocabulary used is relevant to the topic and is cohesively related; and (d) the manner in which messages are shared is concise and avoids ambivalence and obscurity.

Initiation of the speech act (as the message-sender) includes topic selection and introduction and/or change of topic. This communicative act should contain new, relevant, and what is judged to be sincerely wanted information. The message-sender therefore needs to determine what, if any, information is shared by the various message-receivers. Thus, topical or referential identification involves searching one's long-term memory for information that is judged to be relevant, interesting, and wanted or already known by the partner (Chapey, 1994). For some aphasic patients, inappropriate initiation is observed (Avent et al., 1998; Penn, 1988). However, they are reported to be relatively good at being sensitive to their partners' interests and previous knowledge (Penn, 1988).

Maintenance of communication involves turn-taking or the variation of roles as message-sender and message-receiver. The role of the message-receiver is to comprehend the message that is communicated. Comprehension is indicated by one or a combination of the following: nonverbal responses (e.g., nodding the head, leaning forward), a short and usually affirmative verbal response such as "yes," and visual orientation rather than gaze avoidance (Davis, 1981). To assist the message-sender, the message-receiver must also monitor and evaluate the message and provide feedback concerning the effectiveness and acceptability of the communication exchange.

The message-sender usually retains his or her role by gaze avoidance and a hand gesture that is not maintained or not returned to a resting state through a phonetic clause juncture (Rosenfeld, 1978). When a message-sender wants a reaction or response, he or she signals "with a pause between clauses" or "with a rising or falling pitch at the end of a phonemic clause" (Davis, 1981, p. 171). The message-receiver maintains his or her role by visual orientation to the message-sender.

Nonverbal cues are usually used by partners to signal a wish to maintain or change roles (Harrison, 1974; Rosenfeld, 1978). Because role switching typically occurs as a result of the message-sender's desire to relinquish the role, the message-receiver needs to formulate a judgment concerning the message-sender's willingness to switch roles. When role switching occurs in the absence of the speaker's readiness to switch, it may be accompanied by overloudness and a shift of the head away from the speaker. Although the pause time in turn-taking may be lengthened (Lesser & Milroy, 1993; Prutting & Kirchner, 1987), most aphasic patients continue to display appropriate turn-taking skills, often relying primarily upon the use of nonverbal behaviors such as nodding or eye gaze (Penn, 1988; Schienberg & Holland, 1980).

Repair and/or revision are also part of the discourse maintenance and regulations. Discourse repair involves the message-sender's sensitivity to cues provided by the message-receiver and the ability to respond to such cues by repeating and/or modifying the message when necessary. Moves by both communication partners to identify and repair sequences and to respond to regulatory devices such as requests for clarification are essential to the maintenance of communication (Fey & Leonard, 1983; Schegloff et al., 1977). The most common form of repair in normal interactions is the self-initiated self-repair, and it typically occurs within the turn in which the communication breakdown has transpired.

Because of their well-documented difficulties in conveying accurate and nonambiguous information (a product of their language content and form deficits) (e.g., Avent et al., 1998; Prutting & Kirchner, 1987), repair and revisions strategies play an important role in and are frequently used when communicating with aphasic patients (Ferguson, 1994; Milroy & Perkins, 1992). Furthermore, the linguistic impairments of the aphasic patients may limit their ability to identify communication breakdowns, to repair them, or both. Although some aphasic patients retain the ability to initiate and make repairs (e.g., Klippi, 1996), this process typically takes longer to resolve than during normal interactions, and may be accomplished collaboratively rather than solely by one partner. The type of repair used varies between aphasic-family and aphasic-clinician interactions (Lindsay & Wilkinson, 1999) and among types of discourse activity (Heeschen & Schegloff, 1999). Further, some of these types of repair can be detrimental to communication interactions; for example, the partner may use repairs excessively to work on errors if these errors have not obscured the meaning of the aphasic patient's message (Booth & Perkins, 1999; Murray, 1998). This strategy can foster the perception that the aphasic patient is a noncompetent partner as well as change the interactional roles from that of partners to that of a student-teacher or patient-clinician.

Maintenance of communication interaction may also involve a response that sustains a topic. For example, contingent utterances share the same topic as the preceding utterance and add information to the prior communication act. It is an elaboration of preceding messages. Thus, sequential organization of topics is also a component of communication maintenance. For example, in procedural and narrative discourse, a sufficient number of steps and episodes, respectively, must be elaborated on or communicated in a logical order.

Individuals with aphasia have been shown to demonstrate a variety of difficulties in the maintaining of communication interactions. Although mildly aphasic patients frequently demonstrate appropriate discourse maintenance skills, patients with more severe language impairments use fewer contingent utterances than do non-brain-damaged adults (Ulatowska et al., 1992). They have also been found to produce somewhat lengthy and digressive or tangential responses (Penn, 1988). In terms of sequential organization, fewer complete episodes and more missing episodes are observed in aphasic patients' story retellings compared with those of non-brain-damaged adults (Uryase et al., 1991). Although Ulatowska et al. (1983a,b) found that aphasic patients omit story episodes and procedural steps and include some inaccurate information, they also note that those episodes and steps which were conveyed are those considered essential to the story or procedure. Furthermore, most of these episodes and events are presented in the correct sequence.

TABLE 4–15

Tests of Pragmatic and Functional Language Abilities

Instruments	Source
Structured Tests	
Assessment of Language-Related Functional Abilities	Baines et al. (1999)
Communication Activities of Daily Living-2	Holland et al. (1999)
The Amsterdam-Nijmegan Everyday Language Test	Blomert et al. (1994)
Rating Scales and Inventories	
A Questionnaire for Surveying Personal and Communicative Style	Swindell et al. (1982)
ASHA Functional Assessment of Communication Skills For Adults (ASHA FACS)	Frattali et al. (1995)
Assessment Protocol of Pragmatic-Linguistic Skills	Gerber & Gurland (1989)
Communicative/Competence Evaluation Instrument	Houghten et al. (1982)
Communicative Effectiveness Index	Lomas et al. (1989)
Communication Profile	Gurland et al. (1982)
Communicative Profiling System	Simmons-Mackie & Damico (1996)
Everyday Communicative Needs Assessment	Worrall (1992)
Functional Communication Profile	Klein (1994)
Functional Communication Profile	Sarno (1969)
In-patient Functional Communication Interview	McCooey et al. (in press)
Pragmatic Protocol	Prutting & Kirchner (1987)
Profile of Communicative Appropriateness	Penn (1983)
Revised Edinburgh Functional Communication Profile	Wirz et al. (1990)
The Communication Profile: A Functional Skills Survey	Payne (1994)
The Speech Questionnaire	Lincoln (1982)

Therefore, although aphasic patients show many pragmatic strengths in terms of their ability to communicate successfully in discourse activities, they may also display a variety of impairments that may negatively affect the efficiency and success of their discourse interactions. Consequently, assessment in adult aphasia involves an analysis of the patient's ability to initiate and maintain discourse in various contexts and with various partners.

Assessing Pragmatics and Functional Communication

Although assessing pragmatic abilities and assessing functional communication skills are often viewed as one and the same, there are some notable distinctions between the two assessment approaches (Manochiopinig et al., 1992; Worrall, 1995). That is, functional communication refers to the ability to operate and interact in real-life situations in response to specific demands. Both reflect the summation of an individual's linguistic, pragmatic, and cognitive skills. Table 4–15 lists a variety of tests and observational profiles that can be used to examine pragmatic abilities, functional communication skills, or both.

Pragmatics

Pragmatic abilities are primarily assessed using observational profiles or checklists in which the clinician identifies the presence and appropriateness of various pragmatic behaviors. Typically these observations are based upon discourse samples since this level of communication interaction illuminates "the complex associations across linguistic, pragmatic, and cognitive processes as well as the potential dissociations (of) either across or within clinical populations" (Chapman et al., 1998, p. 56). Although some clinicians and payors view such analysis as time consuming, Boles and Bombard (1998) found that such behaviors could be reliably analyzed with 5- to 10-minute discourse samples of aphasic patients when these behaviors occurred at a rate of approximately three times per minute.

Tools such as the Pragmatic Protocol (Prutting & Kirchner, 1983), the Communication Profile (Gurland et al., 1982), the Revised Edinburgh Functional Communication Profile (Wirz et al., 1990), and the Profile of Communicative Appropriateness (Penn, 1983) can be used to rate each patient's use of specific pragmatic skills. For example, the clinician can use approximately 15 minutes of conversation between the aphasic patient and a familiar partner to complete the Pragmatic Protocol and to rate the appropriateness of 30 pragmatic parameters covering a range of speech acts (e.g., requests, comments) and discourse abilities (e.g., topic maintenance, repair/revision skills) in terms of verbal, nonverbal, and paralinguistic domains. When the clinician summarizes Pragmatic Protocol results, he or she compares the overall numbers of appropriate and inappropriate pragmatic behaviors (i.e., calculates a percentage of appropriate behaviors). Such assessment tools clearly provide information that is not obtained from more traditional standardized tests. However, some of the pragmatic tools may have specific psychometric limitations (Ball et al., 1991; Hux et al., 1997; Manochiopinig et al., 1992).

Functional Communication

There are generally two methodologic approaches to examining the functional communication skills: structured tests in which performance of test items is evaluated, and observational profiles based on unstructured or moderately structured communication interactions. Of structured tests available (see Table 4–15), the Communication Activities of Daily Living-2 (CADL-2; Holland et al., 1999) is probably that best known. This test represents a recent revision of the Communicative Abilities in Daily Living (Holland, 1980). Both versions allow for examination of the ability to recognize and produce a variety of speech acts and interactions across both spoken and written language modalities. Evaluations of communicative success are based on both verbal and nonverbal responses. The CADL-2 differs from the earlier version, however, in that it is slightly shorter (i.e., 50 items that take about 25 minutes to complete versus 68 items that take about 35 minutes to complete), and does not include role-playing items.

Strengths of standardized tests of functional communication include their documented reliability and their use in documenting change over time; however, this approach also has been criticized because of its restricted view of how aphasic patients spontaneously interact in real-life functional communication situations (Lomas et al., 1989; Manochiopinig et al., 1992) and because administering one of these tests is more time consuming than completing a rating protocol (Crockford & Lesser, 1994).

Therefore, a number of such observational profiles and rating protocols are used to examine the functional communication abilities of aphasic patients (see Table 4–15). This group of measures includes the Functional Communication Profile (Sarno, 1969), Communicative Effectiveness Index (Lomas et al., 1989), ASHA Functional Assessment of Communication Skills For Adults (ASHA FACS; Frattali et al., 1995), The Communication Profile: A Functional Skills Survey (Payne, 1994), and In-patient Functional Communication Interview (IFCI; McCooey et al., in press). The ASHA FACS has both qualitative and quantitative scales for scoring patient ability to complete a variety of everyday communication activities across four domains: social communication (e.g., "exchanges information on the telephone"), communication of basic needs (e.g., "responds in an emergency"), reading, writing, and number concepts (e.g., "understands simple signs"), and daily planning (e.g., "follows a map").

Unlike several of the other observational profiles, this test has undergone extensive standardization and has good reliability and validity.

Another notable rating scale is Payne's (1994) Communication Profile: A Functional Skills Survey. This protocol uses an interview approach in which the patient rates the relative importance of 26 communication behaviors in his or her daily life related to his or her basic, present health care and social needs (McCooey et al., in press; Code et al., 1999). The normative sample for this instrument includes patients of varying ethnicity, living accommodations, employment history, and income levels, and is therefore culturally sensitive.

A number of researchers propose that clinicians should not rely on the results of a single test or observational profile for the assessment of functional communication abilities. Indeed, Worrall (1995) suggests, "the concept of functional communication is too complex for a single test administration." Consequently, Worrall (1992) developed the Everyday Communicative Needs Assessment. This contains a series of tasks including an interview to evaluate each patient's communicative needs (Table 4–16), a questionnaire to assess the individual's social support system, and observations and ratings of the patient's interactions in his or her natural environment and with his or her daily communicative partners. The Communicative Profiling System, developed by Simmons-Mackie and Damico (1996), is similar and also represents a multi-method approach to examining aphasic patients' conversational abilities and the way these skills are influenced by daily communication partners and environments.

Over the past decade many tools for assessing the functional communication skills of patients with aphasia and other neurogenic communication disorders have been developed (see Table 4–15). However, for many of these tools, further research is needed to determine if they possess the following attributes: "sensitivity to change over time; reliability within and across raters, and over time; sufficient range of performance measured to prevent threshold effects; usefulness across different methods of administration; usefulness during different phases of rehabilitation and relevance to function outside the clinical setting" (Frattali, 1992, p. 79). Considering the recent trend for health care to focus on functional outcomes and measures, this task should be one of our highest priorities.

Goal 9: Determination of Candidacy for Prognosis in Therapy

Formulating prognoses for recovery from aphasia is one of the primary tasks of the speech-language pathologists (Tompkins et al., 1990) and one of the first questions usually asked by aphasic patients, their caregivers, and family. Although relevant and reliable predictors and optimal methods of measuring prognoses are still limited, some of the prognostic indicators commonly suggested in the

TABLE 4–16

Example of an Interview Guide, One Aspect of Worrall's (1992) Everyday Communicative Needs Assessment[a]

1. Finances
— checking and paying bills
— writing cheques
— reading bank statements
— balancing accounts/budgeting
— organizing payment of rent/mortgage
— reading literature (Social Security/Veterans Affairs)
— filling in forms (Social Security, Veterans Affairs, Medicare)
— using an automatic teller machine

2. Using the Phone
— looking up numbers in phone book
— using Yellow Pages
— dialing emergency numbers
— writing down phone messages
— making appointments/business calls
— making social calls

3. Preparing Food
— reading labels on food packets
— measuring ingredients
— reading sell by/use by dates and calculating food freshness
— following recipes
— making choices at mealtimes
— using the microwave and oven

4. General Household Activities
— following washing and ironing instructions on clothes
— following instruction leaflets for household appliances
— setting washing machine
— directing workmen (e.g., plumber)
— dealing with people who come to door (e.g., meter-reader)
— following written instruction re DIY jobs (e.g., shelves)
— writing note for milkman, home help, etc.
— caring for pets
— following instructions for use of gardening products
— gardening

Coding for reasons:
1. immobility
2. aphasia
3. other stroke related problems
4. other

[a]From Worrall, L. (1995). The functional communication perspective. In C. Code & D.J. Muller (eds.), *The Treatment of Aphasia: From Theory to Practice* (pp. 47–69). San Diego, CA: Singular Publishing.

literature include **biographical variables** such as age, gender, education, premorbid intelligence, support systems, usual/necessary activities, and level and type of life participation; **medical variables** such as etiology and duration of aphasia, site and extent of brain lesion, and concomitant physical and mental health problems; and **language and cognitive variables** such as type and severity of aphasia type, and language stimulability.

Biographical Variables

Age

Many authors note that age and outcome correlate significantly (Holland & Bartlett, 1985; Sands et al., 1969); that is, younger aphasic patients demonstrate greater language recovery than older patients. For example, Ogrezeanu and colleagues (1994) show such a correlation for patients younger than 71 years of age. However, several researchers have failed to identify a meaningful relationship between age and aphasia recovery (Basso et al., 1979; Wertz et al., 1981). Consequently, there are most likely many variables such as personal attitude, available support systems, level and type of life participation, and general medical health that confound the influence of age on recovery (Darley, 1977; Johnson et al., 1998). Indeed, Tompkins et al. (1990) note that physiological characteristics such as activity level or general health indicators and "psychosocial factors like personality, social involvement, or life satisfaction...are more predictive of cognitive ability, life adaptation, and morale than is chronological age" (p. 399).

Gender

Some studies show that gender and outcome correlate significantly, favoring males (Holland et al., 1989). Other studies report mixed findings with respect to the influence of gender on prognosis. For example, Basso and colleagues (1982) found better recovery of spoken language in female as opposed to male aphasic patients but did not observe this differential recovery in auditory comprehension skills. However, other researchers have failed to observe any significant differences in the recovery of female and male aphasic patients (Ogrezeanu et al., 1994). Consequently, future research is necessary to shed light on the exact nature of gender as a prognostic variable in language recovery.

Education and Premorbid Intelligence

Although many clinicians use education level as a prognostic factor in aphasia, Tompkins et al. (1990) point out that years of formal education do not necessarily correspond to premorbid intellectual ability. Instead, these authors recommend the use of estimates of premorbid intelligence which weigh and enter standard demographic data including age, education, gender, occupational category, and race into specifically developed equations (Barona et al., 1984; Wilson et al., 1979). These estimates of premorbid functioning may have more predictive power than educational level alone, except in the cases where the patient had been illiterate (Lecours et al., 1988).

Medical Variables

Etiology/Type of Stroke

Prognosis in aphasia is more positive in cases resulting from traumatic as opposed to vascular etiology (Basso et al., 1980; Kertesz & McCabe, 1977). In terms of the type of stroke, if the patient survives a hemorrhagic stroke, he or she is more likely to experience more recovery than the patient who had an ischemic (i.e., thrombotic or embolic) stroke (Holland et al., 1989).

Time Since Onset

The fastest rate of recovery is typically observed during the first few months post-onset when spontaneous physiological recovery processes are taking place. In addition, research and clinical experiences indicate that aphasic patients can continue to make measurable progress for many, many years following the onset of aphasia (Blomert, 1998; Warren & Datta, 1981). Although Sands et al. (1969) found that the longer the time between the onset of aphasia and the beginning of intervention the poorer the prognosis, more recent research suggests that deferred treatment is not necessarily detrimental to language recovery (Sands, 1977; Wertz et al., 1987).

Site and Extent of Lesion

In general, patients with larger dominant-hemisphere lesions or multiple lesions have a poor prognosis (Kertesz et al., 1979). Relations between site of lesion and aphasia outcome are also identified. For example, lesions of the central core of the dominant-hemisphere language area, that served by the middle cerebral artery, even when they are small, frequently result in severe aphasias (Darley, 1982; Holland et al., 1989). Lesions to left temporobasal areas are also associated with less recovery compared with lesions outside of this region (Naeser & Palumbo, 1994). However, despite these generalizations, Darley (1982) notes that some patients with poor prognosis because of the site and extent of lesion have nevertheless recovered well.

Physical and Mental Health Problems

The presence of other physical and mental health problems in addition to aphasia often results in a poorer prognosis (Jorgensen et al., 1995). For example, concomitant motor speech disorders (e.g., apraxia of speech) have been shown to have a negative influence on aphasia recovery (Keenan & Brassell, 1974; Ogrezeanu et al., 1994). In terms of mental health, depression, anxiety, and other psychological problems may negatively affect outcome (Johnson et al., 1998; Paolucci et al., 1998; Sapir & Aronson, 1990). Similarly, aphasic patients with fewer medical problems tend to have a shorter length of hospital stay, which has also been associated with better recovery (Holland et al., 1989).

Medications

Certain drugs can adversely affect an aphasic patient's ability to respond to tasks. For example, dysarthria and stuttering are common adverse reactions to certain antidepressants and anticonvulsant medications (O'Sullivan & Fagan, 1998). Likewise, many anticonvulsant medications may produce undesirable effects such as confusion, fatigue, and decreased arousal levels which can affect patient ability to complete language activities (Vogel & Carter, 1995). Therefore, the clinician needs to know what medication each of their patients takes and the impact of each, separately and in combination.

Neuropsychological and Language Variables

Neuropsychological Variables

Currently, only minimal research has examined the relation between neurocognitive status and language recovery. Results of this research are mixed. That is, some studies like that by Goldenberg and Spatt (1994) show a positive relationship between initial neurocognitive test scores and language recovery (Bailey et al., 1981; Messerli et al., 1976). These researchers found that temporobasal lesions are associated with poor aphasia recovery because such lesions cause a disconnection between deep temporal lobe structures associated with memory abilities and cortical areas associated with language abilities. That is, these lesions result in problems in learning language as well as in acquiring compensatory strategies. In contrast, other studies fail to observe a significant correlation between initial cognitive status and subsequent recovery (Basso, 1987; David & Skilbeck, 1984). Despite some null findings, some clinicians believe that the presence of concomitant attention, memory, and/or executive function deficits negatively affect patients' ability to attend to and remember language, to problem solve, and to learn (e.g., compensatory strategies, generalize) (Helm-Estabrooks, 1998; Johnson et al., 1998). However, further research is necessary in this area.

Aphasia Characteristics

Severity. The initial severity of aphasia is one of the strongest predictors of aphasia outcome (Kertesz & McCabe, 1977; Ogrezeanu et al., 1994; Pedersen et al., 1995); that is, patients with severe language impairments tend to show poorer recovery than those with milder language deficits. More specifically, initial ability to speak has been found to share a definite relationship to the aphasic individual's eventual speech performance (Keenan & Brassell, 1974). Similarly, patients who are severely impaired in auditory recognition and comprehension have an unfavorable prognosis compared with those who are less affected in these language areas (Schuell et al., 1964; Smith, 1971).

Language Profile. Type of aphasia may be predictive of the amount of recovery and the residual pattern of language impairment. For example, patients with global aphasia are expected to have the poorest outcome, particularly those who continue to present with global aphasia beyond three months post-onset (Ogrezeanu et al., 1994; Paolucci et al., 1998; Sarno et al., 1970). In contrast, patients with anomic aphasia are expected to have the best outcome such that approximately half of these patients experience complete recovery by one year post-onset (Kertesz, 1979).

The language improvement that most patients experience often results in a change of aphasia type over time. For example, many patients with global aphasia eventually present with Broca's aphasia as their auditory comprehension and language production abilities recover (Mohr, 1976). In contrast, Broca's, Wernicke's, conduction, and transcortical (sensory, motor, or mixed) aphasias frequently resolve towards anomic aphasia over time (Goodglass, 1992; Ogrezeanu et al., 1994; Rapcsak & Rubens, 1994).

Stimulability

Self-Correction. An aphasic patient's awareness of his or her speech difficulty as well as his or her ability to self-correct relate positively to improvements in speaking abilities (Keenan & Brassell, 1974; Wepman, 1958). That is, patients who have insight into their language disorder as well as an awareness of situations that enhance as well as degrade their communication ability have a better prognosis (van Harskamp & Visch-Brink, 1991).

Cuing. Insight into an aphasic patient's prognosis may also be gained from examining the degree to which his or her language behaviors can be modified. For example, Keenan and Brassell (1974) observe that aphasic patients whose spoken language is initially stimulable to prompts and cues display better recovery of spoken language than do those patients for whom prompting is ineffective. Clinicians might expect that those aphasic patients who can learn to produce their own cues would have better language outcomes or demonstrate better generalization of target language behaviors than aphasic patients who are dependent upon others to provide cues. However, further research is needed to determine if this is indeed the case.

Personality/Social Variables

Personal Attitude

The aphasic patient's desire to improve his or her level of motivation, aspiration, and determination may influence the course and outcome of aphasia therapy (Chapey, 1994; Darley, 1977; Rosenbek et al., 1989). As van Harskamp and Visch-Brink (1991) propose, the "kernal" of therapy is the stimulation of the patient's willingness to participate actively in

the learning process and to practice. These researchers further state that "the patient's motivation is of utmost importance: patients need to exert themselves to make progress" (p. 533). In addition, the level and type of participation in everyday activities and in life may well have a profound effect on prognosis since patients need something to talk about and since such participation can have a positive effect on motivation (Chapey et al., 2000). Indeed, research indicates that personality variables and social support are linked to health generally, to morbidity and mortality, as well as to prognosis in treatment in a variety of health conditions such as stroke (Schut, 1988; Tompkins et al., 1990). Consequently, Tompkins and colleagues (1990) suggest that valid and reliable psychosocial scales that measure personality variables have the potential for enriching our understanding of aphasic patients' responses to treatment and for facilitating prognoses.

Family Attitude

Family interest in the aphasic patient and their desire to see improvement in language ability will also influence the progress made during intervention. For example, a committed support network is needed to help the patient's treatment attendance as well as to encourage the patient's use of treated language behaviors in his or her daily environment (Patterson & Wells, 1995; Payne, 1997). Indeed, in an article assessing factors that predict optimal post-stroke progress, Evans et al. (1991) found that a patient does significantly better when the primary support person is not depressed, is married, is knowledgeable about stroke care, and is from a functional rather than dysfunctional family. These authors suggest that caregiver-related problems can have a collective effect on rehabilitation outcome and that treatment should therefore reduce caregiver depression perhaps through participation in activities and in life (Chapey et al., 2000), minimize family dysfunction, and increase the family's knowledge about stroke care. Tompkins and colleagues (1987, 1990) also stress the importance of developing more reliable and valid measures of social networks and support resources to facilitate statements concerning prognosis.

In summary, it should be noted that no one factor discussed above consistently determines an aphasic patient's progress and success in therapy. Therefore, each patient should be enrolled for a period of trial therapy before a final decision is reached about termination or postponement of intervention.

Goal 10: Specification and Prioritization of Intervention Goals

In an excellent chapter entitled "From Assessment to Intervention: Problems and Solution," Snyder (1983) proposes that making the transition from assessment to intervention is like trying to solve a puzzle. Specifically, she states that "success in solving puzzles seems to require that we have ... only the correct pieces" (p. 160). Snyder (1983) also notes that the assessment process may be lengthy as "it takes time and effort to identify and discard the wrong pieces. Further we need to be able to conceptualize how the pieces fit together and operate as a whole. The puzzle is not really solved unless it fits together and works" (p. 160). There is no one solution to the assessment-intervention puzzle, particularly when working with aphasic patients in whom variability is the norm.

During the data collection phase of assessment, we gather the puzzle pieces and subsequently assemble the puzzle when we attempt to organize, systematize, and condense the data in a meaningful way. The "assembly" phase of assessment involves a sophisticated clinical judgement applied to the information collected. It is an evaluation of the type, frequency, and pattern of behaviors produced by the patient, an identification of influential biographical, medical, and social variables, and an exploration of the interrelatedness of these various behaviors and variables in order to specify and prioritize intervention goals.

Within the context of the WHO model (1998), both the data collection and hypothesis formation phases of assessment target the three components of body structure and function, activities, and participation. Indeed, all three areas are the focus of both assessment and intervention from day one and should not be viewed merely as carryover goals (Chapey et al., 2000) (see Chapters 10–14).

For all three levels, aphasia treatment is a multidimensional process that often requires a succession of methods (Chapey, 1981; 1986; 1994; van Harskamp & Visch-Brink, 1991). However, the usual focus of treatment is on auditory comprehension and spoken language production since these are the most essential components of daily communication for most people (Chapey, 1986; 1994). Reading and writing may be used to facilitate or to cue listening and speaking skills but are not usually the central focus of therapy (Chapey, 1986; 1994). Regardless of the language modality to be targeted in treatment, emphasis is primarily focused on improving the aphasic patient's comprehension and production of meaning and informational content, and generally on improving functional use of language in everyday communication activities and environments. Language forms become the focus of therapy only when they are needed to increase the meaning of language and the functions for which language can be used (Chapey, 1986; 1994). Indeed, too much attention to the formal linguistic aspects of language may impede the communicative act (van Harskamp & Visch-Brink, 1991). Although a typical session may integrate cognitive, linguistic, and pragmatic goals, the facilitation of meaning, of functional language, of activities, and of life participation are viewed as the core of language treatment (Chapey, 1986; 1994).

Specific treatment goals are formulated by analyzing descriptions of the aphasic patient's language and life and

deciding the area that is most in need of intervention (Chapey et al., 2000). Patterns of strengths and weaknesses are identified to determine behaviors that might be used as a base on which to build more functional and more complex responses (Chapey, 1994). For example, in the activities area, treatment is initiated at the level where the patient just begins to experience difficulty in one or more of the following: accuracy, responsiveness, completeness, promptness, and efficiency of behavior (Chapey, 1994; Brookshire, 1972; 1976). In addition, the stimulus variables and response conditions that stimulate more accurate language are defined so that they may be used to facilitate retrieval during therapy (Chapey, 1986; 1994). For example, during assessment, the clinician may note that the patient responds more accurately to visual rather than auditory stimuli or responds more quickly and accurately when using gestures rather than speech; consequently, the clinician can capitalize upon this information when developing treatment goals and activities. In treatment, the clinician starts with and builds on the patient's strengths to optimize initial success (Chapey, 1986; 1994). As Rosenbek and colleagues (1989) note, once the aphasic patient's "strengths have been enhanced, they can be used in combination with weaknesses" (p. 138).

Goals and strategies, then, are chosen on the basis of assessment results that show communicative behaviors that the aphasic patient can already produce either consistently or inconsistently, behaviors that he or she can be stimulated to produce, behaviors at the point where he or she begins to have difficulty, and communicative behaviors and activities that he or she values and will need on a daily basis to participate in activities and in life (Chapey, 1986; 1994). A task hierarchy is then developed (e.g., recognition of familiar one-word utterances, recognition of less familiar one-word utterances, recognition of two- to three-word familiar phrases and commands, etc.), and specific tasks and stimuli are chosen so that they are simple enough to ensure success and yet complex enough to stimulate learning, and so that they pertain to the patient's daily needs and activities (Chapey, 1986; 1994). Thus, tasks and the criterion of performance that is expected are identified.

The actual type of treatment that is selected will depend on what appears to be most appropriate for a specific patient's impairment and what is compatible with a clinician's definition of aphasia (Chapey, 1986; 1999). By far, the largest number of approaches and the most widely accepted approaches can be described as stimulation approaches (Chapey, 1986; 1994). This concept, first suggested by Schuell et al. (1955), emphasizes that the recovery process is a reorganization and retrieval of disrupted language processes rather than the re-learning of highly specific language responses. Specific examples of various approaches to aphasia treatment are presented in subsequent chapters of this text. In many instances, an eclectic, multidimensional approach involving two or perhaps three of these approaches is used (Byng et al., 1990;

Chapey, 1981; 1986; 1994; Holland & Thompson, 1998). This viewpoint recognizes the importance of the expertise, the competence, and the judgment of the clinician in using existing knowledge and appropriate tools and in establishing an individualized regimen for each of his or her aphasic patients (Chapey, 1994). This viewpoint also acknowledges that aphasic patients and their caregivers may present with a variety of difficulties, and that treatment must not only address language impairments, but also the social, emotional, and vocational activity limitations and participation restrictions that may accompany these language impairments (World Health Organization, 1998).

Regardless of approach, the main objective of treatment is to increase success in using language and related behaviors (e.g., drawing, gestures) to exchange information and ultimately to improve communication and participation in real life (Chapey et al., 2000; van Harskamp & Visch-Brink, 1991). That is, the objective is to enable aphasic patients to regain as much language and communication as possible, and to accommodate or compensate for their language and communication impairments as much as possible, so that they can participate in their daily personal, social, and vocational activities to the fullest extent of which they are capable. The object of the rehabilitative process, then, is to increase the productive use of cognitive, linguistic, and pragmatic skills in spontaneous communication, activities, and life participation to the optimum level possible.

FUTURE TRENDS

We still have a great deal to learn about assessment. We can begin this journey by developing more accurate, in-depth, and yet efficient, clinically relevant assessment protocols—standardized and nonstandardized; unstructured, moderately structured, and highly structured; and reliable and modifiable. With respect to the WHO (1998) framework, the vast majority of existing assessment tools focus on delineating the four language modalities of aphasia. Although over the past decade some new aphasia measures have been aimed at identifying personal activity limitations, few tests have been created to quantify and qualify the consequences of aphasia at the society participation level (Chapey et al., 2000; Holland & Thompson, 1998; Simmons-Mackie & Damico, 1996) (see Chapters 10–16). Consequently, there is a need to develop formal tools for assessing possible participation restrictions among our aphasic patients and caregivers, taking into account their psychosocial status and needs, their perceptions of their quality of life, and the degree of their role limitations (Warren, 1999; Zemva, 1999). Many of the tools that have been developed to assess these aspects of participation target populations other than the adult aphasia population and are designed to measure primary health care rather than rehabilitation outcomes (Frattali, 1998b; Hesketh & Sage, 1999). Therefore, most available tools have few items

pertaining to communication abilities and have not been developed to accommodate for the communication limitations of aphasic patients.

There may be several reasons for the fact that the development of such measures has been seriously limited in the past. First, the development of well-conceptualized, thorough, clinically appropriate measures that have relevant service delivery implications is a highly time consuming, extremely arduous, and very expensive task (Chapey, 1992; 1994). Professionals in full-time teaching, clinical positions, or both do not have the ability to allocate large amounts of time necessary for such a task, and colleges, hospitals, and clinics have been unable or unwilling to see the benefit of providing significant amounts of release time for the development of these procedures (Chapey, 1992; 1994). Financial support through grants and other sources has also been severely limited. Few organizations fund research for adult aphasia, and the few that do typically allocate the majority of funds to research aimed at further delineating impairment-level characteristics of aphasia rather than activity- or participation-level assessments and treatments. However, grant money such as that proposed by law PL 101-6713 may provide a welcome stimulus for the development of functional, clinically relevant protocols. Likewise, increased support to federal funding agencies as well as the creation of agencies such as the National Institute on Disability and Rehabilitation Research, the National Centers for Complementary and Alternative Medicine, and the Medical Rehabilitation Research may provide new sources of funding for clinical research. If one believes that creativity is the generation of a number and a variety of responses to the same task (Chapey, 1992; 1994; Guilford, 1967), one would hope that these greater funding opportunities will be used to sponsor a significant number of professionals in a variety of settings to develop different and hopefully better assessment techniques (Chapey, 1994), Encouraging many responses from a variety of perspectives may help us to begin to formulate truly creative solutions to the assessment dilemma—solutions that will allow us to sharpen our clinical acumen (Chapey, 1992; 1994). Subsequently, such measures could be used to compare and contrast the efficacy of various approaches to aphasia treatment, and also to determine the reliability and validity of the various assessment protocols (Chapey, 1994).

One of the strongest factors that has militated against the development of clinically relevant assessment techniques has been the current definition of and pressure for accountability brought about by public and insurance funding of habilitation and rehabilitation (Chapey, 1994). The term "accountability" comes from the words "to account" and means "to furnish a justifying analysis or explanation" (Webster, 1977). Being accountable for one's work is laudable. However, the system of accountability that appears to have emerged is "cost accounting," which does not foster meaningful, functional communication, or reflect current definitions of language, communication, learning (Chapey, 1992; 1994), and activities and life participation.

In fact, there is a misperception that, under current Medicare policy, comprehensive assessments will not receive funding. Although this misperception is most likely reinforced by health care management, insurance companies, and retrospective payment practices, it is contrary to legislation such as the Omnibus Reconciliation Act (Bayles, 1999). Likewise, under the current Prospective Payment System, clinicians must ensure that each patient receives an in-depth assessment so that the most appropriate Resource Utilization Group (RUG) categorization is assigned to the patient; a quick and superficial assessment will no doubt underestimate the extent of a patient's language impairment, activity limitations, and participation restrictions, and consequently result in an inappropriate RUG categorization which results in insufficient funding of treatment services for the patient.

There are other examples of how the emphasis on economy rather than therapy efficacy is affecting current clinical practices. Specifically, government and private health care agencies designate that the behaviors that will be produced by the patient in treatment must be specified in writing in advance (Chapey, 1994). That is, such goals are usually operationally written, behavioral goals such as "By the end of this session, John will name three kinds of fruit." This leads to what Frattali (1992) called a deficit-oriented approach to intervention. Current accountability, then, often involves assessing whether the patient reached criterion, or the expected level of performance. Within this framework of accountability, assessment and intervention target specific language modalities that are discrete, highly measurable, surface-structure behaviors that can be predicted in advance and that primarily reflect short-term outcomes (Chapey, 1992; 1994). Consequently, it encourages a "skills approach" (Chapey, 1992; 1994; Frattali, 1992) to treatment rather than targeting functional communication within a meaningful context and/or activity, or rather than addressing changes in patients' and caregivers' life participation, or perceptions and expectations of themselves and their communicative interactions. All of the latter may be more difficult to measure via long-term outcomes but are far more important to the patient and family.

Defining language and communication in terms of measurable and specific surface structures seems to miss the very core of what language and communication are (Chapey, 1992; 1994). Such definitions ignore the fact that meaning is the essence of language (Goodman, 1971) and that language and communication are like an iceberg—much of what is meant and communicated is below the surface; only a small portion of the communication is spoken or written or heard or read (Chapey, 1992; 1994). Likewise, this approach to aphasia assessment and treatment minimizes or ignores the many societal factors (e.g., perceptions and actions of family, friends, or co-workers) that may interact with the patient's language and communication abilities, and, consequently, the degree of participation restriction they experience (Simmons-Mackie & Damico, 1996). Lastly, this approach fails to acknowledge that the perceptions of the patients and their caregivers are legitimate outcome measures (Blomert, 1995; Chapey, 1977; 1994; Hesketh & Sage, 1999; Whiteneck, 1994).

As a field, we must continue to search for a consensus of what core elements constitute functional communication and we must create a definition that has relevance to functioning in a variety of clinical settings as well as outside of these clinical settings (Frattali, 1998b). Additionally, we must specify what outcomes should be measured to quantify and qualify the effects of aphasia on the societal participation of our patients and their families. Using these definitions, we must develop multidimensional assessment protocols that are thorough (and therefore measure a range of performance and outcomes), reliable, and sensitive to changes over time. The next step will be to apply these definitions to treatment goals and procedures. This is true accountability. We must continue to promote the fact that functional communication is the core activity of daily living, because it is the core of what makes us human (Chapey, 1994). Relatedly, we must advance the importance of determining the effects of aphasia and, the subsequently, treatments for aphasia, on the communicative abilities of our aphasic patients, and also on the social well-being of our patients and their caregivers. We should be committed to make this message clear to political and fiscal policy-makers so that we can deliver the first-rate care that our aphasic patients deserve.

KEY POINTS

1. A thorough language assessment should evaluate cognitive, linguistic, and pragmatic components of language.
2. The goal of assessment is typically multifold in that etiologic (i.e., the determination of the presence of aphasia and concomitant problems), cognitive/linguistic/pragmatic (i.e., the identification of specific language strengths and weaknesses), and treatment goals (i.e., the provision of insight into possible treatment candidacy and treatment procedures) should be specified and accomplished.
3. During assessment, data should be obtained through reported observations as well as direct observations, which may be based on unstructured, moderately structured (e.g., a procedural discourse task), highly structured (e.g., a traditional aphasia battery), or nonstandard (e.g., experimental protocols) observations.
4. Prior to administering any test of aphasia or specific cognitive, linguistic, or pragmatic function, clinicians must examine the psychometric adequacy of the

selected test(s) in term of reliability, validity, and standardization.

5. The integrity of cognitive abilities should be determined because deficits in these areas may negatively affect language skills as well as the ability to acquire new language skills and compensatory strategies.

6. In terms of linguistic abilities, the production and comprehension of language content (i.e., semantics) and form (i.e., phonology, morphology, syntax) must be assessed with stimuli and tasks that vary in terms of length and complexity. All language modalities should be examined including spoken language, listening, reading, and writing abilities, and for more severely impaired patients, gesturing and drawing abilities.

7. Pragmatic abilities across a variety of communication contexts and partners must be assessed to determine if pragmatic abilities are an area of strength that may be capitalized upon during treatment, or whether pragmatic abilities are problematic and need to be remediated during treatment. Additionally, functional communication skills should be assessed to determine how well a patient's cognitive, linguistic, and pragmatic abilities operate and interact in real-life situations and in response to specific daily demands.

8. Following data collection, clinicians must synthesize the assessment data to form hypotheses concerning the nature and extent of the aphasia patient's language deficit. In particular, clinicians should be able to summarize the nature and extent of the patient's language impairment, personal activity limitations, and societal participation restrictions in terms of the WHO model of functioning and disablement.

9. Future developments in the area of language assessment must focus on assuring that patients receive comprehensive assessments despite current health care economic constraints. With reference to the WHO model, there is also a need to develop tools that examine language deficits in terms of not only the extent and nature of language impairment but also the extent and nature of communication activity and participation restrictions.

Suggested Learning Activities

1. Pretend that you have been hired to develop a Speech-Language Pathology Department in a rehabilitation hospital. In particular, your department will specialize in serving only adults with acquired language disorders. Keeping in mind you have a limited budget to purchase assessment tools and materials, list which unstructured, moderately structured, highly structured, and/or nonstandard observational tools you will purchase or collect and justify your choices. How and why might this list of assessment tools and materials differ if your new department was located in an acute care or skilled nursing facility or if you were developing a home health program?

2. Design and justify a battery of tests that would be suitable for assessing the cognitive, linguistic, and pragmatic abilities of a patient who on the basis of a bedside evaluation has been described as mildly aphasic with anomia, and reading and writing difficulties.

3. Pretend that you have received a referral to assess the language abilities of a 79-year-old aphasic patient who has a history of bilateral strokes. With what complicating conditions might you expect this patient to present? How might you identify the presence, nature, and extent of complicating conditions in this patient, and why is it important to identify these conditions prior to your formal language evaluation?

4. Design and justify a battery of assessment procedures that would be suitable for assessing the nature and extent of communication impairments, activity limitations, and participation restrictions of a skilled nursing facility resident with global aphasia. How might your battery differ if the aphasic patient lived at home with a spouse?

5. Design a research study to identify reliable prognostic indicators of aphasia outcome. What biographical, medical, language, cognitive, and personality/social variables will you examine? What assessment tools might you use to measure these variables? How will you measure and quantify aphasia outcome? What types of professionals might be involved in such a research project?

6. Review the research literature, and find and critique one nonstandardized assessment protocol for examining each of the following areas:
   (a) depression
   (b) visual neglect
   (c) divided attention
   (d) auditory short-term memory span
   (e) self-awareness of language problems
   (f) reading comprehension (content)
   (g) understanding of spoken morphosyntax
   (h) written word-finding
   (i) production of spoken morphosyntax
   (j) production of speech acts
   (k) written narrative ability

References

Adamovich, B.B. & Henderson, J.A. (1985). *Cognitive Rehabilitation of Closed Head Injured Patients*. San Diego, CA: College Hill Press.

Albert, M.L. & Bear, D. (1974). Time to understand: A case study of word deafness with reference to the role of time in auditory comprehension. *Brain, 97,* 373–384.

Albert, M.L. & Sandson, J. (1986). Perseveration in aphasia. *Cortex, 22,* 103–115.

Alexander, M.P. & Loverso, F. (1993). A specific treatment for global aphasia. *Clinical Aphasiology, 21,* 277–289.

Alexander, M.P., Benson, D.F., & Stuss, D.T. (1989). Frontal lobes and language. *Brain and Language, 37,* 656–691.

Al-Khawaja, I., Wade, D.T., & Collin, C.F. (1996). Bedside screening for aphasia: A comparison of two methods. *J Neurol, 243,* 201–204.

Allport, D.A. (1986). Distributed memory, modular subsystems and dysphasia. In S. Newman & R. Epstein (eds.), *Current Perspectives in Dysphasia* (pp. 32–60). New York: Churchill Livingstone.

American Speech-Language-Hearing Association (1991). Guidelines for speech-language pathologists serving persons with language, socio-communicative, and/or cognitive-communicative impairments. *ASHA, 33* (Suppl. 5), 21–28.

American Speech-Language-Hearing Association (1995). Functional Communication Measure. ASHA:Rockville, MD.

Annoni, J.M., Khateb, A., Custodi, M.C., Debeauvais, V., Michel, C.M., & Landis, T. (1998). Advantage of semantic language therapy in chronic aphasia: A study of three cases. *Aphasiology, 12,* 1093–1105.

Apel, K., Browning-Hall, J., & Newhoff, M. (1981). Contingent queries in Broca's aphasia. Paper presented at the annual American Speech-Language-Hearing Association convention, Toronto, Canada.

Archibald, Y.M., Wepman, J.N., & Jones, L.V. (1967). Nonverbal cognitive performance in aphasic and nonaphasic brain-damaged patients. *Cortex, 3,* 275–294.

Ardilla, A. (1995). Directions of research in crosscultural neuropsychology. *J Clin Exp Neuropsych, 17,* 143–150.

Arena, R. & Gainotti, G. (1978). Constructional apraxia and visuoperceptive disabilities in relation to laterality of cerebral lesion. *Cortex, 14,* 463–473.

Atkins, C. (1998, April). A treatment plan with real vision. ADVANCE for Occupational Therapists, p. 6.

Avent, J.R., Wertz, R.T., & Auther, L.L. (1998). Relationship between language impairment and pragmatic behavior in aphasic adults. *J Neurolinguistics, 11,* 207–221.

Ayres, A.J. (1966). *Southern California Figure-Ground Visual Perception Test* [manual]. Los Angeles: Western Psychological Services.

Baddeley, A.D. (1986). *Working Memory.* New York: Oxford University Press.

Baddeley, A.D. (1991). *Human Memory: Theory and Practice.* London: Allyn & Bacon.

Badecker, W. & Caramazza, A. (1987). The analysis of morphological errors in a case of acquired dyslexia. *Brain and Language, 32,* 278–305.

Bailey, S., Powell, G., & Clark, E. (1981). A note on intelligence and recovery from aphasia: The relationship between Raven's Matrices scores and change on the Schuell aphasia test. *Br J Dis Comm, 16,* 193–203.

Baines, K.A., Martin, A.W., & Heeringa, H.M. (1999). *Assessment of Language-Related Functional Activities.* Austin, TX: Pro-Ed.

Baker, E., Blumstein, S.E., & Goodglass, H. (1981). Interaction between phonological and semantic factors in auditory comprehension. *Neuropsychologia, 19,* 1–15.

Ball, M.J., Davies, E., Duckworth, M., & Middlehurst, R. (1991). Assessing the assessments: A comparison of two clinical pragmatic profiles. *J Comm Dis, 24,* 367–379.

Barona, A., Reynolds, C., & Chastain, R. (1984). A demographically based index of premorbid intelligence for the WAIS-R. *J Clin Consult Psych, 52,* 885–887.

Basso, A. (1987). Approaches to neuropsychological rehabilitation: Language disorders. In M. Meier, A. Benton, & L. Diller (eds.), *Neuropsychological Rehabilitation* (pp. 234–319). London: Churchill Livingstone.

Basso, A., Capitani, E., & Vignolo, L.A. (1979). Influence of rehabilitation on language skills in aphasic patients. *Arch Neurol, 36,* 190–196.

Basso, A., Capitani, E., & Moraschini, S. (1982). Sex differences in recovery from aphasia. *Cortex, 18,* 469–475.

Basso, A., Capitani, E., Laiacona, M., & Luzzatti, C. (1980). Factors influencing type and severity of aphasia. *Cortex, 16,* 631–636.

Bates, E. (1976). *Language in Context.* New York: Academic Press.

Bates, E., Friederici, A., Wulfeck, B., & Juarez, L. (1988). On the preservation of syntax in aphasia: Cross-linguistic evidence. *Brain and Language, 33,* 323–364.

Bauer, R.M. & Zawacki, T. (1997). Auditory agnosia and amusia. In T.E. Feinberg & M.J. Farah (eds.), *Behavioral Neurology and Neuropsychology* (pp. 267–276). New York: McGraw-Hill.

Baum, S.R. & Pell, M.D. (1997). Production of affective and linguistic prosody by brain-damaged patients. *Aphasiology, 11,* 177–198.

Bayles, K.A. (1999). Doing the right thing right: PPS and evaluation. Special Interest Division 2: *Neurophysiology and Neurogenic Speech and Language Disorders Newsletter, 9,* 30.

Bayles, K.A. & Kaszniak, A.W. (1987). *Communication and Cognition in Normal Aging and Dementia.* San Diego, CA: College-Hill.

Bayles, K.A., Boone, D.R., Tomoeda, C.K., Slauson, T.J., & Kaszniak, A.W. (1989). Differentiating Alzheimer's patients from the normal elderly and stroke patients with aphasia. *J Speech Hear Dis, 54,* 74–87.

Beeson, P.M., Bayles, K.A., Rubens, A.B., & Kaszniak, A.W. (1993). Memory impairment and executive control in individuals with stroke-induced aphasia. *Brain and Language, 45,* 253–275.

Beeson, P.M. & Holland, A.L. (1994). *Aphasia Groups: An Approach to Long-Term Rehabilitation* (Telerounds #19). Tucson, AZ: National Center for Neurogenic Communication Disorders.

Beeson, P.M., Holland, A.L., & Murray, L.L. (1995). Confrontation naming and the provision of superordinate, coordinate, and other semantic information by individuals with aphasia. *Am J Speech-Language Pathol, 4,* 135–138.

Belanger, S.A., Duffy, R.J., & Coelho, C.A. (1996). The assessment of limb apraxia: An investigation of task effects and their cause. *Brain and Cognition, 32,* 384–404.

Bell, B.D. (1994). Pantomime recognition impairment in aphasia: An analysis of error types. *Brain and Language, 47,* 269–278.

Benson, F. (1979). Neurologic correlates of anomia. In H. Whitaker & H.A. Whitaker (eds.), *Studies in Neurolinguistics,* Vol. 4, (pp. 292–328). New York: Academic Press.

Benton, A.L., Smith, K., & Lang, M. (1972). Stimulus characteristics and object naming in aphasic patients. *J Communication Dis, 5,* 19–24.

Benton, A.L., Hamsher, K., Rey, G.J., & Sivan, A.B. (1994). *Multilingual Aphasia Examination* (3rd ed.). San Antonio, TX: The Psychological Corporation.

Benton, A.L., Hamsher, K., Varney, N.R., & Spreen, O. (1993). *Contributions to Neuropsychological Assessment.* New York: Oxford University Press.

Bergner, M., Bobbitt, R., Carter, W., & Gilson, B. (1981). The sickness impact profile: Development and final revision of a health status measure. *Medical Care, 19,* 787–805.

Berndt, R.S. (1998). Sentence processing in aphasia. In M.T. Sarno (ed.), *Acquired Aphasia,* (3rd ed.), (pp. 229–268). New York: Academic Press.

Berndt, R.S., Haendiges, A., & Wozniak, M. (1997). Verb retrieval and sentence processing: Dissociation of an established symptom association. *Cortex, 33,* 99–114.

Bird, H. & Franklin, S. (1995/6). Cinderella revisited: A comparison of fluent and non-fluent aphasic speech. *J Neurolinguistics, 9,* 187–206.

Bishop, D.S. & Pet, R. (1995). Psychobehavioral problems other than depression in stroke. *Top Stroke Rehab, 2,* 56–68.

Bishop, D.V.M. (1983). *Test for Reception of Grammar.* London: Medical Research Council.

Black, K.J. (1995). Diagnosing depression after stroke. *South Med J, 88,* 699–708.

Blomert, L. (1995). Who's the "expert?": Amateur and professional judgment of aphasic communication. *Top Stroke Rehab, 2,* 64–71.

Blomert, L. (1998). Recovery from language disorders: Interactions between brain and rehabilitation. In B. Stemmer & H.A. Whitaker (eds.), *Handbook of Neurolinguistics* (pp. 547–557). New York: Academic Press.

Blomert, L., Kean, M.L., Koster, C., & Schokker, J. (1994). Amsterdam-Nijmegen Everyday Language Test: Construction, reliability, and validity. *Aphasiology, 8,* 381–407.

Blumstein, S.E., Katz, B., Goodglass, H., Shrier, R., & Dworetsky, B. (1985). The effects of slowed speech on auditory comprehension in aphasia. *Brain and Language, 24,* 246–265.

Blumstein, S.E. (1998). Phonological aspects of aphasia. In M.T. Sarno (ed.), *Acquired Aphasia,* (3rd ed.), (pp. 157–185). New York: Academic Press.

Boles, L. (1997). A comparison of naming errors in individuals with mild naming impairment following post-stroke aphasia, Alzheimer disease, and traumatic brain injury. *Aphasiology, 11,* 1043–1056.

Boles, L. (1998). Conversational discourse analysis as a method for evaluating progress in aphasia: A case report. *J Comm Dis, 31,* 261–274.

Boles, L. & Bombard, T. (1998). Conversational discourse analysis: Appropriate and useful sample sizes. *Aphasiology, 12,* 547–560.

Boller, F., Cole, M., Vrtunski, P.B., Patterson, M., & Kim, Y. (1979). Paralinguistic aspects of auditory comprehension in aphasia. *Brain and Language, 7,* 164–174.

Booth, S. & Perkins, L. (1999). The use of conversation analysis to guide individualized advice to carers and evaluate change in aphasia: A case study. *Aphasiology, 13,* 283–304.

Borkowski, J.G. & Burke, J.E. (1996). Theories, models, and measurements of executive functioning. In G.R. Lyon & N.A. Krasnegor (eds.), *Attention, Memory, and Executive Function* (pp. 235–261). Baltimore, MD: Paul H. Brookes.

Boyle, M., Coelho, C.A., & Kimbarow, M.L. (1991). Word fluency tasks: A preliminary analysis of variability. *Aphasiology, 5,* 171–182.

Bracy, C.B. & Drummond, S.S. (1993). Word retrieval in fluent and nonfluent dysphasia: Utilization of pictogram. *J Comm Dis, 26,* 113–128.

Breen, K. & Warrington, E.K. (1994). A study of anomia: Evidence for a distinction between nominal and propositional language. *Cortex, 30,* 231–245.

Brookshire, R.H. (1971). Effects of trial time and inter-trial interval on naming by aphasic subjects. *J Comm Dis, 3,* 289–301.

Brookshire, R.H. (1972). Effects of task difficulty on naming performance of aphasic subjects. *J Speech Hearing Res, 15,* 551–558.

Brookshire, R.H. (1976). Effects of task difficulty on sentence comprehension performance of aphasic subjects. *J Comm Dis, 9,* 167–173.

Brookshire, R.H. (1997). *Introduction to Neurogenic Communication Disorders.* New York: Mosby.

Brookshire, R.H. & Nicholas, L.E. (1994). Speech sample size and test-retest stability of connected speech measures for adults with aphasia. *J Speech Hearing Res, 37,* 399–407.

Brookshire, R.H. & Nicholas, L.E. (1995). Performance deviations in the connected speech of adults with no brain damage and adults with aphasia. *Am J Speech-Language Pathol, 4,* 118–123.

Brookshire, R.H. & Nicholas, L.E. (1997). The Discourse Comprehension Test (rev. ed.). Minneapolis, MN: BRK Publishers.

Brown, L., Sherbenou, R.J., & Johnsen, S.K. (1997). *Test of Nonverbal Intelligence* (3rd ed.). Austin, TX: Pro-Ed.

Brown, V.L., Hammill, D.D., & Wiederholt, J.L. (1995). *Test of Reading Comprehension* (3rd ed.). Austin, TX: Pro-Ed.

Brownell, H.H. (1988). The neuropsychology of narrative comprehension. *Aphasiology, 2,* 247–250.

Brownell, H.H., Gardner, H., Prather, P., & Martino, G. (1995). Language, communication, and the right hemisphere. In H.S. Kirshner (ed.), *Handbook of Neurological Speech and Language Disorders* (pp. 325–349). New York: Marcel Dekker.

Buchman, A.S., Garron, D.C., Trost-Cardamone, J.E., Wichter, M.D., & Schwartz, M. (1986). Word deafness: One hundred years later. *J Neurol Neurosurg Psychiatry, 49,* 489–499.

Burgio, F. & Basso, A. (1997). Memory and aphasia. *Neuropsychologia, 35,* 759–766.

Burns, M.S. (1997). *Burns Brief Inventory of Communication and Cognition.* San Antonio, TX: The Psychological Corporation.

Byng, S., Kay, J., Edmundson, A., & Scott, C. (1990). Aphasia tests reconsidered. *Aphasiology, 4,* 67–91.

Campbell, C.R. & Jackson, S.T. (1995). Transparency of one-handed AmerInd hand signals to nonfamiliar viewers. *J Speech Hearing Res, 38,* 1284–1289.

Cannito, M.P., Hayashi, M.M., & Ulatowska, H.K. (1988). Discourse in normal and pathological aging: Background and assessment strategies. *Sem Speech Language, 9,* 117–134.

Cannito, M.P., Vogel, D., & Pierce, R.S. (1989). Sentence comprehension in context: Influence of prior visual stimulation. *Clin Aphasiol, 18,* 432–443.

Cantor, N. & Sanderson, C. (1999). Life task participation and well-being: The importance of taking part in daily life. In D. Kahneman, E. Diener, & N. Schwarz (eds.), *Well-Being* (pp. 230–243). New York: Russell Sage Foundation.

Caplan, D. (1993). Toward a psycholinguistic approach to acquired neurogenic language disorders. *Am J Speech-Language Pathol, 2*, 59–83.

Caplan, D. & Bub, D. (1990). Psycholinguistic assessment of aphasia. Miniseminar presented at the annual convention of the American Speech-Language-Hearing Association, Seattle, WA.

Caplan, D., Baker, C., & Dehaut, F. (1985). Syntactic determinants of sentence comprehension in aphasia. *Cognition, 21*, 117–175.

Caplan, D. & Hildebrandt, N. (1988). Specific deficits in syntactic comprehension. *Aphasiology, 2*, 255–258.

Caplan, D., Hildebrandt, N., & Makris, N. (1996). Location of lesions in stroke patients with deficits in syntactic processing in sentence comprehension. *Brain, 119*, 993–949.

Caplan, D., Waters, G.S., & Hildebrandt, N. (1997). Determinants of sentence comprehension in aphasic patients in sentence-picture matching tasks. *J Speech Language Hearing Res, 40*, 542–555.

Cappa, S.F., Nespor, M., Ielasi, W., & Miozzo, A. (1997). The representation of stress: Evidence from an aphasic patient. *Cognition, 65*, 1–13.

Carmines, E.G. & Zeller, R.A. (1979). *Reliability and Validity Assessment*. Newbury Park, CA: Sage Publications.

Carramazza, A. & Hillis, A. (1991). Lexical organization of nouns and verbs in the brain. *Nature (London), 349*, 788–790.

Caspari, I., Parkinson, S.R., LaPointe, L.L., & Katz, R.C. (1998). Working memory and aphasia. *Brain and Cognition, 37*, 205–223.

Chapey, R. (1977). Consumer satisfaction in speech-languge pathology. *ASHA, 19*, 829–832.

Chapey, R. (1992). Functional communication assessment and intervention: Some thought on state of the art. *Aphasiology, 6*, 85–93.

Chapey, R. (ed.) (1981). *Language Intervention Strategies in Adult Aphasia*. Baltimore: Williams & Wilkins.

Chapey, R. (1983). Language-based cognitive abilites in adult aphasia: Rationale for intervention. *J Comm Dis, 16*, 405–424.

Chapey, R. (ed.) (1986). *Language Intervention Strategies in Adult Aphasia*. Baltimore: Williams & Wilkins.

Chapey, R. (ed.) (1994). *Language Intervention Strategies in Adult Aphasia*. Baltimore: Williams & Wilkins.

Chapey, R. & Lu, S. (1998). Intercultural variations of specific pragmatic aspects of language: Implifications for the assessment and treatment of aphasia. Unpublished.

Chapey, R., Ellman, R., Duchan, J., Garcia, J., Kagan, A., Lyon, L., & Simmons-Mackie, N. (2000). Life participation approaches to adult aphasia: A statement of values. *ASHA Leader, 5*, 3, Feb. 15.

Chapman, S.B., Highley, A.P., & Thompson, J.L. (1998). Discourse in fluent aphasia and Alzheimer's disease: Linguistic and pragmatic considerations. *J Neurolinguistics, 11*, 55–78.

Chapman, S.B., Levin, H.S., & Culhane, K.A. (1995). Language impairment in closed head injury. In H.S. Kirshner (ed.), *Handbook of Neurological Speech and Language Disorders* (pp. 387–414). New York: Marcel Dekker.

Cherney, L.R. (1998). Pragmatics and discourse: An introduction. In L. R. Cherney, B. Shadden, & C.A. Coelho (eds.), *Analyzing Discourse in Communicatively Impaired Adults* (pp. 1–7). Gaithersburg, MD: Aspen.

Cherney, L.R. & Halper, A.S. (1996). A conceptual framework for the evaluation and treatment of communication problems associated with right hemisphere damage. In A.S. Halper, L.R. Cherney, & M.S. Burns (eds.), *Clinical Management of Right Hemisphere Dysfunction* (pp. 21–29). Gaithersburg, MD: Aspen.

Christopoulou, C. & Bonvillian, J.D. (1985). Sign language, pantomime, and gestural processing in aphasic persons: A review. *J Comm Dis, 18*, 1–20.

Cockburn, J., Wilson, B., Baddeley, A., & Hieorns, R. (1990). Assessing everyday memory in patients with dysphasia. *Br J Clin Psychol, 29*, 353–360.

Code, C., Toffolo, D., & McCooey, R. (1999). Development of an inpatient functional communication interview (IFCI). Poster presentation at the Clinical Aphasiology Conference, Key West, FL.

Coelho, C.A. (1998). Analysis of conversation. In L.R. Cherney, B. Shadden, & C.A. Coelho (eds.), *Analyzing Discourse In Communicatively Impaired Adults* (pp. 123–141). Gaithersburg, MD: Aspen.

Coelho, C.A., Liles, B.Z., Duffy, R.J., Clarkson, J.V., & Elia, D. (1994). Longitudinal assessment of narrative discourse in a mildly aphasic adult. *Clin Aphasiol, 22*, 145–155.

Conlon, C.P. & McNeil, M.R. (1989). The efficacy of treatment for two globally aphasic adults using visual action therapy. *Clin Aphasiol, 19*, 185–195.

Cooper, W.E., Soares, C., Nicol, J., Michelow, D., & Goloskie, S. (1984). Clausal intonation after unilateral brain damage. *Language and Speech, 27*, 17–24.

Craig, H. (1983). Applications of pragmatic language models for intervention. In T.M. Gallagher & C.A. Prutting (eds.), *Pragmatic Assessment and Intervention Issues in Language*. San Diego, CA: College-Hill Press.

Craig, A.H. & Cummings, J.L. (1995). Neuropsychiatric aspects of aphasia. In H.S. Kirshner (ed.), *Handbook of Neurological Speech and Language Disorders* (pp. 483–498). New York: Marcel Dekker.

Crary, M.A., Haak, N.J., & Malinsky, A.E. (1989). Preliminary psychometric evaluation of an acute aphasia screening protocol. *Aphasiology, 3*, 611–618.

Crockford, C. & Lesser, R. (1994). Assessing functional communication in aphasia: Clinical utility and time demands of three methods. *Euro J Dis Comm, 29*, 165–182.

Cronbach, L.J. (1990). Essentials of psychological testing (4th ed.). New York: Harper and Row.

Cropley, A. (1967). *Creativity*. London: Longman.

Crosky, C.S. & Adams, M.R. (1970). The experimental analysis of certain aspects of an aphasic's recovery. *J Comm Dis, 3*, 177–180.

Cummings, J.L. (1987). Dementia syndromes: Neurobehavioral and neuropsychiatric features. *J Clin Psych, 48*, 3–8.

Cummings, J.L. (1990). Introduction. In J.L. Cummings (ed.), *Subcortical Dementia* (pp. 4–16). New York: Oxford University Press.

Cummings, J.L. & Benson, D.F. (1992). *Dementia: A Clinical Approach*. Boston, MA: Butterworth-Heinemann.

Cummings, J.L. & Burns, M.S. (1996). Neurological syndromes associated with right hemisphere damage. In A.S. Halper, L.R. Cherney, & M.S. Burns (eds.), *Clinical Management of Right Hemisphere Dysfunction* (pp. 9–20). Gaithersburg, MD: Aspen.

Cunningham, R., Farrow, V., Davies, C., & Lincoln, N. (1995). Reliability of the assessment of communicative effectiveness in severe aphasia. *Euro J Dis Comm, 30,* 1–16.

Cutting, J. (1978). Study of anosognosia. *J Neurol Neurosurg Psychiatr, 41,* 548–555.

Dabul, B. (1979). *Apraxia Battery for Adults.* Austin, TX: Pro-Ed.

Daniloff, J.K., Noll, J.D., Fristoe, M., & Lloyd, L.L. (1982). Gesture recognition in patients with aphasia. *J Speech Hearing Dis, 47,* 43–49.

Daniloff, J.K., Fritelli, G., Buckingham, H.W., Hoffman, P.R., & Daniloff, R.G. (1986). AmerInd versus ASL: Recognition and imitation in aphasic subjects. *Brain and Language, 28,* 95–113.

Darley, F. (1977). A retrospective view: Aphasia. *J Speech Hearing Dis, 42,* 161–169.

Darley, F. (1982). *Aphasia.* Philadelphia, PA: W.B. Saunders.

Darley, F.A., Aronson, A.E., & Brown, J.R. (1975). *Motor Speech Disorders.* Philadelphia, PA: Saunders.

David, R. & Skilbeck, C.E. (1984). Raven IQ and language recovery following stroke. *J Clin Neuropsych, 6,* 302–308.

David, R.M. (1990). Aphasia assessment: The acid test. *Aphasiology, 4,* 103–107.

Davis, G.A. (1981). Incorporating parameters of natural conversation in aphasia treatment. In R. Chapey (ed.), *Language Intervention Strategies in Adult Aphasia.* Baltimore, MD: Williams & Wilkins.

Davis, G.A. (1993). *A survey of adult aphasia and related language disorders* (2nd ed.). Englewood Cliffs, NJ: Prentice Hall.

Davis, G.A. (1996). Obligations and options in the evaluation of aphasia. Special Interest Division 2: *Neurophysiology and Neurogenic Speech and Language Disorders Newsletter, 6,* 3–8.

De Bleser, R., Cholewa, J., Stadie, N., & Tabatabaie, S. (1997). LeMo, an expert system for single case assessment of word processing impairments in aphasic patients. *Neuropsychological Rehabilitation, 7,* 339–365.

D'Elia, L.F., Satz, P., Uchiyama, C.L., & White, T. (1996). *Color Trails Test.* Odessa, FL: Psychological Assessment Resources.

Delis, D.C., Kaplan, E., & Kramer, J.H. (In press). *Delis-Kaplan Executive Function System.* San Antonio, TX: The Psychological Corporation.

Deloche, G., Hannequin, D., Dordain, M., Perrier, D., Pichard, B., Quint, S., Metz-Lutz, M.N., Kremin, H., & Cardebat, D. (1996). Picture confrontation oral naming: Performance differences between aphasics and normals. *Brain and Language, 53,* 105–120.

Deloche, G., Hannequin, D., Dordain, M., Perrier, D., Cardebat, D., Metz-Lutz, M.N., Pichard, B., Quint, S., & Kremin, H. (1997). Picture written naming: Performance parallels and divergencies between aphasic patients and normal subjects. *Aphasiology, 11,* 219–234.

Denckla, M.B. (1996). A theory and model of executive function: A neuropsychological perspective. In G.R. Lyon & N.A. Krasnegor (eds.), *Attention, Memory, and Executive Function* (pp. 263–278). Baltimore, MD: Paul H. Brookes.

DeRenzi, E. (1997a). Prosopagnosia. In T.E. Feinberg & M.J. Farah (eds.), *Behavioral Neurology and Neuropsychology* (pp. 245–255). New York: McGraw-Hill.

DeRenzi, E. (1997b). Visuospatial and constructional disorders. In T.E. Feinberg & M.J. Farah (eds.), *Behavioral Neurology and Neuropsychology* (pp. 297–307). New York: McGraw-Hill.

DeRenzi, E. & Ferrari, C. (1978). The reporters test: A sensitive test to detect expressive disturbances in aphasics. *Cortex, 4,* 279–293.

Dickerson, F., Boronow, J.J., Ringel, N., & Parente, F. (1996). Neurocognitive deficits and social functioning in outpatients with schizophrenia. *Schizophrenia Research, 21,* 75–83.

DiSimoni, F.G. (1989). *Comprehensive Apraxia Test.* Dalton, PA: Praxis House.

DiSimoni, F.G., Darley, F.L., & Aronson, A.E. (1977). Patterns of dysfunction in schizophrenic patients on an aphasia test battery. *J Speech Hearing Dis, 42,* 498–513.

Docherty, N.M., De Rosa, M., & Andreasen, N.C. (1996). Communication disturbances in schizophrenia and mania. *Arch Gen Psychiatr, 53,* 358–364.

Dore, J. (1974). A pragmatic description of early language development. *J Psycholinguistic Res, 3,* 343–350.

Doyle, P.J., Thompson, C.K., Oleyar, K., Wambaugh, J., & Jackson, A. (1994). The effects of setting variables on conversational discourse in normal and aphasic adults. *Clin Aphasiol, 22,* 135–144.

Doyle, P.J., Tsironas, D., Goda, A.J., & Kalinyak, M. (1996). The relationship between objective measures and listeners' judgments of the communicative informativeness of the connected discourse of adults with aphasia. *Am J Speech-Language Pathol, 5,* 53–60.

Dronkers, N.N. (1996). A new brain region for coordinating speech articulation. *Nature, 384,* 159–161.

Drummond, S.S. (1993). *Dysarthria Examination Battery.* San Antonio, TX: The Psychological Corporation.

Duffy, J.R. (1995). *Motor Speech Disorders: Substrates, Differential Diagnosis, and Management.* New York: Mosby.

Duffy, J.R. & Petersen, R.C. (1992). Primary progressive aphasia. *Aphasiology, 6,* 1–15.

Duffy, J.R. & Watkins, L.B. (1984). The effect of response choice relatedness on pantomime and verbal recognition ability in aphasic patients. *Brain and Language, 21,* 291–306.

Duffy, R.J. & Duffy, J.R. (1984). *Assessment of Nonverbal Communication.* Austin, TX: Pro-Ed.

Dugbartey, A.T., Rosenbaum, J.G., Sanchez, P.N., & Townes, B.D. (1999). Neuropsychological assessment of executive functions. *Sem Clin Neuropsychiatry, 4,* 5–12.

Dunn, L.M. & Dunn, E.S. (1997). *Peabody Picture Vocabulary Test III.* Circle Pines, MN: American Guidance Service.

Edwards, S. (1995). Profiling fluent aphasic spontaneous speech: A comparison of two methodologies. *Euro J Dis Comm, 30,* 333–345.

Edwards, S. (1998). Diversity in the lexical and syntactic abilities of fluent aphasic speakers. *Aphasiology, 12,* 99–117.

Eisenson, J. (1994). *Examining for Aphasia* (3rd ed.). Austin, TX: Pro-Ed.

Elliott, R. & Sahakian, B.J. (1995). The neuropsychology of schizophrenia: Relations with clinical and neurobiological dimensions. *Psychol Med, 25,* 581–594.

Elliott, R., McKenna, P.J., Robbins, T.W., & Sahakian, B.I. (1998). Specific neuropsychological deficits in schizophrenic patients with preserved intellectual function. *Cognitive Neuropsychiatry*, 3, 45–70.

Ellis, A. & Young, A. (1988). *Human Cognitive Neuropsychology*. Hillsdale, NJ: Erlbaum.

Emerick, L.L. (1971). *The Appraisal of Language Disturbance*. Marquette, MI: Northern Michigan University.

Enderby, P. (1983). *Frenchay Dysarthria Assessment*. San Diego, CA: College Hill Press.

Enderby, P. & Crow, E. (1996). *Frenchay Aphasia Screening Test: Validity and Comparability. Disability and Rehabilitation*, 18, 238–240.

Enderby, P., Wood, V., Wade, D., & Langton Hewer, R., (1987). The Frenchay Aphasia Screening Test: A short simple test appropriate for nonspecialists. *Int J Rehab Med*, 8, 166–170.

English, H.B. & English, A.C. (1958). *A Comprehensive Dictionary of Psychological and Psychoanalytic Terms*. New York: McKay.

Erickson, R.J., Goldfinger, S.D., & LaPointe, L.L. (1996). Auditory vigilance in aphasic individuals: Detecting nonlinguistic stimuli with full or divided attention. *Brain and Cognition*, 30, 244–253.

Ernest-Baron, C., Brookshire, R., & Nicholas, L. (1987). Story structure and retelling of narrative by aphasic and non-brain-damaged adults. *J Speech Hearing Res*, 30, 44–49.

Evans, R., Bishop, D., & Haselkorn, J. (1991). Factors predicting satisfactory home care after stroke. *Archives of Phsycial Medicine and Rehabilitation*, 72, 144–147.

Faber, M. & Aten, J.L. (1979). Verbal performance in aphasic patients in response to intact and altered pictorial stimuli. *Clinical Aphasiology*, 10, 177–186.

Farah, M.J. & Feinberg, T.E. (1997). Visual object agnosia. In T.E. Feinberg & M.J. Farah (eds.), *Behavioral Neurology and Neuropsychology* (pp. 239–244). New York: McGraw-Hill.

Faust, M. & Kravetz (1998). Levels of sentence constraint and lexical decision in the two hemispheres. *Brain and Language*, 62, 149–162.

Feinberg, T.E., Heilman, K.M., & Gonzalez-Rothi, L. (1986). Multimodal agnosia after unilateral left hemisphere lesion. *Neurology*, 36, 864–867.

Ferguson, A. (1994). The influence of aphasia, familiarity and activity on conversational repair. *Aphasiology*, 8, 143–157.

Fey, M. & Leonard, L. (1983). Pragmatic skills of children with specific language impairment. In T.A. Gallagher & C.A. Prutting (eds.), *Pragmatic Assessment and Intervention Issues*. San Diego, CA: College Hill Press.

Fischler, I. & Bloom, P. (1979). Automatic and attentional processes in the effect of sentence contexts on word recognition. *Journal of Verbal Learning and Verbal Behavior*, 18, 1–20.

Fitch-West, J. & Sands, E.S. (1998). *Bedside Evaluation Screening Test* (2nd ed.) (BEST2). Austin, TX: Pro-Ed.

Florance, C. (1981). Methods of communication analysis used in family interaction therapy. *Clinical Aphasiology*, 11, 204–211.

Foldi, N.S. (1987). Appreciation of pragmatic interpretations of indirect commands: Comparison of right and left hemisphere brain-damaged patients. *Brain and Language*, 31, 88–108.

Formby, C., Phillips, D.E., & Thomas, R.G. (1987). Hearing loss among stroke patients. *Ear and Hearing*, 8, 326–332.

Fougeyrollas, P., Cloutier, R., Bergeron, H., Cote, J., Cote, M., & St. Michel, G. (1997). *Revision of the Quebec Classification: Handicap Creation Process*. Quebec: International Network on the Handicap Creation Process.

Frattali, C. (1992). Functional assessment of communication: Merging public policy with clinical views. *Aphasiology*, 6, 63–83.

Frattali, C. (1998a). Measuring modality-specific behaviors, functional abilities, and quality of life. In C.M. Frattali (ed.), *Measuring Outcomes in Speech-Language Pathology* (pp. 55–88). New York: Thieme.

Frattali, C. (1998b). Outcomes assessment in speech-language pathology. In A.F. Johnson & B.H. Jacobson (eds.), *Medical Speech-Language Pathology: A Practitioner's Guide* (pp. 685–709). New York: Thieme.

Frattali, C.M., Thompson, C.K., Holland, A.L., Wohl, C.B., & Ferketic, M.M. (1995). *American Speech-Language-Hearing Association Functional Assessment of Communication Skills for Adults*. Rockville, MD: ASHA.

Freed, D.B., Marshall, R.C., & Chuhlantseff, E.A. (1996). Picture naming variability: A methodological consideration of inconsistent naming responses in fluent and nonfluent aphasia. *Clinical Aphasiology*, 24, 193–205.

Gabrieli, J.D., Cohen, N.J., & Corkin, S. (1988). The impaired learning of semantic knowledge following bilateral medial temporal lobe resection. *Brain and Cognition*, 7, 157–177.

Gallagher, T. (1983). Pre-assessment: A procedure for accommodating language variability. In T.M. Gallagher & C.A. Prutting (eds.), *Pragmatic Assessment and Intervention Issues in Language*. San Diego, CA: College-Hill Press.

Gallagher, T. (1998). National initiatives in outcome measurement. In C.M. Frattali (ed.), *Measuring Outcomes in Speech-Language Pathology* (pp. 527–545). New York: Thieme.

Garcia, L.J. & Desrochers, A. (1997). Assessment of language and speech disorders in Francophone adults. *Journal of Speech-Language Pathology and Audiology*, 21, 217–293.

Gardner, H., Albert, M.L., & Weintraub, S. (1975). Comprehending a word: The influence of speed and redundancy on auditory comprehension in aphasia. *Cortex*, 11, 155–162.

Gates, A. & Bradshaw, J.L. (1977). The role of the cerebral hemispheres in music. *Brain and Language*, 4, 403–431.

Gates, G.A., Cooper, J.C., Kannel, W.B., & Miller, N.J. (1990). Hearing in the elderly: The Framingham cohort. *Ear and Hearing*, 11, 247–256.

Gerber, S. & Gurland, G.B. (1989). Applied pragmatics in the assessment of aphasia. *Seminars in Speech and Language*, 10, 270–281.

German, D.J. (1990). *The Test of Adolescent and Adult Word-Finding*. Austin, TX: Pro-Ed.

Gil, M., Cohen, M., Korn, C., & Groswasser, Z. (1996). Vocational outcome of aphasic patients following severe traumatic brain injury. *Brain Injury*, 10, 39–45.

Glosser, G. & Deser, T. (1990). Patterns of discourse production among neurological patients with fluent language disorders. *Brain and Language*, 40, 67–88.

Glosser, G. & Goodglass, H. (1990). Disorders in executive control functions among aphasic and other brain-damaged patients. *Neuropsychology*, 12, 485–501.

Glosser, G., Wiener, M., & Kaplan, E. (1988). Variations in aphasic language behaviors. *Journal of Speech and Hearing Research, 53,* 115–124.

Goldenberg, G. & Spatt, J. (1994). Influence of size and site of cerebral lesions on spontaneous recovery of aphasia and on success of language therapy. *Brain and Language, 47,* 684–698.

Goldstein, K. (1948). *Language and Language Disturbances.* New York: Grune & Stratton.

Golper, L.C. (1996). Language Assessment. In G.L. Wallace (ed.), *Adult Aphasia Rehabilitations* (pp. 57–86). Boston: Butterworth-Heinemann.

Goodglass, H. (1968). Studies on the grammar of aphasics. In S. Rosenberg & J. Koplin (eds.), *Developments in Applied Psycholinguistic Research.* New York: MacMillan.

Goodglass, H. (1992). Diagnosis of conduction aphasia. In S. Kohn (ed.), *Conduction Aphasia.* Hillsdale, NJ: Lawrence Erlbaum.

Goodglass, H. & Berko, J. (1960). Agrammatism and inflectional morphology in English. *Journal of Speech and Hearing Research, 3,* 257–267.

Goodglass, H., Christiansen, J.A., & Gallagher, R. (1993). Comparison of morphology and syntax in free narrative and structured tests: Fluent vs. nonfluent aphasics. *Cortex, 29,* 377–407.

Goodglass, H., Christiansen, J.A., & Gallagher, R. (1994). Syntactic constructions used by agrammatic speakers: Comparison with conduction aphasics and normals. *Neuropsychology, 8,* 598–613.

Goodglass, H. & Kaplan, E. (1983). *Boston Diagnostic Examination for Aphasia.* Philadelphia: Lea and Febiger.

Goodglass, H., Kaplan, E., & Barresi, B. (1998). Innovations in aphasia testing: Preview of the new BDAE. *Brain and Language, 65,* 27–30.

Goodglass, H., Klein, B., Carey, P., & Jones, K.J. (1966). Specific semantic word categories in aphasia. *Cortex, 2,* 74–89.

Goodman, P. (1971). *Speaking and Language: Defense of Poetry.* New York: Random House.

Goodman, R.A. & Caramazza, A. (1986a). *The Johns Hopkins University Dysgraphia Battery.* Baltimore, MD: The Johns Hopkins University.

Goodman, R.A. & Caramazza, A. (1986b). *The Johns Hopkins University Dyslexia Battery.* Baltimore, MD: The Johns Hopkins University.

Gordon, J.K. (1998). The fluency dimension in aphasia. *Aphasiology, 12,* 673–688.

Goren, A.R., Tucker, G., & Ginsberg, G.M. (1996). Language dysfunction in schizophrenia. *European Journal of Disorders of Communication, 31,* 153–170.

Gourevitch, M. (1967). Un aphasique s'exprime par le dessin. *Encéphale, 56,* 52–68.

Gowan, J., Demos, G., & Torrence, E. (1967). *Creativity: Its Educational Implications.* New York: John Wiley and Sons.

Grabowski, J. & Damasio, A. (1997). Definition, clinical features and neuroanatomical basis of dementia. In M. Esiri & J. Morris (eds.), *The Neuropathology of Dementia* (pp. 1–20). Cambridge, MA: University Press.

Grant, D.A. & Berg, E.A. (1993). *Wisconsin Card Sorting Test.* Tampa, FL: Psychological Assessment Resources.

Green, J., Morris, J.C., Sandson, J., McKeel, D.W., & Miller, J.W. (1990). Progressive aphasia: A precursor of global dementia. *Neurology, 40,* 423–429.

Green, W.P., Flaro, L., & Allen, L.M. (1995). *Emotional Perception Test.* Durham, NC: CogniSyst.

Grice, H.P. (1975). Logic and conversation. In P. Cole & J. Morgan (eds.), *Studies in Syntax and Semantics (Vol. 3): Speech Acts* (pp. 41–58). New York: Academic Press.

Grill, J.J. & Kirwin, M.M. (1989). *Written Language Assessment.* Novato, CA: Academic Therapy.

Guilford, J. (1967). *The Nature of Human Intelligence.* New York: McGraw-Hill.

Guilford, J.P. & Hoepfner, R. (1971). *The Analysis of Intelligence.* New York: McGraw-Hill.

Gurland, G.B., Chwat, S.E., & Wollner, S.G. (1982). Establishing a communication profile in adult aphasia: Analysis of communicative acts and conversation sequences. *Clinical Aphasiology, 12,* 18–27.

Haarmann, H.J. & Kolk, H.H.J. (1992). The production of grammatical morphology in Broca's and Wernicke's aphasias: Speed and accuracy factors. *Cortex, 28,* 97–112.

Hall, K.M., Hamilton, B., Gordon, W.A., Zasler, M.D., & Johnston, M.V.F. (1988). *Functional Assessment Measure (FAM).* Santa Clara Valley Medical Center for Rehabilitation Research.

Hammill, D.D. & Larson, S.C. (1996). *Test of Written Language* (3rd ed.). Austin, TX: Pro-Ed.

Hammill, D.D., Pearson, N.A., & Widerholt, J.L. (1996). *Comprehensive Test of Nonverbal Intelligence.* Austin, TX: Pro-Ed.

Hanlon, R.E., Brown, J.W., & Gerstman, L.J. (1990). Enhancement of naming in nonfluent aphasia through gesture. *Brain and Language, 38,* 298–314.

Hanna, G., Schell, L.M., & Schreiner, R. (1977). *The Nelson Reading Skills Test.* Chicago, IL: Riverside Publishing.

Harrison, R.P. (1974). *Beyond words: An Introduction to Nonverbal Communication.* Englewood Cliffs, NJ: Prentice-Hall.

Hart, S. & Semple, J.M. (1990). *Neuropsychology and the Dementias.* New York: Taylor & Francis.

Hartley, L.L. (1995). *Cognitive-Communicative Abilities Following Brain Injury.* San Diego, CA: Singular Publishing Group.

Hartley, L.L. & Levin, H.S. (1990). Linguistic deficits after closed head injury: A current appraisal. *Aphasiology, 4,* 353–370.

Head, H. (1920). Aphasia and kindred disorders of speech. *Brain, 43,* 87–165.

Heaton, R.K., Grant, I., & Matthews, C.G. (1992). *Comprehensive Norms for an Expanded Halstead-Reitan Battery: Demographic Corrections, Research Findings and Clinical Applications with a Supplement for the Wechsler Adult Intelligence Scale-Revised.* Odessa, FL: Psychological Assessment Resources.

Heeschen, C. & Schegloff, E.A. (1999). Agrammatism, adaption theory, conversation analysis: On the role of so-called telegraphic style in talk-in-interaction. *Aphasiology, 13,* 365–406.

Heilman, K.M., Watson, R.T., & Rothi, L.G. (1997). Disorders of skilled movements: Limb apraxia. In T.E. Feinberg & M.J. Farah (eds.), *Behavioral Neurology and Neuropsychology* (pp. 227–235). New York: McGraw-Hill.

Helm-Estabrooks, N. (1991). *Test of Oral and Limb Apraxia.* Austin, TX: Pro-Ed.

Helm-Estabrooks, N. (1992). *Aphasia Diagnostic Profiles.* Austin, TX: Pro-Ed.

Helm-Estabrooks, N. (1998). A "cognitive" approach to treatment of an aphasic patient. In N. Helm-Estabrooks & A.L. Holland (eds.), *Approaches to the Treatment of Aphasia* (pp. 69–89). San Diego, CA: Singular Publishing.

Helm-Estabrooks, N. (In press). *Cognitive Linguistic Quick Test.* San Antonio, TX: The Psychological Corporation.

Helm-Estabrooks, N. & Albert, M.L. (1991). *Manual of Aphasia Therapy.* Austin, TX: Pro-Ed.

Helm-Estabrooks, N., Fitzpatrick, P.M., & Barresi, B. (1982). Visual action therapy for global aphasia. *Journal of Speech and Hearing Disorders, 47,* 385–389.

Helm-Estabrooks, N., Ramsberger, G., Morgan, A.R., & Nicholas, M. (1989). *Boston Assessment of Severe Aphasia.* Chicago: Riverside.

Henderson, L.W., Frank, E.M., Pigatt, T., Abramson, R.K., & Houston, M. (1998). Race, gender, and educational level effects on Boston Naming Test scores. *Aphasiology, 12,* 901–911.

Henderson, V.W. (1995). Naming and naming disorders. In H.S. Kirshner (ed.), *Handbook of Neurological Speech and Language Disorders* (pp. 165–185). New York: Marcel Dekker.

Hesketh, A. & Sage, K. (1999). For better, or worse: Outcome measurement in speech and language therapy. *Advances in Speech-Language Pathology, 1,* 37–45.

Hofstede, B.T.M. & Kolk, H.H.J. (1994). The effects of task variation on the production of grammatical morphology in Broca's aphasia: A multiple case study. *Brain and Language, 46,* 278–328.

Holbrook, M. & Skilbeck, C.E. (1983). An activities index for use with stroke patients. *Age and Aging, 12,* 166–170.

Holland, A.L. (1975). Aphasics as communicators: A model and its implications. Paper presented at the annual American Speech-Language-Hearing Association convention, Washington, D.C.

Holland, A.L. (1980). Communicative abilities in daily living. Austin, TX: Pro-Ed.

Holland, A.L. (1982). When is aphasia aphasia? The problem of closed head injury. *Clinical Aphasiology, 11,* 345–349.

Holland, A.L. (1991). Assessing pragmatic skills in aphasia. Presentation at the annual convention of the Canadian Association of Speech-Language Pathologists and Audiologists, Montreal, Canada.

Holland, A.L. (1996). Pragmatic assessment and treatment for aphasia. In G.L. Wallace (ed.), *Adult Aphasia Rehabilitation* (pp. 161–174). Boston, MA: Butterworth-Heinemann.

Holland, A.L. & Bartlett, C.L. (1985). Some differential effects of age on stroke-produced aphasia. In H.K. Ulatowska (ed.), *The Aging Brain: Communication in the Elderly* (pp. 141–155). San Diego, CA: College-Hill.

Holland, A.L., Frattali, C.M., & Fromm, D. (1999). *Communication Activities of Daily Living* (2nd ed.). Austin, TX: Pro-Ed.

Holland, A.L., Fromm, D., & Swindell, C. (1986). The labeling problem in aphasia: An illustrative case. *Journal of Speech and Hearing Disorders, 51,* 176–180.

Holland, A.L., Greenhouse, J., Fromm, D., & Swindell, C.S. (1989). Predictors of language restitution following stroke: A multivariate analysis. *Journal of Speech and Hearing Research, 32,* 232–238.

Holland, A.L. & Thompson, C.K. (1998). Outcomes measurement in aphasia. In C.M. Frattali (ed.), *Measuring Outcomes in Speech-Language Pathology* (pp. 245–266). New York: Thieme.

Holtzapple, P., Pohlman, K., LaPointe, L.L., & Graham, L.F. (1989). Does SPICA mean PICA? *Clinical Aphasiology, 18,* 131–144.

Hough, M.S., Vogel, D., Cannito, M.P., & Pierce, R.S. (1997). Influence of prior pictorial context on sentence comprehension in older versus younger aphasic subjects. *Aphasiology, 11,* 235–247.

Houghton, P.M., Pettit, J.M., & Towey, M.P. (1982). Measuring communication competence in global aphasia. *Clinical Aphasiology, 12,* 28–39.

Howard, D. & Patterson, K.E. (1992). *Pyramids and Palm Trees.* Bury St. Edmunds: Thames Valley Test Company.

Howard, D., Patterson, K.E., Franklin, S., Orchard-Lisle, V., & Morton, J. (1985). Treatment of word retrieval deficits in aphasia. *Brain, 108,* 817–829.

Hua, M., Chang, S., & Chen, S. (1997). Factor structure and age effects with an aphasia test battery in normal Taiwanese adults. *Neuropsychology, 11,* 156–162.

Huber, W., Poeck, K., Weniger, D., & Willmes, K. (1983). *Der Aachener Aphasie Test.* Gottingen: Hogrefe.

Huber, W., Poeck, K., & Willmes, K. (1984). The Aachen Aphasia Test. In F.C. Rose (ed.), *Progress in Aphasiology.* New York: Raven Press.

Hux, K., Sanger, D., Reid, R., & Maschka, A. (1997). Discourse analysis procedures: Reliability issues. *Journal of Communication Disorders, 30,* 133–150.

Ivnik, R.J., Malec, J.F., Smith, G.E., Tangalos, E.G., & Petersen, R.C. (1996). Neuropsychological test norms above age 55: COWAT, BNT, MAE Token, WRAT-R Reading, AMNART, STROOP, TMT, and JLO. *The Clinical Neuropsychologist, 10,* 262–278.

Jacobs, D.M., Sano, M., Albert, S., Schofield, P., Dooneief, G., & Stern, Y. (1997). Cross cultural neuropsychological assessment: A comparison of randomly selected, demographically matched cohorts of English and Spanish-speaking older adults. *Journal of Clinical and Experimental Neuropsychology, 19,* 331–339.

Jenkins, J.J., Jimenez-Pabon, E., Shaw, R.E., & Sefer, J.W. (1975). *Schuell's Aphasia in Adults: Diagnosis, Prognosis, and Treatment.* New York: Harper and Row.

Jeste, D.V. (1993). Late-life schizophrenia: Editor's introduction. *Schizophrenia Bulletin, 19,* 687–689.

Joanette, Y., Goulet, P., & Hannequin, D. (1990). *Right Hemisphere and Verbal Communication.* New York: Springer-Verlag.

Johnson, A.F., George, K.P., & Hinckley, J. (1998). Assessment and diagnosis in neurogenic communication disorders. In A.F. Johnson & B.H. Jacobson (eds.), *Medical Speech-Language Pathology: A Practitioner's Guide* (pp. 337–353). New York: Thieme.

Johnson, D.J. (1997). Mental status and aging: Cognition and affect. In B.B. Shadden & M.A. Toner (eds.), *Aging and Communication* (pp. 67–95). Austin, TX: Pro-Ed.

Jorgensen, H.S., Nakayama, H., Raaschou, H.O., Vive-Larsen, J., Stoier, M., & Olsen, T.S. (1995). Outcome and time course of recovery in stroke. Part 1: Outcome. The Copenhagen stroke study. *Archives of Physical Medicine and Rehabilitation, 76,* 399–405.

Kagan, A. (1995). Revealing the competence of aphasic adults through conversation: A challenge to health professionals. *Topics in Stroke Rehabilitation, 2,* 15–28.

Kahneman, D. (1973). *Attention and Effort.* Englewood Cliffs, NJ: Prentice-Hall.

Kahneman, D., Diner, E. & Schwartz, N. (1999). *Well-Being.* NY: Russell Sage Foundation.

Kaplan, E., Goodglass, H., & Weintraub, S. (1983). *The Boston Naming Test*. Philadelphia: Lea and Febiger.

Kaufer, D.I. & Cummings, J.L. (1997). Dementia and delirium: An overview. In T.E. Feinberg & M.J. Farah (eds.), *Behavioral Neurology and Neuropsychology* (pp. 499–520). New York: McGraw-Hill.

Kay, J., Byng, S., Edmundson, A., & Scott, C. (1990). Missing the wood and the trees: A reply to David, Kertesz, Goodglass and Weniger. *Aphasiology, 4*, 115–122.

Kay, J., Lesser, R., & Coltheart, M. (1996). Psycholinguistic Assessments of Language Processing in Aphasia (PALPA): An introduction. *Aphasiology. 10*, 159–215.

Kay, J., Lesser, R., & Coltheart, M. (1997). *Psycholinguistic Assessments of Language Processing in Aphasia*. Hove, East Sussex, UK: Psychology Press.

Keefe, R.S.E. & Harvey, P.D. (1994). *Understanding Schizophrenia: A Guide to the New Research on Causes and Treatment*. New York: Free Press.

Keenan, J.S. & Brassell, E.G. (1974). A study of factors related to prognosis for individual aphasic patients. *Journal of Speech and Hearing Disorders, 39*, 257–269.

Keenan, J.S. & Brassell, E.G. (1975). Aphasia Language Performance Scales. Murfreesboro, TN: Pinnacle Press.

Keith, R.W. (1993). SCANA: A Test for Auditory Processing Disorders in Adolescents and Adults. San Antonio, TX: The Psychological Corporation.

Kempler, D., Teng, E.L., Dick, M., Taussig, I.M., & Davis, D.S. (1998). The effects of age, education, and ethnicity on verbal fluency. *Journal of the International Neuropsychology Society, 4*, 531–538.

Kent, R., Weismer, B., Kent, J., & Rosenbek, J. (1989). Toward phonetic intelligibility testing in dysarthria. *Journal of Speech and Hearing Disorders, 54*, 482–499.

Kertesz, A. (1979). *Aphasia and Associated Disorders: Taxonomy, Localization, and Recovery*. New York: Grune and Stratton.

Kertesz, A. (1982). *Western Aphasia Battery*. New York: Grune and Stratton.

Kertesz, A. (1993). *Western Aphasia Battery Scoring Assistant*. San Antonio, TX: The Psychological Corporation.

Kertesz, A. & McCabe, P. (1977). Recovery patterns and prognosis in aphasia. *Brain, 100*, 1–18.

Kertesz, A., Harlock, W., & Coates, R. (1979). Computer tomographic localization, lesion size, and prognosis in aphasia and non-verbal impairment. *Brain and Language, 8*, 34–50.

Kertesz, A., Hudson, L., Mackenzie, I.R.A., & Munoz, D.G. (1994). The pathology and nosology of primary progressive aphasia. *Neurology, 44*, 2065–2072.

Kimelman, M.D.Z. & McNeil, M.R. (1989). Contextual influences on the auditory comprehension of normally stressed targets by aphasic listeners. *Clinical Aphasiology, 18*, 407–419.

Kirshner, H.S. & Webb, W. (1981). Selective involvement of the auditory-verbal modality in an acquired communication disorder: Benefit from sign language therapy. *Brain and Language, 13*, 161–170.

Kirshner, H.S., Tanridag, O., Thurman, L., & Whetsell, W.O. (1987). Progressive aphasia without dementia: Two cases with focal spongiform degeneration. *Annals of Neurology, 22*, 527–532.

Klein, L.I. (1994). *Functional Communication Profile*. East Moline, IL: LinguiSystems.

Klippi, A. (1996). *Conversation as an Achievement in Aphasics*. Helsinki: Suomalaisen Kirjallisuuden Seura.

Koenig, H.G. (1997). Mood disorders. In P.D. Nussbaum (ed.), *Handbook of Neuropsychology and Aging* (pp. 63–79). New York: Plenum Press.

Kolk, H. & Hofstede, B. (1994). The choice for ellipsis: A case study of stylistic shifts in an agrammatic speaker. *Brain and Language, 47*, 507–509.

Korda, R.J. & Douglas, J.M. (1997). Attention deficits in stroke patients with aphasia. *Journal of Clinical and Experimental Neuropsychology, 19*, 525–542.

Labov, W. (1970). The study of language in its social context. *Studium Generale, 23*, 30–87.

Lahey, M. (1988). *Language Disorders and Language Development*. New York: MacMillan.

LaPointe, L.L. & Horner, J. (1978, Spring). The functional auditory comprehension test (FACT): Protocol and test format. *FLASHA Journal*, 27–33.

LaPointe, L.L. & Horner, J. (1998). *Reading Comprehension Battery for Aphasia* (2nd ed.). Austin, TX: Pro-Ed.

Lasky, E.Z., Weidner, W.E., & Johnson, J.P. (1976). Influence of linguistic complexity, rate of presentation, and interphrase pause time on auditory-verbal comprehension of adult aphasic patients. *Brain and Language, 3*, 386–395.

Lebrun, Y. (1987). Anosognosia in aphasia. *Cortex, 23*, 251–263.

Lecours, A.R., Mehler, J., Parente, M.A., & Beltrami, M.C. (1988). Illiteracy and brain damage: III. A contribution to the study of speech and language disorders in illiterates with unilateral brain damage. *Neuropsychologia, 26*, 575–589.

Lee, L. (1971). *Northwestern Syntax Screening Test*. Evanston, IL: Northwestern University Press.

Lemme, M., Hedberg, N., & Bottenberg, D. (1984). Cohesion in narratives of aphasic adults. *Clinical Aphasiology, 14*, 215–222.

Lesser, R. & Milroy, L. (1993). *Linguistics and Aphasia: Psycholinguistic and Pragmatic Aspects of Intervention*. London: Longman.

Levin, H.S., Grossman, R.G., Sarwar, M., & Meyers, C.A. (1981). Linguistic recovery after closed head injury. *Brain and Language, 12*, 360–374.

Lezak, M.D. (1995). *Neuropsychological Assessment* (3rd ed.). New York: Oxford University Press.

Li, E.C., Ritterman, S., Della Volpe, A., & Williams, S.E. (1996). Variation in grammatic complexity across three types of discourse. *Journal of Speech-Language Pathology and Audiology, 20*, 180–186.

Liles, B.Z. (1985). Narrative ability in normal and language disordered children. *Journal of Speech and Hearing Research, 28*, 123–133.

Liles, B. & Coelho, C.A. (1998). Cohesion analysis. In L.R. Cherney, B. Shadden & C.A. Coelho (eds.). *Analyzing Discourse In Communicatively Impaired Adults* (pp. 65–84). Gaithersburg, MD: Aspen.

Lincoln, N.B. (1982). The Speech Questionnaire: An assessment of functional language ability. *International Rehabilitation Medicine, 4*, 114–117.

Lindsey, J. & Wilkinson, R. (1999). Repair sequences in aphasic talk: A comparison of aphasic-speech and language therapist and aphasic-spouse conversations. *Aphasiology, 13,* 305–326.

Lomas, J., Pickard, L., Bester, S., Elbard, H., Finlayson, A., & Zoghaib, C. (1989). The Communicative Effectiveness Index: Development and psychometric evaluation of functional communication measure for adult aphasia. *Journal of Speech and Hearing Disorders, 54,* 113–124.

Lubinski, R. (1994). Environmental systems approach to adult aphasia. In R. Chapey (ed.), *Language Intervention Strategies in Adult Aphasia* (3rd ed.), (pp. 269–291). Baltimore, MD: Williams & Wilkins.

Lubinski, R. (1995). Environmental considerations for elderly patients. In R. Lubinski (ed.), *Dementia and Communication* (pp. 257–278). San Diego, CA: Singular Publishing.

Lucas, E. (1980). *Semantic and Pragmatic Language Disorders: Assessment and Remediation.* Rockville, MD: Aspen.

Luterman, D.M. (1996). *Counseling Persons with Communication Disorders and Their Families.* Austin, TX: Pro-Ed.

Lyon, J.G. & Helm-Estabrooks, N. (1987). Drawing: Its communicative significance for expressively restricted aphasic adults. *Topics in Language Disorders, 8,* 61–71.

Lyon, J.G. (1998). Treating real-life functionality in a couple coping with severe aphasia. In N. Helm-Estabrooks & A.L. Holland (eds.), *Approaches to the Treatment of Aphasia* (pp. 203–240). San Diego, CA: Singular Publishing.

Manochiopinig, S., Sheard, C., & Reed, V.A. (1992). Pragmatic assessment in adult aphasia: A clinical review. *Aphasiology, 6,* 519–533.

Markwardt, F.C. (1998). *Peabody Individual Achievement Test—Revised.* Circle Pines, MN: American Guidance Service.

Marshall, J., Robson, J., Pring, T., & Chiat, S. (1998). Why does monitoring fail in jargon aphasia?: Comprehension, judgment, and therapy evidence. *Brain and Language, 63,* 79–107.

Martin, A.D. (1977). Aphasia testing: A second look at the Porch Index of Communicative Ability. *Journal of Speech and Hearing Disorders, 42,* 547–561.

Mazaux, J.M. & Orgozo, J.M. (1981). *Boston Diagnostic Aphasia Examination: Échelle Française.* Paris: Éditions Scientifiques et Psychologiques.

McCall, D., Cox, D.M., Shelton, J.R., & Weinrich, M. (1997). The influence of syntactic and semantic information on picture-naming performance in aphasic patients. *Aphasiology, 11,* 581–600.

McCooey, R., Toffolo, D., & Code, C. (In press). A socioenvironmental approach to functional communication in hospital in-patients. In L. Worrall & C.M. Frattali (eds.), *Neurogenic Communication Disorders: A Functional Approach.* New York: Thieme.

McNeil, M.R. & Prescott, T.E. (1978). Revised Token Test. Baltimore, MD: University Park Press.

McNeil, M.R., Prescott, T.E., & Chang, E.C. (1975). A measure of PICA ordinality. *Clinical Aphasiology, 4,* 113–124.

McNeil, M.R., Robin, D.A., & Schmidt, R.A. (1997). Apraxia of speech: Definition, differentiation, and treatment. In M.R. McNeil (ed.), *Clinical Management of Sensorimotor Disorders* (pp. 311–344). New York: Thieme.

Menn, L. & Obler, L.K. (1990). *Agrammatic Aphasia.* Amsterdam: Benjamins.

Menn, L., Ramsberger, G., & Helm-Estabrooks, N. (1994). A linguistic communication measure for aphasic narratives. *Aphasiology, 8,* 343–359.

Messerli, P., Tissot, A., & Rodriguez, R. (1976). Recovery from aphasia: Some factors for prognosis. In Y. Lebrun & R. Hoops (eds.), Recovery in aphasics (pp. 124–135). Amsterdam: Swets and Zeitlinger.

Mesulam, M.M. & Weintraub, S. (1992). Primary progressive aphasia. In F. Boller (ed.), *Heterogeneity of Alzheimer's Disease* (pp. 43–66). Berlin: Springer-Verlag.

Meyers, J.E. & Meyers, K.R. (1995). *Rey Complex Figure Test and Recognition Trial.* Odessa, FL: Psychological Assessment Resources.

Mills, R., Knox, A., Juola, J., & McFarland, W. (1979). Cognitive loci of impairments of picture naming by aphasic subjects. *Journal of Speech and Hearing Research, 22,* 73–87.

Milroy, L. & Perkins, L. (1992). Repair strategies in aphasic discourse: Towards a collaborative model. *Clinical Linguistics and Phonetics, 6,* 27–40.

Mitchum, C.C. (1993). Traditional and contemporary views of aphasia: Implications for clinical management. *Topics in Stroke Rehabilitation, 1,* 14–36.

Mitchum, C.C., Haendiges, A.N., & Berndt, R.S. (1993). Model-guided treatment to improve written sentence production: A case study. *Aphasiology, 7,* 71–109.

Mitchum, C.C., Ritgert, B.A., Sandson, J., & Berndt, R.S. (1990). The use of response analysis in confrontation naming. *Aphasiology, 4,* 261–280.

Mohr, J.P. (1976). Broca's area and Broca's aphasia. In H. Whitaker & H. Whitaker (eds.), *Studies in Neurolinguistics* (Vol. 1) (pp. 201–235). New York: Academic Press.

Molloy, D.W. & Lubinski, R. (1995). Dementia: Impact and clinical perspectives. In R. Lubinski (ed.), *Dementia and Communication* (pp. 2–21). San Diego, CA: Singular Publishing Group.

Muma, J. (1978). *Language Handbook: Concepts, Assessment, Intervention.* Englewood Cliffs, NJ: Prentice-Hall.

Murray, L.L. (1996). Relation between resource allocation and word-finding in aphasia. Paper presented at the annual conference of the American Speech-Language-Hearing Association, Seattle, WA.

Murray, L.L. (1998). Longitudinal treatment of primary progressive aphasia: A case study. *Aphasiology, 12,* 651–672.

Murray, L.L. & Holland, A.L. (1995). The language recovery of acutely aphasic patients receiving different therapy regimens. *Aphasiology, 9,* 397–405.

Murray, L.L., Holland, A.L., & Beeson, P.M. (1997). Auditory processing in individuals with mild aphasia: A study of resource allocation. *Journal of Speech, Language, and Hearing Research, 40,* 792–809.

Murray, L.L., Holland, A.L., & Beeson, P.M. (1998). Spoken language of individuals with mild fluent aphasia under focused and divided attention conditions. *Journal of Speech, Language, and Hearing Research, 41,* 213–227.

Myers, P.S. (1999). *Right Hemisphere Damage: Disorders of Communication and Cognition.* San Diego, CA: Singular Publishing Group.

Naeser, M.A. & Palumbo, C.L. (1994). Neuroimaging and language recovery in stroke. *Journal of Clinical Neurophysiology, 11,* 150–174.

National Head Injury Foundation Task Force (NHIF) on Special Education (1989). *An educators manual: What Educators Need to Know About Students with Traumatic Brain Injury.* Southborough, MA: NHIF.

Neils, J., Baris, J.M., Carter, C., Dellaira, A.L., Nordloh, S., Weiler, E., & Weisiger, B. (1995). Effects of age, education, and living environment on Boston Naming Test performance. *Journal of Speech and Hearing Research, 38,* 1143–1149.

Neils-Strunjas, J. (1998). Clinical assessment strategies: Evaluation of language comprehension and production by formal test batteries. In B. Stemmer & H.A. Whitaker (eds.), *Handbook of Neurolinguistics* (pp. 71–82). New York: Academic Press.

Neisser, U. (1967). *Cognitive Psychology.* New York: Appleton-Century-Crofts.

Nelson, H.E. (1984). *New Adult Reading Test (NART).* Windsor, England: NFER-Nelson.

Newcombe, F., Oldfield, R.C., Ratcliff, G.G., & Wingfield, A. (1971). Recognition and naming of object-drawing by men with focal brain wounds. *Journal of Neurosurgery and Psychiatry, 34,* 329–340.

Newhoff, M., Tonkovich, J.D., Schwartz, S.L., & Burgess, E.K. (1985). Revision strategies in aphasia. *Journal of Neurological Communication Disorders, 2,* 2–7.

Nicholas, L.E. & Brookshire, R.H. (1986). Consistency of the effects of rate of speech on brain-damaged adult's comprehension of narrative discourse. *Journal of Speech and Hearing Research, 29,* 462–470.

Nicholas, L.E. & Brookshire, R.H. (1987). Error analysis and passage dependency of test items from a standardized test of multiple-sentence reading comprehension for aphasic and non-brain-damaged adults. *Journal of Speech and Hearing Disorders, 52,* 358–366.

Nicholas, L.D. & Brookshire, R.H. (1992). A system for scoring main concepts in the discourse of non-brain-damaged and aphasic speakers. *Clinical Aphasiology, 21,* 87–99.

Nicholas, L.D. & Brookshire, R.H. (1993). A system for quantifying the informativeness and efficiency of the connected speech of adults with aphasia. *Journal of Speech and Hearing Research, 36,* 338–350.

Nicholas, L.E. & Brookshire, R.H. (1995a). Comprehension of spoken narrative discourse by adults with aphasia, right-hemisphere brain damage, or traumatic brain injury. *American Journal of Speech-Language Pathology, 4,* 69–81.

Nicholas, L.E. & Brookshire, R.H. (1995b). Presence, completeness, and accuracy of main concepts in the connected speech of non-brain-damaged adults and adults with aphasia. *Journal of Speech and Hearing Research, 38,* 145–156.

Nicholas, L.E., MacLennan, D.L., & Brookshire, R.H. (1986). Validity of multiple-sentence reading comprehension tests for aphasic adults. *Journal of Speech and Hearing Disorders, 51,* 82–87.

Nicholas, M., Obler, L.K., Albert, M.L., & Helm-Estabrooks, N. (1985). Empty speech in Alzheimer's disease and fluent aphasia. *Journal of Speech and Hearing Research, 28,* 405–410.

Nickels, L.A. (1995). Getting it right? Using aphasic naming errors to evaluate theoretical models of spoken word production. *Language and Cognitive Processes, 10,* 13–45.

Nickels, L.A. & Howard, D. (1995). Aphasic naming: What matters? *Neuropsychologia, 33,* 1281–1303.

Obler, L.K. & Albert, M.L. (1979). *The Action Naming Test.* Boston, MA: VA Medical Center.

Odell, K.H. & Flynn, M. (1998). Treatment outcomes in individuals with right hemisphere-brain damage. Presented at the annual conference of the American Speech-Language Hearing Association, San Antonio, TX.

Odell, K.H., Bair, S., Flynn, M., Workinger, M., Osborne, D., & Chial, M. (1997). Retrospective study of treatment outcome for individuals with aphasia. *Aphasiology, 45,* 415–432.

Ogrezeanu, V., Voinescu, I., Mihailescu, L., & Jipescu, I. (1994). "Spontaneous" recovery in aphasics after single ischaemic stroke. *Romanian Journal of Neurology and Psychiatry, 32,* 77–90.

O'Sullivan, T. & Fagan, S.C. (1998). Drug-induced communication and swallowing disorders. In A.F. Johnson & B.H. Jacobson (eds.), *Medical Speech-Language Pathology: A Practitioner's Guide* (pp. 176–191). New York: Thieme.

Ottenbacher, K.J., Hsu, Y., Granger, C.V., & Fiedler, R.C. (1996). The reliability of the Functional Independence Measure: A quantitative review. *Archives of Physical Medicine and Rehabilitation, 77,* 1226–1232.

Owens, R.E. (1984). *Language Development: An Introduction.* Toronto: Charles E. Merrill.

Paolucci, S., Antonucci, G., Pratesi, L., Traballesi, M., Lubich, S., & Grasso, M.G. (1998). Functional outcome in stroke inpatient rehabilitation: Predicting no, low, and high response patients. *Cerebrovascular Diseases, 8,* 228–234.

Paradis, M. & Libben, G. (1987). *The Assessment of Bilingual Aphasia.* Hillsdale, NJ: Erlbaum.

Paradis, M. & Libben, G. (1993). *Evaluacion de la Afasia en los Bilingues.* Barcelona, Spain: Masson.

Parkerson, G.R., Gehlbach, S.H., & Wagner, E.H. (1981). The Duke-UNC Health Profile: An adult health status measure. *Medical Care, 19,* 787–805.

Patterson, K., Coltheart, M., & Marshall, J.C. (1985). *Surface Dyslexia.* London, England: Erlbaum.

Patterson, R. & Wells, A. (1995). Involving the family in planning for life with aphasia. *Topics in Stroke Rehabilitation, 2,* 39–46.

Payne, J.C. (1994). *Communication Profile: A Functional Skills Survey.* San Antonio, TX: Communication Skill Builders.

Payne, J.C. (1997). *Adult Neurogenic Language Disorders: Assessment and Treatment. A Comprehensive Ethnobiological Approach.* San Diego, CA: Singular Publishing.

Payne-Johnson, J.C. (1992). An ethnocentric perspective on African American elderly persons and functional communication assessment. *The Howard Journal of Communication, 3,* 194–203.

Pedersen, P.M., Jorgensen, H.S., Nakayama, H., Raaschou, H.O., & Olsen, T.S. (1995). Aphasia in acute stroke: Incidence, determinants, and recovery. *Annals of Neurology, 38,* 659–666.

Pedersen, P.M., Jorgensen, H.S., Nakayama, H., Raaschou, H.O., & Olsen, T.S. (1997). Hemineglect in acute stroke: Incidence and prognostic implications. *American Journal of Physical Medicine and Rehabilitation, 76,* 122–127.

Penn, C. (1983). Syntactic and pragmatic aspects of aphasic language. Unpublished Ph.D. Dissertation, University of the Witwatersrand, South Africa.

Penn, C. (1988). The profiling of syntax and pragmatics in aphasia. *Clinical Linguistics and Phonetics, 2,* 179–207.

Peterson, L.N. & Kirshner, H.S. (1981). Gestural impairment and gestural ability in aphasia: A review. *Brain and Language, 14,* 333–348.

Ponsford, J. & Kinsella, G. (1991). The use of a rating scale of attentional behavior. *Neuropsychological Rehabilitation, 1,* 241–257.

Porch, B.E. (1967). *Porch Index of Communicative Ability. (Vol. 1) Theory and Development.* Palo Alto, CA: Consulting Psychologists Press.

Porch, B. (1971). Multi-dimensional scoring in aphasia testing. *Journal of Speech and Hearing Research, 14,* 776–792.

Porch, B.E. (1981). *Porch Index of Communicative Ability. (Vol. 2) Administration, Scoring, and Interpretation* (3rd ed.). Palo Alto, CA: Consulting Psychologists Press.

Porteus, S.D. (1959). *Porteus Maze Test and Clinical Psychology.* Palo Alto, CA: Pacific Books.

Powell, G.E., Bailey, S., & Clark, E. (1980). A very short form of the Minnesota Aphasia Test. *British Journal of Social and Clinical Psychology, 19,* 189–194.

Prinz, P. (1980). A note on requesting strategies in adult aphasics. *Journal of Communication Disorders, 13,* 65–73.

Prutting, C. (1979). Process/pra/ses/n: The action of moving forward progressively from one point to another on the way to completion. *Journal of Speech and Hearing Research, 14,* 776–792.

Prutting, C.A. & Kirchner, D. (1983). Applied pragmatics. In T.M. Gallagher & C.A. Prutting (eds.), *Pragmatic Assessment and Intervention Issues in Language* (pp. 29–64). San Diego, CA: College-Hill Press.

Prutting, C.A. & Kirchner, D. (1987). A clinical appraisal of the pragmatic aspects of language. *Journal of Speech and Hearing Disorders, 52,* 105–199.

Purdue Research Foundation (1948). *Examiners Manual for the Purdue Pegboard.* Chicago: Science Research Associates.

Puskaric, N.J. & Pierce, R.S. (1997). Effects of constraint and expectation on reading comprehension in aphasia. *Aphasiology, 11,* 249–261.

Rapcsak, S.Z. & Rubens, A.B. (1994). Localization of Lesions in Transcortical Aphasia. In A. Kertesz (ed.), *Localization and Neuroimaging in Neuropsychology* (pp. 297–329). San Diego, CA: Academic Press.

Raven, J.C., Court, J.H., & Raven, J. (1984). *Coloured Progressive Matrices.* London: H.K. Lewis.

Records, N.L. (1994). A measure of the contribution of a gesture to the perception of speech in listeners with aphasia. *Journal of Speech and Hearing Research, 37,* 1086–1099.

Reitan, R.M. (1991). *Aphasia Screening Test* (2nd ed.). Tucson, AZ: Reitan Neuropsychology Laboratory.

Research Foundation, SUNY. (1990). *Guide for Use of the Uniform Data Set for Medical Rehabilitation.* Buffalo, NY: Research Foundation, State University of New York.

Rey, G.J. & Benton, A.L. (1991). *Examen de Afasia Multilingue: Manual de Instrucciones.* Iowa City, IA: AJA Associates.

Ripich, D.N (1995). Differential diagnosis and assessment. In R. Lubinski (ed.), *Dementia and Communication* (pp. 188–222). San Diego, CA: Singular Publishing Group.

Robertson, I.H., Ward, T., Ridgeway, V., & Nimmo-Smith, I. (1994). *The Test of Everyday Attention.* Gaylord, MI: Northern Speech Services.

Robinson, K.M. & Grossman, M. (1997). Hypothesis-driven treatment of naming deficits. *Topics in Stroke Rehabilitation, 4,* 1–14.

Robinson, R.G. & Benson, D.F. (1981). Depression in aphasic patients: Frequency, severity and clinicopathological correlations. *Brain and Language, 14,* 282–291.

Robinson, R.G., Bolla-Wilson, K., Kaplan, E., Lipsey, J.R., & Price, T.R. (1986). Depression influences intellectual impairment in stroke patients. *Journal of Psychiatry, 148,* 541–547.

Rochon, E., Saffran, E., Berndt, R., & Schwartz, M. (1998). Quantitative production analysis: Norming and reliability data. *Brain and Language, 65,* 10–13.

Rogers, M.A. & Alarcon, N.B. (1997). Assessment and management of primary progressive aphasia: A longitudinal case study over a five year period. Presentation at the Clinical Aphasiology Conference, Big Fork, Montana.

Rosenbek, J., LaPointe, L., & Wertz, R. (1989). *Aphasia: A Clinical Approach.* Austin, TX: Pro-Ed.

Rosenfeld, N.M. (1978). Conversational control function of nonverbal behavior. In A.W. Siegman & S. Feldstein (eds.), *Nonverbal Behavior and Communication.* Hillsdale, NJ: Lawrence Erlbaum.

Ross, K.B. & Wertz, R.T. (1999). Comparison of impairment and disability measures for assessing severity of, and improvement in, aphasia. *Aphasiology, 13,* 113–124.

Ross-Swain, D. (1996). *Ross Information Processing Assessment* (2nd ed.). Austin, TX: Pro-Ed.

Rothi, L.J.G., Mack, L., Verfaellie, M., Brown, P., & Heilman, K.M. (1988). Ideomotor apraxia: Error pattern analysis. *Aphasiology, 2,* 381–387.

Rothi, L.J.G., Raymer, A.M., Maher, L., Greenwald, M., & Morris, M. (1991). Assessment of naming failures in neurological communication disorders. *Clinics in Communication Disorders, 1,* 7–20.

Rothi, L.J.G., Raymer, A.M., & Heilman, K.M. (1997). Limb praxis assessment. In L.J.G. Rothi & K.M. Heilman (eds.), *Apraxia: The Neuropsychology of Action* (pp. 61–73). East Sussex, UK: Psychology Press.

Ryalls, J. & Behrens, S. (1988). An overview of changes in fundamental frequency associated with cortical insult. *Aphasiology, 2,* 107–115.

Ryff, C. & Singer, B. (1998). The contours of postive human health. *Psychological Inquiry, 9(1),* 1–29.

Saffran, E.M., Berndt, R.S., & Schwartz, M.F. (1989). The quantitative analysis of agrammatic production: Procedure and data. *Brain and Language, 37,* 440–479.

Saffran, E.M. & Schwartz, M.F. (1994). Of cabbages and things: Semantic memory from a neuropsychological perspective—A tutorial. In C. Umilta & M. Moscovitch (eds.), *Attention and Performance XV* (pp. 507–536). Cambridge, MA: MIT Press.

Sall, M. & Wepman, J.M. (1945). A screening survey of organic impairment. *Journal of Speech and Hearing Disorders, 10,* 283–286.

Sambunaris, A. & Hyde, T.M. (1994). Stroke-related aphasias mistaken for psychotic speech: Two case reports. *Journal of Geriatric Psychiatry and Neurology, 7,* 144–147.

Sands, E. (1977). Early initiation of speech and language therapy and degree of language recovery in adult aphasics. (Doctoral Dissertation, New York University), *Dissertation Abstracts International, 38,* 5871.

Sands, E., Sarno, M., & Shankwilder, D. (1969). Long term assessment of language function in aphasia due to stroke. *Archives of Physical Medical Rehabilitation, 50,* 202–207.

Sapir, S. & Aronson, A.E. (1990). The relationship between psychopathology and speech and language disorders in neurologic patients. *Journal of Speech and Hearing Disorders, 55,* 503–509.

Sarno, M. (1969). *The Functional Communication Profile: Manual of Directions.* New York: Institute of Rehabilitation Medicine.

Sarno, M.T., Silverman, M., & Sands, E. (1970). Speech therapy and language recovery in severe aphasia. *Journal of Speech and Hearing Research, 13,* 607–623.

Schegloff, E., Jefferson, G., & Sacks, H. (1977). The preference for self-correction in the organization of repair in conversation. *Language, 53,* 361–382.

Schienberg, S. & Holland, A.L. (1980). Conversational turn-taking in Wernicke's aphasia. *Clinical Aphasiology, 10,* 106–110.

Schuell, H. (1965a). *Differential Diagnosis of Aphasia with the Minnesota Test.* Minneapolis, MN: University of Minnesota Press.

Schuell, H. (1965b). *The Minnesota Test for Differential Diagnosis of Aphasia.* Minneapolis, MN: University of Minnesota Press.

Schuell, H., Carroll, V., & Street, B. (1955). Clinical treatment of aphasia. *Journal of Speech and Hearing Disorders, 20,* 43–53.

Schuell, H., Jenkins, J., & Jiminez-Paron, E. (1964). *Aphasia in Adults.* New York: Harper and Row.

Schuell, H., Jenkins, J., & Landis, L. (1961). Relationship between auditory comprehension and word frequency in aphasia. *Journal of Speech and Hearing Research, 4,* 30–36.

Schut, L.J. (1988). Dementia following stroke. *Clinical Geriatric Medicine, 4,* 767–784.

Schwanenflugel, P. & Shoben, E. (1985). The influence of sentence constraint on the scope of facilitation for upcoming words. *Journal of Memory and Language, 24,* 232–252.

Schwartz, M., Saffran, E., & Marin, O. (1980). The word order problem in agrammatism I: Comprehension. *Brain and Language, 10,* 249–262.

Schwartz-Cowley, R. & Stepanik, M.J. (1989). Communication disorders and treatment in the acute trauma center setting. *Topics in Language Disorders, 9,* 1–14.

Searle, J. (1969). *Speech Acts.* London: Cambridge University Press.

Seron, X., Van Der Kaa, M.A., Remitz, A., & Van Der Linden, M. (1979). Pantomime interpretation and aphasia. *Neuropsychologia, 17,* 661–668.

Shadden, B. (1998b). Obtaining the discourse sample. In L.R. Cherney, B. Shadden, & C.A. Coelho (eds.). *Analyzing Discourse in Communicatively Impaired Adults* (pp. 9–34). Gaithersburg, MD: Aspen.

Shadden, B. (1998a). Information analysis. In L.R. Cherney, B. Shadden, & C.A. Coelho (eds.). *Analyzing Discourse in Communicatively Impaired Adults* (pp. 85–114). Gaithersburg, MD: Aspen.

Shadden, B.B., Burnette, R.B., Eikenberry, B.R., & DiBrezzo, R. (1991). All discourse tasks are not created equal. *Clinical Aphasiology, 20,* 327–342.

Shewan, C.M. (1979). *Auditory Comprehension Test for Sentences.* Chicago: Biolinguistics Clinical Institutes.

Shewan, C.M. (1988a). Expressive language recovery in aphasia using the Shewan Spontaneous Language Analysis (SSLA) system. *Journal of Communication Disorders, 21,* 155–169.

Shewan, C.M. (1988b). The Shewan spontaneous language analysis (SSLA) system for aphasic adults: Description, reliability, and validity. *Journal of Communication Disorders, 21,* 103–138.

Shewan, C.M. & Canter, G. (1971). Effects of vocabulary, syntax and sentence length on auditory comprehension in aphasic patients. *Cortex, 7,* 209–226.

Shewan, C.M. & Kertesz, A. (1980). Reliability and validity characteristics of the Western Aphasia Battery (WAB). *Journal of Speech and Hearing Disorders, 45,* 308–324.

Shewan, C.M. & Kertesz, A. (1984). Effects of speech and language treatment on recovery from aphasia. *Brain and Language, 23,* 272–299.

Shipley, K.G. & McAfee, J.G. (1998). *Assessment in Speech-Language Pathology: A Resource Manual.* San Diego, CA: Singular Publishing.

Siegel, G. (1959). Dysphasic speech responses to visual word stimuli. *Journal of Speech and Hearing Research, 2,* 152–160.

Simmons-Mackie, N.N. & Damico, J.S. (1996). Accounting for handicaps in aphasia: Communicative assessment from an authentic social perspective. *Disability and Rehabilitation, 18,* 540–549.

Sinyor, D., Amato, P., Kaloupek, D.G., Becker, R., Goldenberg, M., & Coopersmith, H. (1986). Post-stroke depression: Relationship to functional impairment, coping strategies, and rehabilitation outcome. *Stroke, 17,* 1102–1107.

Sivan, A.B. (1992). *Benton Visual Retention Test.* San Antonio, TX: The Psychological Corporation.

Skelly, M. (1979). *AmerInd Gestural Code Based on Universal American Indian Hand Talk.* New York: Elsevier.

Sklar, M. (1983). *Sklar Aphasia Scale.* Los Angeles, CA: Western Psychological Services.

Smith, A. (1971). Objective indices of severity of chronic aphasia in stroke patients. *Journal of Speech and Hearing Disorders, 36,* 167–207.

Smollan, T. & Penn, C. (1997). The measurement of emotional reaction and depression in a South African stroke population. *Disability and Rehabilitation, 19,* 56–63.

Snyder, L.S. (1983). From assessment to intervention: Problems and solutions. In J. Miller, D. Yoder, & R. Schiefelbush (eds.), *Contemporary Issues in Language Intervention.* Rockville, MD: American Speech-Language-Hearing Association.

Sohlberg, M.M. (1992). *The Profile of Executive Control System.* Gaylord, MI: Northern Rehabilitation Services.

Spencer, K.A., Tompkins, C.A., & Schulz, R. (1997). Assessment of depression in patients with brain pathology: The case of stroke. *Psychological Bulletin, 122,* 132–152.

Spreen, O. & Benton, A.L. (1977). *Neurosensory Center Comprehensive Examination for Aphasia (Rev. e.).* Victoria, BC: University of Victoria, Neuropsychology Laboratory.

Spreen, O. & Strauss, E. (1991). *A Compendium of Neuropsychological Tests.* New York: Oxford University Press.

Spreen, O. & Risser, A.H. (1998). Assessment of aphasia. In M.T. Sarno (ed.), *Acquired Aphasia* (3rd ed.), (pp. 71–156). New York: Academic Press.

Square-Storer, P. & Roy, E.A. (1989). The apraxias: Commonalities and distinctions. In P. Squarer-Storer (ed.). *Acquired Apraxia of Speech in Aphasic Adults.* Hillsdale, NJ: Lawrence Erlbaum.

Squire, L.R. (1987). *Memory and Brain.* New York: Oxford University Press.

Stachowiak, F.J., Huber, W., Poeck, K., & Kerschensteiner, M. (1977). Text comprehension in aphasia. *Brain and Language, 4,* 177–195.

Starkstein, S.E. & Robinson, R.G. (1988). Aphasia and depression. *Aphasiology, 2,* 1–20.

State University of New York at Buffalo (1993). *Guide for the Uniform Data Set for Medical Rehabilitation (Adult FIM) Version 4.0.* Buffalo, NY: Author.

Stern, R.A. (1998). *Visual Analog Mood Scales.* Odessa, FL: Psychological Assessment Resources.

Stoicheff, M.L. (1960). Motivating instructions and language performance of dysphasic subjects. *Journal of Speech and Hearing Research, 3,* 75–85.

Stone, S.P., Halligan, P.W., & Greenwood, R.J. (1993). The incidence of neglect phenomena and related disorders in patients with an acute right or left hemisphere stroke. *Age and Ageing, 22,* 46–52.

Stringer, A.Y. (1996). *A Guide to Adult Neuropsychological Diagnosis.* Philadelphia, PA: F.A. Davis Company.

Swindell, C.S. & Hammons, J. (1991). Post-stroke depression: Neurologic, physiologic, diagnostic, and treatment implications. *Journal of Speech and Hearing Research, 34,* 325–333.

Swindell, C.S., Pashek, G.V., & Holland, A.L. (1982). A questionnaire for surveying personal and communicative style. *Clinical Aphasiology, 12,* 50–63.

Syder, D., Body, R., Parker, M., & Boddy, M. (1993). *Sheffield Screening Test for Acquired Language Disorders.* Manual: NferNelson.

Tanner, D.C. & Culbertson, W. (1999). *Caregiver-Administered Communication Inventory.* Oceanside, CA: Academic Communication Associates.

Tanner, D.C. & Culbertson, W. (1999). *Quick Assessment for Aphasia.* Oceanside, CA: Academic Communication Associates.

Tatemichi, T.K., Desmond, D.W., Stern, Y., Paik, M., Sano, M., & Bagiella, E. (1994). Cognitive impairment after stroke: Frequency, patterns, and relationship to functional abilities. *Journal of Neurology, Neurosurgery, and Psychiatry, 57,* 202–207.

Teresi, J.A. & Holmes, D. (1997). Methodological issues in cognitive assessment and their impact on outcome measurement. *Alzheimer Disease and Associated Disorders, 11* (Suppl. 6), 146–155.

Thompson, C.K., Shapiro, L.P., Tait, M.E., Jacobs, B.J., Schneider, S.L., & Ballard, K.J. (1995). A system for the linguistic analysis of agrammatic language production. *Brain and Language, 51,* 124–129.

Thurstone, L.L. & Thurstone, T.G. (1962). *Primary Mental Abilities (Rev.).* Chicago: Science Research Associates.

Tombaugh, T.N. & Hubley, A.M. (1997). The 60-item Boston Naming Test: Norms for cognitively intact adults aged 25 to 88 years. *Journal of Clinical and Experimental Neuropsychology, 19,* 922–932.

Tompkins, C.A. (1995). *Right Hemisphere Communication Disorders: Theory and Management.* San Diego, CA: Singular Publishing Group.

Tompkins, C.A., Bloise, C.G.R., Timko, M.L., & Baumgaertner, A. (1994). Working memory and inference revision in brain-damaged and normally aging adults. *Journal of Speech and Hearing Research, 37,* 896–912.

Tompkins, C.A. & Flowers, C. (1985). Perception of emotional intonation by brain-damaged adults: The influence of task processing levels. *Journal of Speech and Hearing Research, 28,* 527–538.

Tompkins, C.A., Jackson, S., & Shulz, R. (1990). On prognostic research in adult neurologic disorders. *Journal of Speech and Hearing Research, 33,* 398–401.

Tompkins, C.A., Rau, M., Schulz, R., & Rhyne, C. (1987). Post-stroke depression in primary support persons: Predicting those at risk. *ASHA, 29,* 79.

Toppin, C.J. & Brookshire, R.H. (1978). Effects of response delay and token relocation on Token Test performance of aphasic subjects. *Journal of Communication Disorders, 2,* 57–68.

Torrance, E.P. (1966). *Torrance Test of Creative Thinking.* Princeton, NJ: Personnel Press.

Tough, J. (1977). *The Development of Meaning: A Study of Children's Use of Language.* New York: Halstead Press.

Trahan, D.E. & Larrabee, G.J. (1988). *Continuous Visual Memory Test.* Odessa, FL: Psychological Assessment Resources.

Treisman, A. (1965). Effect of verbal context on latency of word selection. *Nature, 206,* 218–219.

Trupe, E.H. (1984). Reliability of rating spontaneous speech in the Western Aphasia Battery: Implications for classification. *Clinical Aphasiology, 14,* 55–69.

Trupe, E.H. (1986). Training severely aphasic patients to communicate by drawing. Paper presented at the annual convention of the American Speech-Language-Hearing Association, Detroit, MI.

Tseng, C.H., McNeil, M.R., & Milenkovic, P. (1993). An investigation of attention allocation deficits in aphasia. *Brain and Language, 45,* 276–296.

Tyler, L.K. & Cobb, H. (1987). Processing bound grammatical morphemes in context: The case of an aphasic patient. *Language and Cognitive Processes, 2,* 245–262.

Ulatowska, H.K., Allard, L., Reyes, B.A., Ford, J., & Chapman, S. (1992). Conversational discourse in aphasia. *Aphasiology, 6,* 325–331.

Ulatowska, H.K., Doyel, A.W., Freedman-Stern, R.F., Macaluso-Hayes, S., & North, A.J. (1983a). Production of procedural discourse in aphasia. *Brain and Language, 18,* 315–341.

Ulatowska, H.K., Freedman-Stern, R.F., Doyel, A.W., Macaluso-Hayes, S., & North, A.J. (1983b). Production of narrative discourse in aphasia. *Brain and Language, 19,* 317–334.

Uryase, D., Duffy, R.J., & Liles, B.Z. (1991). Analysis and description of narrative discourse in right-hemisphere-damaged adults: A comparison with neurologically normal and left-hemisphere-damaged aphasic adults. *Clinical Aphasiology, 19,* 125–137.

Van Harskamp, F. & Visch-Brink, E. (1991). Goal recognition in aphasia therapy. *Aphasiology, 5,* 529–539.

Van Zomeren, A.H. & Brouwer, W.H. (1994). *Clinical Neuropsychology of Attention.* NY/London: Oxford University Press.

Varley, R. (1995). Lexical-semantic deficits following right hemisphere damage: Evidence from verbal fluency tasks. *European Journal of Disorders of Communication, 30*, 362–371.

Varney, N.R. (1982). Pantomime recognition defect in aphasia: Implications for the concept of asymbolia. *Brain and Language, 15*, 32–39.

Varney, N.R. (1998). Neuropsychological assessment of aphasia. In G. Goldstein, P.D. Nussbaum, & S.R. Beers (eds.), *Neuropsychology* (pp. 357–378). New York: Plenum Press.

Vilkki, J. (1988). Problem solving deficits after focal cerebral lesions. *Cortex, 24*, 119–127.

Vogel, D. & Carter, J.E. (1995). *The Effects of Drugs on Communication Disorders*. San Diego, CA: Singular Publishing.

Wallace, G. & Hammill, D.D. (1997). *Comprehensive Receptive and Expressive Vocabulary Test: Adult*. Austin, TX: Pro-Ed.

Wang, L. & Goodglass, H. (1992). Pantomime, praxis, and aphasia. *Brain and Language, 42*, 402–418.

Warden, M.R. & Hutchinson, T.J. (1993). *The Writing Process Test*. Chicago: Riverside.

Ward-Lonergan, J. & Nicholas, M. (1995). Drawing to communicate: A case report of an adult with global aphasia. *European Journal of Disorders of Communication, 30*, 475–491.

Warren, R.G. (1999). Creating value with measurement: Moving toward the patient. *Topics in Stroke Rehabilitation, 5*, 17–37.

Warren, R.L. & Datta, K.D. (1981). The return of speech four and one-half years post head injury. *Clinical Aphasiology, 11*, 301–308.

Webb, W.G. (1995). Language batteries in aphasia. In H.S. Kirshner (ed.), *Handbook of Neurological Speech and Language Disorders* (pp. 431–444). New York: Marcel Dekker.

Webb, W.G. & Love, R.J. (1983). Reading problems in chronic aphasia. *Journal of Speech and Hearing Disorders, 48*, 164–171.

Webster's New Collegiate Dictionary (1977). Springfield, MA: Mirriam-Webster.

Webster-Ross, G., Cummings, J.L., & Benson, D.F. (1990). Speech and language alterations in dementia syndromes: Characteristics and treatment. *Aphasiology, 4*, 339–352.

Weidner, W.E. & Lasky, E.Z. (1976). The interaction of rate and complexity of stimulus on the performance of adult aphasic subjects. *Brain and Language, 3*, 34–40.

Wechsler, D. (1997a). *Wechsler Adult Intelligence Scale* (3rd ed.). San Antonio, TX: The Psychological Corporation.

Wechsler, D. (1997b). *Wechsler Memory Scale* (3rd ed.). San Antonio, TX: The Psychological Corporation.

Ween, J.E., Verfaellie, M., & Alexander, M.P. (1996). Verbal memory function in mild aphasia. *Neurology, 47*, 795–801.

Weiner, M., Bennett, J.A., & Shilkret, R. (1984). Writing and writing difficulties from one perspective. Unpublished manuscript, Clark University, Worcester, MA.

Weintraub, S., Rubin, N.P., & Mesulam, M.M. (1990). Primary progressive aphasia: Longitudinal course, neuropsychological profile, and language features. *Archives of Neurology, 47*, 1329–1335.

Welch, L.W., Doineau, D., Johnson, S., & King, D. (1996). Educational and gender normative data for the Boston Naming Test in a group of older adults. *Brain and Language, 53*, 260–266.

Weniger, D. (1990). Diagnostic tests as tools of assessment and models of information processing: A gap to bridge. *Aphasiology, 4*, 109–113.

Wepman, J. (1958). The relationship between self-correction and recovery from aphasia. *Journal of Speech and Hearing Disorders, 23*, 302–305.

Wertz, R.T., Collins, M.J., Weiss, D., Kurtzke, J.F., Friden, T., Brookshire, R.H., Pierce, J., Holtzapple, P., Hubbard, D.J., Porch, B.E., West, H.A., Davis, L., Matovitch, V., Morley, G.K., & Resurreccion, E. (1981). Veteran's Administration cooperative study on aphasia: A comparison of individual and group treatment. *Journal of Speech and Hearing Research, 24*, 580–594.

Wertz, R.T., Deal, J.L., & Robinson, A.J. (1984). Classifying the aphasias: A comparison of the Boston Diagnostic Aphasia Examination and the Western Aphasia Battery. *Clinical Aphasiology, 14*, 40–47.

Wertz, R.T., Weiss, D., Aten, J., Brookshire, R.H., Garcia-Bunuel, L., Holland, A.L., Kurtzke, J.F., LaPointe, L.L., Milianti, F.J., Brannegan, R., Greenbaum, H., Marshall, R.C., Vogel, D., Carter, J., Barnes, N., & Goodman, R. (1987). A comparison of clinic, home and deferred language treatment for aphasia: A VA cooperative study. *Archives of Neurology, 43*, 653–658.

Westbury, C. & Bub, D. (1997). Primary progressive aphasia: A review of 112 cases. *Brain and Language, 60*, 381–406.

Whiteneck, G.G. (1994). Measuring what matters: Key rehabilitation outcomes. *Archives of Physical Medicine and Rehabilitation, 75*, 1073–1076.

Whurr, R. (1996). *The Aphasia Screening Test* (2nd ed.). San Diego, CA: Singular Publishing Group.

Wickens, C.D. (1989). Attention and skilled performance. In D. Holding (ed.), *Human Skills* (pp. 72–105). New York: John Wiley & Sons.

Wiederholt, J.L. & Bryant, B.R. (1992). *Gray Oral Reading Tests* (3rd ed.). Austin, TX: Pro-Ed.

Wiig, E.H. & Semel, E. (1984). *Language Assessment and Intervention for the Learning Disabled* (2nd ed.). Toronto: Charles E. Merrill.

Wilcox, M.J. & Davis, G.A. (1977). Speech act analysis of aphasic communication in individual and group settings. *Clinical Aphasiology, 7*, 166–174.

Wilcox, M.J., Davis, G.A., & Leonard, L.L. (1978). Aphasic's comprehension of contextually conveyed meaning. *Brain and Language, 6*, 362–377.

Wilkinson, G.S. (1993). *Wide Range Achievement Test* (3rd ed.). Wilmington, DE: Wide Range.

Williams, M. (1994). *Criterion-Oriented Test of Attention*. Woodsboro, MD: Cool Spring Software.

Williams, M. (1994). *Williams Inhibition Test*. Woodsboro, MD: Cool Spring Software.

Williams, M. (1996). *The Naming Test*. Woodsboro, MD: Cool Spring Software.

Williams, S.E. & Canter, G.J. (1987). Action naming performance in four syndromes of aphasia. *Brain and Language, 32*, 124–136.

Wilson, B.A., Alderman, N., Burgess, P., Emslie, H., & Evans, J.J. (1996). *Behavioral Assessment of the Dysexecutive Syndrome*. Gaylord, MI: Northern Rehabilitation Services.

Wilson, B.A., Cockburn, J., & Baddeley, A. (1985). The Rivermead Behavioral Memory Test. Gaylord, MI: Northern Rehabilitation Services.

Wilson, B.A., Cockburn, J., & Halligan, P. (1987). *The Behavioral Inattention Test*. Gaylord, MI: Northern Rehabilitation Services.

Wilson, B.A. & Wearing, D. (1995). Prisoner of consciousness: A state of just awakening following herpes simplex encephalitis. In R. Campbell, & M.A. Conway (eds.), *Broken Memories: Case Studies of Memory Impairment* (pp. 14–30). Cambridge, MA: Blackwell Publishers.

Wilson, R.H., Fowler, C.G., & Shanks, J.E. (1981). Audiological assessment of the aphasic patients. *Seminars in Speech, Language, and Hearing, 2,* 299–314.

Wilson, R.S., Rosenbaum, G., & Brown, B. (1979). The problem of premorbid intelligence in neuropsychological assessment. *Journal of Clinical Neuropsychology, 1,* 49–53.

Wirz, S.L., Skinner, C., & Dean, E. (1990). *Revised Edinburgh Functional Communication Profile.* Tucson, AZ: Communication Skill Builders.

World Health Organization (1980). *International Classification of Impairments, Disabilities and Handicaps: A Manual for Classification Relating to the Consequences of Disease.* Geneva, Switzerland: WHO.

World Health Organization (1998). *Towards a Common Language for Functioning and Disablement: ICIDH-2 the International Classification of Impairments, Activities, and Participation.* Geneva, Switzerland: WHO.

Worrall, L. (1992). *Everyday Communicative Needs Assessment.* Available from the Department of Speech and Hearing, The University of Queensland: Queensland 4072, Australia.

Worrall, L. (1995). The functional communication perspective. In C. Code & D.J. Muller (eds.), *The Treatment of Aphasia: From Theory to Practice* (pp. 47–69). San Diego, CA: Singular Publishing.

Ylvisaker, M. & Feeney, T.J. (1998). *Collaborative Brain Injury Intervention: Positive Everyday Routines.* San Diego, CA: Singular.

Yorkston, K. & Beukelman, D. (1980). An analysis of connected speech samples of aphasic and normal speakers. *Journal of Speech and Hearing Disorders, 45,* 27–36.

Yorkston, K.M., Beukelman, D.R., & Traynor, C. (1984). *Assessment of Intelligibility of Dysarthric Speech.* Austin, TX: Pro-Ed.

Yorkston, K.M., Beukelman, D.R., Strand, E.A., & Bell, K.R. (1999). *Management of Motor Speech Disorders in Children and Adults.* Austin, TX: Pro-Ed.

Zachman, L., Huisingh, R., Barrett, M., Orman, J., & Blagden, C. (1989). *The WORD Test Adolescent.* East Moline, IL: LinguiSystems.

Zachman, L., Jorgensen, C., Huisingh, R. & Barrett, M. (1983). *Test of Problem Solving.* Moline, Ill: LinguiSystems.

Zemva, N. (1999). Aphasic patients and their families: Wishes and limits. *Aphasiology, 13,* 219–224.

Zingeser, L.B. & Berndt, R.S. (1988). Grammatical class and context effects in a case of pure anomia: Implications for models of language production. *Cognitive Neuropsychology, 5,* 473–516.

APPENDIX 4-1
Preinterview or Referral Form for Collecting Family and Medical History and Status Information

Name _____ Birthplace _____

Address _____ Birthdate _____

Phone Number _____ Date of Report _____

Dear Respondent: The following questions are asked to help us understand the above person, and plan assessment and treatment activities. Please answer them as fully as possible. If you need more space, use the back of the sheet. Thank you in advance for your time and assistance.

1. What do you feel is the patient's problem? _____

_____

2. What caused the aphasia (head injury, stroke, illness)? _____

_____

3. What was the date of injury or of the onset of the illness (head injury, stroke, illness)? _____

_____

4. Who is the patient's physician? _____

   What is the physician's address? _____

   What is the physician's phone number? (_____) _____

5. What was the patient's handedness (before stroke or disease onset)? Right _____ Left _____ Ambidextrous _____

6. Does the patient wear glasses? _____

   Can the patient see well enough to read? _____

   Does the patient have any other visual problems, such as right or left visual field cut or cataracts? _____

7. Does the patient have a hearing loss? _____

   Does the patient wear a hearing aid? _____. If yes, in the right ear _____, left ear _____, or both _____?

8. How would you describe the patient's general health? _____

   _____

   _____

9. Please list the patient's current medications and dosages (if known):

   _____

   _____

   _____

   _____

10. Does the patient have a history of any of the following?

			Onset Date and Current Status
Stroke	Yes	No	_____
Aphasia	Yes	No	_____
Other Communication Disorder	Yes	No	_____
Right- or Left-Sided Weakness	Yes	No	_____
Dementia (e.g., Alzheimer's Disease)	Yes	No	_____
Memory Impairment	Yes	No	_____
Other Neurological Disease	Yes	No	_____
Head Injury	Yes	No	_____
Seizure Disorder	Yes	No	_____
Clinical Depression	Yes	No	_____
Psychiatric Problems	Yes	No	_____
Alcohol Abuse/Problems	Yes	No	_____
Other Substance Abuse	Yes	No	_____
Other Major Illness	Yes	No	_____

11. List members of the immediate family:

Name	Age	Relationship	Phone Number	Check If Living in Same Environment as Patient
_____	_____	_____	_____	_____
_____	_____	_____	_____	_____
_____	_____	_____	_____	_____
_____	_____	_____	_____	_____

12. If the patient is living at home, are there others living in the home besides the immediate family? _____

_____

   If the patient is not living at home, where does he/she live? _____

_____

13. Are there relatives on the patient's side of the family who have had a similar problem with speech
and language? If so, who? _____

14. What is the patient's native language? _____

   If not English, at what age did the patient learn English? _____

   What other languages does the patient speak? _____

15. What is the patient's highest level of education? _____

16. What (is/was) the patient's primary occupation? _____

   Who (is/was) the patient's employer? _____

   Is the patient presently working? _____

   Describe the patient's work history (for example, kind of employment and approximate dates).

_____

_____

17. Patient's mother's name _____ Living _____ Deceased _____

   Patient's father's name _____ Living _____ Deceased _____

18. Marital status: single _____   widowed _____   separated _____

                     married _____   divorced _____   remarried _____

19. Does the patient have children _____ or grandchildren _____ ?

   If so, please complete the information below.

Children	Name	Address	Age
	_____	_____	_____
	_____	_____	_____
	_____	_____	_____
	_____	_____	_____
Grandchildren	_____	_____	_____
	_____	_____	_____
	_____	_____	_____
	_____	_____	_____
	_____	_____	_____

20. (Answer question 20 if appropriate.) What is the spouse's name? _____

   What (is/was) the spouse's occupation? _____

   Who (is/was) the spouse's employer? _____

   Is the spouse presently working? _____

   What is the spouse's native language? _____

   If not English, when did the spouse learn English? _____

   What other languages does the spouse speak? _____

21. Does the patient need to be taken care of at all times? _____

    If so, who performs this function? _____

22. To what extent can the patient care for himself (dress, feed, and wash himself)? _____

23. Has the patient's speech and language problem affected the family in any way? If so, how? _____

    _____

24. Describe the patient's ability to communicate. _____

    _____

    _____

25. When did you first notice that the patient had difficulty talking or understanding? _____

    _____

26. How much does he or she talk or write now? _____

    _____

27. How much of this speech or writing does the family understand? _____

    _____

28. To what degree do other adults understand the patient's communication? _____

    _____

29. How do you think he or she feels about his or her communication abilities? _____

    _____

30. What strategies have you found useful to help with the patient's communication? _____

    _____

31. Is he or she attempting to communicate verbally?   Yes   No

    Is he or she attempting to communicate in writing?   Yes   No

    Is he or she attempting to communicate using gestures?   Yes   No

    Can he or she tell you his or her name and address?   Yes   No

    Can he or she write his or her name and address?   Yes   No

    Is his or her speech intelligible?   Yes   No

    Is his or her writing intelligible?   Yes   No

    Can he or she say short sentences?   Yes   No

    Can he or she write short sentences?   Yes   No

    Can he or she repeat or copy words?   Yes   No

    Is there automatic speech (e.g., "Hello," "Thank you," "I'm fine.")?   Yes   No

    Can he or she understand conversational speech?   Yes   No

    Can he or she read and understand the newspaper?   Yes   No

32. Have you read or heard anything about aphasia? _____ If yes, what did you hear and where did you hear it?

    _____

    _____

33. Below are words that describe a person's personality and behavior. Circle those words that you feel apply to the patient's present status.

happy	fights often	sad	enthusiastic	patient
very friendly	warm	independent	energetic	intense
moody	critical	dependent	prefers to be alone	jealous
authoritarian	supportive	impatient	shy	receptive
bossy	at ease	responsive	cooperative	relaxed
active	indifferent	distractible	outgoing	directive
tense	listless	cold	can't sleep	affectionate
even tempered	quarrelsome	vigorous	easily fatigued	curious

has temper tantrums   exhibits control of emotions
follows the lead of others   exhibits self help
waits for recognition   has many fears
has few fears   initiates activities
walks in sleep   seeks social relationships
demands attention   willing to try unknown
stays with an activity

34. In general, the (spouse-patient) or (family-patient) relationship is (circle one):

comfortable   strained   hostile   indifferent

35. What are the patient's interests or favorite activities? _____

_____

_____

36. Does the patient watch TV? _____ If so, what are his or her favorite programs? _____

_____

37. Does the patient read much? _____ If so, what type of reading material does he or she enjoy? _____

_____

38. Has the patient been seen for:

	Dates	Agency	Address
a. speech therapy	_____	_____	_____
b. audiology	_____	_____	_____
c. physical therapy	_____	_____	_____
d. occupational therapy	_____	_____	_____
e. psychological counseling	_____	_____	_____
f. other rehabilitation	_____	_____	_____

APPENDIX 4-2
Various Auditory Retention and Comprehension Tasks (Chapey, 1994)

Auditory Retention and Comprehension Tasks

Task	Example	Input [a]	Output [a]
	Auditory Retention Tasks		
Recognition or repetition of digits	Point to: 8, 4, 2	A	G
	Say after me: 9, 3, 7	A	V
Recognition or repetition of words	Touch the red square and blue circle	A	G
	Say after me: man, cup, hat, dog	A	V
Recognition or repetition of noun phrases	Point to: The man	A	G
	Say after me: The man	A	V
Recognition or repetition of verb phrases	Point to: Ate the lunch	A	G
	Say after me: Ate the lunch	A	V
Recognition or repetition of sentences	Point to: The man ate the sandwich	A	G
	Say after me: The man ate the sandwich	A	V
	Auditory Comprehension Tasks		
Recognition of objects named	Point to the hat	A	G
Recognition of events named	Point to running	A	G
Recognition of relationships named	Point to family	A	G
Recognition of two or more objects, two or more events, or two or more relationships named	Point to the quarter and the comb	A	G
	Point to washing and to eating	A	G
	Point to family and to in front of	A	G
Recognition of categories named	Point to fruit	A	G
Recognition of two or more categories named	Point to clothing and to food	A	G
Recognition of objects when given the function of the object	Point to the one that is used for writing	A	G
Recognition of two objects when given the function of the objects	Point to the one that is used to buy things and the one that is used to comb hair	A	G
Recognition of an event described	Point to the one that shows what we do every night (sleep)	A	G
Recognition of two events described	Point to the one that shows food being prepared and the one that shows going to work	A	G
Recognition of semantically similar objects, events, relationships (2,3,4)	Point to the ones that go together: shopping, walking, cooking	A	G
Recognition of rhyme words	Point to a picture that rhymes with the word peas	A	G
Recognition of antonyms	Point to the opposite of up	A	G
Recognition of synonyms	Point to a word that means the same as sob	A	G
Following directions	Ring the bell	A	G
Understanding concrete sentences	Is this a cup?	A	G
Understanding abstract sentences	Will a stone sink in water?	A	G
Understanding complex or abstract relationships in sentences (adapted from Wiig and Semel [1976])			
a. Comparative relationship	Are towns larger than cities?	A	G/V
b. Possessive relationship	Does the hat belong to the girl?	A	G/V
c. Spatial relationship	Is the man walking in front of the cat?	A	G/V
d. Temporal relationship	Does lunch come before breakfast?	A	G/V
e. Inferential relationship	The man cut the steak. Did the man use a knife?	A	G/V

continued

continued

f. Familial relationship	Is your mother's brother your aunt?	A	G/V
g. Part-whole relationship	Does milk come from cows?	A	G/V
h. Object to action relationship	Can a car be driven?	A	G/V
i. Cause-effect relationship	Can smoke cause fire?	A	G/V
j. Sequential relationship	Were the Indians in this country before the white men came?	A	G/V
k. Degree relationship	Are inches larger than feet?	A	G/V
l. Antonym relationship	Is day the opposite of night?	A	G/V
m. Synonym relationship	Does sob mean the same as cry?	A	G/V
Comprehension of content categories			
a. Existence	Point to the hat	A	G/V
b. Nonexistence	Point to: "The pie is all gone"	A	G/V
c. Recurrence	Point to: "The man returns"	A	G/V
d. Rejection	Point to: "He doesn't want a bath"	A	G/V
e. Denial	Point to: "The cup is not yellow"	A	G/V
f. Possession	Point to the woman's coat	A	G/V
g. Attribution	Point to the large red circle	A	G/V
Understanding paragraphs	(Read paragraph) Questions: In this story, did Lucky find a bird?	A	G/V

[a] A = auditory; G = gestural; V = verbal.

APPENDIX 4-3
Various Tasks Used to Assess Auditory Comprehension of Syntax (Chapey, 1994)

Tasks Used to Assess Auditory Comprehension of Syntax

Task	Example	Input [a]	Output [a]
	Understanding Substantive Words		
Pronouns			
a. Personal	Point to: "She ate the cake"	A	G
b. Reflexive personal	Point to: "She kept it to herself"	A	G
c. Indefinite	Point to: "Is there any left"	A	G
d. Demonstrative	Point to: "This is the cake"	A	G
e. Interrogative	Point to: "Which one won the race"	A	G
f. Negative	Point to: "Nobody is interested"	A	G

continued

continued

Adjectives(attribution)			
a. Color	Point to the blue one	A	G
b. Size	Point to the large one	A	G
c. Shape	Point to the square one	A	G
d. Length	Point to the short one	A	G
e. Height	Point to the tall one	A	G
f. Width	Point to the narrow one	A	G
g. Age	Point to the new one	A	G
h. Taste	Point to the sour one	A	G
i. Speed	Point to the slow one	A	G
j. Temperature	Point to the cold one	A	G
k. Distance	Point to the one that is near	A	G
l. Comparatives	Point to the larger one	A	G
m. Superlatives	Point to the largest one	A	G
Adverbs			
'ly' adverbs	Point to the friendly one	A	G
	Understanding Relational Words		
Prepositions			
a. Locative	Put the hat in the box	A	G
b. Directional	Push the book under the table	A	G
c. Temporal	Do you go to church on Sunday?	A	G
Conjunctions	Point to ice cream and cake	A	G
Articles	Point to a cake	A	G
	(Picture of a boy hitting a girl)		
a. Active declarative	The boy has hit the girl	A	G/V
b. Yes/no question	Did the boy hit the girl?	A	G/V
c. Wh question	Whom has the boy hit?	A	G/V
d. Negative	The boy has not hit the girl	A	G/V
e. Negative question	Has the boy not hit the girl?	A	G/V
f. Passive	The girl has been hit by the boy	A	G/V
g. Passive question	Has the girl been hit by the boy?	A	G/V
h. Negative passive	The girl has not been hit by the boy	A	G/V
i. Negative passive question	Has the girl not been hit by the boy?	A	G/V
j. Complex sentences	Is this sentence complete or incomplete: "The nurse who comes in the morning"	A	G/V

[a]A = auditory; G = gestural; V = verbal.

[1]Another option is LeMo, a computer-assisted system that allows assessing according to a neuropsychological approach at the single-word level (De Bleser et al., 1997); although currently only a German version is available, the development of other language versions has begun.

Section II

Principles of Language Intervention

Chapter 5

Research Principles for the Clinician

Connie A. Tompkins and Amy P. Lustig

OBJECTIVES

Most clinicians value the intuitive, artistic nature of our endeavors. But many also recognize that effective clinical management cannot proceed by intuition alone. As Kearns (1993) suggests, "failure to apply scientific thinking and measurement during the clinical process is surely as misguided as leaving our empathy, clinical intuition, and caring attitudes behind as we enter the clinical arena" (p. 71). This chapter advocates a scientific approach to clinical decision-making, emphasizing primarily the clinician's role as a consumer of research information. Other sections recount the advantages of a systematic approach to treatment planning and implementation and suggest ways in which clinicians can contribute to the professional database. Finally, some future trends are considered in the application of research principles to clinical intervention.

PERSPECTIVES AND DEFINITIONS

Setting the Stage: Key Concepts and Terms

The Research Process

For the purposes of this chapter, **research** can be viewed as a process of asking and answering questions, which is structured by a set of criteria and procedures for maximizing the probability of attaining **reliability, validity,** and **generality** of results (Silverman, 1985). Each of these factors affects the confidence one can have in the findings and conclusions reported for a research effort.

Reliability refers to the stability, consistency, or repeatability of results. The most well-known types include inter- and intra-observer reliability, and test-retest reliability. When standardized instruments or nonstandard probes are used to document performance, these or related indicators (e.g., parallel/alternate forms reliability) should be reported

and evaluated. Standard error plays an important role in the measurement of reliability. Standard error reflects the precision of any particular statistic (mean, median, correlation, proportion, difference between means, etc.) by estimating the random fluctuations that would be obtained if that same index was derived on repeated occasions. A statistic called the standard error of measurement estimates the consistency with which a particular test would measure performance on repeated administrations. The larger the standard error relative to the magnitude of obtained scores, the more difficult it is to tell whether any single score is truly different from some other score (e.g., whether there is a change after treatment). It is beyond the scope of this chapter to elaborate on the calculation and interpretation of standard error statistics, but Kerlinger (1973) is a good source for those who want more information.

Two less familiar forms of reliability also require brief mention. The first, **internal consistency reliability,** reflects the homogeneity of test items, and by inference, the extent to which those items measure the same construct. Items that are summed to generate a "total score" index of a single construct, such as "word-finding ability," or "communicative adequacy," should have acceptable levels of internal consistency. If the items that are added together do not measure the same thing, combining them into a single score is like comparing the proverbial apples and oranges. Second, **procedural reliability** data reflect the consistency of implementation of the experimental conditions or treatment procedures in a research study. Also known as reliability of the independent variable, procedural reliability is often neglected in the language intervention literature. We will return to this concept in another section of the chapter.

Validity refers to "truth" of measurement. The definition of validity is illustrated by the following question: Are we measuring what we think we are measuring? Although many assume that validity once documented is a fixed property of tests and measures, inferences about a measure's validity vary with its application. That is, claims of validity for any particular measure will be influenced by factors such as the conclusions one wishes to draw, the individuals who are tested, and the procedures that are employed.

For tests and other measurement instruments, the familiar types of validity are content, criterion (predictive and concurrent), and construct validity. Two other validity concepts are important for designing and evaluating research. **Internal validity** reflects how confidently one can attribute observed changes to the experimental treatments or conditions themselves, rather than to artifacts or confounding variables (Campbell & Stanley, 1966). **External validity** involves the generality or representativeness of results and conclusions (Campbell & Stanley, 1966), and concerns the extent to which findings can be expected to apply to particular populations, settings, or measurement and treatment variables.[a] It is important to remember that reliability is necessary for, but does not guarantee, validity. Ventry and Schiavetti (1980) give an example of a scale that is consistently off by 1/2 pound: it is a reliable (consistent) instrument, but not a valid one.

Treatment Outcomes and Their Measurement

Outcomes measurement in recent years has seen increasing emphasis on the multidimensional consequences of health problems and health care provision. The idea is that a positive **outcome** (which can be defined simply as the result of an intervention) encompasses social, psychological, and attitudinal changes in addition to the traditional concerns with physical and physiological improvements (Donabedian, 1980). Probably the best-known working framework for outcomes measurement (WHO, 1999;) distinguishes among three levels of functioning: body structure and functioning; activity limitation; participation restriction. Measurement at the impairment level addresses specific anatomical, physiological, or psychological deficits, such as agrammatic output in aphasia. The concept of disability or activity limitation is concerned with the effect of an impairment on an individual's activities and daily life skills (e.g., agrammatism, apraxia of speech, and dysarthria may affect the ability to talk on the phone, to order a meal in a restaurant, or to read aloud to grandchildren). And assessment of handicap or participation restriction reflects the effects of a health condition on social roles and life situations. A handicap would be apparent if, for example, severely dysarthric speech restricted a teacher's ability to perform his or her job, or diminished a grandmother's ability to bond with her grandchildren.

According to Frattali (1998a), both efficacy research and outcomes research contribute to outcomes measurement. **Efficacy research** uses rigorously specified, well-controlled protocols to evaluate a treatment under optimal conditions, whereas **outcomes research** is conducted in typical or routine circumstances. Because well-designed efficacy research minimizes potential confounds, its internal validity can be extremely high, rendering a high degree of confidence in its results. **Outcomes research** yields a lesser

degree of confidence but may provide insights into processes and phenomena that cannot easily or validly be isolated and controlled.

Finishing our terminological survey, outcomes measurement can be aimed at documenting the efficacy, efficiency, effectiveness, and/or effects of treatment (see Frattali, 1998a, for a full discussion). There is little consensus about the meanings of these terms. Some link the terms *treatment effectiveness* and *treatment efficacy* with the conditions under which the data are gathered, suggesting that outcomes research yields evidence on the effectiveness of treatment, and only efficacy research can meet the standard for treatment efficacy data (see Frattali, 1998a). Robey and Schultz (1998) fold in another distinction, using the term *efficacy* to refer to the benefits derived from treating an individual patient (under ideal conditions), and *effectiveness* to indicate the benefits for a broader population (under typical conditions). So for Robey and Schultz, demonstrating treatment efficacy is a prerequisite for establishing treatment effectiveness. However, in this chapter we follow Frattali and others in using the term **treatment effectiveness** as a higher-order concept concerning whether a treatment works (Kendall & Norton-Ford, 1982), regardless of the research method used to generate the evidence. From this perspective, both efficacy and outcomes research can be used to investigate treatment effectiveness, but with different degrees of control and consequent confidence in results (Frattali, 1998a).

Science as a State of Mind

Knowledge of methods to maximize reliability and validity is essential for conducting and evaluating research, and a later section of this chapter examines some reliability and validity concerns related to language intervention studies. But as Chial (1985) reminds us, a commitment to science is also a state of mind. Some principles at the heart of a scientific orientation are summarized in Table 5–1.

An additional principle, central to a discipline like clinical aphasiology, is a concern for **clinical significance,** which calls for evaluating the relevance or meaningfulness of changes that are reported for research and treatment efforts. Is a statistically significant performance change of 5% following intervention a clinically important difference? What about a two-fold increase in the number of times a client initiates a conversation with an unfamiliar person? There is no easy answer, as the importance of a change depends on factors like the specific processes or behaviors being targeted, the client's needs and level of functioning, and the nature of the treatment goals.

The question of clinical significance can be formalized to some extent with reference to the WHO model. Improvements in a communicative "disability" or "handicap" most likely would be considered more relevant, meaningful, and

---

[a] The factors that compromise internal and external validity in research also affect the validation of a test instrument; for examples consult Franzen (1989).

TABLE 5–1

Some Key Principles and Values of Science

Testability:	propositions and questions are specific enough to be evaluated
Replicability:	procedural specificity and detail are sufficient to allow findings to be reproduced
Objectivity:	dogmatism and bias are rejected; counterevidence and alternative interpretations are sought
Systematicity:	theories and experiments are evaluated and developed in a logical, orderly way
Tentativeness:	the possibility and sources of error are recognized; the elusiveness of answers is understood
Concern for protection of human subjects:	the welfare of those participating in research projects is paramount

important than changes at the impairment level. We return to these issues later in the chapter.

Science and Clinical Decision-Making

While some clinicians may shudder at the thought of "doing research," effective diagnosis and treatment are modeled on the principles that guide scientific inquiry. Parallels often have been drawn between research and clinical processes (e.g., Kent, 1985b; Silverman, 1985; Warren, 1986). For example, Nation and Aram (1984) suggest that careful diagnosis is like conducting a "mini research project" (p. 54). Table 5–2 illustrates the scientific nature of the diagnostic process (after Nation & Aram) by setting out the chain of diagnostic steps that correlate with scientific problem solving. This theme is far from new. Decades ago, for example,

TABLE 5–2

Scientific Steps in the Diagnostic Process

1. Define and delimit the problem
2. Develop hypotheses to be tested; know what evidence is needed to evaluate them
3. Develop procedures to test hypotheses systematically
4. Collect the data: minimize bias and maximize validity
5. Analyze the data: score and organize objectively
6. Interpret the data: evaluate meaningfulness; support or reject hypotheses
7. Generalize from data: reason from the evidence to draw tentative conclusions

Source: After Nation & Aram, 1984.

Johnson et al. (1963) emphasized diagnosis as a hypothesis-testing process, guided by principles of critical thinking, special observation skills, and impartial, precise, and reliable observation.

Clinically accountable treatment, which can be documented as efficacious and/or effective, is guided by these same procedures and principles. Each session, the accountable clinician defines a problem, develops and tests hypotheses, collects data that are as sound as possible, evaluates the results, and then determines the next questions to pursue. Using a hypothesis testing model, we would gather initial information about our clients from a range of sources, form our best guesses about the nature of functional strengths and weaknesses and what can be done to ameliorate them, and then test and refine these hypotheses. In delivering and evaluating our treatment, we would systematically manipulate the demands of our tasks, such as the level and type of information processing required, against the background of our knowledge about a client's communicative needs, compensatory abilities, premorbid skills, environmental supports, and the like.

Silverman's (1985) position on the scientific approach to clinical management makes a fitting summary to this section. He emphasizes four principles: specifying clear objectives; posing answerable or testable hypotheses and questions; observing systematically; and remaining aware of the tentative nature of the findings. We add a fifth: justifying the choice of measures and treatments as appropriate to clients' needs and clinical goals. If we strive to adopt these principles, our clinical efforts should be more precise, and our clients can only benefit.

The Value of Science to Clinicians

So why should clinicians care about research and science? At least five reasons are immediately evident. First, as noted just above, the principles and skills of science are essential to accountable clinical practice. Diagnosis and treatment have long been viewed as exercises in hypothesis-testing; in every session, the good clinician develops pertinent questions or hypotheses, postulates relationships, decides how to assess them (reliably and validly), and collects and interprets the data. Second, all of us must think critically to be wise consumers in life. For the purposes of this chapter, the need for critical thinking applies to the published data and continuing education information that we consume professionally. Without critical evaluation, it is too easy to accept at face value anything that is published or presented at a professional conference, especially by someone who is known as an authority. Third, clinicians always have had an ethical responsibility to evaluate the impact of their services. In this vein, Rosenbek et al. (1989) assert that "untested treatments are immoral, therefore clinical practice must include clinical experimentation" (p. 12). Fourth, and relatedly, clinicians can make important contributions to the database that should form the foundation of diagnostic and treatment activities. Research is sorely needed to evaluate the effects, effectiveness, and efficiency of various assessment and treatment approaches, with results documented at multiple levels of outcome. Recent drastic reductions in reimbursement for services and increasing requirements to collect and report outcomes data (e.g., HCFA Outcomes and Assessment Information Set [OASIS] for home care patients; JCAHO ORYX initiative for the accreditation of hospitals and long-term care facilities) only underscore the urgency of generating a solid evidence base to justify clinical interventions. Finally, a scientific approach kindles informed curiosity and keeps us growing and thinking professionally. A scientific attitude may help to stave off "burnout"; searching for another question or pursuing a different hypothesis definitely help to keep life interesting. The next sections of this chapter will highlight clinicians as both consumers and potential producers of research.

THE CLINICIAN AS RESEARCH CONSUMER

As clinicians, the research consumer role is one of the most important that we can adopt. Participating in continuing education efforts or scouring the Internet for the latest developments, while laudable, are worth little if we simply soak up or disseminate the information without critical evaluation.

Some Questions to Ask in Evaluating Research

The literature is replete with contributions that describe general principles for evaluating published material and presentations. Some of the most important considerations are recapitulated here, in the form of 12 questions for the consumer, with examples and elaboration specific to neurologic or aging populations. Most of these questions can be asked of both "basic" and "treatment efficacy" research; they are culled primarily from Kent (1985a), Silverman (1985), and Ventry and Schiavetti (1980)[b].

1. Are convincing rationales and hypotheses provided? The weight one gives to rationales and hypotheses will vary depending on their sources, which can include critical examination of literature, knowledge of normal and disordered processes, and clinical observation and intuition. Most sound rationales and hypotheses originate from more than one of these roots. While a rationale such as "I wonder what would happen if . . ." clearly needs support and development from other sources, in most instances, each of us must decide whether a convincing case is presented for the questions asked or the hypotheses provided.

2. Are the research questions answerable? From the perspective of research evaluation, an answerable question is one

that is explicitly specified. A well-specified question is like an appropriately written behavioral objective. There is an obvious difference between clinical goals such as "improving auditory comprehension" and "achieving 85% comprehension of Yes/No questions about implied main ideas in spoken eighth-grade level paragraphs." The latter is more measurable. To take another example, the standard efficacy question, "Does aphasia treatment work?" lacks operational specificity, and probably is impossible to answer in any one or several studies. A more answerable question would indicate the nature of the treatment, the types of patients to whom it is to be applied, and the criteria for determining if it has "worked."

3. Do the participants represent the group(s) they are meant to represent? Using an example from aphasia, Darley (1972) emphasized long ago that researchers must define and operationalize what they mean by "aphasia." The occurrence of one or more dominant hemisphere "strokes" certainly is not sufficient evidence to render the diagnosis of aphasia. Neither, alone or in combination with etiological information, is poor performance on an aphasia test; low scores could reflect a number of other pre- or post-morbid conditions. Damage to the central nervous system also causes several varieties of non-aphasic language disturbance (e.g., language of confusion; language of generalized intellectual impairment in dementia; Wertz, 1985). This diagnostic distinction is more than a simple semantic one. We would not expect traditional aphasia treatments to benefit someone with an isolated dysarthria or someone whose language impairments are embedded in an assortment of other cognitive problems such as confusion and severe memory disorder. To address this question, a research report should describe the criteria, rationales, and reliability for judgments about essential diagnoses and characteristics. For qualitative or subjective judgments in particular, it is desirable to have independent verification by someone who is unaware of, or "blind" to, each participant's specific status, and who does not have a stake in the outcome of the study.

4. Are participants sufficiently described for assessing the believability, replicability, and generality of results? Again drawing on aphasia to illustrate, a number of variables may influence results in treatment studies, such as duration of aphasia, severity of deficits, aphasia type, etiology, prior neurologic and psychiatric history, sensory and motor status, and literacy (Rosenbek et al., 1989; Shewan, 1986). Similar sets of factors affect research with other neurologically impaired populations, and some of the same variables are relevant for characterizing communication behaviors of normally aging adults. Of course, it is also important that component skills or prerequisites for processing and responding to treatment or probe stimuli (e.g., visual and auditory perceptual abilities) are specified and measured.

Brookshire (1983) suggests a minimum list of descriptors for aphasic clients in his treatise on the subject of

---

[b] Some of these issues have been elaborated further by Tompkins (1992).

TABLE 5–3

Some Useful Descriptive Information About Neurologically Impaired Persons

Brookshire (1983) re: aphasia:	Age Education Gender Premorbid handedness Source of subjects	Etiology Time post-onset Severity of aphasia Type of aphasia Lesion location
Rosenbek (1987):	Risk factors Smoking Drinking Obesity Diabetes Hypertension	Other medical factors Medications Seizures
Rosenbek et al. (1989):	Willingness to practice Ability to learn Ability to generalize Ability to retain	
Tompkins et al. (1990):	Physiologic indices of aging Estimated premorbid intelligence Auditory processing abilities	Personality/attitudinal variables Social integration/social support

subjects. Others (e.g., Rosenbek,1987; Rosenbek et al., 1989; Tompkins et al., 1990) have offered additional possibilities and discussed novel ways to operationalize some of the tried-and-true descriptors (see Table 5–3). It is not practical, or even necessary, to expect all of these variables to be described in every study. However, having a greater number of well-operationalized descriptors such as these may make it easier for consumers to determine how to apply results, and for investigators to attempt replication and extension of reported findings. As Brookshire (1983) notes, including characteristics such as those discussed here also is important for the internal validity of a study. If such factors are not reported, readers cannot rule out the possibility that the results have been influenced in unintended ways. Detailed subject information is critical as well to begin formulating hypotheses about why certain participants do not respond as expected, or about which individuals might benefit most from particular interventions.

5. Are procedures, conditions, and variables adequately specified? This question most obviously refers to replicability, but inadequate specification also may raise internal validity concerns that diminish confidence in the results. Research reports should clearly present the essential aspects of procedures and conditions, and the operational definitions of the dependent (outcome) and independent (predictor) variables. For aphasia treatment trials, some important characteristics of the independent variable (the treatment) include the type and training of the clinician, amount of treatment, type of treatment, intensity of treatment, and nature of the no-treatment comparison condition (Rosenbek

et al., 1989; Shewan, 1986). Treatment procedures, criteria or decision rules, and responses also should be described as precisely as possible. In addition, if several conditions are contrasted, clear operational distinctions should be provided and validated.

6. Are procedures, conditions, and variables reliable and valid? Let us focus first on reliability issues. As noted earlier, the reliability (and validity) question can be asked of standardized measures. But often, psychometrically sound measures are not appropriate or available, and investigators develop or modify dependent measures of their own. When these specialized measures are used, researchers should provide the best data they can to address reliability concerns. Test-retest and standard error information are crucial. Without them, it is impossible to determine whether changes on the outcome measures might be due to unstable measurements rather than the intervention. An estimate of test-retest characteristics can be made from multiple assessments taken in a baseline (pre-intervention) phase of single-subject experiments, and repeated measures can be taken for a similar purpose prior to implementing experimental procedures or treatments in a group study. The appropriate standard error statistic can be calculated and evaluated as well.

Just as crucial are inter-observer and intra-observer reliability for dependent and independent variables, assessed in each phase of a study. Dependent variable reliability data are needed to ensure that scoring of outcome measures is objective and repeatable. Without evidence of acceptable agreement between independent judges, and of consistent scoring by the same judge, the research consumer has to question whether idiosyncratic decisions or unintentional bias could have affected the results. Independent variable reliability data are essential to demonstrate that all aspects of the independent variable (in this case, the treatment) have been delivered consistently and as intended. Thus, research reports should document evidence of procedural reliability for various aspects of an intervention, such as the timing and selection of cues or prompts, and the accuracy and delivery of feedback (see examples in Bourgeois, 1992; Massaro & Tompkins, 1993).

A variety of issues and procedures in observer reliability assessment have been discussed by Kearns and his colleagues (Kearns, 1990; 1992; Kearns & Simmons, 1988; McReynolds & Kearns, 1983). One caveat is that certain well-known correlation coefficients that often are reported to document reliability (e.g., Pearson r; Spearman ρ) are not the best choices for this purpose. These statistics only index the degree of association between two sets of scores, without taking into account exact score agreement. But two sets of scores can be highly associated (i.e., people who score high one time also score high the second time) and still be significantly different (see Wertz et al. 1985). If exact score agreement is of concern, as would be the case for reliability assessment, there are several other correlations that are appropriate, including variants of the intraclass correlation coefficient (Shrout & Fleiss, 1979). Another point to keep in mind is that levels of chance agreement should be considered when evaluating the acceptability of reliability indices (see Kearns, 1990; 1992).

We turn now to **validity** issues to continue illustrating Question 6. One specific concern relates again to the abundance of specially designed, nonstandardized measures in aphasiology research and treatment. While it is unreasonable to expect such measures to have known validity, readers should expect at minimum some evidence and logical arguments about the choice of items included, and about their internal consistency reliability. From a broader perspective, a validity assessment should ask whether the reported observations were appropriate for answering the questions asked, and whether the investigator observed and described what he or she wished to[c] (Silverman, 1985). Along these lines, readers should scrutinize the choice of outcome measures in light of stated goals. For example, if the goal of study is to assess knowledge of particular syntactic constructions in aphasia, how appropriate would it be to rely on a test that requires spoken production of those constructions? The answer depends on a lot of factors, but one might question the validity of this plan because problems of response formulation and execution could mask intact syntactic knowledge. The validity of the connection between treatment and outcome measures also is paramount. As a hypothetical example, one might question whether reading comprehension, as an outcome goal, would be expected to improve by a treatment that focused on oral reading of single words. Readers should look for investigators to justify the link between their independent and dependent variables.

Let us return for a moment to an earlier maxim: reliability is necessary (though not sufficient) for ensuring validity. So the validity of a treatment also depends in part on demonstrating procedural reliability, or compliance with the experimental protocol[d]. Wertz (1992) raises the issue of compliance in treatment studies, but his point applies to other kinds of research as well. Deviations from a protocol part way through a study, such as modifying selection criteria to include more participants, relaxing the amount of treatment or practice provided, or changing the clinician, can vitiate the validity of a research effort[e].

A special validity problem in studies of people with aphasia and related impairments is how to account for "spontaneous recovery" in evaluating treatment outcome. This is discussed in Question 9 below.

7. Is the behavior sample adequate? Four senses of *adequacy* are considered here. The first concerns repeated measurement with the same instrument or task, which was emphasized above. Typically, one-shot measurement is not sufficient. Repeated measurements may be needed to assess the stability of pre-treatment baseline performance, to gather data to approximate test-retest reliability before initiating a treatment or experimental manipulation, and/or to observe the timing or pattern of changes over the course of a study. The second sense of adequacy refers to the number of observations in each task. Generally, the more observations or items included in a measure, the more reliable that measurement will be. Brookshire and Nicholas (1994) demonstrated this point, showing that discourse measures based on single (short) speech samples were less stable than those based on a combination of samples. The third sense of adequacy refers to collecting multiple indicators at each measurement occasion, including measures that index treated behaviors and conditions as well as untreated behaviors and conditions. Multiple measurements are needed in treatment studies to assess whether an effect has generalized beyond that which is specifically trained (and perhaps as a control for "spontaneous recovery"; see Question 9). Finally, the generality of results is enhanced by comprehensive assessments in multiple environments or contexts.

8. Are precautions taken to reduce potential, even unknowing, bias? It is well documented that both examiners' and participants' expectations can introduce critical biases in a research investigation. Hence the emphasis in medical

---

[c] Under these guidelines, it should be clear that Question 3 above bears on the validity of subject selection.

[d] Assessing procedural reliability also would be important for studies comparing treatments; treatment delivery would need to be monitored to ensure that the treatments retained their intended distinctions.

[e] But a later section of this chapter will point out the flexibility of single-subject experimental designs, as long as modifications are analytically motivated and systematically applied.

research on "double-blind" studies, which keep both investigators and participants unaware of whether any individual participant is assigned to a treatment or control group. In language intervention studies, beyond keeping investigators blind to each participant's group (and even diagnosis) whenever possible, another control for experimenter bias is to have different examiners provide treatment and evaluate treatment data. An additional check on examiner bias is achieved when independent interobserver reliability is demonstrated to be high for selecting participants, adhering to procedures, scoring outcomes, and judging the existence and magnitude of treatment effects. The influence of participant expectations ("placebo effects") can be evaluated through simultaneous measurement of treated and untreated "control" behaviors. If all respond similarly over the course of treatment, it is possible that something other than the treatment was responsible for the changes. Question 9 elaborates on this approach as a check on the influence of spontaneous recovery.

9. Are the data interpreted appropriately? Two facets of this question are considered. One element concerns whether the results could be due to something other than the factors that interest the investigator. This is an issue of internal validity. Threats to internal validity probably can never be ruled out entirely, but an investigator should acknowledge and discuss their possible influence, and be appropriately cautious in providing interpretations and conclusions.

It is beyond the scope of this chapter to review all threats to internal validity (see discussions in Campbell & Stanley, 1966 and Ventry & Schiavetti, 1980; for a more general reference on alternative interpretations, see Huck & Sandler, 1979), but several major ones are discussed here from the perspective of language intervention research. One that is important in group treatment trials is the composition of no-treatment control groups. A randomly assigned control group is essential for demonstrating efficacy in group studies (Wertz, 1992). But since it has generally been believed that it is unethical to deny treatment, this crucial condition is rarely met.[f] Rather, control groups typically are self-selected, consisting of patients who, for example, live in remote areas without access to treatment, elect not to participate, or cannot pay for treatment. A self-selected control group may differ from the treatment group in critical ways that are relevant to the response to treatment. The consequence is that differences in outcome between treatment and control groups may not be attributable to the treatment per se. A related difficulty centers around differential dropout from a study. Clients drop out of treatment studies for a variety of reasons: they may be too ill or too severely impaired to participate; they may have improved enough so that they no longer want treatment;

they may not be aware of a continued need for treatment; or they may not like the treatment they are receiving. Any of these sorts of factors may make the groups unequal, biasing the results of the study.

Another difficult problem for the internal validity of language intervention research is a possibility of concurrent other treatments and/or prior treatments interacting with the treatment of interest. Perhaps the other treatments paved the way, bringing the client to the point at which he/she was ready to profit from the intervention under study. This is one example of an order effect. More generally, the order and sequence with which conditions are applied may influence reported results. Sequence and order effects may even affect results on a day-to-day basis. For example, if conditions are arranged in a fixed order or sequence, fatigue or warm-up effects may adversely affect some performances and not others. Conditions should be randomized or counterbalanced in group studies, and in across-subject replications of single-subject designs.

The influence of spontaneous or physiological recovery is nature's version of an "interacting treatments" problem. Physiological improvement brings about behavior changes that can be extremely difficult to separate from changes we would like to attribute to our treatments. Some researchers have tried to skirt the issue by conducting their treatment investigations in neurologically stable patients, years beyond the presumed effects of spontaneous recovery. One limitation of this approach is that no one knows the duration and timeline of spontaneous recovery (particularly for those with traumatic brain injuries). Another concern is that most language and communication treatment is delivered in the period shortly after onset of the disabling condition, so it is imperative to evaluate interventions for those who may still be undergoing neurological restitution.

For a large group treatment trial, random assignment to treatment and control groups is one solution. Then the effects of spontaneous recovery are assumed not to differ between groups (Wertz, 1992). However, random assignment does not ensure equality. Another approach is to measure several "control behaviors" that are approximately equal in difficulty to the target behaviors, but that the treatment is not expected to influence. If the recovery curve is steeper for treated than for untreated functions, treatment may be responsible for the changes.[g] Multiple baseline designs (McReynolds & Kearns, 1983), which track untreated behaviors while others are treated, can provide evidence of this sort for individual participants. Each time treatment is applied to a previously untreated behavior, the slope of change for that behavior should accelerate if treatment is exceeding the influence of

---

[f] Wertz et al. (1986) solved this dilemma by including a deferred treatment group, whose progress during the no-treatment phase could be analyzed as control data. Elman and Bernstein-Ellis (1999) used a similar approach in a study of the efficacy of group treatment for aphasia.

[g] However, another dilemma is that it is not known whether the rate, timing, or extent of spontaneous recovery is comparable for different behaviors or functions. Lesser change in an untreated function may simply represent a difference in the "recovery schedule," or in the complexity of the treated and untreated behaviors.

spontaneous recovery. Single-subject experimental designs that allow reversal and reinstitution of treatment effects for the same behavior in the same individuals (McReynolds & Kearns, 1983) also can provide convincing evidence of the influence of treatment over spontaneous recovery.

A general attention effect presents a related issue in interpreting the results of intervention studies. It might be argued that apparent treatment effects have resulted from the time and attention given the client, rather than from the content or process of treatment. Again, the simultaneous measurement of treated and untreated behaviors can help to address this issue. Also, this threat can be diluted by taking repeated measurements in a pre-treatment baseline phase, where participants are being given time and attention.

Another set of potential problems in attributing results to the experimental conditions involves the influence of factors that have demonstrated relationships to language and cognitive performance in non-neurologically impaired individuals. Some of these include age, hearing ability, medical risk factors, education/premorbid intelligence, and literacy (see Tompkins, 1992, for elaboration). It is important to remember that not all "errors" are due to a patient's neurological condition. A good example of this point comes from Yorkston and her colleagues (Yorkston et al., 1990; Yorkston et al., 1993), who demonstrated that certain measures of word usage and grammatical complexity differed according to socioeconomic status in non-brain-damaged adults. Similarly, Tompkins et al. (1993) reported that several connected speech attributes thought to characterize adults with right hemisphere brain damage did not distinguish their speech samples from those of normally aging adults. And, in a study of 180 normal native Spanish speakers, Ardila and Rosselli (1996) found significant relationships between performance on a picture description task and the variables of age, gender, and education. The lesson is that findings for people with neurological impairments must be evaluated against the appropriate control data and expectations.

The last statement exemplifies the second facet of the interpretive question: given what we already know, does the interpretation ring true? Evaluating interpretations at this level requires knowledge of or access to current theory and data, and a sense of their validity and replicability.

10. Are maintenance and generalization programmed and probed in treatment studies? This question is related to earlier issues regarding adequate behavior samples and multidimensional outcomes. It is important to plan treatments to maximize the likelihood of their generalizing (see Kearns, 1989; Thompson, 1989), and to assess whether treatment effects in fact do generalize to untrained exemplars and to other ecologically valid measures, situations, and conversational partners. Kearns (1993) indicates that generalization planning involves "comprehensive, multifaceted evaluation; the establishment of generalization criteria; incorporation

of treatment strategies that might facilitate generalization; continuous measurement and probing for functional, generalized improvements; and, when necessary, extending treatments to additional settings, people and conditions until targeted levels of generalization occur" (p. 71). If generalization beyond the treated tasks is not apparent, the clinical significance of treatment effects is in doubt. Similarly, maintenance of treatment gains should be assessed. It is rare for long-term maintenance data collected much more than a few weeks after the end of treatment to be provided in language intervention studies. One exception is found in Freed et al. (1997), who monitored maintenance of intervention gains for 13 weeks after the end of treatment. Evaluating maintenance of gains over extended time intervals should become a priority.

11. Are individual participant characteristics related to the reported outcomes? Individual performance can be analyzed in group data, and factors that appear to contribute to success or failure can be evaluated. Most clinical manipulations, like pause insertion or speech rate reduction, affect some people and not others (e.g., Nicholas & Brookshire, 1986). In order to apply findings to other individuals, it is important to try to identify what characterizes those with good and poor response.

12. Is there some attempt to evaluate the meaningfulness or importance of changes attributed to the experimental manipulations? We return to the issue of clinical significance here, and raise the related concept of "effect size." Metter (1985) suggested that some neurologists' skepticism about aphasia treatment efficacy stems from concerns about the relevance of specific improvements in treated deficits to real-life functional goals. Goldstein (1990) reviews several approaches for examining clinical significance, including normative comparisons of target performance and subjective evaluations of changes effected. Results of these types of assessments currently appear in some language intervention research. For example, normative comparison data in the aphasia literature have been gathered by assessing the frequency of requests for information by neurologically intact adults in conversations with unfamiliar partners (Doyle et al. 1989), and by examining non-brain-damaged adults' usage of social conventions (Thompson & Byrne, 1984). Studies by Doyle et al. (1987) and Massaro and Tompkins (1993) exemplify two varieties of subjective evaluation, assessing listeners' ratings of the adequacy of selected communication parameters following language intervention. Whitney and Goldstein (1989) used a hybrid approach, in which subjective evaluations were made of aphasic adults' speech samples intermixed with samples from non-brain-damaged control speakers.

When a research procedure or clinical intervention is not expected to lead directly to a functional outcome, several other measures of "importance" can be reported. Analysis of effect size has a precise statistical meaning (e.g., Cohen,

1977), but the idea is to determine how "large" or meaningful some statistically significant difference really is. Wertz (1991) suggests evaluating the size of a difference between groups of scores by examining their distributions for overlap or separation. This could be done by calculating the 95% confidence intervals for each set of scores, using standard error estimates. Another way to assess the importance or strength of an experimental effect is to set a predetermined difference criterion—for example, designating a change of at least one standard deviation unit, or a doubling or tripling of baseline performance, as clinically meaningful. To convey some indication of the strength of an observed group effect, researchers can report the number or percentage of participants in a group study whose performance conforms to the overall average pattern and/or who achieve the designated criterion for meaningful change.

THE CLINICIAN AS RESEARCHER

As a prelude to this section, it is important to acknowledge that recent changes in the service delivery climate have made it virtually impossible for most clinicians to participate in rigorous research efforts. But despite some very real practical limitations, we think there is value in the perspective and information that follows. We are convinced that the most important thing we can do as a discipline to garner credibility for our services is to accumulate the soundest evidence base possible to justify their efficacy and effectiveness. While it is clearly necessary to collect outcomes data for treatments as they are typically delivered, it also is critical to conduct efficacy research that goes beyond what is dictated by the current clinical climate, as a means to determine what would be possible under less constrained circumstances. The small number of researchers in our discipline simply cannot tackle these problems alone. Thus, we hope that clinicians who read this will be inspired to take part, at some level, in these crucial evidence-gathering efforts.

Contributing to the Scientific Database

Clinicians can contribute meaningfully to their professional literature, although there will almost certainly be obstacles along the way (see, e.g., Schumacher & Nicholas, 1991; Warren et al., 1987). Two avenues are probably most feasible for interested clinicians, particularly if they seek collaborative relationships with established researchers. The first is for clinicians to evaluate the effectiveness of their own interventions, in some cases through efficacy research, but more likely by collecting outcomes data. The second is to contribute more generally to information in the field, helping to provide much-needed data through original studies or replications and extensions of existing work.

Clinicians Evaluating Their Own Interventions

Treatment Efficacy Investigations

Single-subject or within-subject experimental designs (e.g., McReynolds & Kearns, 1983) are the most appropriate designs for clinicians who wish to be involved in evaluating treatment efficacy. Derived from behavioral psychology, single-subject experimental designs are not glorified case studies. Well-conceived single-subject designs are built around important components of scientific inquiry, such as operational definitions, attention to reliability and validity, and control of extraneous variables. The designs incorporate repeated measurements of observable, operationally defined target behaviors, with independent scoring of a portion of those behaviors by more than one examiner, to demonstrate objectivity and consistency. Stable pre-intervention baseline data, collected on the clearly specified dependent variables, are used as reference points for evaluating the efficacy of replicable interventions conducted with well-defined participants. The effects of these interventions are evaluated continuously within and across design phases (e.g., baseline, treatment, return to baseline, or maintenance); across behaviors; and/or across patients. Although tightly controlled and well suited to maximize internal validity, the designs allow flexibility in treatment when a need for modification becomes apparent (Connell & Thompson, 1986; Kearns, 1986a; McReynolds & Thompson, 1986).

Those unfamiliar with single-subject designs may equate them with pretest-posttest studies, but the two are quite dissimilar. In a pretest-posttest design, a target behavior (e.g., some aspect of reading comprehension) is assessed once prior to treatment, an intervention is applied, and then the target behavior is measured again. While this design often is used to gather "outcomes data," it generates only a weak form of evidence about a treatment's effects because of inherent threats to internal validity; any number of factors other than the treatment of interest could have caused a change from the first measurement to the second. In fact, some would not grant the status of "evidence" to the results of pretest-posttest studies (for further discussion see Campbell & Stanley, 1966; Ventry & Schiavetti, 1980).

Single-subject experimental designs are discussed in detail in a number of sources (e.g., Connell & Thompson, 1986; Kearns, 1986a; McReynolds & Kearns, 1983; McReynolds & Thompson, 1986). Kent (1985a) provides a useful table illustrating a variety of research questions, along with some of the single-subject designs that are appropriate for addressing those questions. Examples of studies using these designs with neurologically impaired adults also are available in the aphasiology literature (e.g., Ballard & Thompson, 1999; Bellaire et al., 1991; Doyle et al., 1991; Freed et al., 1997; Kearns, 1986b; Kearns & Potechin Scher, 1989; Massaro & Tompkins, 1993; McNeil et al., 1998; Thompson & Byrne, 1984; Thompson &

Shapiro, 1995; Yoshihata et al., 1998; Whitney & Goldstein, 1989).

Despite the strength of these designs for examining treatment efficacy, there remain relatively few published examples. The difficulty of implementing controlled research in a clinical environment is no doubt largely responsible for this situation. In describing their efforts to evaluate a treatment approach for a fluent aphasic patient, clinicians Schumacher and Nicholas (1991) recount a variety of problems that they faced when conducting research in their clinical setting. They question the feasibility of single-subject research in the clinical arena, unless a clinician is provided with release time for research, or with assistance for collecting and analyzing data. Warren et al. (1987) suggest that the major difference between typical clinical procedure and rigorous study is the time required to conduct behavior probes for no-treatment tasks and phases. In addition, designing and implementing generalization probes outside the treatment setting takes time and planning. Beyond feasibility problems, the often highly specific treatments used in single-subject research do not necessarily generalize to the needs of other clients (e.g., Franklin, 1997).

These barriers notwithstanding, we agree with Schumacher and Nicholas (1991) and Warren et al. (1987), who clearly believe that clinicians can generate worthwhile research in certain conditions. Those who have the drive to tackle a research problem, and who consult with knowledgeable researchers before starting, could probably evaluate a number of questions in their clinical settings, particularly if they enlist assistance in scoring, checking scoring reliability, and the like. If several clinicians in one location are interested, they can share these tasks, or graduate students from local university programs can be recruited and trained to assist. Some of the kinds of studies that clinicians can probably implement most readily are described below.

Treatment Outcomes Research

In an ideal world, ethical considerations would motivate and support the collection of credible evidence about treatment effectiveness. In the real world, emerging regulations and accreditation requirements will ensure the accumulation of at least some level of treatment outcomes data. ASHA's National Outcomes Measurement System (NOMS) provides one vehicle for collecting and analyzing outcomes data. With a goal of developing a national database for speech-language pathologists and audiologists, the NOMS project advocates the use of 11 pre- and post-treatment functional measures, scored on 7-point scales, to provide some estimate of treatment effectiveness. Demographic and consumer satisfaction data also are being collected. The NOMS database presumably will serve as a resource for selecting interventions and advocating for or justifying reimbursement for clinical services.

As indicated above, treatment outcome studies are conducted in the typical setting without stringent controls, yielding less confidence in results than would rigorously designed studies. However, clinicians can enhance the rigor of their treatments, their data-gathering efforts, and the resultant outcomes data by attending to the scientific principles discussed thus far.[h] To recapitulate, these include operationally specifying the nature of the client's abilities and the treatment plans; maximizing reliability and validity of measurement and treatment implementation; collecting an adequate behavior sample, including repeated measurements; attempting to control or account for extraneous factors like spontaneous recovery; programming for and measuring generalization to untreated behaviors and settings; assessing the maintenance of behavior change after treatment ends; examining potential factors related to success or failure; and assessing social validity to determine whether any changes effected have "made a difference."

Clinicians Contributing More Generally to the Professional Literature

Several avenues are probably most feasible for clinicians who wish to contribute to our clinical evidence base: evaluating outcomes (or efficacy) related to established treatment programs; replicating or extending existing studies; analyzing factors that may be important in interpreting assessment data or in implementing treatments; and gathering comparative performance data from persons without neurologic impairments. Each of these is considered briefly.

Evaluating Outcomes of Established Programs

Numerous treatment programs exist, and are recommended to clinicians, with only a cursory evidence base—if any. Clinicians are well situated to evaluate these sorts of programs. One model of this kind of work is provided by Conlon and McNeil (1991), who examined the efficacy of Visual Action Therapy (Helm-Estabrooks et al., 1982) for globally aphasic adults. Another example comes from Freed and colleagues (1997), who assessed the long-term effectiveness of PROMPT treatment (Chumpelik, 1984) for a client with apraxia of speech and aphasia. When attempting to evaluate these kinds of programs, clinicians may note that the specification of treatment procedures is inadequate to allow consistent treatment delivery. In this case, a good deal of planning and work must go into the project up front to specify stimulus choices, cuing/prompting criteria and hierarchies, scoring procedures, and the like. However, after that it becomes a much simpler matter to carry out the treatment program and to use it with other potential candidates.

---

[h] Of course, as Kent and Fair (1985) warn, equating science with effective clinical problem-solving may dilute or trivialize the meaning of the former, and misrepresent or overlook some of what occurs in the latter.

An example of this approach can be found in Massaro and Tompkins (1993), who operationalized a Feature Analysis treatment program (Szekeres et al., 1987) that has been recommended for traumatically brain-injured patients, and gathered some data about the program's efficacy with two patients.

Conducting Replication and Extension Studies

Replication and extension studies are particularly lacking in the speech-language pathology research base. But they are important in part because so much of our research has been done on small samples of participants, who exhibit a limited range of characteristics. Attempting to replicate the findings from an already published project with another sample of participants, or to extend the study using different participants, stimuli, or settings, is an excellent way for a clinical researcher to begin. Some examples of replication and extension studies can be found in Beard and Prescott (1991); Bloise and Tompkins (1993); and Kimelman and McNeil (1987). Bastiaanse et al. (1996) also reported a study replicating a treatment approach used in two previous investigations for word-finding problems. The work of Kearns and Potechin Scher (1989) and Byng et al. (1994) presents an even less frequent phenomenon: replication and extension by the original investigators. Typically, page limits on publications preclude researchers from providing complete methodological detail, so anyone wishing to replicate a study would need to contact the original authors for specific materials and procedures.

Analyzing Factors that Influence Delivery and Interpretation of Assessments of Treatments

Questions about the content, procedures, or interpretation of assessment tools have motivated a variety of clinical research. These kinds of questions typically stem from clinical observation; as such, they are good candidates for the interested clinical investigator. In one example, Nicholas et al. (1986) evaluated a number of reading comprehension batteries, and documented the extent to which the comprehension questions could be answered without reading the associated passages. In other work, Nicholas et al. (1989) revised and standardized the administration and scoring procedures for the **Boston Naming Test,** to improve their specification. The authors reported extended normative data for their revision as well. Investigations also have focused on determining the psychometric properties of abbreviated versions of standardized assessment instruments, such as DiSimoni et al.'s (1980) evaluation of a shortened form of the **Porch Index of Communicative Ability** (Porch, 1981). Another set of inquiries has focused on whether hypothetically important elements of treatment programs have an effect in practice. For example, several studies have examined whether the "new information" principle of PACE therapy (Promoting Aphasics' Communicative Effectiveness; Davis & Wilcox,

1985) has observable effects on narratives elicited from aphasic adults (Bottenberg & Lemme, 1991; Brenneise-Sarshad et al., 1991).

Gathering Normative Comparison Data

Judgments of our clients' abilities and performance should be made against a backdrop of knowledge about the non-neurological factors that may influence performance on language and cognitive tasks. Among the possible influences, noted earlier, are factors like age, education, literacy, socioeconomic status, physical health, or hearing impairment; however, few relevant data are available. Clinicians can design protocols to gather group data as a partial response to this need. Some examples are provided by Parr (1992), who examined everyday reading and writing practices of normal adults; Hansen and McNeil (1986), who studied writing with the nondominant hand; Elman et al. (1991), who documented the influence of education on judgments of non-neurologically impaired adults' writing and drawing samples; Tompkins et al. (1993), who assessed some characteristics of performance in normally aging adults' picture descriptions; and Yorkston et al. (1990; 1993), who reported on the discourse performance of non-brain-damaged participants who were similar in terms of socioeconomic status to the "typical" traumatically brain-injured patient.

In any context, practical concerns affect the kinds of questions or problem areas that one can study. Time demands and the need for consultation and support personnel have already been emphasized; having equipment and facilities on hand also is important. For group data collection, the availability of appropriate participants is a major issue. Funding also is a likely concern, but it should be possible to run some studies, particularly those evaluating established treatments, as part of routine clinical practice (see, e.g., Kearns, 1986b; and Massaro & Tompkins, 1993). In the end, personal interests and the perceived value of the research may be the most important motivators for clinicians deciding to embark on the research enterprise.

Some Competencies for Researching Clinicians

A clinician-investigator should be able to formulate answerable questions that have practical significance, and to make the necessary observations, with acceptable levels of validity and reliability, to offer tentative answers. This presumes current knowledge in the content area (e.g., the nature of neurological disorders and their treatment; the nature of normal language and cognition) as well as familiarity with guidelines for evaluating research. Persistence and tolerance for imperfection are important personality characteristics, because, as Warren (1986) reminds us, there is no perfect design for any study. Compromises are always necessary, in research as well as in clinical endeavors. Clinicians probably will feel more confident about the effects of particular compromises in their research plans after consulting with an expert.

Initiating a Research Project

When clinicians decide that they have the appropriate interests, competencies, and supports, they can begin developing their research projects. The first step is to hone the idea that sparked interest in the investigation. This can be accomplished by consulting with experts and by reviewing the available literature, to see what aspects of the research problem have not been addressed adequately, or at all. Computerized databases such as PsycLIT, PsychINFO, and Medline, and abstract journals such as Psychological Abstracts and Index Medicus will help interested readers locate the relevant literature. Publications from the Clinical Aphasiology Conference (e.g., Lemme, 1993; Prescott, 1989; 1991a; 1991b; and recently in dedicated issues of the journal *Aphasiology*) are particularly valuable references for those who wish to study neurologic disorders of language and communication in adults.

While reviewing the relevant literature, the reader should try to determine what factors point to the need for further investigation in an area of interest. For example, control for spontaneous recovery or examiner bias may be in doubt; the operationalization of the dependent measures may be debatable; the findings may have limited generality given the size and characteristics of the participant sample; or the durability and meaningfulness of results may not be addressed. A project can be developed to rectify particular issues of concern, or to replicate and extend findings in research that is essentially sound.

Planning can proceed by focusing on the questions that have been outlined for research consumers. Brainstorming with others about the best ways to operationalize and measure variables, or about how to minimize factors that might confound the results, is a valuable activity. And again, it is usually helpful to run the initial ideas and plans by someone with research expertise. Pilot-testing the methods on at least a few people is recommended as well; even experienced investigators generally identify wrinkles that remain to be ironed out during initial feasibility testing.

Finally, in the planning phase, investigators should contact their institution's Research and Human Rights Committee, Institutional Review Board, or similar committee, to ascertain what procedures they should follow to obtain approval for the project. Typically, these committees ask for a description of the aims, procedures, and risks and benefits of the proposed research, along with specific precautions taken to protect participants' rights. A detailed consent form, spelling out these elements for the participants, also is essential.

Opportunities for Funding and Consultation Assistance

Funding may be an important consideration, either for partial salary coverage in order to obtain release time to plan and conduct a project, or for paying research assistants or participants. There are a variety of funding opportunities that may be available for clinician-investigators, depending on their level of expertise. Several are outlined below; interested readers should contact the organizations listed for further information.

1. The American Speech-Language-Hearing Foundation (ASHF) has for a number of years sponsored New Investigator awards for those who have recently completed their latest degree program.
2. The American Speech-Language-Hearing Association (ASHA) publishes two research fact sheets, which can be obtained by phone request (800-498-2071) or Fax-on-Demand (703-531-0866). **Research Facts: Grantsmanship** primarily provides information about grants available from the National Institutes of Health, including those for new investigators. **Research Facts: Resources for Grantwriting and Funding** provides a directory of grants, foundations, and agencies that have funded clinical research efforts in communication disorders, as well as a list of relevant publications and Web sites.
3. ASHA maintains two electronic resources as well. The Science and Research web page (www.ASHA.org) includes information on federal and private funding sources. And the ASHA Research Listserv provides a weekly update on opportunities for funding, fellowships, conferences, and workshops. Requests to subscribe to this online mailing list can be sent to asha-research-digest-request@postman.com.
4. Graduate students in our program have received individual grant support from the Alzheimer's Disease and Related Disorders Association, the American Association of University Women, and the Sigma Xi Research Society.
5. The National Institutes of Health (NIH) Small Grants Program (R03) provides two years of funding to support pilot projects and feasibility research for investigators with limited research experience. Language researchers would most likely apply for NIH funding from the National Institute on Deafness and Other Communication Disorders (NIDCD), but some projects might be fundable by the National Institute on Aging (NIA) or the National Institute of Mental Health (NIMH).
6. Finally, internal institutional funding may be available. Some hospitals and rehabilitation centers sponsor competitions for funding, or release time, to encourage staff research efforts. Many universities grant seed monies for pilot projects that are expected to lead to larger efforts; a clinician-investigator's project, sponsored by a faculty member, might be partially fundable in this way. And the Department of Veteran's Affairs Merit Review program, which provides funds for initiating research efforts, is open to new investigators both inside and outside that system.

The value of consulting assistance has been emphasized repeatedly in this chapter. The way to get the most out of a consultative relationship is to consult before beginning a project, rather than trying to salvage mistakes later. But best-laid plans being what they are, a good consultant also may be able to help rescue some elements of an errant project after the fact. A clinician-investigator should not be afraid to seek help with a project by contacting people with the appropriate expertise.

There are a variety of avenues for identifying potential consultants. For example, the American Speech-Language-Hearing Foundation has put on several workshops on treatment efficacy research and, in recent years, ASHA has sponsored several travel fellowships that give new and minority investigators the opportunity to present research, completed or in progress, at the Science and Research Career Forum and the Research Symposium that coincide with ASHA's annual convention. Attending such conferences is valuable for both continuing education and networking purposes, but even reading any published conference proceedings can point clinicians towards experts who might be willing to serve as research consultants. University faculty members or master clinicians who publish their work would be good contacts as well. Also, good sources of possible expert consultants are professional journals, which list their authors and reviewers; and the Research Facts booklets and on-line Grants Digest, maintained by ASHA's Research Division.

Selling the Administration on Your Research Plans

Investigators in most clinical settings would need administrative approval and support for their research efforts. Silverman (1985) provides arguments related to increasing the institution's accountability to various consumers, such as clients, payers, and the community; maximizing the effectiveness of service delivery; and garnering recognition and grant support. Warren (Warren et al., 1987), a clinician and an administrator, also points out the value of efficacy data for demonstrating accountability to quality assurance evaluators and third-party payers. The costs involved are justifiable with relation to the enhanced confidence with which outcomes can be linked to treatments provided.

FUTURE TRENDS IN THE CLINICAL APPLICATION OF RESEARCH PRINCIPLES

Level of Outcome and Clinical Significance

Clinical significance and meaningfulness of outcomes have been recurrent themes in this chapter. Third-party payers' requirements for functional treatment goals indicate that these concerns are paramount from a reimbursement perspective as well. It is anticipated that the future will see much more attention to documenting the clinical importance of changes effected by interventions.

To date, research and clinical intervention in aphasia has focused most often at the level of impairment rather than on social communicative functioning. As suggested earlier, this may have contributed to the poor opinion of our profession held by some neurologists and other medical personnel. It is certainly critical to implement and evaluate interventions that target more ecologically valid outcomes, such as conversational proficiency, whenever possible. But one obvious dilemma in doing so is that there are almost assuredly intermediate or prerequisite steps to clinically relevant outcomes. As such, it is probably legitimate to focus for some period of time on the impairment level, especially in the initial stages of treatment. When treatments are not intended or expected to result immediately in clinically significant gains, it will be incumbent upon investigators to specify the eventual pathway from their treatment focus to the desired end result, indicating why or how their treatment goal should be an important step along the way to some meaningful outcome.

Another problem in targeting ecologically valid outcomes is that they are difficult to operationalize, and consequently to measure. A variety of generic rating scales are used to quantify "functional outcome" (see Frattali, 1998b), but in many cases, their reliability, validity, and sensitivity to change have been questioned. The (**Functional Assessment of Communication Skills;** ASHA-FACS Frattali et al. 1995), which provides a more extensive and specific evaluation of communicative disability for adults with aphasia and traumatic brain injury, is a good supplement to these general assessments. The **Communicative Activities in Daily Living** (CADL-2; Holland et al., 1999) is another option for assessing functional communication. Two other ways to demonstrate the functionality of treatment outcomes are to achieve generalization to everyday settings and tasks and to document social validity. If generalized, meaningful effects can be shown to have staying power, so much the better. To examine the durability of clinically important changes, investigators should begin to assess clinical significance or social validity using data from several phases of treatment studies, including those collected during maintenance probes.

Social validity assessments are relatively new, so standards and criteria for conducting them are still evolving. The future will see more attempts to develop a rigorous technology for determining social validity. The concerns of reliability, validity, and generality are paramount here as they are in any measurement effort. Questionnaires and rating scales should be constructed so that the resulting data are sound.

Silverman (1985) discusses several other critical factors such as the design of the social validity tasks, numbers, and characteristics of raters including their knowledge of subject group or time of sample, and selection of the scaling method. One of the salient questions (Goldstein, 1990; Campbell & Dollaghan, 1992; Tompkins, 1992) has to do with the choice of the "gold standard" for a normative comparison approach to determining clinical significance. When patients are severely impaired, an appropriate standard might be one that approximates the communicative performance of a milder, but functional, aphasic communicator. For mildly involved patients, a normal criterion may be appropriate. Whatever the comparison group, though, we foresee more care in specifying individual participant variables that should be relevant, including some of those identified above. The common practice of matching comparison and treatment subjects only for chronological age and gender will be recognized as insufficient.

As procedural issues are being sorted out, much more work also will be needed to assess the correspondence between these sorts of social validity data and other measures of communication performance in natural environments. The assessment of real-life behaviors, experiences, and phenomena is at the core of a nontraditional research approach that complements the scientific orientation described earlier in this chapter. This "qualitative research" approach (see, e.g., Denzin & Lincoln, 1998; Strauss & Corbin, 1998) involves detailed data-gathering through extensive interviewing and observation of communicative behaviors and social interactions in a variety of authentic contexts. The investigator relies on "disciplined subjectivity" (Heron, 1996, p. 143) to interpret the accumulated information and generate hypotheses about processes that are at work. Simmons-Mackie & Damico (1996) emphasize the goodness-of-fit between the qualitative research perspective and the assessment of 'handicap' in aphasia. They describe a Communicative Profiling System that uses qualitative methods to evaluate communication behaviors and strategies, contextual influences on communication, and the available network of communication partners. Conversation Analysis (Goodwin & Heritage, 1990; Shiffrin, 1994), a qualitative research method derived from discourse studies, provides another frame of reference for evaluating communicative success in aphasia. This approach has been employed in several recent investigations (e.g., Ferguson, 1993; Milroy & Perkins, 1992) to explore dynamic aspects of conversational collaboration. Some treatment studies (e.g., Perkins, 1995; Perkins et al., 1999) have combined quantitative and qualitative methods in an effort to establish a more complete clinical picture than would be obtained by either approach alone. While lacking elements of rigor identified earlier in this chapter and particularly susceptible to (unintended) examiner bias, qualitative approaches can provide a rich source of ideas for those who are interested in documenting, describing, and characterizing meaningful outcomes.

Evaluating Effectiveness of Nontraditional Treatment Approaches

Even before funding pressures prompted increasing exploration of alternatives to direct individual language treatment,

some interest in nontraditional options was evident. We expect to see heightened attention to establishing the effectiveness of nontraditional intervention approaches, including those that involve communication partners, provide therapy in a group context, or rely on computerized treatment delivery.

Targeting communication partner behaviors, instead of or in addition to those of the individuals with communication disorders, remains a relatively untapped but potentially important direction in treatment research. After all, communication is an interactive process, and its success hinges on the interplay between participants. Turning some attention to the neurologically intact member of a communicative dyad would have considerable ecological validity. And with clients receiving less direct treatment, it will become more imperative to rely on communication partners as intervention agents.

Some research has already explored communication partner interventions for adults with aphasia. For example, Simmons et al. (1987) evaluated an intervention to diminish inappropriate partner behaviors, such as interrupting before the participant with aphasia has time to respond. Additionally, Flowers and Peizer (1984) and Simmons-Mackie and Kagan (1999) reported systems designed to quantify partner strategies and to identify those that were more or less successful in communicative exchanges, so that they could be addressed in treatment. Measures of conversational burden (e.g., Marshall et al., 1997; Packard & Hinckley, 1999) also have been used to describe dynamic partner interactions, and to isolate variables such as topic initiation that can be manipulated in therapy.

Relatedly, the future also may see more efforts to train communication partners as intervention agents (e.g., Bourgeois, 1991). This approach may accomplish several goals simultaneously: it can bring the intervention to the natural environment, free some of the clinician's time, and allow more treatment to be delivered than would otherwise be feasible or affordable. It also may empower communication partners by giving them some specific things to do in the event of communication breakdown. One such model, Supported Conversation for Adults with Aphasia (SCA) has been developed by Kagan (1995; 1998). SCA offers individuals, including those with severe aphasia, the opportunity to interact with volunteer partners who are trained to support conversational-level communication using a range of methods and expressive modalities.

Obviously, there can be a number of pitfalls to either of these approaches. A clinician would have to invest time to train the communication partners, and to monitor delivery of treatment and/or evaluation of responses. Personalities and prior patterns of interaction between communication partners also may mitigate against these methods, or diminish their effectiveness. In addition, it may be difficult to get reimbursement for services that target communication partners, unless creative outcome measures are employed. And of course, rigorous evaluation of effectiveness will be necessary, as it is for any language intervention approach. Despite these possible drawbacks, the potential benefits of interventions that involve the neurologically intact communication partner are likely to spur further exploration in the future.

Another nontraditional intervention approach, group treatment, has the potential to enhance generalization of treatment gains because the group context provides a relatively natural setting within which to target both linguistic and communicative goals. Group therapy for aphasia is increasingly being considered a viable adjunct to individual treatment, and in many cases may serve as the primary therapeutic milieu. This undoubtedly is due in part to reimbursement constraints, but there is emerging evidence that group aphasia therapy can effect positive outcomes. The seminal Veteran's Administration cooperative study comparing the effects of individual and group aphasia treatment (Wertz et al., 1981) as well as other more recent studies (e.g., Avent, 1997; Bollinger et al., 1993; Elman & Bernstein-Ellis, 1999; Marshall, 1993) have demonstrated improvements on both standardized and referential language measures, as well as in functional communication abilities, for individuals at all severity levels in various group treatment approaches. Kearns (1994) reviews factors to be considered in providing and evaluating group therapy for individuals with aphasia, and a number of other current references discuss methods for delivering and assessing group aphasia treatment (e.g., Elman, 1999; Marshall, 1999). One obstacle to analyzing the effectiveness of group treatment, specifically, is the complexity of implementing rigorous data collection for multiple participants, who may have multiple goals.

Computer-aided approaches to aphasia treatment are in their infancy, but the future promises to see expansion of efforts in this area as well. Recent studies (e.g., Katz & Wertz, 1997) show some promise of efficacy for improvements in language performance resulting from computer-delivered therapy, as well as generalization of learned skills to noncomputer language contexts. The potential advantages of such an approach, such as cost-effectiveness and the opportunity to tailor modality-specific tasks for individual patients, must be weighed against possible disadvantages such as a lack of procedural flexibility and limited opportunities for communicative interaction and exchange for the person with aphasia. A more complete discussion of merits and drawbacks of computer-aided aphasia rehabilitation was published by Roth and Katz (1998). As for the other nontraditional treatment approaches that are discussed here, computer-delivered aphasia therapy must be subjected to rigorous evaluation over time to establish its effectiveness and efficacy.

▶ *Acknowledgment*–Preparation of this chapter was supported in part by Grant # DC01820 from the National Institute on Deafness and Other Communication Disorders (NIDCD).

KEY POINTS

1. Research and clinical decision-making processes have a number of parallels.

2. A scientific orientation to clinical management has value for a variety of reasons; not the least of these is that clinical accountability is enhanced by following the hypothesis-testing approach that guides scientific inquiry.

3. Clinicians should become critical consumers of the research database.

4. Reliability, validity, and generality of results are important concepts in the evaluation of research. Clinical significance should be addressed as well in evaluating research and treatment efforts.

5. Outcomes measurement comprises both "efficacy research," which involves rigorous, controlled experimental documentation of the effects of treatment, and "outcomes research," which documents the results of treatment in typical circumstances. Outcomes research yields less confidence in results but is important for evaluating phenomena that cannot easily be isolated or controlled.

6. As used in this chapter, the term "treatment efficacy" refers to evidence that is generated from efficacy research, while "treatment effectiveness" refers more broadly to evidence about how well a treatment works, regardless of the rigor of the research method.

7. Outcomes assessment also can be characterized with reference to a multidimensional model of the consequences of health conditions, such as the World Health Organization classification scheme of impairment (body structure and functioning), disability (activity limitation), and handicap (participation restriction).

8. A set of principles, reviewed and illustrated in the chapter, can be used to evaluate both basic and applied research. These focus on issues germane to study rationale, design, and interpretation.

9. Clinicians can satisfy empirical, ethical, and practical concerns by becoming involved in clinical research, and their participation in this process is crucial to the development of a sufficient evidentiary database. Clinicians may best be able to contribute by collecting treatment outcomes data, participating in treatment efficacy studies, replicating and extending existing studies, evaluating published assessment tools and treatment approaches, and/or gathering normative comparison data.

10. Several public and private funding resources are available to both new and experienced clinician-investigators.
11. Established researchers can offer valuable consultation and collaboration to support clinician-investigators in their research endeavors.
12. The future is expected to see increasing emphasis on evaluating the functional and social consequences of treatment, as well as on documenting the effectiveness of nontraditional treatment approaches involving communication/conversation partners, group treatment, and computer-based interventions.

References

Ardila, A. & Rosselli, M. (1996). Spontaneous language production and aging: Sex and educational effects. *Int J Neurosci, 87* (1–2), 71–78.

Avent, J. (1997). Group treatment in aphasia using cooperative learning methods. *J Med Speech-Language Pathol, 5,* 9–26.

Ballard, K.J. & Thompson, C.K. (1999). Treatment and generalization of complex sentence production in agrammatism. *J Speech, Language, Hearing Res, 42,* 690–707.

Bastiaanse, R., Bosje, M., & Franssen, M. (1996). Deficit-oriented treatment of word-finding problems: Another replication. *Aphasiology, 10,* 363–383.

Beard, L.C. & Prescott, T.E. (1991). Replication of a treatment protocol for repetition deficit in conduction aphasia. In T.E. Prescott (ed.), *Clinical Aphasiology*, Vol. 19 (pp. 197–208). Austin, TX: Pro-Ed.

Bellaire, K.J., Georges, J.B., & Thompson, C.K. (1991). Establishing functional communication board use for nonverbal aphasic subjects. In T.E. Prescott (ed.), *Clinical Aphasiology*, Vol. 19 (pp. 219–227). Austin, TX: Pro-Ed.

Bloise, C.G.R. & Tompkins, C.A. (1993). Right brain damage and inference revision, revisited. In M.L. Lemme (ed.), *Clinical Aphasiology*, Vol. 21 (pp. 145–155). Austin, TX: Pro-Ed.

Bollinger, R.L., Musson, N.D., & Holland, A.L. (1993). A study of group communication intervention with chronically aphasic persons. *Aphasiology, 7,* 301–313.

Bottenberg, D. & Lemme, M.L. (1991). Effect of shared and unshared listener knowledge on narratives of normal and aphasic adults. In T.E. Prescott (ed.), *Clinical Aphasiology*, Vol. 19 (pp. 109–116). Austin, TX: Pro-Ed.

Bourgeois, M.S. (1991). Communication treatment for adults with dementia. *J Speech Hearing Res, 34,* 831–844.

Bourgeois, M.S. (1992). Evaluating memory wallets in conversations with patients with dementia. *J Speech Hearing Res, 35,* 1344–1357.

Brenneise-Sarshad, R., Nicholas, L.E., & Brookshire, R.H. (1991). Effects of apparent listener knowledge and picture stimuli on aphasic and non-brain-damaged speakers' narrative discourse. *J Speech Hearing Res, 34,* 168–176.

Brookshire, R.H. (1983). Subject description and generality of results in experiments with aphasic adults. *J Speech Hearing Dis, 48,* 342–346.

Brookshire, R.H. & Nicholas, L.E. (1994). Test-retest stability of measures of connected speech in aphasia. In M.L. Lemme (ed.), *Clinical Aphasiology*, Vol. 22 (pp. 119–134). Austin, TX: Pro-Ed.

Byng, S., Nickels, L., & Black, M. (1994). Replicating therapy for mapping deficits in agrammatism: Remapping the deficit? *Aphasiology, 8,* 315–341.

Campbell, D.T. & Stanley, J.C. (1966). *Experimental and Quasi-Experimental Designs for Research.* Chicago: Rand McNally.

Campbell, T.F. & Dollaghan, C. (1992). A method for obtaining listener judgments of spontaneously produced language: Social validation through direct magnitude estimation. *Top Language Dis, 12,* 42–55.

Chial, M.R. (1985). Scholarship as process: A task analysis of thesis and dissertation research. In R.D. Kent (ed.), *Seminars in Speech and Language: Vol. 6. Application of Research to Assessment and Therapy* (pp. 35–54). New York: Thieme-Stratton.

Chumpelik, D. (1984). The PROMPT system of therapy: Theoretical framework and applications for developmental apraxia of speech. *Sem Speech Language, 5,* 139–156.

Cohen, J. (1977). *Statistical Power Analysis for the Behavioral Sciences.* New York: Academic Press.

Conlon, C.P. & McNeil, M.R. (1991). The efficacy of treatment for two globally aphasic adults using visual action therapy. In T.E. Prescott (ed.), *Clinical Aphasiology*, Vol. 19 (pp. 185–195). Austin, TX: Pro-Ed.

Connell, P.J. & Thompson, C.K. (1986). Flexibility of single-subject experimental designs. Part III: Using flexibility to design or modify experiments. *J Speech Hearing Dis, 51,* 214–225.

Darley, F.L. (1972). The efficacy of language rehabilitation in aphasia. *J Speech Hearing Dis, 37,* 3–21.

Davis, G.A. & Wilcox, M.J. (1985). *Adult Aphasia Rehabilitation: Applied Pragmatics.* San Diego: College-Hill.

Denzin, N.K. & Lincoln, Y.S. (eds.) (1998). *The Landscape of Qualitative Research: Theories and Issues.* Thousand Oaks: Sage.

DiSimoni, F.G., Keith, R.L., & Darley, F.L. (1980). Prediction of PICA overall score by short versions of the test. *J Speech Hearing Res, 23,* 511–516.

Donabedian, A. (1980). *Explorations in Quality Assessment and Monitoring. Volume 1: The Definition of Quality and Approaches to its Assessment.* Ann Arbor, MI: Health Administration Press.

Doyle, P.J., Goldstein, H., & Bourgeois, M.S. (1987). Experimental analysis of syntax training in Broca's aphasia: A generalization and social validation study. *J Speech Hearing Dis, 52,* 143–155.

Doyle, P.J., Goldstein, H., Bourgeois, M.S., & Nakles, K. (1989). Facilitating generalized requesting behavior in Broca's aphasia: An experimental analysis of a generalization training procedure. *J Appl Behav Anal, 22,* 157–170.

Doyle, P.J., Oleyar, K.S., & Goldstein, H. (1991). Facilitating functional conversational skills in aphasia: An experimental analysis of a generalization training procedure. In T.E. Prescott (ed.), *Clinical Aphasiology*, Vol. 19 (pp. 229–241). Austin, TX: Pro-Ed.

Elman, R. (1999). *Group Treatment of Neurogenic Communication Disorders: The Expert Clinician's Approach.* Boston: Butterworth-Heinemann.

Elman, R.J., Roberts, J.A., & Wertz, R.T. (1991). The effect of education on diagnosis of aphasia from writing and drawing performance by mildly aphasic and non-brain-damaged adults. In T.E. Prescott, (ed.), *Clinical Aphasiology*, Vol. 20 (pp. 101–110). Austin, TX: Pro-Ed.

Elman, R.J. & Bernstein-Ellis, E. (1999). The efficacy of group treatment in adults with chronic aphasia. *J Speech, Language, Hearing Res, 42*, 411–419.

Ferguson, A. (1993). Conversational repair of word-finding difficulty. In M. Lemme (ed.), *Clinical Aphasiology*, Vol. 21 (pp. 299–310). Austin, TX: Pro-Ed.

Flowers, C.R. & Peizer, E.R. (1984). Strategies for obtaining information from aphasic persons. In R.H. Brookshire (ed.), *Clinical Aphasiology: Conference Proceedings* (pp. 106–113). Minneapolis: BRK Publishers.

Franklin, S. (1997). Designing single case treatment studies for aphasic patients. *Neuropsych Rehab, 7*, 401–418.

Franzen, M.D. (1989). *Reliability and Validity in Neuropsychological Assessment*. New York: Plenum.

Frattali, C.M. (1998a). Outcomes measurement: Definitions, dimensions, and perspectives. In C.M. Frattali (ed.), *Measuring Outcomes in Speech-Language Pathology* (pp. 1–27). New York: Thieme.

Frattali, C.M. (1998b). Measuring modality-specific behaviors, functional abilities, and quality of life. In C.M. Frattali (ed.), *Measuring Outcomes in Speech-Language Pathology* (pp. 55–88). New York: Thieme.

Frattali, C.M., Thompson, C.K., Holland, A.L., Wohl, C.B., & Ferketic, M.M. (1995). *Functional Assessment of Communication Skills for Adults*. Rockville, MD: American Speech-Language Hearing Association.

Freed, D.B., Marshall, R.C., & Frazier, K.E. (1997). Long-term effectiveness of PROMPT treatment in a severely apractic-aphasia speaker. *Aphasiology, 11*, 365–372.

Goldstein, H. (1990). Assessing clinical significance. In L.B. Olswang, C.K. Thompson, S.F. Warren, & N.J. Minghetti (eds.), *Treatment Efficacy Research in Communication Disorders* (pp. 91–98). Rockville, MD: American Speech-Language-Hearing Foundation.

Goodwin, C. & Heritage, J. (1990). Conversation analysis. *Annual Review of Anthropology, 19*, 283–307.

Hansen, A.M. & McNeil, M.R. (1986). Differences between writing with the dominant and nondominant hand by normal geriatric subjects on a spontaneous writing task: Twenty perceptual and computerized measures. In R.H. Brookshire (ed.), *Clinical Aphasiology*, Vol. 16 (pp. 116–122). Minneapolis: BRK Publishers.

Helm-Estabrooks, N., Fitzpatrick, P.M., & Barresi, B. (1982). Visual action therapy for global aphasia. *J Speech Hearing Dis, 47*, 385–389.

Heron, J. (1996). *Cooperative Inquiry: Research into the Human Condition*. London: Sage.

Holland, A., Frattali, C., & Fromm, D. (1999). *Communication Activities of Daily Living* (2nd ed.). Austin, TX: Pro-Ed.

Huck, S.W. & Sandler, H.M. (1979). *Rival Hypotheses: Alternative Interpretations of Data Based Conclusions*. New York: Harper & Row.

Johnson, W., Darley, F.L., & Spriestersbach, D.C. (1963). *Diagnostic Methods in Speech Pathology*. New York: Harper & Row.

Kagan, A. (1995). Revealing the competence of aphasic adults through conversation: A challenge to health professionals. *Top Stroke Rehab, 2*, 15–28.

Kagan, A. (1998). Supported conversation for adults with aphasia: Methods and resources for training conversational partners. *Aphasiology, 12*, 816–830.

Katz, R.C. & Wertz, R.T. (1997). The efficacy of computer-provided reading treatment for chronic aphasic adults. *J Speech Hearing Res, 40*, 493–507.

Kearns, K.P. (1986a). Flexibility of single-subject experimental designs. Part II: Design selection and arrangements of experimental phases. *J Speech Hearing Dis, 51*, 204–214.

Kearns, K.P. (1986b). Systematic programming of verbal elaboration skills in chronic Broca's aphasia. In R.C. Marshall (ed.), *Case Studies in Aphasia Rehabilitation* (pp. 225–244). Austin, TX: Pro-Ed.

Kearns, K.P. (1989). Methodologies for studying generalization. In L.V. McReynolds & J. Spradlin (eds.), *Generalization Strategies in the Treatment of Communication Disorders*. Toronto: B.C. Decker.

Kearns, K.P. (1990). Reliability of procedures and measures. In L. Olswang, C. Thompson & S. Warren (eds.), *Treatment Efficacy Research in Communication Disorders* (pp. 71–90). Rockville, MD: American Speech-Language-Hearing Foundation.

Kearns, K.P. (1992). *Methodological Issues in Treatment Research: A Single-Subject Perspective. Aphasia Treatment: Current Approaches and Research Opportunities* (pp. 7–16). Washington, DC: National Institute on Deafness and Other Communication Disorders.

Kearns, K.P. (1993). Functional outcome: Methodological considerations. In M.L. Lemme (ed.), *Clinical Aphasiology*, Vol. 21 (pp. 67–72). Austin, TX: Pro-Ed.

Kearns, K.P. (1994). Group therapy for aphasia: Theoretical and practical considerations. In R. Chapey (ed.), *Language Intervention Strategies in Adult Aphasia* (3rd ed.), (pp. 304–321). Baltimore: Williams & Wilkins.

Kearns, K.P. & Potechin Scher, G. (1989). The generalization of response elaboration training effects. In T.E. Prescott (ed.), *Clinical Aphasiology*, Vol. 18 (pp. 223–245). Boston: College-Hill.

Kearns, K.P. & Simmons, N.N. (1988). Interobserver reliability and perceptual ratings: More than meets the ear. *J Speech Hearing Res, 31*, 131–136.

Kendall, P. & Norton-Ford, J. (1982). Therapy outcome research methods. In P. Kendall & J. Butcher (eds.), *Handbook of Research Methods in Clincal Psychology* (pp. 429–460). New York: John Wiley and Sons.

Kent, R.D. (1985a). Science and the clinician: The practice of science and the science of practice. In R.D. Kent (ed.), *Seminars in Speech and Language: Vol. 6. Application of Research to Assessment and Therapy* (pp. 1–12). New York: Thieme-Stratton.

Kent, R.D. (ed.). (1985b). *Seminars in Speech and Language: Vol. 6. Application of Research to Assessment and Therapy*. New York: Thieme-Stratton.

Kent, R.D. & Fair, J. (1985). Clinical research: Who, where, and how? In R.D. Kent (ed.), *Seminars in Speech and Language: Vol. 6. Application of Research to Assessment and Therapy* (pp. 23–34). New York: Thieme-Stratton.

Kerlinger, F.N. (1973). *Foundations of Behavioral Research* (2nd ed.). New York: Holt, Rinehart & Winston.

Kimelman, M.D.Z. & McNeil, M.R. (1987). An investigation of

emphatic stress comprehension in adult aphasia: A replication. *J Speech Hearing Res, 30,* 295–300.

Lemme, M.L. (ed.). (1993). *Clinical Aphasiology,* Vol. 21. Austin, TX: Pro-Ed.

Marshall, R.C. (1993). Problem-focused group treatment for clients with mild aphasia. *Am J Speech-Language Pathol, 3,* 31–37.

Marshall, R.C. (1999). *Introduction to Group Treatment for Aphasia: Design and Management.* Boston: Butterworth-Heinemann.

Marshall, R.C, Freed, D.B, & Phillips, D.S. (1997). Communicative efficiency in severe aphasia. *Aphasiology, 11,* 373–384.

Massaro, M. & Tompkins, C.A. (1993). Feature analysis for treatment of communication disorders in traumatically brain-injured patients: An efficacy study. *Clinical Aphasiology,* Vol. 22 (pp. 245–256). Austin, TX: Pro-Ed.

McNeil, M.R., Doyle, P.J., Spencer, K.A., Goda, A.J., Flores, D., & Small, S.L. (1998). Effects of training multiple form classes on acquisition, generalization and maintenance of word retrieval in a single subject. *Aphasiology, 12,* 561–574.

McReynolds, L. & Kearns, K.P. (1983). *Single-Subject Experimental Design in Communicative Disorders.* Baltimore: University Park Press.

McReynolds, L.V. & Thompson, C.K. (1986). Flexibility of single-subject experimental designs. Part I: Review of the basics of single-subject designs. *J Speech Hearing Dis, 51,* 194–203.

Metter, E.J. (1985). Issues and directions for the future: Speech pathology: A physician's perspective. In R.H. Brookshire (ed.), *Clinical Aphasiology,* Vol. 15 (pp. 22–28). Minneapolis: BRK Publishers.

Milroy, L. & Perkins, L. (1992). Repair strategies in aphasic discourse: Towards a collaborative model. *Clinical Linguistics & Phonetics, 6,* 27–40.

Nation, J.E. & Aram, D.M. (1984). *Diagnosis of Speech and Language Disorders* (2nd ed.). Boston: College-Hill.

Nicholas, L.E. & Brookshire, R.H. (1986). Consistency of the effects of rate of speech on brain-damaged adults' comprehension of narrative discourse. *J Speech Hearing Res, 29,* 462–470.

Nicholas, L.E., Brookshire, R.H., MacLennan, D.L., Schumacher, J.G., & Porazzo, S.A. (1989). Revised administration and scoring procedures for the Boston Naming Test and norms for non-brain-damaged adults. *Aphasiology, 3,* 569–580.

Nicholas, L.E., MacLennan, D.L., & Brookshire, R.H. (1986). Validity of multiple-sentence reading comprehension tests for aphasic adults. *J Speech Hearing Dis, 51,* 82–87.

Packard, M. & Hinckley, J.J. (1999). Measuring conversational burden in adults with moderate and severe aphasia. (Poster presentation, Clinical Aphasiology Conference, Key West, FL.)

Parr, S. (1992). Everyday reading and writing practices of normal adults: Implications for aphasia assessment. *Aphasiology, 3,* 273–284.

Perkins, L. (1995). Applying conversation analysis to aphasia: Clinical implications and analytic issues. *Euro J Dis Comm, 30,* 372–383.

Perkins, L., Crisp, J., & Walshaw, D. (1999). Exploring conversation analysis as an assessment tool for aphasia: The issue of reliability. *Aphasiology, 13,* 259–281.

Porch, B. (1981). *The Porch Index of Communicative Ability.* Palo Alto: Consulting Psychological Press.

Prescott, T.E. (ed.). (1989). *Clinical Aphasiology,* Vol. 18. Boston: College-Hill.

Prescott, T.E. (ed.). (1991a). *Clinical Aphasiology,* Vol. 19. Austin, TX: Pro-Ed.

Prescott, T.E. (ed.). (1991b). *Clinical Aphasiology,* Vol. 20. Austin, TX: Pro-Ed.

Robey, R.R. & Schultz, M.C. (1998). A model for conducting clinical-outcome research: An adaptation of the standard protocol for use in aphasiology. *Aphasiology, 12,* 787–810.

Rosenbek, J.C. (1987). Unusual aphasias: Some criteria for evaluating case studies in aphasiology. In R.H. Brookshire (ed.), *Clinical Aphasiology,* Vol. 17 (pp. 357–361). Minneapolis: BRK Publishers.

Rosenbek, J.C., LaPointe, L.L., & Wertz, R.T. (1989). *Aphasia: A Clinical Approach.* Austin, TX: Pro-Ed.

Roth, V.M. & Katz, R.C. (1998). The role of computers in aphasia rehabilitation. In B. Stemmer & H.A. Whitaker (eds.), *Handbook of Neurolinguistics* (pp.585–596). San Diego: Academic Press.

Schumacher, J.G. & Nicholas, L.E. (1991). Conducting research in a clinical setting against all odds: Unusual treatment of fluent aphasia. In T.E. Prescott (ed.), *Clinical Aphasiology,* Vol. 19 (pp. 267–277). Austin, TX: Pro-Ed.

Shewan, C.M. (1986). The history and efficacy of aphasia treatment. In R. Chapey (ed.), *Language Intervention Strategies in Adult Aphasia* (2nd ed.), (pp. 28–43). Baltimore: Williams & Wilkins.

Shiffrin, D. (1994). *Approaches to Discourse.* Oxford: Blackwell.

Shrout, P.E. & Fleiss, J.L. (1979). Intraclass correlations: Uses in assessing rater reliability. *Psychological Bulletin, 86,* 420–428.

Silverman, F.H. (1985). *Research Design and Evaluation in Speech-Language Pathology and Audiology* (2nd ed.). Englewood Cliffs, NJ: Prentice-Hall.

Simmons, N.N., Kearns, K.P., & Potechin, G. (1987). Treatment of aphasia through family member training. In R.H. Brookshire (ed.), *Clinical Aphasiology,* Vol. 17 (pp. 106–116). Minneapolis: BRK Publishers.

Simmons-Mackie, N. & Damico, J.S. (1996). Accounting for handicaps in aphasia: Communicative assessment from an authentic social perspective. *Disability & Rehabilitation, 18,* 540–549.

Simmons-Mackie, N. & Kagan, A. (1999). Communication strategies used by 'good' versus 'poor' speaking partners of individuals with aphasia. *Aphasiology, 9–11,* 807–820.

Strauss, A. & Corbin, J. (1998). *Basics of Qualitative Research: Techniques and Procedures for Developing Grounded Theory.* Thousand Oaks: Sage.

Szekeres, S.F., Ylvisaker, M., & Cohen, S.B. (1987). A framework for cognitive rehabilitation therapy. In M. Ylvisaker & E.R. Gobble (eds.), *Community Re-entry for Head Injured Adults* (pp. 87–136). Boston: College Hill Press.

Thompson, C.K. (1989). Generalization research in aphasia: A review of the literature. In T.E. Prescott (ed.), *Clinical Aphasiology,* Vol. 18 (pp.195–222). Boston: College-Hill.

Thompson, C.K. & Byrne, M.E. (1984). Across setting generalization of social conventions in aphasia: An experimental analysis of "loose training." In R.H. Brookshire (ed.), *Clinical Aphasiology: Conference Proceedings 1984* (pp. 132–144). Minneapolis: BRK Publishers.

Thompson, C.K. & Shapiro, L.P. (1995). Training sentence production in agrammatism: Implications for normal and disordered language. *Brain & Language, 50,* 201–224.

Tompkins, C.A. (1992). Improving aphasia treatment research: Some methodological considerations. In *Aphasia Treatment: Current approaches and research opportunities* (pp. 37–46). Washington, DC: National Institute on Deafness and Other Communication Disorders.

Tompkins, C.A., Boada, R., McGarry, K., Jones, J., Rahn, A.E., & Ranier, S. (1993). Connected speech characteristics of right hemisphere damaged adults: A re-examination. In M.L. Lemme (ed.), *Clinical Aphasiology,* Vol. 21 (113–122). Austin, TX: Pro-Ed.

Tompkins, C.A., Jackson, S.T., & Schulz, R. (1990). On prognostic research in adult neurogenic disorders. *J Speech Hearing Res, 33,* 398–401.

Ventry, I.M. & Schiavetti, N. (1980). *Evaluating Research in Speech Pathology and Audiology: A Guide for Clinicians and Students.* Reading, MA: Addison-Wesley.

Warren, R.L. (1986). Research design: Considerations for the clinician. In R. Chapey (ed.), *Language Intervention Strategies in Adult Aphasia* (2nd ed.), (pp. 66–80). Baltimore: Williams & Wilkins.

Warren, R.L., Gabriel, C., Johnston, A., & Gaddie, A. (1987). Efficacy during acute rehabilitation. In R.H. Brookshire (ed.), *Clinical Aphasiology,* Vol. 17 (pp. 1–11). Minneapolis: BRK Publishers.

Wertz, R.T. (1985). Neuropathologies of speech and language: An introduction to patient management. In D.F. Johns (ed.), *Clinical Management of Neurogenic Communication Disorders* (2nd ed.), (pp. 1–96). Boston: Little-Brown.

Wertz, R.T. (1991). Predictability: Greater than p < .05. In T.E. Prescott (ed.), *Clinical Aphasiology,* Vol. 19. (pp. 21–30). Austin, TX: Pro-Ed.

Wertz, R.T. (1992). *A Single Case for Group Treatment Studies in Aphasia. Aphasia Treatment: Current Approaches and Research Opportunities* (pp. 25–36). Washington, DC: National Institute on Deafness and Other Communication Disorders.

Wertz, R.T., Collins, M.J., Weiss, D., Kurtzke, J.F., Friden, T., Brookshire, R.H., Pierce, J., Holtzapple, P., Hubbard, D.J., Porch, B.E., West, J.A., Davis, L., Matovitch, V., Morley, G.K., & Resurreccion, E. (1981). Veterans Administration Cooperative Study on Aphasia: A comparison of individual and group treatment. *J Speech Hearing Res, 24,* 580–594.

Wertz, R.T., Shubitowski, Y., Dronkers, N.F., Lemme, M.L., & Deal, J.L. (1985). Word fluency measure reliability in normal and brain damaged adults. Paper presented at the American Speech-Language-Hearing Association convention, Washington, DC.

Wertz, R.T., Weiss, D.G., Aten, J.L., Brookshire, R.H., Garcia-Bunuel, L., Holland, A.L., Kurtzke, J.F., LaPointe, L.L., Milianti, F.J., Brannegan, R., Greenbaum, H., Marshall, R.C., Vogel, D., Carter, J., Barnes, N.S., & Goodman, R. (1986). Comparison of clinic, home, and deferred language treatment for aphasia: A Veterans Administration cooperative study. *Archives of Neurology, 43,* 653–658.

Whitney, J.L. & Goldstein, H. (1989). Using self-monitoring to reduce disfluencies in speakers with mild aphasia. *J Speech Hearing Dis, 54,* 576–586.

World Health Organization (1999). *International Classification of Functioning and Disability.* Beta-2 draft, Geneva: WHO.

Yorkston, K.M., Farrier, L., Zeches, J., & Uomoto, J.M. (1990). Discourse patterns in traumatically brain injured and control subjects. Paper presented at the American Speech-Language-Hearing Association convention, Washington, DC.

Yorkston, K.M., Zeches, J., Farrier, L., & Uomoto, J.M. (1993). Lexical pitch as a measure of word choice in narratives of traumatically brain injured and control subjects. *Clinical Aphasiology,* Vol. 21 (165–172). Austin, TX: Pro-Ed.

Yoshihata, H., Toshiko, W., Chujo, T., & Kaori, M. (1998). Acquisition and generalization of mode interchange skills in people with severe aphasia. *Aphasiology, 12,* 1035–1045.

Chapter 6

Aphasia Treatment: Recovery, Prognosis, and Clinical Effectiveness

Leora R. Cherney and Randall R. Robey

OBJECTIVES

The objectives of this chapter are to (1) describe the typical time course and pattern of recovery in individuals with aphasia; (2) review current information regarding the neuroanatomical and neurophysiological mechanisms underlying recovery; (3) discuss the contributions of the right and left hemispheres to recovery from aphasia; (4) identify neurologic and personal factors affecting prognosis; (5) differentiate types of scientific evidence and clinical outcomes; and (6) discuss scientific evidence obtained through tests of aphasia treatment efficacy and effectiveness.

Clinicians who treat individuals with aphasia have frequently sought to uncover indicators of recovery. Reliable information regarding what factors are associated with positive recovery as well as what factors are associated with negative recovery impact several clinical decisions and actions, including determining prognosis, counseling significant others, and identifying candidates for treatment. In a recent review, Basso (1992) has differentiated between neurological factors and anagraphical factors. Neurological factors are related to etiology, size and site of lesion, and severity and type of aphasia. In addition, through modern neuroimaging technologies, there has been an increased focus on pathophysiological indicators of recovery and the long-term cerebral changes related to resolving aphasia. Anagraphical factors include personal characteristics such as age, sex, handedness, and health status. One of the difficulties encountered in research on recovery from aphasia and prognosis is that many of these factors are interrelated. For example, site of lesion determines to some extent the type of aphasia; size of lesion and type of aphasia have some implications for severity; and type of aphasia may not be independent of age. Nonetheless, clinicians have relied on the extensive literature examining the effects of these factors on recovery to guide their clinical decision-making.

The range of clinical decisions extends beyond prognosis and candidate identification. Once the decision to treat is warranted, clinicians must settle on justifiable treatment(s), a weekly schedule of treatment, and the duration of treatment. The purpose of this chapter is to review the information base underpinning the broad range of clinical decisions from prognosis to treatment schedules. The chapter proceeds in two major sections. First, studies related to recovery are reviewed, with particular emphasis on the factors that may be considered when determining prognosis. Second, the scientific base underlying treatment-related decisions is reviewed, with a focus on the sequence of advancements that has been made in research methodology in this area. However, the sectioning has been imposed merely for organization purposes and it will be readily apparent that these topics are not mutually exclusive, and, in fact, interact with one another.

RECOVERY

Time Course of Recovery

Two different stages in the recovery of function have been differentiated, an early stage and a late stage (Kertesz, 1988). The early stage, which is when maximum language recovery takes place, coincides with the period of spontaneous recovery, and is considered by investigators to occur within 1–3 months post onset of aphasia (Kertesz & McCabe, 1977; Vignolo, 1964). Spontaneous recovery drops precipitously by 6–7 months post onset (Vignolo, 1964), with little or no spontaneous recovery occurring after one year (Kertesz & McCabe, 1977; Kertesz et al., 1979). Therefore, spontaneous recovery has a decelerating curve, steepest in the first month post onset, subsequently flattening out, and finally reaching a plateau between 6 and 12 months post-onset (Basso, 1992; Benson & Ardila, 1996).

A recent prospective study of 330 patients with aphasia supports a pattern of recovery from aphasia consistent with that of spontaneous recovery (Pederson et al., 1995). Patients with aphasia were evaluated on admission to the hospital, weekly during their hospital stay, and then at 6 months post-discharge. The investigators found that stationary language function was reached in 84% of the patients within two weeks, and in 95% of the patients within six weeks from stroke onset. Similarly, Pashek and Holland (1988), in their longitudinal study of 43 individuals with aphasia, noted that improvement most frequently began at about 1–2 weeks post onset; furthermore, by three months, the clinical status of most of the patients approximated the clinical status that was measured at 12 months.

Late or long-term recovery may take place months or even years after stroke onset. However, the degree of recovery can vary greatly from patient to patient. For example, Hanson et al. (1989) conducted a retrospective study that followed 35 males with aphasia from 3–55 months post onset. Patients were evaluated with the Porch Index of Communicative Abilities (PICA) on five factors—speaking, writing, comprehension, gesturing, and copying. Language performance continued to evolve over years, with some patients improving significantly, others stabilizing, and others (10 of 35) regressing. No medical factor could be found to account for the regression, but it was noted that language decline occurred in those patients with relatively milder aphasia.

Pattern of Recovery

Despite individual variation in rate and extent of recovery, there seem to be some general patterns of recovery that have been identified for each type of aphasia. Kertesz and McCabe (1977) studied the evolution of aphasia using the Western Aphasia Battery aphasia quotients obtained serially at 45 days, and at 3, 6, and 12 months. They found that 39 of 93 patients (41.9%) changed aphasia type as they recovered. Similarly, Pashek and Holland (1988) followed 43 subjects from the acute stage (within 5 days post onset) and subsequently at 3, 6, and 12 months post onset. Using descriptive criteria to define aphasia type, they found that approximately 60% of the sample evolved and were reclassified, with each type of aphasia showing a pattern of evolution. They noted that change most frequently began at about 2 weeks post onset, with most types of aphasia evolving within the first month (except conduction aphasia, which typically showed a change at about 6 months post onset) to that of anomic aphasia. Patients who presented initially with a fluent aphasia continued to demonstrate a fluent type of aphasia. Anomic aphasia was often the end-point attained by patients regardless of whether they initially presented with fluent or nonfluent aphasia (Kertesz & McCabe, 1977; Pashek & Holland, 1988).

McDermott et al. (1996) have provided further information about the evolution of the different aphasia types. They followed 39 patients and evaluated them regularly with the Western Aphasia Battery. They confirmed that the direction of evolution appears to operate under some constraints,

and that aphasia subtypes differ in their evolution. Like Pashek and Holland (1988), they found that patients who presented initially with a fluent aphasia continued to demonstrate a fluent type of aphasia. For example, of 7 patients with Wernicke's aphasia, 2 evolved to conduction aphasia, and 5 to anomic aphasia. Of 3 patients with transcortical sensory aphasia, 1 remained unchanged while 2 evolved to anomic aphasia. Of 3 patients with conduction aphasia, 2 remained unchanged and 1 evolved to an anomic aphasia.

The investigators also noted that aphasia severity may interact with the evolution of aphasia (McDermott et al., 1996). Patients with nonfluent or fluent aphasia who evolved from one aphasia type to another were less severe than those who did not evolve. However, magnitude of change, and not initial severity, was the critical variable underlying aphasia evolution. Those patients who evolved from one aphasia type to another had greater aphasia quotient changes from the first test session to the second than those who did not, suggesting that improvement in language performance is a necessary condition for evolution of aphasia type. Specifically, it was found that an aphasia quotient change of 20 points or more predicated aphasia type evolution in about two-thirds of the patients with both fluent and nonfluent aphasia.

Several studies have investigated the evolution of typology in patients with severe or global aphasia. Pashek and Holland (1988) found that age was a factor in the evolution from global aphasia. There was a trend for younger patients to evolve to a Broca's aphasia, while older patients remained global or evolved to a Wernicke's aphasia.

Nicholas et al. (1993) followed 24 subjects with severe aphasia, of which 17 were global. Patients were scheduled for evaluation with the Boston Assessment of Severe Aphasia (BASA) at 1–2 months, 6, 12, 18, and 24 months post onset, but not all subjects were tested at all time periods. The greatest amount of improvement occurred in the first 6 months. While most of the patients with global aphasia showed improvements on the BASA, they did not change classification and remained global.

From a study of 54 patients with global aphasia, Ferro (1992) concluded that there are five different types of global aphasia, depending on the site of lesion, and each type has different outcomes. Patients with global aphasia resulting from large fronto-temporal-parietal lesions with or without subcortical damage had the poorest prognosis and remained global at follow-up. In contrast, the best prognosis was found for those patients with large subcortical infarcts. None of these patients remained global; one patient was not aphasic at follow-up, while the others evolved to transcortical motor aphasia or anomic aphasia. The other three possible localizations for the infarcts that cause acute global aphasia are as follows: frontal lesions with or without subcortical involvement; posterior parietal infarct, with or without subcortical involvement; and a double lesion composed of a frontal and temporal cortical infarct. These patients showed a variable degree of recovery, improving to Broca's or transcortical aphasia. Ferro (1992) also found that the first three months was the crucial period for improvement, in contrast to the findings of Sarno and Levita (1971), who suggested that the greatest changes for global aphasia were evident in the 6–12 month period post stroke.

Several longitudinal studies have considered the pattern of recovery as it relates to the individual language modalities, and a consistent trend has emerged. Typically, a higher percentage of patients improve in comprehension as opposed to production, and a higher percentage improve in oral as opposed to written language (Kenin & Swisher, 1972; Hanson & Cicciarelli, 1978; Lomas & Kertesz, 1978; Prins et al., 1978). Basso et al. (1982) found that improvements of oral and written comprehension and production were usually associated. However, in some patients who do not receive rehabilitation, comprehension may be the only modality to improve.

These results are supported by Mazzoni et al. (1992), who assessed a selected sample of 45 patients, none of whom received language therapy, over a 7-month period of time. The investigators found that comprehension had the best recovery, independent of type and severity of aphasia. In addition, differences in language recovery were evident in relation to type of aphasia. For patients with fluent aphasia, oral expression and written expression improved steadily throughout the 7 months. Auditory comprehension improved for 4 months, while reading comprehension improved over the first month. For patients with nonfluent aphasia, significant improvement was evident in auditory comprehension over a 4-month period of time. Expression showed less recovery, often because it was negatively influenced by the presence of oral apraxia, while no significant changes were evident in written language. Similarly, Hanson et al. (1989) contend that recovery of language modalities may be dependent on the category of the aphasia. However, they caution that differences in recovery between aphasia categories may become apparent only after 2 years post onset.

Severity of Aphasia

The initial severity of the aphasia is an important factor to consider in the recovery from aphasia, not only because of its direct impact on outcome (Basso, 1992; Marshall et al., 1982, 1983; Paolucci et al., 1996), but also because of its interaction with other factors affecting recovery. Indeed, Pederson et al. (1995) have stated that initial aphasia severity is the single most important factor for ultimate language function. Furthermore, in their investigation of the time course of recovery, they found that patients with more severe aphasia demonstrated a longer period of language recovery than patients with less severe aphasia. More specifically, 95% of patients with severe aphasia reached maximum function within 10 weeks; 95% of patients with

moderate aphasia reached maximum function within 6 weeks, while only 2 weeks was required for 95% of those with a mild aphasia to achieve maximum function.

Mazzoni et al. (1992) also found that initial severity was related to outcome of each language modality. For a moderately severe group of 21 patients, both oral expression and written expression improved uniformly over 7 months; auditory and reading comprehension showed no significant improvement, because performance on these modalities was at a near normal level initially. For a severely impaired group of 24 patients, auditory comprehension and to a lesser extent, reading comprehension improved significantly, while no significant improvement was observed for oral expression or written expression. Similarly, Mark et al. (1992) found that initial severity as measured by performance on language tests, rather than neuroradiologic characteristics, correlated strongly with outcome for a group of patients with global aphasia.

Neural Mechanisms of Recovery

The preceding discussion has focused primarily on providing a descriptive account of recovery from aphasia. However, it is important to consider, also, the neural mechanisms contributing to recovery. While these are not completely understood, technological advances in the area of brain imaging have allowed researchers to address those factors that play a role in early and long-term recovery.

Bach-Y-Rita (1990) has summarized the possible neural mechanisms that occur in both the immediate period after a stroke and during long-term recovery. Spontaneous recovery, which occurs naturally without special treatment, may be due, in part, to the resolution of local factors such as the reduction of cerebral edema, the absorption of damaged tissue, and improvement of local circulation. However, these factors probably do not play a role in long-term recovery of function (Bach-Y-Rita, 1990).

Rather, of greater interest to the rehabilitation professional, are those factors associated with brain plasticity. Brain plasticity, which permits enduring functional changes to occur, refers to the capacity to modify structural organization and functioning. According to Bach-Y-Rita (1990), several mechanisms may contribute to brain plasticity: 1) Diaschisis refers to depressed function at a distance from the lesion, due to the sudden interruption of synaptic connections. Diaschisis may occur within the left hemisphere as well as in the contralateral one (Feeney & Baron, 1986; Andrews, 1991). Some long-term recovery may occur with the dissipation of diaschisis, although its mechanisms are not well understood. 2) Regenerative and collateral sprouting refers to changes in connections between neurons from intact cells to denervated regions. Collateral sprouting has been demonstrated in some neural structures including the thalamus and cerebellum. While collateral sprouting may be a mechanism of functional recovery, it also may be a maladaptive response, leading to abnormal function. Further studies are needed to clarify its importance to recovery from central nervous system lesions. 3) Unmasking of preexisting but functionally depressed pathways or substitution may be the most important mechanism for recovery. It occurs when axons and synapses which are present but not used for the particular function under study can be called on when the usually dominant system fails.

Cappa and Vallar (1992) have summarized the current thinking about the neurophysiologic mechanisms underlying recovery from aphasia. They acknowledge that improvements in language function in the early period following a stroke may reflect regression of neurological dysfunction in areas outside the structural lesion (diaschisis) both in the contralateral hemisphere and in non-perisylvian left hemispheric regions. After this early stage of recovery (1–2 months), rate and extent of recovery are largely dependent on the site and size of the area of structural damage in the left perisylvian language areas as shown by CT or MRI. In addition, some participation of right hemisphere in the long-term phase of recovery is likely. However, complete recovery can be expected only if some crucial structures in the left hemisphere, e.g., Wernicke's area, are not completely destroyed.

In the following sections, research investigating the effects of the size and site of lesion is presented. This is followed by a discussion of the role of the right hemisphere in recovery from aphasia, and a review of selected neurophysiologic studies implicating the right hemisphere and/or the importance of intact left hemisphere structures for recovery.

Lesion Size and Site

A basic assumption about recovery from aphasia has been that lesion size exerts a negative influence on recovery (Kertesz et al., 1979, 1993; Selnes et al., 1983; Ludlow et al., 1986; Demeurisse & Capon, 1987; Ferro, 1992; Mazzoni et al., 1992; Goldenberg & Spatt, 1994). Furthermore, lesion size may affect each modality differentially. For example, Selnes et al. (1983) found that there was a significant negative correlation between lesional volume and recovery of comprehension for large but not smaller lesions. According to Mazzoni et al. (1992), patients with small lesions demonstrated significant recovery in oral expression and written expression; comprehension changes were not significant because comprehension was relatively unimpaired initially. Patients with medium-sized lesions improved significantly in all modalities except written expression, while those with large lesions demonstrated improvement in auditory comprehension only. However, Basso (1992) asserts that while the negative effect of extent of lesion on initial severity of aphasia is unquestionable, once initial severity has been taken into account, the effect of lesion size on recovery is not clear-cut.

In a series of studies that looked at location and extent of lesion on CT scans and the severity of impairment in different groups of aphasic individuals, Naeser and colleagues (1987, 1989, 1990) indicated that rather than total lesion size, it is the size of the lesion within specific areas that may affect recovery from aphasia. In their study of 10 patients with Wernicke's aphasia (Naeser, 1987), there was no correlation between total temporoparietal lesion size and severity of auditory comprehension. However, a correlation was found between the amount of temporal lobe damage within Wernicke's area and severity of auditory comprehension. If damage was in half or less of Wernicke's area, patients exhibited good comprehension at 6 months post onset. If the lesion involved more than half of Wernicke's area, patients exhibited poor comprehension, even at 1 year post onset. Furthermore, anterior-inferior temporal lobe extension into the middle temporal gyrus area was associated with particularly poor recovery.

Similarly, Kertesz et al. (1993) correlated outcome measures of aphasia severity and comprehension with lesion extent in 22 patients with Wernicke's aphasia. Like Naeser et al. (1987), they found that the extent of involvement within specific structures, rather than overall lesion size, contributed to the prediction of language recovery. The angular gyrus and the anterior mid temporal area were important for overall language recovery, while the extent of involvement of angular gyrus contributed most significantly to recovery of auditory comprehension at 1 year. With regard to rate of recovery, involvement of the supramarginal gyrus was associated with poor recovery rates of both overall language and auditory comprehension. Partial sparing of the posterior superior temporal gyrus was associated significantly with the highest recovery rates for comprehension.

The importance of lesion extent within specific structures has also been demonstrated with regard to spontaneous language output (Naeser et al., 1989). Twenty-seven patients with aphasia were divided into two groups based on the severity of their spontaneous speech. The more severe group presented with no speech or only stereotypies where no meaningful verbal information was conveyed; the less severe group presented with Broca's aphasia characterized by reduced, hesitant, poorly articulated, agrammatic speech. CT scan analysis revealed no single neuroanatomical area that contained an extensive lesion that could be used to distinguish the more severe from the less severe group. However, the two groups were separable on the basis of the CT scan when the extent of the lesion in two subcortical white matter areas were combined. The two subcortical white matter pathway areas which, when damaged, severely limited spontaneous speech were the most medial and rostral portion of the subcallosal fasciculus, and the periventricular white matter near the body of the lateral ventricle, deep to the lower motor/sensory cortex area for the mouth.

The involvement of Wernicke's area is an important factor to consider also in recovery from global aphasia. Naeser et al. (1990) examined CT scans of 14 patients with global aphasia. Based on the CT scan information, patients were divided into two groups. One group had large cortical/subcortical frontal, parietal, and temporal lobe lesions that included more than half of Wernicke's area. The other group had large cortical/subcortical frontal and parietal lesions; Wernicke's area was spared, although the lesion extended to the subcortical temporal lobe including the temporal isthmus. Language assessment was conducted initially at 1–4 months post onset and then again after 1 year post onset. Significantly more recovery in auditory comprehension had taken place at 1–2 years post onset for the group that did not have lesions involving Wernicke's area. There was no significant difference between the two groups in recovery of spontaneous speech, word repetition, and naming, where severe deficits continued.

None of the studies discussed above have examined the effects of lesion size in patients who are more than 3 years post onset. However, in two recent studies, it has been shown that in some patients with aphasia, a visible expansion in lesion size can be observed on CT scans after at least 3 years (Naeser et al., 1998; van Zagten et al., 1996). The increase in lesion size in the left hemisphere had no adverse effect on language, as long as the expansion was unilateral and gradual (Naeser et al., 1998). While the physiological mechanisms underlying the lesion expansion are not understood, these results provide further support for the contention that lesion size alone is not necessarily an important factor to consider for recovery (Heiss et al., 1993, 1999).

Most studies on the effects of lesion size and location have not considered how these factors impact language therapy outcome. Recently, Goldenberg & Spatt (1994) investigated if size/site of lesion had differential effects during spontaneous recovery as compared to a period of intensive treatment (since language therapy may employ mechanisms that are different from those at work during spontaneous recovery). They followed 18 patients with aphasia across a period of 8 weeks of spontaneous recovery, 8 weeks of intensive language therapy, and a follow-up period of 8 weeks without treatment. Consistent with previous findings, they found that lesion size negatively influenced recovery in all phases, but lesion location was more important to consider. Patients with lesions to the temporobasal regions showed a similar amount of spontaneous recovery than patients without such lesions, but less improvement during therapy and less total recovery.

Neurophysiologic Studies of Recovery

The neuroimaging CT and MRI studies discussed previously have allowed quantification of site and size of lesions, focusing primarily on the structural damage related to the aphasia.

More recently, technological advances such as PET, SPECT, and functional MRI have permitted investigators to focus on the functional consequences of the lesion. Basically three approaches have been used to yield information about brain function and recovery following onset of aphasia (Mimura et al., 1998). One approach has been to quantify the relationship between characteristics of different aphasia types of varying severity to regional cerebral blood flow (CBF) and/or cerebral metabolism in order to find a functional pattern for language deficits. A second approach has been to correlate longitudinally clinical aphasia recovery status to dynamic changes evidenced by functional neuroimaging. Thirdly, increases in CBF and/or cerebral metabolism in specific brain regions have been investigated using activation methods, searching for a precise increased CBF locus associated with language functions.

Results of these neurophysiologic studies are not always comparable because of differences in the imaging techniques and the task paradigms that are used. For example, task paradigms have included reading sentences (Thulborn et al., 1999), verb retrieval (Warburton et al., 1999), and word repetition (Ohyama et al., 1997). Furthermore, patient differences such as variability in time post onset and type and severity of aphasia also prevent direct comparison of study results. Nonetheless, there is a rapidly accumulating body of literature that is beginning to shed some light on our understanding of the process of recovery. Several recent studies have been selected as illustrative and are described below in relation to the roles of the right and left hemispheres in recovery.

Roles of the Right and Left Hemispheres in Recovery

One of the mechanisms underlying late recovery and the functional reorganization of language during recovery pertains to the role of the right hemisphere. Numerous studies have demonstrated that right hemisphere participation in recovery from aphasia is likely and that the right hemisphere may play a crucial role in recovery from aphasia. For example, case studies have been documented in which individuals become aphasic after a left hemisphere stroke, demonstrate some recovery of language, and then have a right hemisphere stroke with subsequent worsening of language function (Basso et al., 1989; Cappa & Vallar, 1992). Dichotic listening studies have shown an increased left ear advantage in aphasic patients (Moore & Papanicolaou, 1988). Evoked potential studies have demonstrated increased participation of the right hemisphere during language tasks (Papanicolaou et al., 1988), while regional cerebral blood flow studies (rCBF) in recovered aphasics reveal increased right hemisphere participation in language functions (Knopman et al., 1984).

Silvestrini et al. (1998) used bilateral transcranial Doppler ultrasonography to measure blood flow velocity in the two middle cerebral arteries during a rest period and during execution of a word-fluency task. Subjects were 26 stroke patients with Broca's aphasia and 25 healthy controls. Flow velocity changes (the percentage of increase from rest to the word-fluency task) were measured within 21 days of onset and then again after 2 months. At this time, patients were classified into two groups based on the extent of their recovery. The good recovery group included 16 patients, while the poor recovery group included 10 patients. It is noteworthy that the two groups were comparable on initial performance of the word-fluency task obtained prior to 21 days; furthermore, lesion size also was not significantly different.

At the initial evaluation, flow velocity changes on the right side were comparable between the two patient groups and between the patient groups and healthy controls. However, flow velocity change in the left hemisphere middle cerebral artery was significantly less in the poor recovery group as compared to the good recovery group and control subjects. Therefore, the presence of an activation of areas within the lesioned left hemisphere soon after stroke onset seems to be a predictor of recovery from aphasia.

When flow velocity changes were compared between the first and second evaluations, the poor recovery group showed a hemodynamic pattern on both sides that was similar. In contrast, the flow velocity change for the good recovery group was similar at both times in the left middle cerebral artery, but significantly greater on the right side at the time of the second evaluation. These results support the involvement of cerebral areas contralateral to the lesion in language recovery from aphasia (Silvestrini et al., 1995, 1998).

A PET study by Cappa et al. (1997) also provides support for the role of the right hemisphere in recovery of aphasia. Eight patients with mild aphasia were assessed within 2 weeks of stroke onset and then 6 months later. At initial testing, analysis of regional glucose metabolism showed hypometabolism in structurally unaffected regions both in the left and right hemispheres (diaschisis). It is likely that this functional depression contributed to the severity of the clinical picture in the acute period after stroke. At the second PET study, when some recovery of language function had occurred, glucose metabolism increased significantly on both sides. However, no metabolic recovery was found in left temporo-parietal, visual associative, and premotor/motor cortices, while normalization of contralateral regions was evident. Specifically, glucose metabolism of the recovered aphasics and the control subjects did not differ significantly in the right hemisphere. Therefore, the investigators concluded that language recovery is associated with regression of functional depression in structurally unaffected areas, in particular in the right hemisphere.

Recently, Thulborn et al. (1999) used functional MRI to follow two patients during recovery from acute stroke and aphasia. Both patients, as well as a group of six normal adults, participated in a simple sentence reading paradigm for functional MRI. This included a rest condition of 30 seconds, followed by silent reading of simple sentences (mean length of 5.5 words). Each sentence was followed by a question requiring a true/false answer which the patient indicated by one or two finger switches. In the normal individuals, the activation pattern represented a large-scale network that included left side asymmetrical activation of Broca's and Wernicke's areas, and symmetrical involvement of the frontal eye fields.

The first patient was evaluated at 5 hours, 76 hours, and 6 months after the abrupt onset of a middle cerebral artery stroke affecting Broca's area. Recovery from aphasia occurred rapidly with a shift of activation within 3 days from Broca's area to the homologous region in the right hemisphere. Rightward lateralization continued so that by 6 months the dominance was totally right sided. Wernicke's area, which was structurally undamaged, was completely left dominant at 76 hours, and remained strongly left dominant at 6 months. For the second patient, who had a stroke involving Wernicke's area, functional MRI data was available prior to the stroke, with additional evaluations repeated at 3 and 9 months post onset. Activation of Wernicke's area changed progressively from a strong left hemisphere dominance before the stroke, to weak right dominance at 3 months and considerable right hemisphere dominance at 9 months. In both patients, no new nodes of activation other than those observed in normal subjects were identified. These results support the hypothesis that clinical recovery is associated with spontaneous redistribution of function to the right hemisphere, followed by consolidation of this pattern over subsequent months of recovery from aphasia.

Other studies have implicated not only the contralateral hemisphere, but also structures in the ipsilateral hemisphere (Demeurisse & Capon, 1987; Metter et al., 1992). Weiller et al. (1995) assessed six recovered patients who had an initial diagnosis of severe Wernicke's aphasia. Regional CBF was measured under three conditions that included rest, silent generation of verbs to spoken nouns, and silent repetition of pseudowords. The increased activation in the left frontal language areas and right perisylvian regions and additional activation in right lateral prefrontal cortex imply that both hemispheres may contribute to recovery from aphasia.

Thomas et al. (1997) have suggested not only that both hemispheres contribute to recovery from aphasia, but also that lateralization patterns change over time and vary with aphasia subtype. They used cortical DC-potential distribution monitoring during language processing to compare patterns of lateralization between normal subjects and individuals with aphasia. The patients were tested twice, initially during the acute phase and later when recovery from aphasia was evident, an average of 12.2 months later. Normal individuals demonstrated a strong lateralization shift toward the left frontal region and central regions at both testing times. At initial testing, the individuals with aphasia did not demonstrate this strong left lateralization. However, the absence of lateralization was not because of dampening of activation in the left frontal hemisphere, but rather because of increased activation in the right hemisphere. At the second testing, all but one of the patients had changed their frontal lateralization pattern. Patients with Broca's aphasia shifted back towards a left hemisphere lateralization; those with Wernicke's aphasia shifted toward the right.

Some studies have investigated recovery of specific language modalities such as oral expression or auditory comprehension. Mlcoch et al. (1994) investigated the relationship between diminished regional cerebral blood flow (rCBF) on SPECT and the recovery of fluent speech in 14 nonfluent aphasic patients. Measurements of speech fluency were acquired initially and at 3 months after infarction. Only the inferior frontal area was significantly associated with recovery of fluent speech. This region was hypoperfused in 4 of 5 patients with poor recovery while 8 of the 9 patients with good speech fluency recovery demonstrated normal rCBF to the inferior frontal region.

In a study of 22 patients with aphasia caused by a single left middle cerebral artery lesion, Karbe et al. (1995) demonstrated that the degree of regional left hemispheric hypometabolism measured early after stroke with positron emission tomography predicts the long-term prognosis of aphasia. Specifically, early cerebral metabolic rates of glucose in the left superior temporal cortex correlated with Token Test scores obtained at 2 years post onset, while early cerebral metabolic rates of glucose in the left prefrontal cortex correlated with word fluency scores.

Similarly, Heiss et al. (1997) studied six stroke patients with clinically significant aphasia at 4 weeks and again at 12–18 months after onset of a left hemispheric stroke. The regional cerebral metabolic rate of glucose (rCMRglc) was measured repeatedly by PET at rest and during word repetition, and severity of speech impairment was assessed by a neuropsychologic test battery. The patterns of speech-associated activation of glucose metabolism were related to improvement in language performance. Three patients experienced significant recovery as measured by improved Token test scores whereas three patients had poor outcome. Good recovery was related to activation of left hemispheric speech areas surrounding the infarct, especially left superior temporal gyrus. In contrast, the three patients with persistent aphasia showed rCMRglc recruitment in right hemispheric regions and were unable to activate left hemispheric speech areas on follow-up. These results indicate that favorable outcome is related to partial sparing of speech areas of the dominant hemisphere that can be (re-) activated. Furthermore, the investigators suggest that predominant recruitment of contralateral areas is not an indicator of recovery from aphasia. Rather, it indicates nonspecific involvement of widespread networks in the effort to perform a complex task.

In another study, Karbe et al. (1998) obtained PET activation data within 3–4 weeks post-stroke, and then again at more than a year post-onset. Individuals were examined both at rest and during a word repetition task. Initially, metabolic activations in the left cortex, specifically the left superior temporal and left precentral areas, were significantly reduced or even lost; however, corresponding right superior temporal and right precentral areas showed typical activation patterns similar to those of the 10 controls. Additional activation of supplementary motor area was seen, more on the left than on the right. Some patients also activated the right inferior frontal cortex (right hemisphere counterpart of Broca's area). At follow-up more than 1 year post stroke, the additional activation of the right hemisphere regions had disappeared, while the left hemispheric superior temporal activation had recovered. The investigators concluded that a good long-term outcome seemed to depend mainly on repair of left superior temporal cortex function, whereas recruitment of right hemisphere regions was significantly less effective. These findings are consistent with previous studies which also demonstrated that recovery of left superior temporal activation sometimes occurred several months after stroke and that this repair or reorganization of the language areas of the cortex was important for a good outcome of aphasia (Karbe et al., 1995, 1997).

Heiss et al. (1999) conducted a prospective PET study of a larger group of 23 aphasic patients and a control group of 11 volunteers. The aphasic patients were divided into three groups depending on site of lesion. There were 7 subjects with major parts of the infarct in the anterior middle cerebral artery territory (frontal group), 7 patients with major parts of the infarct in the posterior middle cerebral artery territory (temporal group), and 9 patients with infarcts affecting the basal ganglia and parts of subcortical white matter, but not cortical regions (subcortical group). Language testing and PET measurement under a word-repetition task were applied twice, 2 and 8 weeks after the acute stroke. During the interim period of 6 weeks, all groups of patients showed improvement. However, different overall outcomes at 8 weeks were evident, with the subcortical group demonstrating minimal disturbances, the frontal group showing moderate disturbances, and the temporal group showing persisting severe aphasia. Results of the PET measurements indicated a differential pattern of activation at each testing time dependent on site of lesion. The subcortical and frontal groups showed similar patterns. They activated the right inferior frontal gyrus and right superior temporal gyrus at baseline and regained left superior temporal gyrus activation at follow-up. The temporal group, which had more limited recovery, activated the left Broca's area and supplementary motor area at baseline; at follow-up the precentral gyrus bilaterally, as well as the right superior temporal gyrus were activated, but they could not reactivate the left superior temporal gyrus. According to the investigators, these differential activation patterns suggest a hierarchy within the language-related network, and stress the inferior role of the right hemisphere language-related network for recovery from poststroke aphasia. They suggest that efficient restoration of language is only achieved if the left temporal areas are preserved and can be reintegrated into the functional network. However, if important left hemispheric regions are destroyed, right hemisphere areas may contribute.

Warburton et al. (1999) also concluded that even limited salvage of peri-infarct tissue in the left hemisphere will have an important impact on rehabilitation and recovery. They compared regional brain activations in response to a verb retrieval task in normal subjects and in six aphasic subjects who had shown some recovery and were able to attempt the task. PET scans using oxygen-15–labelled water as tracer to index regional cerebral blood flow were conducted at rest and during the verb retrieval task. There was little evidence of a laterality shift of word retrieval functions to the right temporal lobe after the left hemisphere lesion. Rather, left inferolateral temporal activation was seen in all patients except one—and he was inefficient at the task.

Mimura et al. (1998) studied the relationship between post-stroke recovery from aphasia and changes in cerebral blood flow, both prospectively and retrospectively, using single photon emission computed tomography (SPECT) scans. Prospectively, 20 patients were evaluated at 3 months and 9 months post onset. A significant correlation between severity of initial language deficits and initial CBF on the left side was found, but not on the right side. In addition, the change in left CBF (but not right) correlated with change in language performance between 3 and 9 months. In the retrospective study, 16 patients with middle cerebral artery territory stroke received language testing and SPECT at a mean of 82.8 months post onset. Language test scores from 6 months post onset were also reviewed. It was found that left CBF did not differentiate good recovery from poor recovery groups. However, right CBF in frontal and thalamic regions and left CBF in frontal regions was higher in the patients who demonstrated good language recovery than in those who showed poor language recovery. The results of these complementary studies indicate that language recovery in the first year post onset is linked to functional recovery in the dominant hemisphere; subsequent language recovery may be related to slow and gradual compensatory functions in the contralateral hemisphere, particularly in the frontal and thalamic areas.

In a review of the mechanisms of recovery in aphasia, Del Toro (1997) notes that much of the data pertaining to cerebral changes and behavioral recovery are largely correlational and the link between specific neuroplasmic changes and recovery from aphasia remains obscure. She also reminds us that the aphasia we observe after a stroke is not just a result of a lesion in the language-dominant hemisphere, but also the result of what the left and the right hemisphere are doing in response to that lesion. As further studies yield new information or confirm previous information, we will move closer to understanding the neural mechanisms that mediate recovery. This is an important issue because better knowledge of these mechanisms may lead to better management of the patient with aphasia and better prediction of outcome.

Personal Factors Affecting Prognosis

Although personal and biographical factors appear to play only a minor role in recovery from aphasia as compared to neurological factors (Benson & Ardila, 1996), these factors should not be ignored. Indeed, factors of age, handedness, and gender have been studied experimentally, with some conflicting evidence regarding their effects.

Age

Some studies that have addressed the effects of age on recovery suggest that younger patients have a more favorable outcome than older ones (Vignolo, 1964; Sands et al., 1969; Gloning et al., 1976; Marshall et al., 1982). Other studies have not found age to have a significant effect on recovery (Sarno & Levita, 1971; Keenan & Brassell, 1974; Messerli et al., 1976; Kertesz & McCabe, 1977; Basso et al., 1979; Sarno, 1992; Heiss et al., 1993; Pederson et al., 1995).

In a review of prognostic factors in aphasia, Basso (1992) cautions that the interaction of age with type of aphasia must be considered because patients with fluent aphasia may be older than patients with nonfluent aphasia (Obler et al., 1978; Basso et al., 1980; De Renzi et al., 1980; Miceli et al., 1981; Code & Rowley, 1987; Ferro & Madureira, 1997). Since type of aphasia may be the prognostic factor rather than age, any studies of the effects of age on recovery must control for type of aphasia.

Similarly, the effects of age on recovery must be considered in relation to etiology. Advanced age may be associated with etiological factors predicting poor outcome (Henley et al., 1985). For example, patients with aphasia resulting from open or closed head injury appear to recover better than patients with aphasia resulting from stroke (Kertesz & McCabe, 1977; Basso et al., 1982; Benson & Ardila, 1996). This may be explained in part by age differences, since trauma usually affects younger individuals. Individuals with hemorrhagic strokes, who usually are somewhat younger than patients with occlusive strokes, typically have a good prognosis for language recovery after the mass effect is eliminated; in contrast, the prognosis for occlusive strokes is more limited depending on the site of the infarction (Rubens, 1977; Basso, 1992; Benson & Ardilla, 1996).

The effects of age on recovery should also be considered in relation to general health status. For example, in a prospective study of outcome following ischemic stroke, older individuals with a more severe initial stroke demonstrated poorer general outcome at 3 months post onset (Macciocchi et al.,

1998). The study also indicated that there was a correlation of age with comorbidities such as medical, psychosocial, and psychiatric disorders, which may not emerge as independent predictors of outcome. Such factors as history of prior stroke, as well as history of hypertension, diabetes, or cardiac disease, have been associated with poorer outcome after stroke, and the impact of these comorbid disorders may be greater in older persons. These findings are consistent with those of Marshall et al. (1982, 1983) who found that general health was a predictive variable of speech and language performance (Marshall & Phillips, 1983). Similarly, the duration of hospitalization may be related to age and general health status, and therefore indirectly related to language outcome (Holland et al., 1989).

Gender

It has been proposed that gender differences may influence the pattern of recovery in aphasia (McGlone, 1977, 1980). In two studies investigating the effects of sex on recovery from aphasia, females had a better prognosis than males for oral expression (Basso et al., 1982) and for auditory comprehension (Pizzamiglio et al., 1985). However, other studies have found no significant difference in recovery for males and females (Sarno et al., 1985; Pederson et al., 1995; Kertesz & McCabe, 1977; Pickersgill & Lincoln, 1983). Therefore, at this time, there appears to be no converging evidence favoring either (Basso, 1992).

Handedness

Some authors have proposed that left-handers and ambidextrous and mixed-handers have a more bilateral representation for language processing, and therefore recover more rapidly than right-handers from aphasia (Subirana, 1958; Luria, 1970; Gloning, 1977). Furthermore, it has been suggested that recovery from aphasia is more frequent among patients with familial sinistrality (Luria, 1970). However, better prognosis for non-right-handers is not supported by the data from more recent studies (Pickersgill & Lincoln, 1983; Basso et al., 1990; Borod et al., 1990). An issue affecting the interpretation of these studies is that handedness may be evaluated by different methods and different criteria for considering a hand as dominant may be adopted. Therefore, like gender, the findings about the effect of handedness on recovery are inconclusive.

Psychosocial Factors

Emotional and psychosocial changes accompany aphasia (Starkstein & Robinson, 1988; Hermann & Wallesch, 1993; Hemsley & Code, 1996). For example, post-stroke depression was found in 25% of stroke patients during the acute stages; this incidence rose to 31% at 3 months post onset, decreased to 16% by 12 months post onset, and then rose again over the next 2 years to 29%, a proportion higher than at the acute stage (Astrom et al., 1993). However, little is known of the interactions between these changes and recovery from aphasia. Many factors, such as motivation, are not easily amenable to experimental study. Nonetheless, emotional and psychosocial well-being may play a significant role in recovery from aphasia and preliminary evidence suggests a relationship between mood state and progress in rehabilitation (Starkstein & Robinson, 1988; Hermann & Wallesch, 1993; Code & Muller, 1992). In this regard, Hemsley and Code (1996) found unique patterns of individual emotional and psychosocial adjustment over time in patients with aphasia and their significant others, even in patients where aphasia type and severity were similar. Therefore, in terms of prognosis, they caution that psychosocial and emotional adjustment and its impact on communication and rehabilitation progress cannot be anticipated.

In summary, many studies have focused on the prognostic indicators that may help predict outcome in patients with aphasia. Several of these studies and their key findings have been discussed. As Tompkins (1990) has noted, "expanding our search for relevant predictors, and for optimal methods of measuring them, is a challenge for future work in this area." Since it appears that no single factor alone can predict outcome, clinicians must rely on information about each variable and make inferences about how they, in combination, affect the extent to which language recovery will occur. Clinicians also must decide if the expectation that treatment will effect positive change is justified. Furthermore, they must decide how much treatment should be administered and for how long. The next section reviews the information base for warranting these treatment decisions.

THE IMPACT OF TREATMENTS FOR APHASIA

The historical record of clinical outcomes for treatments of aphasia is but a part of the rich history of aphasiology. Several authors have composed extensive accounts of the larger history (e.g., LaPointe, 1983; Lecours et al., 1983; Lecours & Lhermitte, 1983; Sarno, 1991; Shewan, 1986; Weisenburg & McBride, 1935; Whitaker, 1998) and no attempt at replicating those achievements will be made in this work. However, because the historical record regarding treatment effectiveness is helpful for building context, selected publications written in English (a constraint rather than a choice) are recounted here.

For over a century, aphasiologists have examined the effects of intervention (e.g., Bateman, 1890) to answer a basic question: "Does treatment work?" The answer is clearly "Yes." However, getting to that answer took hundreds of clinical/experimental efforts conducted over nearly the same number of years. The evolutionary process leading to the answer is a story of advancements in research methodology. This review is organized by that sequence of advancements in research methods: case studies, frequency-of-occurrence studies, pre-post studies, non-randomized control studies, randomized control studies, single-subject studies, and syntheses of research. Notice that within each line of research, the typical progression of normal science is evident. That is, early studies show some variance in conclusions, but as researchers refine their questions and techniques, a consensus among research findings emerges.

Today, aphasiologists face a variety of specific questions from several interested parties: patients, families, referral sources, clinicians, researchers, reimbursing agencies, research funding agencies, and legislators. For example, aphasiologists must determine if treatment will bring about (or is bringing about) desired and valued ends for a particular patient receiving a particular treatment protocol. But the same question applies to a particular treatment administered to a particular clinical population, a particular schedule for treatment, a particular service-delivery model, a class of services provided at a particular service-delivery site, a class of services provided under a policy for federal reimbursement, and so forth. For that matter, what are desired and valued ends? Does treatment establish a certain level of performance on one or more treatment objective(s)? Does a certain treatment protocol establish some level of performance on a test of language impairment (WHO, 1980)? Does it establish some level of handicap status (WHO, 1980), some level of disability status (WHO, 1980), or some level of quality-of-life status? The work required for answering many of these and related questions has just begun.

Each of the parties having an interest in aphasia-treatment outcome asks different questions for different purposes. Answering these different questions requires different forms of evidence and so different research methodologies. All of these methodologies fall under the covering term *clinical outcome research*. At the core of clinical outcome research is the difference between observations made prior to the administration of a treatment and observations made sometime after the administration of treatment (Hopkins, 1998; Sederer et al., 1996). As Frattali (1998a, 1998b) and Kane (1997) point out, measurements of outcome can take many forms (e.g., physiology, impairment, disability, handicap, quality of life, consumer satisfaction, or disposition regarding a return to the workforce, among others). However, because the term *efficacy* is often misused, it is important to note that not all forms of clinical-outcome data constitute evidence of treatment efficacy (Frattali, 1998b; Robey & Schultz, 1998).[1]

The central criterion for establishing efficacy is not what is measured (e.g., impairment, disability) but how it is measured. Efficacy data result from carefully conducted measurements of a large sample of rigorously selected patients

(from a clearly defined clinical population) who are randomly assigned to various treatment (specific treatment protocols delivered by highly trained clinicians) and no-treatment conditions (see Robey & Schultz, 1998, for a full description). These requirements on research design preserve what Cook and Campbell (1979) term *internal validity*: assurance that the observed result (e.g., a change from pre-test to post-test) can be attributed to manipulation of the independent variable (i.e., treatment). The purpose of efficacy data is not to demonstrate change in one or some patients but to assess the potential of a certain treatment protocol for effecting change when administered to members of a clearly defined clinical population. As a result, clinical records, program evaluation data, and payer-accountability data don't constitute efficacy data. That fact does not, however, diminish the value of those data; indeed, those forms of data are precisely what is needed to answer several of the above questions. However, recognizing the distinction may help reduce some confusion regarding the focus of this chapter. Similarly, an explanation of the term *effectiveness* may be helpful. Effectiveness results from research efforts to index changes brought about by a treatment in actual clinical practice (see Robey & Schultz, 1998, for a full description). By way of contrast, a treatment is efficacious to the degree that it possesses demonstrated potential for bringing about beneficial change in a target population and a treatment is effective to the degree that the potential is realized in routine clinical practice. Logically and ethically, then, only efficacious treatments are submitted to effectiveness testing.

A few of the experimental results reviewed in the following sections are efficacy studies and many are effectiveness studies. Most studies center on language impairment and associated handicap (the reported measures of functional communication preceded broad acceptance of that World Health Organization construct). In most of the reports, the descriptions of treatment protocols are too lengthy for inclusion here and the reader is referred to the original articles for descriptions of treatment procedures.

The story of assessing the effects of treatments for aphasia starts in reports of case studies. Although case studies do not yield the necessary evidence for establishing the efficacy or effectiveness of a treatment, they represent for aphasiologists the beginnings of the long march to efficacy and effectiveness data.

Case Studies

In an early work, Bateman (1890) summarized the aphasia of several individuals, the interventions provided them, and a general accounting of outcome. On the basis of his experience, Bateman concluded that behavioral treatments seemed effective in restoring some degree of premorbid function. Similarly, Mills (1904) described the acute communicative behavior, intervention efforts, and communicative

---

[1] The authors are indebted to Dr. Carol M. Frattali (personal communication, March 12, 1999) for the insight underpinning this paragraph.

behavior at various points in recovery for each of five aphasic individuals.

The case study reported by Franz (1905) differs from those of Bateman and Mills in that Franz provided a very detailed accounting of a regimen for improving the naming and repetition behaviors of a single aphasic adult. Franz quantified changes in patient performance and developed hypotheses regarding cerebral mechanisms for recovery. In a later work, he reported three extensive case studies, each of which is a detailed history of communicative behavior with treatment results quantified on a session-by-session basis (Franz, 1924). Franz's understanding of (a) the variability with which individuals demonstrate aphasic signs, (b) the need for individualized treatment plans, (c) the value of monitoring and assessing the impact of treatment, and (d) the need to adapt treatment accordingly were pioneering achievements.

Several case studies of treatment results are to be found in the descriptions of broader clinical services. For instance, a brief description of treatments for 16 individuals with aphasia is included in a comprehensive profile of 200 head-injured veterans seen at the U.S. General Hospital in Cape May, New Jersey (Frazier & Inham, 1920). The status of some aphasic patients had been stable for several months, yet each patient responded to treatment. Similarly, Weisenburg and McBride (1935) described several cases in their care and concluded that intervention speeds recovery and is effective in changing specific communication difficulties. Furthermore, Weisenburg and McBride's (1935) cases documented successful applications of compensatory strategies. In reviewing 18 treated aphasic individuals, Anderson (1945) also concluded that intensive treatment brought about beneficial change.

Kennedy (1947) described the treatment of a veteran with aphasia resulting from head injury and subsequent medical complications. Kennedy's treatment was initiated nearly 2 years after the incident, at which time the patient's verbal responses were limited to two utterances. Treatment was provided each day for 3 hours. After 8 months, Kennedy described the patient's communication as considerably improved in verbal expression and auditory comprehension.

Goldstein (1948), who saw as many as 2000 patients with head wounds (World War I soldiers and veterans) and followed about 50 of them for as long as 10 years, provides us with a rich source of case studies on treatment and recovery. Furthermore, Goldstein's work is a remarkable document in the aphasia-treatment literature. His disciplined formulation of individual-specific communication-oriented treatment objectives as an extension of thorough examination combined with a forthright accounting of outcome formed the basis for a modern era of clinical aphasiology.

Since 1948, nearly 100 case studies of aphasia treatment have appeared in the literature and, as a practical matter, they are not reviewed here. Indeed, case studies, while enormously useful for detailing unusual cases and procedures, do not yield scientifically rigorous evidence for deciding the efficacy or effectiveness of treatments. Nevertheless, in the early years of clinical aphasiology before the broad acceptance of modern research standards, these case studies provided the necessary evidence for warranting (a) an expansion of clinical services and (b) a movement of the discipline toward scientifically valid means for assessing the outcomes of those services.

Group Studies

In the first half of the 20th century, statisticians derived the statistical procedures necessary for inferring results obtained from groups of subjects to the populations from which they were sampled (e.g., Student, 1908) and established a logic for incorporating those mathematics in a scientifically conservative system for testing hypotheses (e.g., Neyman, 1943). In the second half of the century, aphasiologists began applying hypothesis testing logic and inferential statistics in experimental efforts to better understand the effects of intervention as well as those of spontaneous recovery. The number of studies conducted in the past 50 years (more than 200) is simply too large for comprehensive and exhaustive review. Therefore, this chapter centers largely on major studies addressing the direct intervention of speech-language pathologists in terms of overall language impairment and overall functional communication.

Frequency of Occurrence Data

The first efforts in combining results obtained from several aphasic individuals to form a covering conclusion were straightforward extensions of case studies; researchers began counting types of outcomes (e.g., improvement, no improvement). Butfield and Zangwill (1946) examined four dimensions of recovery (i.e., speech, reading, writing, and calculation) to assess the treatment approach described by Goldstein (1948). They assessed 70 aphasic individuals and judged each to be much improved, improved, or unchanged. Beyond their findings, the important contribution of Butfield and Zangwill was to significantly advance the state of aphasia-treatment research by separating their patients into two groups: those treated before 6 months post onset (MPO) and those treated after 6 MPO. Thus began a series of developments in research design for comparing the effects of treatment apart from those of spontaneous recovery.

The percentage of positive outcomes reported by Butfield and Zangwill (1946) (i.e., improved and much-improved counts combined) ranged from approximately 70% to 80% across the four dimensions. Similarly, in two articles on a single group of patients, Godfrey (1959) and Godfrey and Douglass (1959) reported that 80% of their patients seemed to respond positively to treatment. Moreover, the total of generally favorable outcomes reported by Marshall et al. (1982) and Broman et al. (1967) were 70% and approximately 75% of patients, respectively.

In an early effort at documenting the effects of treatment, Marks et al. (1957) studied cases of acquired aphasia seen in a civilian practice where etiology was, presumably, mostly of a vascular nature. Fifty percent of the treated recoveries were judged positive and 50% were judged negative. However, the subjects were heterogeneous with respect to months post onset, and the amount and duration of treatment varied from subject to subject.

The results of Vignolo (1964) marked an important turning point in aphasia-treatment research. Vignolo conducted an extensive exploration of relationships between several clinical dimensions and treatment outcome. Vignolo's definitions and partitioning of independent variables continue to influence the character of aphasia-treatment research. In particular, two aspects of Vignolo's research design fundamentally changed the research paradigm: the inclusion of a no-treatment control group and an examination of treatment duration. Although group membership was not randomly assigned, Vignolo's results provided insight to the effect of treatment relative to the effect of untreated spontaneous recovery. In general, outcomes for rehabilitated patients exceeded those of non-rehabilitated patients but the difference did not achieve statistical significance. However, when Vignolo segregated outcomes attributed to less than 6 months of treatment and outcomes attributed to 6 months or more of treatment, the benefit of treatment became more apparent than in the general analysis.

Like Vignolo (1964), Basso et al. (1979) constituted a no-treatment control group from patients who could not or would not be seen for ongoing treatment. However, the treated subjects of Basso et al. (1979) received 6 months or more of Schuell-Wepman-Darley Multimodality (SWDM) treatment (see Duffy, 1994) in three sessions lasting 45–50 minutes each week. Performance was assessed in each of the four major modalities. In each modality, the proportion of aphasic individuals who improved with treatment far exceeded the proportion of improved individuals in the control group. The authors concluded that treatment has a positive effect if provided 3 times per week for at least 6 months (Basso et al., 1979).

Lesser and Watt (1978) examined the effects of untrained volunteers providing aphasic individuals with psychosocial support as well as opportunities for conversation. Although the social benefit of the program was clear, patients did not change remarkably on indices of communicative function.

In a recent analysis of frequency-of-occurrence data, Popovici and Milhäilescu (1992) studied individuals with Broca aphasia. Subjects were assigned to either a control or an experimental group, but not on a random basis. Members of the experimental group received a variation of Melodic Intonation Therapy (MIT; Sparks et al., 1974) and members of the control group received other forms of treatment (not described). Both groups responded to treatment, with a slight advantage experienced by those receiving MIT.

Pre-Treatment Versus Post-Treatment Data

Because categorical data yield a relatively gross index of treatment effect, researchers soon made a very logical move to a much more sensitive index of change: the magnitude of difference between pre-treatment measurements and post-treatment measurements. Initially, researchers assessed pre-versus-post data sets on their own merit. Gradually, however, researchers began interpreting the change scores in the context of analogous data obtained from untreated control subjects.

No Controls

Wepman (1951) was among the first researchers to examine pre-post data. In studying 68 head-injured veterans, 'speech performance' was measured before and after treatment as part of a large test battery comprising several indices of educational performance. At this early point in the paradigm, Wepman found statistically significant changes in speech performance.

Broida (1977) examined the pre-post data of a heterogeneous group of aphasic individuals who were 1 to 6 years post onset. Fifty minutes of individual treatment was administered 3 to 5 times per week for a period of 2 to 21 months. Like Wepman, Broida also found a statistically significant improvement in overall language impairment.

Sarno and Levita (1979) studied 34 carefully selected aphasic individuals who received three to five sessions of treatment per week during the first 6 MPO. Measurements were made at 1, 2, 3, 6, and 12 MPO. They found that globally aphasic individuals made their greatest gains on indices of language performance and functional communication during the 6–12 MPO period. Nonfluent aphasic individuals achieved their greatest gains during the first 6 MPO; however, improvements on indices of language performance and functional communication continued, at a decelerated rate, through the second 6 MPO. Fluent aphasic individuals also demonstrated their greatest gains during the first 6 months post onset. Although performance on the index of functional communication continued throughout the second 6 MPO, little change was noted on the index of language performance during the same period.

Wertz et al. (1981) randomly assigned subjects to one of two treatment groups: individual treatment and group treatment. Subjects received 8 hours of treatment each week. Measurements were made at 15, 26, 37, and 48 weeks post onset. Inclusion and exclusion criteria were exceptionally rigorous to preserve internal validity. All pre-post differences were significant. Of particular interest were significant gains achieved between 26 and 48 weeks post onset, well past the period of spontaneous recovery. With few exceptions, average test scores for the individual-treatment group exceeded those of the group-treatment group. Group differences in overall score for the Porch Index of Communicative Abilities (Porch, 1981) achieved statistical significance at the 26- and 37-week post-onset measurements; differences on other indices did not achieve statistical significance. In contrast, Avent et al. (1998) conducted a retrospective study through an examination of pragmatic-communication data collected in the Veterans Administration cooperative study. They found no differences in changed performance between individuals treated in group or individual sessions.

Sarno and Levita (1981) examined carefully selected individuals with global aphasia at 4, 8, 12, 26, and 52 weeks post onset. Patients received three to five sessions each week of what Sarno and Levita termed traditional/pedagogical treatment. All patients improved throughout the year, but remained severely aphasic. The greatest gains in scores of language performance and functional communication were obtained in the second 6 months post onset. Sarno and Levita (1981) did not report a statistical analysis of their data; however, their overall scores on the Functional Communication Profile (Sarno, 1969) at 8 and 52 weeks post stroke demonstrate a significant effect.

Aten et al. (1982) administered 2 hours of functional communication treatment to a group of individuals with chronic nonfluent agrammatic aphasia over a 12-week period. Significant gains were observed in functional communication but not in overall language impairment. The gains in functional communication were maintained on a follow-up measurement.

Cherney et al. (1986) provided Oral Reading for Language in Aphasia to a heterogeneous group of aphasic individuals 3 to 5 times per week for 20 to 80 sessions. From pre-test to post-test, they found significant differences on a composite index of language impairment.

For 12 weeks, Brindley et al. (1989) administered 25 hours of treatment per week to 10 Broca aphasic individuals. They contrasted change during this period to change measured during (a) a 12-week period prior to the treatment period as well as (b) a 12-week period following the treatment period. During the first and last 12-week periods, patients received 1 to 2 hours of treatment per week provided by their attending speech-language pathologists (rather than by the experimentalists). Brindley et al. (1989) found that the intensive treatment schedule brought about significant gains on indices of language performance and functional communication relative to the less intensive schedule. Furthermore, the gains were maintained throughout the third 12-week period.

Aftonomos et al. (1997) administered a computer-based treatment (Lingraphia System) to 23 chronic aphasic

individuals 1–3 times per week for 16 weeks, on average. They documented significant change in several tests of linguistic impairment. Aftonomos et al. (1999) administered the same type to a heterogeneous group of aphasic individuals for, on average, 2 hours per week (plus self-directed work) for 20 weeks. They found significant improvements in measures of language impairment and functional communication.

In a retrospective study, Odell et al. (1997) analyzed the charts of 20 systematically selected former patients. Odell et al. applied Functional Communication Measure (FCM; American Speech-Language-Hearing Association, 1995) criteria to the information found in those records. Ten of the records constituted a severe-impairment group having a composite (median) FCM of 0 to 2. The remaining ten records constituted a moderate-impairment group having a composite (median) FCM of 3 to 5. On average, patients in the severe-impairment group received 40 half-hour sessions of unspecified treatment. Similarly, members of the moderate-impairment group received 22 such sessions. Although both groups gained a median of 1 FCM level over their initial composite scores, the authors note that the results of this uncontrolled retrospective analysis are psychometric in nature (i.e., the utility of FCMs) rather than clinical (i.e., outcomes attributed to treatment).

Hinckley and Craig (1998) conducted a series of three retrospective studies on treatment for naming ability. In each study, chronically aphasic individuals (three separate samples) received two 6-week periods of treatment on a 23-hour-per-week basis (15 hours of individual treatment, 5 hours of group treatment, and 3 hours of computer work; see the article for descriptions of each). In between these two blocks of treatment, one group received no treatment, another group received less than 3 hours per week of individual treatment, and a third group received 3 to 5 hours of individual treatment per week. Hinckley and Craig found that improvements were always greatest during the intensive treatment block and that gains were durable. Furthermore, they concluded that treatment administered 1 to 2 times per week has little more effect than no treatment.

No-Treatment Controls

Following Vignolo's (1964) demonstration of the value of no-treatment control subjects, the methodology was soon adopted in pre-post studies. However, acting on a principle that to purposefully withhold treatment constituted an ethical breach, many experimenters filled no-treatment control groups with patients who chose not to participate in treatment or who were unable to attend treatment sessions. Not until 1986 was the dilemma resolved when Wertz and colleagues demonstrated a research method for accomplishing randomized no-treatment control.

Non-Random Assignment

West and Stockel (1965) conducted a classic two-period cross-over experiment testing the effects of the psychotropic drug meprobamate on aphasia. Although they found no treatment effect, this early example of advanced research design deserves special mention.

Sarno et al. (1970) compared three groups of severely aphasic individuals: those receiving programmed instruction, those receiving non-programmed instruction (clinicians in this group were given instructions and target behaviors which were identical to those of the programmed-instruction group), and no-treatment control subjects. On average, patients received 56 half-hour treatment sessions over a 17-week period. Significant differences were observed on only 2 of 10 target behaviors and non-programmed instruction brought about larger changes than did programmed instruction. In general, the results of Sarno et al. (1970) highlighted for all researchers the importance of (a) intensive treatment, (b) controlling for MPO, and (c) selection criteria. The findings of Sarno et al. (1970) should be taken in the context of Sarno and Levita (1979) and Sarno and Levita (1981).

In one of the first studies to impose extensive inclusion/exclusion criteria, Hagen (1973) assigned aphasic individuals to a period of either treatment or no treatment. Performance measurements were made at 3, 6, 12, and 18 MPO. Aphasic individuals began the experimental protocol at 3 MPO. For 3 months, no one received treatment. At 6 MPO, one group began receiving 4 hours of individual treatment, 8 hours of group treatment, and 6 hours of 'independent therapy' on a weekly basis for a period of 12 months. Plots of group means showed a superior recovery on most, but not all, indices of language function.

Levita (1978) reported a no-treatment controlled study of individuals treated with one-half hour of individual treatment combined with 1 hour of group treatment on a daily basis from 4 to 12 weeks post onset. However, the results seem to be of a post-test-only comparison (independent of pre-test results) and so the outcome seems of limited value.

Shewan and Kertesz (1984) reported a highly controlled study of treatment and language recovery. Patients in three experimental groups received 3 hours of treatment per week for as long as 1 year. One group of patients received Language Oriented Treatment (LOT; Shewan & Bandur, 1986), another group received SWDM treatment. A third group of patients received communication stimulation and psychological support from nurses trained by a speech-language pathologist. On average, the gains experienced by subjects receiving LOT or SWDM exceeded the gains experienced by control subjects. That is, the effects of treatment during the period of spontaneous recovery significantly exceeded the effects of spontaneous recovery alone.

Prins et al. (1989) compared two treated groups to a group of untreated individuals and found no appreciable difference. However, at pre-test, the untreated individuals performed at a higher level than did either treatment group. Because performance in the treated groups increased to the level of the untreated group at post-test, the finding of no difference is an equivocal one.

Poeck et al. (1989) reported an exceptional experimental effort to establish the effects of treatment apart from the associated effects of spontaneous recovery. Experimental subjects received 9 hours of treatment (5 hours of individual LOT plus 4 hours of group treatment) per week. Treatment was initiated for one group between the 1st and 4th months post onset and lasted for 6 to 8 weeks. In a second group, treatment was initiated between the 4th and 12th months post onset; the treatment period extended for 7–12 months. Subjects in the third group began treatment at some point after 1 year post onset. The first two groups were compared with analogous control groups; the third was not. On average, performances of the treated groups significantly exceeded those of controls on an index of overall communication.

Poeck et al. (1989) also examined individual results. Using a conservative statistical correction for the effects of spontaneous recovery, they found that 78% of the early-treatment group achieved scores that could not be attributed to spontaneous recovery (likely an underestimate given the conservative nature of the procedure). They also found that 46% of the 4–12 months post-onset group exceeded gains that could be attributed to spontaneous recovery.

Mackenzie (1991) provided a small group of chronically aphasic individuals 5.5 hours of group treatment per day for 5 days in each of 4 consecutive weeks. The 4 weeks of treatment was preceded and followed by a 4-week period of no treatment. A non-brain-damaged control group did not play a major role in the study. On the basis of a qualitative analysis, Mackenzie generally endorsed intense treatment schedules.

Random Assignment

Lincoln et al. (1984) compared 164 randomly assigned no-treatment control subjects to 163 subjects receiving 2 hours of treatment per week (undefined heterogeneous treatments formulated as appropriate by attending speech-language pathologists) starting at 10 weeks post onset and lasting until 34 weeks post onset. However, only 27 patients completed, or nearly completed, the treatment sequence. Lincoln et al.'s main finding was no appreciable difference separating the results of the treatment and the no-treatment groups. Although Lincoln et al. (1984) excluded subjects with very mild aphasia, subjects who were untestable, and subjects with severe dysarthria, their inclusion of subjects with histories of previous strokes and 'other disabilities' is a substantial concern in terms of internal validity (i.e., assurance that the presence or absence of an effect is exclusively attributable to manipulation of the independent variable). The design decision to recruit all aphasic subjects regardless of neurological/medical history combined with (a) heterogeneous and uncontrolled decisions on treatment type, and (b) substantial attrition may have influenced the general finding. This is not to say that Lincoln et al.'s findings should be set aside. Rather, as the authors indicate, the effectiveness test of this intervention model was not positive (generalization to different models may not be warranted), and seeking different methods for assessment, treatment, and research design seems appropriate.

Wertz et al. (1986) and Marshall et al. (1989) reported a most carefully controlled study of aphasia treatment. Stringent and thorough inclusion and exclusion criteria (e.g., a single cerebral vascular accident confined to the left hemisphere without co-morbid neurological conditions) minimized possibilities for alternate explanations of observed effects (i.e., minimized threats to internal validity). Wertz et al. studied three groups. The comparison of the first two groups constitutes a classic two-period crossover design. Group A (not Wertz et al.'s term) received treatment by a speech-language pathologist for the 12 weeks of the first period and then crossed over to a 12-week no-treatment period. In contrast, group B received no treatment in the 12 weeks of period 1 and then crossed over to a 12-week period treatment. An additional group, C, received treatment from volunteers who were trained by the attending speech-language pathologist who designed and monitored treatment.

At the crossover point, group A measurements significantly differed from group B measurements. At the end of period 2, group B had achieved gains comparable to those of group A in period 1. Throughout period 2, group A measures continued to improve, albeit at a decelerated rate. Lesser gains were observed in group C but the difference did not achieve statistical significance. Like Wepman (1951) and Vignolo (1964), Wertz et al. (1986) changed the character of aphasia treatment research. Wertz et al. (1986) demonstrated that deferred treatment, ultimately, does not deny a patient the beneficial effects of treatment. An early-recovery no-treatment control group can be constituted randomly with treatment implemented once the comparison of interest is accomplished.

Katz and Wertz (1997) randomly assigned carefully selected aphasic individuals (1 to 22 MPO) to one of three groups: computer reading, nonverbal computer stimulation, and no-treatment control. Individuals in the first two groups received 3 hours of intervention per week for 26 weeks. Interactions with reading software, rather than interactions with software in general, accounted for significant improvements on indices of language impairment.

Elman and Bernstein-Ellis (1999) randomly assigned carefully selected chronically aphasic individuals to treatment or deferred-treatment groups. Members of the treatment group received 4 months of group treatment on a 5-hour-per-week basis. Members of the deferred-treatment group engaged in social interactions (to assess that differences with treated individuals were not simply the result of socialization versus no socialization) while the first group was in treatment. Measurements of linguistic impairment and functional communication were made throughout the study and in a post-treatment follow-up. No changes were evident as a result of deferred treatment. However, both groups demonstrated changes on the Western Aphasia Battery (WAB; Kertesz, 1982) and the Communication Activities of Daily Living (CADL; Holland, 1980), but not on a shortened version of the Porch Index of Communicative Ability (Disimoni et al., 1980).

Other External Control Groups

Meikle et al. (1979) randomly assigned aphasic individuals to either conventional treatment by a speech-language pathologist or treatment provided by a volunteer who was trained and consulted by a speech-language pathologist. It seems that some of the aphasic individuals had an accompanying dementia or may have had prior neurologic histories. MPO ranged from 4 to 268. All patients received treatment in sessions of 45 minutes 3 to 5 times each week for a period of from 7 to 84 weeks. Despite the fact that the difference scores were nearly twice as great for the speech-language-pathology group, the difference did not achieve statistical significance.

David et al. (1982) randomly assigned heterogeneous (i.e., narrow exclusion criteria) aphasic individuals to one of two treatment groups: treatment by speech-language pathologists or treatment by volunteers. Each group received 30 hours of treatment in a period of 15 to 20 weeks (i.e., ≤2 hours per week). The treatment provided by the speech-language pathologists was not defined. At post-test, David et al. found no difference between the two groups.

Hartman and Landau (1987) randomly assigned aphasic individuals at 1 MPO (some of whom displayed 'other neurologic symptoms') to either conventional therapy or emotionally supportive counseling. Both services were provided by speech-language pathologists. Two sessions of undescribed length were offered each week for 6 months. Although the treatment group demonstrated greater gains than did the counseling group, the difference did not achieve statistical significance.

Huber et al. (1997) randomly assigned carefully selected aphasic individuals (who were 1 to 6 MPO) to one of two treatment groups in a double-blind study. Each group received 5 hours of individual treatment and 5 hours of group treatment each week for 6 weeks. Each day, members of one group received 4.8 g of Piracetam (facilitates specific neurotransmitter transmission; increases cerebral blood flow and perfusion); a placebo was administered to members of the other group. On measures of language impairment, the group receiving combined behavioral and pharmacological treatment showed greater gains.

Beyond Language Impairment and Functional Communication

For the most part, the effects of treatments for aphasia have been assessed in terms of language impairment and functional communication. However, a few studies have assessed treatment outcomes in other important dimensions. For instance, Aronson et al. (1956) administered a *consumer satisfaction* survey to aphasic individuals receiving group treatment. Gil et al. (1996) studied post-treatment *handicap* (or *participation restriction*; WHO, 1997) in terms of employment status of individuals who became aphasic as a result of traumatic brain injury. They found that 84% of individuals who were aphasic secondary to severe traumatic brain injury achieved gainful employment. Boysen and Wertz (1996) conducted a first-approximation *cost-effectiveness* analysis of aphasia treatment. They described the importance and the challenges of conducting cost-effectiveness research.

Sarno (1997) conducted an extensive *quality of life* (QOL) trial of aphasia treatment. Over the period from 3 MPO to 12 MPO, patients were seen for treatment a minimum of 3 times per week (averaged 6 times per week) for individual, group, and computer-based treatments. Sarno (1997, p. 765) concluded, "This suggests that when post-stoke aphasic patients are provided with intensive, long-term aphasia rehabilitation services which address language, communication strategies, functional communication, coping skills, and psychosocial issues for the first year, all of these areas show continuous improvement with a consequently positive impact on QOL."

Single-Subject Studies

Davis (1978) and LaPointe (1978) introduced to aphasiology a new means for assessing the effect of treatment for aphasia: single-subject research. Since then, over 100 single-subject aphasia-treatment studies have appeared in the literature. For the most part, these studies have incorporated rigorous research design controls (e.g., withdrawal periods, multiple baselines across behaviors, multiple baselines across subjects, generalization probes, extinction probes, and social validation measures) in testing scientifically evolved hypotheses (Kearns & Thompson, 1991; Robey et al., 1999).

For instance, single-subject studies have been used to test differential effects of treatment on several dimensions:

Treatment for certain clinical pictures, for example:

• Alexander and Loverso (1993)	Severe aphasia
• Bernstein-Ellis, Wertz, and Shubitowski (1987)	Mild aphasia
• Boyle (1991)	Chronic alcoholism
• Garrett and Beukleman (1995)	Severe aphasia
• McNeil, Small, Masterson, and Fossett (1995)	Primary progressive aphasia
• Peach (1987)	Conduction aphasia
• Schneider, Thompson, and Luring (1996)	Primary progressive aphasia
• Whitney and Goldstein (1989)	Mild aphasia

Treatment to reduce certain signs of aphasia pictures, for example:

• Boyle (1989)	Phonemic paraphasia
• Boyle and Coelho (1995)	Naming
• Hillis (1989)	Naming
• Lowell, Beeson, and Holland (1995)	Naming
• Raymer, Thompson, Jacobs, and Le Grand (1993)	Naming

Treatment to establish certain communicative behaviors, for example:

• Kearns and Salmon (1984)	Auxiliary and copula verb generalization
• Thompson, McReynolds, and Vance (1982)	Locatives in multiword utterances
• Thompson and Shapiro (1994)	Sentence production
• Thompson, Shapiro, Tait, Jacobs, and Schneider (1996)	Wh question production
• Wambaugh and Thompson (1989)	Wh question production

Treatment to establish alternative forms of communication, for example:

• Bellaire, Georges, and Thompson (1991)	Communication board
• Coelho (1991)	Manual sign acquisition
• Kearns, Simmons, and Sisterhen (1982)	Gestural sign

In addition, many single-subject studies have assessed the effectiveness of specific treatment protocols, for example:

• Ballard and Thompson (1999)	Linguistic Specific Treatment
• Conlon and McNeil (1991)	Visual Action Therapy
• Doyle, Goldstein, and Bourgeois (1987)	Helm Elicited Language Program for Syntax Stimulation
• Gaddie, Kearns, and Yedor (1991)	Response Elaboration Treatment
• Kearns and Scher (1989)	Response Elaboration Treatment
• Salvatore (1985)	Helm Elicited Language Program for Syntax Stimulation
• Steele, Weinrich, Kleczewska, Carlson, and Wertz (1987)	Computer-based visual communication
• Steele, Weinrich, Wertz, Kleczewska, and Carlson (1989)	Computer-based visual communication

To achieve a stable series of baseline observations, single-subject studies are largely conducted mostly on aphasic individuals who are well post ictus. As a result, the magnitude of effects reported in this body of literature likely underestimates the magnitude of effects possible for individuals with acute aphasia. Nevertheless, effect sizes of single-subject studies reporting recoverable data are remarkably large (Robey et al., 1999).

Syntheses of Research Findings

Literature Reviews

As in all scientific endeavors, the evidence required for answering a research question (e.g., Does treatment bring about desired ends beyond those expected as a direct result of spontaneous recovery?) is not a single experimental outcome but the concert of all experimental outcomes addressing the question. Aphasiologists have often assessed the value of treatment by assimilating many separate clinical findings in published reviews of salient literature. In early examples, Bateman (1890) and Weisenburg and McBride (1935) concluded that the majority of evidence supported the notion that intervention brought about greater improvement than occurred in the absence of intervention. In the years following World War II, services for aphasic patients progressively expanded and aphasiologists increasingly needed to answer basic questions about the value of their treatments (Darley, 1972). Critical reviews of literature provided the answers.

In an exceptionally thorough and insightful analysis of literature, Darley (1982) concluded that treatment, generally considered, brought about important and valued changes beyond what could be expected without treatment. Eisensen (1984) also conducted an extensive literature review and made the same general conclusion. Two years later, Shewan (1986) reported an extremely thorough analysis of literature and came to the conclusion that language therapy is efficacious. Although Sarno's (1991) review does not include a judgment on the value of treatment per se, it is a remarkable work in literature analysis.

Basso (1992) compared the outcomes in two groups of treatment-versus-control studies: those in which treatment was provided for a relatively short duration (generally less than 6 months) and those in which treatment was provided for a relatively long duration (generally more than 6 months). Basso (1992) found that long-duration treatment studies (e.g., Basso et al., 1979; Hagen, 1973; Marshall et al., 1982; Sarno & Levita, 1979) yielded larger treatment effects than did short-duration treatment studies (e.g., Levita, 1978; Sarno et al., 1970; Vignolo, 1964).

In a definitive analysis of literature, Holland et al. (1996) applied criteria on clinical evidence set forth by the American Academy of Neurology (AAN, 1994) and determined that, "...it must be concluded that, generally, treatment for aphasia is efficacious" (Holland et al., 1996, p. S34). Recently, Albert (1998) reviewed aphasia-treatment literature for neurologists and explained the value of incorporating speech-language pathology services in the care of aphasic individuals.

Meta-Analyses

A new development in the field of statistics is a set of procedures termed meta-analysis. Meta-analysis has become the preferred methodology for synthesizing a body of research throughout the behavioral sciences. Fundamentally, a meta-analysis consists of extracting certain quantities from primary studies, converting them all to a common metric indexing departure from the null hypothesis, and averaging those quantities to arrive at a composite index of the tenability of the null hypothesis (for a more complete explanation, see Robey & Dalebout, 1998). Said differently, meta-analysis is a means for synthesizing a body of research to determine the weight of scientific evidence regarding a particular research question.

Greenhouse et al. (1990) reported the first meta-analysis of aphasia-treatment literature. Greenhouse et al. analyzed 13 pre-post tests of aphasia treatment and found an average weighted effect size of 0.80 corresponding to a medium-to-large effect. In addition, the authors explored many dimensions of meta-analysis as it is applied to aphasia-treatment literature: methodology, operational decisions, problem solving, and reflections on the experience. Whurr et al. (1992) calculated effect sizes for 45 studies and obtained an average effect size of 0.59 separating treated and untreated subjects. On the basis of 21 studies, Robey (1994) conducted a meta-analysis of between effects (i.e., treatment versus control) and within effects (i.e., pre-test versus post-test) with time post-onset controlled for each set of effects. The results indicated that the recovery of treated individuals was, on average, nearly twice as extensive as the recovery of untreated individuals when treatment was begun before 3 MPO. Furthermore, treatment brought about an appreciable improvement in performance when begun after the third MPO. Robey (1994) also found that the effect sizes for treated-versus-untreated comparisons exceeded Cohen's (1988) criterion for a medium-sized effect when treatment was initiated before the third MPO and exceeded the criterion for a small-sized effect in the chronic stage when treatment was initiated after 12 MPO.

In a meta-analysis of 55 studies, Robey (1998) obtained results confirming of the 1994 findings. Furthermore, Robey (1998) found that, in general, (a) greater amounts of treatment brought about larger treatment effects, (b) the average effect size for SWDM was larger than the overall average, and (c) large gains are achieved by severely aphasic persons. Recently, Robey et al. (1999) conducted a meta-analysis of single-subject aphasia-treatment research and found that although variety in types of treatment did not warrant averaging, individual treatment effects were generally large and robust.

Conclusion

The conservatism of science constrains decisions regarding tests of hypotheses to a binary choice: on the basis of experimental evidence, a research hypothesis is deemed tenable or untenable. Independent experiments, particularly those conducted in the exploratory phase of a research paradigm, likely yield evidence on both sides of a question.

As a research paradigm matures, scientists refine hypotheses and test them with ever-improving experimental methodologies. Gradually, the body of experimental findings converges on one or another choice in the binary decision set. In an extensive record of clinical findings, aphasiologists have produced many findings in several forms of scientific evidence regarding the questions of treatment efficacy and effectiveness. The body of evidence resulting from each line of research supports the conclusion that treatment of aphasia, particularly intensive treatment, is effective. The overwhelming majority of findings in the total record support the conclusion that treatments for aphasia, generally considered, are both efficacious and effective. Furthermore, as experimental methodologies have improved (e.g., indexing the magnitude of change in communication behavior from pre-test to post-test, controlling for time post onset, setting clear exclusion and inclusion criteria to establish homogeneous groups, no-treatment control groups having the prospect of deferred treatment, random assignment, and controls on the type(s), amount, and duration of treatment), findings have been unambiguous and lead to a certain conclusion: treatment, particularly treatment administered on an intense schedule, brings about large and important changes in language impairment and functional communication. The precision of Holland et al.'s (1996) conclusion merits repetition, "...people who become aphasic following a single, left-hemisphere thromboembolic stroke and who receive at least 3 hours of treatment each week for at least 5 months, regardless of time post-onset of stroke, make significantly more improvement than people with aphasia who are not treated." (Holland et al., 1996, p. S30).

Moving beyond the conclusion that treatment for aphasia, generally considered, brings about large and important changes in language impairment and functional communication raises two large challenges for aphasiologists. One of those challenges is to assess more fully the changes brought about by treatment in terms of disability, handicap, quality of life, consumer satisfaction, and costs relative to benefits (Robey & Schultz, 1998). The pioneering work of Sarno (1997) is a large contribution in meeting the challenge. The second challenge is to conduct these multi-dimensional assessments of efficacy, and then effectiveness, on specific types of treatment. Given the effort required to answer the general question, establishing the efficacy and effectiveness for each of many forms of treatments could readily become an unwieldy undertaking—all things left to vary freely.

An initiative of the American Psychological Association (APA) could prove helpful in meeting the second challenge. As an extension of the APA initiative, Chambless and Hollon (1998) describe criteria for assessing the efficacy of a particular treatment. In full, the Chambless and Hollon criteria for establishing efficacy are much too extensive for complete review here. However, the core of the criteria focus on research designs and replications of findings. The major criterion for establishing efficacy through group-design research is two or more independent findings of treatment exceeding no-treatment control and achieving statistical significance. Alternatively, efficacy can be established through two or more independent findings of equivalence between an experimental treatment and a treatment for which efficacy has already been established (e.g., best-treatment control, standard treatment control; see Robey & Schultz, 1998). In case of contradictory findings among three or more studies, the preponderance of evidence must be positive if a treatment is to achieve status as efficacious. The major criterion for designating a treatment efficacious on the basis of evidence from single-subject research is two or more independent findings (i.e., from different research settings) of superior treatment-period performances in a treatment-versus-no-treatment comparison achieving statistical significance in at least three subjects (each site). In the presence of conflicting results, the preponderance of outcomes must favor the experimental treatment over the control.

It is not our purpose to advocate that aphasiologists adopt the APA criteria for establishing efficacy. However, as aphasiologists take on the numerous and difficult tasks of establishing efficacy in a series of certain treatments, certain treatment schedules, treatments for certain populations, and so forth, the wisdom of setting a priori consensus thresholds for achieving success (or not) ought not go unnoticed.

FUTURE TRENDS

1. Progressive refinements and advancements in imaging technology make possible ever more detailed assessments of pathology, surviving anatomy, and physiology. In large samples, those forms of information combined with salient history and thorough assessments of communication behavior at certain points in recovery will undoubtedly clarify indicators and moderators of recovery.

2. That concert of information will enhance the clinical decisions of aphasiologists regarding prognosis and treatment scheduling.

3. Demonstrated efficacy and effectiveness is imperative in health care delivery. From that perspective, aphasiologists must continue to test the efficacy and effectiveness of well-defined treatment protocols through well-controlled experiments. The most informing of these tests will assess theory-driven protocols that are practical and efficient in bringing about large and important changes in the lives of aphasic individuals and their care-givers.

4. The test of a certain protocol must focus not only on changes in impairment from pre-test to post-test, but also the effects of certain treatment schedules, certain models of service delivery, direct comparisons of specific treatment protocols, indications and contraindications

of candidacy for a protocol, and the permanence of change brought about by a protocol.

5. The scope of clinical experiments must continue to broaden through assessments of treatment effects expressed in terms of disability (activity limitation), handicap (participation limitation), quality of life, consumer satisfaction, and costs versus benefits.

6. As in all forms of scientific inquiry, initial findings will be strengthened through independent replications of critical tests.

KEY POINTS

1. Despite individual variation in rate and extent of recovery, there seem to be some general patterns of recovery that have been identified for each type of aphasia. Furthermore, there is a consistent trend in the pattern of recovery as it relates to the individual language modalities.

2. The neural mechanisms contributing to recovery from aphasia are not completely understood. Technological advances in the area of brain imaging (e.g., PET, SPECT, functional MRI) have moved researchers closer to understanding the neural mechanisms that mediate early and late recovery.

3. Rate and extent of recovery are dependent to a large extent on the site and size of the area of structural damage in the left perisylvian language areas as shown by CT or MRI.

4. In addition, right hemisphere participation in recovery from aphasia is likely and numerous studies have demonstrated that the right hemisphere may play a crucial role in recovery from aphasia.

5. Other studies have implicated not only the unaffected contralateral hemisphere, but also the integrity of structures in the ipsilateral hemisphere. Even limited salvage of peri-infarct tissue in the left hemisphere will have an important impact on rehabilitation and recovery.

6. There appears to be no single factor alone that can predict outcome in patients with aphasia. Personal and biographical factors such as age, handedness, and gender have been studied experimentally, with some conflicting evidence regarding their effects.

7. Efficacy data results from carefully conducted measurements of a large sample of rigorously selected patients (from a clearly defined clinical population) who are randomly assigned to various treatment and no-treatment conditions. Effectiveness results from research efforts to index changes brought about by a treatment in actual clinical practice. Logically and ethically, then, only efficacious treatments are submitted to effectiveness testing.

8. In an extensive record of clinical findings, aphasiologists have produced many findings in several forms of scientific evidence regarding the questions of treatment efficacy and effectiveness. The body of scientific evidence resulting from each line of research supports the conclusion that treatments for aphasia, generally considered, are both efficacious and effective.

9. As experimental methodologies have improved (e.g., indexing the magnitude of change in communication behavior from pre-test to post-test, controlling for time post onset, setting clear exclusion and inclusion criteria to establish homogeneous groups, no-treatment control groups having the prospect of deferred treatment, random assignment, and controls on the type(s), amount, and duration of treatment), findings have been unambiguous and lead to the conclusion that treatment brings about large and important changes in language impairment and functional communication. Careful and extensive reviews of literature and meta-analyses affirm that conclusion.

10. Typically, the effects of treatments for aphasia are assessed in terms of language impairment and functional communication. More studies are needed to assess and compare treatment outcomes in other important dimensions such as consumer satisfaction, handicap, cost-effectiveness, and quality of life (QOL).

References

Aftonomos, L.B., Appelbaum, J.S., & Steele, R.D. (1999). Improving outcomes for persons with aphasia in advanced community-based treatment programs. *Stroke, 30,* 1370–1379.

Aftonomos, L.B., Steele, R.D., & Wertz, R.T. (1997). Promoting recovery in chronic aphasia with interactive technology. *Archives of Physical Medicine and Rehabilitation, 78,* 841–846.

Albert, M.L. (1998). Treatment of aphasia. *Archives of Neurology, 55,* 1417–1419.

Alexander, M.P. & Loverso, F.L. (1993). A specific treatment for global aphasia. In M.L. Lemme (ed.), *Clinical Aphasiology, Vol. 21.* Austin, TX: Pro-Ed.

American Academy of Neurology. (1994). Definitions and quality of evidence ratings. *Neurology, 44,* 567.

American Speech-Language-Hearing Association (1995). *Functional Communication Measure.* Rockville, MD: ASHA.

Anderson, J.O. (1945). Eighteen cases of aphasia studied from the viewpoint of a speech pathologist. *Journal of Speech Disorders, 10,* 9–34.

Andrews, R.J. (1991). Transhemispheric diaschisis: A review and comment. *Stroke, 22,* 943–949.

Aronson, M., Shatin, L., & Cook, J.C. (1956). Socio-psychotherapeutic approach to the treatment of aphasic patients. *Journal of Speech and Hearing Disorders, 21,* 352–364.

Astrom, M., Adolfsson, R., & Asplund, K. (1993). Major depression in stroke patients: A three year longitudinal study. *Stroke, 24,* 976–982.

Aten, J.L., Caligiuri, M.P., & Holland, A.L. (1982). The efficacy of functional communication therapy for chronic aphasic patients. *Journal of Speech and Hearing Disorders, 47,* 93–96.

Avent, J.R., Wertz, R.T., & Auther, L.L. (1998). Relationship between language impairment and pragmatic behavior in aphasic adults. *Journal of Neurolinguistics, 11,* 207–221.

Bach-Y-Rita, P. (1990). Brain plasticity as a basis for recovery of function in humans. *Neuropsychologia, 28(6),* 547–554.

Ballard, K.J. & Thompson, C.K. (1999). Treatment and generalization of complex sentence production in agrammatism. *Journal of Speech, Language, and Hearing Research, 42,* 690–707.

Basso, A. (1992). Prognostic factors in aphasia. *Aphasiology, 6,* 337–348.

Basso, A., Capitani, E., Laiacona, M., & Luzzatti, C. (1980). Factors influencing type and severity of aphasia. *Cortex, 16,* 631–636.

Basso, A., Capitani, E., & Moraschini, S. (1982). Sex differences in recovery from aphasia. *Cortex, 18,* 469–475.

Basso, A., Capitani, E., & Vignolo, L.A. (1979). Influence of rehabilitation language skills in aphasia. *Archives of Neurology, 36,* 190–196.

Basso, A., Farabola, M., Grassi, M.P., Laiacona, M., & Zanobia, M.E. (1990). Aphasia in left-handers: Comparison of aphasia profiles and language recovery in non-right-handed and matched right-handed patients. *Brain and Language, 38,* 233–252.

Basso, A., Gardelli, M., Grassi, M.P., & Mariotti, M. (1989). The role of the right hemisphere in recovery from aphasia: Two case studies. *Cortex, 25(4),* 555–566.

Bateman, F. (1890). *On Aphasia, or Loss of Speech, and the Localisation of the Faculty of Articulate Language* (2nd ed.). London: J. & A. Churchill, Jarrod and Sons.

Bellaire, K.J., Georges, J.B., & Thompson, C.K. (1991). Establishing functional communication board use for nonverbal aphasic subjects. In M.L. Lemme (ed.), *Clinical Aphasiology, Vol. 19.* Austin, TX: Pro-Ed.

Benson, D.F. & Ardila, A. (1996). *Aphasia: A Clinical Perspective.* New York: Oxford University Press.

Bernstein-Ellis, E., Wertz, R.T., & Shubitowski, Y. (1987). More pace, less fillers: A verbal strategy for a high-level aphasic patient. In R.H. Brookshire (ed.), *Clinical Aphasiology, Vol. 17.* Minneapolis, MN: BRK Publishers.

Borod, J.C., Carper, J.M., & Naesser, M. (1990). Long-term language recovery in left-handed aphasic patients. *Aphasiology, 4,* 561–572.

Boyle, M. (1989). Reducing phonemic paraphasias in the connected speech of a conduction aphasic subject. In T.E. Prescott (ed.), *Clinical Aphasiology, Vol. 18.* Austin, TX: Pro-Ed.

Boyle, M. (1991). Anomia, dysfluency, and chronic alcoholism: Prognostic considerations. In T.E. Prescott (ed.), *Clinical Aphasiology, Vol. 20* (pp. 129–135). Austin, Texas: Pro-Ed.

Boyle, M., Coelho, C.A. (1995). Application of semantic feature analysis as a treatment for aphasic dysnomia. *American Journal of Speech-Language Pathology, 4,* 94–98.

Boysen, A.E. & Wertz, R.T. (1996). Clinical costs in aphasia treatment: How much is a word worth? In M.L. Lemme (ed.), *Clinical Aphasiology, Vol. 24.* Austin, TX: Pro-Ed.

Brindley, P., Copeland, M., Demain, C., & Martyn, P. (1989). A comparison of the speech of ten chronic Broca's aphasics following intensive and non-intensive periods of therapy. *Aphasiology, 3,* 695–707.

Broida, H. (1977). Language therapy effects in long term aphasia. *Archives of Physical Medicine and Rehabilitation, 58,* 248–253.

Broman, T., Lindholm, A., & Mein, B. (1967). Rehabilitation of aphasics. *Acta Neurologica Scandinavia, 43,* 125.

Butfield, E. & Zangwill, O.L. (1946). Re-education in aphasia: A review of 70 cases. *Journal of Neurology, Neurosurgery and Psychiatry, 9,* 75–79.

Cappa, S.F. & Vallar, G. (1992). The role of the left and right hemispheres in recovery from aphasia. *Aphasiology, 6(4),* 359–372.

Cappa, S.F., Perani, D., Grassi, F., Bressi, S., Alberoni, M., Franceschi, M., Bettinardi, V., Todde, S., & Fazio, F. (1997). A PET follow-up study of recovery after stroke in acute aphasics. *Brain and Language, 56,* 55–67.

Chambless, D.L. & Hollon, S.D. (1998). Defining empirically supported therapies. *Journal of Clinical and Consulting Psychology, 66,* 7–18.

Cherney, L.R., Merbitz, C.T., & Grip, J.C. (1986). Efficacy of oral reading in aphasia treatment outcome. *Rehabilitation Literature, 47,* 112–118.

Code, C. & Muller, D.J. (1992). *The Code-Muller Protocols: Assessing Perceptions of Psychosocial Adjustment to Aphasia and Related Disorders.* London: Whurr.

Code, C. & Rowley, D. (1987). Age and aphasia type: The interaction of sex, time since onset and handedness. *Aphasiology, 1(4),* 339–345.

Coelho, C.A. (1991). Manual sign acquisition and use in two aphasic subjects. In M.L. Lemme (ed.), *Clinical Aphasiology, Vol. 19.* Austin, TX: PRO-ED.

Cohen, J. (1988). *Statistical Power Analysis for the Behavioral Sciences.* Hillsdale, NJ: Lawrence Erlbaum.

Conlon, C.P. & McNeil, M.R. (1991). The efficacy of treatment for two globally aphasic adults using visual action therapy. In M.L. Lemme (ed.), *Clinical Aphasiology, Vol. 19.* Austin, TX: Pro-Ed.

Cook, T.D. & Campbell, D.T. (1979). *Quasi-Experimentation: Design and Analysis Issues for Field Settings.* Boston: Houghton Mifflin.

Darley, F.L. (1982). *Aphasia.* Philadelphia: W.B. Saunders.

Darley, F.L. (1972). The efficacy of language rehabilitation in aphasia. *Journal of Speech and Hearing Disorders, 37,* 3–21.

David, R., Enderby, P., & Bainton, D. (1982). Treatment of acquired aphasia: Speech therapists and volunteers compared. *Journal of Neurology, Neurosurgery, and Psychiatry, 45,* 957–961.

Davis, G.A. (1978). The clinical application of withdrawal, single-case research designs. In R.H. Brookshire (ed.), *Clinical Aphasiology, Vol. 8.* Minneapolis, MN: BRK Publishers.

Del Toro, J.F. (1997). Plasticity and recovery from brain damage in adulthood: What can recovery from aphasia teach us? *Newsletter of the American Speech Language Hearing Association, Special Interest Division 2: Neurophysiology and Neurogenic Speech and Hearing Disorders, 7(3),* 8–15.

De Renzi, E., Faglioni, P., & Ferrari, P. (1980). The influence of sex and age on the incidence and type of aphasia. *Cortex, 16,* 627–630.

Demeurisse, G. & Capon, A. (1987). Language recovery in aphasic stroke patients: Clinical, CT, and CBF studies. *Aphasiology, 1,* 301–315.

Disimoni, F., Keith, R., & Darley, R. (1980). Prediction of PICA overall score by short version of the test. *Journal of Speech and Hearing Research, 23,* 511–516.

Doyle, P.J., Goldstein, H., & Bourgeois, M.S. (1987). Experimental analysis of syntax training in Broca's aphasia: A generalization and social validation study. *Journal of Speech and Hearing Disorders, 52,* 143–155.

Duffy, J.R. (1994). Schuell's stimulation approach to rehabilitation. In R. Chapey (ed.), *Language Intervention Strategies in Adult Aphasia* (3rd ed.). Baltimore: Williams & Wilkins.

Eisenson, J. (1984). *Adult Aphasia* (2nd ed.). Englewood Cliffs, NJ: Prentice-Hall.

Elman, R.J. & Bernstein-Ellis, E. (1999). The efficacy of group communication treatment in adults with chronic aphasia. *Journal of Speech, Language, and Hearing Research, 42,* 411–419.

Feeney, D.M. & Baron, J.C. (1986). Diaschisis. *Stroke, 17,* 817–830.

Ferro, J.M. (1992). The influence of infarct location on recovery from global aphasia. *Aphasiology, 6(4),* 415–430.

Ferro, J.M. & Madureira, S. (1997). Aphasia type, age and cerebral infarct localisation. *Journal of Neurology, 244(8),* 505–509.

Franz, S.I. (1905). The reeducation of an aphasic. *The Journal of Philosophy, Psychology and Scientific Methods, 2,* 589–597.

Franz, S.I. (1924). Studies in re-education: The aphasias. *The Journal of Comparative Psychology, 4,* 349–429.

Frattali, C.M. (1998a). Outcome assessment in speech-language pathology. In A.F. Johnson & B.H. Jacobson (eds.), *Medical Speech-Language Pathology: A Practitioner's Guide.* New York: Thieme. 685–709

Frattali, C.M. (1998b). Outcomes measurement: Definitions, dimensions, and perspectives. In C.M. Frattali (ed.), *Measuring Outcomes in Speech-Language Pathology.* New York: Thieme.

Frazier, C.H. & Inham, S.D. (1920). A review of the effects of gunshot wounds of the head. *Archives of Neurology and Psychiatry, 3,* 17–40.

Gaddie, A., Kearns, K.P., & Yedor, K. (1991). A qualitative analysis of response elaboration training. In M.L. Lemme (ed.), *Clinical Aphasiology, Vol. 19.* Austin, TX: Pro-Ed.

Garrett, K.L. & Beukleman, D.R. (1995). Changes in the interaction patterns of an individual with severe aphasia given three types of partner support. In M.L. Lemme (ed.), *Clinical Aphasiology, Vol. 23.* Austin, Texas: Pro-Ed.

Gil, M., Cohen, M.G.M., Korn, C.,& Groswasser, Z. (1996). Vocational outcome of aphasic patients following severe traumatic brain injury. *Brain Injury, 10,* 39–45.

Gloning, K. (1977). Handedness and aphasia. *Neuropsychologia, 15,* 355–358.

Gloning, K., Trappl, R., Heiss, W.D., & Quatember, R. (1976). Prognosis and speech therapy in aphasia. In Y. LeBrun & R. Hoops (eds.), *Recovery in Aphasia* (pp. 57–64). Amsterdam: Swets & Zeitlinger.

Godfrey, C.M. (1959). A dysphasia rehabilitation clinic. *Canadian Medical Association Journal, 80,* 616–618.

Godfrey, C.M. & Douglass, E. (1959). The recovery process in aphasia. *Canadian Medical Association Journal, 80,* 618–624.

Goldenberg, G. & Spatt, J. (1994). Influence of size and site of cerebral lesions on spontaneous recovery of aphasia and on success of language therapy. *Brain and Language, 47,* 684–698.

Goldstein, K. (1948). *Aftereffects of Brain Injuries in War.* New York: Grune & Stratton.

Greenhouse, J.B., Fromm, D., Iyengar, S., Dew, M.A., Holland, A.L., & Kass, R.E. (1990). The making of a meta-analysis: A quantitative review of the aphasia treatment literature. In K.W. Wachter & M.L. Straf (eds.), *The Future of Meta-Analysis.* New York: Russell Sage Foundation.

Hagen, C. (1973). Communication abilities in hemiplegia: Effects of speech therapy. *Archives of Physical Medicine and Rehabilitation, 54,* 454–463.

Hanson, W.R. & Cicciarelli, A.W. (1978). The time, amount, and pattern of language improvement in adult aphasics. *British Journal of Disorders of Communication, 13,* 59–63.

Hanson, W.R., Metter, E.J., & Riege, W.H. (1989). The course of chronic aphasia. *Aphasiology, 3(1),* 19–29.

Hartman, J. & Landau, W.M. (1987). Comparison of formal language therapy with supportive counseling for aphasia due to acute vascular accident. *Archives of Neurology, 44,* 646–649.

Heiss, W.D., Karbe, H., Weber-Luxenburger, G., Herholz, K., Kessler, J., Pietrzyk, U., & Pawlik, G. (1997). Speech-induced cerebral metabolic activation reflects recovery from aphasia. *Journal of Neurological Sciences, 145(2),* 213–217.

Heiss, W-D, Kessler, J., Karbe, H., Fink, G.R., & Pawlik, G. (1993). Cerebral glucose metabolism as a predictor of recovery from aphasia ischemic stroke. *Archives of Neurology, 50,* 958–964.

Heiss, W-D, Kessler, J., Thiel, A., Ghaemi, M., & Karbe, H. (1999). Differential capacity of left and right hemispheric areas for compensation of poststroke aphasia. *Annals of Neurology, 45,* 430–438.

Hemsley, G. & Code, C. (1996). Interactions between recovery in aphasia, emotional and psychosocial factors in subjects with aphasia, and their significant others and speech pathologists. *Disability and Rehabilitation, 18(11),* 567–584.

Henley, S., Pettit, S., Todd-Pokropek, A., & Tupper, A. (1985). Who goes home? Predictive factors in stroke recovery. *Journal of Neurology, Neurosurgery, and Psychiatry, 48(1),* 1–6.

Herrmann, M. & Wallesch, C.W. (1993). Depressive changes in stroke patients. *Disability and Rehabilitation, 15,* 55–66.

Hillis, A.E. (1989). Efficacy and generalization of treatment for aphasic naming errors. *Archives of Physical Medicine and Rehabilitation, 70,* 632–636.

Hinckley, J.J. & Craig, H.K. (1998). Influence of rate of treatment on the naming abilities of adults with chronic aphasia. *Aphasiology, 12,* 989–1006.

Holland, A.L. (1980). *Communicative Abilities in Daily Living: A Test of Functional Communication for Adults.* Baltimore: University Park Press.

Holland, A.L., Fromm, D.S., DeRuyter, F., & Stein, M. (1996). Treatment efficacy: Aphasia. *Journal of Speech and Hearing Research, 39,* S27–S36.

Holland, A.L., Greenhouse, J.B., Fromm, D., & Swindell, C.S. (1989). Predictors of language restitution following stroke: A multivariate analysis. *Journal of Speech and Hearing Research, 32,* 232–238.

Hopkins, A. (1998). The measurement of outcomes of health care.

In M. Swash (ed.), *Outcomes in Neurological and Neurosurgical Disorders*. Cambridge, UK: Cambridge University Press.

Huber, W., Willmes, K., Poeck, K., Van Vleymen, B., & Derbert, W. (1997). Piracetam as an adjuvant to language therapy for aphasia: A randomized double-blind placebo-controlled pilot study. *Archives of Physical Medicine and Rehabilitation, 78,* 245–250.

Kane, R.L. (1997). Approaching the outcomes question. In R.L. Kane (ed.), *Understanding Health Care Outcome Research.* Gaithersburg, MD: Aspen Publishers.

Karbe, H., Herholz, K., Kessler, J., Wienhard, K., Pietrzyk, U.K.E., & Heiss, W.D. (1997). Recovery of language after brain damage. In H.J. Freund, B.A. Sabel, & O.W. Witte (eds.), *Brain Plasticity: Advances in Neurology, Vol. 73,* (pp. 347–358). Philadelphia: Lippincott-Raven.

Karbe, H., Kessler, J., Herholz, K., Fink, G., & Heiss, W.D. (1995). Long-term prognosis of post-stroke aphasia studies with positron emission tomography. *Archives of Neurology, 52,* 186–190.

Karbe, H., Thiel, A., Luxenburger, G.W., Herholz, K., Kessler, J., & Heiss, W-D. (1998). Brain plasticity in post-stroke aphasia: What is the contribution of the right hemisphere? *Brain and Language, 64,* 215–230.

Katz, R.C. & Wertz, R.T. (1997). The efficacy of computer-provided reading treatment for chronic aphasic adults. *Journal of Speech, Language, Hearing Research, 40,* 493–507.

Kearns, K.P. & Salmon, S.J. (1984). An experimental analysis of auxiliary and copula verb generalization in aphasia. *Journal of Speech and Hearing Disorders, 49,* 152–163.

Kearns, K.P. & Scher, G.P. (1989). The generalization of response elaboration training effects. In T.E. Prescott (ed.), *Clinical Aphasiology, Vol. 18.* Austin, TX: Pro-Ed.

Kearns, K.P. & Thompson, C.K. (1991). Analytical and technical directions in applied aphasia analysis: The Midas touch. In T.E. Prescott (ed.), *Clinical Aphasiology, Vol. 19.* Austin TX: Pro-Ed.

Kearns, K.P., Simmons, N.N., & Sisterhen, C. (1982). Gestural sign (Amer-Ind) as a facilitator of verbalization in patients with aphasia. In R.H. Brookshire (ed.), *Clinical Aphasiology, Vol. 12.* Minneapolis, MN: BRK Publishers.

Keenan, J. & Brassell, E. (1974). A study of factors related to prognosis for individual aphasic patients. *Journal of Speech and Hearing Disorders, 39,* 257–269.

Kenin, M. & Swisher, L. (1972). A study of pattern of recovery in aphasia. *Cortex, 8,* 56–68.

Kennedy, L. (1947). Remedial procedures for handling aphasic patients. *Archives of Neurology and Psychiatry, 57,* 646–649.

Kertesz, A. & McCabe, P. (1977). Recovery patterns and prognosis in aphasia. *Brain, 100,* 1–18.

Kertesz, A. (1982). *Western Aphasia Battery.* New York: Grune & Stratton.

Kertesz, A. (1988). Recovery of language disorders: Homologous contralateral or connected ipsilateral compensation? In S. Finger, T.E. LeVere, C.R. Almli, & D.G. Stein (eds.), *Brain Recovery: Theoretical and Controversial Issues* (pp. 307–321). New York: Plenum.

Kertesz, A., Harlock, W., & Coates, R. (1979). Computer tomographic localization, lesion size and prognosis in aphasia and nonverbal impairment. *Brain and Language, 8,* 34–50.

Kertesz, A., Lau, W.K., & Polk, M. (1993). The structural determinants of recovery in Wernicke's aphasia. *Brain and Language, 44,* 153–164.

Knopman, D.S., Rubens, A.B., Selnes, O.A., Klassen, A.C., & Meyer, M.W. (1984). Mechanisms of recovery from aphasia: Evidence from serial xenon 133 cerebral blood flow studies. *Annals of Neurology, 15,* 530–535.

LaPointe, L.L. (1978). Multiple baseline designs. In R.H. Brookshire (ed.), *Clinical Aphasiology, Vol. 8.* Minneapolis, MN: BRK Publishers.

LaPointe, L.L. (1983). Aphasia intervention with adults: Historical, present and future approaches. In J. Miller, D.E. Yoder, & R. Schiefelbusch (eds.), *Contemporary Issues in Language Intervention.* Rockville, MD: American Speech-Language-Hearing Association.

Lecours, A.R. & Lhermitte, F. (1983). Historical review: From Franz Gall to Pierre Marie. In A.R. Lecours, F. Lhermitte, & B. Bryans (eds.), *Aphasiology.* London: Baillière Tindall.

Lecours, A.R., Cronk, C., & Sébahoun-Balsamo, M. (1983). Historical review: From Pierre Marie to Norman Geschwind. In A.R. Lecours, F. Lhermitte, & B. Bryans (eds.), *Aphasiology.* London: Baillière Tindall.

Lesser, R. & Watt, M. (1978). Untrained community help in the rehabilitation of stroke sufferers with language disorder. *British Medical Journal, 2,* 1045–1048.

Levita, E. (1978). Effects of speech therapy on aphasics' responses to functional communication profile. *Perceptual and Motor Skills, 47,* 151–154.

Lincoln, N.B., McGuirk, E., Mulley, G.P., Lendrem, W., Jones, A.C., & Mitchell, J.R.A. (2 June 1984). Effectiveness of speech therapy for aphasic stoke patients: A randomized controlled trial. *The Lancet, 1(8388),* 1197–1200.

Lomas, J. & Kertesz, A. (1978). Patterns of spontaneous recovery in aphasic groups: A study of adult stroke patients. *Brain and Language, 5,* 388–401.

Lowell, S., Beeson, P.M., & Holland, A.L. (1995). The efficacy of a semantic cueing procedure on naming performance of adults with aphasia. *American Journal of Speech-Language Pathology, 4,* 109–114.

Ludlow, C.L., Rosenberg, J., Fair, C., Buck, D., Schesselman, S., & Salazar, A. (1986). Brain lesions associated with nonfluent aphasia fifteen years following penetrating head injury. *Brain, 109* (Pt 1): 55–80.

Luria, A.R. (1970). *Traumatic Aphasia.* The Hague: Mouton.

Macciocchi, S.N., Diamond, P.T., Alves, W.M., & Mertz, T. (1998). Ischemic stroke: Relation of age, lesion location, and initial neurologic deficit to functional outcome. *Archives of Physical Medicine and Rehabilitation, 79(10),* 1255–1257.

Mackenzie, C. (1991). An aphasia group intensive efficacy study. *British Journal of Disorders of Communication, 26,* 275–291.

Mark, V.W., Thomas, B.E., & Berndt, R.S. (1992). Factors associated with improvement in global aphasia. *Aphasiology, 6(2),* 121–134.

Marks, M., Taylor, M., & Rusk, H. (1957). Rehabilitation of the aphasic patient: A survey of three year's experience in a rehabilitation setting. *Neurology, 7,* 837–843.

Marshall, R.C. & Phillips, D.S. (1983). Prognosis for improved verbal communication in aphasic stroke patients. *Archives of Physical Medicine and Rehabilitation, 64(12)*, 597–600.

Marshall, R.C., Tompkins, C.A., & Phillips, D.S. (1982). Improvement in treated aphasia: Examination of selected prognostic factors. *Folia Phoniatrica, 34*, 305–315.

Marshall, R.C., Wertz, R.T., Weiss, D.G., Aten, J.L., Brookshire, R.H., Garcia-Buñuel, L., Holland, A.L., Kurtzke, J.F., LaPointe, L.L., Millianti, F.J., Brannegan, R., Greenbaum, H., Vogel, D., Carter, J., Barnes, N.S., & Goodman, R. (1989). Home treatment for aphasic patients by trained nonprofessionals. *Journal of Speech and Hearing Disorders, 54*, 462–470.

Mazzoni, M., Vista, M., Pardossi, L., Avila, L., Bianchi, F., & Moretti, P. (1992). Spontaneous evolution of aphasia after ischaemic stroke. *Aphasiology, 6*, 387–396.

McDermott, F.B., Horner, J., & DeLOng, E.R. (1996). Evolution of acute aphasia as measured by the Western Aphasia Battery. *Clinical Aphasiology, 24*, 159–172.

McGlone, J. (1977). Sex differences in the cerebral organization of verbal function and cognitive impairment in stroke: Age, sex, aphasia type and laterality differences. *Brain, 100*, 775–793.

McGlone, J. (1980). Sex differences in human brain asymmetry: A critical survey. *Behavioral Brain Sciences, 3*, 215–263.

McNeil, M.R., Small, S.L., Masterson, R.J., & Fossett, T.R.D. (1995). Behavioral and pharmacological treatment of lexical-semantic deficits in a single patient with primary progressive aphasia. *American Journal of Speech-Language Pathology, 4*, 76–87.

Meikle, M., Wechsler, E., Tupper, A., Benenson, M., Butler, J., Mulhall, D., & Stern, G. (1979). Comparative trial of volunteers and professional treatments of dysphasia after stroke. *British Medical Journal, 2*, 87–89.

Messerli, P., Tissot, A., & Rodriguez, J. (1976). Recovery from aphasia: Some factors of prognosis. In Y. LeBrun & R. Hoops (eds.), *Recovery in Aphasia* (pp. 124–135). Amsterdam: Swets & Zeitlinger.

Metter, E.J., Jackson, C.A., Kempler, D., & Hanson, W.R. (1992). Temporoparietal cortex and the recovery of language comprehension in aphasia. *Aphasiology, 6*, 349–358.

Miceli, G., Caltagirone, C., Gainotti, G., Masullo, C., Silveri, C., & Villa, G. (1981). Influence of age, sex, literacy and pathologic lesion on incidence, severity and type of aphasia. *Acta Neurologica Scandinavica, 64*, 370–382.

Mills, C.K. (1904). Treatment of aphasia by training. *Journal of the American Medical Association, 43*, 1940–1949.

Mimura, M., Kato, M., Kato, M., Sano, Y., Kojima, T., Naeser, M., & Kashima, H. (1998). Prospective and retrospective studies of recovery in aphasia: Changes in cerebral blood flow and language functions. *Brain, 121*, 2083–2094.

Mlcoch, A.G., Bushnell, D.L., Gupta, S., & Milo, T.J. (1994). Speech fluency in aphasia: Regional cerebral blood flow correlates of recovery using single-photon emission computed tomography. *Journal of Neuroimaging, 4(1)*, 6–10.

Moore, B.D. & Papanicolaou, A.C. (1988). Dichotic-listening evidence of right hemisphere involvement in recovery from aphasia following stroke. *Journal of Clinical and Experimental Neuropsychology, 10*, 380–386.

Naeser, M.A., Palumbo, C.L., Helm-Estabrooks, N., Stiassny-

Eder, D., & Albert, M.L. (1989). Severe nonfluency in aphasia. *Brain, 112*, 1–38.

Naeser, M.A., Palumbo, C.L., Prete, M.N., Fitzpatrick, P.M., Mimura, M., Samaraweera, R., & Albert, M.L. (1998). Visible changes in lesion borders on CT scan after five years poststroke, and long-term recovery in aphasia. *Brain and Language, 62*, 1–28.

Naeser, M.A., Gaddie, A., Palumbo, C.L., & Stiassny-Eder, D. (1990). Late recovery of auditory comprehension in global aphasia. *Archives of Neurology, 47*, 425–432.

Naeser, M.A., Helm-Estabrooks, N., Haas, G., Auerbach, S., & Srinivasan, M. (1987). Relationship between lesion extent in 'Wernicke's area' on computed tomographic scan and predicting recovery of comprehension in Wernicke's aphasia. *Archives of Neurology, 44*, 73–82.

Neyman, J. (1943). Basic ideas and some recent results of the theory of testing statistical hypotheses. *Journal of the Royal Statistical Society, 106*, 292–327.

Nicholas, M.L., Helm-Estabrooks, N., Ward-Lonergan, J., & Morgan, A.R. (1993). Evolution of severe aphasia in the first two years post onset. *Archives of Physical Medicine and Rehabilitation, 74*, 830–836.

Obler, L.K., Albert, M., Goodglass, H., & Benson, D.F. (1978). Aphasia type and aging. *Brain and Language, 6*, 318–322.

Odell, K.H., Bair, S., Flynn, M., Workinger, M., Osborne, D., & Chial, M. (1997). Retrospective study of treatment outcome for individuals with aphasia. *Aphasiology, 11*, 415–432.

Ohyama, M., Senda, M., Kitamura, S., Ishii K., Mishina, M., & Terashi, A. (1996). Role of the nondominant hemisphere and undamaged area during word repetition in poststroke aphasics: A PET activation study. *Stroke, 27(5)*, 897–903.

Paolucci, S., Antonucci, G., Gialloreti, L.E., Traballesi, M., Lubich, S., Pratesi, L., & Palombi, L. (1996). Predicting stroke inpatient rehabilitation outcome: The prominent role of neuropsychological disorders. *European Neurology, 36(6)*, 385–90.

Papanicolaou, A.C., Moore, B.D., Deutsch, G., Levin, H.S., & Eisenberg, H.M. (1988). Evidence for right hemisphere involvement in recovery from aphasia. *Archives of Neurology, 45*, 1025–1029.

Pashek G.V. & Holland, A.L. (1988). Evolution of aphasia in the first year post-onset. *Cortex, 24(3)*, 411–423.

Peach, R.K. (1987). A short-term memory treatment approach to the repetition deficit in conduction aphasia. In R.H. Brookshire (ed.), *Clinical Aphasiology, Vol. 17*. Minneapolis, MN: BRK Publishers.

Pederson, P.M., Jorgensen, H.S., Nakayama, H., Raaschou, H.O., & Olsen, T.S. (1995). Aphasia in acute stroke: Incidence, determinants, and recovery. *Annals of Neurology, 38*, 659–666.

Pickersgill, M.J. & Lincoln, N.B. (1983). Prognostic indicators and the pattern of recovery of communication in aphasic stroke patients. *Journal of Neurology, Neurosurgery and Psychiatry, 46(2)*, 130–139.

Pizzamiglio, L., Mammucari, A., & Razzano, C. (1985). Evidence for sex differences in brain organization in recovery in aphasia. *Brain and Language, 25*, 213–223.

Poeck, K., Huber, W., & Willmes, K. (1989). Outcome of intensive language treatment in aphasia. *Journal of Speech and Hearing Disorders, 54*, 471–479.

Popovici, M. & Mihäilescu, L. (1992). Melodic intonation in the rehabilitation of Romanian aphasics with bucco-lingual apraxia. *Romanian Journal of Neurology and Psychiatry, 30,* 99–113.

Porch, B.E. (1981). *Porch Index of Communicative Abilities, Vol. II: Administration, Scoring, and Interpretation* (3rd ed.). Palo Alto, CA: Consulting Psychologists Press.

Prins, R.S., Schoonen, R., & Vermeulen, J. (1989). Efficacy of two different types of speech therapy for aphasic stroke patients. *Applied Psycholinguistics, 10,* 85–123.

Prins, R.S., Snow, C.E., & Wagenaar, E. (1978). Recovery from aphasia: Spontaneous language versus language comprehension. *Brain and Language, 6,* 192–211.

Raymer, A.M., Thompson, C.K., Jacobs, B., & Le Grand, H.R. (1993). Phonological treatment of naming deficits in aphasia: model based generalization analysis. *Aphasiology, 7,* 27–53.

Robey, R.R. (1994). The efficacy of treatment for aphasic persons: A meta-analysis. *Brain and Language, 47,* 585–608.

Robey, R.R. (1998). A meta-analysis of clinical outcomes in the treatment of aphasia. *Journal of Speech, Language, and Hearing Research, 41,* 172–187.

Robey, R.R. & Dalebout, S.D. (1998). A tutorial on conducting meta-analyses of clinical outcome research. *Journal of Speech-Language-Hearing Research, 41,* 1227–1241.

Robey, R.R. & Schultz, M.C. (1998). A model for conducting clinical outcome research: An adaptation of the standard protocol for use in aphasiology. *Aphasiology, 12,* 787–810.

Robey, R.R., McCallum, A.F., & Francois, L.K. (1999). A Meta-Analysis of Single-Subject Research on Treatments for Aphasia. A paper presented before the 1999 Clinical Aphasiology Conference, Key West, FL.

Robey, R.R., Schultz, M.C., Crawford, A.B., & Sinner, C.A. (1999). Single-subject clinical-outcome research: Designs, data, effect sizes, and analyses. *Aphasiology, 13,* 445–473.

Rubens, A.B. (1977). The role of changes within the central nervous system during recovery from aphasia. In M.A. Sullivan & M.S. Kommers (eds.), *Rationale for Adult Aphasia Therapy* (pp. 28–43). University of Nebraska Medical Center.

Salvatore, A. (1985). Experimental analysis of a syntax stimulation training procedure. In R.H. Brookshire (ed.), *Clinical Aphasiology, Vol. 15* (pp. 214–221). Minneapolis, MN: BRK Publishers.

Sands, E., Sarno, M.T., & Shankweiler, D. (1969). Long-term assessment of language function in aphasia due to stroke. *Archives of Physical Medicine and Rehabilitation, 50,* 202–206.

Sarno, M.T. (1969). *The Functional Communication Profile: Manual of Directions; Rehabilitation Monograph 42.* New York: New York Institute of Rehabilitative Medicine.

Sarno, M.T. (1991). Recovery and rehabilitation in aphasia. In M.T. Sarno (ed.), *Acquired Aphasia* (2nd ed.). San Diego: Academic Press.

Sarno, M.T. (1992). Preliminary findings in a study of age, linguistic evolution and quality of life in recovery from aphasia. *Scandinavian Journal of Rehabilitation Medicine Supplement, 26,* 43–59.

Sarno, M.T. (1997). Quality of life in aphasia in the first post-stroke year. *Aphasiology, 11,* 665–679.

Sarno, M.T., Buonaguro, A., & Levita, E. (1985). Gender and recovery from aphasia after stroke. *Journal of Nervous and Mental Disease, 173,* 605–609.

Sarno, M.T. & Levita, E. (1971). Natural course of recovery in severe aphasia. *Archives of Physical Medicine and Rehabilitation, 52,* 175–178.

Sarno, M.T. & Levita, E. (1979). Recovery in treated aphasia in the first year post-stroke. *Stroke, 10,* 663–670.

Sarno, M.T. & Levita, E. (1981). Some observations on the nature of recovery in global aphasia after stroke. *Brain and Language, 13,* 1–12.

Sarno, M.T., Silverman, M., & Sands, E. (1970). Speech therapy and language recovery in severe aphasia. *Journal of Speech and Hearing Research, 13,* 607–623.

Schneider, S.L., Thompson, C.K., & Luring, B. (1996). Effects of verbal plus gestural matrix training on sentence production in a patient with primary progressive aphasia. *Aphasiology, 10,* 297–317.

Sederer, L.I., Dickey, B., & Hermann, R.C. (1996). The imperative of outcomes assessment in psychiatry. In L.I. Sederer & B. Dickey (eds.), *Outcomes Assessment in Clinical Practice.* Baltimore: Williams & Wilkins.

Selnes, O.A., Knopman, D.S., Niccum, N., Rubens, A.B., & Larson, D. (1983). Computed tomographic scan correlates of auditory comprehension deficits in aphasia: A prospective recovery study. *Annals of Neurology, 5,* 558–566.

Shewan, C.M. (1986). The history and efficacy of aphasia treatment. In R. Chapey (ed.), *Language Intervention Strategies in Adult Aphasia* (2nd ed.). Baltimore: Williams & Wilkins.

Shewan, C.M. & Bandur, D.L. (1986). *Treatment of Aphasia: A Language-Oriented Approach.* San Diego: College-Hill Press.

Shewan, C.M. & Kertesz, A. (1984). Effects of speech language treatment in recovery from aphasia. *Brain and Language, 23,* 272–299.

Silvestrini, M., Troisi, E., Matteis, M., Cuppini, L.M., & Caltagirone, C. (1995). Involvement of the healthy hemisphere in recovery from aphasia and motor deficit in patients with cortical ischemic infarctions: A transcranial Doppler study. *Neurology, 45,* 1815–1820.

Silvestrini, M., Troisi, E., Matteis, M., Razzano, S.T., & Caltagirone, C. (1998). Correlations of flow velocity changes during mental activity and recovery from aphasia in ischemic stroke. *Neurology, 50,* 191–195.

Sparks, R., Helm, N., & Albert, M. (1974). Aphasia rehabilitation resulting from melodic intonation therapy. *Cortex, 10,* 303–316.

Starkstein, S.E. & Robinson, R.G. (1988). Aphasia and depression. *Aphasiology, 2,* 1–20.

Steele, R.D., Weinrich, M., Wertz, R.T., Kleczewska, M.K., & Carlson, G.S. (1989). Computer-based visual communication in aphasia. *Neuropsychologia, 27,* 409–426.

Steele, R.D., Weinrich, M., Kleczewska, M.K., Carlson, G.S., & Wertz, R.T. (1987). Evaluating performance of severely aphasic Patients on a computer-aided visual communication system. In R.H. Brookshire (ed.), *Clinical Aphasiology, Vol. 17* (pp. 46–54). Minneapolis, MN: BRK Publishers.

Student [William Sealy Gosset] (1908). The probable error of a mean. *Biometrika, 6,* 1–15.

Subirana, A. (1958). The prognosis of aphasia in relation to the factor of cerebral dominance and handedness. *Brain, 81,* 415–425.

Thomas, C., Altenmuller, E., Marckmann, G., Kahrs, J., & Dichgans, J. (1997). Language processing in aphasia: Changes in lateralization patterns during recovery reflect cerebral plasticity in adults. *Electroencephalography and Clinical Neurophysiology, 102(2),* 86–97.

Thompson, C.K. & Shapiro, L.P. (1994). A linguistic-specific approach to treatment of sentence production deficits in aphasia. In M.L. Lemme (ed.), *Clinical Aphasiology, Vol. 22.* Austin, TX: Pro-Ed.

Thompson, C.K., McReynolds, L.V., & Vance, C.E. (1982). Generative use of locatives in multiword utterances in agrammatism: A matrix-training approach. In R.H. Brookshire (ed.), *Clinical Aphasiology, Vol. 12.* Minneapolis, MN: BRK Publishers.

Thompson, C.K., Shapiro, L.P., Tait, M.E., Jacobs, B.J., & Schneider, S.L. (1996). Training wh-question production in agrammatic aphasia: Analysis of argument and adjunct movement. *Brain and Language, 52,* 175–228.

Thulborn, K.R., Carpenter, P.A., & Just, M.A. (1999). Plasticity of language-related brain function during recovery from stroke. *Stroke, 30(4),* 749–754.

Tompkins, C.A., Jackson, S.T., & Schulz, R. (1990). On prognostic research in adult neurologic disorders. *Journal of Speech and Hearing Research, 33,* 398–401.

Van Zagten, M., Boiten, J., Kessels, F., & Lodder, J. (1996). Significant progression of white matter lesions and small deep (lacunar) infarcts in patients with stroke. *Archives of Neurology, 53,* 650–655.

Vignolo, L.A. (1964). Evolution of aphasia and language rehabilitation: A retrospective exploratory study. *Cortex, 1,* 344–367.

Wambaugh, J.L., Thompson, C.K. (1989). Training and generalization of agrammatic aphasic adults' Wh-interrogative productions. *Journal of Speech and Hearing Disorders, 54,* 509–525.

Warburton, E., Price, C.J., Swinburn, K., & Wise, R.J. (1999). Mechanisms of recovery from aphasia: Evidence from positron emission tomography studies. *Journal of Neurology, Neurosurgery, and Psychiatry, 66(2),* 155–161.

Weiller, C., Isensee, C., Rijntjes, M., Huber, W., Muller, S., Bier, D., Dutschka, K., Woods, R.P., Noth, J., & Diener, H.C. (1995). Recovery from Wernicke's aphasia: A positron emission tomographic study. *Annals of Neurology, 37,* 723–732.

Weisenburg, T., & McBride, K.E. (1935). *Aphasia: A Clinical and Psychological Study.* New York: The Commonwealth Fund.

Wepman, J.M. (1951). *Recovery From Aphasia.* New York: The Ronald Press Co.

Wertz, R.T., Collins, M.J., Weiss, D., Kurtzke, J.F., Friden, T., Brookshire, R.H., Pierce, J., Holtzapple, P., Hubbard, D.J., Porch, B.E., West, J.A., Davis, L., Matovich, V., Morley, G.K., & Resurreccion, E. (1981). Veterans Administration cooperative study on aphasia: A comparison of individual and group treatment. *Journal of Speech and Hearing Research, 24,* 580–594.

Wertz, R.T., Weiss, D.G., Aten, J.L., Brookshire, R.H., Garcia-Buñuel, L., Holland, A.L., Kurtzke, J.F., LaPointe, L.L., Milianti, F.J., Brannegan, R., Greenbaum, H., Marshall, R.C., Vogel, D., Carter, J., Barnes, N.S., & Goodman, R. (1986). Comparison of clinic, home, and deferred language treatment for aphasia: A Veterans Affairs cooperative study. *Archives of Neurology, 43,* 653–658.

West, R. & Stockel, S. (1965). The effect of meprobamate on recovery from aphasia. *Journal of Speech and Hearing Research, 8,* 57–62.

Whitaker, H.A. (1998). History of neurolinguistics. In B. Stemmer & H.A. Whitaker (eds.), *Handbook of Neurolinguistics.* San Diego: Academic Press.

Whitney, J.L. & Goldstein, H. (1989). Using self-monitoring to reduce disfluencies in speakers with mild aphasia. *Journal of Speech and Hearing Disorders, 54,* 576–586.

Whurr, R., Lorch, M.P., & Nye, C. (1992). A meta-analysis of studies carried out between 1946 and 1988 concerned with the efficacy of speech and language treatment for aphasic patients. *European Journal of Disorders of Communication, 27,* 1–17.

World Health Organization. (1980). *International Classification of Impairments, Disabilities, and Handicaps.* Geneva: WHO.

World Health Organization. (1997). *International Classification of Impairments, Activities, and Participation* (ICIDH-2). Geneva: WHO.

Chapter 7

Delivering Language Intervention Services to Adults with Neurogenic Communication Disorders

Brooke Hallowell and Roberta Chapey

OBJECTIVES

The objectives of this chapter are to (1) describe the contexts in which clinicians serve adults with neurogenic communication disorders; (2) describe the many professional roles of the aphasiologist; (3) discuss key legislative issues that affect service delivery; (4) present an overview of the means by which clinicians and service providing agencies are reimbursed for services; (5) stimulate discussion of the active ways in which clinicians may serve as advocates for patients in the current service delivery climate; and (6) discuss future trends in service delivery.

INTRODUCTION

In no time in the history of aphasiology has the context in which clinicians work so influenced the delivery of intervention services to persons with neurogenic communication disorders. Throughout the world, changes in health care policy, reimbursement schemes, national health plans, political climates, insurance mechanisms, clinical licensure, and professional training are having dramatic impacts on our access to patients, as well as on the services we may deliver to them. In the United States, particularly, recent impacts of managed care in the private sector and evolving federal health policies are significantly impacting the practice of aphasiology.

In this chapter we discuss the contexts in which aphasiologists work and the multiple roles they play. Legislative issues and other factors affecting reimbursement for clinical services are then presented in terms of their implications for the delivery of services to persons with aphasia. Strategic actions in which aphasiologists may engage to further the effectiveness of services, patients' access to care, and the financial stability of service-providing agencies are highlighted. The nature of the "ultimate excellent clinical aphasiologist" is explored in light of the demands of the current health care climate.

SERVICE DELIVERY CONTEXTS FOR LANGUAGE INTERVENTION

Speech-language pathologists rehabilitate adult patients with aphasia in a variety of settings such as hospitals, rehabilitation centers, skilled nursing facilities, nursing homes, clinics, private offices, and the patient's own home.

Hospitals

Most major community hospitals have a comprehensive program for stroke rehabilitation, including a basic rehabilitation team comprised of a physician, a rehabilitation nurse, a social worker, a physical therapist, an occupational therapist, and a speech-language pathologist. Optimally, a physiatrist, a psychologist, and a rehabilitation counselor are also members of this team. The acute, immediately post-stroke or post-trauma patient is frequently placed in an acute medical area and may receive speech-language evaluation, intervention, and counseling at the bedside. Recent trends in reducing the length of time patients are allowed to remain in acute care contexts, though, have limited acute care clinicians to a primary focus on screening and diagnostic services rather than on concerted intervention (Katz et al., in press). Acute care clinicians are also involved in educating patients' significant others about the nature of aphasia.

In most instances, convalescent stroke and trauma patients are placed near rehabilitation services, in a specific area that is properly equipped for rehabilitation and staffed by personnel with special training in rehabilitation. Adequate space and equipment are usually provided to ensure high-quality evaluation, treatment, and counseling services, which are rendered for both inpatients and outpatients. The advantage of providing speech-language services in this setting is that a hospital may provide integrated, coordinated, comprehensive team management for stroke and aphasia. The same may be said for rehabilitation centers.

Rehabilitation Centers

A rehabilitation center may be a component of a hospital or may exist as a separate, independent facility that has a close working relationship with one or more hospitals. In either case, there are usually both inpatient and outpatient services that provide comprehensive team rehabilitation (Sahs & Hartman, 1976). For patients who have recovered from the acute stages of stroke or trauma, the decision as to whether they should receive sub-acute rehabilitation as outpatients or inpatients or be transferred to another facility depends on several variables, such as the extent of disability; overall health status; geographic location of potential placement sites and access to transportation; the degree of need for integrated comprehensive intervention in nursing, speech-language pathology, physical therapy, and occupational therapy; insurance coverage; the patient's financial resources; and the degree of family support and involvement.

Skilled Nursing Facilities

The distinctions among terms such as long-term care center, nursing home, skilled nursing facility, and even rehabilitation center, have become less and less clear in recent years. Since the late 1980s, rehabilitative care has gravitated away from acute care hospitals, and toward facilities that were once merely considered long-term care centers or "rest homes" (facilities to which most residents traditionally had been admitted with the anticipation that they would stay there for the rest of their lives). Rather than staying in the hospital until they are rehabilitated to the point of being able to return to their homes, most stroke and trauma patients are now discharged from acute care centers to subacute care centers, often outside the hospital context. A majority of skilled nursing facilities now offer comprehensive rehabilitative services, both for short-term patients who are expected to return to their homes, as well as for long-term residents. Consequently, over the past 10 years, most United States residents have seen the signs for "nursing homes" in their local neighborhoods change to signs for "skilled nursing and rehabilitation centers" and the like.

Nursing Homes and Long-Term Care Centers

Even in long-term care contexts that do not specialize in short-term rehabilitation, speech-language therapy, occupational therapy, and physical therapy services are generally offered. In most instances, these homes also provide ongoing environmental stimulation and attempt to meet the patient's social and emotional needs. Speech-language clinicians in these contexts often work on a contractual basis with the nursing home, either as independent professionals or as employees of a rehabilitation company that contracts with multiple nursing homes in a given area. Thus, nursing home clinicians frequently work on an itinerant basis, providing speech-language services to two or more facilities.

Many long-term care centers have varied types of residential facilities that differ according to the levels of care needed by residents. They range from apartments, for adults capable of living independently but wishing to be close to central social and medical facilities, to nursing home rooms, in which residents are provided constant skilled medical and rehabilitative care. In the United States, federal programs do not generally cover the cost of long-term care. Some Medicaid programs cover long-term nursing home expenses, but only for individuals whose savings are minimal enough to qualify for such programs. Thus, financial concerns are often at the forefront for residents of long-term care facilities and their adult children. During the past 10 years, many new long-term care insurance programs have become available. Although potentially costly, they do help individuals plan carefully for long-term care expenses they may incur as they grow older.

Routine help in the home and in adult day-care centers can forestall or eliminate institutionalization for many elderly people. For elderly individuals who receive care from a family member, approximately half of their assistance is provided by a spouse and half from adult children such as a daughter or daughter-in-law (Frady et al., 1985). However, as the general population continues to age, the number of adult children available to provide such care will be reduced (Chapey, 1994). Today, as never before, there is a need to foster comprehensive, coherent, and realistic policies on retirement income, health care, and long-term care within our communities, within industry, and within our government.

Independent Speech and Hearing Centers

One type of independent speech and hearing clinic is the freestanding not-for-profit agency. Another is the speech and hearing clinic housed within a university training program in communication sciences and disorders, in which student clinicians are supervised in the provision of services. A third type of speech and hearing center is the office of the independent speech-language pathologist in private practice.

In all of these settings, services are provided for persons of all ages with any variety of communication disorders. Typically, all three types of settings have suitable rooms and proper equipment in order to provide appropriate assessment, intervention, and counseling services to patients. Outpatient services are the primary offering, although many free-standing agencies provide contractual services through hospitals, nursing homes, rehabilitation centers, and home health agencies as well. Although independent agencies do not generally have formal rehabilitation teams, individual speech-language clinicians often refer patients to other rehabilitation professionals when appropriate and establish close communication with other professionals who are working with a given patient. In addition, many private practices are established in partnership with other rehabilitation personnel, or are located in buildings that house such personnel.

Home Health

Many stroke and aphasia patients return to their homes after the acute medical emergency has subsided, or after a period of therapy at a rehabilitation center. When this happens, community-based home health care agencies provide a variety of services to the patient through a well-structured, closely coordinated program. Indeed, home care services to the elderly have grown rapidly because of the pressure on hospitals to reduce costs (ASHA, 1986; Task Force on Treatment Outcomes and Cost Effectiveness, 1996). Insurers like such services because they are cost-effective, and most elderly consumers prefer to receive services in their own home (ASHA, 1986). According to Kerr (1992), community-based programs provide reasonable prices and high-quality care and have better long-term results than residential facilities. Skills mastered in treatment programs do not have to be transferred to the home environment because they are taught where they will be used. In addition, independence and self-reliance are fostered.

The range of home health services may include visiting physician care; visiting nurse service; physical, occupational, and speech-language therapy and evaluation; psychiatric, psychological, and social work evaluation and therapy; special assistive devices; financial help for medical/rehabilitation and maintenance requirements; dietary counseling; and homemaker or household assistance.

THE MANY ROLES OF THE APHASIOLOGIST

Regardless of the professional setting in which the clinician is employed, the clinical aphasiologist performs many of the same functions. The most common functions of this clinician are identification and selection of clients; assessment; intervention; consultation and collaborative care; counseling; administration; quality assurance; contract negotiation; education; marketing; fundraising; advocacy; ethical decision-making; and research.

Identification and Selection of Clients

The ways in which patients are located or referred vary from setting to setting. In most instances, persons with aphasia are identified when a physician or another member of a rehabilitation team refers them to the aphasiologist. Such referrals are dependent on team members' abilities to recognize the language impairment, and their interest in reporting the problem to the speech-language clinician.

In some residential settings, the clinician screens each individual who enters the facility (Chapey et al., 1979). The purpose of screening is generally to identify those who have language, speech, and/or swallowing problems. Once persons with aphasia have been identified, a more detailed assessment is performed. Enrollment in a diagnostic and/or treatment program depends on many factors, including the patient's willingness and desire to participate; the attitudes and support of the patient's significant others; authorization from the patient's primary physician; the clinician's existing caseload demands; transportation to and from the clinical setting; and insurance coverage and other economic factors.

Assessment

Assessment and intervention are the most important functions of the aphasiologist. The purpose of assessment is to provide an in-depth description of each client's cognitive, linguistic, and communicative behavior, and to define the factors that should be taken into account in order to stimulate the patient's use of language. The diagnostic process, as well as some of the influences of health care reform on the way we engage in the diagnostic process, are discussed in detail elsewhere in this text.

Intervention

Rehabilitation, ideally, is a complex, dynamic, comprehensive process of patient care, beginning at the time of onset and continuing until the "maximum physical, psychological, social (language), and vocational functions for each individual have been achieved" (Sahs & Hartman, 1976, p. 205). The term intervention is frequently used to refer to the process of facilitating rehabilitation through skilled treatment, or therapy.

Through intervention, aphasiologists attempt to heighten each patient's potential to function maximally within his or her environment, to facilitate meaningful relationships, and to restore self-esteem, dignity, and independence (Wepman, 1972a). As we will consider in this chapter, many factors in the service delivery arena may interfere with patients' access to intervention. Thus, the maximum benefits for which patients have potential are not always achieved. Persons with neurogenic communication disorders, like all persons with disabilities, should be treated by highly qualified clinicians using the best techniques available to meet their holistic needs with quality and dignity (Keith, 1975).

Language intervention is also a complex, flexible, organized, goal-directed, dynamic process, aimed at restoring the individual's previously learned language through treatment and/or training. Intervention "must be individually patterned, uniquely presented, and continuously tailored to signs of progress and signs of failure" (Darley, 1982, p. 238). It is a process that is designed to change communicative behavior, not only within the domain of the clinical setting, but in all communicative contexts.

Intervention is not confined to language and communication alone. The clinician helps patients to maintain and strengthen activities, participation in life, and social contacts, set and achieve life goals, gain a positive attitude, increase morale, gain insight into impairments, and develop feelings of acceptance, optimism, and emotional stability. Intervention is an innovative process that responds to the neurological, linguistic, and social and life participation goals and needs of each client (Wepman, 1972b), with a focus on the regaining of functional skills for communication in everyday life.

Due to increasing restrictions on frequency and duration of treatment for many patients requiring rehabilitation services, there is a growing need for stimulation and facilitation of communication outside of the clinical environment from the earliest stages of treatment. Likewise, it is increasingly important to include caregivers and patients' significant others in direct treatment sessions. Numerous technological tools are now available to supplement skilled treatment sessions, as described by Katz and Hallowell (1999) and by Katz (see Chapter 34). While such tools may help to enrich the intervention process, it is essential to recognize that their limitations, when used without a clinician, preclude their use as a solution to problems of reduced frequency and duration of skilled intervention.

Consultation and Collaborative Care

Most clinical aphasiologists function as members of rehabilitative assessment-intervention teams. In this capacity, they share knowledge and information with other professionals, such as occupational therapists, physical therapists, physicians, nurses, social workers, and dietitians, as well as with family members. This necessitates team development and collaborative decision making (see Chapter 8). Interdisciplinary consultation includes in-service training programs and presentations to professional groups. Team discussions may be related to coordination or execution of clinical services, case management of specific clients, the nature of aphasia and other conditions, assessment and intervention related to medical, behavioral, and/or psychological problems, documentation and insurance coverage, personal, occupational and community activities, life participation, and discharge planning. True collaboration, in which the expertise of all team members is oriented toward holistically rehabilitating individuals to their fullest potential, improves case management through knowledge, understanding, and cooperation.

Counseling

The role of counselor or adviser involves exchanging ideas or opinions and conducting discussions with the patient, members of the family, other professionals, or the community. The specific content of individual or group counseling depends on the individuals involved, but most often involves patients and their significant others. Topics such as the causes of stroke, the life-affecting impacts of stroke and aphasia, types of rehabilitation services available, as well as death and dying may be discussed.

Administration

Traditionally, administration or management has encompassed record keeping and report writing, scheduling clients, and ordering supplies. In the past, many aphasiologists practiced in clinical capacities with few other management responsibilities. In most of today's service delivery environments, though, clinicians play greatly expanded administrative roles. Even those without administrative or management titles, per se, are expected to engage in other activities that are not strictly clinical, such as marketing, advocacy, and quality assurance.

Documentation

Records and reports play a significant role in an aphasiology treatment program. The primary purposes for keeping records are to generate an account of the clinical services provided, to support the planning of future assessment and intervention goals, and to justify reimbursement for services provided. The system of record keeping chosen should be one that can be interpreted easily by other professionals. Some of the specific types of records and reports that may be used are assessment records, session plans (including goals, methods, type of therapy, and an evaluation of the client's responses), conference records, release of information forms, referral forms, master schedules, statistical summaries of cases, progress reports, and periodic disposition reports. The primary purposes of preparing reports are to disseminate and maintain information. Accurate, clear, and timely records and reports are essential to (1) providing a continuity of service; (2) maintaining a cumulative account of each individual's assets, limitations, and progress in therapy; (3) evaluating the effectiveness, quality, efficiency, and productivity of clinicians and treatment programs; (4) monitoring consumer satisfaction; (5) developing and justifying programs; and (6) ensuring that clinicians and their employers are financially reimbursed for their services.

Thorough documentation is the vehicle that permits authorization (and sometimes pre- and re-authorization) for diagnosis and treatment, and determines reimbursement by third-party payers (i.e., insurance companies, managed care organizations, and federal health programs). Thus, clinical aphasiologists should be competent writers and should be well trained in the fine art of clinical documentation. Speech-language documentation must contain (1) a complete history; (2) a clear statement of the problem; (3) a plan of action to address the problem, including long-term and short-term goals that are describable and quantifiable; (4) descriptions of tasks and modalities to be used in treatment; and (5) a prognostic statement and indication of expected results of intervention—preferably in terms of skills and abilities that facilitate functional behavior, independence, and improved quality of life. No matter how excellent actual clinical services may be, clinicians and/or their employing agencies are regularly denied reimbursement from insurance companies or other third-party payers when documentation does not address each of these areas.

As treatment continues, progress should be recorded in detail. Changes in an individual's intellectual, emotional, life participation, and social status as they relate to communicative improvement should be described. Has motivation changed? Have there been changes in pre-existing conditions?

Documentation should be logical and sequential. Each report should be strongly tied to preceding and subsequent reports. Whenever possible, statements from patients and their families or significant others should be a component of progress notes or revisions of goals and procedures. Visual aids such as graphs and charts may add clarity to reports (Slominski, 1985a).

In most managed care contexts and in contexts serving Medicare and Medicaid patients, standardized diagnostic and treatment reporting and billing forms are becoming the norm. Responses to these forms require clinicians to summarize vast amounts of information related to patient care in small designated spaces on pre-printed forms. In some cases clinicians from many disciplines are required to input their data on the same form. Such interdisciplinary coordination requires concerted effort to complete treatment and diagnostic records in a timely manner.

Aphasiologists, like clinicians in most health care disciplines, may enjoy the advantages of new technological developments that facilitate report writing and record keeping. For example, report writing templates may be generated through word processing programs (e.g., Microsoft Word or WordPerfect) or commercially available programs (c.f., Hallowell & Katz, 1999). Further, in some settings, voice activation report writing software now allows for hands-free dictation of reports, notes, and letters. Additionally, computerized versions of forms required by the Health Care Financing Administration (HCFA) allow for computerized completion and easy transfer of information from one form to another (c.f., Parrot Software, 1999). Some large hospitals and rehabilitation centers use report writing software that links multiple workstations and integrates input from multiple disciplines. Such software may also be used to coordinate diagnostic, treatment, billing, and patient scheduling functions within and across disciplines (Hallowell & Katz, 1999). Further technological facilitation of report writing is available through voice activation software that allows for hands-free dictation of reports, notes, and letters.

Billing and Coding

Financial reimbursement from third-party payers depends on thoughtful, strategic billing practices. Clinicians are often responsible for the primary billing practices, including the tracking of time spent in treatment and diagnostic services, the coding of services according to coding schemes acceptable to each third-party payer, the completion of billing forms, and the submission of billing forms along with diagnostic and treatment reports to third-party payers. Even in those hospitals, rehabilitation centers, and other agencies that employ clerical professionals who are responsible for billing paperwork, clinicians must provide the factual input that will determine the content of billing records.

In most employment contexts, it is important for clinicians to be familiar with numerical coding systems used by third-party payers. The two coding systems most commonly used in speech-language pathology are the International Classification of Diseases, 9th revision, Clinical Modification (ICD-9-CM) (Centers for Disease Control, 1999) and the Physicians Current Procedural Terminology, 4th edition (CPT™) (American Medical Association, 1999). Most public and private payers require ICD-9 codes for diagnoses and CPT codes for "procedures," or specific services rendered. These codes serve to standardize billing codes for uniformity among service providers and third-party payers.

ICD-9 diagnostic codes are used to classify medical diagnoses across disciplines and clinical settings. They are required by most insurance companies and by all programs of the U.S. Public Health Service and HCFA (i.e., Medicare and Medicaid). ICD-9 codes consist of three digits. Sometimes, additional information is conveyed by adding two more digits to the right of a decimal point. A new edition of ICD codes, the ICD-10 codes, are in draft status and are under review by users and HCFA at the time of publication of the current text. The diagnostic codes currently in use may be obtained through HCFA (HCFA, 1998), and through publications available through the American Speech-Language-Hearing Association (ASHA, 1997).

CPT codes are used to standardize the coding of health care services across disciplines and clinical settings. They consist of five digits. The codes are published annually by the American Medical Association, and are also available through ASHA (ASHA, 1997). Numerous software packages and Internet resources are available for help in automation of billing and coding practices.

Appealing Denials for Treatment Authorization or Reimbursement

In many cases, requests for treatment authorization or for reimbursement of services already provided are denied by third-party payers. As managed care practices have expanded dramatically over the past few years, many agencies have seen their denial rates for evaluations and treatment authorizations grow significantly, some by as much as six times from 1996 to 1998 (Henri & Hallowell, 1999c). Typical reasons for which an insurance company may deny authorization or reimbursement include (1) lack of a physician's order for services; (2) improper documentation or coding of diagnostic and/or treatment information; (3) failure to demonstrate that the patient has adequate rehabilitation potential to justify services; (4) failure to demonstrate the functional impacts that treatment will have on the functional communication, medical management, independence, and quality of life of the individual being served; (5) non-coverage of certain services by the patient's specific health care plan; and (6) exhaustion of services allowed by a given health care plan.

Whenever authorization or reimbursement is denied, clinicians may make an appeal to reverse the denial. In a majority of the cases reported in the United States, appeals for reimbursement are successful (Henri & Hallowell, 1999c). Documentation that supports a letter of appeal may include a copy of written diagnostic or treatment authorization from the primary care physician, progress notes, and discharge reports. The likelihood of success in the appeals process depends, in large part, on the quality of documentation, as well as in the persistence of the clinician or other professionals pursuing the appeal. Excellent documentation, and ongoing educational and advocacy efforts between clinicians and third-party payers, may help to reduce the likelihood of denials occurring in the first place.

If an appeal to overturn a denial for treatment authorization or reimbursement is unsuccessful, the clinician may be instrumental in having the patient or his or her significant other(s) file a complaint with the insurance company. Likewise, individuals with employer-sponsored insurance may file complaints with the human resources department of their employers. A more confrontational measure is to inform the third-party payer that a complaint will be filed with the state's insurance commissioner. It is important to avoid undermining relationships with insurers, though, and to maintain a cooperative, rather than adversarial, spirit throughout the process of reversing a denial whenever possible (Henri & Hallowell, 1999c).

Scheduling

Scheduling involves preparing a timed plan for the week, month, and/or year. Scheduling for the year involves accounting for legal holidays and professional conventions and conferences, and providing time for in-service training sessions and vacation time for staff members. In planning a weekly schedule, time must be reserved for traveling, holding conferences, writing reports, preparing sessions, coordinating activities, performing in-service education, and reading current professional literature. For most clinicians,

the largest amount of time is ideally invested in patient assessment and intervention. Scheduling of individual patients is dependent on such things as the patient's health and prognosis, transportation, clinicians' expertise, current clinical caseloads, insurance coverage, and additional financial considerations.

Ordering Supplies

Relevant equipment, materials, and supplies are often ordered by the clinician, depending on their perceived usefulness and the availability of funds for such purchases. Items that are frequently obtained include standard tests, textbooks, workbooks, prepared treatment materials, tape recorders and audiotapes, videotape recorders and videotapes, computers, software, and paper.

Negotiating Contracts with Third-Party Payers

To be listed on an insurance company's preferred provider list, or to provide services for members of a preferred provider plan, clinicians must have a contract with the corresponding insurance company. In many cases, professionals with administrative titles are the designated officials who engage in developing and negotiating the details of such contracts. Sometimes clinicians negotiate contracts, too, especially those who work in private practice, small speech-language hearing centers, community agencies, and university clinics (Henri et al., 1996).

Currently, there is keen interest among many clinicians in joining specialty provider networks. Provider networks enable clinicians to team together, thus expanding patient and referral bases for network members, and decreasing the costs of marketing, billing, and other management functions through shared expenses (Davolt, 1999). Like contracting with HMOs, contracting with networks may be highly beneficial, and even necessary to some clinicians' and agencies' fiscal survival; but it involves complex professional risks, and requires keen business savvy on the part of clinicians. The employment of professional consultants for help in this arena is often well worth its cost.

Education

In the role of educator, the aphasiologist may supervise student clinicians and paraprofessionals and/or teach in university training programs. The aphasiologist may also present in-service training to administrators, home health aides, other health care staff, and family members. Further, continuing self-education is essential to advanced professional competence. Reading professional journals and attending conferences, workshops, and courses helps to enrich professional development. Patient education may involve empowering individuals by informing them about the array of medical, communicative, activity, life participation, environmental, and social choices available to them. The more individuals are involved in making decisions about their own care, the more positive and participatory they become. In addition, informing patients about their rights and discussing issues such as hope and its role in recovery, stress management, and self-esteem may be beneficial to treatment (Chapey, 1994).

Ideally, the clinical aphasiologist also educates the public, fostering awareness of means of preventing stroke and traumatic brain injury. "Every year millions of people suffer and die of illnesses that could be cured or eliminated by altering patterns of personal behavior" (Ewart, 1991, p. 931). Clinicians may empower individuals for improvement by stimulating a sense of self-control, mastery, and power to effect change. Through education, they also encourage collective empowerment within the community, and development of strategies to promote better health patterns.

Marketing

Marketing is the process of defining what a potential customer wants or needs, producing that service, and letting others know the service is for sale (Matthews, 1988). It involves (1) detailed analysis of the customers' perceptions, wants, and needs; (2) analysis of the competition and other external factors that will affect service delivery; (3) development of products and services; (4) public relations; (5) publicity (such as brochures, newsletters, education pamphlets, and slide shows); and (6) advertising (Chapey, 1994; Matthews, 1988).

In this era of health care reform, few service-providing agencies, be they hospitals, long-term care facilities, rehabilitation centers, not-for-profit clinics, home health agencies, or private practices, can assume that a steady flow of patients who can pay for diagnostic and treatment services will appear at their doors. Service providers must now dedicate resources to marketing efforts to ensure that their agencies remain fiscally stable, that patients with communication disorders have access to treatment, and that communication disorders professionals continue to be employed (Cohn, 1994; Henri et al., 1996). Clinicians often participate in collaborative marketing efforts, including the development and dissemination of publicity materials, meetings with physicians and other referral sources, conferences with insurance company representatives, and offering of in-services to the case managers and reviewers who make coverage and reimbursement decisions for managed care organizations (MCOs).

Quality Assurance

Deep budget cuts and increased competitiveness require health care professionals to deliver better products and services with greater efficiency (Roth, 1999). Quality is a competitive advantage. While quality assurance programs were once considered to be in the domain of management staff, most service-providing agencies now depend upon the contributions of all staff members in holistic, strategic quality assurance efforts (Underhill, 1991). Total quality management (TQM) is a notion that has received a great deal of attention in all types of businesses throughout the world over the past two decades. It involves delivering a service or making a product, engaging employees in every process, assessing customer satisfaction, and modifying operations strategically based on outcomes and consumer feedback. The emphasis is on productivity, flexibility, efficiency, effective communication, and consumer-driven services (Chapey, 1994).

TQM involves building quality into the whole of an organization, not just in specific aspects, components, or departments (Labovitz, 1991). Enterprises with successful TQM programs have well-defined objectives and guidelines for every participant, and are led by informed and active people. Ideally, these institutions invest in the notions that (1) it is people who are critical to success, thus employees at all levels should be empowered (Chapey, 1994); (2) customers must receive the best possible services; (3) excellence must be pursued in all areas of operation; and (4) strong investments in research and development are essential to quality, as are high readiness and receptiveness to change (Bernowski, 1991; Chapey, 1994).

Many regulatory agencies, including the Joint Commission on Accreditation of Healthcare Organizations (JCAHO) and the Professional Services Board (PSB) of ASHA, require accredited clinical facilities to demonstrate continuous quality improvement programs (Roth, 1999). Such programs, generally employing multiple facets of TQM and related quality management strategies, involve the ongoing and systematic monitoring, analysis, and improvement of services to yield improved patient outcomes. Regulatory agencies that accredit MCOs (e.g., the National Committee on Quality Assurance [NCQA]) also require quality assurance programs on the part of MCOs (NCQA, 1999). In all organizations, communication lines must be open before TQM concepts are introduced (McLaurin & Bell, 1991). Good communication is vital to the success of the total quality process (Chapey, 1994; Varian, 1991).

Within health care in general and speech-language pathology in particular, there is a need to define what makes a TQM program. We need to define our customers in very specific terms. Who are we serving? Insurance companies, facilities, the state, the patient? What are their specific needs? How can we become more responsive to these needs? What constitutes success in a TQM facility? What is our vision? What are our goals? To be excellent, we must stay close to our customers, learn their preferences, and cater to them (Peters & Waterman, 1982). We need to assess consumer satisfaction and ask how we can make their schedules better, use our facilities better for their benefit, and use our human resources better in order to be the preferred provider of

TABLE 7–1

Survey of Facility and Organizational TQM

How do you define the service that you provide?

What is the vision of your organization? Was it arrived at collaboratively? Does everyone share that constancy of purpose?

Is this facility/organization built on quality, excellence, and service?

Is the culture of the organization characterized by ethical behavior, expectations of excellence, and respect for fellow employees?

Do you have specific goals for quality, as you do for other key areas, such as fiscal containment?

Are you continuously striving for quality improvement and perfection?

What rewards do you provide for quality improvement accomplished by employees?

Is the employment environment conducive to excellence?

Is this facility an enjoyable place to work?

Are people having fun working at this facility and working toward quality? Is it a fear-free environment?

Does the organization provide necessary continuing education and training?

How many layers of management are there?

Are upper-level managers readily accessible to the employees?

Has the company created a democratic environment (no titles on doors, no executive washrooms)?

Does the organization empower people?

Do the people closest to the customer make the decisions?

Do subordinates always have to check with supervisors before performing tasks?

Is there a "we" orientation or mindset of collaboration and not competition?

Is there true congeniality among the employees? Is there mutual trust?

Does your company delegate responsibility as aggressively as possible?

Has your organization lost its direction and momentum?

Is it clear that people are the organization's greatest asset?

How does this facility communicate to its employees that they are respected ? That they are the top priority? That they make a difference?

How does this organization promote growth of employees from within?

Does this facility recruit the most motivated, highly educated, competent professionals?

Do employees use their creative energies to satisfy and delight customers?

Do all employees think about conducting their business in a perfect way?

Are there vehicles within the organization that continually strive for work simplification, work elimination, and business process improvement?

Do people across this organization feel that everyone else is working as hard as they are?

Does the credit for the prosperity of the facility/organization go to the people?

What vehicles do you use to get people to take pride in their work?

Are all members of the organization involved in the quality effort?

How is superior performance rewarded?

Do individuals accomplish their tasks in a timely, effective, and high-quality manner?

Have you created a customer-centered culture?

How often do you administer a consumer satisfaction survey? What were the results of this customer satisfaction study? What areas are you targeting for improvement as a result of this investigation? How have you translated customer needs into designing your service?

Is your purchaser confident in your (the supplier's) quality systems?

Is there a customer/supplier partnership?

Are service delivery, marketing, billing, and customer service processes reviewed and analyzed regularly to determine if they can be improved?

Do you search for changes in services to create a competitive advantage?

Have you determined your customer's prioritized expectations related to service (such as ease of use, timeliness, and outcomes)?

cognitive, linguistic, and communicative services for our patients (see Table 7–1) (Chapey, 1977; 1994).

In the field of communication sciences and disorders we must create reliable and valid quality assurance measures to assess patients' perceptions of the outcomes and efficacy of our treatments. In addition, we need to advocate for our professional integrity by promoting the importance of adequate professional training, certification, and licensure for professionals who work in the area of neurogenic communication disorders. Our clients have complex, multifaceted disabilities and deserve to interact with qualified professionals (Chapey, 1994).

Health care and containment of health care costs will continue to be a prime political issue in the upcoming decades. The winners in service delivery competition "will not necessarily be the cheapest health care facilities, but those that meet customer needs by delivering quality care" (Labovitz, 1991, p. 46). We need to integrate TQM into our decisions regarding the kind of changes we believe are essential to the highest quality service (Chapey, 1994).

Fundraising

Reduced rates for clinical services under managed care, in combination with reduced frequency and intensity of many covered services, is resulting in generally decreased revenues associated with clinical services. Thus, many service-providing agencies are increasingly reliant on finding additional means of financial support. Not-for-profit agencies, in particular, which are charged with providing services to clients regardless of their ability to pay, are dependent on alternative means of generating income to support clinical revenues. Many for-profit agencies have established their own not-for-profit foundations, or are partnering with existing foundations that help support the provision of services to persons whose access might otherwise be limited. Thus, clinicians are often involved in supporting fundraising efforts.

Fundraising efforts may include collaboration in developing fundraising materials, establishing and expanding a donor base of individuals, clients, foundations, and corporations that support the concerns of people with communication disorders; participating in annual fund campaigns, special events (e.g., benefit concerts, dinners, and sporting events); meeting with donors and potential donors about special clinical programs and needs; collaborating with fundraising professionals on planned giving programs; and establishing partnerships with corporations and fraternal organizations (Henri & Hallowell, 1999a; 1999c).

Ethical Decision-Making

During the 21st century, health care workers will increasingly be interacting with patients, family, and other health care workers, and making decisions about the right to life, euthanasia, do-not-resuscitate (DNR) orders, the quality of life, and the right to health care access. Agonizing questions we will have to face include: Who has the right to decide how long a patient lives? How much of our limited financial resources should be used to delay death? Should we provide rehabilitative services to people who are near death? How much emphasis should we give a patient's estimated prognosis when we decide whether or not to provide services?

In addition, clinicians face other conflicts of interest related to their own financial gains (Council on Ethical and Judicial Affairs, American Medical Association, 1995). During the past two decades, many rehabilitation companies in the United States have offered financial bonuses to clinicians based upon the amount of time they have engaged in billable service. Henri and Hallowell (1997) enumerate and describe the ways in which incentive systems may affect the quality and ethics of patient care by speech-language pathologists:

1. Seeing high-fee patients too long or beyond the point of expecting further reasonable progress
2. Seeing low-fee patients too briefly or at such a frequency and intensity that progress is unlikely
3. Admitting patients to treatment who are unlikely to benefit from skilled therapy, i.e., patients who have limited rehabilitation potential. Related to this would be admitting persons to treatment as a result of overstating the likelihood of improvement
4. When documenting progress for billing, "stretching the truth," i.e., misrepresenting actual progress or other forms of dishonesty
5. Misrepresenting the actual time spent in treatment
6. Avoiding non-billable activities that are important to quality of service, e.g., in-services, informal discussions with team members, staff meetings (p. 9).

Although there is an enormous amount of research across disciplines and industries documenting the effectiveness of incentive systems, ethical implications of incentive systems are virtually ignored in most of the research literature. A recent study (Hallowell et al., 1999) suggests that students exiting graduate school and entering the clinical workforce are susceptible to such conflicts of interest, which appear to be related to the students' sense of financial need. The study also demonstrates that practicing clinicians across the country confront a multitude of ethical conflicts related not only to financial bonuses, but also to more dire personal needs. For example, an increasing number of clinicians are threatened with the loss of their jobs if they do not achieve a certain minimum level of billable clinical productivity per week. Consequently, many report a sense of ongoing ethical pressure in balancing their needs for job security with the ethical nature of treatment, billing, and caseload management decisions. As recent world-wide trends in health care restructuring have reduced financial gains through the provision of rehabilitation services (Katz et al., in press; Penn, 1993), clinicians must be well prepared to face with solid moral fortitude personal conflicts of interest related to professional decisions.

Research

Some aphasiologists pursue careers in research at colleges, universities, or at private, state, or federal research agencies. A national shortage of doctoral-level personnel in communication sciences and disorders in the United States is now yielding rich opportunities for careers in higher education

(Geffner, 1997). Furthermore, the need for faculty members who specialize in neurogenic communication disorders is greater than the need for those in most other specialties within the profession. According to the results of annual surveys of graduate programs in communication sciences and disorders (Petrosino et al., 1997), the anticipated doctoral faculty openings in adult neurogenic disorders outnumbered those in every other specialty within speech-language pathology from 1991 through 1998. Additionally, the survey results indicate that the number of new doctoral program graduates in adult neurogenic disorders is far below the number needed to fill the corresponding open positions.

Many clinicians with interests in scholarly work find personal and professional rewards in continuing their graduate and post-graduate training in research. For some seasoned clinicians, those interests lead to significant career changes as they return to school for doctoral study. Others know from the start of their graduate studies that they want to engage in academic careers, and thus continue their doctoral studies soon after their master's-level training.

Even clinicians who are not invested in research careers should be good consumers of and contributors to research. Minifie (1983) aptly claims that the destiny of our field is imminently tied to practitioners assuming a greater role in developing the clinical science, and that mediocrity comes from a division between clinical and research programs. Research is inseparable from clinical service.

There is a greater need now than in any time in the history of aphasiology to demonstrate the effectiveness of our interventions. It is essential to establish "how much and what kind of treatment is best and what changes constitute important treatment outcomes" (Thompson & Kearns, 1991, p. 52). As third-party payers are demanding published, empirically based evidence of treatment efficacy and functional treatment outcomes to justify reimbursement for our services, every clinical aphasiologist has a responsibility to document his or her clinical successes and failures. Consequently, clinicians must be familiar with techniques of scientific research design, measurement, and analysis, and with specific behavioral, cognitive, communicative, and/or linguistic models of intervention (Thompson & Kearns). Clinicians who are not well versed in research design, and those whose schedules do not permit time to perform extensive reviews of literature, collect data, and write for publication, may establish constructive partnerships with doctoral-level researchers in nearby academic institutions.

While the kind and quality of research that is undertaken depends on the availability of facilities and subjects and on the cooperative atmosphere provided by the administration and staff, it also largely depends on the commitment of the individual clinician to analyze the effectiveness of his or her work. An essential component of quality research is the creation of an environment that is conducive to risk taking. Thus, the quality, motivation, and personal relationships of the research staff, and the style of management that is either supportive of creativity or critical of new ideas, will influence the quality of research that is conducted (Ringel, 1982).

Advocacy

Increasing competition for limited health care resources requires that speech-language pathologists be active advocates on behalf of their profession and their patients. Some specific means by which aphasiologists may advocate for their patients were discussed above in terms of appealing denials for authorization and reimbursement, marketing, quality assurance, education, negotiating contracts, and participating in research. Although it may seem obvious to the aphasiologist that speech and language services are essential to the total care of a patient, it is often necessary to demonstrate that fact to consumers and their significant others, colleagues in other disciplines, referral sources, insurance company representatives, and legislators. Consumer advocacy is usually effective. However, consumers who have communication disorders, especially aphasia, are often unable to advocate independently for the services they need. It is important for the clinician to provide patients and their significant others the information necessary to be effective self-advocates. Aphasiologists may provide guidance concerning how to approach primary care physicians and insurers, reverse prior authorization or treatment denials, write letters to legislators and insurance commissioners, or even testify before state and regional committees that monitor the performance of MCOs (Henri & Hallowell, 1999b; 1999c).

In the United States, numerous legislative advocacy campaigns to support the provision of services to persons with communication disorders are supported by ASHA, which provides free advocacy materials on the Internet and through mailings. Numerous state and local professional organizations provide training and materials to support legislative advocacy, too. Although it is not often part of the clinicians' job description to be engaged in local, regional, and national advocacy, many clinicians feel compelled to do so, recognizing its importance. They may engage in letter-writing campaigns to legislators, election campaigns to support political representatives who support the provision of services to persons with communication disorders, and consumer education projects. Each individual's advocacy efforts contribute to the gains of all patients and professionals in our discipline.

LEGISLATIVE ISSUES AFFECTING SERVICE DELIVERY

In the United States, several pieces of federal and state legislation have been passed to ensure that persons of all ages with special conditions have access to adequate and appropriate levels of service. It is important for speech-language clinicians to be familiar with federal and state laws and rules and regulations that support access to special services. The Social Security Act, for example, contains several titles (i.e., chapters or subsections) that ensure reimbursement for speech-language pathology and audiology services (Henri & Hallowell, 1999b). Those pertinent to serving adults with aphasia include Title 18 (Medicare), Title 19 (Medicaid), Title 20 (the Social Services Subsidy, which supports social work services that, in turn, may help families access speech-language pathology and audiology services). Many of these reimbursement mechanisms have mixed histories serving populations with chronic or degenerative conditions (Smith & Ashbaugh, 1995).

Several other pieces of federal legislation also support services to adults with aphasia. The Americans with Disabilities Act does not ensure funding, but may require employers to make available certain resources in cases where communication disorders have demonstrable impacts on an individual's ability to perform job duties. Other such federal acts include the Individuals with Disabilities Education Act, the primary funding vehicle for states' special education programs, and the Rehabilitation Act, which funds rehabilitation services, including speech-language pathology and audiology, for persons ranging in age from 16 to 64 (Henri & Hallowell, 1999b).

THE ECONOMICS OF LANGUAGE INTERVENTION SERVICES

The delivery of diagnostic and intervention services is heavily influenced by economics. Professional clinicians are paid for the services they provide. Income generated through clinical services very rarely comes from fees paid by patients directly to providers. Rather, provider agencies are reimbursed by third-party payers. Third-party payers are usually insurance companies, federal health care plans, or special not-for-profit foundations. Most often, clinicians receive salaries or hourly wages from their employers. Those who are self-employed generally pay themselves a fixed salary or a portion of the profits from their practice's annual revenues.

Third-Party Payers

In most countries, health care services are covered through nationalized health programs. In the United States, however, individuals are insured primarily through private health insurance programs, the majority through plans offered by employers as part of a benefits package. In many cases, those who are insured by their employers make some financial contribution to maintain their insurance plans. Often, employees have some choices regarding the type and extent of medical coverage they would like, with less costly plans providing fewer medical benefits.

In addition to private insurance programs, there are two federal health programs that influence service delivery to adults in the United States: Medicare and Medicaid. Medicare provides for speech-language pathology coverage to adults over 65 years of age and for persons under the age of 65 who have long-term disabilities (those lasting more than 2 years). Medicare plans are generally administered through private insurance companies that serve as interfaces between service providers and the Medicare program. Medicaid provides for services to persons who meet definable levels of low income and specific asset standards. Medicaid programs are administered by individual states. Additionally, individuals who have served in the United States armed forces are eligible for health care services provided through the Veterans Health Administration in the Department of Veterans Affairs (VA), most often at VA hospitals and clinics.

Reimbursement Schemes

Traditionally—that is, prior to about 1996—most insurance companies throughout the United States reimbursed service providers for specific services rendered and/or for units of time during which clinicians engaged in billable services with covered individuals. This reimbursement arrangement is known as "fee-for-service." Now, however, far-reaching measures known collectively as "managed care" have modified the traditional modes of reimbursement. Some of these managed care modes have existed for a long time, especially in certain geographic pockets of the United States. They now characterize the majority of reimbursement arrangements in the United States. Examples of alternative reimbursement modes are discounted fee-for-service, case rate, per diem, and capitation. There are many permutations to each of these modes.

Discounted fee-for-service arrangements involve the establishment of reduced rates for patients who are members of a specific plan. In order to provide services to a plan's members, providers must agree to those rates. Third-party payers are billed for units of billable time or for specific services rendered.

In a *case rate* arrangement, the provider is paid a specific fee for treating a patient with a particular diagnosis, regardless of the duration of care or the number of services rendered. The case rate is based on actuarial analyses of the likely needs of patients according to their diagnoses. The standard Medicare diagnosis-related group (DRG) system and the new Medicare prospective payment system (PPS) are examples of this type of arrangement.

In a *per diem* arrangement, the third-party payer pays the provider a specific amount of money for each day during which a patient is in the provider's care. The type and number of services does not generally influence the per diem rate.

Capitation involves a fixed amount of money that is paid to a provider, based on the number of people enrolled in a specific plan, not on the actual services rendered. Capitation rates are based on actuarial analyses of the likely needs of individuals who are insured through a specific plan. If those individuals require more services than are covered by the capitation revenue, then providers must absorb the remaining cost of caring for the enrolled individuals. Thus, capitation arrangements can be highly risky for providers. Still, capitation is the fastest-growing type of payment system (Task Force on Treatment Outcomes and Cost Effectiveness, 1996).

Managed Care

The rapid proliferation of managed care practices in the United States is having a dramatic influence on virtually all aspects of service delivery to persons with aphasia and other communication disorders (Ad Hoc Committee on Managed Care of the American Speech-Language-Hearing Association, 1994). Managed care has been defined in myriad ways in the health care literature. Sometimes it is defined with a focus on managed care's goals of preventing illness, maximizing health outcomes, coordinating care, and reducing unnecessary care (Henri & Hallowell, 1999c). Other definitions highlight specific cost-control and cost-cutting tactics that are characteristic of managed care modes of service delivery. Regardless of the specific way one defines managed care, the three main goals most frequently stated are assurance of the quality and coordination of care, access to care for persons who need it, and cost control (Henri & Hallowell, 1999c). Unfortunately, the health care literature and the popular media are replete with accounts of how the overwhelming focus on cost control in managed care often leads to compromises in quality and access.

Because of great variability in managed care proliferation according to geographic location within the country, and because of variability in the definition of what constitutes managed care, specific estimates of managed care market penetration in the United States are variable. A majority of privately insured citizens receive service though a managed care arrangement. Likewise, a large and growing proportion of Medicare and Medicaid patients receive federally sponsored benefits through managed care plans (Inglehart, 1995; Stollman, 1995). If one considers the cost-control mechanisms that are implemented across virtually all health care contexts, the actual rate of managed care penetration across the country is now near 100%. These cost-control mechanisms, enumerated by Henri and Hallowell (1999c), include

...increasingly stringent utilization review; preadmission certification for hospital stays; required preauthorization for services; negotiated reduced reimbursement rates; designation of a restricted list of "preferred providers;" the designation of physicians as "gatekeepers" of patients' health care expenditure allotments; salaried employment of physicians by payer organizations; payment of incentives to physicians not to refer patients for specialty (e.g., rehabilitation) services; use of red-flag diagnostic or treatment categories to deny reimbursement; and restrictions on frequency, intensity, and duration of care (p. 4).

During the expansion of managed care in the United States, there has been a general, parallel trend in health care restructuring all over the globe. Even in those countries that rely extensively on nationalized health care systems, there have been upheavals in organizational structures and a proliferation of severe cost-cutting tactics in both federal and private programs (Katz et al., in press).

Managed Care Organizations

MCOs are insurance companies or programs that operate in managed care modes. Given that the definition of managed care varies according to one's professional context and point of view, one might argue that the definition of an MCO does, too. Generally, though, MCOs are characterized by (1) use of specific types of cost-saving reimbursement schemes, as described above; (2) promotion of health and wellness through preventive care and patient education; (3) concerted efforts to coordinate the type and number of services received by each enrollee; and (4) reduced enrollment fees for enrollees and/or the employers who pay for enrollees' insurance coverage.

There are many types of MCOs. The two most common examples are preferred provider organizations and health maintenance organizations. A preferred provider organization (PPO) is one that contracts with specific providers who agree to offer services to the PPO's enrollees at rates that are significantly below what the same providers would normally charge in a fee-for-service arrangement. Providers generally agree to reduced rates in the form of discounted fees-for-service, capitation schemes, case rates, or per diem allowances. Very low fees, usually in the form of co-payments, serve as an incentive for enrollees to use preferred providers. Members of a plan may use "out-of-network" providers, but at much higher rates and with greater restrictions on the type and extent of services allowable.

A health maintenance organization (HMO) is a type of MCO in which comprehensive services are provided through one health care facility or a network of facilities. Many of the clinicians who work for HMOs, including physicians, nurses, rehabilitation therapists, social workers, etc., are salaried by the HMO. They generally do not bill a third-party payer for services. Reimbursement schemes in HMOs are generally based on prospective payment models. The primary care physician of each enrollee is considered a gatekeeper of all health care resources, having the authority to determine the frequency, intensity, and duration of any services allowable for each patient. Since the gatekeeper almost always receives financial rewards for spending less of the available financial resources on services to patients, he or she has inherent conflicts of interest related to the determination of services to be provided (Begley, 1987; Grey, 1990a; Grey, 1990b; Rodwin, 1995).

Consequences of Managed Care for Intervention in Aphasia

Restructuring of health care systems to reduce costs has transferred control of the access to, and duration of, care from clinicians to administrators. Although efforts to control rising health care costs are laudable, such efforts often threaten patients' access to care and the quality of care they receive (Henri & Hallowell, 1996; Purtillo, 1995; Randall, 1994).

The key areas of challenge to professional practice in neurogenic communication disorders are the same as those summarized by Henri and Hallowell (1999c) for the professions of speech-language pathology and audiology in general:

(a) consumers' access to our services;
(b) the quality, intensity, duration, and frequency of care that we can provide;
(c) the fiscal stability of our service-providing agencies;
(d) the livelihood of our professionals;
(e) the maintenance of our professional integrity; and
(f) problems of consumers' access to our services (p. 4).

Let us briefly review each of these key areas as they pertain to adults with neurogenic communication disorders.

Consumer Access

Consumers' access to diagnostic and treatment services is threatened by decreased referrals from managed care's gatekeepers, usually physicians, who often receive financial incentives to decrease the amount of service offered. For persons with neurogenic disorders, managed care's emphasis on acute-care service delivery models is particularly troublesome. One of the principal ways in which clinicians are held accountable for the outcomes of their services in such models is through the documentation of patients' ongoing improvements throughout treatment, with a logical point of discharge based on maximal progress (Henri & Hallowell, 1999c). Since persons with chronic and/or multiple disabilities, and/or with degenerative conditions (Fox et al., 1993; Smith & Ashbaugh, 1995), and persons who are elderly (Clement et al., 1994; Oberlander, 1997) often do not fit the acute-care patterns of quick and steady gains toward recovery and discharge, such individuals are experiencing more and more difficulty in receiving our services. Furthermore, MCOs are less likely to provide full coverage for such persons

(Iglehart, 1995). Restrictions on coverage for conditions diagnosed prior to enrollment enable MCOs to reduce expenditures associated with the care of costly conditions (Clement et al., 1994; Fisher, 1994; Henri & Hallowell, 1999a; Hiller & Lewis, 1995; Perkins, 1998).

Members of cultural and ethnic minorities and of low-income populations have restricted access to care as well (Henri & Hallowell, 1999c; Leigh, 1994; Stenger, 1993), perhaps because they are "less likely to enjoy employer-sponsored health care plans, are less likely to afford their own health care coverage, and may be less likely to advocate for their own health care coverage needs" (Henri & Hallowell, 1999c, p. 6). Ironically, such individuals tend to have disproportionately greater needs for rehabilitation services (Screen & Anderson, 1994).

MCO clauses emphasizing the relatively new concept of "evidence-based medical necessity" further threaten patient access to speech-language services. Under such clauses, if providers cannot present a solid body of well-controlled research to support the effectiveness of any intervention administered, then they will not be reimbursed for providing that intervention. An additional repercussion of medical necessity clauses is the emphasis on the importance of treatment of medical impairments rather than of disabling conditions that influence quality of life. A disconcerting example of this repercussion is that many clinicians are finding it easier to obtain authorization and reimbursement for dysphagia services than for language intervention. Given that many clinicians who treat aphasia also treat dysphagia, there is an alarming trend to prioritize treatment for swallowing problems over problems of communication (Hallowell & Clark, 2000).

Quality, Intensity, Duration, and Frequency of Care

Despite the supposed focus on "quality" in MCOs, several factors related to managed care modes of delivery have eroded the quality of care clinicians can deliver. First, a prominent cost-containment feature of managed care plans is the restriction of duration and frequency of treatments (Gill, 1995), which limits clinicians' abilities to foster significant functional gains, even in patients with good rehabilitation potential (Sarno, 1998). Second, insurance companies are increasingly intervening in matters that traditionally have been in the hands of clinicians, such as treatment planning and discharge decision making. This trend has led to decision-making that is more financially than clinically sound. Third, interruptions in the continuity of care have been on the uprise due to delays in authorization and re-authorization for services. Fourth, although the use of assistants and aides in the treatment of communication and swallowing disorders is relatively new in the United States, concerns about the overuse and misuse of these less expensive (but less qualified) personnel and the potential consequences for further reductions in the quality and outcomes of care are growing (Henri & Hallowell, 1999c).

Quality assurance is a stated aim in the literature of virtually every MCO. MCO accrediting agencies, such as the NCQA, require that MCOs meet high standards of quality assurance and quality improvement practices. So how can it be that there are such a preponderance of complaints about managed care in the popular media, as well as evidence of decreasing quality in the research literature? One reason is that overall comparative standards among HMOs may be lower than standards under more traditional models. Another is that MCOs tend to minimize their quality under pressure to reduce their own administrative cost improvement efforts (Fisher, 1994). Recent research on the quality of health care suggests accreditation of HMOs may be misleading because a large proportion of enrollees who are not satisfied with their care withdraw from membership, thus eliminating their participation in consumer satisfaction surveys (Health Advocate, 1998).

Fiscal Stability of Service-Providing Agencies

Many of the features that characterize managed care threaten the fiscal stability of the agencies that support the delivery of care. Reduced reimbursement levels, increased reimbursement processing time, increases in the frequency of reimbursement denials, increased administrative costs, reductions in coverage, and reduced access for some patient populations are all factors that threaten agencies' clinical revenues. A recent surge in staffing reductions, modifications of salaried contracts to hourly contracts based on billable services, implementation of rigorous clinical productivity standards, and dramatic dissolution of numerous rehabilitation companies and private practices is indicative of the current fiscal pressure on providers.

Because the majority of persons with aphasia are older than the age of 65, two of the most drastic threats to United States agencies that support intervention for aphasia have been Medicare's new prospective payment system (PPS) implemented progressively in 1998 and 1999 and Medicare's payment cap for outpatient rehabilitation services implemented in 1999 (Moore, 1999). Both of these measures were implemented by HCFA following congressional passage of the Balanced Budget Act of 1997.

PPS affects in-patient services in long-term care facilities in particular. Rather than being reimbursed for actual costs incurred, or for actual services rendered, facilities are paid a flat daily rate based on the conditions of individual residents. The rates are calculated with complex formulas involving resource utilization group (RUG) classifications and case mix data. RUG classifications are based on studies of the actual time clinicians from multiple disciplines spent caring for patients with a variety of conditions as

assessed through a standardized assessment scheme, known as the Minimum Data Set (MDS) (now in its third version). Case mix data are based on RUG classifications of a facility's residents.

Medicare's payment cap for outpatient rehabilitation services originally involved a $1500 limit on payments for both speech-language pathology and physical therapy services, combined. Initiated in 1999, the cap dramatically reduced the frequency and duration of treatment that clinicians could provide, and required clinicians across disciplines to make difficult and often arbitrary decisions about the priority of one treatment over another. Although it is too soon for controlled studies of the fiscal effects of PPS and the Medicare cap on the care of patients with neurogenic communication disorders to appear in the research, tremendous financial losses were felt by long-term care facilities and rehabilitation providers throughout the United States. The decrease in access to services for persons with neurogenic communication disorders was equally, if not more, devastating. Following a strong advocacy campaign, this cap was at least temporarily rescinded in November 1999.

Livelihood of Professionals

Given the financial losses to service-providing agencies discussed above, it is not surprising that clinicians, too, are experiencing the effects of managed care in terms of reduced salaries and employment opportunities. Restructuring, re-engineering, consolidation, and downsizing movements in hospitals, speech and hearing centers, private practices, and rehabilitation companies have had direct and personal impacts on many speech-language clinicians (Henri & Hallowell, 1999c).

Professional Integrity

Under managed care, many insurance companies, as well as service-providing agencies, are attempting to reduce costs by addressing the expense of employing highly educated and skilled clinicians, such as fully certified and licensed speech-language pathologists. One way they may do this is to employ less costly assistants, technicians, and aides (ASHA, 1996a; Gerard, 1990; Holzemer, 1996). Another is to employ "multiskilled" or "transdisciplinary" professionals who are trained in a variety of medical and rehabilitative diagnostic and treatment methods that were once exclusively in the domain of specific clinical disciplines (ASHA, 1996c). Both of these strategies have resulted in a decrease in the level of skill, education, training, licensure, certification, and overall competence of clinical practitioners, and have yielded tremendous inconsistencies in the quality of care across treatment settings. Although there are merits to some of the arguments for the use of support and/or cross-trained personnel in some environments, it is essential that clinicians advocate for the integrity of their professions (Henri & Hallowell, 1999c), as well as for their specialized expertise in such areas as aphasiology.

Positive Impacts of Managed Care

Not all of managed care's influences on services available to persons with neurogenic communication disorders are negative. Some of managed care's touted virtues of prevention, cost-saving, accessibility, and accountability have, in fact, impacted our professional practices in positive ways.

Prevention, Access, and Cost

The emphasis of most MCOs on preventive care and health maintenance should ideally reduce the number of people who are affected by stroke, traumatic brain injury, infectious processes, etc., and thus may help to prevent some communication disorders. Additionally, the reduced cost of insurance coverage for most people who enroll in MCOs enhances the accessibility of coverage. While we lament the decline in revenues for our clinical services, we must also recognize that the continuous escalation of health care costs from the 1960s through the early 1990s could not continue. Many practitioners and agencies representing the whole array of health care disciplines are known to have abused the lucrative insurance billing opportunities within the traditional indemnity fee-for-service modes of operation. Certainly, some reductions in reimbursement and coverage are truly outrageous, having no relevance to patients' actual needs or to actual expenses incurred in offering our services; the Medicare $1500 cap shared among speech-language pathologists and physical therapists was a good but unfortunate example. Even in the realm of aphasiology, there have been ongoing abuses of systems that allow for continuous high-cost hourly billing for frequent sessions and long-lasting treatment programs that are not necessarily optimal in terms of achieving positive functional outcomes.

Accountability and Enhancement of Research

A related and critically important positive impact of health care restructuring is that it demands increased accountability of clinicians, service-providing agencies, and clinical professions (Wolfe, 1994). Scientific evidence of our treatment efficacy and treatment outcomes is being far more carefully scrutinized than ever. This scrutiny has increased awareness of our great need for a richer empirical base of research with which to justify our interventions. Thus, we have been driven to improve the quantity and quality of clinical research in our discipline (Boston, 1994; Sarno, 1998).

Another facet of our heightened accountability is that clinicians are now required to ensure that services provided address important life-affecting changes in clients and patients, and that those services are necessary. Clinicians were once typically trained to think of treatment in terms of clinical performance–based objectives (i.e., those pertaining to grammatical structures, articulator placement, or speech sound discrimination), remote from practical communication in real-world contexts. Now we have been challenged to reformulate our diagnostic and treatment methods to better address "functional outcomes," a concept that is addressed repeatedly in this book.

It is troublesome that the new evidence-based medical necessity clauses of some MCOs impose unreasonable restrictions on the types of evidence required to justify treatments. It is also troublesome that such clauses often encourage denial of the communicative, cognitive, and psychosocial needs of patients, in favor of the treatment of physical impairments that are not always as life-affecting. Still, clinicians in the past were probably far too liberal in providing services that were not necessarily based in solid scientific research and theory. Further, the resources they had in the treatment outcomes and efficacy literature to support their treatment approaches were lacking.

The fact that third-party payers and government-sponsored health care plans now require solid evidence to justify reimbursement has stimulated concerted research and publication efforts on the part of our professional organizations, researchers, and clinicians (Task Force on Treatment Outcomes & Cost Effectiveness, 1996). Some university research and teaching programs in communication sciences and disorders have reorganized research priorities over the past 10 years, such that clinical research is valued in academic cultures more than it had been previously. Likewise, private, state, and federal funding opportunities for research involving treatment outcomes and treatment efficacy have increased (Henri & Hallowell, 1999c). The continued expansion of controlled research regarding our clinical practices will undoubtedly help us not only justify our services, but also learn better ways to diagnose, treat, and make valid prognostic statements about neurogenic communication disorders.

One additional benefit of managed care, reported by health care administrators, is that clinical professionals are increasingly aware of the financial impact of their individual and agency-wide services on the financial well-being of their employing agencies. In contexts where clinicians once performed clinical duties without engaging in the monitoring of clinical revenues, clinicians now frequently play a vital role in business and financial planning teamwork within their agencies. This change appears to have increased clinicians' sense of ownership for their agency's operations. Likewise, employers report being impressed with the improved business savvy of their clinical employees (Henri & Hallowell, 1999c; 1997).

Gender Influences on Salary and Status

Wage rates are influenced primarily by the sex composition of specific occupations (U.S. Department of Labor Women's

Bureau, 1999). Signer (1988) observes that low salary and low status are linked to the preponderance of women in a profession. Women consistently make less money than men in almost every industry (Isaacs, 1995; Schwartz, 1988). According to a recent U.S. Department of Labor report, women's median weekly full-time wage and salary earnings in 1998 were 76% of those of men with the same experience (U.S. Department of Labor, Bureau of Labor Statistics, 1999). Since women make up 75% of the health care work force (Butler et al.,) salaries are low throughout the health care professions.

Not surprisingly, there is also a strong relationship between gender and status. The health labor force is notorious for its hierarchical status and power differences between high-ranking and low-ranking workers (Butler et al., Signer, 1988). For example, in 1988, 88.8% of the members of ASHA were reported to be women; however, 17% of male members were directors and heads of programs, whereas only 6.2% of female members were administrators (Signer, 1988). Because women sometimes contribute only secondarily to income, they may not assert their right to a salary commensurate with their training and professional status. The lower salaries in our profession are also tied to inadequate marketing of our scope of practice and the perceived value of our services (Holley, 1988).

THE ULTIMATE EXCELLENT APHASIOLOGIST

What constitutes the ultimate excellent clinical aphasiologist? What factors characterize the very best clinicians? There certainly are not definitive answers to these questions, as the skills and qualities needed for excellence differ according to the contexts in which we work, the patients and colleagues with whom we work, and the nature of our specific professional responsibilities. One must recognize that the degree of excellence perceived is relative to the person who perceives it. A list of prescriptive features indicating what constitutes the "best" aphasiologist may not be appropriate, as diversity in expertise, skills, knowledge, affect, and culture among clinicians is certainly desirable. Still, there are numerous ideal characteristics that we might all aspire to possess.

The excellent aphasiologist is competent. Competent clinicians have a graduate education, national and regional certification in speech-language pathology (in the United States, this means a Certificate of Clinical Competence (CCC) granted by ASHA and, where appropriate, a state license as a speech-language pathologist). They have clinical practice experience under the supervision and mentorship of seasoned excellent aphasiologists (Kovach & Moore, 1992). They also demonstrate outstanding oral and written communication skills; use only high-caliber assessment and intervention techniques; foster maximum self-determination on the part of patients (Cormier & Cormier, 1991); maintain

an effective climate that contributes positively to the therapeutic relationship (Rogers, 1969); provide inspiration, motivation, encouragement, and leadership to patients and colleagues; are flexible and adapt well to change; and integrate the personal, scientific, and artistic parts of themselves to achieve a balance of interpersonal, intellectual, and technical competence.

The excellent aphasiologist is knowledgeable. Knowledgeable clinicians are able to reason scientifically, incorporate new findings, and generate new applications. They use knowledge effectively and think and learn independently. They are committed to interdisciplinary study, and have formal and informal training in the arts and sciences, including not only speech-language pathology and audiology, but also cognitive sciences, psychology, linguistics, education, medicine (especially neurology), statistics, computer science, manual communication and other modern languages, business and health administration, economics, gerontology, sociology, anthropology, music, and counseling. They have training and experience in the effective management of communication problems resulting not only from stroke, but also those associated with traumatic brain injury, dementia, infectious processes, neoplasm, and confusional states. Their knowledge base is constantly expanding as they read the current professional literature, take advantage of continuing education opportunities, and learn from their colleagues and patients. They have a profound sense of inquiry, and are open to questioning and exploration (Rogers, 1969). They complement their knowledge with keen insight in managing simple and complex cases (Falck, 1972).

The excellent aphasiologist is sensitive to issues of gender, age, culture, race, and sexual orientation. Sensitive clinicians appreciate multiculturalism and multilingualism, and familiarize themselves with, and celebrate, differences and similarities among their patients and colleagues (American Speech-Language-Hearing Association, 1988; 1992b). Some have been raised in bilingual or multilingual environments. Others strive to learn additional languages in order to expand opportunities for communication and, when possible, to provide services in more than one language. They are aware of the relative lack of persons from culturally diverse populations in the profession of communication sciences and disorders (American Speech-Language-Hearing Association, 1992b; Terrell et al., 1991) and support "innovative and aggressive efforts to recruit, train, support and retain" multicultural clinicians (Wallace & Freeman, 1991, p. 60). Sensitive clinicians are aware of biases—their own and those of others—and examine the basis for any unreasoned distortion of judgment. They strive to resolve their own prejudices through education, exposure, and sensitivity training (ASHA, 1989b; 1992; Lebrun, 1988; Paradis, 1983; 1987).

The excellent aphasiologist is ethical. Ethical clinicians are aware of conflicts of interest and work to resolve personal wants and needs without compromising the appropriateness of their actions (Hirsch, 1994). They are unfailingly honest. They follow their professional codes of ethics, obey all laws, and adhere to their own personal solid moral codes.

The excellent aphasiologist is professional. His or her primary goal is high-quality, first-rate patient care. Effective clinicians have a rationale for everything they do, and communicate that rationale, whenever possible, to patients and the patients' clinicians from other disciplines. They foster responsible participation in the selection of goals, in ways of reaching those goals, and in the development of appropriate attitudes and skills, such as personal responsibility for learning and improvement (Chapey, 1994). They critique, assess, monitor, and edit their own behavior. They interact effectively with the entire rehabilitation team. They treat colleagues with respect, courtesy, fairness, and good faith (Cormier & Cormier, 1991). They maintain records and reports accurately and completely and keep them up to date. They consistently protect clients' privacy and confidentiality, initiate proper referrals and recommendations, and exhibit proper follow-through. They have definite but malleable professional and personal goals and defined ways of reaching those goals.

The excellent aphasiologist is a warm, caring, patient, thoughtful, interesting person. Excellent clinicians fit Ringel's definition of "gifted scientists" who are "individualistic, open-minded, freedom-loving, highly motivated, fiercely independent, imaginative, nonconformist and usually critical of the status quo" (Ringel, 1982, p. 401). They are also genuinely motivated to help others (Minifie, 1983), and have a terrific sense of humor, a love of people, a commitment to service, and a passion for patient and professional advocacy. They have numerous weaknesses and failures, and acknowledge and grow through them with grace. Although aware of their assets, they are humble.

The excellent aphasiologist is emotionally healthy. Healthy clinicians serve as a role models to clinicians in training, colleagues, consumers, and others in terms of health maintenance, stress management, lifestyle balance, and self-esteem. They have familiarized themselves with books on healthy interpersonal interaction/intimacy such as "Getting Love Right" by Terrance Gorski (1993), and avoid professional burnout, actively balancing their psychological resources with the demands of their jobs.

FUTURE TRENDS

Demographic trends will certainly continue to play an important role in aphasia intervention. With post World War generations growing older and living longer than ever before, and with fewer children being born, attention to issues affecting older adults is steadily growing. Public and private retirement and medical programs will necessarily evolve with increasing focus on the elderly over the next few decades (Mechanic, 1999). The aging of the population brings with it increased risks for catastrophic disease, illness, and disability (Kaplan et al., 1999), including adult aphasia. Enhanced consumer education and new methods to prevent stroke and traumatic brain injury will help address these risks.

Other demographic trends, such as the growth of racial, ethnic, and linguistic minority populations in the United States, will continue to stimulate our constructive actions to meet the needs of the members of such populations. Increases in certain patient populations, such as those with HIV/AIDS, in our caseloads (ASHA 1989a; ASHA Committee on Quality Assurance, 1990; Flower & Sooy, 1987; Larsen, 1998) will require that we engage in ongoing research pertaining to relatively new areas of clinical practice.

As new formulae for practice under changing modes of service delivery continue to evolve, we will continue to see further positive effects on our professions, such as more efficient and increasingly outcomes-focused treatments, new types of employment opportunities, and improved interdisciplinary teamwork in the coordination of patient care, co-treatment, and discharge planning. At the same time, we are likely to see more women in leadership roles (Chapey, 1994).

Over the next few decades, we will draw on the evolving empirical research base to enhance our methods for improving our patients' quality of life, independence, and medical management. We will take advantage of technological advancements that will influence virtually every one of our many professional roles. We will also continue to adapt constructively to reduced patient access, both through advocacy for improved access, and through the use of alternative models of intervention and caregiver training.

As the research base on treatment efficacy, cost effectiveness, and outcomes continues to grow, we will become increasingly sophisticated about the appropriate patterns of practice associated with patients' specific diagnostic characteristics. More and more clinical agencies will implement "clinical pathways," or optimal plans for diagnostic and treatment services that take into account the nature and severity of patients' deficits and time post-onset. Likewise, guidelines concerning the common best practices given a patient's diagnosis, such as ASHA's "Preferred Practice Patterns" (ASHA 1993; 1996b), will undoubtedly continue to be refined.

The specialty of neurogenic communication disorders will benefit from clinicians who are dedicated to fostering all of the characteristics that constitute the "ultimate excellent aphasiologist." The active role that aphasiologists play as advocates for our clients and profession is critical to maximizing our effectiveness.

▶ *Acknowledgment*–This work was supported in part by a grant DC00153-01A1 from the National Institute on Deafness and Other Communication Disorders. Thanks to Jessica DeSimone, Kirsten C. Carr, and Jacquie Kurland for editorial assistance.

1. Compare and contrast the type of collaborative care and teamwork in which aphasiologists are likely to be engaged within their varied employment contexts.

2. For each of the varied employment contexts, consider which of the many roles of the aphasiologist are most emphasized.

3. Discuss the ways in which employment in each of the different service delivery contexts might affect the quality of life of clinicians.

4. In what ways is excellence in documentation critical to the success of the aphasiologist?

5. Describe the ways in which recent service delivery trends have influenced where (in what type of service delivery context) persons with neurogenic communication disorders receive treatment.

6. How do reductions in stays in acute care hospitals impact what the speech-language clinician accomplishes in the acute care context?

7. How do reductions in the frequency and duration of treatment programs for patients with aphasia influence intervention?

8. List specific ways in which aphasiologists may engage actively in quality assurance, marketing, contract negotiation, and fundraising.

9. Describe what you think are the most critical ethical issues for aphasiologists. What might be done to alleviate some of the ethical dilemmas and conflicts of interest that clinicians face in the workplace?

10. In what ways might the full-time clinician without doctoral training participate in research?

11. Make an outline of both positive and negative service delivery trends that are influencing intervention for adults with aphasia and related disorders. For each of the negative trends, list and discuss specific ways in which you may act strategically as an advocate to lessen the negative effects for your patients and your profession. List and discuss the specific ways in which you might capitalize on each of the positive trends to improve service for your patients.

12. Consider this hypothetical case: You are an SLP who is treating Mr. Comet, a 48-year-old man who recently suffered a CVA. He is enrolled in an HMO. Mr. Comet's physician, his primary medical provider, has a contract with the patient's HMO. She had authorized one evaluation and six treatment sessions to address speech and language problems secondary to CVA. You have exhausted those authorized sessions. Now the physician refuses to authorize any further treatment from your discipline. You have ample evidence that Mr. Comet's communication deficits are having a significant impact on his safety, his medical management, his ability to live independently, and his quality of life. You are confident that he is an appropriate candidate for treatment and that you have effective strategies to implement in a treatment program for him. What specific steps will you take to advocate effectively for Mr. Comet's continued access to your services?

13. How would you describe the ultimate excellent clinical aphasiologist? What are your own strengths and weaknesses relative to your view of the ideal clinician?

References

Ad Hoc Committee on Managed Care of the American Speech-Language-Hearing Association. (1994). *Managing Managed Care: A Practical Guide for Audiologists and Speech-Language-Hearing Pathologists.* Rockville, MD: American Speech-Language-Hearing Association.

American Medical Association. (1999). *Coding Current Procedural Terminology, CPT*™ *2000.* Chicago, IL: American Medical Association.

American Speech-Language-Hearing Association. (1986). The delivery of speech-language and audiology services in home care. *ASHA, 28*(5), 49–52.

American Speech-Language-Hearing Association. (1988). Definition: Bilingual speech-language pathologists and audiologists. *ASHA, 30*(5), 53.

American Speech-Language-Hearing Association. (1989a). AIDS/HIV: Implications for speech-language pathologists and audiologists. *ASHA, 31*(6–7), 33–37.

American Speech-Language-Hearing Association. (1989b). Committee on the status of racial minorities. Definition: bilingual speech language pathologists and audiologists. *ASHA, 31*(3), 93.

American Speech-Language-Hearing Association. (1992a). ASHA's proposed long-range strategic plan. *ASHA, 34*(5), 32–36.

American Speech-Language-Hearing Association. (1992b). Our multicultural agenda. *ASHA, 34*(5), 37–53.

American Speech-Language-Hearing Association. (1993). Preferred practice patterns for the professions of speech-language pathology and audiology. *ASHA, 35*(3), (Suppl. 11).

American Speech-Language-Hearing Association (1996a). Guidelines for the training, credentialing, use, and supervision of speech-language pathology assistants. *ASHA, 38*(Suppl. 16), 21–34.

American Speech-Language Hearing Association. (1996b). *Preferred Practice Patterns for the Professions of Speech-Language Pathology and Audiology.* Rockville, MD: American Speech-Language Hearing Association.

American Speech-Language-Hearing Association. (1996c). Technical report of the Ad Hoc Committee on Multiskilling. *ASHA, 38*(Suppl. 16), 53–61.

American Speech-Language-Hearing Association. (1997). *Private Health Plans Handbook for Speech-Language Pathology and Audiology.* Rockville, MD: American Speech-Language Hearing Association.

American Speech-Language-Hearing Association Committee on Quality Assurance. (1990). AIDS/HIV: Implications for speech-language pathologists and audiologists. *ASHA, 32*, 46–48.

Begley, C.E. (1987). Prospective payment and medical ethics. *Journal of Medicine and Philosophy, 12*, 107–122.

Bemowski, K. (1991, May). Big Q at big blue. *Quality Progress, 24*, 17–21.

Butler, I., Carpenter, E., Kay, B., & Simmons, R. *Sex and Status in the Workforce*. Washington, DC: American Public Health Association.

Boston, B.O. (1994). Destiny is in the data: A wake-up call for outcome measures. *American Speech-Language and Hearing Association, 36*, 35–38.

Centers for Disease Control. (1999). *ICD9-CM*. [on-line]. Available: ftp://ftp.cdc.gov/pub/Health_Statistics/NCHS/Publications/ICD9-CM

Chapey, R. (1977). Consumer satisfaction in speech-language pathology. *ASHA, 19*, 829–832

Chapey, R. (1994). Introduction to language intervention strategies in adult aphasia. In R. Chapey (ed.), *Language Intervention Strategies in Adult Aphasia* (pp. 3–26). Baltimore, MD: Williams & Wilkins, 3–26.

Chapey, R., Lubinski, R., Salzberg, A., & Chapey, G. (1979). Survey of speech, language and hearing services in nursing home settings. *Long-Term Care Health Services Administration Quarterly, 3*, 307, 316.

Clement, D.G., Retchin, S.M., Brown, R.S., & Stegall, M.H. (1994). Access and outcomes of elderly patients enrolled in managed care. *Journal of the American Medical Association, 271*(19), 1487–1492.

Cohn, R. (1994). Strategies for positioning in the managed health care marketplace. *Journal of Hand Therapy, 7*, 5–9.

Cormier, W.H. & Cormier, L.S. (1991). *Interviewing Strategies for Helpers*. Pacific Grove, CA: Brooks/Cole.

Council on Ethical and Judicial Affairs, American Medical Association. (1995). Ethical issues in managed care. *Journal of the American Medical Association, 273*(4), 330–335.

Darley, F.L. (1982). *Aphasia*. Philadelphia: W.B. Saunders.

Davolt, S. (1999). Network providers find strength in numbers. *ASHA Leader, 4*(10), 1, 8.

Ewart, C. (1991). Social action theory for a public health psychology. *American Psychologist, 46*(9), 931–942.

Falck, V. (1972). The role and function of university training programs. *ASHA, 14*, 307–310.

Fisher, R.S. (1994). Medicaid managed care: The next generation? *Academic Medicine, 69*(5), 317–322.

Flower, W. & Sooy, D. (1987). AIDS: An introduction for speech-language pathologists and audiologists. *ASHA, 29*, 25–30.

Fox, H.B., Wicks, L.B., & Newacheck, P.W. (1993). State Medicaid health maintenance organization policies and special-needs children. *Health Care Financing Review, 15*, 25–37.

Frady, M., Gerdau, R., Lennon, T., Sherman, W., & Singer, S. (1985, December 28). Growing old in America. ABC News Close-Up.

Geffner, D. (1997). Growing the field: Who will teach future generations? *ASHA, 39*, 37–38, 40–42.

Gerard, R. (1990). Preparing a multiskilled work force for the 21st century hospital. *Journal of Biocommunication, 17*(4), 24–26.

Gill, H.S. (1995). The changing nature of ambulatory rehabilitation programs and services in a managed care environment. *Archives of Physical Medicine and Rehabilitation, 76*, SC10–SC15.

Gorski, T. (1993). *Getting Love Right: Learning the Choices of Healthy Intimacy*. New York: Fireside/Simon & Schuster.

Grey, J.E. (1990a). Conflict of interest (part 1). *Healthcare Forum, 33*, 25–28.

Grey, J.E. (1990b). Conflict of interest (part 2). *Healthcare Forum, 33*, 96–99.

Hallowell, B. & Clark, H. (2000). (unpublished manuscript). A national survey of current management practices in aphasia rehabilitation.

Hallowell, B., Henri, B.P., & Miller, P. (1999). (unpublished manuscript). The influence of financial incentives on billing and caseload management decisions in speech-language pathology.

Hallowell, B. & Katz, R.C. (1999). Technological applications in the assessment of acquired neurogenic communication and swallowing disorders in adults. *Seminars in Speech, Language, and Hearing, 20*(2), 149–167.

Health Advocate (1998, Winter). Medicare HMOs with high rates of voluntary disenrollment fully accredited. *Health Advocate, 191*, Los Angeles, CA: National Health Law Program, 8.

Health Care Financing Administration. (1998). *ICD-9-CM: International Classification of Diseases, 9th Revision, Clinical Modification, Vols. 1, 2, and 3* (5th ed.). Los Angeles, CA: Practice Management Information Corp.

Henri, B. P. & Hallowell, B. (1996). Action planning for advocacy: Issues for speech-language pathologists and audiologists in the face of the expansion of managed care. HEARSAY: *Journal of the Ohio Speech and Hearing Association, 11*(1), 61–64.

Henri, B.P. & Hallowell, B. (1997). Ethics and clinical productivity pressures under managed care. *Newsletter of Special Interest Division 11 (Administration and Supervision) of the American Speech-Language-Hearing Association*. Rockville, MD: American Speech-Language-Hearing Association.

Henri, B.P. & Hallowell, B. (1999a). Funding alternatives to offset the consequences of managed care. *Newsletter of Special Interest Division 2 (Neurophysiology and Neurogenic Speech and Language Disorders) of the American Speech-Language-Hearing Association*. Rockville, MD: American Speech-Language-Hearing Association.

Henri, B.P. & Hallowell, B. (1999b). Improving access to speech-language pathology and audiology services. In R. Lubinski & S. Frattali (eds.), *Professional Issues in Speech-Language Pathology and Audiology*, (2nd ed.). San Diego: Singular Publishing Group.

Henri, B.P. & Hallowell, B. (1999c). Relating managed care to managing care. In B.S. Cornett (ed.), *Clinical Practice Management in Speech-Language Pathology: Principles and Practicalities*. Gaithersburg, MD: Aspen Publishers, Inc.

Henri, B.P., Hallowell, B., & Johnson, C. (1996). Advocacy and marketing to support clinical services. In R. Kreb (ed.), *A Practical Guide to Treatment Outcomes and Cost Effectiveness* (pp. 39–48). Rockville, MD: American Speech-Language-Hearing Association Task Force on Treatment Outcomes and Cost Effectiveness.

Hiller, M.D. & Lewis, J.B. (1995). Managed health care benefit plans: What are the ethical issues? *Trends in Health Care, Law & Ethics, 10*(1, 2), 109–112, 118.

Hirsch, B.D. (1994). Risky business: Financial incentives in managed care warrant regulation. *Texas Medicine, 90*(12), 30–33.

Holley, S. (1988). Marketing your services. *ASHA, 30*(9), 37–38.

Holzemer, W.L. (1996). The impact of multiskilling on quality of care. *International Nursing Review, 41*(1), 21–25.

IBM (1999). *About IBM.* [on-line]. Available: http://www.ibm.com/ibm/

Inglehart, J.K. (1995). Health policy report—Medicaid and managed care. *The New England Journal of Medicine, 332*(25), 1727–1731.

Isaacs, E. (1995). Gender discrimination in the workplace: A literature review. *Communications of the ACM, 38*(1), 58–59.

Kaplan, G.A., Haan, M.N., & Wallace, R.B. (1999). Understanding changing risk factor associations with increasing age in adults. *Annual Review of Public Health, 20*, 89–108.

Katz, R.C. & Hallowell, B. (1999). Technological applications in the treatment of acquired neurogenic communication and swallowing disorders in adults. *Seminars in Speech, Language, and Hearing, 20*(3), 251–269.

Katz, R., Hallowell, B., Code, C., Armstrong, E., Roberts, P., Pound, C., & Katz, L. (in press). A multinational comparison of aphasia management practices. *International Journal of Language and Communication Disorders.*

Keith, R. (1975). The effectiveness of treatment in aphasia: Discussion. In R.H. Brookshire (ed.), *Clinical Aphasiology Conference Proceedings.* Minneapolis, MN: BRK Publishers.

Kerr, P. (1992, April 3). Cutting costs of brain injuries. *New York Times,* pp. D1–D2.

Kovach, T. & Moore, S. (1992). Leaders are born through the mentoring process. *ASHA, 34*(1), 33–34.

Labovitz, G. (1991). The total quality health care revolution. *Quality Process, 24*(9), 45–50.

Larsen, C.R. (1998). *HIV-1 and Communication Disorders: What Speech and Hearing Professionals Need to Know.* San Diego: Singular Publishing Group.

Lebrun, Y. (1988). Multilingualism and aphasia. *Review of Laryngology, Otology and Rhinology, 109*(4), 299–306.

Leigh, W.A. (1994). Implications of health-care reform proposals for Black Americans. *Journal of Health Care for the Poor and Underserved, 5*(1), 17–32.

Matthews, C. (1988). Marketing your services: Strategies that work. *ASHA, 30*, 22–25.

Mechanic, D. (1999). The changing elderly population and future health care needs. *Journal Of Urban Health, 76*(1), 24–38.

McLaurin, D. & Bell, S. (1991). Open communication lines before attempting total quality. *Quality Process, 24*(6), 25–28.

Minifie, F. (1983). ASHA from adolescence onward. *ASHA, 25*, 17–24.

Moore, M. (1999). Nursing homes shaken from effects of Medicare reform. *ASHA Leader, 4*(10), 1,4.

NCQA. (1999). *NCQA consumer page.* [on-line]. Available: http://www.ncqa.org/Pages/Main/index.htm

Oberlander, J.B. (1997). Managed care and Medicare reform. *Journal of Health Politics, Policy and Law, 32*(2), 595–627.

Paradis, M. (1983). Readings on aphasia. In M. Paradis (ed.), *Bilinguals and Polyglots.* Quebec: Didier.

Paradis, M. (1987). *The Assessment of Bilingual Aphasia.* Hillsdale, NJ: Lawrence Erlbaum.

Parrot Software (1999). *HCFA 700 & 701 Forms.* [on-line]. Available: http://www.parrotsoftware.com

Penn, C. (1993). Aphasia therapy in South Africa: Some pragmatic and personal perspectives. In A.L. Holland & M.M. Forbes (eds.), *Aphasia Treatment: World Perspectives* (pp. 25–54). San Diego, CA: Singular Publishing Group.

Perkins, J. (1998). *Managed Care Update.* Los Angeles, CA: National Health Law Program.

Peters, T. & Waterman, R. (1982). *In Search of Excellence.* New York: Warner Books.

Petrosino, L., Lieberman, R.J., & McNeil, M.R. (1997). *1996-97 National Survey of Undergraduate and Graduate Programs.* Minneapolis, MN: Council of Graduate Programs in Communication Sciences and Disorders.

Purtillo, R.B. (1995). Managed care: Ethical issues for the rehabilitation professions. *Trends In Health Care, Law & Ethics, 10*(1/2), 105–108.

Randall, V.R. (1994). Impact of managed care organizations on ethnic Americans and underserved populations. *Journal of Health Care for the Poor and Underserved, 5*(3), 224–236.

Ringel, R. (1982). Some issues facing graduate education. *ASHA, 24*, 399–404.

Rodwin, M.A. (1995). Conflicts in managed care. *The New England Journal of Medicine, 332*(9), 604–607.

Rogers, C. (1969). Freedom to learn. Columbus, OH: Charles E. Merrill.

Roth, C.R. (1999). Developing and implementing a quality improvement plan in an acute care hospital setting. *Newsletter of Special Interest Division 2 (Neurophysiology and Neurogenic Speech and Language Disorders) of the American Speech-Language-Hearing Association, 9*(2), 24–28.

Sahs, A.L. & Hartman, E.C. (1976). *Fundamentals of Stroke Care.* Washington, DC: U.S. Department of Health, Education and Welfare.

Sarno, M.T. (1998). Recovery and rehabilitation in aphasia. In M.T. Sarno (ed.), *Acquired Aphasia* (pp. 595–631). San Diego: Academic Press.

Schwartz, J. (1988, January). Closing the Gap. *American Demographics, 10,* 56.

Screen, M.R. & Anderson, N.B. (1994). Legal and ethical issues in communication disorders affecting multicultural populations. In *Multicultural Perspectives in Communication Disorders* (pp. 51–64). San Diego: Singular Publishing Group.

Signer, M. (1988). The value of women's work. *ASHA, 30,* 24–25.

Slominski, T. (1985a). Medicare and speech pathology: Reimbursement strategies (an audiocassette tape). Gaylord, MI: Northern Speech Services.

Smith, G. & Ashbaugh, J. (1995). *Managed Care and People with Developmental Disabilities: A Guidebook.* Alexandria, VA: National Association of State Directors of Developmental Disabilities Services, Inc.

Stenger, A. (1993). Who will advocate for patients? *Postgraduate Medicine, 94*(7), 108–110.

Stollman, J. (1995). Medicaid, a new frontier for managed care. . . but it's a very tough sell. *Medical Group Management Journal, 42*(2), 38–45.

Task Force on Treatment Outcomes and Cost Effectiveness. (1996). *Curriculum Guide to Managed Care.* Rockville Pike, MD: American Speech-Language-Hearing Association.

Terrell, S., Mueller, P., & Conley, L. (1991). Sister programs: Historically black and majority white universities. *ASHA, 33*(9), 45–48.

Thompson, C. & Kearns, K. (1991). Analytical and technical directions in applied aphasia analysis: The Midas touch. In T. Prescott (ed.), *Clinical Aphasiology* (pp. 41–54). Austin, TX: Pro-Ed.

Underhill, B. (1991). "Total" remains bread and butter of total quality management. Letter to editor. *Quality Process, 24,* 8.

U.S. Department of Labor Bureau of Labor Statistics (1999). What women earned in 1998. *Issues in Labor Statistics.* [on-line]. Available: http://www.bls.gov/opub/ils/pdf/opbils30.pdf

U.S. Department of Labor Women's Bureau (1999). *Facts on Working Women: Earnings Differences Between Women and Men.* [on-line]. Available: http://www.dol.gov

Varian, T. (1991). Communicating total quality inside the organization. *Quality Progress, 6,* 30–31.

Wallace, G. & Freeman, S. (1991). Adults with neurological improvement from multicultural populations. *ASHA, 33*(67), 58–60.

Wepman, J. (1972a). Aphasia therapy: A new look. *Journal of Speech and Hearing Disorders, 37,* 203–214.

Wepman, J. (1972b). Aphasia therapy: Some relative comments and some purely personal prejudices. In M. Sarno (ed.), *Aphasia: Selected Readings.* New York: Appleton-Century-Crofts.

Wolfe, S.M. (1994). Quality assessment of ethics in health care: The accountability revolution. *American Journal of Law and Medicine, 20(1 & 2),* 105–128.

Chapter 8

Teams and Partnerships in Aphasia Intervention

Lee Ann C. Golper

INTRODUCTION: IT TAKES A VILLAGE

In almost every service arena throughout the world—from emergency rooms to community mental health clinics—team intervention is recognized as the optimal approach to health services delivery (Cifu & Steward, 1999; Collins et al., 1999; Heikkila et al., 1999; Hogh et al., 1999; Ko, 1999; Lott et al., 1999; Rosin et al., 1996). This approach necessitates bringing together the knowledge and skills of individuals from many disciplines in order to ensure complex problems receive the comprehensive attention they require (Allen et al., 1978). As aphasic individuals move from their hospital beds to their homes, their concerns often shift from surviving the acute event to issues related to finances or changes in their family dynamics. No one discipline can encompass the whole life-changing condition "aphasia." It takes a village. Developing collaborations with others is particularly important throughout the recovery continuum following the onset of aphasia since many patients with aphasia have medical, physical, psychosocial, emotional, recreational, vocational, and financial concerns that may or may not be directly complicated by their communication impairment. Indeed, such issues can supersede the language deficits. Those of us who work with individuals who have communication disorders have long been proponents of family-centered team intervention (Rosin et al., 1996). We rarely evaluate or treat any type of communication disorder without having some amount of collaboration with the patients' families and with other disciplines.

OBJECTIVES

The objectives of this chapter are (1) to define and examine typical team organizational designs found in health care delivery; (2) to review basic elements in group processes that lead to successful teams and some of the potential barriers to developing effective teams; (3) to consider how the team designs may differ depending upon the setting and how priorities and the primary decision-makers change across the continuum of recovery from aphasia; (4) to examine related issues, including collaborative evaluations, documentation, outcomes studies, family and patient education, professional education, and research; and (5) to suggest the overriding aim of the rehabilitation team throughout the recovery continuum with adult aphasia should be directed at educating and empowering patients and families to become collaborative partners, to make use of community resources, and ultimately to lead their own "team aphasia."

DEFINITION: WHAT IS A TEAM?

Teams are groups of people collaborating in some way to reach a common goal. Teams can be made up of two people or fifty people. They can have face-to-face meetings or use more indirect communication. They can be formal and structured in a hierarchy, or loosely organized groups of peers. Usually, teams have at least one designated leader. Teams may have leaders who are authoritarian, controlling their actions, or have leaders who function more as facilitators, advising from the sidelines. They may be made up of people from a single discipline or multiple disciplines and can have professional and nonprofessional members. They can be designed to include the patient and family as active participants or can be restricted to an exclusive panel of specialist-consultants. Teams can have smaller teams within them, such as the nursing care team within the rehabilitation care team. Whatever the composition, structure, or purpose, it is important to remember that teams are human enterprises. Teams are made up of people and personalities and they are often "caldrons of bubbling emotions." (Goleman, 1998, p. 101). No team will look or function exactly like any other. Appreciating that there are no ideal blueprints for teams and the design can vary depending on the setting, let's examine a couple of typical models for team processes in health services delivery.

MODELS

The models of team processes most commonly found in health care delivery are either *multidisciplinary* or *interdisciplinary* teams. In education, particularly early intervention, *transdisciplinary* teams are more common. These team models mainly differ in their role delineations and communication processes. Occasionally, the terms multidisciplinary, interdisciplinary, and transdisciplinary seem to be used interchangeably at times in reference to teams. Thus, it may be helpful to consider the differences between them. In a multidisciplinary model, specialists with clearly defined roles work side by side, each addressing different problems, or different aspects of a given problem. Multidisciplinary teams are probably a good way to characterize how disciplines typically function in acute care setting, such as on an inpatient medicine or surgery unit. In that setting, various disciplines have defined roles and work cooperatively together, but for the most part they work in parallel, rather than partnerships, with one another. In multidisciplinary teams, individual members bring discipline-specific skills and the members' responsibilities are clearly defined and understood (Tuchman, 1996). Opportunities for communication between and among the disciplines may be cursory, and shared goals may be lacking (Allen et al., 1978).

Interdisciplinary teams are, by contrast, intended to be interactive and highly collaborative. There is greater emphasis on communication processes in interdisciplinary teams, as compared with multidisciplinary teams (Tuchman, 1996). True interdisciplinary teams allow for at least some amount of blurring between traditional professional boundaries. In interdisciplinary teams, different professional disciplines not only work together in a cooperative manner, they also collaborate in partnerships to implement the treatment procedures. In an interdisciplinary format, goals are discussed as "our goals," rather than "OT goals" or "PT goals."

There is very good evidence to suggest the most effective model for rehabilitation services teams is an interdisciplinary design. In their review of 79 studies looking at factors affecting outcomes in stroke, Cifu and Stewart (1999) examined the effects of interdisciplinary versus multidisciplinary teams on patient outcomes. They conducted a meta-analysis of 11 well-defined Level I studies, including 8 studies where patients were randomized to either a multidisciplinary medical stroke unit or an interdisciplinary rehabilitation unit. These analyses demonstrate that interdisciplinary team intervention is associated with decreased mortality, improved functional outcomes, shorter lengths of stays, and decreased costs (Cifu & Stewart, 1999). It may be that a key feature to successful outcomes in stroke rehabilitation is not so much having several different disciplines involved in patient care but, rather, having good communication and intervention partnerships established.

Teams that are truly *transdisciplinary* tend to be more common in early childhood intervention settings (Rosin et al., 1996). In these settings team members have had specific transdisciplinary orientation and training and are encouraged to practice *role release*. Role release refers to the elimination of traditional professional boundaries in intervention practices (Tuchman, 1996). A transdisciplinary approach to intervention requires incorporating the knowledge and skills from many discipline areas into one multi-skilled practice (Allen et al., 1978). Transdisciplinary teams are most advantageous when intervention requires interfacing a number of related professional disciplines. Although true transdisciplinary teams are rare in hospitals and other health care settings, the transdisciplinary team model is promoted by the Individuals with Disabilities Education Act (IDEA) of 1990, PL 101-476 (Rosin, 1996).

In health services settings issues such as clinical privileges and licensure restrictions may interfere with forming transdisciplinary teams. In addition, there may be resistance from staff who are not in favor of "cross training." There is a movement in health service delivery today toward encouraging *cross-training* between disciplines and *multi-skilling* within disciplines. Cross-training refers to situations where staff are trained to do all or parts of each other's jobs. Cross-training discourages "that's not my job" thinking and encourages staff to feel a part of a team process. For example, ward clerks may be cross-trained with patient transport personnel so they can cover for each other when needed. Multi-skilling implies having skills that exceed the boundaries of the traditional scopes of practice within a given discipline. An example would be training a speech-language pathologist to draw blood, perform range of motion exercises, or take blood pressures. Multi-skilling is sometimes viewed as creating minimally skilled technicians with specific skill sets across several areas but without the depth of knowledge needed to make independent decisions. Cross-training and multi-skilling, unfortunately, are concepts that developed in an attempt to save costs. Thus, the notions of cross-training and multiskilled staff are sometimes viewed with skepticism among licensed professionals.

TEAM PROCESSES
Group Communication

Much of what we call "interdisciplinary patient care" is just group problem-solving to develop partnerships in interventions through good communication. The key element is communication. Eliciting group problem-solving and group actions involves more than getting people together who have mutually supportive "roles and goals" in patient care. How well a group of people work together to help one another help patients and their families depends largely on how well communication is managed within the team. Groups of people work together most effectively when there are two basic elements in place: 1) group communication processes that encourage interactions, cooperation, and mutual respect, and 2) focused activities aimed at meeting specific objectives or performance measures (Manion et al., 1996).

Researchers looking at small group communication in health care settings have found the communication characteristics will vary along a continuum, depending upon the nature and purpose of the group (Northouse & Northouse, 1998). Our behavior and the manner in which we participate in groups shifts when the focus of the group is more toward *content-oriented* activities as opposed to *process-oriented* activities (Loomis, 1979). A content-oriented activity is one that is directed toward some *objective* (e.g., discharge planning) or some *performance measure* (e.g., improved functional rating scores). Team activities that are skewed toward content over process are common in health care settings where everyone feels pressured to make an economic use of time, or in situations where weekly patient care team conferences are viewed by the participants as merely a mandated necessity. Typically, content-oriented patient care teams spend little time in idle chatting or group process, but move to the objectives of the meeting. In these settings, reporting information to the group to ensure everyone has a general notion about what the various disciplines are doing with the patient is essentially the extent of the communication. There is not much attention paid to processes that promote good interactions among team members. At meetings that are highly content oriented, the team members might make their reports in turn, take their respective notes, and then move on to the next task. When communication is focused more on tasks without attending to group participation, it is difficult to engender good interactive collaborations within the team.

At the other end of the continuum, process-oriented communication is directed toward developing relationships, cooperation, or mutual goals. Process-oriented communication includes group activities such as sharing feelings, brainstorming solutions, supporting one another, and building alliances. Communication itself may be the main purpose. Therapy groups, such as aphasia group therapy or various support groups, are good examples of groups engaged mostly in process-oriented activities.

Interdisciplinary teams need to strike a balance between content and process. Although interdisciplinary patient care teams are not "support groups," intervention plans often require negotiations between or among disciplines. Consequently, it is important to incorporate process-oriented communication into the group's activities, even when time is limited and there are several tasks to accomplish in a short amount of time. In interdisciplinary management, trust and collaboration are essential. Developing good communication processes at the outset of team development tends to discourage polarities. The team members may refer to these activities, affectionately, as "sharing and caring." Time spent building and maintaining mutual trust and open communication between team members is absolutely essential to a successful interdisciplinary team.

CREATING A COHESIVE TEAM

One of the ways corporations and other groups develop a sense of cohesion within a team is to do things like take periodic retreats or engage in similar activities to promote good interpersonal relationships. Team retreats can be anything from wilderness survival treks to an afternoon away from the office. Usually, retreats are intended to accomplish both group relationship building and goal setting. Managers and group process facilitators also use devices like personality inventories, such as the Meyers-Briggs Inventory (Meyers-Briggs & Briggs, 1980) as a way for the group members to identify and inventory their individual work styles and consider how these styles differ from on another. Another method to aid in developing group cooperation and reliance is to involve the members in problem-solving games that require teamwork solutions. Here is an example. A group of healthcare providers is divided up into teams of four members and each team is given five sheets of standard, $8\frac{1}{2}'' \times 11''$ paper. Each team is then asked to solve this problem, "Imagine that the carpet in this room is a raging river and each of your pieces of paper is a stepping stone. Using only your five 'stepping stone' sheets of paper, how can all the members of your team cross the river?" Since just laying down the five sheets of paper end to end would not allow the group to reach the other side of the room, the solution to the problem requires teamwork. The four-member teams cross the room by laying down the sheets of paper ahead of them in a row; and as each member moves forward one step, the last sheet rotates from the member at the tail of the line to the member at the front to take the next step. Thus, each team member moves forward until everyone has reached the opposite "shore." These activities are intended to convey a simple message about teamwork, which is plan together, work together, look out for one another, and we will get to the goal.

In most health care teams, retreats, personality assessments, and group problem-solving games may not be very practical, but there are less elaborate ways to create a sense of membership and trust within the group. Simply engaging in "ice breakers" during the formative team meetings may be sufficient. For example, have members tell the group something about themselves, like: What is the one junk food they would want to have if stranded on a desert island? What was their greatest achievement in high school? What is one of their most embarrassing moments. Just taking a few minutes to get the group talking to one another and revealing personal information helps to set aside the roles and goals of the team to create a degree of familiarity and comfort among team members and improve interactions in patient care.

BARRIERS TO COMMUNICATION

We have made a case for infusing non-task-directed communication ("sharing and caring") processes into team meetings as helpful when developing a cohesive interdisciplinary team. What are some of the barriers to maintaining good communication? Aside from time—never having enough of it to maintain good group communication processes—there are a couple of factors inherent to medical settings specifically that present problems. First is the traditional top-down *professional hierarchies* that exist in health service delivery, with physicians sitting at the capstone of the pyramid (Northouse & Northouse, 1998). The second relates to the *ethnocentrisms* and fears of encroachment that exist between professions (Ducanis & Golin, 1979).

Decision-Makers Versus Leaders

Physicians

When physicians are a part of the health service team, they often assume a *de facto* leadership of the group because they are the primary decision-makers in the health care world. That primacy is appropriate in hospitals during the acute and subacute phase of recovery, where concerns center mainly on the medical status of the patient. But when medical issues are no longer a major concern, the physician's hold on the decision-making processes ought to diminish. Unfortunately, for several reasons related to medical legal responsibilities and their "gatekeeping" role, physicians maintain decision-making power even when they are no longer directly treating the patients.

Throughout the continuum of care, physicians are expected to take the ultimate legal responsibility for patient care decisions. Additionally, the adult aphasic patient's primary care physicians are usually the "gatekeepers" and are required to "certify" or "authorize" the necessity of rehabilitation services on behalf of the insurance payer, the managed provider, or Medicare. Because these payer groups nearly always require a physician's order for a patient to receive covered therapy services by a nonphysician, physicians continue to be the decision-makers long after the medical issues have resolved. Even when the team members consider themselves to work on a par with one another, or when a nonphysician heads up the team, typically the only member empowered to authorize the care plan is the physician. And, even though facility policies may say something like "the values, goals, and wishes of the patient and families must be addressed in the care plan," in practice, the values, goals, and wishes of the person writing the orders can intrude. How physicians view their role with relation to the team can help or hinder good group cohesion and communication.

Effective Team Leaders

What makes a good leader? There are volumes of answers to that question in management texts and articles, but the general consensus is that effective leaders have an ability (either innate or acquired) to get others to focus their energies on a goal. That ability is not necessarily endowed by status, degrees, or intelligence. Evidence is emerging to suggest the most important characteristic of a good leader is "emotional intelligence" (Goleman, 1998). Goleman (1998) lists five components of emotional intelligence that he felt were more important to effective leadership than I.Q., technical skills, and other cognitive abilities. These traits included *self-awareness* (the ability to recognize your own mood, emotions, and drives); *self-regulation* (the ability to control impulses and moods); *motivation* (having a passion for work beyond money or status); *empathy* (the ability to understand the emotions of others); and *social skill* (a special proficiency in managing interpersonal relationships).

Professional Ethnocentrism

Good interdisciplinary teams are those with members who appreciate and respect the competencies of other disciplines (Sampson & Marthas, 1977). Mutual respect is the cornerstone of successful partnerships with other disciplines. Most of us bring fairly ingrained notions about our professional boundaries, and we often have prejudices about the training and professional standards of others. To work together collaboratively, we may have to reexamine and relinquish some of the notions established during our professional training. Just like developing good group communication processes, breaking down professional ethnocentrisms may require specific attention. Ducanis and Golin (1979) discuss the problems with interprofessional ethnocentrisms as a major obstacle to interdisciplinary teams. They suggested teams engage in an explicit examination of attitudes and develop an ongoing dialogue aimed at maintaining good relationships. They designed an instrument referred to as the "Interprofessional Perception Scale" which they suggested might provide a way to get members of different disciplines to examine their interprofessional attitudes. With this scale, members of various professional groups (such as physical therapy, speech-language pathology, nursing, respiratory therapy, etc.) assess their preconceived notions of another professional group by responding to a list of subjective statements and relating them to that group. These include statements such as, for example, "physical therapists are well trained," "physical therapists have good relations with my profession," "physical therapists are very defensive about their professional prerogatives," and so forth (Ducanis & Golin, 1976; p. 34). The members of the various professional groups represented on the team, other than the target group (in this example, physical therapists) indicate if each statement is "true" or "false."

In addition, they indicate how they think members of the target group (physical therapy) would answer about themselves, and then how the members of that profession would say the other professional group respondents answered. What Ducanis and Golan are suggesting is that it is important to acknowledge our prejudices and appreciate that we all bring preconceived attitudes, not necessarily justified by fact or experience, and these attitudes can hinder developing open communication, mutual trust, and cooperation in teams. Interdisciplinary teams function best when each member discipline appreciates not only their own strengths and limitations but also appreciates the contributions other disciplines bring (Allen et al., 1978).

Communication Patterns

In their review of group process in the health professions, Sampson and Marthas (1977) found three types of communication channels to be common in health services. The most common type of communication pattern was referred to as the "chain structure," in which communication occurs up and down a line in some established professional hierarchy. In this structure the physician is at the top of the chain and ward clerks, therapy aides, and patient care techs are at the bottom. This type of communication structure discourages much direct contact with decision-makers. The second pattern is referred to as the "wheel structure," in which information is fed to a central person, typically the unit's head nurse or the physician. In this structure, the central conduit of information (a nurse, social worker, physician, or ward clerk) is the only person to have the whole picture at any one time. The wheel structure is probably a good way to describe much of the communication that occurs with multidisciplinary teams. Last is the "circle structure," in which messages flow within a connected circle of disciplines. This pattern is most consistent with the type of communication needed to maintain effective interdisciplinary and transdisciplinary teams.

Weak Links and Poor Team Processes

There are several other potential barriers to successful communication and team intervention. Specifically, since teams are made up of human beings, individual members will vary in their ability to be open, receptive, cooperative, and professionally dedicated to the goals of the team. Therefore, there will probably be at least one or two "weak links" in any team. For example, if the speech-language pathologist (SLP) collaborates with the recreational therapist to work on functional communication abilities during recreation activities, but the recreation therapist is the sort of employee who frequently calls in sick, the SLP will have difficulty implementing his or her goals effectively. Weak links deplete the energies of the group and create resentments. Poor team processes can also present problems. Planning meetings

at times when key members cannot be present, or trying to cover too much at one sitting, are examples of poor processes. Not having adequate background information provided ahead of a meeting can lead to inefficiencies. Teams may be too large or too small for the demands placed on them. Teams can have the wrong mix of members or may not have the right combination of expertise and shared responsibilities. Teams also need to be designed to fluidly shift activities among members and adjust to changes in workload and priorities (Sampson & Marthas, 1977). When process problems are apparent, it may be a good idea to charter a team to figure out what's wrong with the team. By using tools from a "continuous quality improvement" (CQI) or a "total quality improvement" (TQI) problem-solving approach, the team can identify and correct process problems.

WHO ARE YOUR PARTNERS?
Patient's Primary Physician

Patients with aphasia may have various physician specialists involved in their care. Their primary physician could be an internist (specialist in internal diseases), neurologist (specialist in diseases of the nervous system), cardiologist (specialist in diseases of the heart and vascular system), physical medicine and rehabilitation physician, or physiatrist (specialist in rehabilitation medicine), neurosurgeon (neurologic surgical specialist), geriatrician (specialist in geriatric medicine), family practice physician, general practitioner, or some other physician coming from a general or specialized area of medicine or surgery. Even though the interests, background, and training of physicians will vary, they bring to the interdisciplinary team a comprehensive knowledge of diseases, disease processes, and disease treatment. They understand how biologic functions and diseases involving one organ system can impair another. They can interpret laboratory data and other findings. They can determine when findings are within normal or abnormal limits for a given individual. They prescribe drugs and perform invasive procedures for which there may be some risk of injury to the patient. In most situations physicians are given the medical-legal responsibility for care decisions, as well as financial oversight authority. Physicians may have a good or a not-so-good grasp of the linguistic and other cognitive problems the aphasic patient has, and they may have a good or a not-so-good sense of the psychosocial issues the adult aphasic patient and the family are likely to face. There is very little in medical training that prepares physicians to characterize the psycholinguistic deficits, quality of life changes, or the functional communication handicap brought on by aphasia. Although the physician may know the patient and family well (which is perhaps not as likely in today's health care delivery systems as it was previously), he or she may not have spent any amount of time in conversation with the family about what their priorities are, much less in conversation with the aphasic patient. The physician is the team member best prepared to identify and manage the medically related issues. Physicians will rely on the other specialists, such as speech-language pathologists, to characterize and plan remediation in the arenas in which the patient's physician lacks sufficient familiarity.

Nurses

Nurses come in a lot of varieties. Some may have post-graduate degrees in some specialty area (doctorates, masters degrees, or Advanced Practice degrees). They may be Registered Nurses (RNs) with or without bachelor's degrees. They may be Licensed Practical Nurses (LPNs), or nurses' aides, personal care aides, and personal care technicians. Rehabilitation nurses have specific training and expertise in developing and implementing a rehabilitation nursing care plan. Depending upon where they fit in the hierarchy of skills and training, as well as which state they are licensed in, nursing staff are the professionals who will administer the prescribed medications and perform medical procedures according to the physician's order or oversight. They maintain ongoing monitoring of the patient's vital signs and the patient's general mental and physical status. They also ensure all of the basic care needs (nutrition, hydration, elimination, comfort, hygiene, and so forth) of the patient are met. In an inpatient facility, nurses have the most ongoing and frequent contact with the patients and families. As a group, nurses are with patients more than any other member of the team, 24 hours a day. Nurses are also trained and skilled in teaching the patient and family to manage their own care, and they are especially good at reinforcing both the team's instructions to the patient and family and the functional independence goals of the team.

Case Managers and Medical Social Workers

Case managers are usually nurses and most often are RNs. In general, case managers are interested in ensuring the requirements of the patient's health care coverage (insurance, managed care, Medicare, etc.) are met. If coverage requires a certain number of hours, or minutes, of therapy per week, or that the patient be seen "daily," meaning seven days a week, the case manager makes sure the therapy team can provide that level of service. When the speech-language pathologist sees a therapy need that exceeds the aphasic patient's insurance coverage, the case manager can be a very helpful advocate for the patient and the team.

Medical social workers sometimes have responsibilities in case management. Usually, however, their primary roles are 1) to provide counseling to patients and families for the psychosocial issues that arise, 2) to provide assistance with practical matters, such as financial concerns, and 3) to arrange for discharges appropriate to the needs of the aphasic adult and the family. The medical social worker is often the first person the speech-language pathologist will turn to when family adjustment and coping problems are apparent, or when financial assistance is needed.

Pharmacists

Not all facilities or settings will have pharmacists as participants on their care teams. Hospitals are probably the places where pharmacists are most likely to be involved as formal members of unit teams. In hospitals, pharmacists routinely participate in care planning meetings and ward rounds. Pharmacists play a key role in determining appropriate therapeutic drug dosages for individual patients based on age, gender, weight, and other medical conditions. They monitor for errors in medication orders, for potential drug complications and side effects, and for polypharmacy effects (taking too many drugs and potentially causing negative interaction effects). They participate in teaching the patient and family self-management of medications, and can work with the speech-language pathologist to address safe self-medication.

Dietitians

Inpatient facilities typically have a dietitian or dietary technician attached to their care team. They follow the patient's nutrition and hydration status, monitoring parameters such as body weight, renal chemistry panels, serum albumin, daily intake of food and water, and general appetite. They also monitor the patient's alertness and well-being. The speech-language pathologist may work with the dietitian, particularly if the aphasic patient has a concomitant problem managing oral intake, or if there are other issues related more directly to the aphasia, such as difficulties ordering preferred items from the facility menu.

Psychologists

Neuropsychologists, geropsychologists, or general clinical psychologists may be a part of the core care team, or may be consultants to the team. In comprehensive rehabilitation facilities, psychologists are an integral part of the rehabilitation team. In units such as head injury programs, where cognitive and behavioral issues tend to be principal concerns, psychologists may be the team leaders. Psychologists conduct and participate in the team assessments of cognitive, emotional, and behavioral areas. They collaborate with the team to design and implement the cognitive, emotional, and behavioral therapies. They work with families and, when needed, collaborate with medical social workers to link families and patients to community mental health services. Depending upon the individual's training and specialty area, the psychologist can be a very close partner with the speech-language pathologist in developing a profile of the cognitive and other deficits and collaborating on interpretations of test findings.

Recreation Therapy

Rehabilitation units and other facilities, such as skilled nursing units, are usually required to have someone on staff to conduct a recreation and resident activities program. These individuals may have bachelors or associate degrees in recreation therapy or may be Certified Activities Directors, who may not have completed professional degrees but have completed a course and passed a state-certifying examination in this area. These individuals are responsible for planning and scheduling the daily activity calendar of patients. Speech-language pathologists will work closely with the recreation therapy staff to ensure the aphasic patients have activities they can engage in as fully as possible in the unit's recreation activities, without experiencing a communication disadvantage. Recreation therapy is more than just keeping patients busy. Recreation therapy groups can be the first place where the aphasic patient and the family resume shared activities; thus, these groups offer excellent opportunities for partnerships with the speech-language pathologist. By engaging patients and their families in recreation activities together that do not require much language facility (such as playing cards or dominoes) the team can demonstrate to the family the aphasic patient's residual nonlanguage abilities. By involving aphasic patients in recreation tasks that have some demand for communication (targeted to be just within the patient's ability range) the speech-language pathologist can demonstrate the value of applying the communication-facilitating strategies they are developing in therapy to everyday social activities.

Occupational Therapists and Physical Therapists

Occupational therapists (OTs) and physical therapists (PTs) have uniquely different professional preparation and perspectives on rehabilitation, but also have some overlapping areas in their scopes of practice, which sometimes leads the general public and health care personnel to refer to all therapies (including speech-language therapy) as "Physical Therapy." In general, occupational therapists are concerned with the patient's functional daily living abilities, safety, and independence in self-care and related areas. OTs ensure the patients can take care of their grooming and hygiene, can don and doff clothes, and can functionally transfer in and out of a wheelchair, in and out of bed, in and out of a tub or shower, etc., for optimal independence and self-care. Most OTs have experience in the assessment and treatment of perceptual-motor abilities and the visuo-spatial abilities and visuo-perceptual abilities associated with brain injuries. Some OTs have had specialized training in "Low Vision Rehab" with patients who have visuo-sensory losses. They are

a valuable partner for the speech-language pathologist in designing a plan for improving a patient's functional impairments involving visual, visual perceptual, visuo-motor, visual recognition, or perceptual-motor deficits, as with conditions such as apraxias and neglect syndromes, or with visual field cuts. OTs also are very adept at designing or providing assistive devices to improve functional independence. In some settings, OTs may be involved in kitchen and recreation evaluations, or they may be involved in an assessment of the patient's ability to safely return to driving. Many of these areas are going to be crucial for the patient to return to a maximal level of independence. The speech-language pathologist and OT often work in partnerships when communication problems interact with other functional losses, or to combine the objectives of both therapies into sessions. For example, the OT might be asked to have the patient point to the items of clothing he or she names before beginning the dressing routine.

Physical therapists (PTs) have a key role with stroke rehabilitation whenever weakness, incoordination, or balance problems are present. For the most part PTs are focused on the patient's mobility, strength, balance, transfers, endurance, range of movement, and exercise or activity tolerance. PTs and OTs may also be involved in other areas of rehabilitation with the aphasic patient, such as splinting, cardiac rehabilitation, or bladder continence control. Physical therapists, like all other members of the team, are concerned with maximizing functional independence. Physical therapy addresses not only the neuromuscular weakness, coordination, and balance problems found in patients with neurologic damage, but also the associated functional living problems. For example, the goal of physical therapy may be something like "the patient will walk 50 feet without assistance," but in addition, "the patient will be able to carry a basket of clothes the distance from his bedroom to the laundry room." Speech-language pathologists might partner with the PT to incorporate functional language-facilitating activities into the physical therapist's directions and requests. Similarly, the SLP might incorporate a PT objective into therapy sessions, such as asking the patient to transfer from the bed to a chair before beginning therapy.

Speech-Language Pathologist

The speech-language pathologist (SLP) brings to the team knowledge and skills in the evaluation and remediation of the aphasic person's communication and related cognitive impairments. This text provides a comprehensive review of the breadth of the SLP's expertise in aphasia intervention. The SLP is the member of the team who provides theory-driven and evidence-based language intervention. The SLP evaluation usually includes a psycholinguistic assessment of the aphasic patient's language deficits, and an assessment of related cognitive impairments. Test findings, along with all of the evaluations, behavioral data, and observational input provided by other members of the care team—in collaboration with the patient and family in identifying the communication goals—forms the basis of the SLP's intervention program.

Therapy Assistants

In rehabilitation, it is increasingly common to find therapy assistants. Certified Occupational Therapy Assistants (COTAs), Physical Therapist Assistants (PTAs) and Speech-Language Pathology Assistants (SLP-As) may be a part of the team, and in some cases work *en par* with the professional therapists. In most states these individuals have to have met qualifying examinations to be licensed in their discipline area after completing required education and training (usually either a bachelors degree or an associate degree). Therapy assistants usually are restricted by the State Boards of Examiners to the implementation of treatment procedures only under specific conditions, including under the supervision and direction of professional therapists. Therapy assistants sometimes are viewed as "therapy extenders"—implementing the plans that are established by the physical therapists, occupational therapists, or speech-language pathologists. They do not conduct new patient evaluations, make differential diagnoses, or design the plans of treatment. Therapy assistants have to demonstrate specific competencies before they can treat patients independently. In addition to assistants, therapy aides, or rehab techs, are fairly common in rehabilitation settings. These individuals may be students or others without degrees in rehabilitation therapy specialties but with specific training to lend help to the therapists and assistants in patient care and other clinical duties (e.g., setting up equipment).

Other Allied Professionals

Professionals from a variety of disciplines, such as audiologists, biomedical engineers, vocational counselors, and chaplains, may be members of the heath care team with aphasic adults. If the aphasic patient has a hearing impairment, the audiologist can become a central member of the team. If the patient requires special adaptive equipment or augmentative communication systems or other purposes, the biomedical engineer will help the team select the instruments and design the access switches. If there is potential for the aphasic adult to return to a previous vocation, similar vocation, or even a new vocation, a rehabilitation vocation counselor is the individual best equipped to direct the patient and family toward potential alternatives. When the patient and family have spiritual needs that require specialized attention, a member of the facility's pastoral care or chaplaincy service will help the team address those concerns.

TEAMS ACROSS THE CONTINUUM

Changing Priorities

As aphasic patients move from the crisis of the acute event through various care settings, and eventually, hopefully, reentering their home life and community, there will be shifts in primary concerns and priorities for intervention, and correspondingly there will be changes in the major decision-makers.

Table 8–1 illustrates how priorities can change across settings and through the continuum of recovery with adult aphasia. Team designs and the primacy of different individuals in the hierarchy of decision making will also change (see Table 8–2). Obviously, these scenarios are intended to illustrate a point. Not every facility, setting, or individual patient will necessarily follow this pattern. Shifts in priorities, team designs, and decision-makers across the recovery continuum are considered here merely to emphasize that intervention extends beyond any one setting or team. Intervention rolls through many settings from the hospital bed to the nursing home or rehab facility, from outpatient therapy to home health agency, from the rehab team to independent living. In fairly short order the support systems provided by the multidisciplinary or interdisciplinary teams will end. Patients and families need to be prepared for the time when decision-making responsibilities will fall squarely on their shoulders. As soon as the aphasic patient's medical condition has stabilized and the patient enters rehabilitation, the overarching goal of all of the rehabilitation professionals they encounter should be directed toward functional independence and encouraging the aphasic patient and the family to take control of their own lives.

Changing Rehabilitation Outcome Goals

As illustrated by a schema described by Sundance and Cope (1995) rehabilitation outcome goals move through a continuum as the patient progresses from a destabilized state during the acute phase up through later phases of community reintegration and productive activity. These authors conceptualized the continuum of treatment to span the following stages.

Level 0 = Physiologic Instability—this is the stage of the acute onset of illness in which medical stabilization is the main concern and diagnostic evaluations are completed.

Level I = Physiologic Stability—at this stage there will be limited attention given to functional rehabilitation restoration while mainly addressing medical stabilization.

Level II = Physiologic Maintenance—at this point rehabilitation primarily is aimed at establishing adequate and safe systems of nutrition and hydration, and prevention of complications, such as aspiration pneumonia, skin breakdown, joint mobilization problems, and bowel and bladder control problems. Secondarily, rehabilitation at this phase will be aimed at communication, self-care, mobilization, and cognitive and

TABLE 8–1

Shifts in Priorities Across Settings and the Recovery Continuum With Aphasic Adults

Setting	Typical Priorities
Acute care	1. Physiologic and medical stability 2. Emotional issues 3. Physical limitations 4. Communicative and other cognitive limitations 5. Discharge plan
Sub-acute nursing	1. Physiologic and medical status 2. Physical limitations 3. Communicative and other cognitive limitations 4. Functional independence 5. Discharge plan
Inpatient rehab	1. Communication and other cognitive limitations 2. Physical limitations 3. Functional independence 4. Psychosocial and emotional issues 5. Discharge plan
Outpatient rehab	1. Functional independence 2. Communication and other cognitive limitations 3. Physical limitations 4. Psychosocial and emotional issues 5. Financial and vocational issues
Home health	1. Functional independence 2. Communication and other cognitive limitations 3. Physical limitations 4. Financial and vocational issues 5. Psychosocial and emotional issues
Home and community re-entry	1. Psychosocial and emotional issues 2. Financial and vocational issues 3. Functional independence 4. Physical limitations 5. Communication and other cognitive limitations

behavioral issues, depending on the patient's responsiveness.

Level III = Primary Functional Goals—at this point functional deficit-specific goals are established to facilitate discharge to home or to improve residential integration.

Level IV = Advanced Functional Goals—at this stage, rehabilitation is directed toward community reintegration.

Level V = Productive Activity—at this point rehabilitation outcomes are directed at returning the aphasic adult to productive activities within his or her level of ability (Sundance & Cope, 1995; Landrum et al., 1995; Paradigm Health Corporation, 1993).

Changing Settings

Acute Care Setting

Initially, the team's efforts are directed toward moving the patient out of physiologic instability toward a level of physiologic stability and maintenance (Sundance & Cope, 1995). In the acute setting, the first priorities are 1) ensuring the aphasic patient survives the acute event with minimal residual neurologic damage and 2) diminishing risks for complications. Some patients are ready to participate in rehabilitation services within a few days of the acute event and onset of aphasia. Unfortunately, most acute stroke clinical care pathways anticipate discharge in 3 to 5 days from admission, making interdisciplinary team rehabilitation virtually impossible. With just a few days' involvement with the patient before discharge, the team's emphasis tends to be on patient and family education and appropriate discharge planning. As is the case with nearly any hospitalization with an acute event, the aphasic person's family is under tremendous emotional stress. They may not be in the best frame of mind to absorb new information or make decisions. The family will, however, be sensitive to the verbal messages, body

TABLE 8–2

Team Designs and Decision-Makers Across Settings and the Recovery Continuum
With Aphasic Adults

Setting	Team Design	Primary Decision-Makers
Acute care	Multidisciplinary	Physician
Sub-acute unit	Interdisciplinary	1. Physician 2. Patient care team 3. Patient and family
Inpatient rehab unit	Interdisciplinary	1. Physician 2. Rehab team 3. Patient and family
Outpatient rehab facility	Multidisciplinary Community support networks & partnerships	1. Physician 2. Rehab team 3. Patient and family
Home health	Multidisciplinary Community support networks & partnerships	1. Physician 2. Home health rehab team 3. Patient and family
Home and community re-entry	Community support networks & partnerships	Patient and family

language, and attitudes of all the team members participating in caring for the patient. It is especially important that family and patients be approached with a professional, supportive, and reassuring attitude (vanVendendaal et al., 1996). Education and verbal messages need to be brief and consistent. Information needs to guide and not overwhelm. The family should not be expected to fully grasp the consequences of the neurologic damage, so a supercilious lecture on recovery from aphasia full of grim predictions intended to correct the family's "unrealistic expectations" is completely inappropriate and unnecessary at this point. The messages need to be accurate but also hopeful.

As we suggested earlier, unless the patient is admitted to an acute "stroke unit" where an interdisciplinary team is in place, the typical model for team care in an acute setting is more likely to look like a multidisciplinary than interdisciplinary model. Consequently, care planning discussions, if they take place at all, focus on sharing assessment findings with other team members, and making discharge recommendations to the physician and medical social worker. Group discussions of observations of the patient are an important part of decision-making during this time. Often, the patient's responsiveness will vary during the day, so team discussions of observations on cognitive and communicative status will help the speech-language pathologist gauge the reliability of communication assessments. Finally, because the patient and family are under stress, it may be better to channel information through as few people as possible and principally through the physician, the primary nurse, or

the social worker, and allow them to work with the family. Other professionals should be available to address their particular concerns; however, it is important for the team to keep messages consistent and to not overwhelm the patient or family.

Sub-Acute Nursing Setting

Usually, after the medical and acute physiologic conditions have stabilized, patients are transferred to some kind of sub-acute setting, where physiologic maintenance may still be the main outcome goal. These settings can be a skilled nursing facility, recuperative care unit, transitional care unit, or the like. Prevention of complications continues to be a concern along with communication, cognitive and emotional issues, mobility, and independence. Emotional issues, such as anxiety and depression on the part of the family, continue to be major concern, and the psychosocial effects of the aphasia and other impairments will begin to be felt by the patient and the family. Psychosocial concerns can include such things as changes in body image and losses in the level of independence, uncertainties about the future and the recovery processes, frustration with communication and impaired movement, emotional lability, changes in family dynamics and a sense of a lack of control over events happening to them, irritability, self-centeredness, unrealistic expectations or denial, and dependency (Churchill, 1993; Flick, 1999). Patients also may display post stroke depression and anxiety. These emotional problems usually respond to a combination of medication and reassurance. At the sub-acute phase, the patient's residual physical impairments, if any, often are more of a concern to the family and to the patient than communication and other cognitive impairments, possibly because mobility is linked to independence. Integral to improving the psychosocial and emotional status of the patient is the implementation of rehabilitation for physical, self-care, and cognitive/communicative problems. If the patient's physical tolerance and cognitive status allows, the earliest possible involvement in rehabilitation should be encouraged (Flick, 1999). Intervention at this phase is usually in a residential program setting where teams tend to be interdisciplinary (Cifu & Steward, 1999). It is important that everyone working with the patient and family have the same goals in mind and that no one professional group exerts ownership over their goals or procedures. Although different members of the team have a slightly different center of concern, the entire team is responsible for achieving the intervention goals. When possible, intervention procedures are shared and implemented in partnerships between team and family members.

Inpatient Rehab Setting

Some patients transfer directly to a rehab setting from their acute care ward, and some continue rehabilitation following a stay in a sub-acute nursing unit. Typically, once the patient reaches the rehab setting the major medical issues have resolved and some of the acute emotional reactions and psychosocial issues have become slightly less of a priority than the residual effects of the stroke (such as hemiparesis, aphasia, and other cognitive problems). There may be significant, chronic medical issues to consider, such as pain management, depression, blood pressure management, blood coagulation management, seizure control, or incontinency, but the patient is typically felt to be generally medically stable. Typically, on an inpatient rehab unit the family sees the patient working for several hours a day with a team of experts attempting to maximize the functional status. Also, most likely, the patient has experienced some amount of recovery at this point. In such settings, the family and the patient are usually highly confident some improvement will result; consequently, the concerns about psychosocial and emotional issues may be temporarily set aside, or less acute. In a rehab setting there is a "full court press" to address the specific deficit effects of the stroke. Aggressive speech-language therapy for the aphasia will be implemented, in addition to 3 or 4 hours of occupational and physical therapy daily. The focus on everyone's part is placed on maximizing the patient's abilities for home or residential facility integration, with the overriding goal of maximizing independence. Again, inpatient team intervention tends to be interdisciplinary and collaborative goals are emphasized. Because there is an expectation for positive results from all of this intensive therapy and team activity, one of the problems

that arises with the inpatient rehabilitation setting is that patients and families may see the end of rehabilitation as the end of recovery (Flick, 1999). Therefore, psychological stresses may begin to emerge at about the time the inpatient rehabilitation stay is nearing an end. The end of formal treatment can signal a concern for "is this is as good as it gets?" which creates anxiety for both the family and the patient.

Outpatient Rehab Setting

In this setting daily contact with non-therapist, allied disciplines such as pharmacists, social workers, dieticians, nurses, and even physicians is not typical. Therapists from different disciplines may work in the same clinic area, but the team intervention model is more likely to be closer to the multidisciplinary design. Much like the hierarchy of concerns when patients enter inpatient rehab facilities, the interventions in outpatient rehab settings are impairment-specific, for the most part, but with the overriding goal to improve self-care and independence for home and community integration and toward some resumption of productive activity. Because the patient is typically coming to therapy from home at this juncture, psychosocial, emotional, financial, and vocational concerns may be uppermost on the minds of the patient and family. In this setting especially, caregivers are likely to express frustration with communicating with the aphasic person and sadness over the loss of companionship. Issues such as lifestyle changes, social isolation, and financial difficulties may surface after the patient goes home (Flick, 1999); thus, these should be addressed as part of the outpatient rehab program. Since this arena of treatment can tend to be more multidisciplinary than interdisciplinary, due mostly to difficulties with scheduling collaborative therapies and the unavailability of support professionals, a mechanism to address these special issues easily may be lacking. Explicit referrals and consultations with allied professionals will need to be set up. Similar to a home health–based setting, encouraging the patient and family to link with community support networks well ahead of the completion of formal outpatient therapy is essential.

RELATED ISSUES

Team Evaluations and Team Treatments

One of the frequent concerns expressed when team evaluations and treatments are considered is the belief that "only one discipline can bill for this time." That may be the case in any fee-for-service visits, where charges are made per procedure and payers usually will not pay for two procedure charges in the same unit of time. Other types of reimbursement schemes, however, might support collaborative interdisciplinary team evaluations and treatment. For example, when a pre-established payment is made for a certain amount of treatment time (as with Medicare's DRGs or prospective payment system for Part A coverage or with inpatient insurance *per diems*) there are no *payer restrictions* on having more than one discipline involved in a given evaluation or therapy session. The issue may be provider costs. The facility may resist having more people involved patient care than are necessary. Increased staff time translates to increased costs to the provider facility; therefore, it may be necessary to justify collaborative evaluations and interventions and nonbillable staff time (such as team meetings) as a facility cost *savings*. Collaborative evaluations may accomplish a more comprehensive assessment in a shorter time frame than evaluations that are done independently. In the earlier discussion of "who are your partners" several examples of collaborative evaluations and interventions were mentioned. It's a bit like the parable of the seven blind men and the elephant, where a different interpretation emerges depending upon which part of the elephant you are touching. Team evaluations with more than one discipline participating can yield a much better composite picture than independent assessments.

Collaborative interventions can reduce redundancies, reduce the time taken for communications, and more efficiently ease transfers and discharges, which reduce the lengths of stays. Reducing the lengths of stays often saves costs to the facility and prevents the risks of nosocomial infections and other hospital-stay related complications.

Documentation

Documentation is another important area for collaborations. Some of the current practices in health care in the U.S. today strongly encourage multidisciplinary documentation. For example, Clinical Care Pathways are increasingly used to guide day-to-day care plans, particularly in inpatient facilities. The documentation for these pathways flows across multiple disciplines and some items may be shared between or among disciplines (e.g., patient education) (Ignativicius & Housman, 1995). To be in compliance with the Joint Commission on Accreditation of Health Care Organizations (JCAHO) (JCAHO, 1998) or the Commission on Accreditation of Rehabilitation Facilities (CARF) (CARF, 1997) standards, it is expected that the family and patient education be conducted in a multidisciplinary manner.

Clinical Preparation and Research

Training programs and research are also ripe for interdisciplinary collaborations. The time to initiate good interdisciplinary relations to prevent potential problems related to professional ethnocentrisms, discussed earlier, is during the professional clinical preparation. It is important that students have a good exposure to different team interventions as a part of their professional training. Collaborative research also has exciting possibilities. When different disciplines collaborate in research we discover a new way of looking at old notions, and test the extent to which our data apply to other areas.

COMMUNITY SUPPORT NETWORKS AND PARTNERSHIPS

Every aphasic adult who completes formal therapy under the care of an array of disciplines or just a couple of disciplines eventually reaches an outcome: the rest of life. In outcome-oriented rehab (Landrum et al., 1995; Schmidt, 1999), the intervention services of the health care delivery team are, from the initiation of care, conceptualized, organized, and delivered with an eye on the quality of the rest of life for that aphasic person. Landrum et al. (1995) and Schmidt (1999) observe that all too often the team fails to consider the resources the patient and family have available to them, much less how to incorporate those resources and social support networks into their future until the end of the patient's stay.

Schmidt (1999) suggests the following resources should be identified with the patient and family very early in the continuum of rehabilitation therapy services: 1) *Health services funding resources* (what will the insurance coverage provide for this person to support his or her needs now and in the future?); 2) *financial resources* (what are the additional financial resources available to this patient and family?); 3) *family resources* (what are the caregiver and other resources available to this family unit?); and 4) *community resources* (what community and social support services are available to this family?) It is important that every member of the rehabilitation team understand the global impact that aphasia and other problems resulting from brain damage will have on the individual and the family unit. The intervention team should anticipate and incorporate that perspective into each phase of therapy. The team needs to not only be focused on the future themselves, but to also keep the patient and family clearly focused on the future as well. Schmidt (1999) suggests starting with the endpoint and aligning expectations throughout the continuum of recovery. The team should be supportive and also encourage and empower aphasic adults and their families to use their available resources to reintegrate into their homes and communities and return to productive activity. One of the projects for the team can be to help the family develop an individualized resource directory for community services. This can include such things as elder care services, day treatment programs, Meals on Wheels, community or university-based aphasia therapy programs, church activities, support groups, recreation opportunities, and the like. The team can also help the aphasic patient and the family plan post-therapy goals, such as continuing language-reinforcing tasks at home (word processor letters, reading selected sections of the newspaper) and family or community activities (attending a reunion, participating with a church project). These kinds of planned activities may help to carry forward formal treatment into functional living in the future.

The outcome of *survival* following a major neurologic event, such as a stroke, is, literally, life. After formal therapy ends, the patient and the family may need to maintain contact with a support team, and that should not be discouraged. However, one of the overarching goals of rehabilitation should be to identify the potential risks and concerns prior to the end of treatment and help the patient and family establish the community support networks they will need and to then be prepared to lead their own "team aphasia."

SUMMARY

This chapter examined concepts in team collaborations mainly within the context of therapeutic interventions for aphasia in health care facilities and other rehabilitation settings. The notion of team intervention is extended to family-centered partnerships as early as possible in the continuum of care and to community support partnerships after formal therapy has ended. In an examination of the differences between *interdisciplinary*, *multidisciplinary*, and *transdisciplinary* teams in health care settings, the importance of good communication is stressed. We have also emphasized how becoming comfortable with a certain amount of blurring of professional scopes of practice may be necessary for the success of interdisciplinary teams. In team dynamics, there needs to be a balance of both content (activities, goals, and products) and process (communication, affiliation, and collaboration). We considered how team processes may be hindered by a number of factors that can be barriers to communication. We looked at how professional hierarchies in health care settings tend to place the physician in the role of primary decision-maker, especially in the more acute phases of care. We consider how the structure of teams tends to vary in different settings, and how the priorities and primary decision-makers might shift over the recovery continuum. The principal goal of this chapter is to emphasize the value of team collaborations and partnerships both in the formal rehabilitation program itself and in the transition to the home and community. We suggest one of the overarching goals of therapy should be to empower patients and families to become independent decision-makers. When therapy has ended, the leaders in "team aphasia" are ultimately the patient and the family.

FUTURE TRENDS

Teams and family-centered and community partnerships have an important future in patient care in all arenas, but especially in aphasia intervention. An interdisciplinary team approach is supported by research examining evidence-based treatment (Cifu & Steward, 1999). Team intervention is also strongly encouraged by legislative and certifying bodies (CARF, 1997; JCAHO, 1998; Rosin et al., 1996), and by third-party payers. All of the current trends and influences in health care delivery today suggest the "lone professional" practice is diminishing and collaborations in patient care are here to stay.

KEY POINTS

1. Typical team organizational designs in health services delivery are defined and examined.
2. The basic elements in group processes that lead to successful interdisciplinary teams are reviewed, and barriers to communication when developing effective teams are examined.
3. Depending on the setting and the aphasic patient's or family's priorities across the continuum of recovery, team design might differ.
4. Related issues, such as evaluations, documentation, and outcomes research are reviewed.
5. If the goal is to bring about the best quality of life after the onset of aphasia, the patient and family are, ultimately, the most important players on the team.

Review/Reflection

1. What are the advantages and disadvantages of having more than one discipline involved in intervention with aphasia?
2. What are the similarities and differences between multidisciplinary, interdisciplinary, and transdisciplinary teams?
3. Which professional group tends to be the decision-makers in health care in the U.S., and why?
4. What do case managers and social workers bring to the team?
5. What do nurses contribute to the rehabilitation team?
6. How might teams differ in the acute phase of rehabilitation as compared with the sub-acute and chronic phases of recovery?
7. During which time frames are patients and families most likely to become more concerned about psychosocial and financial issues than medical issues?
8. List the ways team intervention is encouraged by trends and influences in health service delivery.
9. What are some of the processes that could be employed to develop trust and cooperation in teams?
10. Describe some specific objectives teams might incorporate into the therapy plan to ultimately empower patients and families to take control of "team aphasia" after formal rehabilitation has ended.

References

Allen, K.E., Holm, V.A., & Scheifelbusch, R.L. (1978). *Early Intervention—A Team Approach*. Baltimore, MD: University Park Press.

Cifu, D.X. & Steward, D.G. (1999). Factors affecting functional outcome after stroke: A critical review of rehabilitation interventions. *Archives of Physical Medicine and Rehabilitation, 80* (5 Suppl. 1), S-35–39.

Churchill, C. (1993). Social problems after stroke. *Physical Medicine Rehabilitation: State of the Art Review,* 7(1), 213–23.

Collins, D., Moore, P., Mitchell, D., & Alpress, F. (1999). Role and confidentiality in multidisciplinary athlete support programs. *British Journal of Sports Medicine, 33*(3), 208–211.

Commission on Accreditation of Rehabilitation Facilities (1997). *Medical Rehabilitation Accreditation Manual.* Tucson, AZ: CARF Publications.

Ducanis, A.J. & Golin, A.K. (1979). *The Interdisciplinary Health Care Team: A Handbook.* Rockville, MD: Aspen Publishers, Inc.

Flick, C.L. (1999). Stroke rehabilitation: 4. Stroke outcome and psychosocial consequences. *Archives of Physical Medicine and Rehabilitation, 80* (5 Suppl. 1), S-21–26.

Goleman, D. (1998). What makes a leader? *Harvard Business Review,* Nov-Dec, 93–102.

Heikkila, V.M., Korpelainen, J., Turkka, J., Lallanranta, T., & Summala, H. (1999). Clinical evaluation of driving in stroke patients. *Acta Neurologica Scandinavia, 99*(6), 349–399.

Hogh, P., Waldmar, G., Knudsen, G.M., Bruhn, P., Mortensen, H., Wildschiodtz, G., Bech, R.A., Juhler, M., & Paulson, O.B. (1999). A multidisciplinary memory clinic in a neurologic setting. *European Journal of Neurology, 6*(3), 279–288.

Ignatitivicius, D.D. & Housman, K.A. (1995). *Clinical Pathways for Collaborative Practice.* Philadelphia: W.B. Saunders.

Joint Commission on Accreditation of Hospitals (1998). *JCAHO Standards for Hospitals.* Oakbrook, IL: JCHAO Publications.

Landrum, P.K., Schmidt, N.D., & McLean, A. Jr. (eds.) (1995). *Outcome-Oriented Rehabilitation: Principles, Strategies, and Tools for Effective Program Management.* Gaithersburg, MD: Aspen.

Loomis, M.E. (1979). *Group Processes for Nurses.* St. Louis: C.V. Mosby.

Lott, C., Hennes, H.J., & Dick, W. (1999). Stroke—a medical emergency. *Journal of Accident and Emergency Medicine, 16*(1), 2–7.

Manion, J., Lorimer, W., & Leander, W.J. (1996). *Team-Based Health Care Organizations: Blueprint for Success.* Gaithersburg, MD: Aspen Publishers, Inc.

Meyers-Briggs, I. & Briggs, P. (1980). *Gifts Differing.* Palo Alto, CA: Consulting Psychologists Press.

Northouse, L.L. & Northouse, P.G. (1998). *Health Communication: Strategies for Health Professionals.* Stamford, CT: Appleton & Lange.

Paradigm Health Corporation Publications (1993). Paradigm Health Corp., 1001 Galaxy Way, Suite Number 400, Concord, CA 94520.

Rosin, P., Whitehead, A.D, Tuchman, L.I., Gesien, G.S., Begun, A.L., & Irwin, L. (1996). *Partnerships in Family-Centered Care: A Guide to Collaborative Early Intervention.* Baltimore: Paul H. Brookes Publishing Co.

Sampson, E.E. & Marthas, M.S. (1977). *Group Process for the Health Professions.* New York: John Wiley & Sons.

Schmidt, N.D. (1999). Predicting the future. *Advance for Directors of Rehabilitation, 8*(8), 31–33.

Sundance, P. & Cope, D.N. (1995). Outcome Level I: Physiologic stability—acute management. In P.K. Landrum, N.D. Schmidt, & A. McLean Jr., (eds.) *Outcome-Oriented Rehabilitation: Principles, Strategies, and Tools for Effective Program Management.* Gaithersburg, MD: Aspen.

Tuchman, L.I. (1996). The team and models of teaming. In P. Rosin, A.D. Whitehead, L.I. Tuchman, G.S. Gesien, A.L. Begun, & L. Irwin (eds.). *Partnerships in Family-Centered Care: A Guide to Collaborative Early Intervention.* Baltimore: Paul H. Brookes Publishing Co.

Rosin, P. (1996). The diverse American family. In P. Rosin, A.D. Whitehead, L.I. Tuchman, G.S. Gesien, A.L. Begun, & L. Irwin. *Partnerships in Family-Centered Care: A Guide to Collaborative Early Intervention.* Baltimore: Paul H. Brookes Publishing Co.

van Vendendaal, H., Grinspin, D.R., & Andriaanse, H.P. (1996). Educational needs of stroke survivors and their family members as perceived by themselves and by health professionals. *Patient Education Council, 28,* 265–76.

Chapter 9

Aphasia Assessment and Treatment for Bilingual and Culturally Diverse Patients

Patricia M. Roberts

Clinical work with patients from different backgrounds is challenging. In addition to the literature on aphasia, the clinician should be familiar with research in three fields: 1) bilingualism, 2) culture, and 3) comparative aphasiology. Studies of bilingualism examine how people learn and use two or more languages or dialects, and compare their performance to that of unilingual speakers. In this literature, and in the present chapter, the term bilingual includes bilinguals (those who speak two languages) and multilinguals or polyglots (those who speak more than two languages). This avoids cumbersome "bilingual and/or multilingual/polyglot" constructions in sentences. Although there may be differences between bilinguals and multilinguals, our current knowledge base has not identified these, making this short-hand acceptable. The literature on culture and cultural diversity examines the customs, beliefs, and behavior of different groups defined by race, national origin, socioeconomic status (SES), or other common factor, and their impact on the clinical process or outcome. Comparative aphasiology refers to the study of aphasia in different languages. All three fields fall within what is called the study of culturally and linguistically diverse (CLD) patients. A specialty within the CLD field is CLD neurogenics, or multicultural neurogenics, which focuses on neurogenic communication disorders. This chapter addresses CLD issues in aphasia, those relating to culture and also to bilingualism.

Prior to 1990, bilingual aphasia is rarely mentioned in English textbooks, and cultural issues, if mentioned at all, are given little attention. Yet, "bilingualism, far from being exceptional, is a problem which affects the majority of the world's population" (Mackey, 1967, p. 11).[1] Paradis echoed this view, within a clinical perspective: "Bilingualism is not just a rare, occasional occurrence in the language/speech

pathology clinic, but a phenomenon every clinic must be prepared to cope with" (1995c, p. 219).

In recent years, there has been a growing recognition in the English-language aphasiology literature of the importance of addressing the needs of the patients from all linguistic and cultural backgrounds. This recognition may be due to three interrelated factors.

First, the combined effects of immigration patterns and birth rates have produced large populations of linguistically and culturally diverse (CLD) adults in many areas of the United States, Canada, the United Kingdom, and Australia. Recognizing this, policy statements by influential bodies require or recommend that CLD issues be given more attention in research and/or in speech-language pathology training (ASHA, 1985; ASHA, 1989; ASHA, 1991; Australian Association of Speech and Hearing, 1994; Australian Institute of Multicultural Affairs, 1985; Cole, 1989; Martin et al., 1998). Publications in medicine and (neuro)psychology have also called for more study of CLD groups (e.g., Ardila, 1995; Frayne et al., 1996; National Institutes of Health, 1990; NINCD, 1992; Rowland, 1991).

Second, in the 1980s and 1990s researchers found that language and cultural background have an impact on performance on some neuropsychological tests (Ellis, 1992; Mungas, 1996; Puente & McCaffrey, 1992) and on the clinical process. In the same period, it became clear that aphasia in languages other than English and aphasia in bilinguals presented features not addressed in the English aphasiology literature. Third, the number of publications in bilingual aphasia and comparative aphasiology grew large enough to draw attention to the field.

OBJECTIVES

The goals of this chapter are as follows: (1) to highlight how culture may influence the clinical process, and to provide references and a framework for detailed study of this area; (2) to provide a brief overview of the key terminology and concepts in bilingualism and bilingual aphasia; (3) to

---

[1] In the French version of the same paper, Mackey refers to bilingualism as a "phenomenon." The English wording may or may not express his intended meaning.

summarize some of the findings from psycholinguistic studies which are most relevant for clinical work with bilingual, aphasic adults; and (4) to outline issues in the assessment and treatment of bilingual aphasia. These include test reliability and interpretation; available tests in different languages; patterns of impairment and recovery; setting treatment goals; choice of language(s) for treatment; use of interpreters; and generalization across languages.

In all areas, the goal is to highlight key issues. A comprehensive literature review and detailed analyses of specific languages or cultural groups are impossible in a single chapter. The focus is on issues that have the most direct bearing on clinical work and on issues that have received little attention in the speech pathology CLD literature to date. In some cases, only recent work is cited. In the recent studies and review articles, the reader will find references that could not be included here due to space limitations. While language and culture are closely related, the challenges they present to clinicians working with aphasic clients are quite different. In this chapter, therefore, they will be considered separately.

CULTURE

Avoiding Stereotypes While Recognizing Differences

According to Grosjean (1982): "anthropologists commonly agree that culture consists of a number of components: the human's way of maintaining life, and perpetuating the species, along with habits, customs, ideas, sentiments, social arrangements, and objects. Culture is the way of life of a people or a society, including its rules of behavior, its economic, social, and political systems; its language; its religious beliefs; its laws; and so on. Culture is acquired, socially transmitted, and communicated in large part by language." (p. 157)

Figure 9–1 illustrates the interaction between cultural factors, domains/topics, pragmatics, and linguistic knowledge to produce communication. The items within each ring are examples of relevant factors, not a complete list. Depending on the communicative situation, the importance of each ring may grow or shrink. For example, asking someone where the nearest bus stop is has far less cultural content than asking someone out on a date.

Most discussions of culture focus at a macro level. That is, they look at cultures as a whole. There are many books which describe various cultures, to assist health care workers and/or teachers in working with people from these cultures (e.g., Asante & Gudykunst, 1989; Battle, 1998; Brislin, 1994; Brislin et al., 1986; Fawcett & Carino, 1987; Galens et al., 1995; Lynch & Hanson, 1992; Taylor, 1986). These books describe various societies in terms of specific characteristics, often prefaced by a historical sketch of how a particular group came to live in a given country or region. Most sketches include the following characteristics: 1) views of health and wellness; 2) attitudes toward disability; 3) family structure and roles within the family; 4) how status is determined; 5) views of time; 6) religious views and practices; 7) food preferences and customs; 8) language(s) and dialect(s) spoken and some of their key characteristics; and 9) nonverbal aspects of communication.

There are many sources of information on different cultures, and many different cultures which could be relevant for readers in different settings. Therefore, specific cultural profiles will not be presented here. Instead, the following section offers some caveats and comments for clinicians to consider as they read cultural guidebooks (e.g., Galens et al., 1995; Lynch & Hanson, 1992).

The problem with brief cultural sketches is that they tend not to recognize individual variations. Therefore, they can easily create or reinforce ethnic and racial stereotypes. One author, for example, describes the Japanese immigrant family as characterized by interdependency, hierarchical relationships, and empathy and contrasts this with the Anglo-American family which, the author implies, does not share these characteristics (Tempo & Saito, 1996, p. 114). Another cultural guide states that some devout Muslims do not plan more than a few weeks ahead because they believe that only Allah knows the future (Davis et al., 1998). If true, this would mean that they do not plan for their own education, finances, vacations, buying/selling a house, and other important events. There is no indication of how many Muslims might share this fatalistic approach. Nor does the author remind us that some people of other faiths share a similar fatalistic view of the future. Such inaccurate, sweeping generalizations do little to help us understand each other.

A different approach to culture can help to minimize stereotyping. Gollnick and Chin (1990) suggest viewing individuals as coming from individual (micro)cultures within a broader (macro)culture. This view encourages clinicians to look beyond race or ethnicity to see what factors influence a specific patient's behavior. The microcultural variables Gollnick and Chin identify are 1) ethnic or national origin, 2) religion, 3) gender/sex, 4) age, 5) exceptionality, 6) urban-suburban-rural, 7) geographic region, and 8) social class.

These eight factors, and the individual patient's views and behavior can help us to look beyond ethnic groups and see that, despite their different race and nationality, a 55-year-old Chinese lawyer from Hong Kong may have more in common with a 52-year-old Anglo architect from Chicago than he does with a 22-year-old Hong Kong street vendor. A number of authors have reminded us of the importance of individual differences within cultural groups (e.g., Kayser, 1998; Pontón & Ardila, 1999; Wallace, 1997) but this point is often neglected. We must be particularly careful to guard against cultural stereotypes and generalizations when a patient's appearance (skin color, hair, features) identifies them as having a specific background.

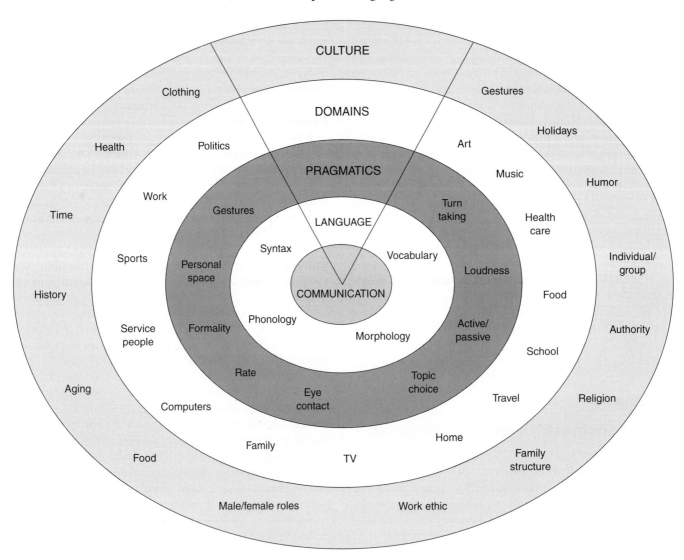

Figure 9–1. Communication within a cultural context.

The descriptions in many books stress the differences between CLD groups and the so-called mainstream culture. The differences can be important. However, we must not lose sight of the many similarities across cultures, and of individual variability within each cultural group. Holland and Penn (1995) describe Native American and African views in which disability is due to evil spirits. These views may lead some patients and families to reject rehabilitation efforts. The cases are used to support Holland and Penn's recommendation that treatment "should [not] be imposed upon patients whose cultural belief systems do not recognize therapy as a need" (p. 154). This is true not only for CLD patients but for all patients. Some white, middle class, Anglo-Saxon clients also reject therapy. What are often cited as "cultural variables" apply to all patients. They are factors clinicians can use to assess their possible impact on the clinical process.

They allow us to tailor the assessment and treatment to meet individual needs of each patient, not only those labeled CLD.

Acculturation is another factor in working with CLD patients. Acculturation refers to the process by which people from one cultural background adopt the cultural values and practices of a different culture. Usually, it applies to immigrants adopting the prevailing culture of their new country. Some authors propose seeing people as being on a continuum of acculturation or a series of levels of acculturation (Langdon, 1992b; Marin, 1992; Valle, 1994). Culture is a multilayered, multifaceted thing. A given person may be at a different level of acculturation in different areas of their lives, adopting "mainstream" values and habits around work and retaining more customs and values from their national group around religious or family matters. Within the same family, different members may have different views on work, religion, gender roles, or health, and different levels of acculturation.

Finally, many immigrants, especially those who have chosen to move from one country to another, may have left their country of birth because they reject aspects of its prevailing culture. Immigrants and their children may embrace the values of their new country. Thus, knowing that someone is a recent immigrant from Haïti, Pakistan, or Russia does not mean that they share the prevailing religious, political, or family values of those countries. This is demonstrated in a study by Erickson et al. (1999). Thirty young women, all born in Korea but living in the United States, identified many folk beliefs about illness and disability as being typical of Korean culture. However, their own beliefs closely matched those of the mainstream American culture.

It is important for clinicians working with CLD clients to read about and learn about the cultural backgrounds of their patients. These descriptions provide tools for problem solving and clues about what to watch for in our interactions. These descriptions suggest questions: Why is this client late? Does the patient want a relative to be in the room during our sessions? Can the patient attend an appointment on Friday? However, descriptions about racial, linguistic, or political groups cannot be used to predict what any individual may believe or do.

The Need for Data

Many recommendations in the CLD literature are based on the authors' clinical experience, or their opinion. While some provide valuable insights, others are incorrect. For example, one writer, commenting on the problems associated with translating English tests into other languages, stated that the phrase "no if's and's or but's" probably cannot be translated into any other language (Teng, 1996, p. 78). It is possible to translate this into a number of languages (French is one) though it would not necessarily have the status of a fixed expression in these languages, which it does in English. Some recommendations in the CLD literature are untested. Suggestions such as "Better clinical results may be obtained if music consistent with the African American culture is played while the client waits" (Terrell et al., 1998, p. 37) need to be tested. The clinician should also weigh the possible benefits of suggested changes in the clinical environment or clinical process in relation to their cost.

Clinical Chameleons?

In some cases, a center may serve a single client group such as Hispanic, African American, or Chinese. This makes it possible to link the clinical environment to that culture (e.g., decor, music, clinical tools). In many cities, however, a clinic serves clients from different cultures. This makes it impossible to tailor the environment to any one group. It also means that the clinician and the client will often not be from the same linguistic or cultural background. Therefore, compromises will have to be made.

To work with CLD clients, clinicians should be as knowledgeable as possible about customs and views that may affect the clinical process. It is possible to change many aspects of our testing and treatment. Possible changes include using appropriate greetings, having other family members attend with the patient, asking the appropriate person in the family group when decisions must be made, asking indirect questions, and allowing more or less time for informal conversation as part of each appointment. It is also possible to learn to interpret signals such as eye contact or punctuality within a range of cultural contexts. It is not possible, however, for a clinician to fully master all the culture-specific behaviors needed in a setting in which a range of people are seen. Inevitably, when clinical services are offered by a professional who does not share the patient's macro- or microcultural background, some things may seem "foreign." The client, family, and the clinician can all work to avoid misunderstandings. Ways the clinician can do this include stating explicitly what the assessment or treatment involves, what role the patient, family, and clinician will play, and giving choices where it is possible to do so. If read with a critical eye, the literature on different cultures provides a starting point for clinical problem solving. It provides the clinician with tools to use in their exciting and challenging work with patients from different backgrounds.

BILINGUALISM

Debates About Defining Bilingualism

The word "bilingual" has different meanings for different people. In fact, Hakuta has said that the difficulty defining bilingualism makes it "fruitless to estimate the proportion of the world's population that is bilingual" (Hakuta, 1986, p. 4). Other authors have stated that at least half the world's population is bilingual (Grosjean, 1997; Harris & Nelson, 1992). In bilingualism research, there is no consensus about the definition of "bilingual." In some studies, the bilingual subjects are in the process of learning a second language, while in others, the subjects have spoken both languages well since early childhood.

The problems defining bilingualism lead to differences in how the term is used. For some authors, one can speak two languages but not be bilingual if the second language (L2) is a "foreign" language which is not needed for day-to-day life (Baker, 1993; Duncan, 1989; Grosjean, 1992; Paradis, 1997). Thus, Americans who speak French are seen as bilingual by some authors (Frenck-Mestre & Pynte, 1997), but would be called L2 speakers by others. For other authors (see Baetens Beardsmore, 1982), bilingualism is defined in terms of language use, not in terms of knowledge. The problem in basing definitions of bilingualism on patterns of use is that these can change, while the level of knowledge of the language does not. For example, if a bilingual speaker moved from Texas, where she regularly used English and Spanish, to South Dakota where she only spoke English, would she stop being bilingual?

This lack of consensus about what "bilingual" means is important to keep in mind when interpreting and comparing studies, and when deciding to whom the results of a particular study generalize. If the participants were in the process of learning a second language, the results may nor may not apply to people already proficient in their second language, even though they may all be called bilingual.

Most authors, especially in studies of adult bilinguals, define bilingualism in terms of level of linguistic knowledge. They see bilingualism as a **continuum,** not a bilingual/unilingual dichotomy (Hakuta, 1986; Paradis, 1998; Paradis & Libben, 1987). Many studies refer to more fluent or less fluent bilinguals or compare groups with different levels of bilingualism.

The bilingualism continuum is multidimensional. A person may have different levels of proficiency in the different language modalities (auditory and written comprehension, verbal expression, and written expression) and in different linguistic components (morphology, syntax, phonology, lexical semantics). Although some authors have viewed 'true' bilinguals as those who have equal proficiency in their two languages, such people are the exception, if they exist at all. Most bilinguals have unequal abilities in their two languages (Grosjean, 1989, 1997; Kohnert et al., 1998). Even people who appear to have native or near-native proficiency in their second language (L2) display subtle differences in their performance on both production and comprehension tasks (e.g., Cutler et al., 1992; Hyltenstam, 1992).

People rarely experience all activities and all types of interactions in both their languages. Therefore, their vocabulary, use of idioms, and mastery of formal and informal registers is rarely equivalent in the two languages. There are domains of use such as family, religion, and work, each with its own vocabulary and linguistic patterns (Baker, 1995; Baker, in press; Fishman, 1965; Miller, 1984; Reyes, 1998). Someone who uses only one language at work may not know work-related vocabulary in his other language. Grosjean (1997, 1998) has termed this the **complementary principle**—each language is used for certain purposes in specific situations. The two do not duplicate each other if it has not been necessary for that individual to use both languages in a particular context.

Another feature of bilingualism is its instability over time. A person's level of bilingualism may increase or decrease with use or disuse. Language **attrition**—also called language loss—is a common process (for a recent review, see Seliger & Vago, 1991). Attrition may affect different language modalities and linguistic components differently. Expressive use of vocabulary is particularly vulnerable to forgetting (Weltens & Grendel, 1993), while comprehension is less so. The type and degree of attrition vary with the age of acquisition, amount of use, and level of proficiency attained in each language and not simply with years of residency in a particular country (Bahrick et al., 1994; Bettoni, 1991). Some aspects of linguistic knowledge that may be particularly vulnerable to attrition are infrequently used words, distinctions that exist in the weaker language, but not in the language which is becoming dominant, bound items (as opposed to free), and irregularities (see Seliger & Vago, 1991; Sharwood Smith, 1989; Weltens & Grendel, 1993). Because of language attrition, a person's first language (L1) or native language is not always his or her stronger language.

In considering how to define bilingualism, it is important to acknowledge **dialects.** In some cases, a speaker of two dialects of the same language may be seen as bilingual, especially when the dialects are not mutually intelligible, as is the case for some dialects of Italian, Arabic, and Chinese, for example. There is no standard for determining at what point a dialect is different enough from its base language to become a language in its own right. Some pairs of languages are more similar and more mutually intelligible than are some pairs of dialects.

Another factor to keep in mind is that, in regions with a history of extensive interaction between speakers of different languages, the languages themselves change. For example, there are different varieties of English learned by native English speakers in Singapore, Hawaii, India, Canada, and Scotland. The term "world Englishes" is often used to designate these varieties. Within the United States and the United Kingdom, there are also many varieties of English spoken, often linked to regional, racial, or socioeconomic differences. The same is true of Spanish, French, and Arabic, all of which have creole, pidgin, and regional varieties spoken in countries where a second language has influenced each of them. Clinical assessments must measure language abilities in relation to the patient's dialect.

Code-switching is one feature of how bilinguals communicate. Code-switching is the use of a word, phrase, or sentence in one language, when speaking another. It is sometimes used when the speaker does not know how to say what he wants to in the language being spoken or when one language has a word or phrase which expresses his intended meaning better than the other. Code-switching is also triggered by the topic, by shared group membership or experiences, and other factors. Code-switching occurs more often in some speakers, and some groups, than in others, and follows different patterns (see Hamers & Blanc, 1989, and Jacobson, 1998, for recent overviews).

Bilingualism creates a unique speaker-hearer, unlike a unilingual speaker of either language (Fishman, 1965; Grosjean, 1998, 1989; Selinker, 1972, 1992). Bilingual speakers may differ from unilingual speakers in how they use both their first and second languages. Each language influences the other. Extensive exposure to a new language can change a person's native language. The most obvious change occurs when words from L2 become accepted as words within L1. In North America this has happened with English terms such as "modem" or "back-up," which are often used in Spanish or French conversations about computers. When speakers live in bilingual environments, or in predominantly L2 environments, their lexicon, their phonology, and their syntax may all come to show the influence of L2 on L1 (Anisfeld et al., 1969; Bettoni, 1991; Clyne, 1991; Oesch-Serra, 1992; Grosjean & Py, 1991).

In L2, there are usually signs of the speaker's L1. These occur at the phonological, syntactic, and lexical levels, in comprehension and in expression (Chitri & Willows, 1997; Frenck-Mestre & Pynte, 1997; Hyltenstam, 1992; Kilborn, 1992; Roberts et al., 2000; Wulfeck et al., 1986). There are two models which attempt to explain this cross-language interference: Selinker's *interlanguage* and the *competition model* of MacWhinney and Bates.

Selinker (Selinker, 1972, 1992) coined the term **interlanguage** to refer to the influence of one language on another. Interlanguage refers to errors made by L2 speakers which can be linked to the influence of their L1 (for a recent review of interlanguage during acquisition, and how interlanguage becomes permanent, see Gass & Selinker, 1994). The most well-known examples of interlanguage are perhaps in pronunciation. For example, some Spanish speakers roll their R's when speaking English, and some native Chinese speakers substitute /r/ for /l/.

The **competition model** (e.g., MacWhinney & Bates, 1989; MacWhinney, 1997) sees the patterns of the two languages as competing for control. Within a spreading activation framework, related nodes and possible alternatives compete for activation. The 'winner' is the alternative that is easiest to activate. Frequency of use (more frequent items are more easily activated), complexity (simple patterns are more easily activated), and saliency or distinctiveness are among the features which make a word or a syntactic comprehension strategy from one language more likely to be used than its equivalent in the other language.

Types of Bilingualism

Many typologies of bilingualism have been proposed. Perhaps the most widely used is the compound/coordinate/subordinate distinction (for overviews see Baetens Beardsmore, 1982, or Hamers & Blanc, 1989). Popular until the early 1980s, it held that coordinate bilinguals have separate lexicons for each language, linked to language-specific concepts, while compound bilinguals have a single linguistic and conceptual system that contains both languages. The compound/coordinate typology has been discarded by most researchers. It is based on an outdated and overly simple view of lexical, semantic, and conceptual systems (Altenberg, 1989; Diller, 1974; Green, 1993; Obler et al., 1995; Paradis, 1995b). Also, the experimental methods used and the interpretation of the results supposedly identifying compound and coordinate subjects are questioned by many (e.g., Durgunoglu & Roediger, 1987; Grosjean, 1998; Kirsner et al., 1993; Paradis, 1995b). Recent studies also suggest that different types of lexical representations may exist for different types of words, with concrete nouns, for example, sharing more of the elements of their representations than other types of words (de Groot, 1993). Because of these problems with the compound/coordinate model, most studies group their subjects by age of acquisition of the two languages and by level of proficiency in each language. In clinical work, too, when and how well the patient learned their languages are key factors.

Various models of how the two languages are organized and processed have been proposed (e.g., de Bot, 1992; de Bot & Schreuder, 1993; Green, 1998; Grosjean, 1997; Kroll & de Groot, 1997; Paradis, 1997; Paradis & Libben, 1987). Experimental evidence is still being gathered on these models. It seems clear, however, that the question "do bilinguals store their languages in one system or two" is overly simple. For many, the question of how languages are processed has now become more relevant than how they are stored (Hummel, 1993). The links and/or the strength of links between languages, and processing strategies used, vary with level of proficiency in each language, the type of word, perhaps the degree of similarity between the two languages, and other factors. Studies to date show that the two languages are connected. This finding has direct consequences for clinical work, as described below.

Age of Acquisition

Many studies support modified versions of Lenneberg's thesis that there is a critical period for language acquisition. Recent work shows **sensitive periods** of varying length for different language components, such as syntax and phonology. During these sensitive periods, a child can acquire native-like proficiency in a second language (L2). Language learning is still possible later, but more conscious effort is required and the L2 will show the influence of L1, in at least some linguistic components (Harley & Wang, 1997; Hurford, 1991; Scovel, 1989).

On a clinical level, this means that the later a patient began to learn a given language, the more imperfect their mastery of that language is likely to be. We can expect to see more interlanguage, more influence of L1 on L2 in late learners. However, individual differences in ability to learn new languages, and patterns of use of each language will also play a big role in determining the level of proficiency. Whether, or how, age of acquisition influences the cognitive organization of the two languages and the processes involved in comprehension and production is not yet known.

Localization of Languages in Bilinguals

Localization of language in the brain has been studied since the earliest studies of aphasia. Scientists are only beginning to explore the localization of two languages in the bilingual brain. Localization has been studied in terms of left and right hemisphere functions and also within the left hemisphere. Despite the claims of some early research, it is now clear that functions which are in the left hemisphere of unilinguals are also in the left hemisphere of bilinguals (Paradis, 1990b, 1998). This is apparently the case even for tone languages such as Chinese and Thai (Gandour, 1998; Naeser & Chan, 1980). Damage to the left hemisphere affects linguistic tones, which serve a lexical role. Comprehension and production of tones is dissociable (Gandour, 1998; Packard, 1986), just as comprehension and expression for nontonal elements can be.

Subcortical aphasia similar to that reported in unilinguals has been documented following lesions in the L putamen, L caudate nucleus, internal capsule, and thalamus in one trilingual and three bilingual Italian patients (Aglioti & Fabbro, 1993; Fabbro & Paradis, 1995). There are also cases of subcortical aphasia in Mandarin, Cantonese, and Thai (Gandour, 1998).

Within the left hemisphere, some early studies suggested that an imperfectly learned language (L2) is distributed over a wider area of cortex than a more automatic, well-learned language (L1) (Ojemann & Whitaker, 1978; Rapport et al., 1983). However, these studies have been criticized on methodological grounds (see Paradis 1998). Other studies using sodium Amytal injections have found that the two languages occupy at least partially different cortical regions (Berthier et al., 1990). It is difficult to obtain specific localizations using this method, and the interpretation of results can be difficult (Paradis, 1990a, 1995a; Pulvermuller & Schumann, 1995).

The pioneering techniques of sodium amytal and sticking electrodes into the cortex have been replaced by more precise functional MRI (fMRI) and PET studies. Initial PET studies of English/French bilingual adults who learned French at an average age of 7 years found that the two languages activate overlapping regions in the left hemisphere (Klein et al., 1994, 1995). "Within- and across-" language searches [synonym generation, translation of single words] involve similar distributed networks even when there are differences in the accuracy and latencies across the tasks, strongly suggesting that word generation in the two languages makes demands on overlapping neural substrates (Klein et al., 1995, p. 31).

However, translation from L1 (English) to L2 (French) in these subjects activated the putamen, but backward translation (L2 to L1) did not (Klein et al., 1995).

A similar but not identical result is reported by Kim et al. (1997) using 12 adults who spoke six different pairs of languages. Using fMRI, Kim et al. found overlapping areas of activation for L1 and L2 in Wernicke's area, for all subjects. For the 6 early bilinguals, the two languages also activated similar regions in and near Broca's area. Less overlap in Broca's area was observed for the 6 subjects who began L2 acquisition later (mean age, 11). Also using fMRI, Chee et al. (1999) found that single word production in Mandarin/English bilingual adults activated the same regions within the left hemisphere in both languages. This was true for early bilinguals (began L2 by age 6) and for late bilinguals (began L2 after age 12).

Unlike the previous studies, Perani and colleagues have used a receptive language task in a series of studies. Using French/English and Italian/English bilingual adults, these studies have shown that the left hemisphere areas activated when listening to stories in L1 and L2 vary with the age of acquisition and with the level of proficiency in L2 (Dehaene et al., 1997; Perani et al., 1996; Perani et al., 1998).

Overlapping areas of activation during language tasks does not mean that the same neuronal networks are involved in both languages. Clinically, there is evidence that the vocabulary or the syntax of only one language may be available at certain times, suggesting that different languages draw on different micro-anatomical regions or circuits. This variability is similar to what we see in unilingual patients who can produce some words or sentence types but not others.

We are only beginning to map the localization of the bilingual's two languages. The range of tasks used in the brain mapping studies to date is limited. Few language pairs, and few individuals have been studied with fMRI and PET. There is a risk that individual differences in anatomy and localization will be incorrectly interpreted (Dehaene et al., 1997; Steinmetz & Seitz, 1991). How neural representation of the two languages relates to symptoms, prognosis, or rehabilitation for aphasia has not yet been addressed. As more studies are done, language localization will be an important line of research for clinicians to follow.

Functional Links Between Languages

Understanding how languages are stored neuroanatomically is important. Just as important for clinical work is understanding how the two languages are functionally connected. What are the links or relationships between languages that may be exploited in treatment?

In exploring how the two languages are organized, researchers have studied cross-language priming (facilitation) and cross-language interference. These studies use single words, usually nouns. Therefore, the results apply to the bilingual lexicon, and not necessarily to other aspects of language. Nonetheless, there are dozens of studies showing that reading or hearing a word in one language can facilitate or interfere with responses in another language. The tasks studied include reading aloud, lexical decision, translating single words, and categorizing words. (For reviews see Altarriba, 1992; Chen, 1992; de Groot, 1993; Kirsner et al., 1993; Kroll & Sholl, 1992; Snodgrass, 1993, and recent studies such as Van Hell & de Groot, 1998; Costa et al., 1999). In most studies, the priming or interference is stronger in one direction than the other. The strength and the direction of between-language effects are influenced by factors such as the length of time (in milliseconds) between the prime and the target, the level of proficiency of the subjects in each language, age of acquisition, and the stimuli used. All of these factors, except the first, come into play in clinical work.

In addition to the usual factors that make stimuli easier or harder such as frequency, or length of the words, two factors specific to bilinguals have been identified. First, the number of **"neighbors"** (words with similar spelling) in one language affects lexical decision speed in the other language (Grainger & Dijkstra, 1992). Second, the similarity of the words in each language is a factor. Synonyms with a very similar form in different languages are called **cognates** (e.g., lemon and limòn). Several studies show that priming between languages is greater for cognates than for noncognates (see above reviews).

Clinically, these findings suggest that cues in one language may assist word finding in the other, that interference across languages should be monitored, and that in selecting stimuli, the clinician should be aware of possible cross-language phenomena, including the bilingual neighborhood effect, and the influence of cognates.

The literature on culture and on bilingualism has implications for clinical work. The remainder of this chapter will outline these, and examine the challenges facing clinicians who assess and treat bilingual aphasia.

ISSUES IN ASSESSING BILINGUAL APHASIA

To plan appropriate treatment, one must conduct a valid, comprehensive, and reliable assessment. This is difficult to do in bilingual aphasia. There are problems related to culture, level of bilingualism, available tests, interpreters, and test-retest reliability, as outlined below. The assessment of a bilingual patient also includes determining of the impact of the aphasia on each language.

Culture

Cultural factors can influence the level of cooperation with the assessment. These may include the perceived appropri-

ateness of the clinician's age, gender, race, body language, tone of voice, or dress. How the testing tasks are presented (direct commands versus indirect), and the patient's understanding of why he is being tested and of what is expected of him are also important.

Prior to the assessment, the clinician should learn enough about a patient's background to know what aspects of the clinical process might be problematic. For inpatients, it is often helpful to observe the patient and family, and to consult with the social worker and nurses to learn more about the macro- and microcultural history of the patient, and about the patient's and family's reaction to the communication disorder.

During the assessment and treatment, give the patient and family members choices, when possible, based on cultural factors. For example, ask them whether another clinician may be seen as more appropriate because of his or her age or gender. Offer these choices in a way that makes it more likely the patient/family will feel comfortable expressing their preference. One way to do this is to have another person ask them if they would prefer another clinician, rather than asking yourself. Or, have another clinician see them once or twice and observe whether their talkativeness, compliance, or performance improves.

Throughout the assessment, it is important to interpret the client's behavior in context. Before interpreting behaviors, especially apparently negative ones, consider all possible reasons for the behavior, including cultural ones. Different conversation topics are seen as appropriate or inappropriate in different cultures (e.g., Chapey & Lu, 1999; Lu, 1996). Being late may indicate a lack of motivation, a different view of time, transportation problems, anxiety about coming to the clinic.... Other behaviors which are easily misunderstood include eye contact, greetings, notifying the clinic to cancel an appointment, asking or not asking questions, indicating yes/no, accepting/refusing food, giving/receiving gifts, gestures, choice of topics for conversation, and being active or passive in the treatment process.

Dealing with CLD patients and families can be a wonderful experience. Flexibility, a nonjudgmental view, and good clinical problem-solving skills are essential qualities. Cheng (1996) emphasizes how difficult intercultural communication is, and how easily misunderstandings can occur. But working with CLD clients can, with a little flexibility on all sides, work well. Published case summaries demonstrate this (Holland & Penn, 1995; Wallace, 1997; Whitworth & Sjardin, 1993). For aphasia assessment and treatment to work, the clinician need not master all aspects of the patient's culture. The clinician and the patient do not have to be from the same culture. Our goals should be to understand the aspects of each patient's beliefs, values, and communication style that will have the most impact on the clinical process. We can then be creative in reaching a way of interacting that the patient finds culturally acceptable, while still allowing the clinician to offer assessment and treatment that are clinically appropriate. This goal applies to all patients, not only those whose language background, race, or heritage are different from ours.

Level of Bilingualism

Decisions about testing and treatment must take into account the patient's pre-morbid level of bilingualism. The psycholinguistic studies of bilingualism show that the speed and accuracy on many language tasks, the effects of cues, and the amount of interference between languages are all influenced by the level of proficiency in each language. Unfortunately, it is impossible to know precisely what the patient's pre-morbid abilities were. Using the psycholinguistic literature as a guide, one can use four types of information to arrive at an estimate.

1) Self-ratings: Adults can reliably rate their abilities in each language for various types of tasks (Albert & Obler, 1978; Hamers & Blanc, 1989; Le Blanc, 1995). Some authors use a 5-point or 7-point scale, obtaining separate ratings for each language. Others ask subjects to directly compare their abilities in each language (de Groot & Poot, 1997; Roberts & Le Dorze, 1997, 1998). Both types of self-rating correlate with group performance on a number of tasks used in clinical work including verbal fluency (Lafaury & Roberts, 1998; Roberts & Le Dorze, 1997) and picture naming (Kohnert et al., 1998; Roberts & Bois, 1999).

One group study has used self-rating of premorbid abilities by aphasic adults (Roberts & Le Dorze, 1998). While this identified groups of balanced bilinguals, how well self-ratings correlate with individual performance on a given task or aphasia test has not been examined.

2) Ratings by family members: Information provided by the patient can be supplemented by asking the family to assess the patient's level of bilingualism. Ratings of the patient's abilities may be influenced by the family member's own level of bilingualism. To obtain an accurate view, ask more than one person, and take their own bilingualism into account in interpreting their ratings. A wife who speaks little English may overestimate her husband's abilities. A child who grew up speaking English may be very critical of an immigrant parent's less than perfect abilities.

In trying to establish the patient's pre-morbid level of bilingualism, it is best to avoid the use of the word "bilingual." For many people, bilingual means perfect and equal proficiency in both languages. When asked if the patient is bilingual, they will say "No," and the patient will be incorrectly identified thereafter as unilingual. It is important to ask sufficiently detailed questions before deciding on a rating, and to ask the questions in terms the patient/family can understand. Instead of "How was his auditory comprehension in _____," ask "Could he understand the news on the radio? people talking at work? people who spoke quickly? people with different accents?..."

3) Patterns of use for each language: Knowing what language was used in what situation helps to determine the importance of each language for the patient, what language(s) will be needed post-stroke, and what vocabulary may be used for which types of treatment tasks.

Baker (1995) has shown the importance of assessing domains of use. In a study of 72 immigrants from six different countries, most of whom had lived in Australia for over 10 years (>60/72), there was a wide range of patterns of use of L1 and English. Length of residence in Australia and even level of ability in English did not correlate with patterns of use. Subjects identified 10 domains of use: family, friends, shopping, religion, medical, dealing with tradespeople, hobbies, business/work, dealing with the legal/government system, and public transportation. Within these domains, 38 specific tasks were identified. Baker's list of tasks makes a good starting point for a language use questionnaire. Paradis has also published a comprehensive questionnaire as part of the Bilingual Aphasia Test (Paradis & Libben, 1987).

4) Acquisition history: Knowing how and at what age the patient was exposed to each language may suggest treatment approaches. For example, one might refer to "grammar rules" or the names of verb tenses if English (L2) was learned in a classroom but not if it was acquired informally. The acquisition history and patterns of use both provide indirect evidence about level of proficiency. Early acquisition and extensive use across different domains often suggest a high level of proficiency. If there are discrepancies between the family's assessment of the patient's abilities and the patient's use of his languages, these can be explored.

Information on language proficiency, use, and acquisition is important in deciding what areas to assess, interpreting the results (separating pre-morbid characteristics from the effects of the aphasia), and in planning treatment. For example, if a patient says "now talk hard—no talk good," this could indicate nonfluent aphasia or could be close to his pre-stroke level of English. Only by gathering information about the patients' pre-morbid bilingualism can the clinician accurately assess their post-stroke language performance, and plan appropriate treatment. This information, however, does not allow us to predict patterns of impairment (L1 vs. L2) or recovery, nor to establish a prognosis specifically focused on the bilingualism. "No correlation has been found between pattern of recovery and neurological, etiological, experimental or linguistic parameters: not site, size or origin of lesion, type or severity of aphasia, type of bilingualism, language structure type, or factors related to acquisition or habitual use" (Paradis, 1995c, p. 211).

Using Interpreters

When a patient must be assessed or treated in a language that the clinician does not master (see ASHA 1989 guidelines for the level of proficiency needed for clinical work), an interpreter can be used. Interpreters should be used only if there is no speech-language pathologist (SLP) available who speaks the patient's language(s). This is because of the disadvantages associated with using interpreters. These include difficulties locating an interpreter who is able to spend the time required and who is able to fit into the constraints of the patient's schedule, and the time needed to train interpreters in test administration, interviewing, and therapy techniques. In the session, interpreters may inadvertently alter the test stimuli or protocol. Because the SLP does not speak the language being tested, he may not always be aware that this has happened. Furthermore, the clinician cannot be certain that the interpreter is reporting all the relevant aspects of the patient's performance such as the nature of errors. There may be direct costs for the interpreter's time, which are not covered by health insurance.

When demand justifies it, a clinic may hire interpreters for specific languages as full or part-time staff. The Royal College of Speech-Language Therapists has guidelines for the use of support staff or "bilingual coworkers" in this role with children (Martin et al., 1998), most of which apply to adults. There are also training resources to draw on (e.g., Gentile et al., 1996; Kayser, 1995; Langdon, 1992a; Wallace, 1997).

When a professional interpreter or aide trained to fill this role is not available, members of the patient's community or family can be used if they are trained by the SLP for this role. Family members who have close ties to the patient may find it distressing to see the full extent of the deficits exposed. They may also be more inclined to provide cues or assistance to the patient. Friends and members of the patient's religious or community groups can often be more detached. The person chosen as interpreter must also be acceptable to the patient, available for the time needed to complete the assessment, and available for regular treatment sessions.

Given the time and expense required, and given the problems in achieving reliable results in assessment, is it worth using an interpreter? The consensus in the current literature is that patients must be assessed in all languages they use on a regular basis, or for a specific purpose (Baker, in press; Paradis, 1995c, 1998; Wallace, 1997). Without this assessment, the diagnosis and the treatment goals may be inappropriate. The resources and policies of each clinic will determine whether this standard is reached for all patients.

Testing in Various Languages

To adequately assess bilingual aphasia, we need a range of tests that are reliable and valid with norms for bilinguals from specific groups. Such tests should be as free of cultural bias as possible. Unfortunately, we do not yet have such a range of tests, although progress is being made.

There are two broad tools designed specifically for CLD patients. One is a test designed to assess communication and related abilities after a stroke or head injury: Reliable Assessment Inventory of Neuro-behavioral Organization (see Wallace, 1997). Available in English and Spanish, it also includes culturally appropriate alternate stimuli and allows for dialectal variations. To assess the patient's or family's perception of the impact of aphasia on the patient's communication the ASHA Functional Assessment of Communication Skills (Frattali et al., 1995) may be used. Its test items are designed to be suitable for use with patients from a wide range of cultural backgrounds. It falls to the individual clinician, however, to translate the questions.

Beyond these two tests, clinicians working with bilingual patients have three choices: the Bilingual Aphasia Test, tests published in and designed for unilingual speakers of other languages, or in-house translations/adaptations of published tests or therapy tasks.

The Bilingual Aphasia Test

The Bilingual Aphasia Test (BAT) developed by Paradis and his colleagues is specifically designed for bilinguals. It exists in over 60 languages, and tests all language modalities. It also has a section which tests translation abilities between more than 100 pairs of languages. Detailed descriptions of the BAT's rationale, development, and administration instructions are available in English (Paradis & Libben, 1987) and in Spanish (see Paradis & Libben, 1993, in Appendix 9–1).

Each version of the BAT uses vocabulary and pictures which are culturally appropriate. The content is modified somewhat to assess different features in different languages. Scoring and administration procedures have been designed to facilitate administration and scoring of the test by non-speech pathologists. Each version has been normed on a sample of native speakers of each language.

According to Paradis and Libben (1987), normal speakers of each language, or L2 speakers with 400 or more hours of instruction should score 100% on most subtests. However, a study by Manuel-Dupont et al. (1992) suggests that local norms for the BAT are needed. In this study, a group of 14 Spanish/English bilingual adults (mean education, 14.5 years, Cuban background) did not score within the expected range for normals on 6 of 24 subtests in Spanish (L1) and on 2 subtests in English (L2).

Tests in Other Languages and Dialects

Clinicians assessing aphasia in unilinguals can draw on a wide range of tests, some aimed at detecting mild impairments, others at severe ones. Some tests assess a specific aspect of language, such as reading, in detail. No such range of tests exists for bilingual aphasia. However, there are tests developed in different languages, some of which have versions in more than one language. Appendix 9–1 lists a number of these tests, and some of the normative studies on them.

To use tests designed for one group to assess members of another group (for example, a test from Italy to test English/Italian-speaking immigrants in North America or Australia), clinicians need studies of their reliability and validity (Ardila, 1995; Baker, 1993). A number of studies have been done. They illustrate how complex this area is, and how much is yet to do. The following (incomplete) review highlights some of the issues.

Armstrong et al. (1996) found that the *Arizona Battery for Communication Disorders in Dementia* (Bayles & Tomoeda, 1991) is suitable for use with speakers of British English. The authors do not recommend changing any stimulus items. They recommend using the American norms.

A number of studies on the *Boston Naming Test* (BNT) (Kaplan et al., 1983) yield a more complex picture. In Spanish and French versions of the BNT, the item difficulty is not the same as in English (see Roberts et al., 2000, for a review). When the BNT is used in English with different cultural groups, results are mixed. Worrall et al. (1995) found 2 of the 60 items are not familiar to Australians. Whether there is cultural bias beyond these 2 items, and how the group means of Australian adults compare with those in American studies cannot be determined from Worrall et al.'s study since the education level for the Australian subjects is not stated. Thus, it is not possible to separate the effects of age or education from cultural factors, or from simple variations across samples.

In studies of African American performance on the BNT, some have shown no difference in BNT scores across races when age and education are controlled (Henderson et al., 1998). Other studies find that African Americans score below Whites (e.g., Lichtenberg et al., 1994). However, small sample size and failure to control for or to report education limit the usefulness of these findings.

The unmodified BNT was sensitive to age and education in English-speaking Australian subjects (Worrall et al., 1995) and in 45 unilingual French Canadian subjects (Doucet & Roberts, 1999). This suggests that despite cultural factors, the test is fairly robust. However, studies of bilingual adults (Kohnert et al., 1998; Roberts et al., 2000) show that the unilingual norms clearly do not apply. Thus, different cut-off scores must be established for different age and educational levels within each linguistic group.

There are fewer studies of other tests, but some work has been done. Molrine and Pierce (1998) found that on the *Boston Diagnostic Aphasia Examination* (BDAE) (Goodglass & Kaplan, 1983), the *Western Aphasia Battery* (WAB) (Kertesz, 1982), and the *Minnesota Test for Differential Diagnosis of Aphasia* (MTDDA) (Schuell, 1965), the scores of African Americans were below those of European Americans (N = 24 of each) on only 3 of 26 subtests of expressive language. For upper SES subjects, these were Animal Naming (BDAE, WAB), and paragraph retelling (MTDDA), and, for middle SES, word reading (BDAE).

With 12 subjects for each SES level and only a single category used in the verbal fluency test (Animal Naming), these results are preliminary.

Huntress (1979, quoted in Wallace & Tonkovich, 1997, p. 153) found statistically significant but not clinically significant differences in performance on the MTDDA in a group of 15 African Americans, matched for age, education, and income to a group of white subjects. If credit had been given for responses that were correct, but given in nonstandard English, the scores for the African American group would have been higher. Thus, this study also suggests that test performance can be very similar across CLD groups.

More studies of CLD test performance are needed, with complete data on the age, education, and language history of participants. This information is critical to allow comparison across studies and appropriate generalization of the findings. The studies done to date illustrate that the answer to the question "can existing tests be used with CLD populations?" is complex. We cannot reject all tests initially normed on white, middle class, native English speakers as unsuitable for use with other groups. Some tests, and many subtests in existing batteries, are proving to be appropriate. Other tests need specific stimuli, or scoring procedures changed. Still others may prove entirely inappropriate. Through rigorous validation and normative studies, we will learn which is which.

Informal Assessments and In-House Translations

Until we have more data and more norms for various patient groups, clinicians will continue their current practice of using published tests or in-house translations of various tasks on CLD patients, without norms to guide them. The use of nonstandardized evaluation tools is widespread (Katz et al., 2000) and is not limited to CLD patients. Clinical judgment is an important component in interpreting these results. There are, however, pitfalls associated with using ad hoc translations of subtests or tasks.

Tasks can change in nature and in difficulty when they are translated. For example, counting and reciting the months of the year are different tasks in English, but not in Mandarin (Chinese), since the months are called "one-month, two-month, three-month..." (Naeser & Chan, 1980). Spelling is a challenge in English, but not in Spanish or Italian because of their highly regular phoneme-grapheme correspondence. Because of this, spelling is a familiar task to people educated in English, but may not be for people educated in Spanish or Italian (Ardila, 1998). Spelling, of course, exists only in languages that use an alphabet-based writing system. In naming, nouns that are high frequency and short in one language can be low frequency and multisyllabic in other language. For bilinguals, frequency of use may be much more idiosyncratic and less predictable in bilinguals than in unilinguals. Because knowledge is dependent on domains of use, we cannot assume that all bilinguals know "simple" vocabulary in both languages. Also, bilinguals show lower name agreement for some pictures than do unilinguals (Goggin et al., 1994; Roberts & Bois, 1999), which may have implications for how naming and other lexical retrieval tasks are scored.

A further challenge in assessing CLD patients is that some symptoms of aphasia vary across languages. This has been shown in syntactic deficits (Bates & Wulfeck, 1989; Bates et al., 1991; Menn, 1989; Menn et al., 1995; Menn & Obler, 1990; Nilipour & Paradis, 1995; Sasanuma, 1986) and for deep and surface dyslexia (Ardila, 1998; Luzzatti et al., 1998; Sasanuma, 1986). The noun/verb dissociation, commonly seen in aphasia in English and several European languages, is difficult to assess in Chinese, where many words are noun-verb compounds (Bates et al., 1991; Chen & Bates, 1998). There are also studies of reading deficits which suggest that the frequency and/or the types of errors vary across languages, making the deep dyslexia and surface dyslexia patterns described for English inapplicable to some other languages (Ardila, 1998; Ferreres & Miravalles, 1995; Sasanuma, 1986). Other studies report patterns similar to those reported in English-speaking patients (Weekes et al., 1998). These studies demonstrate that one cannot apply all English-based definitions of symptoms or syndromes to other languages. Some apply, some do not. Assessment results must be interpreted with caution, and must take into account the features of the patient's (other) language or dialect. For bilinguals, competition between the processing strategies or the elements of the two languages and interlanguage must both be considered when determining what is a clinical symptom and what is a pre-morbid feature of bilingualism. There are also error types that are possible in some languages but not in others (e.g., correct phonemes, but incorrect tones; wrong gender or case for nouns; creating a false cognate word to cover a word-finding problem). Symptom lists generated to describe one language do not address all possible symptoms in other languages.

Test–Retest Reliability

When a patient is tested twice, once in each language, the question of test-retest (TRT) reliability arises. To interpret possible between-language differences, we need to know the normal variability on retesting within a single language. Roberts and Le Dorze (1994) have shown that on semantic verbal fluency, individual scores may increase or decrease by more than 30%. Brookshire and Nicholas (1994) found significant variability on retesting using the picture description task from the BDAE. More accurate scores and less TRT variability are obtained when results of several connected speech tasks or several verbal fluency categories are combined (Brookshire & Nicholas, 1994; Monsch et al., 1992). On the BNT, most unilingual English speakers scored within 1 point on retesting, but some changed by 3 or 4 points (Roberts et al., 2000). Until there is more data on the variability of

individual scores within a given language, clinicians should be cautious in interpreting different scores between languages (see Roberts, 1998, for more on this), and doubly so when using tests which do not have norms for the specific educational, age, and cultural/linguistic group of the patient being tested.

Clinicians can sample or test some tasks twice in each language for each patient to provide an indication of within-language variability that can guide the interpretation of between-language differences. Using the complete test, not the shortened version, a longer language sample and more exemplars in informal evaluations may yield more reliable results.

Patterns of Impairment and Recovery in Bilingual Aphasia

One purpose of the assessment is to determine the impact of the aphasia on each language. The patterns of impairment and recovery in bilingual aphasia have been described in individual, usually exceptional patients since the 19th century (Paradis, 1983). These patterns have been identified and given labels by Paradis (Paradis, 1989, 1993a, 1998; Paradis & Libben, 1987). To facilitate clinical use of these patterns, I have modified Paradis' list somewhat, separating impairment from recovery, and expanding and commenting on the definitions.

Types of *Impairment* in Bilingual Aphasia

1. Parallel impairment: The two languages are impaired in the same manner and to the same degree. Parallel impairment is determined in relation to premorbid proficiency. If the patient mastered both languages equally premorbidly, the level of ability will be equal post-onset. If one language was stronger than the other, it remains so in cases of parallel impairment. Because aphasia can affect some aspects of language more than others (comprehension vs. expression, or oral vs. written language), the most accurate way to use this label is to rate each modality separately. There may be parallel impairment in auditory comprehension, but differential impairment in reading comprehension, for example.

2. Differential impairment: One language is more severely damaged by the aphasia than the other one. Thus, a difference in proficiency may exist between languages which were approximately equal premorbidly. Or, a premorbid difference may have been erased by the stroke. For example, Spanish may have been stronger than English pre-stroke, but post-stroke, the two are equal. This is not parallel impairment, because the aphasia has had a greater impact on Spanish.

3. Differential aphasia: This refers to the type of aphasia, not to the degree of deficit. Differential aphasia exists

when symptoms differ across languages. In a case reported by Albert and Obler (1978), a multilingual patient appeared to have Broca's aphasia in one language and Wernicke's aphasia in another. The validity of published reports of differential aphasia has been questioned (Dronkers et al., 1995; Paradis, 1997, 1998).

4. Blended or mixed pattern: "Patients systematically mix or blend features of their languages at any or all levels of linguistic structure (i.e., phonological, morphological, syntactic, lexical, and semantic) inappropriately" (Paradis, 1989, p. 117). In these cases, it is as if the patient no longer recognizes what words or features belong in each language, and creates a new blended pattern using both languages. The patient uses this blended language even when speaking to unilinguals. This is not the same as code switching or mixing, which is normal behavior in many bilinguals, when speaking to another bilingual. Initially called mixed impairment, Paradis now labels this as blending (1998), to avoid possible confusion with mixed aphasia.

5. Selective aphasia: Only one language is affected; the other remains at its premorbid level (Paradis & Goldblum, 1989).

Types of *Recovery* in Bilingual Aphasia

1. Parallel recovery: Both languages improve at the same rate and to the same degree, relative to premorbid levels.
2. Differential recovery: One language recovers better than the other.
3. Successive recovery: "One language does not begin to reappear until another has been maximally recovered" (Paradis, 1989, p. 117). In practice, one cannot determine when maximum recovery has been reached, but the label of successive recovery applies when one language appears to have reached a plateau before any real progress occurs in the other language.
4. Antagonistic recovery: As one language improves, the other regresses. In some cases, the pattern alternates, with first one language improving, then the other (Nilipour & Ashayery, 1989; Paradis et al., 1982; Paradis & Goldblum, 1989). This variant is also called alternating antagonism, or see-saw recovery.
5. Selective recovery: Only one language shows improvement (Aglioti & Fabbro, 1993).

In theory, these types seem clear. In practice, because of the problems inherent in testing bilingual aphasia and in determining the premorbid mastery of each language, it can be difficult to distinguish among the first three types of impairment. Some authors use the label "differential impairment" when one language is better than the other, even when this reflects premorbid proficiency (e.g., Nilipour, 1988). According to Paradis' definition, these should be

labeled as parallel. Some published cases of differential aphasia have been reclassified since the authors failed to take into account different symptom presentation in different languages, or did not use appropriate tests and bilingual norms (see Gomez-Tortosa et al., 1995; Kohnert et al., 1998; Paradis, 1993b, 1997; Silverberg & Gordon, 1979).

Before labeling a recovery or impairment pattern, one must carefully consider the symptom pattern of the specific languages, the patient's dialect, sociocultural factors (what is a normal pattern for the patient's peer group), and the nature of the test used (Paradis, 1995c). Given the complementary principle and that bilinguals usually have different premorbid levels of proficiency in their languages and different levels in different language modalities, and given that aphasia can differentially affect each language modality, ratings of impairment should be done separately for auditory comprehension, reading, verbal expression, and written expression. The case of an English/Nepalese bilingual illustrates how the "strong" language can vary across tasks (Byng et al., 1984).

The few studies done thus far also highlight the need to proceed cautiously in classifying bilingual aphasia by syndrome type. Dronkers et al. (1995) have shown that the aphasia classification of a patient can change when credit is given for regional dialect. The issue of classifying aphasia is complex. Many non-CLD patients are assigned to different syndromes using the WAB and the BDAE in English (Crary et al., 1992). It is not surprising, therefore, that attempts to classify CLD patients by syndrome will often lead to unreliable results. Of course, it is not necessary to label an aphasia syndrome or patterns of bilingual impairment or recovery. Treatment and counseling generally target symptoms and residual abilities, not labels. Still, to the extent that labels are used, they must be used cautiously, and seen as representing tendencies or general patterns—not absolute truths.

The syndrome types described in English-, Italian-, French-, and German-speaking patients appear to exist in a wide range of languages. There are no data about whether the incidence of these syndromes in bilingual patients is similar to that in unilingual patients. Perecman (1989) suggested that the incidence of jargon aphasia might be higher in bilinguals than in unilinguals, but there is no large study to support or refute this.

Many authors have attempted to explain non-parallel recovery. The literature contains proposals that the prognosis for recovery should be better for the native language (Ribot), the best known language (Pitres), the most automatic (Pick), the most emotionally important (Minkowski), the language of the initial hospital environment, and the language with stronger literacy. After reviewing the various theories and their supporting case reports, Paradis (1989) concludes: "no single principle or hierarchy of principles has emerged to explain the whole array of recovery patterns. Neither primacy, nor automaticity, habit strength, stimulation pre- or post-onset, appropriateness, need, affectivity, severity of the aphasia, type of bilingualism or type of aphasia could account for the non-parallel recovery patterns observed" (p. 127).

The literature offers little information on the incidence of each type of impairment. Clinical experience suggests that parallel impairment and parallel recovery are by far the most common patterns, especially after the first few weeks. There is some support for this view in the literature (Chary, 1986, quoting Nair & Virmani; Junqué et al., 1995; Lhermitte et al., 1966; Paradis, 1977; Vaid & Genesee, 1980). There are also a number of published cases of parallel impairment and recovery (e.g., Dronkers et al., 1995; Mimouni et al., 1995; Nilipour, 1988; Roberts et al., 1997; Sasanuma & Park, 1995). There are more published reports of non-parallel patterns because of a tendency to write up the unusual or interesting patterns. We need studies of unselected, consecutive cases with detailed language histories and thorough testing to determine the incidence of parallel and non-parallel recovery.

ISSUES IN INTERVENTION

Treatment for bilingual aphasia has been neglected in the literature. Little published information exists on the effects of treatment and even less on appropriate methods. Two types of studies provide some guidance: studies of the effects of treatment in various languages and a small number of studies of the symptoms of bilingual aphasia. The principles that guide unilingual treatment are also relevant to bilingual treatment. The following section presents some of these, along with a liberal dose of suggestions based on clinical experience. Most findings and suggestions presented below have not yet been tested formally, though they have proved helpful/effective in clinical practice.

Effects of Treatment in Bilinguals

On the one hand, bilingual treatment studies are few in number, and vary widely in the level of detail and hence in their value in supporting clinical practice. On the other hand, the studies that have been done, and the unilingual treatment studies in a range of languages suggest that treatment principles that work in unilinguals often work in bilinguals as well. A study by Wiener et al. (1995) documented the treatment outcomes, length of stay, and reasons for discharge for 54 unilingual and 55 bilingual patients in a New York City rehabilitation center. The authors expected to find that the bilingual patients were underserved (shorter treatment, fewer types of treatment) and made less improvement than the unilingual patients. Instead they found that "bilingual patients showed recovery that was virtually equivalent to that of unilinguals" (p. 55).

The few studies of treatment of bilingual aphasia show that treatment effects can generalize from one language to another. There are reports that when only one language is used in treatment or practice, one or more untreated languages improve (Holland & Penn, 1995; Penn & Beecham, 1992). The treated language may improve more than the untreated one (de Luca et al., 1994; Fredman, 1975; Wender, 1989). This finding has been replicated in single case studies (Roberts et al., 1997; Watamori & Sasanuma, 1976, 1978) and in group studies (Junqué et al., 1989; Junqué et al., 1995).

Other studies, however, have found equal improvement in the two languages following treatment in one language (Sasanuma & Park, 1995) or greater gains in the untreated language (L2) (Roberts, 1992). In both of these studies, the subjects (N=2 in Sasanuma & Park, and N=1 in Roberts) were 3 months or less post-CVA when treatment began. Therefore, the effects of spontaneous recovery cannot be separated from treatment effects. There are at least two other reports of greater gains in the untreated language (L1) (Durieu, 1969, and Linke, 1979, cited in Paradis, 1993b).

Some authors have interpreted a lack of generalization from one language to another as support for the view that the two languages are stored in separate systems. However, we know that some unilingual patients do not generalize from treated to untreated stimuli. This does not mean that the two sets of stimuli are stored in "different systems." As we learn more about within-language generalization, we will be better able to interpret between-language generalization, and vice versa.

Treatment

Treatment Methods

The studies just cited show that a general stimulation approach can be used in bilingual patients who speak English and Japanese (Watamori & Sasanuma, 1976, 1978) and Japanese and Korean (Sasanuma & Park, 1995). Howard's phonemic cueing technique was used with a chronic French-English bilingual (Roberts et al., 1997). Other studies give limited information about the treatment method (de Luca et al., 1994; Fredman, 1975; Junqué et al., 1995; Junqué et al., 1989; Wender, 1989).

Other sources, however, show that a number of aphasia treatment methods have been used in a range of different languages. PACE therapy has been used in Italian, German, Dutch, and Japanese (Carlomagno, 1994; Sasanuma, 1993). Melodic Intonation Therapy has been used with French-speaking (Van Eeckhout et al., 1992; Belin et al., 1996) and Dutch-speaking patients (cited in Visch-Brink et al., 1993). Examples of cognitive neuropsychological approaches, cueing techniques, and Blissymbols in a range of languages can be found in sources specifically highlighting international work (e.g., Holland & Forbes, 1993), but also scattered throughout the English language journals and books.

In adapting a technique developed in one language for use in another, the specific characteristics of each language must be borne in mind. Some cues that have great value in one language, such as word order in English may have little value in another. Also, there are cues that are not possible in English that may be important to use in other languages—the gender of nouns in Spanish, for example, to assist word retrieval, or the auxiliary used to conjugate verbs in French or Italian. In some languages, rehabilitation strategies unique to that language must be developed, as for kana/kanji reading and writing in Japanese (see Sasanuma, 1986, 1993).

Another possible pitfall in adapting therapy techniques is establishing appropriate hierarchies of difficulty for tasks and stimuli. The syntactic difficulty of different sentence types must be determined in a language-specific context. In choosing stimuli based on word frequency cultural variations can be important. Also, controlling for cognate words in a naming or other lexical task is important for some language pairs. There is evidence that cognate words are more easily retrieved than noncognates in bilingual aphasic adults (Ferrand & Humphreys, 1996; Roberts & Deslauriers, 1999; Stadie et al., 1995).

The fact that a treatment approach has been used with speakers of different languages does not guarantee that it is appropriate for bilingual speakers of those languages. Studies are needed. But, until these studies are done, unilingual treatment studies offer some guidelines about changes needed to adapt a method from one language to another. They also demonstrate that the principles the method is based on can apply to both languages. A high level of linguistic competence is needed to adapt most treatment strategies into different languages.

Setting Goals in Treatment

The principles for unilingual treatment apply to bilinguals: goals should be realistic, meaningful to the patient, and tailored to the individual patient's deficits. The factors relevant in unilingual work apply to bilinguals. Some additional factors must be considered, however.

Realistic goals are based on the patient's pre- and post-morbid proficiency and patterns of use. Improving a patient's L2 or reversing the attrition that has occurred in a little-used L1 are not part of our clinical mandate. Given how little is known about prognosis in bilinguals, our goals must be even more modest, and our comments to the family about prognosis more guarded than for unilinguals. As the recovery progresses and as the treatment brings changes or fails to bring changes in targeted aspects of communication, our goals will change, and our prognosis along with them.

The patient's need for each language in various situations is a key factor in setting goals. Even when therapy is carried out in both languages, this does not mean that all tasks should be. For example, if the patient used only one language for reading, the treatment goals should reflect this.

In tailoring the goals to the patient's deficits, processing and self-cueing strategies are important factors. These often reflect the interaction of the two languages. Research based on MacWhinney and Bates' competition model has shown that some bilinguals use processing strategies from one language to interpret the other. An L1 English speaker may rely on word order as a cue for thematic roles when processing sentences in L2, even when L2 does not use word order to mark them (e.g., Liu et al., 1992). It is important for the clinician to consider factors from both languages, and the possible interaction of languages in interpreting error patterns.

In overcoming word retrieval problems, there are strategies that are unique to bilinguals. First, when unable to say what he or she wants to in one language, the patient may simply switch to his or her other language. This is an obvious and appropriate strategy, if the listener is bilingual. Some patients use it spontaneously. For others, explicit teaching may be needed. If the listener has even some grasp of this other language, enough of the message may be understood to move the exchange along. In language pairs with cognates, saying or writing a cognate word in one language will often allow even a unilingual speaker of the other language to understand the word. This switching behavior when talking to a bilingual listener has been documented in aphasic patients (Marty & Grosjean, 1998; Munoz et al., 1999; Springer et al., 1998), and is seen daily in clinical settings.

A second strategy that bilinguals use spontaneously is producing a word from one language to self-cue its retrieval in another (Roberts & Deslauriers, 1999; Roberts et al., 2000). This can be encouraged or explicitly taught if it is an effective strategy for the patient.

Choice of Language(s) of Treatment

Regardless of the treatment goals and methods, the languages used in treatment should reflect premorbid use and proficiency. Although there are anecdotal reports suggesting that treatment in more than one language is harmful (e.g., Chlenov, 1948; Wald, 1958, 1961, cited in Paradis, 1993b), there is no recent, controlled study on this issue. If the patient displays a blended pattern of impairment, treatment may need to be restricted to one language. For most patients, however, in light of the research showing that the two languages interact, and that bilinguals regularly use their languages as a whole system, with both languages always active to some degree, there is little support for limiting treatment to one language. Clinical experience shows that most patients can work in one of three ways:

1) working on one language with the clinician, and the other language at home or with a volunteer. This may be

the only way to work on a language the clinician does not speak.

2) alternating languages. This involves a block of sessions in one language, followed by a block in the other. Each block can be 5 to 10 sessions or longer, with regular probes to see whether treatment gains in one language generalize to the other language.

3) separate the languages by modality, reflecting the patient's premorbid patterns of use. For example, work on writing in one language and auditory comprehension in both languages.

In the rare cases where a patient "loses" a language he or she used extensively, he or she may want to work on this language, but be unable to. Clinical experience suggests that it is pointless to attempt to work in a language until the patient can access it fairly consistently. Work in the other language(s), provide passive exposure to the "lost" language, and probe it regularly to see if it reappears. When/if it does, the balance of languages in treatment can be adjusted to include this language. The case described by Roberts (1998) illustrates this approach. A fully bilingual teacher spoke English only at home, but could speak only French after his stroke for a period of more than 1 month. Despite his need to regain English to communicate with his unilingual wife, treatment in English was impossible initially. A basic principle of aphasia treatment is that the patient should be reasonably successful at the therapy tasks. This case illustrates the application of that principle to bilingual work.

The questions of what pattern of languages to use in treatment, and of generalization between languages are closely linked. Both are complex and both require study. To the extent that treatment generalizes from one language to another, treatment in only one language may be ethically appropriate. However, when generalization does not occur, treatment may be necessary in both languages needed by the patient.

FUTURE TRENDS

While it is difficult to predict where the next decade will take us, two trends seem clear. First, there is growing interest in CLD issues in general and in bilingual aphasia in particular. In the 1990s, the number of books, articles, and conference presentations reflects this. This trend will likely continue. There are also more studies with a clinical focus in recent years. Clinicians need many more such studies to guide their assessment and treatment.

Second, bilingual aphasia and aphasia seem to be less and less separate from each other. The literature on bilingual aphasia has been separate from the "mainstream" aphasia literature. Different authors are quoted. Different questions have been addressed. As more clinician-researchers become aware of bilingual aphasia and of how little is known about it, the two streams are beginning to draw closer together. For example, when considering whether treatment generalizes from one language to another, studies can draw on models of bilingual language, and on the treatment literature on generalization within a single language. When assessing a patient in more than one language, the studies of within-language test-retest variability can guide interpretation of between-language results.

Other future trends will depend, in part, on how we meet the challenges inherent in studying CLD patients. The first challenge is objectivity. We must be open to results that contradict our own, or society's expectations about a particular group. Test performance and treatment outcomes for some CLD patients may be better than for other patients, or worse, or there may be no difference beyond minor sampling differences. As the calls for more focus on CLD issues are answered by studies with hard data, we must interpret these data objectively. We must give equal weight to the similarities across groups and to the differences. We must be very cautious in saying why a result was obtained.

The second challenge is experimental rigor. Factors related to bilingualism and culture are difficult to control in studies already complex because of the many neurological and linguistic variables related to the aphasia. Given the difficulty in finding patients with similar linguistic, cultural, and neurological status, there will probably be more collaborative studies. This will help ensure adequate sample sizes and representative results. Appropriate experimental control, and the publication of replications will help us to correctly interpret the results.

The third challenge is cultural and linguistic competence. With study, and interaction with people of various cultures, clinicians can become culturally aware and learn to adapt their methods to reduce cultural stumbling blocks on the clinical path. Linguistic competence represents a greater challenge. ASHA and the Royal College of Speech and Language Therapists have both set very high language standards for clinicians who work with CLD clients. The near-native proficiency in the language of treatment that ASHA requires for bilingual speech-language pathologists is achieved, usually, only by acquisition of both languages during childhood. A significant challenge for the profession is to recruit and train people who meet these standards.

The final challenge is time. A bilingual patient takes more time than a unilingual one. Finding, adapting, or developing tests and treatment material, finding and training interpreters, and testing in two languages instead of one are among the factors that take more time. Working in two languages in treatment also adds to the time required, especially for cases where the gains in one language do not generalize to the other and the patient needs to regain use of both languages. Given the increased interest in CLD issues, we may hope to see experimental support for specific treatment methods, and more tests to support our clinical work. However, without adequate time, these positive developments will not benefit the patients. Clinicians in many settings are subject to limits in the number of sessions they may provide or in the length of stay the patient is allowed. These constraints and pressures to see more patients in shorter times will make it increasingly difficult to give bilingual patients the care they need. Research documenting the best methods and their impact will support our efforts to obtain essential services for CLD patients.

KEY POINTS

Clinicians who work with CLD patients should read as widely as possible in the literature on culture and on bilingualism. Among the points that are clinically important are the following:

1. Language and culture are closely tied.
2. It is important to consider the possible influence of cultural factors on clinical work, using the patient's background to suggest factors that may be relevant, and interpreting behavior within the appropriate cultural context. It is equally important to avoid cultural stereotypes and assumptions. Each client is a unique individual from a specific microculture, within a macroculture.
3. Bilingualism is a continuum, with different levels of ability for different linguistic tasks and different domains of use. Bilingual abilities change over time with patterns of use or disuse.
4. A bilingual is a unique speaker-hearer, with abilities in each language that often reflect the influence of the other.
5. The languages of a bilingual are stored in the left hemisphere, as they are for unilinguals, in largely but perhaps not completely overlapping cortical and subcortical regions.
6. Lexical items are connected across languages, with between-language facilitation and interference both occurring in neurologically intact adults. Cognates appear more closely linked than noncognates. These between-language factors should be considered in interpreting aphasic error patterns and in planning treatment.
7. It can be difficult to assess bilingual patients for many reasons, including availability of tests, local norms, the need for interpreters, and a lack of data on individual test-retest reliability on aphasia tests.
8. Interpretation of test results should be done in light of the patient's premorbid level of bilingualism, dialect(s), patterns of use, and the features and unique symptom hierarchy of each language tested.
9. Five patterns of impairment and five patterns of recovery have been identified, with parallel patterns believed to be the most common.
10. A number of treatment principles and methods have been successfully used in a range of languages.

However, we need much more research into treatment methods for bilingual aphasia and into cross-language generalization.

References

Aglioti, S. & Fabbro, F. (1993). Paradoxical selective recovery in a bilingual aphasic following subcortical lesions. *Cognitive Neuroscience and Neuropsychology, 4,* 1359–1362.

Albert, M. & Obler, L. (1978). *The Bilingual Brain.* New York: Academic Press.

Altarriba, J. (1992). The representation of translation equivalents in bilingual memory. In R.J. Harris (ed.), *Cognitive Processing in Bilinguals* (pp. 157–174). New York: Elsevier.

Altenberg, E.P. (1989). The bilingual's lexicon: A theoretical discussion. *CUNY Forum: Papers in Linguistics, 14,* 1–6.

American Speech-Language-Hearing Association (1991). Multicultural action agenda. *ASHA, 33(5),* 39–41.

American Speech-Language-Hearing Association: Committee on the Status of Racial Minorities (1989). Bilingual speech-language pathologists and audiologists. *ASHA, 31,* 93.

American Speech-Language-Hearing Association (1985). Clinical management of communicatively handicapped minority language populations. *ASHA, 27,* 29–32.

Anisfeld, M., Anisfeld, E., & Semogas, R. (1969). Cross-influence between the phonological systems of Lithuanian-English bilinguals. *Journal of Verbal Language and Verbal Behavior, 8,* 257–261.

Ardila, A. (1995). Directions of research in cross-cultural neuropsychology. *Journal of Clinical and Experimental Neuropsychology, 17,* 143–150.

Ardila, A. (1998). Semantic paralexias in the Spanish language. *Aphasiology, 12,* 885–900.

Armstrong, L., Borthwick, S.E., Bayles, K.A., & Tomoeda, C.K. (1996). Use of the Arizona Battery for Communication Disorders of Dementia in the UK. *European Journal of Disorders of Communication, 31,* 171–180.

Asante, M.K. & Gudykunst, W.B. (1989). *Handbook of International and Intercultural Communication.* Newbury Park: Sage Publications.

Australian Association of Speech and Hearing (1994). *Speech Pathology in a Multicultural, Multilingual Society.* Melbourne: AASH.

Australian Institute of Multicultural Affairs (1985). *Ageing in a Multicultural Society.* Canberra: AIMA.

Baetens Beardsmore, H. (1982). *Bilingualism: Basic Principles.* Clevendon: Multilingual Matters.

Bahrick, H.P., Hall, L.K., Goggin, J.P., Bahrick, L.E., & Berger, S.A. (1994). Fifty years of language maintenance and language dominance in bilingual Hispanic immigrants. *Journal of Experimental Psychology: General, 123,* 264–283.

Baker, R. (1993). The assessment of language impairment in elderly bilinguals and second language speakers in Australia. *Language Testing, 10,* 255–276.

Baker, R. (1995). Communicative needs and bilingualism in elderly Australians of six ethnic backgrounds. *Australian Journal on Ageing, 14(2),* 81–88.

Baker, R. (In press). The assessment of functional communication in culturally and linguistically diverse populations. In L. Worrall & C. Frattali (eds.), *Neurogenic Communication Disorders: A Functional Approach* (pp. 81–100). New York: Thieme Medical Publishers.

Bates, E., Chen, S., Tzeng, O., Li, P., & Opie, M. (1991). The noun-verb problem in Chinese aphasia. *Brain and Language, 41,* 203–233.

Bates, E. & Wulfeck, B. (1989). Comparative aphasiology: A cross-linguistic approach to language breakdown. *Aphasiology, 3(2),* 111–142.

Bates, E., Wulfeck, B., & MacWhinney, B. (1991). Cross-linguistic research in aphasia: An overview. *Brain and Language, 41,* 123–148.

Battle, D.E. (ed.) (1998). *Communication Disorders in Multicultural Populations* (2nd ed.). Newton, MA: Butterworth-Heinemann.

Bayles, K.A. & Tomoeda, C.K. (1991). *Arizona Battery for Communication Disorders of Dementia.* Tucson, AZ: Canyonlands Publishing.

Belin, P., Van Eeckhout, P., Zilbovicius, M., & Remy, P. (1996). Recovery from non-fluent aphasia after melodic intonation therapy: A PET study. *Neurology, 47,* 1504–1511.

Berthier, M.L., Starkstein, S., Lylyk, P., & Leguarda, R. (1990). Differential recovery of languages in a bilingual patient: A case study using selective amytal test. *Brain and Language, 38,* 449–453.

Bettoni, C. (1991). Language variety among Italians: Anglicisms, attrition and attitudes. In S. Romaine (ed.), *Language in Australia.* Cambridge: Cambridge University Press.

Brislin, B.W., Cushner, K., Cherrie, C., & Yong, M. (1986). *Intercultural Interactions: A Practical Guide.* Beverly Hills, CA: Sage Publications.

Brislin, R.W. (1994). *Intercultural Training: An Introduction.* Thousand Oaks, CA: Sage Publications.

Brookshire, R.H. & Nicholas, L.E. (1994). Test-retest stability of measures of connected speech in aphasia. In M.L. Lemme (ed.), *Clinical Aphasiology, Vol. 22* (pp. 119–134). Austin, TX: Pro-Ed.

Byng, S., Coltheart, M., Masterson, J., Prior, M., & Riddoch, J. (1984). Bilingual biscriptal deep dyslexia. *Quarterly Journal of Experimental Psychology, 36A,* 417–433.

Carlomagno, S. (1994). *Pragmatic Approaches to Aphasia Therapy* (Hodgkinson, G., Trans.). London: Whurr Publishers.

Chapey, R. & Lu, S. (1999). Cross-cultural variations in specific pragmatic aspects of ordinary conversation: Implications for the assessment and treatment of aphasia in intercultural contexts. Manuscript. City University of New York.

Chary, P. (1986). Aphasia in a multilingual society. In J. Vaid (ed.), *Language Processing in Bilinguals: Psycholinguistic and Neurolinguistic Perspectives* (pp. 183–197). Hillsdale, NJ: Lawrence Erlbaum Associates.

Chee, M.W.L., Tan, E.W.L., & Thiel, T. (1999). Mandarin and Chinese single word processing studied with functional magnetic resonance imaging. *Journal of Neuroscience, 19,* 3050–3056.

Chen, H.C. (1992). Lexical processing in bilingual or multilingual speakers. In R.J. Harris (ed.), *Cognitive Processing in Bilinguals* (pp. 253–264). New York: Elsevier.

Chen, S. & Bates, E. (1998). The dissociation between nouns and verbs in Broca's and Wernicke's aphasia: Findings from Chinese. *Aphasiology, 12,* 5–36.

Cheng, L.L. (1996). Beyond bilingualism: A quest for communicative competence. *Topics in Language Disorders, 16,* 9–21.

Chitiri, H.-F. & Willows, D.M. (1997). Bilingual word recognition in English and Greek. *Applied Psycholinguistics, 18,* 138–156.

Clyne, M. (1991). *Community Languages: The Australian Experience.* New York: Cambridge University Press.

Cole, L. (1989). E pluribus unum: Multicultural imperatives for the 1990's and beyond. *ASHA, 31(2),* 65–70.

Costa, A., Miozza, M., & Caramazza, A. (1999). Lexical selection in bilinguals: Do words in the bilingual's two lexicons compete for selection? *Journal of Memory and Language, 41,* 365–397.

Crary, M.A., Wertz, R.T., & Deal, J.L. (1992). Classifying aphasia: Cluster analysis of Western Aphasia Battery and Boston Diagnostic Examination results. *Aphasiology, 6,* 29–36.

Cutler, A., Mehler, J., Norris, D., & Segui, J. (1992). The monolingual nature of speech segmentation by bilinguals. *Cognitive Psychology, 24,* 381–410.

Davis, P.N., Gentry, B., & Hubbard-Wiley, P. (1998). Clinical practice issues. In D.E. Battle (ed.), *Communication Disorders in Multicultural Populations* (2nd ed.), (pp. 427–452). Boston: Butterworth-Heinemann.

de Bot, K. (1992). A bilingual production model: Levelt's "speaking" model adapted. *Applied Linguistics, 13(1),* 1–24.

de Bot, K. & Schreuder, R. (1993). Word production and the bilingual lexicon. In R. Schreuder & B. Weltens (eds.), *The Bilingual Lexicon* (pp. 191–214). Philadelphia: John Benjamins.

de Groot, A.M.B. (1993). Word-type effects in bilingual processing tasks: Support for a mixed-representational system. In R. Schreuder & B. Weltens (eds.), *The Bilingual Lexicon* (pp. 27–52). Philadelphia: John Benjamins.

de Groot, A.M.B. & Poot, R. (1997). Word translation at three levels of proficiency in a second language: The ubiquitous involvement of conceptual memory. *Language Learning, 47(2),* 215–264.

Dehaene, S., Dupoux, E., Mehler, J., Cohen, L., Paulesu, E., Perani, D., Van de Moortele, P.F., Lehericy, S., & Le Bihan, D. (1997). Anatomical variability in the cortical representation of first and second language. *NeuroReport, 8,* 3809–3815.

de Luca, G., Fabbro, F., Vorano, L., & Lovati, L. (1994). Valuazione con il Bilingual Aphasia Test (BAT) della rieducazione dell'afasico multilingue. Paper presented to the 4th meeting on Disturbi cognitivi, comportamentali e della comunicazione nelle lesioni cerebrali acquisite, Udine, Italy. July. Proceedings. pp. 51–68.

Diller, K.C. (1974). Compound and coordinate bilingualism: A conceptual artifact. *Word, 26,* 254–261.

Doucet, N. & Roberts, P.M. (1999, May). Performance des adultes francophones québécois au Boston Naming Test. Presented to the Association Canadienne Française pour L'avancement des Sciences. Ottawa, Canada.

Dronkers, N., Yamasaki, Y., Ross, G.W., & White, L. (1995). Assessment of bilinguality in aphasia: Issues and examples from multicultural Hawaii. In M. Paradis (ed.), *Aspects of Bilingual Aphasia* (pp. 57–66). Tarrytown, NY: Elsevier.

Duncan, D.M. (1989). Issues in bilingualism research. In D.M. Duncan (ed.), *Working with Bilingual Language Disability* (pp. 18–35). New York: Chapman and Hall.

Durgunoglu, A.Y. & Roediger, H.L. (1987). Test differences in accessing bilingual memory. *Journal of Memory and Language, 26,* 377–391.

Ellis, N. (1992). Linguistic relativity revisited: The bilingual word length effect in working memory during counting, remembering numbers and mental calculation. In R.J. Harris (ed.), *Cognitive Processing in Bilinguals* (pp. 137–156). New York: Elsevier.

Erickson, J.G., Devlieger, P.J., & Sung, J.M. (1999). Korean-American female perspectives on disability. *American Journal of Speech-Language Pathology, 8,* 99–108.

Fabbro, F. & Paradis, M. (1995). Differential impairments in four multilingual patients with subcortical lesions. In M. Paradis (ed.), *Aspects of Bilingual Aphasia* (pp. 139–176). Tarrytown, NY: Elsevier.

Fawcett, J.T. & Carino, B.V. (1987). *Pacific Bridges: The New Immigration from Asia and the Pacific Islands.* New York: Center for Migration Studies.

Ferrand, L. & Humphreys, G.W. (1996). Transfer of refractory states across languages in a global aphasic patient. *Cognitive Neuropsychology, 13,* 1163–1191.

Ferreres, A.R. & Miravalles, G. (1995). The production of semantic paralexias in a Spanish-speaking aphasic. *Brain and Language, 49,* 153–172.

Fishman, J.A. (1965). Who speaks what language to whom and when? *Linguistics, 2,* 67–88.

Frattali, C.M., Thompson, C.K., Holland, A.L., Wohl, C.B., & Ferketic, M.M. (1995). *The American Speech-Language-Hearing Association Functional Assessment of Communication Skills for Adults (ASHA FACS).* Rockville, MD: ASHA.

Frayne, S.M., Burns, R.B., Hardt, E.J., Rosen, A.K., & Moskowitz, M.A. (1996). The exclusion of non-English-speaking persons from research. *Journal of General Internal Medicine, 11,* 39–43.

Fredman, M. (1975). The effect of therapy given in Hebrew on the home language of the bilingual or polyglot adult aphasic in Israel. *British Journal of Disorders of Communication, 10,* 61–69.

Frenck-Mestre, C. & Pynte, J. (1997). Syntactic ambiguity resolution while reading in second and native languages. *Quarterly Journal of Experimental Psychology, 50A,* 119–148.

Galens, J., Sheets, A., & Young, R.V. (1995). *Gale Encyclopedia of Multicultural America.* New York: Gale Research.

Gandour, J. (1998). Aphasia in tone languages. In P. Coppens, Y. Lebrun, & A. Basso (eds.), *Aphasia in Atypical Populations* (pp. 117–142). Mahwah, NJ: Lawrence Erlbaum Associates.

Gass, S.M. & Selinker, L. (1994). *Second Language Acquisition.* Hillsdale, NJ: Lawrence Erlbaum Associates.

Gentile, A., Ozolins, U., & Vasilakakos, M. (1996). *Liaison Interpreting: A Handbook.* Melbourne: Melbourne University Press.

Gollnick, D. & Chinn, P. (1990). *Multicultural Education in a Pluralistic Society.* Columbus, OH: Merrill Publishers.

Goggin, J.P., Estrada, P., & Villarreal, R.P. (1994). Picture-naming agreement in monolinguals and bilinguals. *Applied Psycholinguistics, 15,* 177–193.

Gomez-Tortosa, E., Martin, E.M., Gaviria, M., Charbel, F., & Ausman, J.I. (1995). Selective deficit of one language in a bilingual patient following surgery in the left perisylvian area. *Brain and Language, 48,* 320–325.

Goodglass, H. & Kaplan, E. (1983). *The Assessment of Aphasia and Related Disorders* (2nd ed.). Philadelphia: Lea & Febiger.

Grainger, J. & Dijkstra, T. (1992). On the representation and use of language information in bilinguals. In R.J. Harris (ed.), *Cognitive Processing in Bilinguals* (pp. 207–220). New-York: Elsevier.

Green, D.W. (1998). Motor control of the bilingual lexico-semantic system. *Bilingualism: Language and Cognition, 1,* 67–81.

Green, D.W. (1993). Towards a model of L2 comprehension and production. In R. Schreuder & B. Weltens (eds.), *The Bilingual Lexicon* (pp. 249–277). Philadelphia: John Benjamins.

Grosjean, F. (1982). *Life with Two Languages: An Introduction to Bilingualism.* Cambridge: Harvard University Press.

Grosjean, F. (1989). Neurolinguists beware! The bilingual is not two monolinguals in one person. *Brain and Language, 36,* 3–15.

Grosjean, F. (1992). Another view of bilingualism. In R.J. Harris (ed.), *Cognitive Processing in Bilinguals* (pp. 51–62). New York: Elsevier.

Grosjean, F. (1997). The bilingual individual. *Interpreting, 2,* 163–187.

Grosjean, F. (1998). Studying bilinguals: Methodological and conceptual issues. *Bilingualism: Language and Cognition, 1,* 131–149.

Grosjean, F. & Py, B. (1991). La restructuration d'une première langue: l'intégration de variantes de contact dans la compétence des migrants bilingues. *La Linguistique, 27(2),* 35–60.

Hakuta, K. (1986). *Mirror of Language.* New York: Basic Books.

Hamers, J. & Blanc, M. (1989). *Bilinguality and Bilingualism.* Cambridge: Cambridge University Press.

Harley, B. & Wang, W. (1997). The critical period hypothesis: Where are we now? In A.M.B. de Groot & J.F. Kroll (eds.), *Tutorials in Bilingualism* (pp. 19–52). Mahwah, NJ: Lawrence Erlbaum Associates.

Harris, R.J. & Nelson, E.M. (1992). Bilingualism: Not the exception any more. In R.J. Harris (ed.), *Cognitive Processing in Bilinguals* (pp. 3–14). New York: Elsevier.

Henderson, L.W., Frank, E.M., Pigatt, T., Abramson, R.K., & Houston, M. (1998). Race, gender, and educational level effects on Boston Naming Test scores. *Aphasiology, 12,* 901–911.

Holland, A.L. & Forbes, M.M. (1993). *Aphasia Treatment: World Perspectives.* San Diego: Singular Publishing.

Holland, A.L. & Penn, C. (1995). Inventing therapy for aphasia. In L. Menn, M. O'Connor, L.K. Obler, & A. Holland (eds.), *Nonfluent Aphasia in a Multilingual World* (pp. 144–155). Philadelphia: John Benjamins.

Hummel, K.M. (1993). Bilingual memory research: From storage to processing issues. *Applied Psycholinguistics, 14,* 268–284.

Hurford, J.R. (1991). The evolution of the critical period for language acquisition. *Cognition, 40,* 159–201.

Hyltenstam, K. (1992). Non-native features of near-native speakers: on the ultimate attainment of childhood L2 learners. In R.J. Harris (ed.), *Cognitive Processing in Bilinguals* (pp. 351–368). New York: Elsevier.

Jacobson, R. (1998) (ed.), *Code-Switching Worldwide.* New York: Mouton de Gruyter.

Junqué, C., Vendrell, P., & Vendrell-Brucet, J. (1989). Differential recovery in naming in bilingual aphasics. *Brain and Language, 36,* 16–22.

Junqué, C.,Vendrell, P., & Vendrell, J. (1995). Differential impairments and specific speech phenomena in 50 Catalan-Spanish bilingual aphasic patients. In M. Paradis (ed.), *Aspects of Bilingual Aphasia* (pp. 177–210). Tarrytown, NY: Pergamon.

Kaplan, E., Goodglass, H., & Weintraub, S. (1983). *The Boston Naming Test*. Philadelphia: Lea & Febiger.

Katz, R.C., Hallowell, B., Code, C., Armstrong, E., Roberts, P.M., Pound, C., & Katz, L. (2000). A multi-national comparison of aphasia management practices. *International Journal of Language and Communication Disorders, 35*, 303–314.

Kayser, H. (1995). Interpreters. In H. Kayser (ed.), *Bilingual Speech-Language Pathology: An Hispanic Focus* (pp. 207–221). San Diego: Singular Publishing.

Kayser, H. (1998). Outcome measurement in culturally and linguistically diverse populations. In C.M. Frattali (ed.), *Measuring Outcomes in Speech-Language Pathology* (pp. 225–244). New York: Thieme.

Kertesz, A. (1982). *The Western Aphasia Battery*. New York: Grune & Stratton.

Kilborn, K. (1992). On-line integration of grammatical information in a second language. In R.J. Harris (ed.), *Cognitive Processing in Bilinguals* (pp. 337–350). New York: Elsevier.

Kim, K.H.S., Relkin, N.R., Lee, K.-M., & Hirsch, J. (1997). Distinct cortical areas associated with native and second languages. *Nature, 388*, 171–174.

Kirsner, K., Lalor, E., & Hird, K. (1993). The bilingual lexicon: Exercise, meaning and morphology. In R. Schreuder & B. Weltens (eds.), *The Bilingual Lexicon* (pp. 215–248). Philadelphia: John Benjamins.

Klein, D., Zatorre, R.J., Milner, B., Meyer, E., & Evans, A.C. (1994). Left putaminal activation when speaking a second language: Evidence from PET. *Neuro Report, 5*, 2295–2297.

Klein, D., Zatorre, R.J., Milner, B., Meyer, E., & Evans, A.C. (1995). The neural substrates of bilingual language processing: Evidence from positron emission tomography. In M. Paradis (ed.), *Aspects of Bilingual Aphasia* (pp. 23–36). Tarrytown, New York: Elsevier.

Kohnert, K.J., Hernandez, A.E., & Bates, E. (1998). Bilingual performance on the Boston Naming Test: Preliminary norms in Spanish and English. *Brain and Language, 65(3)*, 422–440.

Kroll, J.F. & de Groot, A.M.B. (1997). Lexical and conceptual memory in the bilingual: Mapping form in two languages. In A.M.B. de Groot & J.F. Kroll (eds.), *Tutorials in Bilingualism: Psycholinguistic Perspectives* (pp. 169–199). Mahwah, NJ: Lawrence Erlbaum Associates.

Kroll, J.F. & Sholl, A. (1992). Lexical and conceptual memory in fluent and non-fluent bilinguals. In R.J. Harris (ed.), *Cognitive Processing in Bilinguals* (pp. 191–204). New York: Elsevier.

Lafaury, P.J. & Roberts, P.M. (1998, November). Cognate words in a verbal fluency task. Paper presented to the annual conference of the American Speech-Language-Hearing Association. San Antonio, TX.

Langdon, H.W. (1992a). *Interpreter/Translator Process in the Educational Setting: A Resource Manual*. Sacramento, CA: Resources in Special Education.

Langdon, H.W. (1992b). The Hispanic population: Facts and figures. In H.W. Langdon (ed.), *Hispanic Children and Adults with Communication Disorders* (pp. 20–56). Gaithersburg, MD: Aspen Publishing.

LeBlanc, R. (1995). La place de l'auto-évaluation dans le domaine des langues secondes. Twenty-five years of second language teaching at the University of Ottawa, PC Version.

Lhermitte, R., Hécaen, H., Dubois, J., Culioli, A., & Tabouret-Kelly, A. (1966). Le problème de l'aphasie des polyglottes: Remarques sur quelques observations. *Neuropsychologia, 4*, 315–329.

Lichtenberg, P.A, Ross, T., & Christensen, B. (1994). Preliminary normative data on the Boston Naming Test for an older urban population. *The Clinical Neuropsychologist, 8*, 109–111.

Liu, H., Bates, E., & Li, P. (1992). Sentence interpretation in bilingual speakers of English and Chinese. *Applied Psycholinguistics, 13*, 451–484.

Luzzatti, C., Laiacona, M., Allamano, N., De Tanti, A., & Inzaghi, M.G. (1998). Writing disorders in Italian aphasic patients: A multiple single-case study of dysgraphia in a language with shallow orthography. *Brain, 121*, 1721–1734.

Lu, S. (1996). Intercultural variations of specific aspects of language. Manuscript. CUNY.

Lynch, E.W. & Hanson, J. (1992). *Developing Cross-Cultural Competence: A Guide for Working with Young Children and Their Families*. Baltimore: Brookes.

Mackey, W.F. (1967). *Bilingualism as a World Problem/Le Bilinguisme: Phénomène Mondial*. Montreal: Harvest House.

MacWhinney, B. (1997). Second language acquisition and the competition model. In A.M.B. de Groot & J.F. Kroll (eds.), *Tutorials in Bilingualism: Psychololinguistic Perspectives* (pp. 113–142). Mahwah, NJ: Lawrence Erlbaum Associates.

MacWhinney, B. & Bates, E. (1989). *The Cross-Linguistic Study of Sentence Processing*. New York: Cambridge University Press.

Manuel-Dupont, S., Ardila, A., Rosselli, M., & Puente, A.E. (1992). Bilingualism. In A.E. Puente & R.J. McCaffrey (eds.), *Handbook of Neuropsychological Assessment* (pp. 193–210). New-York: Plenum Press.

Marin, G. (1992). Issues in the measurement of acculturation among Hispanics. In K.F. Geisinger (ed.), *Psychological Testing of Hispanics, APA Science Volumes* (pp. 235–251). Washington, DC: APA.

Martin, D., Anderson, S., Chaudry, N., Clark, C., Hooke, E., Little, C., Quinn, T., & Raval, A. (1998). *Good Practice for Speech and Language Therapists Working with Clients from Linguistic Minority Communities: Guidelines of the Royal College of Speech and Language Therapists*. London: RCSLT.

Marty, S. & Grosjean, F. (1998). Aphasie, bilinguisme et modes de communication. *Aphasie und verwandte, 12(1)*, 8–28.

Menn, L. (1989). Comparing approaches to comparative aphasiology. *Aphasiology, 3(2)*, 143–150.

Menn, L., O'Connor, M., Obler, L.K., & Holland, A. (1995). *Nonfluent Aphasia in a Multilingual World*. Philadelphia: John Benjamins.

Menn, L. & Obler, L.K. (1990). *Agrammatic Aphasia: A Cross-Language Narrative Sourcebook*. Philadelphia: John Benjamins.

Miller, N. (1984). Language use in bilingual communities. In N. Miller (ed.), *Bilingualism and Language Disability: Assessment and Remediation* (pp. 3–25). San Diego, CA: College-Hill Press.

Mimouni, Z., Béland, R., Danault, S., & Idrissi, A. (1995). Similar language disorders in Arabic and French in an early bilingual aphasic patient. *Brain and Language, 51*, 132–134.

Molrine, C.J. & Pierce, R.S. (1998, November). African American and European American adults' expressive language performance on three aphasia tests. Paper presented to annual American Speech-Language-Hearing conference. San Antonio, TX.

Monsch, A., Bondi, M., Butters, N., Salmon, D., Katzman, R., & Thal, L. (1992). Comparison of verbal fluency tasks in the detection of dementia of the Alzheimer type. *Archives of Neurology, 49*, 1253–1258.

Mungas, D. (1996). The process of development of valid and reliable neuropsychological assessment measures for English- and Spanish-Speaking elderly persons. In G. Yeo & D. Gallagher-Thompson (eds.), *Ethnicity and the Dementias* (pp. 33–46). Washington, DC: Taylor & Francis.

Munoz, M.L., Marquardt, T.P., & Copeland, G. (1999). A comparison of the codeswitching patterns of aphasic and neurologically normal bilingual speakers of English and Spanish. *Brain and Language, 66*, 249–274.

Naeser, M.A. & Chan, S.W.-C. (1980). Case study of a Chinese aphasic with the Boston Diagnostic Aphasia Exam. *Neuropsychologia, 18*, 389–410.

National Institute of Deafness and other Communication Disorders (1992). *Report from the Working Group: Research and Research Training Needs of Minority Persons and Minority Health Issues.* Bethesda, MD: National Institutes of Health.

National Institutes of Health (1990). *National Institutes of Health Guide, 35(19)*, 1–2.

Nilipour, R. (1988). Bilingual aphasia in Iran: A preliminary report. *Journal of Neurolinguistics, 3(2)*, 185–232.

Nilipour, R. & Ashayery, H. (1989). Alternating antagonism between two languages with successive recovery of a third in a trilingual aphasic patient. *Brain and Language, 36*, 23–48.

Nilipour, R. & Paradis, M. (1995). Breakdown of functional categories in three Farsi-English bilingual aphasic patients. In M. Paradis (ed.), *Aspects of Bilingual Aphasia* (pp. 123–138). Tarrytown, NY: Elsevier.

Obler, L.K., Centeno, J., & Eng, N. (1995). Bilingual and polyglot aphasia. In L.K. Obler & A.L. Holland (eds.), *Non-fluent Aphasia in a Multilingual World* (pp. 132–143). Philadelphia: John Benjamins.

Oesch-Serra, C. (1992). Code-switching et marqueurs discursifs: Entre variation et conversation. *Travaux Neuchâtelois de Linguistique, 18*, 155–171.

Ojemann, G. & Whitaker, H.A. (1978). The bilingual brain. *Archives of Neurology, 35*, 409–412.

Packard, J. (1986). Tone production deficits in nonfluent aphasic Chinese speech. *Brain and Language, 29*, 212–223.

Paradis, M. (1977). The stratification of bilingualism. In M. Paradis (ed.), *Aspects of Bilingualism* (pp. 165–175). Columbia, SC: Hornbeam Press.

Paradis, M. (1983). *Readings on Aphasia in Bilinguals and Polyglots.* Montreal: Didier.

Paradis, M. (1989). Bilingual and polyglot aphasia. In F. Boller & J. Grafman (eds.), *Handbook of Neuropsychology, Vol. 2* (pp. 117–140). New York: Elsevier.

Paradis, M. (1990a). Differential recovery of language in a bilingual patient following selective amytal injection: A comment on Berthier et al. (1990). *Brain and Language, 39*, 469–470.

Paradis, M. (1990b). Language lateralization in bilinguals: Enough already! *Brain and Language, 39*, 576–586.

Paradis, M. (1993a). Multilingualism and aphasia. In G. Blanken (ed.), *Linguistic Disorders and Pathologies: An International Handbook* (pp. 278–288). New York: Waller de Gruyter.

Paradis, M. (1993b). Bilingual aphasia rehabilitation. In M. Paradis (ed.), *Foundations of Aphasia Rehabilitation* (pp. 423–419). New York: Pergamon.

Paradis, M. (1995a). Exchange: When the interpretation does not fit the facts, alter the facts, not the interpretation!: A comment on Pulvermüller and Schumann, 1994. *Language Learning, 45*, 725–727.

Paradis, M. (1995b). The need for distinctions. In M. Paradis (ed.), *Aspects of Bilingual Aphasia* (pp. 1–9). Tarrytown, NY: Elsevier.

Paradis, M. (1995c). Bilingual aphasia 100 years later: Consensus and controversies. In M. Paradis (ed.), *Aspects of Bilingual Aphasia* (pp. 211–223). Tarrytown, NY: Elsevier.

Paradis, M. (1997). The cognitive neuropsychology of bilingualism. In A.M.B. de Groot & J.F. Kroll (eds.), *Tutorials in Bilingualism: Psycholinguistic Perspectives* (pp. 331–354). Mahwah, NJ: Lawrence Erlbaum Associates.

Paradis, M. (1998). Acquired aphasia in bilingual speakers. In M. Taylor-Sarno (ed.), *Acquired Aphasia* (3rd ed.). (pp. 531–549). New York: Academic Press.

Paradis, M., Goldblum, M.-C., & Abidi, R. (1982). Alternate antagonism with paradoxical translation behaviour in two bilingual aphasic patients. *Brain and Language, 15*, 55–69.

Paradis, M. & Goldblum, M.C. (1989). Selective crossed aphasia followed by reciprocal antagonism in a trilingual patient. *Brain and Language, 36*, 62–75.

Paradis, M. & Libben, G. (1987). *The Assessment of Bilingual Aphasia.* Hillsdale, NJ: Lawrence Erlbaum Associates.

Penn, C. & Beecham, R. (1992). Discourse therapy in multilingual aphasia: A case study. *Clinical Linguistics & Phonetics, 6*, 11–25.

Perani, D., Dehane, S., Grassi, F., Cohen, L., Cappa, S., Paulesu, E., Dupoux, E., Fazio, F., & Mehler, J. (1996). Brain processing of native and foreign languages. *NeuroReport, 7*, 2439–2444.

Perani, D., Paulesu, E., Galles, N.S., Dupoux, E., Dehaene, S., Bettinardi, V., Cappa, S.F., Fazio, F., & Mehler, J. (1998). The bilingual brain: Proficiency and age of acquisition of the second language. *Brain, 121*, 1841–1852.

Perecman, E. (1989). Bilingualism and jargonaphasia: Is there a connection? *Brain and Language, 36*, 49–61.

Pontón, M.O. & Ardila, A. (1999). The future of neuropsychology with Hispanic populations in the United States. *Archives of Clinical Neuropsychology, 14*, 565–580.

Puente, A.E. & McCaffrey, R.J. (eds.) (1992). *Handbook of Neuropsychological Assessment: A Biopsychosocial Perspective.* New York: Plenum Press.

Pulvermüller, F. & Schumann, J.H. (1995). Exchange: On the interpretation of earlier recovery of the second language after injection of sodium amytal in the left middle cerebral artery or are there relevant facts without interpretation?: A response to Paradis. *Language Learning, 45*, 729–735.

Rapport, R.L., Tan, C.T., & Whitaker, H.A. (1983). Language function and dysfunction among Chinese- and English-speaking polyglots: Cortical stimulation, Wada testing and clinical studies. *Brain and Language, 18*, 342–366.

Reyes, B.A. (1998). Bilingual aphasia: A case study. Communication disorders and sciences in culturally and linguistically diverse populations. Rockville, MD: ASHA SID *14*, 2–7.

Roberts, P.M. (1992, October). Therapy and spontaneous recovery in a bilingual aphasic. Paper presented to the Academy of Aphasia. Toronto, Canada.

Roberts, P.M. (1998). Clinical research needs in bilingual aphasia. *Aphasiology, 12,* 119–130.

Roberts, P.M. (2001). Test-retest reliability on the Boston Naming Test and Graded Naming Test. Unpublished Manuscript. University of Ottawa.

Roberts, P.M. & Bois, M. (1999). Picture-name agreement for French-English bilingual adults. *Brain and Cognition, 40,* 238–241.

Roberts, P.M., Bois, M., & Brunet, M. (2000). Written picture name agreement in French-English bilinguals. Manuscript in preparation. University of Ottawa, Canada.

Roberts, P.M., de la Riva, J., & Rhéaume, A. (1997, May). Effets de l'intervention dans une langue pour l'anomie bilingue. Paper presented to the annual meeting of the Canadian Association of Speech-Language Pathology and Audiology. Toronto.

Roberts, P.M. & Deslauriers, L. (1999). Picture naming of cognate and non-cognate nouns in bilingual aphasia. *Journal of Communication Disorders, 32,* 1–23.

Roberts, P.M., Garcia, L., & Desrochers, A. (2000). Performance of unilingual English and bilingual speakers on the Boston Naming Test. Manuscript in preparation. University of Ottawa.

Roberts, P.M. & Le Dorze, G. (1994). Semantic verbal fluency in aphasia: A quantitative and qualitative study in test-retest conditions. *Aphasiology, 8,* 569–582.

Roberts, P.M. & Le Dorze, G. (1997). Semantic organization, strategy use and productivity in bilingual semantic verbal fluency. *Brain and Language, 59,* 412–449.

Roberts, P.M. & Le Dorze, G. (1998). Bilingual aphasia: Semantic organisation, strategy use, and productivity in semantic verbal fluency. *Brain and Language, 65,* 287–312.

Rowland, D.T. (1991). *Pioneers Again: Immigrants and Ageing in Australia.* Canberra: Australian Government Publishing Service.

Sasanuma, S. (1986). Universal and language specific symptomatology and treatment of aphasia. *Folia Phoniatrica, 38,* 121–175.

Sasanuma, S. (1993). Aphasia treatment in Japan. In A.L. Holland & M.M. Forbes (eds.), *Aphasia Treatment: World Perspectives* (pp. 175–198). San Diego, CA: Singular Publishing.

Sasanuma, S. & Park, H.S. (1995). Patterns of language deficits in two Korean-Japanese bilingual aphasic patients: A clinical report. In M. Paradis (ed.), *Aspects of Bilingual Aphasia* (pp. 111–123). New York: Elsevier.

Schuell, H. (1965). *The Minnesota Test for Differential Diagnosis of Aphasia.* Minneapolis: University of Minnesota Press.

Scovel, T. (1989). *A Time to Speak: A Psycholinguistic Inquiry into the Critical Period for Human Speech.* Cambridge: Newbury House.

Seliger, H.W. & Vago, R.M. (1991). The study of first language attrition: An overview. In H.W. Seliger & R.M. Vago (eds.), *First Language Attrition* (pp. 1–15). New York: Cambridge University Press.

Selinker, L. (1972). Interlanguage. *International Review of Applied Linguistics, 10,* 209–231.

Selinker, L. (1992). *Rediscovering Interlanguage.* New York: Longman.

Sharwood Smith, M.A. (1989). Crosslinguistic influence in language loss. In K. Hyltenstam & L.K. Obler (eds.), *Bilingualism Across the Lifespan: Aspects of Acquisition, Maturity, and Loss* (pp. 185–201). New York: Cambridge University Press.

Silverberg, R. & Gordon, H. (1979). Differential aphasia in two bilingual individuals. *Neurology, 29,* 51–55.

Snodgrass, J.G. (1993). Translating versus picture naming: Similarities and differences. In R. Schreuder & B. Weltens (eds.), *The Bilingual Lexicon* (pp. 83–114). Philadelphia: John Benjamins.

Springer, L., Miller, N., & Bürk, F. (1998). A cross language analysis of conversation in a trilingual speaker with aphasia. *Journal of Neurolinguistics, 11,* 223–241.

Stadie, N., Springer, L., de Bleser, R., & Burk, F. (1995). Oral and written naming in a multilingual patient. In M. Paradis (ed.), *Aspects of Bilingual Aphasia* (pp. 85–100). Tarrytown, NY: Elsevier.

Steinmetz, H. & Seitz, R.J. (1991). Functional anatomy of language processing: Neuroimaging and the problem of individual variability. *Neuropsychologia, 29,* 1149–1161.

Taylor, O. (1986). *Nature of Communication Disorders in Culturally and Linguistically Diverse Populations.* San Diego: College Hill.

Tempo, P.M. & Saito, A. (1996). Techniques of working with Japanese American families. In G. Yeo & D. Gallagher-Thompson (eds.), *Ethnicity and the Dementias* (pp. 109–122). Washington, DC: Taylor and Francis.

Teng, (1996). Cross-cultural testing and the Cognitive Abilities Screening Instrument. In G. Yeo & D. Gallagher-Thompson (eds.), *Ethnicity and the Dementias* (pp. 77–85). Washington, DC: Taylor and Francis.

Terrell, S.L., Battle, D.E., & Grantham, R.B. (1998). African American cultures. In D.E. Battle (ed.), *Communication Disorders in Multicultural Populations* (2nd ed.) (pp. 31–71). Newton, MA: Butterworth-Heinemann.

Vaid, J. & Genesee, F. (1980). Neuropsychological approaches to bilingualism: A critical review. *Canadian Journal of Psychology, 34(4),* 417–445.

Valle, R. (1994). Culture-fair behavioral symptom differential assessment and intervention in dementing illness. *Alzheimer Disease and Associated Disorders, 8(3),* 21–45.

Van Eeckhout, P., Pillon, B., Signoret, J.-L., Deloche, G., & Seron, X. (1992). Rééducation des réductions sévères de l'expression orale: La thérapie mélodique et rythmée. In X. Seron & C. Laterre (eds.), *Rééduquer le Cerveau: Logopédie, Psychologie, Neurologie.* (pp. 109–121). Brussels: Pierre Mardaga.

Van Hell, J.G. & de Groot, A.M.B. (1998). Conceptual representation in bilingual memory: Effects of concreteness and cognate status in word association. *Bilingualism: Language and Cognition, 1,* 193–212.

Visch-Brink, E.G., van Harskamp, F., van Amerongen, N.M., Wielart, S.M., & van de Sandt-Koenderman, M.E. (1993). A multidisciplinary approach to aphasia therapy. In A.L. Holland & M.M. Forbes (eds.), *Aphasia Treatment: World Perspectives* (pp. 227–262). San Diego, CA: Singular Publishing.

Wallace, G.L. (1997). *Multicultural Neurogenics: A Resource for Speech-Language Pathologists Providing Services to Neurologically Impaired Adults from Culturally and Linguistically Diverse Backgrounds.* San Antonio: The Psychological Corporation.

Wallace, G.L. & Tonkovich, J.D. (1997). African Americans: Culture, communication, and clinical management. In G.L.

Wallace (ed.), *Multicultural Neurogenics* (pp. 133–164). San Antonio: Communication Skill Builders.

Watamori, T. & Sasanuma, S. (1976). The recovery process of a bilingual aphasic. *Journal of Communication Disorders, 9,* 157–166.

Watamori, T. & Sasanuma, S. (1978). The recovery process of two English-Japanese bilingual aphasics. *Brain and Language, 6,* 127–140.

Weekes, B.S., Chen, M.J., Qun, H.C., Lin, Y.B., Yao, C., & Xiao, X.Y. (1998). Anomia and dyslexia in Chinese: A familiar story? *Aphasiology, 12,* 77–98.

Weltens, B. & Grendel, M. (1993). Attrition of vocabulary knowledge. In R. Schreuder & B. Weltens (eds.), *The Bilingual Lexicon* (pp. 135–156). Philadelphia: John Benjamins.

Wender, D. (1989). Aphasic victim as investigator. *Archives of Neurology, 46,* 91–92.

Whitworth, A. & Sjardin, H. (1993). The bilingual person with aphasia. In D. Lafond, Y. Joanette, R. Ponzio, R. Degiovani, M.T. Sarno (eds.), *Living with Aphasia: Psychosocial Issues* (pp. 129–149). San Diego: Singular Publishing.

Wiener, D., Obler, L.K., & Taylor-Sarno, M. (1995). Speech/language management of the bilingual aphasic in a U.S. urban rehabilitation hospital. In M. Paradis (ed.), *Aspects of Bilingual Aphasia* (pp. 37–56). Tarrytown, NY: Elsevier.

Worrall, L.E., Yiu, E.M.-L., Hickson, L.M.H., & Barrett, H.M. (1995). Normative data for the Boston Naming Test for Australian elderly. *Aphasiology, 9,* 541–551.

Wulfeck, B., Bates, E., Juarez, L., & Kilborn, K. (1986). Sentence interpretation strategies in healthy and aphasic bilingual adults. In J. Vaid (ed.), *Language Processing in Bilinguals: Psycholinguistic and Neuropsychological Perspectives* (pp. 199–220). Hillsdale, NJ: Lawrence Erlbaum Associates.

APPENDIX 9.1
Tests in Various Languages

Alphabetical List of Tests for Which Published Norms and/or Reports Exist in More Than One Language

( ) indicates a language or version not listed in this appendix.

Aachen Aphasia Test—German, English, Dutch, Italian, Thai
Aphasia Language Performance Scales—(English), Spanish
Aphasia Screening Test—(English), Punjabi
Bilingual Aphasia Test—(English), Spanish, many languages
Boston Diagnostic Aphasia Exam—(English), Chinese, Finnish, French, Spanish, Thai
Boston Naming Test—(English), Dutch, Finnish, French, Spanish
Communication Activities of Daily Living—(English), Japanese
Multilingual Aphasia Exam—English, Spanish
PALPA—(English), Dutch
Token Test (Italian, English), Chinese
Verb and Sentence Test—Dutch, English. German and French in preparation
Western Aphasia Battery—(English), Chinese, Japanese, Thai

Tests and Normative Data in Various Languages

* indicates the test itself. Other entries report norms or development of the test.

Readers are invited to send additions to this listing to the author. Updated lists will be published on her web site.

Chinese: Mandarin & Cantonese

Naeser, M.A. & Chan, S.W.-C. (1980). Case study of a Chinese aphasic with the Boston Diagnostic Aphasia Exam. *Neuropsychologia, 18,* 389–410. (BDAE and Token Test)

Yiu, E. (1992). Linguistic assessment of Chinese-speaking aphasics: Development of a Cantonese aphasia battery. *Journal of Neurolinguistics, 7,* 1–46. (WAB)

Dutch

*Graetz, P., de Bleser, R., & Willmes, K. (1992). *Akense Afasie Test.* Lisse, The Netherlands: Swetz and Zeitlinger. (Aachen Aphasia Test. Also in German, English, Italian, Thai)

Willmes, K., Graetz, P., de Bleser, R., Schulte, B., & Keyser, A. (1991). De akense afasie test. *Logopedie en Foniatrie, 63,* 375–386.

*Bastiaanse, R., Bosje, M., & Visch-Brink, E. (1995). *PALPA—Nederlandse Versie.* Hove, England: Lawrence Erlbaum Associates.

*Bastiaanse, R., Maas, E., & Rispens, J. (1999). *Werkwoordenen Zinnen Test (WEZT) (Verb and Sentence Test—VAST).* Lisse, The Netherlands: Swetz and Zeitlinger. German and French versions are planned.

Marien, P., Mampaey, E., Vervaet, A., Saerens, J., & de Deyn, P.P. (1998). Normative data for the Boston Naming Test in native Dutch-speaking Belgian elderly. *Brain and Language, 65,* 447–467.

English

*Bastiaanse, R., Edwards, S., & Rispens, J. (In press). *The Verb and Sentence Test (VAST).* Thames Valley. Also in Dutch. German and French versions are planned.

*Benton, A.L. & Hamsher, K.D. (1994). *The Multilingual Aphasia Exam (Third Edition).* San Antonio, TX: The Psychological Corporation. Also in Spanish.

Miller, N., de Bleser, R., & Willmes, K. (1997). The English language version of the Aachen Aphasia Test. In W. Ziegler & K. Deger (eds.), *Clinical Phonetics and Linguistics* (pp. 257–265). London: Whurr.

Wallace, G.J. (in preparation). *The Reliable Assessment Inventory of Neurobehavioral Organization (RAINBO)*. In English (various dialects) and Spanish.

Finnish

Laine, M., Goodglass, H., Niemi, J., Koivuselka-Sallinen, P., Tuomainen, J., & Martilla, R. (1993). Adaptation of the Boston Diagnostic Aphasia Examination and the Boston Naming Test into Finnish. *Scandinavian Journal of Logopedics and Phoniatrics, 18,* 83–92.

*Laine, M., Koivuselkä-Sallinen, P., Hänninen, R., & Niemi, J. (1993). *Bostonin Nimentätestin Suomenkielinen Versio [The Finnish version of the Boston Naming Test].* Helsinki: Psykologien Kustannus.

*Laine, M., Niemi, J., Koivuselkä-Sallinen, P., & Tuomainen, J. (1993). *Bostonin Diagnostises Afasiatestistön Suomenkielinen Versio [The Finnish version of the Boston Diagnostic Aphasia Examination].* Helsinki: Psykoligien Kustannus.

French

*Deloche, G., Metz-Lutz ; M.N., Kremin, H., Hannequin, D., Ferrand, I., Perrier, D., Dordain, M., Quint, S., & Cardebat, D. (1990). Test de dénomination orale de 80 images: DO 80. Atelier de Dénomination du Réseau de Recherche Clinique INSERM.

Lemay, M.A. (1988). Protocole d'évaluation des dyslexies acquises. *Rééducation Orthophonique, 26,* 363–376.

*Lemay, M.A. (1990). *Examen des Dyslexies Acquises (EDA).* Montréal: Les Éditions Point Carré.

*Mazaux, J.M. & Orgogozo, J.M. (1981). *Boston Diagnostic Aphasia Examination: Échelle Française.* Paris: Éditions Scientifiques et Psychologiques.

Metz-Lutz, M.N., Kremin, H., Deloche, G., Hannequin, D., Ferrand, I., Perrier, D., Quint, S., Dordain, M., Bunel, G., Cardebat, D., Larroque, C., Lota, A.M., Pichard, B., & Blavier, A. (1991). Standardisation d'un test de dénomination orale: Contrôle des effets de l'âge, du sexe et du niveau de scolarité chez les sujets adulte normaux. *Revue de Neuropsychologie, 1,* 73–95.

*Nespoulos, J.L., Lecours, A.R., Lafond, D., Lemay, A., Puel, M., Joannette, Y., Cot, F., & Rascol, A. (1992). Protocole Montréal-Toulouse d'Examen Linguistique de l'Aphasie. Version M1 beta/1992. Isbergues, France: Éditions L'ortho.

Roberts, P.M. & Doucet, N. (In preparation). Boston Naming Test performance for elderly French Canadians.

Thuillard-Colombo, F. & Assal, G. (1992). Adaptation française du test de dénomination de Boston: Versions abrégées. *Revue Européene de Psychologie Appliquée, 42,* 67–71.

German

*Huber, W., Poeck, K., Weniger, D., & Willmes, K. (1983). *Der Aachener Aphasie Test.* Gottingen: Verlag fur Psychologie Hogrefe. (Aachen Aphasia Test.) Also in English, Dutch, Italian, and Thai.

Stadie, N., Cholewa, J., de Bleser, R., & Tabatabaie, S. (1994). Pas neurolinguistische experten system LeMoI: Theoretischer Rahmen und Konstruktions merkmale des testteils LEXIKON. *Neurolinguistik, 1,* 1–27.

Italian

Basso, A. & Capitani, E. (1979). Un test standardizzato per la diagnosi di acalculia. Descrizione e valori normativi. *AP-Rivista di Applicazioni Psicologiche, 1,* 551–564.

*Luzzati, C., Willmes, K., & de Bleser, R. (1992). *Aachener Aphasie Test: Versione Italiana.* Firenze: O.S. Organizzazioni Speciali. (The Aachen Aphasia Test.) Also in German, Dutch, English, and Thai.

*Miceli, G., Laudanna, A., & Burani, C. (1991). *Batteria per l'Analisi dei Deficit Afasici.* Milan: Associazone Sviluppo Ricerche Neuropsicologiche.

Novelli, G., Papagano, C., Capitani, E., Laiacona, M., Vallar, G., & Cappa, S.F. (1986). Tre test clinici di ricerca e produzione lessicale: Taratura susoggetti normali. *Archivio di Psicologia, Neurologia Psichiatria, 47,* 477–506.

Japanese

Test of Differential Diagnosis of Aphasia (TDDA) described in Sasanuma, S., Itoh, M., Watamori, T., Fukusako, Y., & Monoi, H. (1992). *Treatment of Aphasia.* Tokyo: Igaku-shoin (in Japanese)

*Sugishita, M. (1988). *WAB Aphasia Test in Japanese.* Tokyo: Igaku Shoin.

Watamori, T., Takeuchi, A., Itoh, M., Fukusako, Y., Suzuki, T., Endo, K., Takahashi, M., & Sasanuma, S. (1990). *Test for Functional Abilities—CADL Test.* Tokyo: Ishiyaku (in Japanese).

Korean

Park, H.S., Sasanuma, S., Sunwoo, I.N., Rah, U.W., & Shin, J.S. (1992). The preliminary clinical application of the tentative Korean Aphasia Test Battery Form (1). *Korean Neuropsychology, 10,* 350–357.

Punjabi

Mumby, K. (1990). Preliminary results from using the Punjabi adaptation of the Aphasia Sceening Test. *British Journal of Disorders of Communication, 25(2),* 209–226.

Mumby, K. (1988). An adaptation of the Aphasia Screening Test for use with Punjabi speakers. *British Journal of Disorders of Communication, 23,* 267–292.

Spanish

Allegri, R.F., Mangone, C.A., Villavicencio, A.F., Rymberg, S., Taragano, F.E., & Baumann, D. (1997). Spanish Boston Naming Test norms. *The Clinical Neuropsychologist, 11,* 416–420.

*Benton, A.L. & Hamsher, K.D. (1994). *Examen de Afasia Multilingue (MAE-S).* San Antonio, TX: The Psychological Corporation.

*Goodglass, H. & Kaplan, E. (1974). *Evaluación de la Afasia y de Trostornos Similares.* Buenos Aires, Argentina: Editorial Medical Panamericana. (BDAE)

*Kaplan, E.F., Goodglass, H., & Weintraub, S. (1986). *Test de Vocabulario de Boston.* Madrid: Panamericana. (BNT)

*Keenan, J.S. & Brassel, E.G. (1975). *Aphasia Language Performance Scales.* Spanish version from: Pinnacle Press.

Manuel-Dupont, S., Ardila, A., Rosselli, M., & Puente, A.E. (1992). Bilingualism. In A.E. Puente & R.J. McCaffrey (eds.), *Handbook of Neuropsychological Assessment* (pp. 193–210). New-York: Plenum Press. (Bilingual Aphasia Test: group study)

Paradis, M. & Libben, G. (1993). *La Evaluación de la Afasie en los Bilingues.* Barcelona: Masson. (Bilingual aphasia test description)

Ponton, M.O., Satz, P., Herrera, L., Young, R., Ortiz, F., D'Elia, L., Furst, C., & Namerow, N. (1992). Modified Spanish version of the Boston Naming Test. *The Clinical Neuropsychologist, 6(3),* 334.

Rosselli, M., Ardila, A., Florez, A., & Castro, C. (1990). Normative data on the Boston Diagnostic Aphasia Examination in a Spanish-speaking population. *Journal of Clinical and Experimental Neuropsychology, 12,* 313–322.

Sanfeliu, M.C. & Fernandez, A. (1996). A set of 254 Snodgrass-Vanderwart pictures standardized for Spanish: Norms for name agreement, image agreement, familiarity, and visual complexity. *Behavior Research Methods, Instruments, and Computers, 28,* 537–555.

Taussig, I.M., Henderson, V.W., & Mack, W. (1992). Spanish translation and validation of a neuropsychological battery: Performance of Spanish- and English-speaking Alzheimer's disease patients and normal comparison subjects. *Clinical Gerontologist, 11,* 95–108.

Wallace, G.J. (in preparation). *The Reliable Assessment Inventory of Neurobehavioral Organization (RAINBO).* In English (various dialects) and Spanish.

Thai

Dardarananda, R., Potisuk, S., Grandour, J., Holasuit, S. (1999). *Thai adaptation of the Western Aphasia Battery (WAB).* Chiangmai Medical Bulletin (Thailand).

Gandour, J., Dardarananda, R., Buckingham, H. Jr., & Viriyavejakul, A. (1986). A Thai adaptation of the BDAE. *Crossroads: An Interdisciplinary Journal of Southeast Asian Studies, 2(3),* 1–39.

Holasuit Petty, S. & Gandour, J. (1984). Some auditory language comprehension tests for Thai aphasic patients. *Nursing Newsletter (Thailand), 11(1),* 20–24.

Holasuit Petty, S., Gandour, J., & Jirakupt, S. (1985). A picture arrangement test for eliciting connected discourse from Thai aphasic patients. *Nursing Newsletter (Thailand), 12(4),* 42–48.

Pracharitpukdi, N., Phanthumchinda, K., Huber, W., & Willmes, K. (1998). The Thai version of the German Aachen Aphasia Test (AAT): Description of the test and performance in normal subjects. *Journal of the Medical Association of Thailand, 81(6),* 402–412.

Website for journal is yui@alpha.tu.ac.th

Over 60 Languages

The Bilingual Aphasia Test, M. Paradis and colleagues: Available from Lawrence Erlbaum Associates, Mahwah, NJ. Many languages, and dialects within some languages.

Section III

Psychosocial/ Functional Approaches to Intervention: Focus on Improving Ability to Perform Communication Activities of Daily Living

Chapter 10

Life Participation Approach to Aphasia: A Statement of Values for the Future

LPAA Project Group (in alphabetical order): Roberta Chapey, Judith F. Duchan, Roberta J. Elman, Linda J. Garcia, Aura Kagan, Jon G. Lyon, and Nina-Simmons Mackie

Unprecedented changes are occurring in the way treatment for aphasia is viewed—and reimbursed. These changes, resulting from both internal and external pressures, are influencing how speech-language pathologists carry out their jobs.

Internal influences include a growing interest in treatments that produce meaningful real life outcomes leading to enhanced quality of life. Externally, we are influenced by disability rights activists encouraging adjustments in philosophy and treatment and by consumers frustrated by unmet needs and unfulfilled goals. Most recently, a strong external influence is emanating from the curtailment of funding for our work that has caused a significant reduction in available services to people affected by aphasia.

To accommodate these varied influences on service delivery, it is important to take a proactive stance. We therefore propose a philosophy of service delivery that meets the needs of people affected by aphasia and confronts the pressures from our profession, providers, and funding sources.

Our statement of values has been guided by the ideas and work of speech-language pathologists as well as by individuals in psychology, sociology, and medicine (see the ASHA Web site, www.asha.org/publications/ashalinks.htm, for a detailed reference list). We intend neither to prescribe exact methods for achieving specific outcomes, nor to provide a quick fix to the challenges facing our profession. Rather, we offer a statement of values and ideas relevant to assessment, intervention, policy making, advocacy, and research that we hope will stimulate discussion related to restructuring of services and lead to innovative clinical methods for supporting those affected by aphasia.

DEFINING THE APPROACH

The "Life Participation Approach to Aphasia" (LPAA) is a consumer-driven service-delivery approach that supports individuals with aphasia and others affected by it in achieving their immediate and longer term life goals (note that "approach" refers here to a general philosophy and model of service delivery, rather than to a specific clinical approach). LPAA calls for a broadening and refocusing of clinical practice and research on the consequences of aphasia. It focuses on re-engagement in life, beginning with initial assessment and intervention, and continuing, after hospital discharge, until the consumer no longer elects to have communication support.

LPAA places the life concerns of those affected by aphasia at the center of all decision making. It empowers the consumer to select and participate in the recovery process and to collaborate on the design of interventions that aim for a more rapid return to active life. These interventions thus have the potential to reduce the consequences of disease and injury that contribute to long-term health costs.

THE ESSENCE OF LPAA

We encourage clinicians and researchers to focus on the real-life goals of people affected by aphasia. For example, in the initial stages following a CVA, a goal may be to establish effective communication with the surrounding nursing staff and physicians. At a later stage, a life goal may be to return to employment or participation in the local community.

Regardless of the stage of management, LPAA emphasizes the attainment of re-engagement in life by strengthening daily participation in activities of choice. Residual skill is thus seen as only one of many requisites. For example, full participation is dependent on motivation and a consistent and dependable support system. A highly supportive environment can lessen the consequences of aphasia on one's

TABLE 10–1

Examples of Shift in Focus of Life Participation Approach to Aphasia

LPAA	Examples of Shift in Focus
Assessment includes determining relevant life participation needs and discovering competencies of clients	In addition to assessing language and communication deficits, clinicians are equally interested in assessing how the person with aphasia does *with support*
Treatment includes facilitating the achievement of life goals	In addition to work on improving and/or compensating for the language impairment, clinicians are prepared to work on anything where aphasia is a barrier to life participation (even if the activity is not directly related to communication)
Intervention routinely targets environmental factors outside of the individual	In addition to working with the individual on language or compensatory functional communication techniques, clinicians might train communication partners or work on other ways of reducing barriers to make the environment more "aphasia-friendly"
All those affected by aphasia are regarded as legitimate targets for intervention	In addition to working with the individual who has aphasia, clinicians would also work on life participation goals for family and others who are affected by the aphasia, including friends, service providers, work colleagues, etc.
Clinician roles are expanded beyond those of teacher or therapist	In addition to doing therapy, clinicians might take on the role of: • "communication partner" and give the person with aphasia the opportunity to engage in conversation about life goals, concerns about the future, barriers to life participation, etc. • "coach," "problem solver," or "support person" in relation to overcoming challenges in re-engaging in a particular life activity
Outcome evaluation involves routinely documenting quality of life and life participation changes	In addition to documenting change in language and communication, clinicians would routinely evaluate the following in partnership with clients: • life activities and how satisfying they are • social connections and how satisfying they are • emotional well-being

[a]This chapter was previously published as an article in the ASHA Leader (Feb 15, 2000, pp. 4–6). Reprinted with permission from American Speech Language Hearing Association.

life, whatever the language impairment. A nonsupportive environment, on the other hand, can substantially increase the chance of aphasia affecting daily routines. Someone with mild aphasia in a nonsupportive environment might experience greater daily encumbrances than another with severe aphasia who is highly supported.

In this broadening and refocusing of services, LPAA recommends that clinicians and researchers consider the dual function of communication—transmitting and receiving messages and establishing and maintaining social links. Furthermore, life activities do not need to be in the realm of communication in order to deserve or receive intervention. What is important is to judge whether aphasia affects the execution of activities of choice and one's involvement in them (see Table 10–1 (www.asha.org/publications/ashalinks.htm) for a

few examples of how LPAA may lead to a broadening and refocusing of services).

THE ORIGINS OF LPAA

Functional and Pragmatic Approaches

LPAA draws on ideas underlying functional and pragmatic approaches to aphasia and shares some common values with those who take a broad approach to functional communication treatment by focusing on life participation goals and social relationships. In our view, however, the term "functional" does not do justice to the breadth of this work. In addition, the term is often used narrowly to mean "functional independence in getting a message across." Although LPAA recognizes the value of this type of impairment-level work, it should form part of a bigger picture where the ultimate goal for intervention is re-engagement into everyday society.

Human Rights Issues and Consumers' Goals

LPAA is a means of addressing unmet needs and rights of individuals with aphasia and those in their environment. Indeed, the Americans With Disabilities Act (ADA), signed into law on July 26, 1990, requires that physical and communication access be provided for individuals with aphasia and other disabilities and allows them legal recourse if they are blocked from accessing employment, programs, and services in the public and private sectors.

In 1992, ASHA provided guidelines for a "communication bill of rights" (National Joint Committee for the Communicative Needs of Persons with Severe Disabilities). Its preface states that "all persons, regardless of the extent or severity of their disabilities, have a basic right to affect, through communication, the conditions of their own existence." Communication is defined as "a basic need and basic right of all human beings" (p. 2). ASHA thus views communication as an integral part of life participation.

Emphasis on Competence and Inclusion

LPAA philosophy embraces a view of treatment that emphasizes competence and inclusion in daily life, focusing as much on the consequences of chronic disorders as on the language difficulty caused by the aphasia. Along with other movements in education and health care, LPAA shifts from a focus on deficits and remediation to one of inclusion and life participation (see Fougeyrollas et al., 1997; WHO, ICIDH-2, 1997). Such international changes in focus point to the need to address the personal experience of disability and promote optimal life inclusion and reintegration into society.

Changes In Reimbursement and Service Delivery

Health care and reimbursement in America have undergone an unprecedented overhaul. Financial exigencies have led to an emphasis on medically essential treatments and others seen as likely to save on future health care costs. Many of the incentives in this model result in the provision of efficient short-term minimal care, rather than the longer term, fuller care supported in the past.

LPAA represents a fundamental shift in how we view service delivery for people confronting aphasia. Since LPAA focuses on broader life-related processes and outcomes from the onset of treatment, service delivery and its reimbursement will require novel means that stand outside most current practices. We are confident that cost-sensitive and therapeutically effective models are possible. Our purpose in this introductory article is to prompt a discussion with providers and consumers as to whether life participation principles and values should play a more central role in the delivery and reimbursement of future service delivery for all those affected by aphasia.

THE CORE VALUES OF LPAA

LPAA is structured around five core values that serve as guides to assessment, intervention, and research.

The Explicit Goal Is Enhancement of Life Participation

In the LPAA approach, the first focus of the client, clinician, and policy maker is to assess the extent to which persons affected by aphasia are able to achieve life participation goals, and the extent to which the aphasia hinders the attainment of these desired outcomes. The second focus is to improve short- and long-term participation in life.

All Those Affected by Aphasia Are Entitled to Service

LPAA supports all those affected directly by aphasia, including immediate family and close associates of the adult with aphasia. The LPAA approach holds that it is essential to build protected communities within society where persons with aphasia are not only able to participate but are valued as participants. Therefore, intervention may involve changing broader social systems to make them more accessible to those affected by aphasia.

The Measures of Success Include Documented Life Enhancement Changes

The LPAA approach calls for the use of outcome measures that assess quality of life and the degree to which those affected by aphasia meet their life participation goals. Without a cause to communicate, we believe, there is no practical need for communication. Therefore, treatment focuses on a reason to communicate as much as on communication repair. In so doing, treatment attends to each consumer's feelings, relationships, and activities in life.

Both Personal and Environmental Factors Are Targets of Intervention

Disruption of daily life for individuals affected by aphasia (including those who do not have aphasia themselves) is evident on two levels: personal (internal) and environmental (external). Intervention consists of constantly assessing, weighing, and prioritizing which personal and environmental factors should be targets of intervention and how best to provide freer, easier, and more autonomous access to activities and social connections of choice. This does not mean that treatment comprises only life resumption processes, but rather that enhanced participation in life "governs" management from its inception. In this fundamental way, the LPAA approach differs from one in which life enhancement is targeted only after language repair has been addressed.

Emphasis Is on Availability of Services as Needed at all Stages of Aphasia

LPAA begins with the onset of aphasia and continues until consumers and providers agree that targeted life enhancement changes have occurred. However, LPAA acknowledges that life consequences of aphasia change over time and should be addressed regardless of the length of time post-onset. Consumers are therefore permitted to discontinue intervention, and re-enter treatment when there is a felt need to continue work on a goal or to attain a new life goal.

CONCLUSIONS

Our health care systems are undergoing change and, as a result, so are our professions. How we allow this change to affect our clinical practice, our research directions, and our response to consumer advocacy is up to us. We need to educate policy makers that being fiscally responsible means having a consumer-driven model of intervention focusing on interventions that make real-life differences and minimize the consequences of disease and injury.

While it is clear that the implicit motivation underlying all clinical and research efforts in aphasia is related to increased participation in life, the way of achieving that goal is often indirect. Because LPAA makes life goals primary and explicit, it holds promise as an approach in which such goals are attainable. We invite other speech-language pathologists to join us in discussing and developing life participation approaches to aphasia.

References

Short List of References

Please refer to the ASHA Web site (www.asha.org/publications/ashalinks.htm) for a detailed reference list of the important prior work that has influenced and guided creation of LPAA. The following references are cited in the article:

Fougeyrollas, P., Cloutier, R., Bergeron, H., Cote, J., Cote, M., & St. Michel, G. (1997). *Revision of the Quebec Classification: Handicap creation process*. Lac St-Charles, Quebec: International Network on the Handicap Creation Process.

National Joint Committee for the Communicative Needs of Persons with Severe Disabilities. (1992). Guidelines for meeting the communication needs of persons with severe disabilities. *ASHA, 34* (March, Suppl. 7), 1–8.

World Health Organization. (1997). *International classification of impairments, activities and participation: A manual of dimensions of disablement and functions. Beta-1 draft for field trials*. Geneva, Switzerland: WHO.

Detailed List of References

Alexander, M. (1988). Clinical determination of mental competence: A theory and retrospective study. *Archives of Neurology, 45*, 23–26.

Angeleri, F., Angeleri, V., Foschi, N., Giaquinto, S., & Nolfe, G. (1993). The influence of depression, social activity, and family stress on functional outcome after stroke. *Stroke, 24*, 1478–1483.

Armsden, G. & Lewis, F. (1993). The child's adaptation to parental medical illness: Theory and clinical implications. *Patient Education and Counseling, 22*, 153–165.

Amstrong, E. (1993). Aphasia rehabilitation: A sociolinguistic perspective. In A. Holland & M. Forbes (eds.), *Aphasia treatment: World perspectives* (pp. 263–290). San Diego, CA: Singular Publishing Group.

Astrom, M., Asplund, K., & Astrom, T. (1992). Psychosocial function and life satisfaction after stroke. *Stroke, 23*, 527–531.

Aten, J. (1986). Functional communication treatment. In R. Chapey (ed.), *Language intervention strategies in adult aphasia* (pp. 292–303). Philadelphia: Williams & Wilkins.

Aten, J., Cagliuri, M., & Holland, A. (1982). The efficacy of functional communication therapy for chronic aphasic patients. *Journal of Speech and Hearing Disorders, 47*, 93–96.

Banigan, R. (1998). *A family-centered approach to developing communication*. Boston: Butterworth-Heinemann.

Bastiaanse R. & Edwards, S. (1998). Diversity in aphasiology: A crisis in practice or a problem of definition? *Aphasiology, 12*, 447–452.

Becker, G. (1997). *Disrupted lives: How people create meaning in a chaotic world*. Los Angeles: University of California Press.

Becker, G. (1980). Continuity after a stroke: Implications for life-course disruption in old age. *The Gerontologist, 33*, 148–158.

Becker, G. & Nachtigall, R. (1995). Managing an uncertain illness trajectory in old age: Patients' and physicians' views of stroke. *Medical Anthropology Quarterly, 9*, 165–187.

Bernstein-Ellis, E. & Elman, R. (1999). Aphasia group communication treatment: The Aphasia Center of California approach. In R. Elman (ed.), *Group treatment of neurogenic communication disorders* (pp. 47–56). Woburn, MA: Butterworth-Heinemann.

Bethoux, R., Calmels, P., Gautheron, V., & Minaire, P. (1996). Quality of life of the spouses of stroke patients: A preliminary study. *International Journal of Rehabilitation Research, 19*, 291–299.

Beukelman, D. & Mirenda, P. (1992). *Augmentative and alternative communication: Management of severe communication disorders of children and adults*. Baltimore, MD: Paul H. Brookes.

Biegel, D., Sales, E., Schulz, R., & Rau, M. (1991). *Family caregiving in chronic illness* (pp. 129–146). London: Sage.

Bindman, B., Cohen-Schneider, R., Kagan, A., & Podolsky, L. (1995). Bridging the gap for aphasic individuals and their families: Providing access to service. *Topics in Stroke Rehabilitation, 2*, 46–52.

Blackford, K. (1988). The children of chronically ill parents. *Journal of Psychosocial Nursing and Mental Health Services, 26*, 33–36.

Black-Schaffer, R. & Osberg, J. (1990). Return to work after stroke: Development of a predictive model. *Archives of Physical Medicine and Rehabilitation, 71*, 285–290.

Blomert, L. (1990). What functional assessment can contribute to setting goals for aphasia therapy. *Aphasiology, 4,* 307–320.

Bogdan, R. & Biklen, D. (1993). Handicapism. In M. Nagler (ed.), *Perspectives on disability* (pp. 69–76). Palo Alto, CA: Health Markets Research.

Boland, J. & Follingstad, R. (1987). The relationship between communication and marital satisfaction: A review. *Journal of Sex and Marital Therapy, 13,* 286–313.

Boles L. (1997). Conversation analysis as a dependent measure in communication therapy with four individuals with aphasia. *Asia Pacific Journal of Speech, Language, and Hearing, 2,* 43–61.

Bouchard-Lamothe, D., Bourassa, S., Laflamme, B., Garcia, L., Gailey, G., & Stiell, K. (1999). Perceptions of three groups of interlocutors of the effects of aphasia on communication: An exploratory study. *Aphasiology, 13,* 839–855.

Bourgeois, M. (1997). Families caring for elders at home: Caregiver training. In B. Shadden and M.A. Toner (eds.), *Aging and communication* (pp. 227–249). Austin, TX: Pro-Ed.

Bradburn, N.M. (1969). *The structure of well-being.* Chicago: Aldine.

Brookshire, R. (1994). Group studies of treatment for adults with aphasia: Efficacy, effectiveness, and believability. *ASHA Special Interest Division 2 Newsletter, 4,* 5–13.

Brumfitt, S. (1993). Losing your sense of self: What aphasia can do. *Aphasiology, 7, 6,* 569–591.

Brumfitt, S. & Clark P. (1983). An application of psychotherapeutic techniques to the management of aphasia. In C. Code & D. Müller (eds.), *Aphasia therapy.* London: Whurr.

Byng, S. (1995). What is aphasia therapy? In C. Code & D. Müller (eds.), *The treatment of aphasia: From theory to practice* (pp. 3–17). London: Whurr.

Byng, S. & Black, M. (1995). What makes a therapy? Some parameters of therapeutic intervention in aphasia. *European Journal of Disorders of Communication, 30,* 303–316.

Byng, S., Kay, J., Edmundson, A., & Scott, C. (1990). Aphasia tests reconsidered. *Aphasiology, 4,* 67–91.

Byng, S., Pound, C., & Parr, S. (in press). Living with aphasia: A framework for therapy interventions. In I. Papathanasiou (ed.), *Acquired neurological communication disorders: A clinical perspective.* London: Whurr.

Caplan, D. (1993). Toward a psycholinguistic approach to acquired neurogenic language disorders. *American Journal of Speech-Language Pathology, 2, 1,* 59–83.

Carriero, M.R., Faglia, Z., & Vignolo, L.A. (1987). Resumption of gainful employment in aphasics: Preliminary findings. *Cortex, 26,* 667–672.

Chapey, R. (1992). Functional communication assessment and intervention: Some thoughts on the state of the art. *Aphasiology, 6,* 85–93.

Christensen, J.M. & Anderson, J.D. (1989). Spouse adjustment to stroke: Aphasic versus nonaphasic partners. *Journal of Communication Disorders, 22,* 225–231.

Clark, L. (1997). Communication intervention for family caregivers and professional health care providers. In B. Shadden & M. Toner (eds.), *Aging and communication* (pp. 251–274). Austin, TX: Pro-Ed.

Clinical Forum. (1998). Beyond the "plateau": Discharge dilemmas in chronic aphasia. *Aphasiology, 12,* 207–243.

Cochrane, R. & Milton, S. (1984). Conversational prompting: A sentence building technique for severe aphasia. *The Journal of Neurological Communication Disorders, 1,* 4–23.

Code, C. & Müller, D. (1992). *The Code-Müller Protocols: Assessing perceptions of psychosocial adjustment to aphasia and related disorders.* London: Whurr.

Coles, R. & Eales, C. (1999). The aphasia self-help movement in Britain: A challenge and an opportunity. In R. Elman (ed.), *Group treatment for neurogenic communication disorders: The expert clinician's approach* (pp. 107–114). Woburn, MA: Butterworth-Heinemann.

Csikszentmihalyi, M. (1990). *Flow: The psychology of optimal experience.* New York: HarperCollins.

Csikszentmihalyi, M. (1993). *The evolving self.* New York: Harper-Collins.

Csikszentmihalyi, M. (1997). *Finding flow: The psychology of engagement with everyday life.* New York: HarperCollins.

Damico, J.S., Simmons-Mackie, N., & Schweitzer, L.A. (1995). Addressing the third law of gardening: Methodological alternatives in aphasiology. In M.L. Lemme (ed.), *Clinical aphasiology, Vol. 23* (pp. 83–93). Austin, TX: Pro-Ed.

Darley, F. (1991). I think it begins with an A. In T. Prescott (ed.), *Clinical aphasiology, Vol. 20* (pp. 9–20). Austin, TX: Pro-Ed.

Davis, A. & Wilcox, J. (1985). *Adults' aphasia rehabilitation: Applied pragmatics.* San Diego, CA: College Hill Press.

Davis, A. (1986). Pragmatics and treatment. In R. Chapey (ed.), *Language intervention strategies in adult aphasia* (pp. 251–265). Baltimore: Williams & Wilkins.

Davis, G. & Wilcox, J. (1981). Incorporating parameters of natural conversation in aphasia treatment. In R. Chapey (ed.), *Language intervention strategies in adult aphasia.* Baltimore: Williams & Wilkins.

de Hann, R., Aaronson, N., Limburg, M., Langton Hewer, R., & van Crevel, H. (1993). Measuring quality of life in stroke. *Stroke, 24,* 320–327.

de Hann, R., Horn, J., Limburg, M., van der Meulen, J., & Bossuyt, P. (1993). A comparison of five stroke scales with measures of disability, handicap, and quality of life. *Stroke, 24,* 1179–1181.

Dickson, H.G. (1996). Problems with the ICIDH definition of impairment: Clinical commentary. *Disability and Rehabilitation, 18,* 52–54.

Disability Alliance (1995). *Disability rights handbook.* London: Disability Alliance Educational and Research Associations.

Doolittle, N. (1992). The experience of recovery following lacunar stroke. *Rehabilitation Nursing, 17,* 122–125.

Doolittle, N. (1994). A clinical ethnography of stroke recovery. In P. Benner (ed.), *Interpretive phenomenology: Embodiment, caring and ethics in health and illness.* Thousand Oaks, CA: Sage.

Duchan, J. (1995). *Supporting language learning in everyday life.* San Diego, CA: Singular Publishing Group.

Duchan, J. (1997). A situated pragmatics approach for supporting children with severe communication disorders. *Topics in Language Disorders, 17,* 1–18.

Duchan, J., Maxwell, M., & Kovarsky, D. (1999). Evaluating competence in the course of everyday interaction. In D. Kovarsky, J. Duchan, & M. Maxwell (eds.), *Constructing (in)competence* (pp. 3–26). Mahwah, NJ: Lawrence Erlbaum.

Eldridge, M. (1968). *A history of the treatment of speech disorders.* Edinburgh: Livingstone.

Elman, R. (1995). Multimethod research: A search for understanding. *Clinical Aphasiology, 23,* 77–81.

Elman, R. (1998a). Diversity in aphasiology: Let us embrace it. *Aphasiology, 12(6),* 456–457.

Elman, R. (1998b). Memories of the 'plateau': Health-care changes provide an opportunity to redefine aphasia treatment and discharge. *Aphasiology, 12,* 227–231.

Elman, R. (ed.). (1999). *Group treatment of neurogenic communication disorders.* Woburn, MA: Butterworth-Heinemann.

Elman, R. & Bernstein-Ellis, E. (1995). What is functional? *American Journal of Speech-Language Pathology, 4,* 115–117.

Elman, R. & Bernstein-Ellis, E. (1999a). The efficacy of group communication treatment in adults with chronic aphasia. *Journal of Speech, Language, and Hearing Research, 42,* 411–419.

Elman, R. & Bernstein-Ellis, E. (1999b). Psychosocial aspects of group communication treatment: Preliminary findings. *Seminars in Speech & Language, 20(1),* 65–72.

Enderby, P. (1997). *Therapy outcome measures: Speech-language pathology technical manual.* San Diego, CA: Singular Publishing Group.

Evans, R.L., Dingus, C.M., & Haselkorn, J.K. (1993). Living with a disability: A synthesis and critique of the literature on quality of life, 1985–1989. *Psychological Reports, 72,* 771–777.

Ewing, S. (1999). Group process, group dynamics, and group techniques with neurogenic communication disorders. In R. Elman (ed.), *Group treatment for neurogenic communication disorders: The expert clinician's approach* (pp. 9–16). Woburn, MA: Butterworth-Heinemann.

Ezrachi, O., Ben-Yishay, Y., Kay, T., Diller, L., & Rattock, J. (1991). Predicting employment in traumatic brain injury following neuropsychological rehabilitation. *Journal of Head Trauma Rehabilitation, 6(3),* 71–84.

Ferguson, A. (1994). The influence of aphasia, familiarity, and activity on conversational repair. *Aphasiology, 8,* 143–157.

Ferguson, A. (1996). Describing competence in aphasic/normal conversation. *Clinical Linguistics and Phonetics, 10,* 55–63.

Ferguson, D. (1994). Is communication really the point? Some thoughts on interventions and membership. *Mental Retardation, 32,* 7–18.

Finkelstein V. (1991). Disability: An administrative challenge. In M. Oliver (ed.), *Social work, disabled people and disabling environments* (pp. 19–39). London: Jessica Kinglsey.

Flickinger, E.E. & Amato, S.C. (1994). School-age children's responses to parents with disabilities. *Rehabilitation Nursing, 19,* 403–406.

Florence, C. (1981). Methods of communication analysis used in family interaction therapy. In R. Brookshire (ed.), *Clinical aphasiology conference proceedings* (pp. 204–211). Minneapolis, MN: BRK.

Flowers, C. & Peizer, E. (1984). Strategies for obtaining information from aphasic persons. In R. Brookshire (ed.), *Clinical aphasiology conference proceedings* (pp. 106–113). Minneapolis, MN: BRK.

Fougeyrollas, P., Cloutier, R., Bergeron, H., Cote, J., Cote, M., & St. Michel, G. (1997). *Revision of the Quebec Classification: Handicap creation process.* Lac St-Charles, Quebec: International Network on the Handicap Creation Process.

Fox, L. & Fried-Oken, M. (1996). AAC Aphasiology: Partnership for future research. *Augmentative and Alternative Communication, 12,* 257–271.

Fraser, R. & Baarslag-Benson, R. (1994). Cross-disciplinary collaboration in the removal of work barriers after traumatic brain injury. *Topics in Language Disorders, 15(1),* 55–67.

Frattali, C. (1992). Functional assessment of communication: Merging public policy with clinical views. *Aphasiology, 6,* 63–85.

Frattali, C. (1993). Perspective on functional assessment: Its use for policy making. *Disability and Rehabilitation, 15,* 1–9.

Frattali, C. (1996). Measuring disability. *ASHA Special Interest Division 2 Newsletter-Neurophysiology and Neurogenic Speech and Language Disorders, 6,* 6–10.

Frattali, C. (1997). Clinical care in a changing health system. In N. Helm-Estabrooks & A. Holland (eds.), *Approaches to the Treatment of Aphasia* (pp. 241–265). San Diego, CA: Singular Publishing Group.

Frattali, C. (1998). Measuring modality-specific behaviors, functional abilities, and quality of life. In C. Frattali (ed.), *Measuring outcomes in speech-language pathology* (pp. 55–88). New York: Thieme.

Frattali, C., Thomson, C., Holland, A., Wohl, C., & Ferketic, M. (1995). *The American Speech-Language-Hearing Association functional assessment of communication skills for adults (ASHA FACS).* Rockville, MD: ASHA.

Frattali, C. & Sutherland, C. (1994). Improving quality in the context of managed care. *Managing Managed Care.* Rockville, MD: ASHA.

French, S. (1993). What's so great about independence? In J. Swain, F. Finkelstein, S. French, & M. Oliver (eds.), *Disabling barriers-enabling environments* (pp. 44–48). London: Sage.

French, S. (1994a). Dimensions of disability and impairment. In S. French (ed.), *On equal terms: Working with disabled people* (pp. 17–34). Oxford: Butterworth Heinemann.

French, S. (1994b) The disabled role. In S. French (ed.), *On equal terms: Working with disabled people* (pp. 47–60). Oxford: Butterworth Heinemann.

French, S. (1994c) Researching disability. In S. French (ed.), *On equal terms: Working with disabled people* (pp. 136–147). Oxford: Butterworth Heinemann.

Fuhrer, M.J. (1994). Subjective well-being: Implications for medical rehabilitation outcomes and models of disablement. *American Journal of Physical Medicine and Rehabilitation, 73,* 358–364.

Gainotti, G. (ed.). (1997). Emotional, psychological and psychosocial problems of aphasic patients [Special Issue]. *Aphasiology, 11(7).*

Garcia, L.J., Barrette, J., & Laroche, C. (in press). Perceptions of the obstacles to work reintegration for persons with aphasia. *Aphasiology.*

Garnes, H. & Olson, D. (1995). Parent-adolescent communication and the circumplex model. *Child Development, 56,* 438–447.

Garrett, K. (1996). Augmentative and alternative communication: Applications to the treatment of aphasia. In G. Wallace (ed.), *Adult aphasia rehabilitation* (pp. 259–278). Boston: Butterworth-Heinemann.

Garrett, K. (1999). Measuring outcomes of group therapy. In R. Elman (ed.), *Group treatment for neurogenic communication disorders: The expert clinician's approach* (pp. 17–30). Woburn, MA: Butterworth-Heinemann.

Garrett, K. & Beukelman D. (1995). Changes in the interactive patterns of an individual with severe aphasia given three types of partner support. In M. Lemme (ed.), *Clinical Aphasiology, Vol. 23* (pp. 237–251). Austin, TX: Pro-Ed.

Garrett, K. & Beukelman, D. (1992). Augmentative communication approaches for persons with severe aphasia. In K. Yorkston (ed.), *Augmentative communication in the medical setting* (pp. 245–338). Tucson, AZ: Communication Skill Builders.

Garrett, K. & Ellis, G. (1999). Group communication therapy for people with long-term aphasia: Scaffolded thematic discourse activities. In R. Elman (ed.), *Group treatment for neurogenic communication disorders: The expert clinician's approach* (pp. 85–96). Woburn, MA: Butterworth-Heinemann.

Gerber, S. & Gurland, G. (1989). Applied pragmatics in the assessment of aphasia. *Seminars in Speech and Language, 10,* 263–281.

Goodwin, C. (1995). Co-constructing meaning in conversations with an aphasic man. In E. Jacoby & E. Ochs (eds.), *Research on language and social interaction, 28,* 233–260.

Gordon, J. (1997). Measuring outcomes in aphasia: Bridging the gap between theory and practice...or burning our bridges. *Aphasiology, 11,* 845–854.

Graham, M. (1999). Aphasia group therapy in a subacute setting: Using the American Speech-Language-Hearing Association Functional Assessment of Communication Skills. In R. Elman (ed.), *Group treatment for neurogenic communication disorders: The expert clinician's approach* (pp. 37–46). Woburn, MA: Butterworth-Heinemann.

Granger, C. Hamilton, B., Keith, R., Zielezny, M., & Sherwin, F. (1986). Advances in functional assessment for medical rehabilitation. *Topics in Geriatric Rehabilitation, 1,* 569–574.

Hales, G. (1996). *Beyond disability—Towards an enabling society.* London: Sage.

Hemsley, G. & Code, C. (1996). Interactions between recovery in aphasia, emotional and psychosocial factors in subjects with aphasia, their significant others and speech pathologists. *Disability and Rehabilitation, 18,* 567–584.

Hermann, M. & Code, C. (1996). Weightings of items on the Code-Müller protocols: The effects of clinical experience of aphasia therapy. *Disability and Rehabilitation, 18,* 509–514.

Hermann, M. & Wallesch, C. (1990). Expectations of psychosocial adjustment in aphasia: A MAUT study with the Code-Müller Scale of Psychosocial Adjustment. *Aphasiology, 4,* 527–538.

Hermann, M. & Wallesch, C. (1989). Psychosocial changes and psychosocial adjustments with chronic and severe nonfluent aphasia. *Aphasiology, 3,* 513–526.

Hersh, D. (1998). Beyond the 'plateau': Discharge dilemmas in chronic aphasia, *Aphasiology, 12,* 207–218.

Hinckley, J., Packard, M., & Bardach, L. (1995). Alternative family education programming for adults with chronic aphasia. *Topics in Stroke Rehabilitation, 2,* 53–63.

Hinckley, J. (1998). Investigating the predictors of lifestyle satisfaction among younger adults with chronic aphasia. *Aphasiology, 12,* 509–518.

Hoen, R., Thelander, M., & Worsley, J. (1997). Improvement in psychological well-being of people with aphasia and their families: Evaluation of a community-based programme. *Aphasiology, 11*(7), 681–691.

Holland, A. (1977). Some practical considerations in the treatment of aphasic patients. In M. Sullivan & M. Kommers (eds.), *Rationale for adult aphasia therapy* (pp. 167–180). Omaha, NE: University of Nebraska Press.

Holland, A. (1980). *Communicative abilities in daily living—CADL.* Austin TX: Pro-Ed.

Holland, A. (1982). Observing functional communication of aphasic adults. *Journal of Speech and Hearing Disorders, 47,* 50–56.

Holland, A. (1991). Pragmatic aspects of intervention in aphasia. *Journal of Neurolinguistics, 6,* 197–211.

Holland, A. (1992). Some thoughts of future needs and directions for research and treatment of aphasia. *NIDCD Monograph, Vol. 2* (pp. 147–152).

Holland, A. (1996). Pragmatic assessment and treatment for aphasia. In G. Wallace (ed.), *Adult aphasia rehabilitation* (pp. 161–173). Boston: Butterworth-Heinemann.

Holland, A. (1998a). Some guidelines for bridging the research-practice gap in adult neurogenic communication disorders. *Topics in Language Disorders, 18,* 49–57.

Holland, A. (1998b). Why can't clinicians talk to aphasic adults? Clinical Forum. *Aphasiology, 12,* 844–846.

Holland, A. & Beeson, P. (1999). Aphasia groups: The Arizona experience. In R. Elman (ed.), *Group treatment for neurogenic communication disorders: The expert clinician's approach* (pp. 77–84). Woburn, MA: Butterworth-Heinemann.

Holland, A., Frattali, C., & Fromm, D (1998). *Communicative abilities in daily living—CADL 2.* Austin TX: Pro-Ed.

Holland, A., Fromm, D., DeRuyter, F., & Stein, M. (1996). Treatment efficacy: Aphasia. *Journal of Speech and Hearing Research, 39,* 527–536.

Holland, A. & Ross, R. (1999). The power of aphasia groups. In R. Elman (ed.), *Group treatment of neurogenic communication disorders* (pp. 115–117). Boston, MA: Butterworth-Heinemann.

Holland, A. & Thompson, C. (1998). Outcomes measurement in aphasia. In C. Frattali (ed.), *Measuring outcomes in speech-language pathology* (pp. 245–266). New York: Thieme.

Howard, D. & Hatfield, F. (1987). *Aphasia therapy: Historical and contemporary issues.* Hillsdale, NJ: Lawrence Erlbaum.

Hughes, B. & Paterson, K. (1997). The social model of disability and the disappearing body: Toward a sociology of impairment. *Disability and Society, 12,* 325–340.

Hux, K., Beukelman, D., & Garrett, K. (1994). Augmentative and alternative communication for persons with aphasia. In R. Chapey (ed.), *Language intervention strategies in adult aphasia* (3rd ed.) (pp. 338–357). Baltimore: Williams & Wilkins.

Ireland, C. & Wootton, G. (1993). *Time to talk: ADA counseling project,* Department of health report. London: Action for Dysphasic Adults.

Iskowitz, M. (1998). Preparing for managed care in long-term care. *Advance for Speech-Language Pathologists and Audiologists,* January 12th, 7–9.

Jennings, B., Callahan, D., & Caplan, A. (1988). *Ethical challenges of chronic illness.* Briarcliff Manor, NY: A Hastings Center Report.

Johnson, E. (1993). Open your doors to disabled workers. In M. Nagler (ed.), *Perspectives on disability* (pp. 475–479). Palo Alto, CA: Health Markets Research.

Johnson, R. (1987) Return to work after severe head injury. *International Disability Studies, 9*, 49–54.

Jordan, L. (1998). 'Diversity in aphasiology': A social science perspective, *Aphasiology, 12*, 474–480.

Jordan, L. & Kaiser, W. (1996). *Aphasia—A social approach.* London: Chapman & Hall.

Kagan, A. (1995a). Family perspectives from three aphasia centers in Ontario, Canada. *Topics in Stroke Rehabilitation, 2*, 1–19.

Kagan, A. (1995b). Revealing the competence of aphasic adults through conversation: A challenge to health professionals. *Topics in Stroke Rehabilitation, 2*, 15–28.

Kagan, A. (1998). Supported conversation for adults with aphasia: Methods and resources for training conversation partners. *Aphasiology, 12*, 851–864.

Kagan, A. & Cohen-Schneider, R. (1999). Groups in the 'introductory program' at the Pat Arato Aphasia Centre. In R. Elman (ed.), *Group treatment of neurogenic communication disorders* (pp. 97–106). Woburn, MA: Butterworth-Heinemann.

Kagan, A. & Gailey, G. (1993). Functional is not enough: Training conversation partners for aphasic adults. In A. Holland & M. Forbes (eds.), *Aphasia treatment: World perspectives* (pp. 199–215). San Diego, CA: Singular Publishing Group.

Kagan, A. & Kimelman, D. (1995). 'Informed' consent in aphasia research: Myth or reality? *Clinical Aphasiology, 23*, 65–75.

Kagan, A., Winckel, J., & Shumway E. (1996a). *Pictographic communication resources.* North York, Canada: Pat Arato Aphasia Centre.

Kagan, A., Winckel, J., & Shumway E. (1996b). *Supported Conversation for aphasic adults: Increasing communicative access* (Video). North York, Ontario, Canada: Pat Arato Aphasia Centre.

Kaufman, S. (1988a). Illness, biography, and the interpretation of self, following a stroke. *Journal of Aging Studies, 2*, 217–227.

Kaufman, S. (1988b). Toward a phenomenology of boundaries in medicine: Chronic illness experience in the case of stroke. *Medical Anthropology Quarterly, 2*, 338–354.

Keatley, M.A., Miller, T.I., & Mann, A. (1995). Treatment planning using outcome data. *ASHA, 37(2)*, 49–52.

King, R.B. (1996). Quality of life after stroke. *Stroke, 27*, 1467–1472.

Kovarsky, D., Duchan, J., & Maxwell, M. (eds.). (1999). *Constructing (In)competence: Disabling evaluations in clinical and social interaction.* Hillsdale, NJ: Lawrence Erlbaum.

Kraat, A. (1990). Augmentative and alternative communication: Does it have a future in aphasia rehabilitation? *Aphasiology, 4*, 321–338.

Krefting, L. (1991). Rigor in qualitative research: The assessment of trustworthiness. *The American Journal of Occupational Therapy, 45(3)*, 214–222.

Kwa, V., Limburg, M., & de Hann, R.J. (1996). The role of cognitive impairment in the quality of life after ischemic stroke. *Journal of Neurology, 243*, 599–604.

LaCoste, L.D., Ginter, E.J., & Whipple, G. (1987). Intrafamily communication and familial environment. *Psychological Reports, 61*, 115–118.

Lafond, D., Joanette, Y., Ponzio, J., Degiovani, R., & Sarno, M. (eds.) (1993). *Living with aphasia: Psychosocial issues.* San Diego, CA: Singular Publishing Group.

LaPointe, L. (1997). Adaptation, accommodation, aristos. In L.

LaPointe (ed.), *Aphasia and related neurogenic disorders.* (2nd ed.) (pp. 265–287). New York: Thieme.

LaPointe, L. (1996). On being a patient. *Journal of Medical Speech-Language Pathology, 4*:1.

LaPointe, L. (1989). An ecological perspective on assessment and treatment of aphasia. *Clinical Aphasioiogy, 18*, 1–4.

Le Dorze, G. & Brassard, C. (1995). A description of the consequences of aphasia on aphasic persons and their relatives and friends, based on the WHO model of chronic diseases. *Aphasiology, 9*, 239–255.

LeDorze, G., Croteau, C., & Joanette Y. (1993). Perspectives on aphasia intervention in French-speaking Canada. In A. Holland & M. Forbes (eds.), *Aphasia treatment, world perspectives* (pp. 87–114). San Diego, CA: Singular Publishing Group.

Light, J. (1988). Interaction involving individuals using augmentative and alternative communication systems: State of the art and future directions. *Augmentative and Alternative Communication, 4*, 66–82.

Livneh, H. (1991). On the origins of negative attitudes toward people with disabilities. In R. Marinelli & A. Dell Orto (eds.), *The psychological and social impact of disability* (pp. 181–196). New York: Springer Publishing.

Lomas, J., Pickard, L., Bester, S., Elbard, H., Finlayson, A., & Zoghaib, C. (1989). The Communication Effectiveness Index: Development and psychometric evaluation of a functional communication measure for adult aphasia. *Journal of Speech and Hearing Disorders, 54*, 113–124.

Lomas, J., Pickard, L., & Mohide, A. (1987). Patient versus clinician item generation for quality-of-life measures: The case of language-disabled adults. *Medical Care, 25*, 764–769.

Lord, M. (1993). Away with barriers. In M. Nagler (ed.), *Perspectives on disability* (pp. 471–474). Palo Alto, CA: Health Markets Research.

Lubinski, R. (1981). Environmental language intervention. In R. Chapey (ed.), *Language intervention strategies in adult aphasia* (pp. 223–248). Baltimore: Williams & Wilkins.

Lubinski, R. (1986). Environmental systems approach to adult aphasia. In R. Chapey (ed.), *Language intervention strategies in adult aphasia* (pp. 267–291). Philadelphia, PA: Williams & Wilkins.

Lubinski, R., Duchan, J., & Weitzner-Lin, B. (1980). Analysis of breakdowns and repairs in aphasic adult communication. In R. Brookshire (ed.), *Clinical aphasiology conference proceedings.* Minneapolis, MN: BRK.

Lund, N. & Duchan, J. (1993). *Assessing children's language in naturalistic contexts* (3rd ed.). Englewood Cliffs, NJ: Prentice Hall.

Luterman, D. (1996). *Counseling persons with communication disorders and their families* (3rd ed.). Austin, TX: Pro-Ed.

Lyon, J. (1992). Communication use and participation in life for adults with aphasia in natural settings: The scope of the problem. *American Journal of Speech-Language Pathology, 1*, 7–14.

Lyon, J. (1995a). Drawing: Its value as a communication aid for adults with aphasia. *Aphasiology, 9(1)*, 33–50.

Lyon, J. (1995b). Communicative drawing: An augmentative mode of interaction. *Aphasiology, 9(1)*, 84–94.

Lyon, J. (1996a). Measurement of treatment effects in natural settings. *ASHA Special Interest Division 2 Newsletter-Neurophysiology and Neurogenic Speech and Language Disorders, 6*, 10–15.

Lyon, J. (1996b). Optimizing communication and participation in life for aphasic adults and their prime caregivers in natural settings: A use model for treatment. In G. Wallace (ed.), *Adult aphasia rehabilitation* (pp. 137–160). Newton, MA: Butterworth Heinemann.

Lyon, J. (1997a). Treating real-life functionality in a couple coping with severe aphasia. In N. Helm-Estabrooks & A. Holland (eds.), *Approaches to the treatment of aphasia* (pp. 203–239). San Diego, CA: Singular Publishing.

Lyon, J. (1997b). Volunteers and partners: Moving intervention outside the treatment room. In B. Shadden & M. Toner (eds.), *Communication and aging* (pp. 299–324). Austin, TX: Pro-Ed.

Lyon, J. (1998). *Coping with aphasia.* San Diego, CA: Singular Publishing.

Lyon, J. (in press). Finding, defining, and refining functionality in real-life for people confronting aphasia. In L. Worrall & C. Frattali (eds.), *Neurogenic communication disorders: A functional approach.* New York: Thieme.

Lyon, J. Cariski, D., Keisler, L., Rosenbek, J., Levine, R., Kumpula, J., Ryff, D., Coyne, S., & Levine, J. (1997). Communication partners: Enhancing participation in life and communication for adults with aphasia in natural settings. *Aphasiology, 11,* 693–708.

Lyon, J.G. & Sims, E. (1989). Drawing: Its use as a communicative aid with aphasic and normal adults. *Clinical Aphasiology, 18,* 339–356.

Markus, H. & Nurius, P. (1986). Possible selves. *American Psychologist, 41*(9), 954–969.

Marshall, R. (1993). Problem focused group therapy for mildly aphasic clients. *American Journal of Speech-Language Pathology, 2,* 31–37.

Marshall, R. (1999a). An introduction to supported conversation for adults with aphasia: Perspectives, problems and possibilities. *Aphasiology, 12,* 811–816.

Marshall, R. (1999b). *Introduction to group treatment for aphasia: Design and management.* Woburn, MA: Butterworth-Heinemann.

Marshall, R. (1999c). A problem-focused group treatment program for clients with mild aphasia. In R. Elman (ed.), *Group treatment for neurogenic communication disorders: The expert clinician's approach* (pp. 57–65). Woburn, MA: Butterworth-Heinemann.

Marshall, R., Freed, D., & Phillips, D. (1997). Communicative efficiency in severe aphasia. *Aphasiology, 11,* 373–384.

McClenahan, R., Johnston, M., & Denham, Y. (1992). Factors influencing accuracy of estimation of comprehension problems in patients following cerebro-vascular accident by doctors, nurses and relatives. *European Journal of Disorders of Communication, 27,* 209–219.

Meeuwesen, L., Schaap, C., & Van der Staak, C. (1991). Verbal analysis of doctor-patient communication. *Social Science in Medicine, 32,* 1143–1150.

Milroy, L. & Perkins, L. (1992). Repair strategies in aphasic discourse: Towards a collaborative model. *Clinical Linguistics and Phonetics, 6,* 17–40.

Müller, D. (1984). Psychological adjustment to aphasia. Brief Research Report. *International Journal of Rehabilitation Research, 7,* 195–196.

Müller, D. & Code, C. (1983). Interpersonal perception of psychosocial adjustment to aphasia. In C. Code & D.J. Müller (eds.), *Aphasia therapy* (pp. 101–112). London: Edward Arnold.

National Joint Committee for the Communicative Needs of Persons with Severe Disabilities (1992). Guidelines for Meeting the Communication Needs of Persons with Severe Disabilities. *ASHA, 34* (March, Suppl. 7), 1–8.

Nester, M. (1984). Employment testing for handicapped persons. *Public Personnel Management Journal, 13*(4), 417–434.

Nettleton, S. (1996). *The sociology of health and illness.* Cambridge, UK: Polity Press.

Newhoff, M., Tonkovich, J., Schwartz, S., & Burgess, E. (1985). Revision strategies in aphasia. *Journal of Neurological Communication Disorders, 2,* 2–7.

Nicholas, L. & Brookshire, R. (1993). A system for quantifying the informativeness and efficiency of the connected speech of adults with aphasia. *Journal of Speech and Hearing Research, 36,* 338–350.

Niemi, M., Laaksonen, R., Kotila, M., & Waltimo, O. (1988). Quality of life 4 years after stroke. *Stroke, 19,* 1101–1107.

Nisbet, J. (ed.), (1992). *Natural supports in school, at work and in the community for people with severe disabilities.* Baltimore, MD: Paul H. Brookes.

Oelschlaeger, M. & Damico, J. (1998). Spontaneous verbal repetition: A social strategy in aphasic conversation. *Aphasiology, 12,* 971–988.

Oliver, M. (1996). *Understanding disability: From theory to practice.* London, UK: Macmillan.

Parr, S. (1994). Coping with aphasia: Conversations with 20 aphasic people. *Aphasiology, 8,* 457–466.

Parr, S. (1996a). The road more traveled: Whose right of way? *Aphasiology, 10,* 496–503.

Parr, S. (1996b). Everyday literacy in aphasia: Radical approaches to functional assessment and therapy. *Aphasiology, 10,* 469–479.

Parr, S. & Byng, S. (1998). Breaking new ground in familiar territory. Clinical Forum. *Aphasiology, 12,* 839–844.

Parr, S., Byng, S., & Gilpin, S. (1997). *Talking about aphasia: Living with loss of language after stroke.* Buckingham, UK: Open University Press.

Patterson, J. & Garwick, A. (1992). The impact of chronic illness on families: A family systems perspective. *Annals of Behavioral Medicine, 16,* 131–142.

Patterson, R., Paul, M., Wells, A., Hoen, B., & Thelander, M. (1994). *Aphasia: A new life. Handbook for helping communities.* Stoufville, Ontario, Canada: York-Durham Aphasia Centre.

Peach, R. (1993). Clinical intervention for aphasia in the United States of America. In A. Holland & M. Forbes (eds.), *Aphasia treatment: World perspectives* (pp. 335–369). San Diego, CA: Singular Publishing Group.

Penn C. (1998). Clinician-researcher dilemmas: Comment on 'supported conversation for adults with aphasia.' Clinical Forum. *Aphasiology, 12,* 839–844.

Pessar, L., Coad, M., Linn, R. & Willer, B. (1992). The effects of parental traumatic brain injury on the behavior of parents and children. *Brain Injury, 7,* 231–240.

Petheram, B. & Parr, S. (1998). Diversity in aphasiology: A crisis in practice or a problem of definition? *Aphasiology, 12,* 435–446.

Petheram, B. & Parr, S. (1998). Reply: Plenty of room in the wardrobe: A response to Bastianne, Edwards, Cappa, Elman, Ferguson, Gordon, and Jordan. *Aphasiology, 12,* 481–488.

Pound, C. (1996). New approaches to long term aphasia therapy and support. *Bulletin of the Royal College of Speech and Language Therapists, 532,* 12–13.

Pound, C. (1998). Therapy for life: Finding new paths across the plateau. *Aphasiology, 12,* 222–227.

Prutting, C. & Kirchner, D. (1987). A clinical appraisal of the pragmatic aspects of language. *Journal of Speech and Hearing Disorders, 52,* 105–119.

Ramsburger, G. (1994). Functional perspective for assessment and rehabilitation of persons with severe aphasia. *Seminars in Speech and Language, 15,* 1–16.

Rao, P. (1997). Functional communication assessment and outcome. In B. Shadden & M. Toner (eds.), *Aging and communication* (pp. 197–225). Austin, TX: Pro-Ed.

Rice, B., Paull, A., & Müller, D. (1987). An evaluation of a social support group for spouses of aphasic partners. *Aphasiology, 1,* 247–256.

Robey, R. (1998). A meta-analysis of clinical outcomes in the treatment of aphasia. *Journal of Speech, Language and Hearing Research, 421,* 172–187.

Robillard, A. (1994). Communication problems in the intensive care unit. *Qualitative Sociology, 17,* 383–395.

Rolland, J.S. (1994). In sickness and in health: The impact of illness on couples' relationships. *Journal of Marital and Family Therapy, 20,* 327–347.

Roter, D.L. & Hall, J.L. (1992). *Doctors talking with patients/patients talking with doctors: Improving communication in medical visits.* Westport, UK: Auburn House.

Ryan, E., Bourhis, R., & Knops, U. (1991). Evaluative perceptions of patronizing speech addressed to elders. *Psychology and Aging, 6,* 442–450.

Ryan, E., Meredith, S., MacLean, M., & Orange, J. (1995). Changing the way we talk with elders: Promoting health using the communication enhancement model. *International Journal of Aging and Human Development, 4,* 89–107.

Ryff, C. (1989a). Happiness is everything, or is it? Explorations on the meaning of psychological well-being. *Journal of Personality and Social Psychology, 57(6),* 1069–1081.

Ryff, C. (1989b). In the eye of the beholder: Views of psychological well-being among middle and old-aged adults. *Psychology and Aging, 4,* 195–210.

Ryff, C. (1989c). Scales of psychological well being (short form). *Journal of Personality and Social Psychology, 57,* 1069–1081.

Ryff, C. & Singer, B. (1998). The contours of positive human health. *Psychological Inquiry, 9(1),* 1–29.

Sacchett, C. & Marshall, J. (1992). Functional assessment of communication: Implications for the rehabilitation of aphasic people: Reply to Carol Frattali. *Aphasiology, 6,* 95–100.

Sacks, H., Schegloff, E., & Jefferson, G. (1974). A simplest systematics for the organization of turn-taking for conversation. *Language, 50,* 696–735.

Sandin, K.J., Cifu, D.X., & Noll, S.F. (1994). Stroke rehabilitation: Psychological and social implications. *Archives of Physical Medicine and Rehabilitation, 75,* S-52–S-55.

Sands, E., Sarno, M., & Shankweiler, D. (1969). Long term assessment of language function in aphasia. *Archives of Physical Medicine and Rehabilitation, 50,* 202–206.

Sarno, M. (1965). A measurement of functional communication in aphasia. *Archives of Physical Medicine and Rehabilitation, 46,* 101–107.

Sarno, M. (1969). *The functional communication profile: Manual of directions.* New York: Institute of Rehabilitation Medicine.

Sarno, M. (1993). Aphasia rehabilitation: Psychosocial and ethical considerations. *Aphasiology, 7,* 321–334.

Sarno, M. (1997). Quality of life in aphasia in the first post-stroke year. *Aphasiology, 11(7),* 665–678.

Sarno, M.T. (1991). The psychological and social sequelae of aphasia. In M.T. Sarno (ed.), *Acquired aphasia* (2nd ed.) (pp. 521–582). San Diego, CA: Academic Press.

Sarno, M.T. (1992). Preliminary findings in a study of age, linguistic evolution and quality of life in recovery from aphasia. *Scandinavian Journal of Rehabilitative Medicine,* Suppl. 26, 43–59.

Sarno, M.T. & Chambers, N. (1997). A horticultural therapy program for individuals with acquired aphasias. *Activities, Adaptation and Aging, 22,* 81–91.

Schuling, J., de Haan, R., Limburg, M., & Groenier, K.H. (1993). The Frenchay activities index. *Stroke, 24,* 1173–1177.

Sherman, S. & Anderson, N. (1982). *Ability testing of handicapped people: Dilemma for government, science and the public.* Washington, DC: National Academy Press.

Shewan, C. & Bandur, D. (1986). Language-oriented treatment: A psycholinguistic approach to aphasia. In R. Chapey (ed.), *Language intervention strategies in adult aphasia* (3rd ed.) (pp. 184–206). Philadelphia, PA: Williams & Wilkins.

Shewan, C. (1986). The history and efficacy of aphasia treatment. In R. Chapey (ed.), *Language intervention strategies in adult aphasia.* (2nd ed.). Philadelphia, PA: Williams & Wilkins.

Shontz, F.C. (1991). Six principles relating disability and psychological adjustment. In R. Marinelli & A. Dell Orto (eds.), *The psychological and social impact of disability* (pp. 107–110). New York: Springer Publishing.

Simmons, N. (1986). Beyond standardized measures: Special tests, language in context, and discourse analysis. *Seminars in Speech and Language, 7,* 181–205.

Simmons, N., Kearns, K., & Potechin, G. (1987). Treatment of aphasia through family member training. In R. Brookshire (ed.), *Clinical Aphasiology Conference Proceedings, Vol. 17* (pp. 106–116). Minneapolis, MN: BRK.

Simmons-Mackie N. (1998a). A solution to the discharge dilemma in aphasia: Social approaches to aphasia management. Clinical Forum. *Aphasiology, 12,* 231–239.

Simmons-Mackie N. (1998b). In support of supported communication for adults with aphasia: Clinical Forum. *Aphasiology, 12,* 831–838.

Simmons-Mackie, N. (in press). Social approaches to the management of aphasia. In Worrall, L. & Frattali, C. (eds.), *Neurogenic communication disorders: A functional approach.* New York: Thieme.

Simmons-Mackie, N. & Damico J. (1995). Communicative competence in aphasia: Evidence from compensatory strategies. *Clinical Aphasiology, 23,* 95–105.

Simmons-Mackie, N. & Damico J. (1996a). Accounting for handicaps in aphasia: Communicative assessment from an authentic social perspective. *Disability and Rehabilitation, 18,* 540–549.

Simmons-Mackie, N. & Damico J. (1996b). The contribution of discourse markers to communicative competence in aphasia. *American Journal of Speech Language Pathology, 5,* 37–43.

Simmons-Mackie, N. & Damico J. (1997). Reformulating the definition of compensatory strategies in aphasia. *Aphasiology, 8,* 761–781.

Simmons-Mackie, N. & Damico, J. (1999). Social role negotiation in aphasia therapy: Competence, incompetence and conflict.

In D. Kovarsky, J. Duchan, & M. Maxwell (eds.), *Constructing (in)competence: Disabling evaluations in clinical and social interaction* (pp. 313–341). Hillsdale, NJ: Lawrence Erlbaum.

Simmons-Mackie N., Damico, J., & Damico, H. (1999). A qualitative study of feedback in aphasia therapy. *American Journal of Speech-Language Pathology, 8*, 218–230.

Simmons-Mackie, N. & Kagan, A. (1999). Communication strategies used by 'good' versus 'poor' speaking partners of individuals with aphasia. *Aphasiology, 13*, 807–820.

Slansky, B. & McNeil, M. (1997). Resource allocation in auditory processing of emphatically stressed stimuli in aphasia. *Aphasiology, 11*, 461–472.

Spencer, K., Tompkins, C., Schulz, R., & Rau, M. (1995). The psychosocial outcomes of stroke: A longitudinal study of depression risk. *Clinical Aphasiology, 23*, 9–23.

Stainback, W. & Stainback, S. (eds.) (1990). *Support networks for inclusive schooling.* Baltimore, MD: Paul H. Brookes.

Starkstein, S. & Robinson, R. (1988). Aphasia and depression. *Aphasiology, 2*, 1–20.

Stiell, D. & Gailey, G. (1995). Cotherapy with couples affected by aphasia. *Topics in Stroke Rehabilitation, 2*, 34–39.

Strauss Hough, M. & Pierce, R. (1994). Pragmatics and treatment. In R. Chapey (ed.), *Language intervention strategies in adult aphasia.* Philadelphia, PA: Williams & Wilkins.

Sutherland, A. (1981). *Disabled we stand.* London, UK: Souvenir Press.

Swanson, K. (1993). Nursing as informed caring for the well-being of others. *Journal of Nursing Scholarship, 25*, 352–357.

Taylor, M. (1965). A measurement of functional communication in aphasia. *Archives of Physical Medicine and Rehabilitation, 46*, 101–107.

Thompson, C. (1989). Generalization research in aphasia: A review of the literature. *Clinical Aphasiology, 18*, 195–222.

Thompson, C. (1994). Treatment of nonfluent Broca's aphasia. In R. Chapey (ed.), *Language intervention strategies in adult aphasia.* Baltimore, MD: Williams & Wilkins.

Tippett, D. & Sugarman, J. (1996). Discussing advance directives under the patient self determination act: A unique opportunity for speech-language pathologists to help persons with aphasia. *American Journal of Speech-Language Pathology, 5*, 31–54.

Verbrugge, L.M. & Jette, A.M. (1994). The disablement process. *Social Science and Medicine, 38*, 1–14.

Wahrborg, P. (1989). Aphasia and family therapy. *Aphasiology, 3*, 479–482.

Wahrborg, P. (1991). *Assessment and management of emotional and psychosocial reactions to brain damage and aphasia.* San Diego, CA: Singular Publishing Group.

Wahrborg, P. & Borenstein, P. (1989). Family therapy in families with an aphasic member. *Aphasiology, 3*, 93–98.

Walker-Batson, D., Curtis, S., Smith, P., & Ford, J. (1999). An alternative model for the treatment of aphasia: The Lifelink© approach. In R. Elman (ed.), *Group treatment for neurogenic communication disorders: The expert clinician's approach* (pp. 67–75). Woburn, MA: Butterworth-Heinemann.

Wang, C. (1993). Culture, meaning and disability: Injury prevention campaigns and the production of stigma. In M. Nagler (ed.), *Perspectives on disability* (pp. 77–90). Palo Alto, CA: Health Markets Research.

Warren, R. (1996). Outcome measurement: Moving toward the patient. *ASHA Special Interest Divisions-Neurophysiology and Neurogenic Speech and Language Disorders, 6*, 5–6.

Webster, E., Dans, J., & Saunders, P. (1982). Descriptions of husband-wife communication pre and post aphasia. In R. Brookshire (ed.), *Clinical aphasiology conference proceedings* (pp. 64–74). Minneapolis, MN: BRK.

Weisman, C.S. (1987). Communication between women and their health care providers: Research finding and unanswered questions. *Public Health Reports, 102*, 147–151.

Weniger, D. & Sarno M. (1990). The future of aphasia therapy: More than just new wine in old bottles? *Aphasiology 4*, 301–306.

Wertz, R. (1984). Language disorders in adults: State of the clinical art. In A. Holland (ed.), *Language disorders in adults* (pp. 10–78). San Diego, CA: College Hill Press.

West, J. (1993). "Ask me no questions": An analysis of queries and replies in physician-patient dialogues. In T.A. Dundas & S. Fosher (eds.), *The social organization of doctor-patient communication* (pp. 127–157). Hillsdale, NJ: Ablex Publishing Corporation.

Whiteneck, G.G., Charlifue, S.W., Gerhart, K.A., Overholser, J.D., & Richardson, G.N. (1992). Quantifying handicap: A new measure of long-term rehabilitation outcomes. *Archives of Physical Medicine and Rehabilitation, 73*, 519–526.

Whurr, R., Lorch, M., & Nye, C. (1992). A meta-analysis of studies carried out between 1946 and 1988 concerned with the efficacy of speech and language therapy treatment for aphasic patients. *European Journal of Disorders of Communication, 27*, 1–17.

Wilcox, M. (1983). Aphasia: Pragmatic considerations. *Topics in Language Disorders, 3*(4), 35–48.

Wilcox, M. & Davis, G. (1977). Speech act analysis of aphasic communication in individual and group settings. In R. Brookshire (ed.), *Clinical aphasiology conference proceedings* (pp. 166–174). Minneapolis, MN: BRK.

Wood, L. & Ryan, E. (1991). Talk to elders: Social structure attitudes and address. *Ageing and Society, 11*, 167–188.

World Health Organization (1980). *International classification of impairments, disabilities, and handicaps: A manual for classification relating to the consequences of disease.* Geneva, Switzerland: WHO.

World Health Organization (1997). *International Classification of Impairments, Activities and Participation. A manual of dimensions of disablement and functions. Beta-1draft for field trials.* Geneva, Switzerland: WHO.

Worrall, L. (1992). Functional communication assessment: An Australian perspective. *Aphasiology, 6*, 105–110.

Yalom, I. (1985). *The theory and practice of group psychotherapy.* (3rd ed.). New York: Basic Books.

Zemba, N. (1999). Aphasia patients and their families: Wishes and limits. *Aphasiology, 13*, 219–224.

Zraik, R.I. & Boone, D.R. (1991). Spouse attitudes toward the person with aphasia. *Journal of Speech and Hearing Research, 34*, 123–128.

Chapter 11

Social Approaches to Aphasia Intervention

Nina Simmons-Mackie

Major strides have been made in the past decade in the development of social approaches to aphasia (Byng et al., 2000; Elman & Bernstein-Ellis, 1999a,b; Holland, 1999; Kagan, 1999; Lyon, 1992, 1996; LPAA, 2000; Parr, 1996b; Pound, 1998b; Sarno, 1993a; Simmons-Mackie, 1993, 1994, 1998a,b, 2000). It is the objective of this chapter to explain the rationale, philosophy, and principles of socially motivated approaches and provide examples of assessment and intervention methods that fit into the social model philosophy.

OBJECTIVES

This chapter will 1) introduce and define a social model of aphasia intervention; 2) contrast social approaches with traditional restorative and functional approaches; 3) outline the principles of a social approach to intervention; 4) introduce assessment strategies appropriate to a social model of management; and 5) describe intervention objectives and examples that fit within the philosophy of a social approach.

RATIONALE FOR SOCIAL APPROACHES

The goal of a social approach is to promote membership in a communicating society and participation in personally relevant activities for those affected by aphasia. The ultimate aim of a social approach, enhancing the living of life with aphasia, is consistent with the philosophy of "Life Participation Approaches to Aphasia" (LPAA, 2000). The need for a social approach to aphasia management draws from several sources.

First, aphasia is a chronic disorder with long-term consequences beyond the acute disruption of communication. In spite of linguistic gains, many people with aphasia experience residual communication problems that significantly impact their daily lives. Those affected by aphasia report social isolation, loneliness, loss of autonomy, restricted activities, role changes, and stigmatization (Black-Schaffer & Osberg, 1990; Herrmann et al., 1993; LeDorze & Brassard, 1995; National Aphasia Association, 1988; Parr, 1994; Parr et al., 1997; Sarno, 1993a, 1997). Many of these long-term consequences are not addressed by traditional aphasia intervention. Such untreated psychological and social problems can increase disability, diminish community reintegration, and reduce response to rehabilitation (Sandin et al., 1994). The cycle of diminished participation in various aspects of "life" can take a drastic toll on self-confidence and personal identity.

In addition, funding sources have pressed for more "functionally relevant" outcomes and evidence that our services make a difference in the lives of our clients (Frattali, 1996, 1998a; Johnson, 1999; Warren, 1996). Restructuring in health care has forced us to balance quality outcome with cost of care (Frattali, 1996). Pressure from consumers, desire to improve outcomes, and changes in the health care industry suggest an urgent need for creative approaches that increase the quality of communicative life for those affected by aphasia. A social model provides a philosophical framework for developing interventions that fulfill these requirements.

EXPANDING THE MANAGEMENT FOCUS

In traditional aphasia therapy the emphasis has been on improving linguistic or cognitive processing. These restorative therapies have been effective in changing language performance. Such approaches tend to focus on the "impairment" of the individual with aphasia, and rely on formal tests and treatment probes to determine the level of deficit and degree of change after therapy. Certainly, restoration of communicative processes is an important goal for people with aphasia. However, gaps between changes on linguistic measures and "real life" functional performance of people with aphasia have been noted (Holland, 1998a; Simmons, 1993). Therefore, functional therapies have been developed to address performance of daily activities and communication "in use" (Aten et al., 1982; Frattali, 1998a; Holland, 1991). Functional approaches often focus on the ability to utilize compensatory strategies and perform typical tasks such as using the telephone or making a grocery list. The personal experience of aphasia and individual lifestyle adjustments have rarely been addressed in restorative and functional approaches. For example, in spite of improved linguistic processing and success on "functional" tasks, clients and families continue to report social isolation, loss of confidence, decreased roles, and limited communication opportunities (Parr et al., 1997). Frattali (1998a) argues for expansion of functional approaches to encompass quality of life and social participation. A social model expands intervention to address the living of life with aphasia including lifestyle changes and psychosocial issues.

CONTRASTING MEDICAL AND SOCIAL MODELS

A social model of management requires a shift from the traditional medical model that has been the prevailing paradigm in aphasiology (Sarno, 1993b). The influence of the medical model is evident in our practices. For example, clinicians plan and control treatment since the responsibility for "cure" and authority for decision-making is placed with the "expert." While professional expertise is needed, the marked power differential can create a passive, dependent "patient" who learns to "take the cure" with little participation in life choices (Pyypponen, 1993). In a social model, clients take an active, participatory role in their own health care decisions.

The medical model is also evident in our terminology. Thus, "patients receive treatment" as though treatment is a tonic that will cure aphasia (Pyypponen, 1993; Sarno, 1993a,b). When complete recovery is not the result, individuals with residual aphasia face discharge from treatment with little attention to chronic affects (Hersh, 1998). By contrast, the social model requires a view of aphasia in the long term. The focus shifts to optimally "living with" aphasia with an emphasis on health rather than illness (Pound, 1998b; LPAA, 2000; Lyon, 1992).

"Problems" tend to be located within the individual in a medical model. A social model orients away from defining the problem as situated wholly within the individual. That is, problems result from an interaction between the individual's organic condition and the social and physical environment (World Health Organization, 1997; Fougeyrollas et al., 1997). In a social model disability is a consequence of disabling attitudes and barriers imposed by society, not simply an impairment that resides within the individual (Fourgeyrollas et al., 1997; Pound, 1998b). Thus, aphasia is not only a disorder, but also a situation in which opportunities and rights are not readily available. Both internal problems and external barriers are addressed for optimal return of function and well-being.

DEFINING A SOCIAL APPROACH

The "social" of social approach refers to the broad concept that people are members of society and reside within a sociocultural context. As Goodwin (1995) describes, aphasia is more than a lesion within the skull; aphasia is also located outside of the person in dynamic relationships with others and in the social community. Thus, aphasia is addressed as an element of a social system and communication is viewed as a social act. Through communication we express and create our ideas, and also our personalities, our culture, and our life values. Communication fulfills a critical social goal when it allows us to reveal a healthy identity or "create a positive face" (Goffman, 1967). Because of the social significance of communication, disrupted communication entails social meanings and consequences, hence the importance of a social model.

INTEGRATING PSYCHOSOCIAL WITH COMMUNICATION

When social systems do not support communicative access, psychosocial well-being, and quality of life are diminished (Kagan, 1998). While psychosocial issues associated with aphasia have long been recognized, they have remained on the outskirts of therapy. Remediation of psychosocial problems tends to be divorced from the communication impairment and aphasia therapy. Typically counseling and education are considered the approaches of choice for psychosocial issues. Yet, these services are often unavailable or tangential to the "real" therapy. Also, psychosocial problems such as depression and loneliness are sometimes accepted as a natural and expected consequence of aphasia. Finally, the huge research emphasis on the linguistic dimensions of aphasia appear to have overshadowed psychosocial issues resulting in neglect of "the person" (Byng et al., 2000; Sarno, 1993a,b).

Attention to psychosocial dimensions of aphasia is integrated into communication intervention in a social model (Bouchard-Lamothe et al., 1999; Brumfitt, 1993; Byng et al., in press; Lafond et al., 1993; Muller, 1999; Muller & Code, 1989; Sarno, 1991; Simmons-Mackie, 1998b). Psychosocial issues are not separable from communication. Social affiliation and maintaining a healthy identity are a major goal of human communication (e.g., Brown & Yule, 1983; Fairclough, 1989; Goffman, 1959; Tannen, 1984). We craft our utterances and construct our interactions as a social and emotional endeavor. When communicative interactions are successful, we obtain emotional and social rewards. Through communication we obtain membership in a communicating society. This critical aspect of communication cannot be overlooked. Although often artificially separated in the literature, communication and psychosocial issues are woven together into the fabric of human existence. A social model aims to assist those affected by aphasia in fulfilling psychosocial needs through communication.

DEFINING APHASIA IN A SOCIAL MODEL

The definition of aphasia is expanded within a social model to reflect more than linguistic or cognitive processing deficits. Thus, aphasia is an impairment due to brain damage in the formulation and reception of language, often associated with diminished participation in life events and reduced fulfillment of desired social roles. Kagan (1995) defines aphasia as impairment in communication that masks inherent competence. Byng et al. (2000 p. 53) define functional communication goals in aphasia as "being able to communicate competently, through your own communication skills and those of others and feeling comfortable that you are representing who you are."

PRINCIPLES OF A SOCIAL MODEL

A social approach to aphasia management can best be conceptualized through a set of basic principles. Management within a social model is designed to 1) address both information exchange and social needs as dual goals of communication; 2) address communication within authentic, relevant, and natural contexts; 3) view communication as dynamic, flexible, and multidimensional; 4) focus on the collaborative nature of communication; 5) focus on natural interaction, particularly conversation; 6) focus on personal and social consequences of aphasia; 7) focus on adaptations to impairment; 8) embrace the perspective of those affected by aphasia; and 9) encourage qualitative as well as quantitative measures.

Dual Goals of Transaction and Interaction

Communication is designed to meet two primary goals: the exchange of information (transaction) and the fulfillment of social needs (interaction) (Simmons, 1993; Simmons-Mackie & Damico, 1995). In traditional aphasia therapy clinicians have focused on the transactional aspects of communication. For example, functional therapies have been designed to promote message exchange—to get ideas across in whatever way possible (Davis & Wilcox, 1985). Surprisingly, the social goals of communication have been largely ignored. While certainly the exchange of messages is important, the social goals are equally, if not more, important. Through communication we not only exchange information, but also develop and maintain an identity and sense of self, fulfill emotional needs, provide connections with other people, and promote our membership in groups. Appreciation of the social goals of communication is critical to fully addressing the consequences of aphasia.

Address Communication within an Authentic Context

Communicative change must make a difference in personally relevant contexts of those affected by aphasia. Much traditional aphasia therapy and most formal aphasia tests are conducted in relatively controlled contexts and focus on decontextualized tasks and discrete elements of language (e.g., naming, sentence completions). By contrast, natural communication occurs in a complex, dynamic social context with shifting expectancies, social roles, and goals. When communication is stripped of the natural context, we get a skewed appreciation of a person's communicative life. A full appreciation of communication within natural, personally relevant contexts is imperative to ensuring effective therapy outcomes. "Authentic contexts" are at the forefront of decision making, assessment, and intervention in a social model.

Communication as Dynamic, Flexible, and Multidimensional

Aphasiologists have evaluated communication in terms of "idealized" normal language. We assess "deficits" based on expectations of how a normal speaker would perform. While this helps determine an objective skill level, it potentially deludes us into viewing communication as invariant and static. In reality, informal communication includes dysfluencies, word errors, revisions, and sentence fragments (Button & Lee, 1987; Shiffrin, 1987). Following is a transcription of a question asked to a presenter at a recent aphasia conference: "so is this like one of the uh uh one of those that we've seen before...at least I have...and how can we be sure to make the uh uh reee uh make the shift?" No one seemed disturbed by this question proffered by a well-respected aphasiologist; yet, according to traditional standards the production would not be considered normal. In fact, such deviations are typical of the informal discourse of standard speakers. It is important that clinicians fully appreciate the flexibility and creativity of normal language in use. Many devices that deviate from "idealized language norms" are used in natural conversation to meet communicative goals. Tannen (1984) examines the use of interruptions and joint talk in normal conversation as a means of achieving affiliation in certain cultural groups. Utterances such as "oh," "well," and "you know" are used to bracket information and manage the flow of discourse (Shiffrin, 1987; Simmons-Mackie & Damico, 1996b). Goodwin (1987) describes purposeful "forgetfulness" as a strategy used by couples to bring a spouse into a conversation. Thus, strategies are often employed to serve a goal beyond the accurate and grammatical production of language. Perhaps in the practice of aphasia assessment and intervention, a more open-minded view of behavior and an appreciation of situated pragmatics are needed (Duchan, 1997; Simmons, 1993). Social approaches assume the flexibility and creativity of communication, and social goals are taken into account when assessing communication.

Communication is Collaborative

In a social model the focus is shifted away from the individual with aphasia and onto the collaborative nature of communication (Simmons, 1993). Conversation is a co-constructed activity in which participants negotiate important social actions and work to help each other understand with as little effort as possible (Clark & Wilkes-Gibbs, 1986; Goodwin, 1996; Milroy & Perkins, 1992). Research repeatedly affirms that communication is a collaborative achievement (Goodwin, 1995; Klippi, 1996; Oelschlaeger & Damico, 1998a,b). Social roles are established and maintained through interactive cooperation (Brumfitt, 1993; Simmons-Mackie & Damico, 1999b). Speaking style, content, discourse, structure and even opinions are modified to accommodate to speaking partners and context (Bell, 1984; Giles et al., 1973). A view of communication as a collaborative achievement requires expanding research and management efforts beyond the individual with aphasia to include the communicative skills of those "around" the person with aphasia and the dynamics of interaction.

Focus on Natural Interaction: Conversation

Conversation in its myriad forms has been labeled the primary site of human communication in our society (Clark & Wilkes-Gibbs, 1986). Until recently, very little research has focused on natural conversation in aphasia, assessment rarely includes a sample of natural conversation and few intervention approaches directly target conversation. Furthermore, "functional communication" is often defined in terms of very goal directed, transactional tasks such as cashing a check, asking for directions, or ordering in a restaurant. It is likely that the social chat that surrounds these activities is as important as the task itself. Therefore, success in and enjoyment of conversational interactions is a potentially important objective in aphasia intervention.

Focus on Adaptations and Enablement rather than Impairment and Disability

A social approach involves a positive stance towards life with aphasia. While impairment tends to be the focus of traditional aphasia therapy, successful adaptations to aphasia and ability (rather than disability) are primary in social approaches (LaPointe, 1996). Attention to the prevalence of adaptive strategies used by a person with aphasia can make a difference in our predictions of functional outcomes. In addition, the adaptive skills and attitudes of speaking partners of people with aphasia will influence the success of interactions. Therefore, emphasis expands beyond the adaptation of the individual with aphasia, to adapting society to enable the person's participation.

An overemphasis on deficits might obscure appreciation of adaptive behavior. For example, when asked to describe a client's naming response—"uh uh pen"—clinicians routinely described word-finding problems or processing delays (Simmons-Mackie, 1993). However, the "uh uh" behavior could also be described as a successful floor holding strategy. When communication is disrupted, nonstandard compensations might be required to meet communicative goals. Successful adaptations are often contrary to what are considered normal or preferred behaviors (Booth & Perkins, 1999). For example, one client with chronic aphasia often bombastically announced "I can't talk" when addressed by strangers. Analysis suggested that he preferred to "powerfully" terminate the interaction rather than expose his communicative "weakness." Thus, in order to meet his own identity needs, this man chose what some might consider a pragmatically undesirable behavior. What is deemed "appropriate" is judged in terms of the goal of the behavior and available alternatives. In a social approach the clinician focuses on the adaptive purpose of behaviors, builds on existing adaptations, and takes into account social as well as linguistic goals.

Focus on Social Consequences

As noted, a social model assumes that communication has a critical socio-cultural role. Impaired communication can be associated with social consequences and potential social barriers. Consequences are judged based on the personal experience of the communication problem, which will undoubtedly vary among those affected by aphasia. Thus, one individual with mild aphasia might experience no life changes while another individual with the same impairment might experience significant life changes and personal loss. Aphasia also creates personal and social consequences for family and friends who might experience stigma, embarrassment, energy depletion, and changed roles.

Consequences not only vary among individuals, but also might vary from one context to another. Thus, using a picture board to convey food choices at home might be quite different from using the aid in a restaurant with an unprepared waitress. In part, the personal experience of aphasia depends on cultural attitudes and knowledge regarding disability and expected life roles of those affected by aphasia. Addressing the consequences for all those affected by aphasia will help to promote a healthy social system.

The Perspective of Those Affected by Aphasia

It is difficult to address consequences of aphasia without a full appreciation of how those affected "perceive" these consequences. Consumer perspectives and consumer satisfaction are a priority. Rather than simply deciding what a client "needs," intervention is based on consumer perceptions of life changes, barriers to participation, and important life goals. Recent research confirms that people with aphasia are able to participate in interviews and ratings in order to share their perspectives (e.g., Hoen et al., 1997; Kagan, 1999;

LeDorze & Brassard, 1995; Lyon, 1998b; Parr et al., 1997; Simmons-Mackie & Damico, 1999a). Personal choice and autonomy are driving factors in management. That is, in a social approach those confronting aphasia chart the direction of intervention in concert with clinicians.

Qualitative as well as Quantitative Measures

In a social approach clinicians access the subjective experience of aphasia and describe outcomes relative to the rich authentic context of daily communicative life. Subjective experience and richly contextualized events call for qualitative as well as quantitative approaches to description. Qualitative approaches such as ethnographic interviews, personal narratives, and observational assessment provide important insights to drive management plans (Simmons-Mackie & Damico, 1999a). Qualitative and descriptive methods are gaining attention as viable additions to research and assessment (e.g., Booth & Perkins, 1999; Damico et al., 1999; Perkins et al., 1999; Simmons-Mackie & Damico, 1996a, 1999a).

EFFECTIVENESS OF SOCIAL APPROACHES

Although the social model is a relative newcomer to aphasiology and additional research is needed, a growing database is accumulating to support the notion that social communication, communication opportunities, and well-being are amenable to intervention. For example, improvements in communication, relationships, and social participation have been documented after training communication partners (Boles, 1997; Hickey et al., 1998; Hopper et al., 1999; Kagan, 1999; Lyon, 1998b; Lyon et al., 1997; Rogers et al., 1999; Simmons et al., 1987). There are also reports of positive effects of approaches that modify external barriers or facilitate participation in activities of choice (e.g., Garrett & Beukelman, 1995; Lyon et al., 1997; Simmons-Mackie & Damico, 1996a, 1999a). Elman & Bernstein Ellis (1999a,b) report positive effects of social group therapy for chronic aphasia on both linguistic and psychosocial measures. Integrating psychosocial support and access to social interaction into intervention has also been successful (Hoen et al., 1997; Ireland & Wotten, 1996; Kagan, 1999).

GOALS OF INTERVENTION WITHIN A SOCIAL MODEL

Socially motivated approaches conform to the ultimate goal of Life Participation Approaches to Aphasia—that is, to enhance the living of life with aphasia. In order to achieve the overall goal of living a satisfying life with aphasia, objectives might include 1) enhancing natural communication; 2) increasing successful participation in authentic events;

3) providing support systems within the speaker's community; 4) increasing communicative confidence and positive sense of self; and 5) promoting advocacy and social action.

ASSESSMENT WITHIN A SOCIAL MODEL

Assessment in a social model encompasses a variety of tools that document accomplishment within the goal domains outlined above. Traditional measures such as standardized tests remain appropriate to determine the level and pattern of deficits. However, measures of outcome beyond "linguistic skills" are needed to determine if intervention is making a difference in the lives of those affected by aphasia (Frattali, 1998a,b; Wertz, 1984). For people with aphasia, making a difference probably means returning to work, enjoying dinner with friends, sharing a good joke, or gossiping over coffee. Thus, assessment is designed to provide insight into well-being, personal consequences, and lifestyle effects of aphasia. Examples of assessment tools applicable to a social approach to aphasia are listed in Table 11–1. Measurements might include the perspectives of those affected by aphasia, professional judgements of communication and participation, or actual life accomplishments.

Perspectives of Those Affected by Aphasia

Ethnographic Interviews

Ethnographic interviews have been recommended to determine the personal viewpoints of those affected by aphasia (Simmons-Mackie & Damico 1996a; 1999a). By analyzing interviews before, during, or at the end of intervention, general themes are identified that help focus intervention or document outcomes. Candidates for interviews include both the person with aphasia and others impacted by the aphasia. Ethnographic interviewing and analysis requires training and practice in order to access the authentic perspectives of informants. Readers are directed to Spradley (1979) and Westby (1990) for explanations of the methodology.

Communicative Profiling System (CPS)

An approach to assessment based on qualitative research methods is the Communicative Profiling System described by Simmons-Mackie and Damico (1996a). Interviews, personal journals, and observation are used to identify personally relevant behaviors, social relationships, and situational contexts. Thus, the client and significant others catalog the behaviors that they consider significant to life with aphasia. A social network diagram is devised to represent the people with whom the person with aphasia interacts on a regular basis, as in Figure 11–1. Finally, the contexts or activities that the person participates in on a regular basis are described. Using the layers of description the clinician gains insight into communication patterns and motivations.

TABLE 11–1

Examples of Assessment Tools for a Social Approach to Aphasia

Obtaining Perspectives of Those Affected by Aphasia
Ethnographic Interviews (Simmons-Mackie & Damico, 1996a, 1999a; Spradley, 1979; Westby, 1990)
Communicative Profiling System (CPS) (Simmons-Mackie & Damico, 1996a)
Visual Analog Scales for Subjective Rating of Conversational Burden (Marshall et al., 1997)
Communicative Effectiveness Index (CETI) (Lomas et al., 1989)
Communication Profile (Payne, 1994)
Client/Family Self-Report Opinion or Consumer Satisfaction Surveys (e.g., Patterson & Wells, 1995)
Analysis of Personal Narratives (Barrow, 1999; Frank, 1995; Greenlaugh & Hurwitz, 1999)

Psychosocial, Quality of Life, and Well-Being Measures
Life Satisfaction Index (Neugarten et al., 1961)
Satisfaction with Life Scale (Larsen et al., 1985)
Life Satisfaction Survey (Chubon, 1987)
Ryff Scales (Ryff, 1989)
Affect Balance Scale (Bradburn, 1969)
Present Life Survey (Records et al., 1992)
Psychosocial Well-Being Index (Lyon et al., 1997)
Visual Analogue Mood Scale (Stern et al., 1997)
Code-Müller Protocols (Code & Müller, 1992)
ASHA Quality of Communicative Life Scale (Paul-Brown et al.; in progress)

Professional Judgments of Communication
Conversational Rating Scales (Erlich & Barry, 1989)
Conversational Interaction Rating Scale (Garrett, 1999)
Interactive Communication Scales (Lyon, 1998b)
Discourse Analysis
    Informal Discourse Rating Scale (Garret, 1999; Garret & Pimentel, 1995)
    Content Units (e.g., Yorkston & Beukelman, 1980)
    Correct Information Units (e.g., Nicholas & Brookshire, 1993)
    Lexical Efficiency (Helm-Estabrooks & Albert, 1991)
    Turns, initiations, time, & efficiency (Packard & Hinckley, 1997)
    Functional Scenario ratings (Lyon et al., 1997)
    Communicative effectiveness/content/efficiency
Measure for Rating Conversation Partner's Skill in Supported Conversation for Aphasia (Kagan, 1999)
Measure for Rating Aphasic Adult's Participation in Conversation (Kagan, 1999)
Communicative Effectiveness Ratings (Lyon et al., 1997)
Communicative Effectiveness Index (Lomas et al., 1989)
Everyday Language Test (Blomert et al., 1994)
Pragmatic Assessments (e.g., Penn, 1988)
Observational Assessment
    Catalogue barriers to participation
    Catalogue compensatory strategies
    Descriptive measures of #, success, type of compensatory strategies
Conversation Analysis Profile for People with Aphasia (CAPPA) (Whitworth et al., 1997)

Functional Communication Measures
Functional Assessment of Communication Skills for Adults (ASHA FACS) (Frattali et al., 1995)
Functional Communication Profile (Sarno, 1969)
Communication Profile (Payne, 1994)
CADL-2 (Holland et al., 1998)

Accomplishment or Participation Measures
Frequency counts (e.g., number of social contacts, number of activities, hours of participation)
Community Integration Questionnaire (Corrigan et al., 1998)
Social Network Analysis/Contextual Analysis (Simmons-Mackie & Damico, 1996a, 1999a)
Personal goal attainment scales

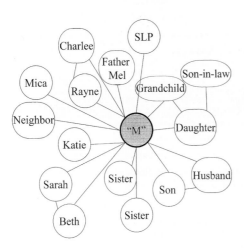

Figure 11–1. Example of a social network analysis for "M", an individual with aphasia (Simmons-Mackie & Damico, 1996a).

Quality of Life (QOL)

Another approach to assessment from the perspective of those affected by aphasia includes gathering self-reports or ratings of life satisfaction. Numerous measures are grouped as "quality of life" tools (Bradburn, 1969; Chubon, 1987; Fuhrer et al., 1992; Larsen et al., 1985; Neugarten et al., 1961; Paul-Brown et al., in progress; Records et al., 1992; Ryff, 1989). Typically, the person with aphasia and/or others affected by the onset of aphasia conduct a rating across one or more dimensions believed to represent aspects of well-being, satisfaction, or quality of life. Since these are highly personal and subjective experiences, those actually affected by aphasia should complete the ratings, and the dimensions rated must be meaningful and important to the person.

Consumer Satisfaction

Consumer satisfaction measures have gained significant attention in health care delivery (Frattali, 1996; Rao et al., 1998). Although most consumer satisfaction assessment relates to aspects of service delivery, Lyon (1998b) has applied the concept of perceived satisfaction directly to ratings of communicative interactions. Using a 5-point ordinal scale, clients or family members rate communicative comfort, confidence, connectedness, and pleasure to track qualitative changes in interaction (Lyon, 1998b).

Professional Judgments

Assessment from the perspective of the professional is another method of measuring outcomes. The speech-language pathologist evaluates performance as compared to defined target goals or expectations of "normal." In fact, most traditional assessment tools involve scoring or ratings completed by the professional to document aspects of communication.

Functional Assessment

Using tests of functional communication clinicians assess performance across a variety of categories or tasks typical of the daily activities of most people (Frattali et al., 1995; Worrall, 1992). For example, the clinician rates observed or reported performance on "talking on the phone" or "reading the newspaper." In a social model, interpretation of such data must be balanced with information on the personal relevance of each task since the importance of functional tasks varies from person to person (Davidson et al., 1999; Payne, 1994; Smith, 1985). Talking on the phone might be deemed highly important to one person, yet minimally important to another, even when their lifestyles appear similar.

Communicative Effectiveness Ratings

Analyzing communicative interactions using communicative effectiveness ratings is a prevalent approach. Aspects of an exchange such as success of message transmission, efficiency, naturalness, or pragmatic appropriateness are rated for baseline or follow-up data. Barrier activities, "simulated" functional scenarios, or samples of natural conversation provide contexts for rating behaviors of interest (Lyon et al., 1997). The interaction, not simply the behavior of the client alone, is an important target of assessment (Leiwo, 1994). Kagan (1999) has devised two scales that provide insight into both the interactional and message transmission skills of the person with aphasia and a communication partner. Communicative effectiveness ratings need not be solely from the perspective of the professional. Clients or others (e.g., family, friend, employer) can rate their own perceptions of communicative effectiveness, as in the Communicative Effectiveness Index (Lomas et al., 1989).

Observational Assessment

Observational data collected by the clinician in natural communication situations is valuable in documenting presence and success of adaptations or compensations. Increases in successful compensations and decreases in unsuccessful behaviors can be documented over the course of treatment. In addition, observation of natural communicative events provides data on barriers to participation.

Analysis of Conversation

Analysis of conversation is particularly relevant if intervention is to address changes in natural social interactions. Conversation Analysis (CA) is a potential tool for documenting communicative interactions (Perkins et al., 1999). Although application of CA principles to outcome measurement is only recently being explored, one tool, the *Conversation Analysis Profile for People with Aphasia*, is available (e.g., Whitworth et al., 1997).

TABLE 11–2

Example of an Inventory of Key Life Activities Pre-Onset of Aphasia at Assessment (2 Years Post-Onset) and After Participation-Focused Intervention

Pre-Onset	Initial Assessment	Outcome Assessment
Teaching 1st grade		Preschool volunteer
Church on Sunday	Church on Sunday	Church on Sunday
Cook for church (Wed)		
Carnival Club Secretary		Carnival Club attendee
Walk 2 miles daily		Walk with friend daily
Prepare family dinner		Host family dinner
Baby sit grandchild	Baby sit grandchild	Baby sit grandchild
Garden Club		
Gardening	Gardening (some)	Gardening (some)
Reading	Reading (news)	Reading (news)
	Television	Television

(Adapted from Simmons-Mackie & Damico, 1999a)

Accomplishment Measures

Participation Measures

Documenting life participation is a potential method of measuring change. If a goal involves increasing the number of social contacts per week or the variety of activities, then simple frequency counts document increases over time. Similarly, hours of participation might serve as a "quick and dirty" measure of increased activity. Measures of social participation such as the "Community Integration Questionnaire" (Corrigan et al., 1998) have been used to determine productive activity and social participation after traumatic brain injury. Lyon (2000) lists "obligated" and "free-time" activities pre- and post-aphasia to provide data on lifestyle changes. Simmons-Mackie & Damico (1996a, 1999a) apply social network analysis and activity inventories to identify social contacts and activities performed on a regular basis. Personally relevant changes in these inventories represent life participation accomplishments. An activity inventory for a person with aphasia who entered therapy 2 years post onset is presented in Table 11–2; it is clear from visual inspection that both the number and quality of activities increased after 'activity-focused' intervention. Similarly, social network maps (as in Figure 11–1) can serve as visual evidence of increased social relationships (Simmons-Mackie & Damico, 1996a, 1999a).

Goal Attainment Scales

Improvement over time can be measured with scales designed to judge movement towards particular individually defined life participation goals (Pound, 1998a,b; Simmons-Mackie, 1999). For example, the individual who wishes to participate in an adult education class works with the therapist to identify requirements to be achieved in order to meet this goal. Relevant scales can be developed to document achievement towards selected life goals. For example, return to work might be documented along an ordinal scale ranging from unemployed (rated as 1) to working full time at full pay with adaptations (rated as 5). Within the goal attainment scale each rating is defined (e.g., a 3 = half time, reduced salary/benefits). While results of such measures are not comparable across patients and do not inherently indicate the "significance" of changes (Hesketh & Hopcutt, 1997), personal goal attainment scales are valuable in combination with other measures.

INTERVENTION WITHIN A SOCIAL MODEL

A social approach to intervention involves the ever-present and explicit goal of enhancing overall quality of life and participation in activities of choice. Individual goals explicitly address practical and personally relevant outcomes. Specific objectives to be discussed below include 1) enhancing communication, 2) increasing participation in events, 3) providing support systems, 4) increasing confidence and positive identity, and 5) promoting advocacy.

Enhancing Communication

To participate fully in life, one important goal of intervention is enhanced communicative interactions. Thus, increasing communicative skill and confidence of the person with aphasia and/or potential communication partners might constitute a focus of therapy.

Expanding Skill and Confidence in Conversation

Skill and confidence in conversation is an appropriate objective of socially motivated intervention. Significant attention to natural conversation is only recently being addressed in the aphasia literature. As Leiwo (1994, p. 480) explains "a genuine social interaction with meaningful discourse topics sets different goals for communication than the more or less artificial metalinguistic tasks, role-playing tasks or discussions that employ stimulus pictures and cards. Different goals evoke different discourse strategies." Research supports Leiwo's statement. For example, traditional therapy discourse includes a pervasive "teaching" discourse structure—the Request-Response-Evaluation (RRE) triad in which the therapist "requests" the client to perform some task (e.g., What is this?), the client "responds" (e.g., pencil), and the therapist "evaluates" the response (e.g., "good job") (Simmons-Mackie & Damico, 1999b; Simmons-Mackie et al., 1999). This RRE structure is not typical of adult social conversation. Natural conversation—the everyday, ordinary talk that serves both social and transactional goals—involves varied discourse structures, creative discourse devices, varying social stances, and shifting social roles. This contrasts markedly with the relatively rigid structure of traditional therapy in which therapist-patient roles tend to be maintained and discourse structures are relatively restricted (Silvast, 1991; Simmons-Mackie & Damico, 1997b, 1999b; Wilcox & Davis, 1977). Even "conversation" between therapist and client often conforms to interview patterns, with therapists asking questions and clients responding (Holland, 1998b; Simmons-Mackie & Damico, 1997b, 1999b). Restricted discourse structures and passive roles provide little occasion for practicing the myriad skills typical of natural conversation. In order for people with aphasia to practice strategies for engaging in conversation then, mediated and supported opportunities should be provided.

Conversation Therapy

One means of enhancing conversational interaction is direct conversation therapy (Simmons-Mackie, 2000). Conversation therapy refers to planned intervention that is explicitly designed to enhance conversational abilities. It does not necessarily involve "conversing" during therapy, although usually a conversational context is appropriate. Conversation therapy is goal directed and individualized. It is not simply having a conversation. The goal of having a conversation is to exchange information and fulfill social needs. The goal of conversation therapy is to improve one's skill and confidence as a conversational participant. Conversation therapy focuses not only on message exchange, but also on social communication skills appropriate to specific communicative events. Thus, aspects of interaction such as power and control, variety of social roles, range of discourse structures, and issues of self-esteem gain equal importance to linguistic form and content. Improving skill in activities such as arguing, joke telling, story telling, and gossiping might be addressed, along with the usual speech act repertoire. Emphasis is placed on gaining confidence as well as building skill in participating in communicative interactions.

Enhanced Compensatory Strategy Training

Improving natural interactions often requires use of compensatory strategies. Traditionally, the individual with aphasia has been taught compensatory strategies designed to enhance message transmission across a variety of situations. For example, strategies such as gesture, writing, asking for repeats, and using augmentative aids are widely used to improve communication in the face of residual aphasia (Simmons, 1993). Training in such message transmission strategies has not always generalized as well as we might expect (e.g., Kraat, 1990; Simmons 1993; Thompson, 1989). One reason is probably related to the social appropriateness of strategies and the necessity for both parties to understand and use strategies. For example, Sachett et al. (1998) demonstrated that communication partners must modify their own communication to accommodate strategy use by the person with aphasia. Simmons-Mackie (1998a) suggests that accommodation theory might explain this to some degree—that is, people in conversation tend to alter their manner of communication to be "like" the other person's style of communication (Bell, 1984; Giles et al., 1973). If a nonaphasic partner does not use writing, then it is less likely that the aphasic speaker will feel comfortable doing so. Furthermore, most compensatory strategies are trained independent of their natural use; thus, natural social contingencies are not present. Also, strategy training has not emphasized creativity and flexibility in generating novel applications during the rapid, dynamic flow of conversation. Therefore, an expanded approach to compensatory strategy training is suggested.

In enhanced compensatory strategy training creativity, generativity, and interactivity are priorities. For example, rather than simply training a corpus of gestures or drawings, the client learns to generate ideas via drawing or gesture within a dynamic interchange. Examples include Lyon's (1995a,b) interactive drawing approach to training drawing as a collaborative effort between communication partners and Demchuk's (1996) creative communication approach in which people with aphasia generate pantomime scenarios using principles drawn from dramatic enactment. In such approaches, creativity and spontaneity are reinforced. Clients are encouraged and supported in generating their own novel strategies, and existing strategies are reinforced and expanded. Therapy is conducted in a richly contextualized interaction. For example, drawing is practiced within a conversational exchange in which both the client and clinician augment verbal productions with drawing. The person with aphasia is considered a partner in identifying and elaborating a strategy repertoire.

Interactive as well as transactional strategies are included in enhanced compensatory strategy management. For example, strategies for shifting the communicative burden or encouraging the nonaphasic partner to continue talking might be important methods for a person with severe aphasia to stay in a conversation. A range of variables are considered in selecting strategies such as the amount of "burden" placed on the partner (e.g., having to guess what a gesture means), stigma associated with the strategy (e.g., does it call attention), naturalness (e.g., performed relatively automatically versus requiring much conscious effort), time constraints (e.g., does it take too long), effect on the "flow" of interaction, and appropriateness in a specific context (e.g., attitudes, cultural norms) (Simmons-Mackie & Damico, 1997a).

We as clinicians must maintain an open mind about potential strategies. That is, many strategies are not "normal," yet they constitute the best available alternative for a given person. For example, avoiding interaction is often considered a "problem" by speech-language pathologists who are anxious for their clients to use their residual communication to participate in society. However, if the client feels that participating is more "punishing" than sitting home alone, then the avoidance behavior serves a necessary social objective. In such a case it might be important to identify "supported" activities that are rewarding and work towards building contexts that satisfy the client's social needs rather than eliminating a strategy without a viable alternative.

Conversational Coaching

Conversational coaching, introduced by Holland (1988), provides for practice of communicative scenarios with the guidance of the speech-language pathologist who serves as a "coach." The approach involves 1) identifying a goal or scenario to target in therapy, 2) planning what is needed, 3) developing a script and resources, 4) practicing with coaching as needed, 5) performing the scenario, and 6) evaluating the outcome. For example, one client wanted to "argue" with her dietician about her unpalatable diet. Planning involved identifying the main ideas, how to begin, possible strategies, useful resources such as pictures and written words, and important details to convey. Together, the client and clinician developed a scripted scenario. Practice sessions revealed a number of potential weak spots and alternative strategies. In addition, manner of delivery was targeted to avoid angering the dietician. In the process, strategies applicable to other situations were identified by the client and her confidence soared. Thus, a scripted scenario not only met a specific communicative need, but also served to build confidence and skill in general. In addition, the format of conversational coaching tends to "equalize" the roles of therapist (coach) and client

(communication player), creating a more "client-centered" approach. Leiwo (1994) also describes an approach that capitalizes on the communicative partnership between therapist and client. "Communicative speech therapy" emphasizes participation in symmetric discourse, encourages the client to take an active role in discourse, and considers "face saving" as a priority. Armstrong (1993) also employs scripts and texts to focus on various social functions and forms of discourse.

Group Therapy

Group therapy is an effective context for improving communication and well-being in aphasia (Elman & Bernstein-Ellis, 1999a,b). Moreover, groups provide an ideal context for conversation therapy. The key to addressing conversational skills within a group format is to focus on interaction rather than practicing didactic, discrete skills. Overlaying a "teaching" style and traditional therapy tasks (e.g., naming, sentence formulation) onto a group is unlikely to fulfill the requirements of conversation therapy. Rather, promoting conversation within a group context requires considerable skill in facilitating participation, equalizing control, and promoting confidence. Several texts are now available with information on managing aphasia groups (e.g., Avent, 1997; Elman, 1999; Marshall, 1998).

Scaffolded and Supported Conversations

One method of promoting conversation which works well in a group or role play context is to employ scaffolding techniques. In order to scaffold communication the clinician or other group members provide cues or facilitators within the natural flow of interaction. In other words, others mediate the participation of a person with aphasia. Damico (1992) proposes suggestions for scaffolding:

1. The clinician follows the communicative contributions of the client rather than controlling or directing the discourse. In other words, the clinician is available to expand and facilitate, but avoids "taking over" (e.g., asking all the questions, dictating topics, requesting performance).
2. Interaction emerges from a meaningful activity. For example, sharing photos of vacations might elicit more interactive communication than asking someone to tell about a trip.
3. Responses are mediated or facilitated within the natural give and take of the interaction. For example, the clinician might use subtle gestural prompts or write key words to support a client during the interaction.
4. Feedback should be appropriate to the communication event. If the communication is understood, then the talk proceeds; if not, then a request for clarification is in order. Thus, clients experience natural contingencies for communicative success and failure, rather than evaluative feedback such as "good talking."

Contrast the following examples of communication. A group of people with aphasia have watched a short excerpt from an "I Love Lucy" show.

Example #1

Clinician:	John, can you tell me about Lucy's job?
John:	(Laughs) Eating.
Clinician:	Well, (laughs) that is what she did, but what was her real job?
John:	(Shrugs)
Clinician:	George, what was her job supposed to be?
George:	Candy.
Clinician:	Good, she worked with candy. Claire what was her job?
Claire:	(gestures)
Clinician:	Right, she was supposed to put the candy in the box.

Example #2

Clinician:	(Laughing) Oh boy! Isn't that Lucy something?
Claire:	(Laughing) (gestures shoving food into her mouth)
Clinician:	(Laughs) (writes eating in large letters while Claire gestures)
John:	Eating, eating (gestures)
Claire:	Too much (laughing and gesturing).
Clinician:	Not too much for me—I could eat it all.
George:	Me too. Eat it all. Candy.
John:	Mmm. I like candy.

The first example is a didactic, clinician-focused interaction in which the therapist attempts to elicit specific responses from the group members. The second example is a scaffolded conversation in which the content and direction flows with the group interaction. The clinician provides a written prompt (eating) and models a verbal production (I could eat it all) within the natural give and take of conversation. Although scaffolded conversation is the intent, it is appropriate for both the clinician and group members to occasionally "step outside" of the interaction to serve as "coaches" and make "meta" comments or suggest potentially useful strategies.

Duchan (1997) expands on the idea of scaffolding discourse to suggest that the therapist support multiple aspects of the interaction. She provides guidelines for interactive therapy with children that can be generalized to adults with aphasia. She suggests that the role of the clinician shifts from that of "interventionist imparting knowledge" to that of "facilitator supporting role change." The supports provided include social (e.g., relating well, creating positive role identity), emotional (e.g., helping one another

save face, feel empowered), functional (e.g., achieving communication goals), physical (e.g., providing accessible materials), discourse (e.g., scaffolding), and event support (e.g., providing contexts, letting participants know what to expect).

Partner Training

Another method of enhancing communication is through trained and knowledgeable communication partners. Training speaking partners actually improves the communication of the person with aphasia (Boles, 1997; Hickey et al., 1998; Hopper et al., 1999; Kagan, 1999; Lyon, 1997, 1998b; Lyon et al., 1997; Rogers et al., 1999; Simmons et al., 1987). In fact, Kagan (1995, 1998) reports that onlookers judge aphasic speakers as more competent when they interact with a trained partner who provides "communication support." Thus, success of the interaction and judgments of competence depend not only on the person with aphasia, but also on the skills of the nonaphasic communication partner.

Partner training accomplishes several objectives. First, speaking partners learn concrete strategies to support communication when aphasia interferes. Second, trained speaking partners who employ augmentative tools provide a context that encourages the aphasic partner to use such modes. Third, training of partners results in altered expectations and perceptions of aphasic speakers. Once partners recognize that people with aphasia can be competent and interesting human beings, they are less likely to avoid interactions or feel bewildered by communicative failures. Finally, partner training can expand opportunities for communication. By alleviating embarrassment, feelings of helplessness, and fear, it is more likely that partners will provide supportive opportunities to communicate.

Direct partner training and feedback are necessary for interactive patterns and techniques to be learned and incorporated into daily use (Rogers et al., 1999; Simmons et al., 1987). Counseling or providing lists of do's and don'ts are insufficient. Moreover, communication partner training does not involve teaching partners to be "therapists" for the person with aphasia. In fact, such an approach often creates a teacher-student interactive relationship that differs in structure and social dynamics from natural adult social interaction. Rather, a successful speaking partner requires an understanding of how to facilitate a satisfying conversation. This includes knowledge of potential compensatory strategies and insight into characteristics of interactive communication. Appendix 11-1 lists examples of compensatory strategies for speaking partners of people with aphasia. In addition to successful communication strategies, partners need to learn how to create an interaction that feels natural and reinforces the confidence and autonomy of the person with aphasia. Research suggests that an empowering attitude might be as important as concrete strategy use for speaking partners of people with aphasia (Simmons-Mackie & Kagan, 1999).

Partner training is appropriate for family members, friends, colleagues at work, and the community at large. Thus, interactions ranging from social conversation with poker buddies to discussion with one's attorney can be facilitated when speaking partners are knowledgeable and skilled.

Increasing Successful Participation in Authentic Communication Events

Without opportunities to communicate, improved language is a trivial accomplishment. For most of us, communication takes place in the context of life activities. For example, people converse while eating lunch with friends, attending art openings, or playing cards. In fact, research suggests that subjective well-being and involvement in social activity are positively associated (Diener, 1984; Fuhrer et al., 1992; Fuhrer, 1994). Among individuals with physical disability "greater life satisfaction was reported by persons who were doing more to maintain customary social relationships…and spending more time in ways customary for their gender, age and culture." (Fuhrer, 1994, p. 362). In a social model the speech-language pathologist is responsible for increasing opportunities for communication outside of the clinical environment and for addressing barriers beyond the impairment of the individual.

One means of increasing participation in relevant communication events is to ensure that relevant life activities are accessible and successful (Lyon, 1996; Lyon, 1997; Lyon et al., 1997; Simmons-Mackie, 1993, 1994, 2000). Thus, activity-focused intervention involves identifying potential activities with the client and intervening to ensure successful participation. The activity need not be "communication centered"; rather, the goal is to enhance life participation. Once an activity of choice is identified, then the clinician in collaboration with those affected by aphasia determine characteristics of the activity that will be addressed to ensure success. This might involve working with the client to build specific skills or strategies and/or modifying the activity to accommodate the person with aphasia. It is particularly helpful for the clinician to participate in the identified activity in order to fully appreciate the requirements and identify an entry point that helps smooth the way for participation.

Prior or existing pastimes as well as new activities are appropriate targets of intervention. It is not the intent to strive for a "pre-aphasia" lifestyle. Rather, a satisfying life with aphasia is the goal. The clinician, client, and others identify activity goals such as hobbies, interests, functional tasks, volunteer jobs, or employment in which the client would like to participate. Through interviews prior interests and future aspirations can be gleaned. An interest survey can identify potential new activities. For example, clients might sort a large variety of activity pictures (e.g., grooming pets, cooking, gardening, painting, walking, etc.) into preference categories. In this way a rough inventory of preferences can serve as a starting point for identifying potential activities. It is important that choices are client motivated and that participation is directly facilitated. Simply identifying an activity and encouraging participation is generally unsuccessful.

Case Example

Moderate Aphasia

TG, a woman with moderate aphasia, expressed interest in returning to her bible class at church. In spite of improvements in communication and expressed desire to return to class, she avoided doing so. A visit to the event with the clinician was initiated. During this visit TG and the clinician met privately with the bible class teacher. At the suggestion of the teacher, TG agreed to pass out coffee and snacks, but insisted that she did not want to participate in the class discussion. The teacher suggested that TG and the clinician explain aphasia to the class. Since TG was visibly alarmed at this prospect, the clinician offered to present to the class. As TG greeted her old friends and served coffee her demeanor changed; the demands of serving did not require sophisticated conversation and allowed her a "soft" initiation back into the group. Interestingly, once the clinician began to talk to the class about aphasia TG "forgot" about her pledge to remain quiet and became absorbed in the discussion. During this discussion the therapist modeled various methods for facilitating interaction and made suggestions to the class members. Over the next few weeks, a variety of additional adaptations were identified. For example, the teacher provided TG with a written lesson script that TG could use to follow the discussion and access difficult words. The class began using a flip chart to write key words during the discussions; all agreed that this facilitated their discussion as much as it helped TG. In effect, the teacher and other class members learned how to support TG's communication and facilitate her re-entry into the class, and TG gained confidence in her ability to participate.

Activity-focused intervention shares similarities with traditional "functional therapies" that address performance of specific activities. However, many functional therapies focus on discrete tasks or generic skills such as writing a grocery list or ordering in a restaurant. Unfortunately, learning specific tasks does not ensure actual participation in the event. Functional approaches can be expanded to be more socially valid by ensuring that intervention is contextually situated and by modifying the environment as well as training the client. Thus, the functional task should be defined to address all parameters that will increase participation. Finally, a satisfying life is rarely limited to performing "chores"; therefore, it is important that an array of chosen life activities provide opportunities for socialization and fulfilling engagement.

In addition to activity-focused intervention, a related method of increasing participation is to identify and eliminate barriers to participation. Disability has been defined as a limitation of access to normal life due to physical or social barriers (French, 1993; Finkelstein, 1991; Byng et al., 2000). Fougeyrollas et al. (1997) have proposed a model of disablement that helps focus intervention on factors that affect participation. In this model both personal (internal) and environmental (external) factors affect one's participation in life (Fougeyrollas et al., 1997). Personal factors pertain to physical and psychological functions such as cognitive, linguistic, motor, or sensory integrity. Personal consequences, such as language processing deficits, are often addressed in traditional rehabilitation. Environmental factors include the physical and social structures of the outside world. Physical barriers include architectural, visual, auditory, or temporal elements that disrupt communication or participation. For example, attempting to communicate in a noisy bank lobby or trying to conduct business when impatient people are waiting in line could be very difficult for a person with aphasia. Societal barriers to communication include attitudinal, political, governmental, economic, and educational factors. Barriers can be observable such as complex written signs in buildings or hidden such as prejudice, negative attitudes, and ignorance. Garcia and colleagues 2000 suggest that sometimes a simple shift in viewpoint will reconfigure an impairment into a barrier that can be removed. For example, a person with aphasia who has difficulty talking on the telephone would be unable to perform a job that depends on phone use. Thus, the "verbal impairment" of the individual prevents job performance. However, if the individual with aphasia could perform the same functions using electronic mail, then "phone use" can be considered a barrier that could be removed to help accommodate the disability. This shift in focus away from the problems of the individual and onto the external barriers is an important paradigm shift required in adopting a social approach (Garcia et al., 2000).

Providing Communicative Support Systems within the Speaker's Community

Related to measures designed to increase participation in relevant activities, is the concept of providing an environment conducive to successful communication and participation. As noted above, this can be accomplished in part by identifying and modifying barriers within the environment. Similarly, it is important to identify methods of "enabling" participation such as providing physical and social accommodations. People with aphasia have a right to accessible communication and services even if this requires accommodations (ADA, 1990; ASHA, 1992). As Kagan and Gailey (1993) suggest, supported communication can be considered the "ramp" that enables people with aphasia to participate.

Trained Partners and Prosthetic Communities

Partner training (as discussed above) not only enhances communication, but also potentially expands opportunities for satisfying interactions. Thus, trained partners within an individual's community serve as "communicative support systems" and enable improved participation. In order to build expanded support systems, intervention might focus on training individuals within existing social networks. For example, a number of successful interventions with family members of the person with aphasia are reported in the literature (Boles, 1997; Hopper et al., 1999; Lyon, 1998b; Rogers et al., 1999; Simmons et al., 1987). However, social life usually extends beyond our immediate family. Therefore, potential communication partners outside of the immediate family might be identified and trained. For example, a friend within the community (e.g., fellow club member, neighbor) might be willing to support community "re-entry."

In addition, the support system might be expanded to include new communication partners such as new acquaintances, aphasia group members, volunteers, or peer mentors. Lyon (1992, 1997) has paired individuals with aphasia with a volunteer and worked on effective communication as a dyad. He also works with the dyad to identify an activity they can share as a means of facilitating life participation. Kagan (1998) and Hoen et al. (1997) describe community-based programs designed to provide opportunities for successful conversation between trained volunteers and people with aphasia. Peer mentors are another source of expanded social networks and supported communication. Peer mentors are individuals with aphasia who agree to visit, serve as social contacts, assist as advocates, help with counseling, or perform other needed services (Cohen-Schneider, 1996; Ireland & Wotton, 1996; Simmons-Mackie, 2000). For example, two people with aphasia might be matched to fulfill some need such as providing a ride to an aphasia group or helping with a project. The helping relationship serves both individuals since "helping others" is often an important missing element after the onset of aphasia.

In addition to training specific individuals to interact with people with aphasia, community training is an important element of a social approach. Community education at religious institutions, community organizations, businesses, medical facilities, or educational institutions increases public knowledge and promotes positive attitudes. Training people within the community in methods of supporting communication could have far-reaching consequences. Gradually, the "community" of people trained to support communication with people with aphasia can be expanded, resulting in aphasia-friendly "prosthetic communities."

Resources as Supports

In addition to trained partners, a variety of resources such as pictures, paper and markers, remnant books, written aids, vocabulary notebooks, maps, or communication boards can support communication. The *Pictographic Communication Resources Manual* is a collection of thematically organized pictures developed specifically to support conversation in aphasia (Kagan et al., 1996b). Garrett & Beukelman (1995) demonstrated that "thematic written support," in which the speaking partner writes key word choices during conversation, promoted increased participation of the person with aphasia. LeDorze (1997) suggested that institutionalized individuals with aphasia frequently remain "anonymous" to caregivers; life story notebooks that provide a brief history, family photos, and key life events can provide a context for sharing information with caregivers. Others have used remnant books or memory albums as resources to initiate topics and sustain talk (e.g., Bernstein-Ellis & Elman, 1995). In addition, changes in the physical environment can support communication (e.g., a surface for writing, changing seating arrangements) (Lubinski, 1981).

Increasing Communicative Confidence and Positive Sense of Self

Human beings place great value on feeling important and successful. In fact, much of our communication is crafted to present a public identity or "face" (Goffman, 1967). Our view of ourselves is "re-evaluated" constantly as we interact with others and obtain verification or contradiction of our perceived self-image and roles (Brumfitt, 1993). Communication and identity are entwined with the social roles we enact. Unfortunately, role change is a major consequence of aphasia. For example, unemployment after aphasia often results in the loss of a significant role and important part of one's "identity." Similarly, each communicative interaction has the potential to disrupt one's self-image as a competent person. The cycle of communication breakdown, changed social roles, and loss of identity can undermine the goals of aphasia therapy.

Therefore, a positive outcome depends on the development of a healthy sense of self with aphasia (Brumfitt, 1993; Byng et al., 2000; Sarno, 1993a,b, 1997). A robust identity not only contributes to improved quality of life, but also directly relates to one's willingness to use residual communication skills. The person who lacks confidence is far less likely to risk participating in social situations. Development of

productive new roles, robust identities, and healthy relationships often depends on external assistance or direction (Rolland, 1994).

Modifying the Structure and Content of Services

In part, a healthy identity can be encouraged by attending to how our services promote or inhibit an empowered identity. Impairment-oriented therapy might actually undermine the development of a healthy identity with aphasia by emphasizing what is wrong and exposing failures (Byng et al., 2000; Simmons-Mackie & Damico, 1999b). The social structure of traditional therapy could also devalue the person with aphasia by reinforcing the roles of "expert" therapist and "impaired" patient (Simmons-Mackie & Damico, 1999b; Simmons-Mackie, 2000). Byng et al. (2000) caution that we must sensitively negotiate work on impairments, keeping in mind the potential effects on the developing sense of self with aphasia. Perhaps by modifying the didactic structure of therapy and moving towards a collaborative partnership approach, we might enhance the client's autonomy and sense of self. Furthermore, moving the emphasis away from the impairment and onto the interaction and external barriers reduces the emphasis on individual problems.

Case Example

Anomic Aphasia

RT, a 55-year-old man with anomic aphasia, contacted a university clinic seeking therapy. RT was 10 years post onset and had functioned for the past 8 years independently. Although unemployed, he managed his own investments and enjoyed travel to visit friends. RT described his disability as "not too bad." His reasons for self-referral were to improve his ability to write letters and to converse in groups. RT attended the university clinic for an initial assessment that entailed administration of several standardized aphasia tests by a young female student clinician. Later, the student clinician and supervisor conducted a detailed counseling session to appraise RT of the test results. The assessment and subsequent conference were typical of a traditional evaluation. RT was visibly upset during the testing and conference. He remarked that he had no idea he was "so bad off" and appeared embarrassed to have "appeared the fool" in front of the "pretty girl." His usually outgoing personality gave way to depression as he faced his self-delusion regarding the extent of his disability.

This example raises an important ethical question: Was the exposure of residual deficits via standard testing in the best interest of this client? Standardized assessment did not allow RT to use many of his compensatory strategies to succeed. The assessment did provide a "window" into the pattern and severity of his language disorder; however, it also markedly impacted RT's self-confidence and sense of self. Traditionally, the importance of linguistic data might outweigh the negative psychosocial impact. However, a social model forces us to reconsider and weigh the overall impact of our practices on the person as a whole. This example is not an argument for eliminating standard tests; rather, it is an argument for carefully considering the client's stated goals and the potential impact of each procedure on communicative, social, and psychological well-being.

Modifying Our Own Language and Attitudes

Our language and attitudes can also empower or enable others. As specialists in language, aphasiologists undoubtedly know the power of words. Duchan (1997) describes "negative rhetoric" associated with medical approaches (e.g., disease causes problems, deficits) and more positive rhetoric often employed in participation approaches (e.g., challenges, supports). Shifting our usage to wording that avoids the biases of the medical model might help focus on living with aphasia over the long term. Thus, wording such as "patient," "treatment," and "discharge" implies a "treat and recovery" course similar to illness. Such terms reinforce the illness model and possibly allow us to shed some of our responsibility for long-term outcome. Substituting goals such as "reintegration" as opposed to "discharge" shifts the emphasis to the chronic nature of aphasia, and promotes a client-centered rather than service-delivery emphasis.

In addition, language can help those affected by aphasia learn that the "person is not the disorder" (Rolland, 1994). Too often the disability and the "self" become one (Goffman, 1963). Language can help externalize the disorder to reinforce that the person is far more than the aphasia. For example, saying "you seem to be having trouble with your bridge club" places the burden on the person, while saying "the aphasia seems to be getting in the way of participating in your bridge club" places the onus on the aphasia. Thus, problems are the disorder, not the person. Attention to service-delivery styles and language use can help ensure that our practices promote a healthy identity as well as improved communication.

Counseling and Psychosocial Support

In addition to examining the structure of therapy and our own language, speech-language pathologists have a responsibility for aspects of counseling (Brumfitt, 1993; Cunningham, 1998; Holland, 1999; Luterman, 1996; Muller, 1999; Wahrborg, 1989). Those affected by aphasia need information and guidance in exploring the effects of aphasia on their lives. The speech-language pathologist is uniquely qualified to help other professionals understand the consequences of aphasia, to teach supported communication, and to ensure that counseling needs are met. In addition, counseling and communication intervention overlap. For example, disability powerfully affects relationships and role boundaries within families and couples (Rolland, 1994). Typically, communication processes are critical for re-establishing a functional, balanced relationship. With aphasia the pre-onset modes of communication within relationships are altered. Focusing intervention at the level of the "couple" can assist both parties in identifying new ways of communicating (Boles, 1997; Lyon, 1998b).

Many aspects of aphasia group therapy fall squarely within the realm of counseling. Thus, psychosocial support groups, caregiver support groups, and self-advocacy groups have been recommended (Byng et al., 2000; Elman, 1999; Holland & Ross, 1999; Chapey, 2001). Groups provide a context for exploring topics related to living with aphasia such as identity, stress management, relationships, and emotions. Caregiver groups help those who experience aphasia as a family member or caregiver to address concrete issues, provide psychological support, and help build new identities. Self-help groups provide a mechanism for people confronting aphasia to define their own needs and assist each other in addressing these needs (Coles & Eales, 1999).

Self-Advocacy

Byng et al. (2000) propose self-advocacy as a means of 1) enhancing self-esteem, 2) developing skills and knowledge, and 3) promoting empowerment. Strategies for promoting self-advocacy include focusing on strengths, building social and political consciousness, promoting a "group" or community identity, gaining a role in community service, and ensuring that people with aphasia are partners in, rather than recipients of, services (Byng et al., 2000; Pound, 1998a). Pound (1998a) described a self-advocacy project in which people with aphasia developed personal portfolios. Like pictorial vitae many of the portfolios depicted "life" before and after the onset of aphasia. Clients reported that this process of examining their lives resulted in significant insights into their own identity and appreciation for their accomplishments since the onset of aphasia.

Self-advocacy groups have addressed topics such as identity and life roles, attitudes towards disability, assertiveness, or development of support networks (Pound, 1998a; Byng et al., 2000). Individuals explore personal values and identify values that are inconsistent with a healthy self with aphasia (Fuhrer, 1994). For example, placing high value on being an expert story teller might be contrary to achieving a satisfactory view of oneself. Instead of the "story teller" the person with aphasia might need to identify other aspects of his/her self upon which to build self-worth (e.g., pet lover, father, spiritual person). Clients can learn that methods of expressing oneself need not be traditional; painting, drawing, poetry, dramatics, and music also serve self-expression and release. Thus, exposure to other people with aphasia can help with the reassessment of life values and objectives.

Caveats of a Social Approach

Communication provides a foundation for maintaining autonomy—the right to make our own decisions, freedom from control by others, and the ability to enforce our own values. Thus, part of our goal is to promote choice, freedom from control, and expression of personal values. However, any therapy approach carries with it the potential for invading rights and privacy. Therapists must avoid imposing their own values and choices in the name of treatment. Expanding and supporting participation is not to be construed as a license to "remake" peoples' lives according to our own prescriptions and values. Work must be conducted in complete collaboration with those affected by aphasia and with an understanding of their values and desires. Confidentiality and sensitivity to intrusion into personal situations and relationships are extremely important. If partners are to be recruited and trained, the clinician ensures that the "help" is not invasive or embarrassing to those involved. Explanations of intervention procedures or "contracts" in simple written and pictograph form might ensure that clients fully understand the methods and objectives of intervention, and participate in the plan and implementation. Part of a successful outcome in aphasia involves enforcing a sense of one's own autonomy and personal rights.

Promoting Advocacy and Social Action

The role of the speech-language pathologist includes not only intervention with those affected by aphasia, but also development of social and political systems that support participation for people with aphasia. Advocacy means that we "practice what we preach" relative to inclusion. For example, people with aphasia can serve as aphasia group leaders or co-facilitate groups. People with aphasia can be "teacher-clients," rather than patients, in university clinics in recognition of their unique and valuable perspectives. People affected by aphasia are qualified to serve on our "boards of advisors" or as co-investigators in research. Aphasia group members can offer services as a "panel of experts" to educate others, such as allied health students or community leaders. Through these expanded roles, accessibility strategies are modeled. Such partnerships offer many advantages, not the least of which is the bold affirmation of the expertise and value of people with aphasia.

Speech-language pathologists and those affected by aphasia play an important role in building public recognition of aphasia and promoting availability of accessible services. Aphasia is a relative "unknown." In fact, in a recent public survey only 5% of those surveyed knew the meaning of the term "aphasia" (Simmons-Mackie & Stiegler, in progress). Aphasia is mentioned in the public press with much lower frequency than other disorders with similar incidence rates (Elman et al., 1999). The impacts of poor public awareness include reduced funding for research and services, lack of understanding and acceptance by the public, and barriers inadvertently reinforced by political and public actions (Elman et al., 1999). Advocacy activities promote the development of a "group identity" for those affected by aphasia and increase public awareness.

Along with public recognition, inclusion of people with aphasia in existing community services is needed. People with aphasia have a right to access information and services such as adult education and leisure programs. Texts that provide information about coping with aphasia can be made available to those confronting aphasia (e.g., Lyon, 1998a). Manuals written in a style that is "accessible" to people with aphasia can outline available resources and benefits (e.g., Parr et al., 1999). Pictographic "consent forms" promote access to health care choices for people with severe aphasia (Kagan & Kimelman, 1995; Kagan et al., 1996a). Organizations such as the National Aphasia Association (United States) and the Action for Dysphasic Adults (United Kingdom) provide support and information. Public education can help inform others of methods (as in Appendix 11-2) for increasing accessibility and participation.

THE FUTURE OF SOCIAL APPROACHES: EXPANDING SERVICE DELIVERY OPTIONS

With the advent of social models and changing health care systems, alternative means of delivering services are being explored and advocated. For example, the prevailing practice of offering treatment for aphasia only during the acute stage has been criticized (Elman, 1998; Lyon, 1992; LPAA, 2000; Simmons-Mackie, 1998b). Rather than shift from treatment to no treatment, a continuum of services should be available throughout the person's life with aphasia (Elman, 1998; Pound, 1998b; Simmons-Mackie, 1998b). Expanding our concept of services in aphasia requires that we recognize that aphasia is both an acute problem and a life-long feature for those affected. As people learn to live with aphasia and as life situations change, the need for and type of services will change. Changed living arrangements, marriage, death of a loved one, or an opportunity for employment can create new goals and challenges. Ideally, those affected by aphasia should have access to support and professional expertise during such life changes.

Services might constitute an array from which clients can select those appropriate to their current life goals (Elman, 1998). Thus, in addition to individual and group therapy, a range of services such as community-based programs, support groups, self-help programs, advocacy services, vocational programs, leisure programs, educational services, and counseling might be appropriate (Müller, 1999). An expanded service-delivery model will likely involve changes in our own services, as well as addition of services outside the domain of speech-language pathology. Expanding services beyond the health care umbrella to include social or community agencies is a possibility. Adult day centers and programs for the elderly might be re-engineered to accommodate those affected by aphasia. Adult education programs such as basic computer and internet training or art classes can be tailored to people with communication disabilities. Although not all of these services should or can be offered by speech-language pathologists, the speech-language pathologist is uniquely situated to ensure that varied services are adequately addressed. Thus, our roles, responsibilities, and payment sources are likely to shift as service delivery adjusts to changing demands.

CONCLUSION

Social approaches to intervention hold promise for promoting inclusion of people affected by aphasia in a communicating society. Creative and socially motivated approaches to the management of aphasia are emerging around the world. Such approaches have arisen from the belief that communication is more than putting words together to get an idea across. Rather, communication is part of the foundation of social structure and human dignity. This philosophy drives efforts to establish effective and efficient methods for enhancing the living of life with aphasia. This opportunity to retool aphasia management in keeping with a social model is both an exciting and daunting prospect.

KEY POINTS

1. Adopting a social model requires a philosophical shift from traditional, medical model approaches.
2. A social model is based on the belief that communication is a social act; through communication we create and express our ideas, our identities, and our life values, and assure our membership in society.
3. In a social approach, communication and psychosocial functioning are considered inseparable.
4. Intervention in a social model focuses not only on the communication and life participation of those affected by aphasia, but also on the communicative, physical, social, and emotional environment.

5. Long-term personal consequences of aphasia are the focus of intervention.
6. Traditional clinician roles and service-delivery models are likely to expand and change with the adoption of social approaches.
7. The ultimate aim of a social approach is to enhance the living of life with aphasia.

Activities for Review/Reflection

1. List all of the activities or events that you participated in over the past week. Consider the effects that aphasia might have on each of these activities or events. Choose one of the activities and consider methods for modifying the activity to support someone with moderate aphasia.
2. Discuss the differences between a medical model of aphasia intervention and a social model of aphasia intervention.
3. Explain the relationship between psychosocial adjustment and communication.
4. What are the principles of a social model as defined in this chapter?
5. Listen to a "real" conversation (e.g., friends, coworkers). Identify examples of the following within the conversation:
   a. Behavior designed to "save face" or project an "identity"
   b. Evidence of "collaboration" in conversation
   c. Behavior that "deviates" from accurate, syntactically complete sentences
   d. Strategies that seem to help manage the interaction rather than add specific "information"
6. Garcia et al. (2000) provide an example of reconfiguring a functional disability (inability to use the phone) into an external barrier (lack of availability of electronic mail) as a means of identifying accommodations for people with aphasia. Think of two examples of "problems" in aphasia that might be "recast" as external barriers.
7. How does assessment in a social model differ from "traditional" assessment (e.g., standardized aphasia tests, probes of language behaviors)?
8. How does traditional therapy discourse usually differ from natural, adult conversation?
9. What is "enhanced compensatory strategy training?"
10. What are four possible benefits of training the communication partner of a person with aphasia?
11. What is an aphasia-friendly "prosthetic community?"
12. Describe one method of enhancing a positive "sense of self" with aphasia.

References

American Speech-Language-Hearing Association (ASHA) (1992, June/July). Communication and the ADA. *ASHA*, 62–65.

Americans with Disabilities Act (ADA) (1990). Public law 101–336(s.933); July 26, US Congressional Record, 36, 104 STAT, 327–379.

Armstrong, E. (1993). Aphasia rehabilitation: A sociolinguistic perspective. In A. Holland (ed.), *Aphasia treatment: world perspectives* (pp. 263–290). San Diego, CA: Singular Publishing.

Aten, J., Caligiuri, M., & Holland, A. (1982). The efficacy of functional communication therapy for chronic aphasic patients. *Journal of Speech and Hearing Disorders*, 47, 93–96.

Avent, J. (1997). *Manual of cooperative group treatment for aphasia.* Boston: Butterworth-Heinemann.

Barrow, R. (1999). *Hearing the story: A narrative perspective on aphasia therapy.* Paper presented at the Dorset Mini-Conference on Aphasia, Dorset, UK.

Bell, A. (1984). Language style as audience design. *Language and Society*, 13, 145–204.

Bernstein-Ellis, E. & Elman, R. (1995, June). *A picture's worth a thousand questions: The use of a photo event journal with a severely aphasic patient and his spouse.* Paper presented at the meeting of the Clinical Aphasiology Conference, Sunriver, OR.

Black-Schaffer, R.M. & Osberg, J.S. (1990). Return to work after stroke: Development of a predictive model. *Archives of Physical Medicine and Rehabilitation*, 71, 285–290.

Blomert, L., Kean, M., Koster, C., & Schokker, J. (1994). Amsterdam-Nijmegen Everyday Language test: Construction, reliability, and validity. *Aphasiology*, 8, 381–407.

Boles, L. (1997). Conversation analysis as a dependent measure in communication therapy with four individuals with aphasia. *Asia Pacific Journal of Speech, Language and Hearing*, 2, 43–61.

Booth, S. & Perkins, L. (1999). The use of conversation analysis to guide individualized advice to careers and evaluate change in aphasia: A case study. *Aphasiology*, 13, 283–304.

Bouchard-Lamothe, D., Bourassa, S., Laflamme, B., Garcia, L.J., Gailey, G., & Stiell, K. (1999). Perceptions of three groups of interlocutors of the effects of aphasia on communication: An exploratory study. *Aphasiology*, 13, 839–856.

Bradburn, N.M. (1969). *The structure of well-being.* Chicago: Aldine.

Brown, G. & Yule, G. (1983). *Discourse analysis.* Cambridge, UK: Cambridge University Press.

Brumfitt, S. (1993). Losing your sense of self: What aphasia can do. *Aphasiology*, 7, 569–591.

Button, J. & Lee, J. (eds.) (1987). *Talk and social organization.* Clevedon, England: Multilingual Matters.

Byng, S., Pound, C., & Parr, S. (2000). Living with aphasia: A framework for therapy interventions. In I. Papathanasiou (ed.), *Acquired neurological communication disorders: A clinical perspective.* (pp. 49–75). London: Whurr.

Chubon, R.A. (1987). Development of a quality-of-life rating scale for use in health care evaluation. *Evaluation and the Health Professions*, 10, 186–200.

Clark, H. & Wilkes-Gibbs, D. (1986). Referring as a collaborative process. *Cognition*, 22, 1–39.

Code, C. & Müller, D. (1992). *The Code-Müller Protocols: Assessing perceptions of psychosocial adjustment to aphasia and related disorders.* London: Whurr.

Cohen-Schneider, R. (1996, November). *Peer support and leadership training program for aphasic adults.* Paper presented at the meeting of the American Speech-Language-Hearing Association, Seattle, WA.

Coles, R. & Eales, C. (1999). The aphasia self-help movement in Britain: A challenge and an opportunity. In R. Elman (ed.), *Group treatment for neurogenic communication disorders: The expert clinician's approach* (pp. 107–114). Woburn, MA: Butterworth-Heinemann.

Corrigan, J., Smith-Knapp, K., & Granger, C. (1998). Outcomes in the first 5 years after traumatic brain injury. *Archives of Physical Medicine and Rehabilitation*, 79, 298–305.

Cunningham, R. (1998). Counseling someone with severe aphasia: An explorative case study. *Disability and Rehabilitation*, 20, 346–354.

Damico, J. (1992). *Whole language for special needs children.* Buffalo, NY: Educom Associates.

Damico, J., Simmons-Mackie, N., Oelschlaeger, M., Elman, R., & Armstrong, E. (1999). Qualitative methods in aphasia research: Basic issues. *Aphasiology*, 13, 651–666.

Davidson, B., Worrall, L., & Hickson, L. (1999, September). *Activity limitations in aphasia: Evidence from naturalistic observations.* Paper presented at the British Aphasiology Conference, London, England.

Davis, A. & Wilcox, J. (1985). *Adults aphasia rehabilitation: Applied pragmatics.* San Diego, CA: College Hill Press.

Demchuk, M. (1996, November). *Creative communication in aphasia.* Paper presented at the meeting of the American Speech-Language-Hearing Association, Seattle, WA.

Diener, E. (1984). Subjective well-being. *Psychological Bulletin*, 95, 542–575.

Duchan, J. (1997). A situated pragmatics approach to supporting children with severe communication disorders. *Topics in Language Disorders*, 17, 1–18.

Elman, R. (1998). Memories of the 'plateau': Health-care changes provide an opportunity to redefine aphasia treatment and discharge. *Aphasiology*, 12, 227–231.

Elman, R. (ed.) (1999). *Group treatment of neurogenic communication disorders: The expert clinician's approach.* Boston: Butterworth-Heinemann.

Elman, R. & Bernstein-Ellis, E. (1999a). The efficacy of group communication treatment in adults with chronic aphasia. *Journal of Speech, Language, and Hearing Research*, 42, 411–419.

Elman, R. & Bernstein-Ellis, E. (1999b). Psychosocial aspects of group communication treatment: Preliminary findings. *Seminars in Speech & Language*, 20(1), 65–72.

Elman, R., Ogar, J., & Elman, S. (1999, June). Aphasia: Awareness, advocacy, and activism. Paper presented at the Clinical Aphasiology Conference, Key West, FL.

Erlich, J. & Barry, P. (1989). Rating communication behaviors in the head injured adult. *Brain Injury*, 3, 193–198.

Fairclough, N. (1989). *Language and power.* London: Longman.

Finkelstein, V. (1991). Disability: An administrative challenge. In M. Oliver (ed.), *Social work, disabled people and disabling environments* (pp. 19–39). London: Jessica Kinglsey.

Fougeyrollas, P., Cloutier, R., Bergeron, H., Cote, H., & St Michel, G. (1997). *Revision of the Quebec Classification: Handicap creation process.* Quebec: International Network on the Handicap Creation Process.

Frank, A. (1995). *The wounded storyteller: Body, illness and ethics.* Chicago: University of Chicago Press.

Frattali, C. (1996). Clinical care in a changing health care system. In N. Helm-Estabrooks & A. Holland (eds.), *Approaches to the treatment of aphasia* (pp. 241–265). San Diego, CA: Singular Publishing.

Frattali, C. (1998a). Assessing functional outcomes: An overview. *Seminars in Speech and Language, 19,* 209–221.

Frattali, C. (1998b). Measuring modality-specific behaviors, functional abilities, and quality of life. In C. Frattali (ed.), *Measuring outcomes in speech-language pathology* (pp. 55–88). New York: Thieme.

Frattali, C., Thompson, C., Holland, A., Wohl, C., & Ferketic, M. (1995). *The American Speech-Language-Hearing Association functional assessment of communication skills for adults (ASHA FACS).* Rockville, MD: ASHA.

French, S. (1993). What's so great about independence? In J. Swain, F. Finklestein, S. French, M. Oliver (eds.), *Disabling barriers—Enabling environments* (pp. 44–48). London: Sage.

Fuhrer, M. (1994). Subjective well-being: Implications for medical rehabilitation outcomes and models of disablement. *American Journal of Physical Medicine and Rehabilitation, 73,* 358–364.

Fuhrer, M., Rintala, D., Hart, K., Clearman, R., & Young, M. (1992). Relationship of life satisfaction to impairment, disability and handicap among persons with spinal cord injury living in the community. *Archives of Physical Medicine and Rehabilitation, 73,* 552–557.

Garcia, L., Barrette, J., & Laroche, C. (2000). Perceptions of the obstacles to work reintegration for persons with aphasia. *Aphasiology, 14,* 269–290.

Garrett, K. (1999). Measuring outcomes of group therapy. In R. Elman (ed.), *Group treatment of neurogenic communication disorders: The expert clinician's approach* (pp. 17–30). Boston: Butterworth-Heinemann.

Garrett, K. & Beukelman, D. (1995). Changes in the interactive patterns of an individual with severe aphasia given three types of partner support. In M. Lemme (ed.), *Clinical aphasiology, Vol. 23* (pp. 237–251). Austin, TX: Pro-Ed.

Garrett, K. & Pimentel, J. (1995). A triangulated model of outcome assessment in aphasia. Paper presented at the American Speech-Language-Hearing Association Annual Convention, Orlando, FL.

Giles, H., Taylor, D., & Bourhis, R. (1973). Towards a theory of interpersonal accommodation through language: Some Canadian data. *Language in Society, 2,* 177–192.

Goffman, I. (1959). *The presentation of self in everyday life.* New York: Doubleday Anchor.

Goffman, I. (1963). *Stigma: Notes on the management of spoiled identity.* New York: Touchstone.

Goffman, I. (1967). *Interaction ritual.* New York: Pantheon Books.

Goodwin, C. (1987). Forgetfulness as an interactive resource. *Social Psychology Quarterly, 50,* 115–131.

Goodwin, C. (1995). Co-constructing meaning in conversations with an aphasic man. In E. Jacoby & E. Ochs (eds.), *Research on language and social interaction* (pp. 233–260). Special issue.

Goodwin, C. (1996). Transparent vision. In E. Ochs, E. Schgloff, & S. Thompson (eds.), *Interaction and grammar* (pp. 370–404). Cambridge, UK: Cambridge University Press.

Greenhalgh, T. & Hurwitz, B. (1999). Why study narrative? *British Medical Journal, 318,* 48–50.

Helm-Estabrooks, N. & Albert, M. (1991). *Manual of aphasia therapy.* Austin, TX: Pro-Ed.

Herrmann, M., Johannsen-Horback, H., & Wallesch, C. (1993). The psychosocial aspects of aphasia. In D. Lafond, R. DeGiovani, Y. Joannette, J. Ponzio, & M. Sarno (eds.), *Living with aphasia: Psychosocial issues* (pp. 17–36). San Diego, CA: Singular Publishing.

Hersh, D. (1998). Beyond the 'plateau': Discharge dilemmas in chronic aphasia. *Aphasiology, 12,* 207–218.

Hesketh, A. & Hopcutt, B. (1997). Outcome measures for aphasia therapy: It's not what you do, it's the way you measure it. *European Journal of Disorders of Communication, 32,* 189–202.

Hickey, E., Alarcon, N., Rogers, M., & Olswang, L. (1998, June). *Social validity measures for family-based intervention for chronic aphasia (FICA).* Paper presented at the Clinical Aphasiology Conference, Asheville, NC.

Hoen, B., Thelander, M., & Worsley, J. (1997). Improvement in psychological well-being of people with aphasia and their families: Evaluation of a community-based programme. *Aphasiology, 11,* 681–691.

Holland, A. (1999). *Counseling adults with neurogenic communication disorders.* [Videotape]. (Available from American Speech-Language-Hearing Association, Rockville, MD, ASHA).

Holland, A. (1988). *Conversational coaching in aphasia.* Paper presented at the Deep South Conference on Communicative Disorders, Baton Rouge, LA.

Holland, A. (1991). Pragmatic aspects of intervention in aphasia. *Journal of Neurolinguistics, 6,* 197–211.

Holland, A. (1998a). Functional outcome assessment of aphasia following left hemisphere stroke. *Seminars in Speech and Language, 19,* 249–260.

Holland, A. (1998b). Why can't clinicians talk to aphasic adults? *Aphasiology, 12,* 844–846.

Holland, A., Frattali, C., & Fromm, D. (1998). *Communicaton Activites of Daily Living (CADL-2).* Austin, TX: Pro-Ed.

Holland, A. & Ross, R. (1999). The power of aphasia groups. In R. Elman (ed.), *Group treatment for neurogenic communication disorders: The expert clinician's approach* (pp. 115–120). Boston: Butterworth-Heinemann.

Hopper, T., Holland, A., & Rewega, M. (1999, June). *Conversational coaching: Treatment effects with an aphasic person and his spouse.* Paper presented at the Clinical Aphasiology Conference, Key West, FL.

Ireland, C. & Wotton, G. (1996). Time to talk: Counseling for people with dysphasia. *Disability and Rehabilitation, 18,* 585–591.

Johnson, A. (1999). Dealing with change in service reimbursement: Managing or caring? *Neurophysiology and Neurogenic Speech and Language Disorders; Special Interest Division 2, 9(1),* 6–8.

Kagan, A. (1995). Revealing the competence of aphasic adults through conversation: A challenge to health professionals. *Topics in Stroke Rehabilitation, 2,* 15–28.

Kagan, A. (1998). Supported conversation for adults with aphasia:

Methods and resources for training conversation partners. *Aphasiology, 12,* 816–830.

Kagan, A. (1999). '*Supported Conversation for Adults with Aphasia*^TM': *Methods and evaluation.* Unpublished thesis. Institute of Medical Science, University of Toronto.

Kagan, A. & Gailey, G. (1993). Functional is not enough: Training conversation partners for aphasic adults. In A. Holland & M. Forbes (eds.). *Aphasia treatment: World perspectives* (pp. 199–215). San Diego, CA: Singular Publishing Group.

Kagan, A. & Kimelman, M. (1995). Informed consent in aphasia research: Myth or reality? In M. Lemme (ed.), *Clinical aphasiology conference, Vol. 23* (pp. 65–76). Austin, TX: Pro-Ed.

Kagan, A., Winckel, J., & Shumway, E. (1996a). *Pictographic Communication Resources.* North York, Canada: Pat Arato Aphasia Centre.

Kagan, A., Winckel, J., & Shumway E. (1996b). Supported Conversation for aphasic adults: Increasing communicative access [Videotape]. (available from Pat Arato Aphasia Centre. North York, Ontario, Canada).

Klippi, A. (1996). *Conversation as an achievement in aphasics. Studia Fennica Linguistica 6.* Helsinki: Finnish Literature Society.

Kraat, A. (1990). Augmentative and alternative communication: Does it have a future in aphasia rehabilitation? *Aphasiology, 4,* 321–338.

Lafond, D., DeGiovani, R., Joanette, Y., Ponzio, J., & Sarno, M.T. (eds.), (1993). *Living with aphasia.* San Diego, CA: Singular Publishing Group.

Lapointe, L. (1996). Adaptation, accommodation, aristos. In L. LaPointe (ed.), *Aphasia and related neurogenic disorders* (2nd ed.). New York: Theime.

Larsen, R., Diener, R., & Emmons, R. (1985). An evaluation of subjective well-being measures. *Social Indicators Research, 17,* 1–17.

LeDorze, G. & Brassard, C. (1995). A description of the consequences of aphasia on aphasic persons and their relatives and friends based on the WHO model of chronic diseases. *Aphasiology, 9,* 239–255.

LeDorze, G. (1997). *Towards understanding communication in communication disorders such as aphasia.* Paper presented at the Nontraditional Approaches to Aphasia Conference, Yountville, CA.

Leiwo, M. (1994). Aphasia and communicative speech therapy. *Aphasiology, 8,* 467–482.

Lomas, J., Pickard, L., Bester, S., Elbard, H., Finlayson, A., & Zoghaib, C. (1989). The Communication Effectiveness Index: Development and psychometric evaluation of a functional communication measure for adult aphasia. *Journal of Speech and Hearing Disorders, 54,* 113–124.

LPAA Project Group (2000). Life participation approaches to aphasia: A Statement of Values for the Future. *ASHA Leader, 3,* 4–6.

Lubinski, R. (1981). Environmental language intervention. In R. Chapey (ed.), *Language intervention strategies in adult aphasia* (1st ed.) (pp. 223–245). Baltimore: Williams & Wilkins.

Luterman, D. (1996). *Counseling persons with communication disorders and their families* (3rd ed.). Austin, TX: Pro-Ed.

Lyon, J. (1992). Communication use and participation in life for adults with aphasia in natural settings: The scope of the problem. *American Journal of Speech-Language Pathology, 1,* 7–14.

Lyon J. (1995a). Drawing: Its value as a communication aid for adults with aphasia. *Aphasiology, 9,* 33–50.

Lyon, J. (1995b). Communicative drawing: An augmentative mode of interaction. *Aphasiology, 9,* 84–94.

Lyon, J. (1996). Optimizing communication and participation in life for aphasic adults and their prime caregivers in natural settings: A use model for treatment. In G. Wallace (ed.), *Adult aphasia rehabilitation* (pp. 137–160). Newton, MA: Butterworth Heinemann.

Lyon, J. (1997). Volunteers and partners: Moving intervention outside the treatment room. In B. Shadden & M.T. Toner (eds.), *Communication and aging* (pp. 299–324). Austin, TX: Pro-Ed.

Lyon, J. (1998a). *Coping with aphasia.* San Diego, CA: Singular Publishing.

Lyon, J. (1998b). Treating real-life functionality in a couple coping with severe aphasia. In N. Helm-Estabrooks & A. Holland (eds.), *Approaches to the treatment of aphasia* (pp. 203–239). San Diego, CA: Singular Publishing.

Lyon, J. (2000). Finding, defining, and refining functionality in real-life for people confronting aphasia. In L. Worrall & C. Frattali (eds.), *Neurogenic communication disorders: A functional approach.* (pp. 137–161). New York: Thieme.

Lyon, J., Cariski, D., Keisler, L., Rosenbek, J., Levine, R., Kumpula, J., Ryff, D., Coyne, S., & Levine, J. (1997). Communication partners: Enhancing participation in life and communication for adults with aphasia in natural settings. *Aphasiology, 11,* 693–708.

Marshall, R. (1998). *Introduction to group treatment for aphasia: Design and management.* Boston, MA: Butterworth-Heinemann.

Marshall, R., Freed, D., & Phillips, D. (1997). Communicative efficiency in severe aphasia. *Aphasiology, 11,* 373–384.

Milroy, L. & Perkins, L. (1992). Repair strategies in aphasic discourse: Towards a collaborative model. *Clinical Linguistics and Phonetics, 6,* 17–40.

Müller, D. (1999). Managing psychosocial adjustment in aphasia. *Seminars in Speech and Language, 20,* 85–92.

Müller, D.J. & Code, C. (1989). Interpersonal perceptions of psychosocial adjustment to aphasia. In C. Code & D. Müller (eds.), *Aphasia therapy* (2nd ed.) (pp. 101–112). London: Cole & Whurr.

National Aphasia Association (1988). Impact of aphasia on patients and family: Results of a needs survey. New York: NAA.

Neugarten, B., Havighurst, R., & Tobin, S. (1961). The measurment of life satisfaction. *Journal of Gerontology, 16,* 134–143.

Nicholas, L. & Brookshire, R. (1993). A system for quantifying the informativeness and efficiency of the connected speech of adults with aphasia. *Journal of Speech and Hearing Research, 36,* 338–350.

Oelschlaeger, M. & Damico, J. (1998a). Spontaneous verbal repetition: A social strategy in aphasic conversation. *Aphasiology, 12,* 971–988.

Oelschlaeger, M. & Damico, J. (1998b). Joint productions as a conversational strategy in aphasia. *Clinical Linguistics and Phonetics, 12,* 459–480.

Packard, M. & Hinckley, J. (1997). *Measuring conversational burden in adults with moderate and severe aphasia.* Paper presented at the American Speech-Language-Hearing Association Annual Convention, Boston.

Parr, S. (1994). Coping with aphasia: Conversations with 20 aphasic people, *Aphasiology, 8,* 457–466.

Parr, S. (1996b). Everyday literacy in aphasia: Radical approaches to functional assessment and therapy. *Aphasiology, 10,* 469–479.

Parr, S., Pound, C., Byng, S., & Long, B. (1999). *The aphasia handbook*. Leicestershire, UK: Ecodistribution.

Parr, S., Byng, S., Gilpin, S., & Ireland, S. (1997). *Talking about aphasia: Living with loss of language after stroke*. Buckingham, UK: Open University Press.

Patterson, R. & Wells, A. (1995). Involving the family in planning for life with aphasia. *Topics in Stroke Rehabilitation, 2*, 39–46.

Paul-Brown, D., Frattali, C., Holland, A., Thompson, C., & Caperton, C. (in progress). *Quality of Communicative Life Scale*. Rockville, MD: American Speech-Language-Hearing Association.

Payne, J. (1994). *Communication profile: A functional skills inventory*. San Antonio, TX: Communication Skill Builders.

Penn, C. (1988). The profiling of syntax and pragmatics in aphasia. *Clinical Linguistics and Phonetics, 6*, 11–25.

Perkins, L., Crisp, J., & Walshaw, D. (1999). Exploring conversation analysis as an assessment tool for aphasia: The issue of reliability. *Aphasiology, 13*, 259–282.

Pound, C. (1998a). *Power, partnerships and perspectives: Social model approaches to long term aphasia therapy and support*. Paper presented at the 8th International Aphasia Rehabilitation Conference, S. Africa.

Pound, C. (1998b). Therapy for life: Finding new paths across the plateau. *Aphasiology, 12*, 222–227.

Pyypponen, V. (1993). The point of view of the clinician. *Aphasiology, 7*, 579–581.

Rao, P., Blosser, J., & Huffman, N. (1998). Measuring consumer satisfaction. In C. Frattali (ed.), *Measuring outcomes in speech-language pathology* (pp. 89–112). New York: Thieme.

Records, N., Tomblin, J., & Freese, P. (1992). The quality of life of young adults with histories of specific language impairment. *American Journal of Speech-Language Pathology, 1*, 44–53.

Rogers, M., Alarcon, N., & Olswang, L. (1999). Aphasia management considered in the context of the WHO model of disablements. In I.R. Odderson & E. Halar (eds.), *Physical Medicine and Rehabilitation Clinics of North America on Stroke*. (pp. 907–923). Philadelphia: WB Saunders.

Rolland, J.S. (1994). In sickness and in health: The impact of illness on couples' relationships. *Journal of Marital and Family Therapy, 20*, 327–347.

Ryff, C. (1989). Scales of psychological well being (short form). *Journal of Personality and Social Psychology, 57*, 1069–1081.

Sachett, C., Byng, S., Marshall, J., & Pound, C. (1998). Drawing together: Evaluation of a therapy programme for severe aphasia. *International Journal of Disorders of Language.*

Sandin, K., Cifu, D., & Noll, S. (1994). Stroke rehabilitation. Psychological and social implications. *Archives of Physical Medicine and Rehabilitation, 75*, S52–S55.

Sarno, M.T. (1969). *Functional Communication Profile*. New York: Institute for Rehabilitation Medicine, NYU Medical Center.

Sarno, M.T. (1991). The psychological and social sequelae of aphasia. In M.T. Sarno (ed.), *Acquired aphasia* (2nd ed.) (pp. 521–582). San Diego, CA: Academic Press.

Sarno, M.T. (1993a). Aphasia rehabilitation: Psychosocial and ethical considerations, *Aphasiology, 7*, 321–334.

Sarno, M.T. (1993b). Ethical-moral dilemmas in aphasia rehabilitation. In D. Lafond, R. DeGiovani, Y. Joannette, J. Ponzio, & M. Sarno (eds.), *Living with aphasia: Psychosocial issues* (pp. 269–277). San Diego, CA: Singular Publishing.

Sarno, M.T. (1997). Quality of life in aphasia in the first post-stroke year. *Aphasiology, 11*, 665–678.

Shiffrin, D. (1987). *Discourse markers*. Cambridge, UK: Cambridge University Press.

Silvast, M. (1991). Aphasia therapy dialogues. *Aphasiology, 5*, 383–390.

Simmons, N. (1993). *An ethnographic investigation of compensatory strategies in aphasia*. Ann Arbor, MI: University Microfilms International.

Simmons, N., Kearns, K., & Potechin, G. (1987). Treatment of aphasia through family member training. In R. Brookshire (ed.), *Clinical aphasiology conference proceedings, Vol. 17* (pp. 106–116). Minneapolis, MN: BRK.

Simmons-Mackie, N. (1993). *Management of aphasia: Towards a social model*. Workshop presented at the Julie McGee Lambeth Conference, Denton, TX.

Simmons-Mackie, N. (1994). *Treatment of aphasia: Incorporating a social model of communication*. Workshop presented at the Aphasia Centre, North York, Toronto, Canada.

Simmons-Mackie, N. (1998a). In support of supported communication for adults with aphasia. *Aphasiology, 12*, 831–838.

Simmons-Mackie, N. (1998b). A solution to the discharge dilemma in aphasia: Social approaches to aphasia management. *Aphasiology, 12*, 231–239.

Simmons-Mackie, N. (2000). Social approaches to the management of aphasia. In L. Worrall, L. & C. Frattali (eds.), *Neurogenic communication disorders: A functional approach*. (pp. 162–187) New York: Thieme.

Simmons-Mackie, N., Damico, J., & Damico, H. (1999). A qualitative study of feedback in aphasia therapy. *American Journal of Speech-Language Pathology, 8*, 218–230.

Simmons-Mackie, N. & Damico, J. (1995). Communicative competence in aphasia: Evidence from compensatory strategies. *Clinical aphasiology, Vol. 23* (pp. 95–105). Austin, TX: Pro-Ed.

Simmons-Mackie, N. & Damico, J. (1996a). Accounting for handicaps in aphasia: Communicative assessment from an authentic social perspective. *Disability and Rehabilitation, 18*, 540–549.

Simmons-Mackie, N. & Damico, J. (1996b). The contribution of discourse markers to communicative competence in aphasia. *American Journal of Speech-Language Pathology, 5*, 37–43.

Simmons-Mackie, N. & Damico, J. (1997a). Reformulating the definition of compensatory strategies in aphasia. *Aphasiology, 8*, 761–781.

Simmons-Mackie, N. & Damico, J. (1997b). *Support for nontraditional approaches to aphasia: Evidence from conversation analysis*. Paper presented at the Nontraditional Approaches to Aphasia Conference, Yountville, CA.

Simmons-Mackie, N. & Damico, J. (1999a, November). *Intervention outcomes: Clinical applications of qualitative methods*. Presentation at the American Speech-Language-Hearing Association Annual Convention, San Francisco, CA.

Simmons-Mackie, N. & Damico, J. (1999b). Social role negotiation in aphasia therapy: Competence, incompetence and conflict. In D. Kovarsky, J. Duchan, & M. Maxwell (eds.), *Constructing (in)competence: Disabling evaluations in clinical and social interaction*. Mahwah, NJ: Erlbaum.

Simmons-Mackie, N. & Kagan, A. (1999). Communication strategies used by 'good' versus 'poor' speaking partners of individuals with aphasia. *Aphasiology, 13*, 807–820.

Simmons-Mackie, N. & Stiegler, L. (in progress). Public awareness of aphasia: A survey.

Smith, L. (1985). Communicative activities of dysphasic adults: A survey. *British Journal of Disorders of Communication, 20,* 31–44.

Spradley, J. (1979). *The ethnographic interview.* New York: Holt, Rinehart & Winston.

Stern, R., Arruda, J., Hooper, C., Wolfner, G., & Morey, C. (1997). Visual analogue mood scales to measure internal mood state in neurologically impaired patients: Description and initial validity evidence. *Aphasiology, 11,* 59–71.

Tannen, D. (1984). *Conversational style: Analyzing talk among friends.* Norwood, NJ: Ablex.

Thompson, C. (1989). Generalization research in aphasia: A review of the literature. In T. Prescott (ed.), *Clinical aphasiology, Vol. 18* (pp. 195–222). Boston: College-Hill Press.

Wahrborg, P. (1989). Aphasia and family therapy. *Aphasiology, 3,* 479–482.

Warren, R. (1996). Outcome measurement: Moving toward the patient. *ASHA Special Interest Divisions-Neurophysiology and Neurogenic Speech and Language Disorders, 6,* 5–6.

Wertz, R. (1984). Language disorders in adults: State of the clinical art. In A. Holland (ed.), *Language disorders in adults* (pp. 1–78). San Diego, CA: College Hill.

Westby, C. (1990). Ethnographic interviewing: Asking the right questions to the right people in the right ways. *Journal of Childhood Communication Disorders, 13,* 101–112.

Whitworth, A., Perkins, L., & Lesser, R. (1997). *Conversation Analysis Profile for People with Aphasia.* London: Whurr.

Wilcox, J. & Davis, A. (1997). Speech act analysis of aphasic communication in individual and group settings. In R. Brookshire (ed.), *Clinical aphasiology conference proceedings* (pp. 166–174). Minneapolis, MN: BRK.

World Health Organization (1997). International Classification of Impairments, Activities and Participation, ICIDH-2. *A manual of dimensions of disablement and functions.* Beta-1 draft for field trials. Geneva, Switzerland: World Health Organization.

Worrall, L. (1992). Functional communication assessment: An Australian perspective. *Aphasiology, 6,* 105–111.

Yorkston, K. & Beukelman, D. (1980). An analysis of connected speech samples of aphasic and normal speakers. *Journal of Speech and Hearing Disorders, 45,* 27–36.

APPENDIX 11-1
Examples of Strategies for Communication Partners of People with Aphasia

Slow the rate of speech
Chunk ideas with pauses between
Insert pauses between topics
Simplify sentence structure
Convey one idea at a time
Place key information at the end of the sentence
Repeat key words
Write key words as referents
Rephrase when not understood
Use direct instead of indirect referents (Mary vs. she)
Use gestures, body lean, and gaze to shift topics
Use verbal terminators to end a topic ("so much for that")
Use verbal introductions to open topics ("Let's talk about...")
Use redundancy ("Where's Spot, the dog?" vs "Where's Spot?")
Use alerting phrases or gestures (touch, "uhh, John")
Emphasize key content with stress and intonation
Tolerate silence of the other person
Use gestures and pantomime to add information while talking
Backchannel to encourage the aphasic speaker (I see, oh yes)
Paraphrase, summarize, or reinterpret to verify, elaborate, and sustain topic

Verify your understanding by paraphrasing, repeating, or questioning as needed
Use "thematic written support" (Garrett & Beukelman, 1995)
Use props (magazines, photo albums, pictures)
Subtly incorporate words that the person with aphasia "didn't get" into your own utterances
Get information from his/her body language—focus on more than the talk
Progress from general to specific in questioning
Provide and use paper and markers to support talk
Draw or write key ideas while talking
Use the augmentative strategies of the person with aphasia to model and establish equality
Use the environment (talk about a picture on the wall)
Establish shared experiences as topics (sports, gardening)
Focus on doing things together versus carrying out discussions
Avoid teaching comments such as "you said that right"
Reflect feelings communicated nonverbally ("Oh boy, that makes you angry")
Establish equality in relationship by following the aphasic individual's lead; acknowledge opinions, etc.

APPENDIX 11-2
Advocacy Strategies for Supporting Participation (adapted from ASHA, 1992)

Build public awareness and understanding of aphasia

Establish attitudes and behaviors that promote inclusion

Promote public knowledge of facilitating behaviors and accommodations

Provide communication aids & materials to support communication

Provide communication in an accessible format (e.g., alternatives such as pictures and written instructions, multiple modality communication, large print)

Encourage environmental adaptations to promote communication (reduced noise, provide alerting systems; make speakers visible to the person with aphasia, alter signage)

Alter information complexity

Prepare for management of emergency or unexpected situations (e.g., written message for transport driver, police, or hospital staff)

Provide accessible information regarding services

Chapter 12

Environmental Systems Approach to Adult Aphasia

Rosemary Lubinski

The concept of "functional" dominated rehabilitation in the 1990s. Rehabilitation specialists are being required by private and government health care insurers, and by consumers themselves, to demonstrate in unambiguous, realistic terms how therapeutic intervention makes a qualitative difference in the everyday life of the patient. Numerous trends in health care have spawned this focus, and the most potent of these is the rapidly escalating costs of rehabilitation, particularly to older adults. From 1984 to 1987 alone, Medicare-covered rehabilitation costs tripled from $405 million to $1.3 billion (Langenbrunner et al., 1989). Hospitals and rehabilitation departments must justify who will benefit from rehabilitation, what methods are most efficacious, and what the expected functional outcomes are. The underlying theme is "Are the outcomes of therapy worth the cost?" In the near future, we can expect to see a functional status prospective payment system for Medicare and Medicaid patients in rehabilitation programs. Such a payment plan is likely to revolutionize aphasia therapy. (See Wilkerson et al., 1992, for an in-depth discussion of functional status payment for rehabilitation.)

Speech-language pathologists have recognized for some time that functional assessment and intervention with adult aphasics must go beyond traditional approaches that focus on isolated cognitive or communicative skills (e.g., Aten, 1986; Aten et al., 1982; Davis, 1986; Davis & Wilcox, 1981; Holland, 1980, 1982; Lubinski, 1981, 1988, 1991; Lyon, 1992; Wertz, 1983). In 1990 ASHA (1990) recently convened an advisory committee that defined functional communication as the "ability to receive a message or to convey a message, regardless of mode, to communicate effectively and independently in a given environment." Following from this definition, functional assessment of communication involves evaluating the ability of individuals and their communicative environment to accommodate to the communication problem, thus achieving the highest level of quality of life possible. For aphasic individuals, accommodation entails improvement of communication skills and coping with changes in their physical and social environment. For the environment,

accommodation involves learning communication strategies that facilitate interaction and ways to maintain or enhance the social role of the aphasic individual. Frattali (1992), in her discussion of functional assessment and public policy, states that functional assessment is at odds with traditional deficit-oriented assessment and treatment. To meet individual and third-party payors' expectations of a functional communication assessment, speech-language pathologists must now reconsider the nature of their assessment protocol and the intervention that ensues from it.

One approach to aphasia assessment and intervention that appears to meet the requirements of a functional approach is that which focuses on aphasic individuals and their communicative environment as a dynamic and interdependent system. Adult aphasics and their environment create a single, inextricably interwoven unit that in turn affects the people, the events, and the relationships occurring around them. While it may be efficient to isolate the communication sequelae of the stroke from individuals and their environment, the process results in a synthetic assessment of the person.

The stroke and its physical, cognitive, emotional, and communicative sequelae now serve as active agents of change for individuals, their social network, and the physical surroundings. Therefore, if communication therapy is to be comprehensive and truly tailored to the individual's needs and resources, a broader perspective on the goals of therapy, the agents of change, and the evaluation of outcomes must be offered.

This chapter aims to present a model of assessment and intervention for adult aphasics that derives from environmental and family systems theory and their application to the aphasia rehabilitation field. The philosophy discussed here is one that can be easily incorporated with other approaches presented in this text. Ideally, the environmental systems approach should complement and enhance other cognitive, linguistic, and communicative approaches while increasing their functionality for aphasic individuals in their physical and social environment.

The environmental systems approach is based on the philosophy that effective and functional therapy emanates from a comprehensive rehabilitative management model that takes into consideration the interrelatedness of individuals, their communication abilities, the effectiveness of communication partners to facilitate communication, and the physical and social environment. While therapeutic goals should rightly focus on the primary communication impairment, the goals must also facilitate and strengthen those strategies that allow aphasic individuals and their significant others to become effective communication problem solvers. If we acknowledge the principle that communication is a dyadic process, we realize that aphasia by its very nature creates problems for both members of that communication team. Although one individual incurs the stroke, each and every individual with whom that person communicates will face a predicament. The natural response by some communication partners is to talk for the aphasic individual; for others it is to anticipate every need; and for yet others it is to avoid communication because of potential problems. Each of these responses results in a loss of opportunity for the aphasic individual to demonstrate intact or improving communication ability. Each response may also result in fewer opportunities for the aphasic individual and partners to consider, initiate, and evaluate productive communication problem-solving strategies. The diminution of communication opportunities negatively affects the social relationships between aphasic individuals and their communication partners and reverberates to larger social systems, including family, friends, and other social groups.

The philosophy underscoring this chapter is congruent with Banja's (1990) definition of rehabilitation that focuses on "empowering a disabled person to achieve a personally fulfilling, socially meaningful and functionally effective interaction with the world" (p. 615). Speech-language pathologists who suspect that their aphasia therapy is incomplete, artificial, and unfulfilling to the client, to significant others, or to themselves might find this approach a starting point for answering these questions. As Lyon (1992) states, "[S]ole preoccupation with the act of communicating has failed, so far, to deliver a solution to the problem of restoring optimal function (i.e., communication use and participation in life) in natural settings" (p. 9). The approach described here helps the speech-language pathologist leave the cloister of the therapy office and enter the environment of the aphasic individual.

SYSTEM DEFINITION

A system is defined as a network of elements that has many simultaneous interactions. The interaction of any two elements produces dynamics that influence all the other elements and interactions possible within that system. In systems theory, the characteristics of the individual elements become important in how they alter the infrastructure of the whole system. Each element of the subsystem affects the entire system either overtly or subtly. In the reality of human systems, individuals are part of multiple subsystems

that influence each other in multidirectional ways (Brubaker, 1987). Further, the system is composed not only of human networks but also of the relationship of persons and their physical surroundings. Thus, in a comprehensive systems approach to aphasia, we might consider microsystems such as the family and macrosystems such as the cultural milieu, the physical setting, and the influence of the clinician and the rehabilitation process.

The application of systems theory to communication disorders and aphasia is not new (e.g., Andrews & Andrews, 1987; Bishop, 1982; Brocklehurst et al., 1981; Hyman, 1972; Kinsella & Duffy, 1979; Norlin, 1986; Rollin, 1987; Watzlawick & Coyne, 1980; Webster & Newhoff, 1981). What makes the present approach different is that the approach is layered rather than singularly focused on the primary system of the family. It begins by exploring the impact of aphasia on the individual, then moves to the primary system of the family, and concludes with a discussion of extended environmental and sociocultural systems. Such a layering provides a practical model for a comprehensive approach to assessment and intervention.

The Individual

The individual is at the core of the systems approach presented in this chapter. By contributing personal characteristics to the environment, the individual becomes a member of it. Basic characteristics include age, race, sex, education, occupation, and family and socioeconomic status. To this basic framework other changing physical, psychological, and emotional characteristics are added. These characteristics have evolved through time and sociocultural experiences. Human beings enrich their environment with these distinctive features, yet must rely on other individuals and subsystems for information, support, and feedback. The individual becomes the generator of social imperatives but must also respond to social conventions.

Ideally, pressure from other individuals or subsystems will never exceed the person's ability to respond competently. This means that individuals must be sensitive to role expectations, match their characteristics to the role, self-evaluate, and modify where possible. The interplay between human beings and their environment is delicate and dynamic, creating challenges for humans' ability to adapt and survive. Lawton (1970) calls this "person-environment congruence."

Family as a Microsystem

For most of us, the family is the fundamental system within which we interact. The nucleus of the family is composed of individuals and their previous, present, and changing personal attributes. These individuals beget multiple networks, including the marital, parental, sibling, and extended family subsystems (Turnbull & Turnbull, 1991). The marital subsystem consists of the husband and wife and the stage of their family life development. McGoldrick and Carter (1982) suggest that families advance through six normative family stages, each with its particular influence on the individuals and the larger unit: (a) between families—the unattached young adult; (b) the joining of families through marriage; (c) the family with very young children; (d) the family with adolescents; (e) the launching of children and moving on; and (f) the family in later life. Jones (1989) states that this development is not a continuous process but one characterized by oscillations and vacillations. For example, one family may be in stage 4 and also in stage 5, while another family in stage 6 may have adult children return home and thus regress to stage 5.

The parental subsystem emerges in the interactions between parents and their child or children, and the sibling subsystem reflects the relationships between children of the family. As parents age and their children grow into adult roles, the relationship between parent and child evolves. Similarly, the children of the family have changing relationships as they mature and enter into new subsystems both within and outside the family.

The core family is also a part of the extended family subsystem of relatives, friends, support groups, and professionals (Turnbull & Turnbull, 1991). The family does not live in isolation but extends to many other individuals and systems. Thus, the characteristics of the family, or any of its components, will affect and be influenced by their relationships with larger social groups such as work, school, church, and leisure organizations.

Each of these subsystems is well organized, has control mechanisms, and has energy that keeps the system going (Gray et al., 1969). Organization means that the system can be recognized by its wholeness. For example, the family is organized by its composition of members and their roles within the boundary of the family. In today's society, the organization of families can take many different forms yet conform to the definition of a family. At least 10 viable family organizations exist: (a) the nuclear family of husband, wife, and children; (b) married individuals with no children; (c) individuals in widowhood with or without children; (d) unmarried individuals with child or children; (e) never-married or divorced individuals; (f) remarried individuals with or without children; (g) companionate relationships; (h) blended nuclear family with children from one or more marriages; (i) any of the above with the presence of a grandparent or other family member; and (j) communes or collective living arrangements.

The roles that individuals have within the family emerge from tasks that need to be accomplished to keep the family in a steady state. Primary or shared roles include the financial well-being of the family, homemaking, education, caregiving, and support. The roles that individuals have are likely to change over time as the needs of the family shift and as individuals change in their ability to handle roles.

The family also has mechanisms to control itself or maintain its organization (Bonder, 1986/1987). There is potential for family disruption as the family and its individuals change over time and are influenced by the myriad systems with which they interact. Families have the self-preservation need to maintain homeostasis. Thus, the family must constantly provide feedback to its members and find ways to maintain the delicate balance of the family system. Homeostasis is generally achieved when individuals have clearly and mutually agreed on roles and an effective communication system to convey information among members. Should internal or external elements from the family cause a change in these roles, the balance of the family system is altered. Fortunately, families can be energized from within their own organization or from external systems such as professional or peer support networks. It is hoped that the resources that the individuals and the family as a system have will be strong enough to adjust family roles, to facilitate role transition with relative ease, and to minimize role strain (Maitz, 1991).

Environment as a Macrosystem

While the family has an enormous role in systems theory, an even broader concept of the environment should be considered. The environment in this chapter is defined as the aggregate of influences that impinge on individuals throughout their life cycle. These influences can be categorized into those arising from an individual's physical and social environment. The combination of these external forces with the internal characteristics of each individual forms a "total environment" for each person.

External Environment

The stimuli that create human beings' external environment can be grouped into two main categories: first, those generated by the physical surroundings and perceived through the senses; second, those stimuli derived from the cultural and economic climate and transmitted through the communication networks of human beings. These stimuli function in tandem, partially defining how humans will behave in any setting.

Physical Environment

The physical environment is composed of natural phenomena perceived through the senses; human contributions such as buildings and objects; and the elements of time and space. These physical stimuli create the backdrop in which human beings function and help determine where they will live, how they will live, and the rules they will develop to maintain order within that environment. The physical environment is not merely a passive stage setting for communication, but can create opportunities or barriers to people and events where communication might flourish.

Sociocultural and Economic Environment

It is through social interaction that individuals learn their roles and the expectations of others in their environment. The sociocultural milieu of an individual is a web of values, standards, and activities that define particular groups. This rule system specifies how one should behave in various roles and situations. From infancy to old age, one assumes a variety of roles. These roles are influenced by the personal characteristics of the individual and the expectations of the environment. Societies prescribe guidelines for how an individual should progress to and from various roles during the life cycle.

Formal social behavior is learned through direct, explicit communication, for example, by the rules and laws of social organizations. By contrast, mores, or traditional customs, are acquired more subtly. These are learned through informal interaction within specific subsystems such as family, work groups, and social activities (Ittelson et al., 1974). These two types of norms determine how much individual involvement, support, independence, personal growth, and expressiveness will be tolerated (Moos, 1976). Thus, each environment creates its own personality, and this unique combination of social formulae forms the social climate for the individual.

Considering that African-American, Hispanic, and Asian populations are increasing faster than the white population in the United States, aphasiologists need to be aware of the heterogeneous characteristics and expectations of numerous cultures (Friedman, 1990). Wallace and Freeman (1991) reported that in their survey of 30 university-related clinics that had a multicultural emphasis, approximately half of the neurological cases from a multicultural background were black, 28% were Hispanic, and 21% were Asians and Pacific Islanders. Most of these neurological cases were cerebral vascular accidents. Unfortunately, the majority of the individuals attended therapy for 2 months or less.

In particular, we need to understand clients' sociocultural background and how it interacts with health care systems, rehabilitation programs, and individuals from outside their usual cultural experiences. This culturally relevant sensitivity will modify our therapy goals, the agents of change, and reasonable outcomes of therapy. Cross (1988) calls this "cultural competence." At a most basic level, cultural competence or multicultural sensitivity to aphasic clients necessitates that we appreciate their health care beliefs and values. Friedman (1990) states that unless health care practitioners take a transcultural perspective in working with minority clients, there will be poor communication and interpersonal tension, leading to inaccurate assessment and intervention. A clinician who does not take into consideration the sociocultural milieu of a client may find that therapy compliance and carryover to outside settings are less than expected. (See Sue & Sue, 1990, and Kavanagh & Kennedy, 1992,

for discussions of communication with culturally diverse populations.)

The economic environment also influences the individual, the family, and the larger society. How health care and rehabilitation are approached may be determined to a great degree by the financial resources of the aphasic individual and his or her significant others (Ingstad, 1990). The nature and extent of one's own finances or third-party insurance to cover extensive and prolonged rehabilitation may mitigate the person's willingness to participate in therapy. While speech-language pathologists are encouraged to be culturally sensitive, they must also be "economically sensitive" to client and family concerns about the cost of therapy and the perceived cost/benefit ratio. Economic sensitivity involves understanding the cost of therapy and its impact on the everyday lives of the individuals involved. Knowing that the family cannot afford extensive therapy or that therapy costs will cut deeply into their savings may influence how therapy is done and progress is evaluated. Finally, aphasic individuals and families will appreciate a speech-language pathologist who acknowledges that financial coverage of therapy may be a burden.

RELATIONSHIP OF COMMUNICATION TO THE ENVIRONMENT

Communication is the reciprocal act of sending and receiving information. This act can assume a variety of forms. Individuals communicate through the transmission of spoken or written symbols, body language signals, vocal cues, and olfaction, as well as through manipulation of objects and space in the environment. The content of communication is limited only by the boundaries of human beings' perception of the external world and the scope of their inner world.

Communication serves human beings generously. First, it is the primary mechanism through which persons learn the rules of their environment and their social role within it. Second, communication helps humans control both their physical environment and their companions. Third, through social discourse, individuals avoid isolation and achieve a sense of belonging. Communication is a therapeutic tool when it helps individuals express their feelings and achieve psychological well-being. All individuals, especially aphasics, experience successful communication and realize its benefits when there is a physical and social environment that supports and reinforces communicative interaction, and a willingness on the part of the individual to enter into this interaction.

External Factors Related to Successful Communication

Successful communication is highly dependent on the adequate transmission and reception of the message. The environment must be structured so that communicating individuals can come within a reasonable and effective physical distance of each other. Distance is determined by one's sensory receptive abilities and sociocultural conventions. The message must also travel between sender and receiver with a minimum of interference and distortion. Thus, the physical environment is an integral component of the communication event.

This is also true for the sociocultural environment. Simon and Agazarian (1967) explain that communicators must first establish "good maintenance." They state that communication will be successful when interactants accept each other. This is similar to Gibb's (1961) concept of a supportive communication climate. For example, an environment that places a premium on evaluation and control of its members will create defensive behavior and communication. "Defensive behavior engenders defensive listening and this in turn produces postural, facial and verbal cues which raise the defense level of the original communicator" (Gibb, 1961, p. 141).

Individual Characteristics Related to Successful Communication

For successful communication to occur, the individual must have the ability to send and receive messages. Language, speech, and hearing mechanisms must be intact and capable of sending and receiving signals. Visual acuity also contributes to effective communication, since it is through vision that one decodes many nonverbal cues. Communication will be unsuccessful when the sender transmits an unintelligible message, when he or she misperceives the availability of the receiver, and/or when the content is ambiguous, inappropriate, or irrelevant. Communication also becomes ineffectual when the individual does not comprehend the signals, receives a distorted signal, is distracted by extraneous stimuli, or loses interest.

Individuals must also contribute a sense of involvement in a situation for successful communication to occur there. They must perceive that their participation is valued by members of the group, and in turn, they must be recognized as a viable communication partner. Although physical accessibility to a variety of social occasions is important, mere presence is insufficient to stimulate interest and involvement. Social acceptance of the individual is a prerequisite for meaningful interaction.

IMPACT OF APHASIA ON SYSTEMS

When an individual suffers brain damage, the equilibrium between the person and his or her environment is disturbed. The equilibrium will be changed by many factors on immediate, short-term, and long-term bases. Few individuals or their families understand or are prepared for the numerous and complex physical, communicative, cognitive, emotional, and social changes the stroke will create. These changes have a far-reaching impact on the individual, the family, larger social groups, and the physical and social environment.

The Challenge of Being an Aphasic Individual

Brain damage and its resulting aphasia impose numerous immediate and long-term challenges for an individual: (a) the immediate health crisis; (b) long-term comorbidities; (c) communication problems; (d) the hurdles of rehabilitation; and (e) reintegration into the home and society.

Immediate Health Crisis

An individual's initial reaction to brain damage is that he or she is in an immediate life-threatening situation. There is a real possibility that the individual will die. Medical intervention and the innate forces related to recovery enable the person to cope with and relieve this initial crisis. The emergency may last for a few days or several weeks until the physical well-being of the person is stabilized. The impact of the illness is realized more fully when the health status is brought under control. The individual will survive, but now his or her physical and communicative abilities have been altered. This is the transition from the illness stage to the disability stage (Safilios-Rothchild, 1970).

Long-Term Comorbidities

Rehabilitation specialists such as speech-language pathologists, physiatrists, physical therapists, and occupational therapists may myopically view the problems of the stroke patient. In reality, physical and psychological problems following a stroke form a complex of their own that reverberates throughout the subsystems of the aphasic individual and to the rehabilitation process itself. These problems must be understood as potential influences on the effectiveness of therapy and cannot be divorced from it.

The majority of stroke patients have some physical sequelae of the stroke including physical/health problems, perceptual disabilities, and dysphagia. In addition, health problems related to the stroke, to the lifestyle, or to the aging process itself are likely concomitants. These may directly affect the family system, communication of the aphasic individual, and rehabilitation efforts. For example, a 75-year-old male stroke patient may also have emphysema, presbycusis, cataracts, macular degeneration, and prostate cancer. Physical and health concerns may have priority over communication rehabilitation for the individual or caregivers. For example, the elderly wife of an aphasic may perceive the major stroke-related difficulty to be her inability to assist in transfer and lifting during toileting. The nurse may be more concerned about increased dependence resulting from decrease in muscle strength, additional time in bed, and decubitus ulcers.

A second long-term comorbidity is the strong relationship between damage to the left hemisphere and psychological reactions (e.g., Starkstein & Robinson, 1988; Wahrborg, 1991). Without doubt, difficulty in expressing oneself and understanding others, physical impairments, and social changes negatively affect the individual's psychological well-being. Tanner and Gerstenberger (1988) discuss the psychological reactions to aphasia as grief arising from loss of person, loss of self, and loss of object. The stroke and its sequelae create obstacles for the maintenance of accustomed relationships with family and other social systems. Members of these social groups are usually unaware of the complex properties of stroke and have few strategies for interacting effectively with the aphasic individual. Loss of self ensues as fewer social roles are available to the aphasic individual because of active withdrawal of opportunities by the family or other social systems or because of loss of physical function to participate. Loss of external objects, such as personal items and familiar settings, can also fuel a grief response within the aphasic individual. The 80-year-old aphasic woman who finds herself institutionalized in a nursing home without her cherished possessions may have little desire to communicate or to interact socially with staff or family.

Perhaps the major psychological reaction of aphasic individuals to their predicament is depression. 30 to 60% of stroke patients exhibit depression sometimes following their insult, and this depression may be long term (e.g., Cullum & Bigler, 1991; Egelko et al., 1989; Robinson & Benson, 1981). Tearfulness and crying appear to be common long-term depressive symptoms. Such symptoms may be mistaken now as primary characteristics and lead to reduced opportunities for communication (Wahrborg, 1991).

Wahrborg (1991) states that the depression following stroke can be categorized as "major poststroke depression" and "reactive poststroke depression." Major poststroke depression is that associated with the proximity of the lesion to the frontal lobe. In contrast, reactive depression is related to the ability to cope with the challenges of stroke and aphasia. Keller et al. (1989) add that depression can also emanate from a combination of the organic biochemical changes and the psychosocial challenges of aphasia. Stern and Bachman (1991) found in a recent study of depressive symptoms following stroke that dysphoria was related to site of lesion but not to the severity of aphasia. It might be added that the depression that some aphasic individuals show may be an extension of premorbid depression. Steger (1976) cautions us to remember that depression in elderly patients may be related to the complex of losses that characterize their life period as well as to the frustration involved in rehabilitation. Even without a stroke, at least 15% of the elderly are depressed, and this prevalence increases to 35% when there is a concurrent medical illness (Jenike, 1988).

The depressive symptoms that aphasic individuals may show can be multiple, ranging from pervasive sadness, dependency, and indecisiveness to physical and cognitive problems. The most extreme symptom includes suicide (Jenike, 1988). The Diagnostic and Statistical Manual of Mental Disorders (DSM-III-R) (American Psychiatric Association, 1987) lists major depression criteria to be related to sleep disturbance, loss of interest in activities that the person once enjoyed, feelings of guilt, loss of energy, decreased concentration, diminished appetite, psychomotor disturbance, and suicide. In general, five of these criteria persisting for at least 2 weeks may indicate clinical depression. Such depression symptomatology may be interpreted, however, by family or professionals as confusion or dementia. Comments by Jenike (1988) on "guarding against fatalistically diagnosing the cognitively impaired depressed individual as irretrievably demented and withholding a treatment as a result" (p. 128) can be applied to depressed aphasic individuals. The aphasic individual with depression is in double jeopardy because of difficulty in verbally expressing feelings. Tanner (1987) states that language is the tool for introspection and therapeutic exchange. Thus, language therapy to improve expression may be essential in addressing depressive symptoms.

Depression is not the only affective disorder exhibited among aphasic individuals. Affective changes can be any of a constellation of reactions including frustration, anger, hostility, anxiety, aggression, withdrawal, denial, regression, boasting, and catastrophic reactions (Wahrborg, 1991). Further, aphasic individuals may also incur other cognitive changes such as dementia including Alzheimer's disease, multiinfarct dementia, and dementia related to Parkinson's disease (see Chapter 35 in this text). Again, these must be differentially diagnosed from the aphasia itself and any other concomitant psychological problems such as depression.

The speech-language pathologist has an important role in identifying affective symptoms and making appropriate referral for accurate differential diagnosis and medical, psychiatric, or pharmaceutical intervention. At times, however, the speech-language pathologist, by the very nature of his or her intimate communicative experiences with the aphasic client, will need to deal directly with the psychological reactions of the aphasic individual to ensure that therapy is effective and functional. Particularly important is the speech-language pathologist's ability to use effective counseling/communicative skills with the aphasic individual. See Tanner (1987) and Tanner et al. (1989) for a more in-depth discussion of psychological reactions and their remediation in brain-damaged individuals.

Communication Difficulties

The inability to communicate successfully may be the most significant problem for aphasic persons and the greatest price they must pay for their illness. Aphasic persons are stigmatized (Goffman, 1964) by their communication problem. Each time they attempt to communicate and fail, they strengthen their negative self-perception. At a time when communication is essential for adjustment and reintegration into family and community, their skill is impaired, and opportunities to interact are often seriously reduced.

Aphasic persons face a crisis each time they cannot quickly and efficiently express or comprehend the symbols of their environment. For example, each time individuals are bombarded by communication that comes too abundantly or quickly, they must choose from among replying unintelligibly, replying inappropriately, or withholding a response. They find it difficult to fulfill their roles as adult communicators within their family and other social groups. Similarly, a crisis occurs each time the individuals are isolated from communication contact by their voluntary withdrawal or by the retreat of significant communication partners. It may be easier to avoid communication and thereby lessen the frustration of failure.

Hurdles of Rehabilitation

Once the immediate health crisis is overcome, a new multidimensional system enters the lives of aphasic individuals and their families: the rehabilitation system. While the focus of this book is specifically on communication rehabilitation, we must remember that aphasia rehabilitation is likely to be only one of several health service programs working with the individual. Helping specialists bring unfamiliar value systems and agendas that may or may not be in concert with the aphasic individual and/or family. Rehabilitation also is influenced by the society's valuation of rehabilitation goals and outcomes. Is society willing to pay for rehabilitation and then meaningfully reintegrate the aphasic individual into the community?

The first hurdle the aphasic individual faces in the communication rehabilitation system is facing the reality that communication is impaired to some degree. Rehabilitation may be viewed as an approach-avoidance process. On one side of the scale is the potential for improvement and return to premorbid status. On the other side of the scale are numerous factors, including unknown amount of effort, fear of failure, stigmatization of being a therapy client, dependency, and imposition on others. In addition, life-long individual and societal conceptions or misconceptions of disability and rehabilitation add to the imbalance. The equation becomes more complicated when the aphasic individual is elderly and "beyond" the typical age when rehabilitation efforts focus on return to a socially important job role (Bozarth, 1981).

The second rehabilitation hurdle the aphasic individual faces is that of being a therapy "client" or "patient." With this new and unfamiliar role comes certain expectations generated by a multilateral group of therapist, family, third-party payors, and the aphasic person. Rabinowitz and Mitsos (1964) state that at this point the client is "enrobed in a distinctive social garment" (p. 9). Traditionally, a "good client" participates enthusiastically, carries out assignments faithfully, respects and refrains from questioning the therapist's judgment of therapy goals and methods, attends therapy promptly and regularly, is appropriately gracious and grateful, verbalizes difficulties, and so on (Rabinowitz & Mitsos, 1964). All this is seen as reflecting the good client's high motivation to improve. In fact, these very behaviors may mask confusion about therapy, indifference, and low motivation. The success of therapy rides on the shoulders of the aphasic client (Safilios-Rothchild, 1970).

According to systems theory, the "client" in actuality is the individual and his or her family. Rather than define a "good client," we might now consider the therapy belief system of these individuals and how this translates to positive or facilitating behaviors. For example, do they believe that therapy is more effective when client and family are actively involved? Do they believe that therapy is a problem-solving process whereby they will learn strategies to repair their communication difficulties? Do they believe that progress can be measured in multiple ways, including improvement in specific communication skills, increased willingness to enter into communication exchanges, increased ability on the part of significant others to facilitate interaction, and decreased depression or stress on the part of the client and family?

Reintegration into Home and Community

Perhaps the most difficult personal challenge for aphasic individuals is reintegration into their home and community. For some aphasic individuals, this process occurs simultaneously with outpatient therapy; for others it occurs after therapy is completed—the "ex-client" stage. Beginning with the immediate health crisis stage and afterward, the aphasic individual's accustomed family and community roles have been altered, assimilated by others, or eliminated. Carver and Rodda (1978) question whether the disabled individual is "assimilated" or "integrated" into his or her environment. With assimilation, the emphasis is on clients appropriately adapting themselves to a relatively unchanged environment. They must fit in. In contrast, in an environment that focuses on integration, there is coadaptation on the part of the physical and social environment systems. The aphasic individual and the environment now work at conforming to each other. An aphasic person who is integrated has opportunities to demonstrate accustomed, meaningful adult roles in a variety of contexts.

As a "client" or "patient," the aphasic individual is expected to passively relinquish former social roles, participate eagerly in rehabilitation, and have an ardent desire to return to normal. A dilemma arises, however, when the aphasic person declines to fulfill this model. The individual may not choose to relinquish family, vocational, or social responsibilities, nor may he or she want to participate enthusiastically in rehabilitation. Society and the individual may become adversaries during rehabilitation. For example, the aphasic person has the choice of (a) accepting the rehabilitant role that requires acceptance of disability and active participation in therapy, (b) participating impassively in therapy, or (c) refusing participation. The aphasic individual may not be able to communicate effectively his or her personal goals and consequently may resort to behaviors that society considers maladaptive or antisocial. Now, in addition to being aphasic, the individual is further stigmatized as uncooperative, unmanageable, or hostile. Consequently, fewer opportunities for reintegrating into the community materialize. Evaluation of aphasic individuals' integration into the community 5 or 10 years poststroke would provide much needed data on what the focus of therapy should be.

Microsystems Impact

Rolland (1988) states that the "family may provide the best lens through which to view other systems" (p. 17). Concurrently with understanding the impact of aphasia on the individual, we must focus on its impact on the family. "Family" is broadly defined here as the network of individuals with whom the aphasic individual is closely involved on a daily basis. This can be an immediate system of spouse and/or children, or can extend to other relatives, friends, and informal or professional caregivers. The majority of the discussion focuses on the immediate family with some discussion of more extended family systems.

Table 12–1 portrays a model for the stages through which the aphasic individual and family will evolve after the stroke. This model begins with the severe illness or crisis stage and evolves to subsequent stages of recuperation, rehabilitation, postrehabilitation, and institutionalization. While this model is presented as a sequential series of stages, in reality some stages are brief, whereas others are lengthy for individual aphasics and their families.

The family's initial concern after the stroke is coping with the sudden life-threatening illness. The family, particularly the spouse, is likely to fear that the stroke will result in death or some unknown type and degree of disability. Not only is this fear directed toward the stroke patient but there is also an amorphous fear about how their own lives will be changed by this crisis event immediately and in the long term. All sorts of feelings cloud this time: obsessive concern, anxiety, helplessness, grief, and guilt. During this time, few changes in family roles are likely to occur because the family's energy is directed toward the immediate health crisis.

Once the stroke patient's health is stabilized, the patient and the family system move into the recuperation stage. The first feeling is one of relief that the stroke patient will live. This is when the family system tries to begin the return to its precrisis state (homeostasis). In actuality, the system changes

that begin to occur are likely to modify the family network forever. The changes that occur emanate from many sources, including the normative stage of the family, their historical ability to cope with problems, the immediate tasks that need to be done and the resources for accomplishing them, and other demands on the family. For example, a mature family that has clear lines of communication, a resource network of family and friends, and a history of successfully coping with problems may face a crisis differently than the family that is disengaged, interacts poorly, and has numerous conflicting demands on its members.

While stroke may occur in younger adults who are in early stages of family development, it is more likely to occur when the family is in the late life cycle. The elder spouse is likely to assume primary caregiving responsibility, although adult children play an increasingly important role in providing assistance to their parent(s). The changing demographics of our society translate into fewer middle-aged children to care for older parents (Gatz et al., 1990). Further, these children, particularly adult daughters, are likely to be employed outside the home and be caught in the "sandwich" of caring for their own children and their parents. The older family, however, has many years of experience in coping with other life problems that may assist in coping with stroke and aphasia. Rolland (1990) states that when disease occurs later in the family life cycle, the "strains are counterbalanced by a firmer relationship base" (p. 239). On the negative side, the spouse of the later-life aphasic may also exhibit health, physical, cognitive, or sensory problems that complicate the caregiving context.

During the recuperation stage, the family is likely to concentrate on activities of daily living such as walking, feeding, dressing, and toileting. These problems require direct and strenuous caregiving on the part of family members. There is a simultaneous awareness that communication is disrupted. The communication difficulties now evident between the aphasic individual and his or her family members confound provision of physical care and their social relationships. Kinsella and Duffy (1979) found that difficulty in communication results in a loss of the intimacy and support found in most marriages.

Most families with a member who has incurred a stroke do not come as units untouched by other life problems. Numerous demands concurrently have an impact on the aphasic family, including those arising from family life stage, prior family dysfunction, and financial, employment, and health problems. For example, Jones and Lubinski (unpublished), in a family systems study of nine poststroke families, found that all families contended with stresses faced by maturing families such as those related to launching children, managing retirement, and coping with needs of elderly parents. Many of the families had histories of alcoholism, problems with children, unemployment, and so on. House et al. (1990) found that stroke patients as compared with controls experienced

TABLE 12–1

Patient Stages, Possible Family Effects, and Potential Family Needs

Patient Stage	Possible Effects on Family	Potential Family Needs
Severe illness or crisis stage	Fear and shock Disequilibrium Anxiety Depression Guilt Helplessness Grief Obsessive concern	Emotional support for entire family, particularly spouse, adult child caregiver, significant other
Recuperation stage	Sense of relief from acute stage Family works toward homeostasis Members assume needed roles and jobs Search for help begins Individuals try to maintain self-image	Continued emotional support Information about family demands, resources, concerns; see ABCX model Informal education about stroke and its effects Family mobilized to work together Facilitative communication strategies modeled while communicating with aphasic adult
Rehabilitation	"Hope" that things will improve Expectation that patient will improve Solidification of new family roles Beginning of isolation from community Physical changes in home Possible logistical problems in attending therapy by patient and/or family member(s) Possible financial problems	Continued emotional support with more emphasis on self-reliance Problem-solving approach to communication difficulties Direct involvement in rehabilitation Discussion of family, individual, and clinician goals and expectations of therapy Definition of and access to community resources Peer support groups Planning for postrehabilitation stage
Postrehabilitation	Possible role-overload for primary caregiver Possible health problems for primary caregiver Long-term changes in family roles Isolation of family from extended groups Possible reduction in intimacy between aphasic and spouse or significant other Over- or underexpectations for continued improvements	Realization and support for caregiver personal needs Peer and extended group support Increase in normative features of home and aphasic person Continued emotional support—referral to community counselors
Institutionalization	Physical/psychological overload Lack of awareness of community alternatives Conflicting feelings of relief and guilt Further role changes Discomfort with setting Reduction in contact with institutionalized family member Preparation for family member deterioration or death	Help in decision making Counseling regarding alternatives Support during decision making and entry Encouragement to visit; strategies for productive visits provided Information regarding impact of institutionalization on family member Modeling of facilitative communication strategies in this setting Work with facility staff to stress importance of communication to aphasic individual Development of new roles in this setting encouraged Participation in activities with aphasic adult within and outside setting encouraged Counseling regarding deterioration and death

a significantly greater number of severe events in the year preceding a stroke. Evans et al. (1991a) found that poststroke patients at risk for poor-quality home care had families with caregivers who were depressed, had little knowledge about stroke care, and had prestroke family dysfunction. They concluded that "caregiver problems can have a collective effect on rehabilitation outcome" (p. 144). In another study of family characteristics related to better treatment adherence poststroke, Evans et al. (1991b) portrayed such families as having clear and direct communication exchange, effective problem-solving ability and strong emotional interest in one another. Kelly-Hayes et al. (1988) found that family and social factors were equal to medical factors in determining final outcome from stroke. Thus, these studies demonstrate that individuals and their families are vitally important in the rehabilitation process, although they bring "baggage" to the rehabilitation situation.

When medical conditions have stabilized and physical recuperation appears possible, therapies are likely to begin. These may be instigated by the medical/rehabilitation system or by the family. For many families, this will be their first encounter with a speech-language pathologist and aphasia therapy. The individual and the family are moving into the rehabilitation stage where the focus is on helping the aphasic individual improve language skills. The family system is also continuing its restructuring during this time. Role changes become more solidified so that even when aphasic individuals return to their family, the modifications are in place without their active involvement. Difficulties in communicating contribute significantly to the need for, yet impede, the aphasic's participation in family role restructuring. Unwittingly, the aphasic individual may become the marginal member of the family.

The extended family of the aphasic is also affected by the stroke and the resulting communication problems. Friends and acquaintances may feel uncomfortable during interactions with the aphasic and may withdraw from former social interaction with the entire family unit or individual members within it. The family may lose some of its opportunities for social connectedness because one member cannot communicate. This results in the disengagement of the family from the mainstream of the community.

Finally, the extended system of the aphasic individual is likely to include some new members such as professional caregivers. Nurses and nursing assistants assume a prominent role in the lives of many aphasic individuals in hospital, home, or long-term care setting. These individuals assume "quasi-family" roles in that they perform intimate caregiving tasks and serve as primary communication partners for the aphasic individual. Family members who are not present for therapy may look to the nursing assistant for feedback on "how therapy is going with Dad." This individual may subtly influence how the aphasic individual and family perceive therapy and its progress.

Macrosystems Impact

The impact of aphasia extends beyond the immediate family to the aphasic individual's larger social and physical environments. For example, a father's aphasia has implications for resuming his coaching role on his son's soccer team and is likely to affect his ability to supervise his office staff. Most persons with whom the aphasic individual is likely to interact have had little or no experience in communicating with someone with this type of problem. Even when communication skills are greatly improved, the impression may be of someone who is less than whole. When communication problems are evident, the individual has more difficulty demonstrating his or her intelligence, social competence, and productive social role, all qualities valued by Western industrialized societies. Safilios-Rothchild (1970) says that such societies do not tolerate "behavioral deviations [such as communication difficulties] that tend to disrupt the smooth functioning and easy flow of interpersonal relations" (p. 127). In general, contact with an adult who has difficulty communicating arouses anxiety. The cultural norm is to mask such aversion. It therefore becomes necessary to avoid contact with the aphasic individual lest their prejudices and own inadequacies in coping with the communication difficulty become evident.

Society appears to have conflicting perceptions of someone with a disability. Rolland (1990) states that our society admires personal responsibility as the means to recovery. On the other hand, Western societies also feel a need to "protect the less fortunate." Protection may lead to elimination of situations where the aphasic individual, and hence society, might face communication frustration or failure. The aphasic individual is now out of mainstream society and part of an unfamiliar minority group. Reintegration into society thus becomes more challenging.

Impact of Rehabilitation Setting and Clinician

The setting offering communication rehabilitation is itself a multifaceted system influenced by many equally complicated factors. Fundamentally, therapy is influenced by the goals of the institution and the agenda set by third-party payors. For example, restrictions set by insurers on agencies that can offer evaluation and therapy services limit patient options. Similarly, a predetermined number of paid therapy sessions may limit scope and direction of therapy. Romano (1989) posits that many rehabilitation programs send mixed messages to the client: On the one hand, decision making is generally removed from the patient, yet on the other the patient is expected to demonstrate independence and self-motivation. The model underlying many rehabilitation programs closely resembles a biomedical model focused on the direct relationship between differential diagnosis and treatment. At present, such a medical model will not support an environmental systems approach to therapy where the emphasis is simultaneously on client, family, and environment.

The speech-language pathologist is one of the most influential factors in the aphasia therapy process. Clinician knowledge, skills, and attitudes about aphasia, aging, and rehabilitation influence who will receive therapy and how it will be delivered. Clinicians bring their own unique traits and histories that act as a "cultural filter" in how we communicate with, assess, and plan therapy for clients (Krefting & Krefting, 1991). In addition, clinicians contribute their professional biases that have accrued from training programs and cultural influences. Agar (1980) states that "whether it is your personality, your rules of social interaction, your cultural bias toward significant topics, your professional training or something else, you do not go into the field as a passive recorder of objective data" (p. 10). Clinicians are influenced by their own known and unknown biases and the expectations of the rehabilitation setting, the client, family, and society.

SYSTEM ASSESSMENT

The first step in the environmental systems rehabilitation program is to identify the impact of the stroke and the resulting aphasia on individuals, their family system, their extended social systems, and their physical and social milieu. Because of time and therapy setting constraints, we need to obtain the most direct information about individuals and their family and assumptions about extended social systems and the broader environment. The fact that we cannot observe aphasic individuals and their family in their home setting with their extended systems should not discourage us from developing ways to assess these components. The value added from such information contributes to a comprehensive, sensitive, and functional assessment.

A qualitative approach to assessment is presented in this chapter. What speech-language pathologists should be interested in is the quality and insight of answers given and how the questions and answers contribute to new thinking by the aphasic individual, the family members, and the speech-language pathologist. The questions presented here should be viewed as vehicles for ongoing discussion with the client and family and not just as initial assessment tools. The assessment process described here should naturally merge with communication therapy for the client and his or her family. A total picture of the client's communicative environment should develop from this layered approach to assessment of multiple systems. This information can be used in goal setting, in reassessment, and in feedback to the client, family, and third-party payors.

Individual Assessment

In addition to the traditional communicative/cognitive evaluation, we must examine (a) aphasic individuals' perception

of their problem(s), (b) the impact of these problems on everyday life, (c) their expectations regarding therapy and its outcomes, and (d) their motivation to improve their communication. The format of questions presented here should be used as a springboard to other issues that arise during interaction with the client and/or family and adapted according to the communication abilities and cultural background of the individual. Moreover, questions for the more expressively impaired aphasic individual should be phrased to elicit "yes/no" or gestural responses. Further, the questions posed here emanate from a typical "middle-class white clinician" interacting with a similar-type client. These questions may need to be rephrased to sensitively meet the "self-disclosure" values of minority groups (see Sue & Sue, 1990). Finally, it is important that during such discussions, the clinician convey a supportive and nonjudgmental attitude toward the client and the family.

Table 12–2 presents a series of questions under three main headings. The first area focuses on how clients define their present situation. Note that the questions target issues broader than communication per se. It is possible that the client perceives difficulties other than communication as primary burdens. Identification of such a perception helps the clinician appropriately modify therapy goals and methods, leading to greater functionality of therapy outcomes. For example, the aphasic who is more concerned about independently performing activities of daily living so that he would not be a burden for his wife on returning home might have his communication therapy focus on vocabulary and ideas associated with these activities.

The second area of questions focuses on the clients' perception of the impact of the stroke and aphasia on their role and interaction with their family and extended systems. If clients perceive that they have a limited role within these systems and few opportunities to communicate, therapy is not likely to be productive. Identification of the complicated demands that the stroke and aphasia have placed on the aphasic leads to more functional therapy outcomes. For example, if the aphasic client perceives that his or her family avoids entering into conversations because of potential communication breakdowns, functional therapy would provide the communication partners with effective repair strategies.

The third area of questions concentrates on the client's motivation to improve. Being a "client" is a foreign role for many, if not most, aphasic adults. It is often a role associated with inadequacy, dependency, and helplessness. We need to know the client's previous experiences of being in a helping situation and what factors contributed to success or failure. The aphasic client who took his child to a speech-language pathologist for speech therapy may have a different conception about his own therapy than the client who is unsure of what a speech-language pathologist does. The final area of questions focuses on what clients would like to improve in

TABLE 12–2

Interview Questions for Aphasic Individual Regarding Stroke and Aphasia[a]

Definition of Present Situation
 1. What concerns you about your speech?
 2. What problems do you have in understanding your spouse (or primary caregiver)?
 3. What problems do you have in understanding other people?
 4. What problems do you have in expressing yourself?
 5. What problems do you have in reading? In writing?
 6. How important is reading (and writing) to you?
 7. In what situations do you have the most difficulty talking (or understanding)?
 8. What other problems do you have besides a communication problem?
 9. What is your greatest concern right now—these other problems (e.g., self-care) or communication? Why?
10. What other therapies are you receiving?

Impact of Aphasia
 1. How do you feel when you have a problem communicating?
 2. How do others react when you have a problem communicating?
 3. Do you ever avoid a situation or a person because of your difficulty communicating? Why? Describe this.
 4. How has your communication problem affected your interaction with your family?
 5. How has your communication problem affected your interaction with others outside your family, such as friends or coworkers?
 6. How has your communication problem affected your social life (employment)?
 7. Who are the primary people you talk with every day?
 8. Do you feel you have enough opportunities to talk about things that interest you? With people who are interesting to you?

Motivation to Improve Communication
 1. Tell me about a typical day of yours. What do you do?
 2. What would you like to improve about your communication?
 3. Why is this important to you?
 4. What have you done on your own that helps you communicate better?
 5. Have you attended speech therapy before? If so, where? What did you work on? How successful was therapy?
 6. Who in your family would you like to work with on your communication? Why this person?
 7. What do you think I can do to help you in therapy?
 8. What would you like to be able to do 6 months from now?
 9. What concerns do you have about coming to speech therapy?
10. What motivates you to improve your speech?

[a]Note that questions should be rephrased to a simpler form or to a yes/no or gesture response format to accommodate the communication ability of the aphasic individual.

therapy and explores their expectations for success. Answers to these questions will help the speech-language pathologist fine-tune therapy goals and make them congruent with the client's personal agenda for therapy.

Microsystems Assessment

While there are numerous models of family assessment adaptable to this environmental systems approach, one model that is especially useful is the ABCX described originally by Hill (1949) and modified by McCubbin and Patterson (1983). This model focuses on how the family deals with the stroke situation over time. Table 12–3 lists the model's components, definitions, and established formal assessment tools. Variable A is composed of the stressor event itself and the present and lingering demands faced by the family. Variable B encompasses the internal and external resources that the family may use to cope with their normative life-stage stressors,

the stroke, and its sequelae. Variable C is the individual family members' definition of the problem as a source of stress. The X variable is the interaction of the above variables, resulting in the ability of the family to make productive changes to meet their challenged system. For a more complete discussion of this model, the reader is referred to Jones, 1989; Lubinski, 1991; and McCubbin and Patterson, 1983.

The ABCX model can be operationalized into an assessment tool in either of two ways. First, a number of assessment instruments are available from the family counseling literature. Jones and Lubinski (unpublished) recently applied these tools to the assessment of nine poststroke mature families and found that speech-language pathologists could easily use these to assess families. Although somewhat time consuming for individual family members to complete, the instruments did provide a uniform means of assessing the ABCX factors.

TABLE 12–3

ABCX Model of Family Stress: Definitions and Tools for Assessment of Families

Variable	Definition	Self-Report Assessment Tools
A	Stressor event and its ensuing demands, negative coping strategies, lingering coexisting family problems	Questionnaire on Resources and Stress for Families with Chronically Ill or Handicapped (Holroyd, 1986) Family Needs Assessment Tool (Rawlins et al., 1990) Family Inventory of Life Events (FILE) (McCubbin et al., 1981) Strain Questionnaire (Lefebre & Sanford, 1985)
B	Internal and external resources to meet demands associated with stressor	Family Assessment Device (FAD) (Epstein et al., 1983) Family Adaptability and Cohesion Scales (FACES III) (Olson et al., 1985) Family Crisis Oriented Personal Evaluation Scale (F-COPES) (McCubbin et al., 1981)
C	Family definition of stressor	Family Definition Rating Scale (Jones, 1989)
X	Stress, crisis, and change exhibited by the family	Subjective analysis of interviews, observation, and above family self-report tools

Speech-language pathologists may feel more comfortable designing their own open-ended questions that reflect this model. For example, Table 12–4 offers a series of questions that probe the first three components of the ABCX model. The questions in the demand area feature the significant events prior to, during, and after the stroke that have caused hardships for individual family members and the family as a whole. Remember that in systems theory, hardships felt by one member are likely to reverberate to others. The questions are presented on a time line, beginning with prestroke hardships and proceeding to current demands. Family members may be surprised that you are interested in areas other than the aphasia, and justification for the line of questioning should be given.

The second area of questions focuses on the internal and external resources the family members bring to the current stroke situation. Through these questions, we learn more about our client's family system: their roles, family subsystems, their problem-solving style, their communication patterns, their flexibility, and their cohesion. We will also attempt to define the type, degree, and receptivity to support from extended systems such as relatives, friends, and community agencies.

The family definition of the problem constitutes the third area of questions. We must not assume that aphasia is the family's primary concern. Despite our own professional bias that communication is essential to personal well-being, we must sensitively appreciate other viewpoints. Should the family perceive other difficulties as paramount, this will lead to adjustments in therapy goals, family education, and involvement in therapy.

The analysis of the above variables helps the speech-language pathologist understand how stress develops for the aphasic person and his or her family (variable X). Many combinations of variables are possible. Some families may have such strong resources that the demands of the stroke or aphasia result in controllable changes within the family system. Other families may have strong resources, but the immediate demands are so great that they feel out of control. Yet other families may have such weak internal or external resources that even a mild problem greatly affects their return to homeostasis.

External Environment Assessment

Two aspects of the external environment can be explored by the speech-language pathologists to further complete the total environmental systems assessments. First, careful assessment of the sociocultural and economic environment provides sensitivity to powerful but amorphous forces affecting compliance and progress in therapy. Second, assessment of the physical environment increases the aphasic client's opportunities to communicate in a setting that enhances rather than obstructs interchange.

Sociocultural and Economic Assessment

Looking at a client's surname or color of skin is no substitute for a more in-depth cultural assessment of the client and family. May (1992) further reminds us that by looking at an individual or family, we cannot assume that they fully ascribe to the dominant belief system of their culture. He states, "Cultures themselves are continually changing as they adapt to new realities" (p. 47). The speech-language pathologist should review the findings offered by other specialists, such as social workers or psychologists, for additional

TABLE 12–4

Interview Questions to Explore ABCX Model of Family Coping as Applied to Adult Aphasics and Their Families[a]

A: Demands
1. What significant events were occurring in your family prior to the onset of your family member's stroke (e.g., other illnesses, death, divorce, job loss, relocation, adult child leaves home)?
2. How did these events affect your whole family when they occurred?
3. How do you think these events affect your family at this time?
4. How do you describe the impact of your family member's stroke on the family at this time?
5. How has your family member's communication difficulty affected the family?
6. Who do you think has been most affected by your family member's stroke? Why? In what way?
7. Who has primary responsibility for the care of your family member?
8. What other demands does this individual have on him/her while caring for your family member (e.g., own illness, work outside home, own family)?
9. What is involved in the care of your family member at this time?
10. How has the care of your family member affected the primary caregiver (e.g., fatigue, competing demands, illness, psychological stress)?
11. How has the care of your family member affected the social life of your family and of the primary caregiver?
12. What financial problems is your family incurring related to the stroke?
13. Do you think there will be any other major changes occurring in your family in the near future (e.g., upcoming marriage, relocation, need for home health care)?

B: Resources
1. How would you describe your family's strengths (e.g., adaptable, cohesive, good communication, opportunities for independence)?
2. How would you describe your family member's ability to cope with difficult situations in the past?
3. When your family faces a problem, what strategies do they use to solve the problem (e.g., family discussion, sharing of responsibilities, seeking outside help)?
4. How successful do you think your family is in solving difficult problems? Why?
5. How willing is your family to seek help from outside sources such as friends, medical personnel, clergy, or community counselors? Describe the circumstances in which outside help was sought previously and their effectiveness in helping the family cope.
6. Who is likely to be the leader of your family at this time? Why?
7. How are major decisions regarding the care of your family member made?
8. Who is (or will be) the primary communication partner of your family member? How willing and available is this individual to attend communication therapy?
9. What information have you received about the nature and impact of a stroke? What information have you received about communication problems following a stroke?
10. Has anyone else in your immediate family ever had a stroke? How did the family cope with this problem?
11. Has anyone else in your immediate family ever had a communication problem after a stroke? Did this person have speech-language therapy?
12. What strategies have you tried so far that facilitate communication with your family member?

C: Problem Definition
1. What do you perceive as the major problem facing your family at present?
2. Why is this problem so critical?
3. What do you think can be done about this problem?
4. If the communication problem is not mentioned, then ask the following: How does your family member's communication problem compare with the one you just mentioned?
5. What are your priorities for your family member's rehabilitation at this time?
6. How important is it to your family member to improve his or her communication at this time? Why?
7. What do you expect of communication therapy for your family member?
8. How much control do you (and other family members) feel over the present situation related to your family member's stroke and rehabilitation?

[a] The individual with aphasia is referred to as "your family member" throughout the interviews.

TABLE 12–5

Questions to Assist in Sociocultural and Economic Assessment of the Aphasic Individual and the Family[a]

Sociocultural Issues
1. Do you (or does your family) identify with a certain ethnic or racial group? If yes, which one?
2. Where were you (your family member) born?
3. If not born in the United States, when did you (your family member) come to this country?
4. Where do you live? Are there individuals from different ethnic or racial groups in the neighborhood?
5. What is the primary language spoken at home? Is there anyone in the home who does not speak English? What is the relationship between this person and you (your family member)?
6. With whom do you (your family member) socialize on a regular basis?
7. Do you (your family member) interact with individuals outside your ethnic or racial group? For what purpose (e.g., work, leisure, religious services)?
8. With whom did you (your family member) discuss the stroke or aphasia? What advice was given to you? Did you try it? How effective was it in helping you talk?
9. Do you think that your religious beliefs affect your (your family member's) participation in therapy? If so, how?

Economic Issues
1. Have you discussed financial planning for therapy with anyone? With whom?
2. Do you have insurance that will cover therapy sessions? What kind?
3. Do you understand the limitations of your insurance to cover therapy sessions?
4. Will therapy costs be a burden to your family?
5. Would you like to speak with a financial counselor in our setting to further discuss therapy costs?

[a]The individual with aphasia is referred to as "your family member" throughout the interviews.

information on sociocultural background. It is also natural that these types of questions could be incorporated into the other areas of the interview such as in discussion of family roles.

Westby (1990) suggests that speech-language pathologists use an ethnographic interview process with multicultural clients. "Ethnographic interviews have the goal of helping the interviewer understand the social situations in which the families exist and how the families perceive, feel about and understand these situations" (p. 105). Basic to this process is the development of rapport, the use of descriptive questions, and careful wording of questions. In general, open-ended questions are most productive. These questions encourage the individuals to express their perceptions and feelings about the communication problem and its relationship to family and culture.

Table 12–5 is adapted from work on cultural assessment for nursing personnel by Friedman (1990). The initial questions elicit information regarding the cultural experiences and values of the individual and family. Again, clients from some cultural groups may be wary of such questions, and thus they should be asked with respect, judgment, and communication sensitivity.

In addition, several questions might be posed to the client or family to assess the economic impact of the stroke and therapy. Answers to these questions may be sought from other sources such as social workers and financial officers of the rehabilitation setting. It is important that the speech-language pathologist, the client, and the family understand the costs of

therapy, the nature and extent of insured coverage, and the options available to supplement existing resources.

Physical Environment Assessment

Once the sociocultural milieu is better understood, we need to focus on the physical environment of our aphasic client. Particular attention should be addressed to (a) the physical accessibility to people and activities that generate communication opportunities, (b) the sensory/cognitive dimensions of the environment that contribute to adequate transmission and reception of verbal and nonverbal messages, and (c) the psychosocial environment to stimulate interaction. Specific environmental profiles to evaluate the physical environment for communication are published elsewhere (Carroll, 1978; Lubinski, 1991). In keeping with the "question format" used in this chapter, Table 12–6 presents questions that explore the nature of the physical and social settings in which the aphasic individual resides. These questions can be adapted to hospital, nursing or rehabilitation facility, home, or other community setting.

The first series of questions explores how well the aphasic individual can access communication opportunities in his or her environment. Identification of factors that impede access to people or activities that promote conversations and cognitive stimulation is basic to carryover of therapy goals. The next two areas of questions focus on the auditory and visual environment. Answers to these questions tell us more about the sensory conditions that may facilitate or impede adequate

TABLE 12–6

Questions Regarding the Physical and Social Environment of the Aphasic Adult[a]

Access Within Physical Environment
1. Describe the living situation where your family member resides.
2. Does your family member spend most of his/her time in one area of the setting or does he/she have access to all areas? Where does he/she spend most of his day?
3. How well can your family member get around this setting? Independently? With help from whom?
4. Does your family member use an assistive device to get around the setting, such as a wheelchair, walker, or cane?
5. Can your family member maneuver easily within the setting? If no, why not?

Auditory Environment
1. How noisy is the situation where your family member spends most of his/her day?
2. Is this situation one where he/she is likely to have conversations?
3. Can noisy situations be controlled (e.g., turn off radio or TV, close door to hall)?
4. Does your family member have a hearing loss?
5. Does your family member have a hearing aid for one or both ears? An assistive listening device?
6. Does your family member wear the hearing aid (or assistive listening device) regularly?
7. Does anyone else in the immediate situation have a hearing loss (e.g., elder spouse)?

Visual Environment
1. Is there sufficient lighting to see clearly in the areas where your family member spends most of his/her day?
2. Is light from the windows or lamps easily available and controlled?
3. Does your family member have any visual difficulties such as cataracts, glaucoma, or macular degeneration?
4. Does your family member wear glasses regularly? Or use any type of visual assistive device such as a magnifying glass?

Psychosocial Environment
1. In what activities does your family member participate on a daily basis?
2. How personally fulfilling are these activities to your family member?
3. Is communication an important part of these activities?
4. Who is available to talk with your family member throughout the day?
5. Who would your family member enjoy talking with if he/she had the opportunity?
6. Who takes a special interest in talking with your family member?
7. What activities does your family member participate in outside his/her everyday setting (e.g., outside the home or nursing facility)?
8. How much does your family member participate in family decision-making activities?
9. How has your family member's social role changed since the stroke?
10. Do family members or other caregivers understand the nature of your family member's communication difficulties? Their impact on his/her quality of everyday life?
11. How well do you think your family member has been reintegrated into the family? Other favorite social groups?

[a]The individual with aphasia is referred to as "your family member" throughout the interviews.

transmission of information for the aphasic person and his or her partners. The final area tells us more about the social role available to the aphasic client. These questions help us understand the aphasic's opportunities for reintegration into family and extended social systems.

SYSTEMS INTERVENTION

Goal Planning for Environmental Systems Intervention

The line between assessment and intervention in a systems approach is less clear than in other approaches to aphasia therapy for several reasons. By the very act of interviewing and assessing, the original systems of the aphasic individual have been modified. For example, the clinician's questions regarding therapy goals force the aphasic individual and family

to assess their priorities and involvement in the therapy process. Second, by asking such questions, there is an implicit assumption that the answers to these questions are meaningful to setting therapy goals. Third, during the process of assessment, the beginning of a therapeutic relationship between client, family, and clinician is being established. Interaction with the clinician during assessment sets the stage for the establishment of trust, communication, cooperation, interactive problem solving, and eventual independence.

Thus, the therapeutic goals for an environmental system approach evolve during the assessment process and therapy itself. Therapeutic objectives might be considered on both a short-term and long-term basis. Short-term environmental goals focus on that which can be accomplished during the severe illness stage, recuperation, and rehabilitation. Long-term goals concentrate on helping the individual and family cope with a communication disability and handicap, changes within the family network, and possible institutionalization. Goals are arrived at through a joint effort of the speech-language pathologist, the aphasic person, and other significant members of the aphasic individual's environment such as family members, rehabilitation specialists, and professional caregivers. An interactive approach encourages the continued reassessment and renegotiation of therapy objectives and the development of self-dependence and self-determination on the part of the client and family.

Effective and functional environmental systems goals must be operationally defined. Their effects must be measurable changes in the behaviors of the significant individuals and in the physical setting. All participants in the environmental systems management program should understand therapy goals, the importance of self-generated goals, and the relationship of goals to eventual therapy success. Goals that emanate from the aphasic individual or significant others are likely to be the most functional. For example, an operational goal for an aphasic client who wants and needs a greater variety of communication partners might be one of the following:

1. To encourage three individuals outside the family to talk with the aphasic person at least once daily for a period of at least 15 minutes.
2. To encourage the spouse of the aphasic individual to invite one or two of her husband's friends home each week for a game of cards.
3. To take the aphasic individual to a social event where he or she has the opportunity to interact with friends and acquaintances at least once weekly.

Focus on the Individual

At the core of the environmental systems approach is the individual with aphasia. Rehabilitation efforts focus primarily on empowering this individual to lead as meaningful a social role as possible in his or her home and extended social groups. The most immediate need is to help the individual retain or achieve status as an active and viable communication partner. This is done by strengthening specific receptive and expressive communication skills whereby individuals can intelligibly and meaningfully contribute their personal ideas and can have their physical and psychological needs appropriately met. Traditionally, this goal is achieved through individual and group speech and language therapy sessions using a variety of approaches, as offered in this text.

There are, however, other immediate goals for the individual that have long-term implications and that go beyond strengthening specific communication skills. These include helping the individual understand (a) what has happened to him or her, (b) the nature of therapy, (c) the goal-setting process, (d) the mutual responsibilities of client and clinician,

(e) how progress can be measured, and (f) the long-term prospectus. Litman (1962), in an early study of physical rehabilitation, found that patients frequently did not know what was involved in the "disability, its limitations, implications and possibilities" (p. 569). The speech-language pathologist may need to modify how these topics are discussed with the aphasic client, depending on the client's communicative, cognitive, and emotional status.

Coping with rehabilitation and residual psychological and communication disabilities is an unfolding process for the aphasic person. The aphasic enters therapy with some degree of knowledge, however limited, regarding aphasia and rehabilitation, and this knowledge base is modified by his or her new experience as an aphasic "client" or "patient." Clients may have one set of expectations when they begin therapy and yet develop another set 6 months later. Clients who are encouraged to understand their circumstances and participate in decision making regarding them are more likely to perceive control over these circumstances and thus participate more actively in the therapeutic process. These individuals are also more likely to be perceived by significant others in their environment as more alert, more competent, and less helpless (Lubinski, 1991). Continued discussion with clients about their perceptions of aphasia and therapy should extend throughout the therapy process.

Specific topics focusing on aphasia and rehabilitation with clients might include:

1. What happened to the brain during the stroke
2. The immediate and long-term effects of the stroke on communication
3. The diagnostic process of delineating communication strengths and weaknesses
4. Tentative short- and long-term goals for therapy
5. The importance of the client's therapy goals and expected outcomes
6. How progress can be measured
7. Other effects of stroke: on social roles, on family, on extended social groups, and so on
8. Depression following stroke
9. Taking control of circumstances
10. Assets and resources to help in the rehabilitation process

The clinician must constantly be alert for signs of depression in the aphasic client. In some situations, referral to a mental health specialist is the appropriate alternative. However, several approaches to relieving symptoms of depression can be incorporated into daily aphasia rehabilitation. In fact, these approaches appear to be cornerstones of a positive approach to clients in general. Tanner et al. (1989) suggest that the speech-language pathologist incorporate frequent positive reinforcement into every session as a means of relieving depression: "Rewards permit the client to concentrate on the positive, not the negative, aspects of the disability" (p. 79). They also suggest that the aphasic client should have opportunities to participate in private time, activities of choice, and group therapy with other aphasic clients.

Other considerations that help relieve depression include clinician willingness to temporarily put aside speech or language goals to allow aphasic patients to vent their feelings. Although some clinicians may feel uneasy when the client discusses such private feelings as inadequacy, loneliness, unhappiness, and guilt, the very act of revealing these feelings may be therapeutic. Revelation of these feelings indicates that the aphasic client has a sense of trust in the speech-language pathologist. This is the time when positive verbal and nonverbal communication skills on the part of the clinician become critical. The reader is referred to several recent resources for an in-depth discussion of communication skills during therapy and counseling (Luteman, 1991; Scheuerle, 1992; Shipley, 1992).

The speech-language pathologist also needs to consider long-term goals for the aphasic client, including strengthening coping skills to deal with residual communication difficulties, achieving independence and socially fulfilling roles in the community, returning to employment, and, for some aphasics, preparing for long-term care. Teamwork with other rehabilitation specialists provides the optimum vehicle for accomplishing these goals. Many hospitals and rehabilitation centers will have teams composed of rehabilitation counselors or psychologists, discharge planners, and vocational counselors in addition to traditional medical and rehabilitation personnel. Speech-language pathologists will need to articulate the communication needs of the aphasic patient and family to these professionals and suggest strategies for incorporating communication goals with the goals of other specialists.

Focus on the Family

Virtually every speech-language pathologist would agree that the family is important in the success of a comprehensive rehabilitation program. Two initial questions should be answered before we discuss how to involve the family: Why is the family so important? What is involvement? Answering these questions leads to defining how family involvement can be operationalized so that therapy is functional and effective for the aphasic individual and the family itself.

Importance of Family in Aphasia Rehabilitation

From the beginning of the recovery period through rehabilitation and discharge, the family performs an important role in the success of the rehabilitation program. The family has been described as "central," "critical," and "focal" to positive outcomes of rehabilitation of any kind. The literature is replete with research and clinical reports that the success of the rehabilitation process may be anchored in the family

(e.g., see articles by Norlin, 1986; Power, 1989; Rau et al., 1986; Rolland, 1988; Rollin, 1987; Watson, 1989). The family is important for at least four reasons.

First, aphasic individuals' initial and continuing impressions of their communication impairment and disability will be grounded in their interactions with their family. The bewilderment, anxiety, and frustration that the family members show during interactions impress on patients the potential gravity of their communication problem. Family members' expectations of, reactions to, and ability to cope with the initial and changing social roles and communication skills may greatly influence how aphasic individuals approach communication rehabilitation. Evans et al. (1992) state that patients make conclusions about their recovery in rehabilitation based on the perceptions of family members.

Second, after hospitalization, most aphasic individuals return to their family living situation (Evans et al., 1992). Thus, the primary communication partners and sources of support for outpatient rehabilitation will be the family. The family can offer instrumental support to meet daily care needs, or expressive support, such as the feelings of caring for and being cared about (Lin, 1986). It is hoped that the family will have strong internal and external resources to meet the level of support needed for the aphasic individual. Support encompasses obtaining therapy, bringing the individual to therapy, reinforcing communication attempts, and participating in family programs. It extends to providing interesting and challenging activities that foster communication and appropriate modification of the physical environment to promote communication interchanges.

The third reason why the family is so critical in rehabilitation is that a positive, well-adapting family promotes compliance with therapy objectives (Evans et al., 1991b). Families come to the stroke rehabilitation event with preconceived beliefs regarding disability, rehabilitation, and their role in the rehabilitation process. If families are not interested in participating in communication therapy themselves, this sends a clear message to the client that the burden for improvement is his or hers alone. Further, families so enmeshed in coping with prior demands and current crises may be too overwhelmed to understand their role in therapy. Des Rosier et al. (1992), in a study of the support needs of well spouses of chronically ill individuals, found that spouses needed personal time and social support from individuals outside the home. Family members' own active participation may be dependent on first receiving physical or psychological support that will help them cope more effectively with the myriad problems facing them.

Fourth, the family serves as an important source of information to the speech-language pathologist. During initial assessment, the family is often the primary resource regarding the premorbid client and family history. Families are also excellent resources regarding goals and progress in therapy. The family is the speech-language pathologist's principal and immediate link to the everyday environment of the aphasic individual.

What is Family Involvement?

Family involvement is defined here as the inclusion of significant family members as active participants in communication assessment, goal setting, and therapy. The environmental systems approach is based on the premise that family members will be consulted, supported, and educated in each stage of recovery from the initial severe illness or crisis stage through disability and possibly institutionalization. The primary goal for the family is to become effective and independent communication problem solvers during everyday interaction. The family should feel a sense of co-responsibility for the communication life of the aphasic individual. This concept is currently defined as "empowerment" and leads to a greater sense of personal control over the course of events (Dunst et al., 1989). Family involvement must go beyond providing progress statements as the client leaves the therapy situation, sending workbooks home for practice, or mentioning the value of family support groups.

Strategies for Involving the Family

The model for working with families presented in Table 12–1 is based on the premise that the family's needs are dynamic and change over time. This is a holistic model that cannot be accomplished by the speech-language pathologist alone but should incorporate other helping professions and extended social groups. Four strategies may be used at each stage of the model: support, education, modeling, and resource referral. Support is generally provided through active, open communication between the speech-language pathologist and the family. Education involves information given about stroke, aphasia, and the therapy process. This may be done through discussion and through supplemental readings for the family. Some popular readings for family members and significant others include Aphasia and the Family (American Heart Association, 1986a); An Adult Has Aphasia (Boone, 1983); Helping the Aphasic to Recover His Speech (Longerich, 1986); Pathways (Ewing & Pfalzgraf, 1991a); Strokes: A Guide for the Family (American Heart Association, 1986b); The Family's Guide to Stroke, Head Trauma, and Speech Disorders (Tanner, 1987); and Understanding Aphasia (Taylor, 1958). In addition, videocassettes on aphasia for home or small-group use can supplement readings: for example, What Is Aphasia? (Ewing & Pfalzgraf, 1991b) and Pathways (Wayne State University Press, 1991). Modeling is done each time the speech-language pathologist talks to the aphasic individual in the presence of family and when family members are present during specific strategy-teaching sessions. Resource referral involves knowing hospital, community, and peer group resources that may be of benefit to the family.

Severe Illness or Crisis Stage

When the individual first has the stroke, the family is likely to be in a state of disequilibrium or crisis. Usual activities halt, and family and individual resources focus on the physical state of the stroke patient. A multitude of deep and conflicting feelings surge among family members, including shock, fear of death and disability, guilt, helplessness, sorrow, and obsessive concern. This is the time when the entire family, and in particular the spouse, needs emotional support. Emotional support involves letting the individuals know that someone in the unfamiliar and impersonal world of the hospital knows who they are and understands the trauma they have experienced. Generally, this is a time when simple introductions, active listening, and comforting nonverbal communication will be important. Such supportive counseling helps establish an atmosphere of trust whereby individual family members can eventually express their feelings and concerns to the speech-language pathologist (Ziolko, 1991). It is not a time to explain the nature of stroke or aphasia, its severity, or its impact. This initial contact alerts the family that there will be a familiar and understanding professional there during the stages of recuperation and rehabilitation.

Recuperation Stage

Once the initial life-threatening stage is completed and the patient moves into recuperation, the family is set on a new course. There is a sense of relief that the patient will survive. There is also the realization that their relative exhibits some physical and communicative difficulties. The search for help begins. Simultaneously, life outside the hospital must return to some semblance of normal; the need for family homeostasis rises. Halm (1990) states that if the family does not try to reestablish equilibrium within a few days or weeks, their efforts will eventually be redirected from "problem neutralization to anxiety reduction" (p. 62). Consequently, family members assume or are assigned new roles within the family. Family members are still highly visible and available in the hospital during their visits to the patient. This becomes an ideal time to gather information about family resources to cope with the stroke, the competing demands on them, and their general coping styles. This is also the time for our initial communication assessment and for our first formal interaction with the family. Although the initial assessment provides only baseline information, family members will be interested in knowing the nature of the communication problem and its prognosis. Common questions include "What's wrong with Dad's speech?" and "Is he going to talk normally again?" During this early contact with the family, the speech-language pathologist must help the family begin to understand their role in the communication rehabilitation process. This is the opportunity to help the family mobilize their resources and problem-solving skills to help the aphasic individual communicate.

This early stage is also the time when general communication-facilitating strategies can be modeled by the speech-language pathologist. Simple strategies include (a) alerting the individual that conversation is to begin, (b) maintaining eye contact while talking, (c) using well-formed short utterances, (d) pausing frequently and using a slow to moderate speaking rate, and (e) generally including the aphasic individual in conversation even if responses are limited to single words or gestures. The speech-language pathologist must also remember that the family will need continued emotional support even though the life-threatening crisis is past.

Rehabilitation

Once the stroke patient is enrolled in a therapy program, the family has a sense of "hope" that things will get better, and they "expect" the patient to invest all of his or her energies into recovery. Success of rehabilitation is partly dependent on a balance of encouragement and realistic expectations. Thus, the speech-language pathologist should discuss with the aphasic individual and the family their expectations and how these coincide with the patient's neurological status and other internal and external factors that affect the outcome of therapy. This is also the time to actively include the family in observing and participating in therapy sessions that focus on communication-facilitating strategies. The family can also be an excellent resource for sharing strategies that they have developed spontaneously to assist in interaction. To work effectively with the family during rehabilitation, we must be available to them during nontraditional therapy times. Spouses and adult children who have jobs will not be able to regularly attend therapy offered during typical daytime hours. Thus, occasional evening and weekend hours for family-centered therapy should be available.

During rehabilitation, the family continues its metamorphoses. New family roles become more solidified. There may be financial and logistical strains associated with therapy. There may be physical changes in the home and the beginning of isolation from the community. The initial support given by extended systems recedes. Spouses and adult daughters are likely to bear the burden of responsibility for managing the household, meeting the physical and rehabilitation needs of their relative, and fitting in their own personal activities. Family members may feel isolated and physically and emotionally exhausted by caregiving stresses. Throughout rehabilitation, open communication between the speech-language pathologist and the family is imperative to ensure that information regarding direct therapy is balanced with family concerns. This is an especially important time when family members should feel a sense of control about therapy decisions.

Other than the direct provision of therapy, perhaps the most important goal during rehabilitation is planning for postrehabilitation. This involves fortifying the critical family communication partners with strategies and the problem-solving mental set that normal, if not functional, communication is possible with their aphasic relative. This also involves helping the family to define their present and expected needs and helping them to access extended systems resources to meet these needs.

Postrehabilitation Stage

At some point, direct rehabilitation with a speech-language pathologist ends, and the stroke patient is likely to have some degree of residual communication disability—from imperceptible to severe. The aphasic individual and the family no longer have the cushion that rehabilitation will result in improvement. Now they must truly rely on their own internal resources and the resources provided by extended systems. The postrehabilitation stage can be less handicapping and isolating if the speech-language pathologist has helped the family plan for this period. Should this not have been a focus, the family may face many years of frustration, resentment, and anger, resulting in fewer and less fulfilling communication opportunities for the aphasic individual. The extended systems of the aphasic individual and the family become particularly important in this stage, as will be described in the next section. With careful planning and guidance, the family should be able to reintegrate the aphasic individual into the family and their extended systems in former or newly created roles.

Long-Term Care

Some aphasic individuals may need to relocate to a long-term care setting such as a nursing facility. The decision to institutionalize the aphasic individual may be made during the recuperation stage or sometime after the individual has returned to the community. This decision is difficult for families and for the aphasic person. It is likely that once the aphasic person enters a long-term care setting he or she will remain there indefinitely. The aphasic person's relationship with the family is altered by the fact that he or she is not able to participate actively in the family, and thus the individual becomes the marginal member of the family. For some families, acceptance of permanent institutionalization may instill guilt feelings; for others, institutionalization may bring a sense of relief. In either case, families continue as an important source of cognitive and social stimulation for the aphasic individual. Counseling for the family of the institutionalized individual concentrates on helping them to understand the meaning of institutionalization, their role in the communication life of the aphasic individual, and strategies for communicating with the individual in that setting. Teamwork with the social worker or nursing staff can be important in helping the family and aphasic individual adjust successfully to long-term care. Finally, families in long-term care facilities may also join family support groups or participate in institution family councils. The value of such groups will be discussed in the next section on extended systems. For more in-depth discussion of the relationship between institutionalization, communication, and aging, the reader is referred to other works by Lubinski (1988, 1991).

Focus on Extended Systems and the Sociocultural Milieu

As stated previously, stroke not only affects the aphasic individual and the immediate family but reverberates to extended systems and to the larger sociocultural milieu. These social networks in turn influence how the aphasic individual and the family seek and receive help. As family structure and physical availability change in our society, extended systems assume important social support functions. These include direct instrumental assistance; psychological and emotional comfort; resource and information sharing, such as offering referrals; and attitude or value transmission (Gourash, 1978). Speech-language pathologists should never underestimate the power of nonimmediate family and friends in the success or failure of the rehabilitation process.

The questions become how to delineate the extended systems of the aphasic individual and family and how to activate these systems to become positive influences in the communication rehabilitation process and after dismissal from therapy. Network mapping can be done through interviewing of the aphasic individual and family members regarding the types and extent of assistance they need and who provides it. The Inventory of Social Support (Trivette & Dunst, 1988) is a formal caregiver self-report tool that identifies social networks and types of assistance given by network members.

During rehabilitation, a natural extended system is composed of the rehabilitation team members and other patients attending therapy simultaneously. Clinicians such as occupational and physical therapists can be catalysts for promoting the communication skills gained in speech-language therapy. They provide opportunities and reinforcement for communication. Similarly, patients who participate in the same therapy programs can become important communication partners for the aphasic individual. The speech-language pathologist might spend some time observing the interactions occurring in other therapies, provide suggestions, and model effective-communication techniques for other therapists and patients who interact with the aphasic individual.

New components to the supportive extended system for the aphasic individual and the family are the "language stimulation therapy group" and the "aphasia family group." One of the best ways to encourage reintegration of the aphasic person and his or her family into the larger sociocultural milieu is through self-help group work. A self-help group is composed of peers who share a common problem and who unite to form a collective identity. Language stimulation therapy

groups may be formed as a part of formal communication therapy or as a postdirect therapy strategy. These groups may be either a homogeneous or heterogeneous collection of aphasic individuals who meet weekly to strengthen communication skills in a more natural interactional setting. Such groups help to make direct therapy more functional, encourage a sharing of knowledge and experiences, and create a new reference group for socialization and support (Cole et al., 1979). Group work may help patients more realistically measure abilities and progress (West, 1981). Aphasic individuals assisting each other assume a helping relationship role for themselves (Glozman, 1981). These groups are usually structured by a speech-language pathologist who has the primary responsibility for the goals and activities of the sessions. Haire (1981) suggests that during such sessions, the tasks should (a) focus on communicative interaction, (b) result in communication success for the aphasic regardless of communication mode or ability, (c) be client originated rather than clinician directed when possible, and (d) be relevant and interesting to the clients. Luterman (1991) finds that structured experience groups effect fewer positive changes than less structured groups. See Chapter 14 in this text for more details on group therapy.

A natural adjunct to the language stimulation group is the aphasia family support or recovery group. This group can be a combination of aphasic individuals and family members or family members alone. At times, family members appreciate having their own reference group where they can exchange ideas and feelings. Mixed groups of aphasic persons and family members may be particularly good for demonstration of communication strategies and resocialization. To be effective, the group should be organized by the members, with the speech-language pathologist serving as an adjunct or informal adviser.

In some cases, the peer group may ask the speech-language pathologist to present a series of talks about aphasia and its disorders. McCormick and Williams (1976) organized a 17-week program that covered such topics as the etiology of stroke, rehabilitation services, physical and medical management, psychological/emotional changes, environmental barriers, diet, relaxation, and role changes. Pasquarello (1990) evaluated a similar type of program and found that family members specifically appreciated the opportunity to share feelings with others and find out how other families coped with a stroke. In another study of support group effectiveness, Halm (1990) found that families perceived that such groups reduced anxiety and instilled hope. Support groups may assist families in locating available services and in advocating for services where they do not exist. Thus, topics chosen for such groups should be less lecture oriented and include more open discussion and problem solving.

Other creative extended systems might be encouraged for the aphasic individual and the family, including family-to-family programs (Williams, 1991). Bissett et al. (1978)

designed a spouse advocate program in which a family member of an aphasic person assisted other aphasic individuals and their families. These individuals, by their unique kinship and empathy with the problem, can offer families special support. Such family-to-family programs are based on the premise that individuals with intimate knowledge of a problem can be excellent resources for other families while gaining positive reward from the helping experience themselves. While such programs are not intended to replace professional counseling, the families can help relieve feelings of isolation and offer practical information about logistics of obtaining funding and other assistive services. Williams (1991) states that family-to-family programs give families a "sense of control, predictability, and opportunity" (p. 305).

Family advocacy groups can take on yet another dimension. Family members may wish to affiliate and become involved with local and national family advocacy groups such as the National Stroke Foundation and the National Head Injury Foundation. These groups serve important functions such as affecting legislation on issues related to stroke and head injury and helping to change the health care and rehabilitation system. Some families assume prominent roles in such organizations.

Finally, extended systems can include other community networks such as adult day-care programs, respite programs, health care assistants in the home, and volunteers. Full-time and part-time adult day-care programs may be associated with hospitals, nursing homes, or senior citizen centers. These programs provide custodial and health care, recreation, and nutrition as well as opportunities for socialization. Respite programs may be based in a community health care setting such as a nursing home whereby the aphasic individual can reside for a limited stay while the family travels or pursues noncaregiving activities. Brief respite programs may also be available within the aphasic individual's home while a family member shops, goes to a physician, or participates in other activities. National and local volunteer programs are available through many organizations such as the Ombudsman Program offered through the American Red Cross. In this program, senior volunteers visit nursing home patients and act as patient and family advocates with nursing home administration. Bell (1990) is an excellent resource for how to build volunteer programs for patients and their families.

The speech-language pathologist should be available to the extended groups in which the aphasic individual and the family are involved. Many of these groups are open to consultation from the speech-language pathologist regarding how to facilitate communication with the aphasic individual. Most of these individuals have limited experience with aphasic individuals and are eager to learn how to communicate more effectively. The goal in working with such groups is to provide strategies for facilitating communication with the aphasic individual. Role playing and problem solving, rather than didactic information regarding the nature and etiology of aphasia, are the most effective means of instruction.

Sociocultural Milieu

What can the speech-language pathologist do to meet the cultural needs of aphasic patients and their families? While this topic could be an entire chapter unto itself, a few guidelines are suggested. The first suggestion is that more individuals from minority groups should be encouraged to become speech-language pathologists. Interaction with a variety of minority individuals and more practica experience with diverse client groups should provide white middle-class speech-language pathologists with greater cultural depth perception. Graduate training programs are encouraged by the American Speech-Language-Hearing Association to incorporate cultural issues into and across coursework and practica. In addition to understanding the communication problems of various cultural groups, coursework should also focus on understanding transcultural concepts and the spectrum of health care values and beliefs outside traditional Western medicine.

Rothenburger (1990) suggests that clinicians must learn to use all senses in interacting with clients of diverse cultures. She places a special emphasis on improving verbal and nonverbal skills that increase interaction sensitivity. Most important, clinicians need to assess their own cultural history and biases and how such perceptions affect service delivery to aphasic individuals and their families. Professional speech-language pathologists could also improve their cultural awareness through increasing interaction with diverse cultural and ethnic groups, attending departmental inservices or professional meetings, and reading literature that focuses on multicultural issues. Barney (1991) suggests that professionals should have built into their quality assessment process methods for assuring that the needs of specific ethnic and racial groups have been addressed appropriately.

Focus on the Physical Environment

No matter what setting the aphasic person lives in, either family home or institution, the physical characteristics of that environment become an important backdrop for communicative interaction. The physical setting should be a source of information and stimulation for the aphasic individual. While it may be impractical to redesign the hospital or family home, some realistic modifications that facilitate communication are possible. The factors that can be manipulated in most environments include (a) lighting and visual cues, (b) acoustic treatment, (c) furniture arrangement, and (d) environmental props. For a more in-depth discussion of these topics, the reader is referred to Calkins (1988) and Lubinski (1991).

Lighting and Visual Cues

Adequate and pleasant illumination creates a visually stimulating environment for aphasic persons and their communication partners. A high proportion of aphasic individuals and their spouses will exhibit visual changes associated with aging, including glaucoma, cataracts, and macular degeneration (Carroll, 1978). These visual changes result in blindness, low or blurred vision, and changes in central or peripheral vision. Thus, rooms that are dimly lit or filled with glare will reduce the aphasic person's ability to comprehend nonverbal cues, take advantage of contextual information, and derive cognitive and social stimulation from the visual environment. When possible, the aphasic person should have visual access to windows facing outdoors or to areas where everyday activities occur, such as the kitchen and living room at home, and the nursing station and lounge areas of the nursing home. Visual access gives the aphasic person a sense of connectedness with the external environment.

The use of color in the aphasic person's environment also plays an important role. Improving visual contrasts through color enhances information and aids in visual discrimination. For example, walls painted in primary colors with contrasting colors for doors aid in identification of one's own room, as do name plates printed in large-size white letters on a contrasting dark surface. Other simple strategies that enhance visual access include eliminating slick, shiny surfaces that provide glare; adding texture to surfaces of walls, furniture, and bedding; and using warm, medium-intensity colors to facilitate orientation. Because some aphasic individuals will be seated in wheelchairs, placement of visual information such as clocks and bulletin boards should be adjusted appropriately for a seated person.

Perhaps the simplest strategy to enhance visual access is to ensure that the aphasic individual has the best vision possible through regular referral for ophthalomological or optometrical evaluations. Use of glasses or other visual assistive devices should be easily accessible to the aphasic individual. Speech-language pathologists should check the patient's chart to note if there are visual field disturbances or if glasses are used prior to evaluations and therapy. Use of large-print materials and access to magnifying glasses or magnifying sheets should be encouraged to facilitate use of pictures or printed materials. Aphasic individuals with severe visual difficulties may benefit from listening to "talking books" or specially adapted televisions for the visually impaired. Finally, visual access is enhanced by coming face to face with the aphasic individual or asking what positioning facilitates facial access.

Acoustic Treatment

The primary goal of enhancing the acoustic environment is to ensure that intact auditory information reaches the aphasic individual. In addition to auditory comprehension difficulties, the aphasic individual may have hearing difficulties related to the aging process or previous life experiences, such as employment in noisy environments. Again, the first step in enhancing the acoustic environment is to begin with a referral for a complete otological and audiological evaluation. Aphasic individuals with a hearing loss should be encouraged to use a hearing aid or other assistive listening device to receive auditory information more adequately. Face-to-face communication also will optimize auditory receptive abilities.

Ambient noise in the environment may reduce the aphasic person's auditory attention and comprehension skills, particularly during conversation. Ideally, areas where the aphasic person frequently communicates should be acoustically treated with sound-absorbing materials to reduce ambient noise and reverberation. Other noise control strategies include turning off the radio or television when talking with the aphasic individual, and closing a door or window to reduce noise from other areas or corridors. Each of these techniques is inexpensive.

Noise abatement, however, does not mean removing all sound from the aphasic person's environment. Everyday sounds are a source of stimulation and conversation. Stimulation from the sounds of daily life, music, radios, and television can stimulate interaction with others in the environment. Auditory stimulation gives the aphasic individual knowledge about his or her surroundings and a sense of belonging.

Furniture Arrangement

The arrangement of furniture determines where, when, and with whom the aphasic person will talk. For example, the aphasic person in a wheelchair may lack access to favorite areas and social groups. Aphasic individuals will be more likely to join a group if they feel they can enter it with a minimum of inconvenience and disruption. Furniture, when possible, should be movable to promote easy access. Circular furniture arrangement also facilitates eye contact with a variety of people. It is crucial that the aphasic person retain control over some personal space in the environment. All individuals require areas and objects that reflect their unique personalities and interests. Finally, furniture arrangement should provide opportunities for privacy and intimate talk with chosen partners.

Environmental Props

Physical props in the environment also stimulate the aphasic person's general orientation and communication. Additions such as personal items, mementos, and favorite pictures into the institutional setting give individuals consistency with their family home and their life-long identity. Other props promote comprehension and way-finding in the environment. For example, clocks, calendars, pictures, and bulletin boards serve as orientation devices. As much as possible, the physical "stuff" of the environment should reflect the person's history and interests while providing multisensory cuing about time and place.

THE CLINICIAN AS A SYSTEMS CATALYST

Lest we forget, the speech-language pathologist (or other rehabilitation specialist) is a new and critically important component in the environmental systems approach to aphasia. From the initial referral and reading of a client's medical chart, the speech-language pathologist has entered the environment of the aphasic and his or her family. The speech-language pathologist brings to this encounter a host of personal and professional characteristics, as well as a health care and rehabilitation value system. The setting in which the speech-language pathologist offers communication therapy and any third-party payors for such service influence the clinician and the therapy offered. While research continues to delineate aphasic characteristics, less attention has been paid to the characteristics that the clinician and the rehabilitation setting contribute to therapy delivery and effectiveness.

McNeny and Wilcox (1991) state that rehabilitation specialists have overt, distinct perspectives on rehabilitation based on their education and experiences, but they also are influenced by less conscious beliefs. McNeny and Wilcox suggest that clinicians who have insight into their underlying feelings and attitudes may understand therapy better. Dunst et al. (1989) suggest that clinician attitudes, beliefs, and behaviors associated with client empowerment can be categorized along a prehelping, helping, and posthelping continuum. During the prehelping stage, the primary characteristics needed to foster client empowerment include (a) seeing the individual and the family as having strengths and abilities rather than deficits and (b) focusing on problem solving as the goal of therapy. During the help-giving stage, positive clinician behaviors include good listening skills, focusing on client definition of needs, and a partnership mentality. Finally, during the posthelping stage, positive clinician responses stress minimizing help seeker indebtedness, accepting of client decisions, and enhancing a sense of self-efficacy on the part of the client and the family.

Particularly in working with families, it may be difficult for the speech-language pathologist to divorce one's own family experiences from interactions with client families. Cultural differences between clinician and aphasic/family also may engender conflicts between these entities. Fatigue, frustration, and lack of positive reinforcement—which are inherent in working with long-term multiply impaired clients who evidence little progress—influence how the clinician approaches the aphasic client and family. All of these factors may lead the clinician to misinterpret or be less sensitive to the actions and beliefs of those within the aphasic environment. Maslach (1982) states that "the kind of person you are dealing with

may influence what you provide, how well you do it, and even whether you will do it at all" (p. 25).

Speech-language pathologists need to become more conscious of how powerful a factor they are in the lives of clients and families. A balance must be struck between rehabilitating specific communication skills and enabling the client and family to be their own clinician. The traditional focus on remediating specific communication skills tends to be clinician-driven, while the focus on enabling stresses that the solutions to communication difficulties can be generated by client and family. The speech-language pathologist as enabler provides information, models and reinforces facilitating communication strategies, and serves as a resource and advocate for the family and the client.

FUTURE TRENDS

Each section of this chapter raises important issues for the speech-language pathologist to consider, from philosophical perspectives of aphasia rehabilitation to practical questions of effective service delivery. The first issue raised was the growing emphasis on functional assessment and rehabilitation. This will be a major challenge for speech-language pathologists and aphasiologists. A major concern is that functional assessment tools possess rigorous psychometric properties if they are to be valid and reliable components of our testing batteries. Functional assessment will mean that speech-language pathologists must include assessment of clients outside traditional therapy settings as well as rely on caregiver report. Functional assessment will need to extend to better instruments for assessment of the family's attitude toward and ability to communicate effectively with the aphasic individual. A comprehensive functional assessment may include components directed toward the individual, the family or primary caregiver, and the physical and social environment.

This chapter challenges us to specifically, rather than incidentally, target some of our treatment toward the family and other significant persons in the lives of our patients. This will mean that our preprofessional and continuing education should include more work on understanding families and the sociocultural and economic milieu of the aphasic person. Specific coursework and practica in counseling should be required. This chapter also reminds us that the physical environment can either enhance or obstruct communication opportunities for our aphasic patients.

Numerous areas of research emanate from this chapter. Although a single research study to investigate the feasibility of the environmental systems approach is impossible, more discrete components could be empirically investigated in either traditional group or single-subject studies. It is likely that to investigate the environment more carefully, we need to move toward ethnometric, descriptive field, and hypothetico-deductivism studies of post-stroke family interaction in their natural settings (Jones &

Lubinski—unpublished). Such studies would open new avenues of research opportunities for practicing clinicians and add to our much needed data on the efficacy of such therapy.

As clinicians we are faced with making many choices with and for our aphasic clients. This chapter encourages you to choose between a narrow philosophy and a broad philosophy of assessment and intervention; between clinician-directed and client/family-enabled therapy; and between progress based on quantity of speech for the aphasic and progress based on quality of communication for the aphasic and his or her partners. The communication life of the aphasic is enhanced when we choose to go beyond words to function and from function to context.

▶ *Acknowledgments*–Sincere appreciation is offered to the following individuals for their invaluable assistance in the preparation of this chapter: J.B. Orange, Ph.D., University of Western Ontario, for his careful reading of the chapter; Terri Cinotti, M.A., State University at Buffalo, for her help in collecting references and in preparing the bibliography; and Kathleen Jones, Ph.D., State University College at Geneso, for introducing me to the family process literature.

References

American Heart Association (1986a). *Aphasia and the family.* Dallas, TX: American Heart Association's Communications Division.

American Heart Association (1986b). *Strokes: A guide for the family.* Dallas, TX: American Heart Association's Communications Division.

American Psychiatric Association (1987). *Diagnostic and statistical manual of mental disorders, III-R.* Washington, DC: APA.

American Speech-Language and Hearing Association (ASHA) (1990). *Functional Communication Scales for Adults Project: Advisory report.* Rockville, MD: ASHA.

Andrews, J. & Andrews, M. (1987). *Family based treatment in communicative disorders.* Sandwich, IL: Janelle Publications.

Agar, M. (1980). *The professional stranger: An informed introduction to ethnography.* New York: Academic Press.

Aten, J. (1986). Functional communication treatment. In R. Chapey (ed.), *Language intervention strategies in adult aphasia.* Baltimore, MD: Williams & Wilkins.

Aten, J., Caliguiri, M., & Holland, A. (1982). The efficacy of functional communication therapy for chronic aphasic patients. *Journal of Speech and Hearing Disorders, 47,* 93–96.

Banja, S. (1990). Rehabilitation and empowerment. *Archives of Physical and Medical Rehabilitation, 71,* 614–615.

Barney, K. (1991). From Ellis Island to assisted living: Meeting the needs of older adults from diverse cultures. *American Journal of Occupational Therapy, 45,* 586–593.

Bell, V. (1990). Tapping an unlimited resource: Building volunteer programs for patients and their families. In N. Mace (ed.), *Dementia care: Patient, family and community.* Baltimore, MD: Johns Hopkins University Press.

Bishop, P. (1982). Psychological issues and behavior in stroke rehabilitation. In J. Basmajian & M. Brandstates (eds.), *Stroke Rehabilitation.* Baltimore, MD: Williams & Wilkins.

Bissett, J., Haire, A., & Nelson, M. (1978). Involving the aphasic's wife in the rehabilitation of other aphasics. Poster session at the Annual Convention of the American Speech and Hearing Association, San Francisco, CA.

Bonder, B. (1986/1987). Family systems and Alzheimer's disease: An approach to treatment. *Physical and Occupational Therapy in Geriatrics, 5,* 13–24.

Boone, D.R. (1983). *An adult has aphasia.* Danville, IL: Interstate Printers and Publishers.

Bozarth, J. (1981). The rehabilitation process and older people. *Journal of Rehabilitation, 45,* 28–32.

Brocklehurst, J., Morris, P., Andrews, K., Richards, B., & Laycock, P. (1981). Social effects of stroke. *Social Science Medicine, 15,* 35–39.

Brubaker, E. (1987). *Working with the elderly: A social system approach.* Newbury Park, CA: Sage.

Calkins, M. (1988). *Design for dementia: Planning environments for the elderly and confused.* Owing Mills, MD: National Health Publishing.

Carroll, K. (1978). *Human development in aging: The nursing home environment.* Minneapolis, MN: Ebenezer Center for Aging and Human Development.

Carver, V. & Rodda, M. (1978). *Disability and the environment.* New York: Schocken Books.

Cole, S., O'Conner, S., & Bennett, L. (1979). Self-help group for clinic patients with chronic illness. *Primary Care, 6,* 325–340.

Cross, T. (1988). *Cultural competence continuum—Focal point 3(1).* Portland, OR: Research and Training Center to Improve Services for Seriously Emotionally Handicapped Children and Their Families.

Cullum, C.M. & Bigler, E. (1991). Short- and long-term psychological status following stroke. *Journal of Nervous and Mental Diseases, 179,* 274–278.

Davis, G. (1986). Pragmatics and treatment. In R. Chapey (ed.), *Language intervention strategies in adult aphasia.* Baltimore, MD: Williams & Wilkins.

Davis, G. & Wilcox, M. (1981). Incorporating parameters of natural conversation in aphasia treatment. In R. Chapey (ed.), *Language intervention strategies in adult aphasia.* Baltimore, MD: Williams & Wilkins.

Des Rosier, M., Catanzaro, M., & Piller, J. (1992). Living with chronic illness: Social support and the well spouse perspective. *Rehabilitation Nursing, 17,* 87–91.

Dunst, C., Trivette, C., Gordon, N., & Pletcher, L. (1989). Building and mobilizing informal family support networks. In G. Singer & L. Irvin (eds.), *Support for care giving families.* Baltimore, MD: Paul Brookes.

Egelko, S., Simon, D., Riley, E., Gordon, W., Ruckdeschel-Hibbard, M., & Diller, L. (1989). First year after stroke: Tracking cognitive and affective deficits. *Archives of Physical and Medical Rehabilitation, 70,* 297–302.

Epstein, N., Baldwin, L., & Bishop, D. (1983). The McMaster family assessment device. *Journal of Marital Family Therapy, 9,* 171–180.

Evans, R., Bishop, D., & Haselkorn, J. (1991a). Factors predicting satisfactory home care after stroke. *Archives of Physical and Medical Rehabilitation, 72,* 144–147.

Evans, R., Bishop, D., Haselkorn, J., Hendricks, R., Baldwin, D., & Connis, R. (1991b). From crisis to recovery: The family's role in stroke rehabilitation. *Neurological Rehabilitation, 1,* 69–78.

Evans, R., Griffith, J., Haselkorn, J., Hendricks, R., Baldwin, D., & Bishop, D. (1992). Poststroke family function: An evaluation of the family's role in rehabilitation. *Rehabilitation Nursing, 17,* 127–132.

Ewing, S. & Pfalzgraf, B. (1991a). *Pathways: Moving beyond stroke* (video). Detroit, MI: Wayne State University Press.

Ewing, S. & Pfalzgraf, B. (1991b). *What is aphasia?* (video). Detroit, MI: Wayne State University Press.

Frattali, C. (1992). Functional assessment of communication: Merging public policy with clinical views. *Aphasiology, 6,* 63–83.

Friedman, M. (1990). Transcultural family nursing: Application to Latino and Black families. *Journal of Pediatric Nursing, 5,* 214–221.

Gatz, M., Bengston, V., & Blum, M. (1990). Caregiving families. In J. Birren & K. Schari (eds.), *Handbook of psychology of aging* (3rd ed.). San Diego, CA: Academic Press.

Gibb, J. (1961). Defensive communication. *Journal of Communication, 11,* 141–148.

Glozman, J. (1981). On increasing motivation to communication in aphasics rehabilitation. *International Journal of Rehabilitation Research, 4,* 78–81.

Goffman, E. (1964). *Stigma.* Englewood Cliffs, NJ: Prentice-Hall.

Gourash, M. (1978). Help-seeking: A review of the literature. *American Journal of Community Psychology, 6,* 499–517.

Gray, W., Dyhl, F., & Rizzo, N. (1969). *General systems theory and psychiatry.* Boston, MA: Little, Brown.

Haire, A. (1981). Principles for organizing group treatment. In R. Brookshire (ed.), *Clinical aphasiology* (pp. 146–149). Minneapolis, MN: BRK.

Halm, M. (1990). Effects of support groups on anxiety of family members during critical illness. *Heart and Lung, 19,* 62–70.

Hill, R. (1949). *Families under stress.* New York: Harper & Row.

Holland, A. (1980). *Communicative abilities of daily living.* Baltimore, MD: University Park Press.

Holland, A. (1982). Observing functional communication of aphasic adults. *Journal of Speech and Hearing Disorders, 47,* 50–56.

Holroyd, J. (1974). The questionnaire on resources and stress: An instrument to measure family response to a handicapped family member. *Journal of Community Psychology, 2,* 92–94.

House, A., Dennis, M., Mogridge, L., Hawton, K., & Warlaw, C. (1990). Life events and difficulties preceding stroke. *Journal of Neurology, Neurosurgery, and Psychiatry, 53,* 1024–1028.

Hyman, M. (1972). Social psychological determinants of patients' performance in stroke rehabilitation. *Archives of Physical and Medical Rehabilitation, 53,* 217–226.

Ingstad, B. (1990). The disabled person in the community: Social and cultural aspects. *International Journal of Rehabilitation Research, 13,* 187–194.

Ittelson, W., Proshansky, H., Rivlin, L., & Winkel, G. (1974). *An introduction to environmental psychology.* New York: Holt, Rinehart, & Winston.

Jenike, M. (1988). Depression and other psychiatric disorders. In M. Albert & M. Moss (eds.), *Geriatric neuropsychology.* New York: Holt, Rinehart, & Winston.

Jones, K. (1989). Impacts of cerebrovascular accidents on family systems. Unpublished doctoral dissertation, State University of New York at Buffalo, NY.

Jones, K. & Lubinski, R. (a-unpublished manuscript). Communication disorders research: Building scientific alliances in research for clinical relevance.

Jones, K. & Lubinski, R. (b-unpublished manuscript). Methodology for investigating impacts of strokes on family systems.

Kavanagh, K. & Kennedy, P. (1992). *Promoting cultural diversity.* Newbury Park, CA: Sage.

Keller, C., Tanner, D., Urbina, C., & Gerstengberger, D. (1989). Psychological responses in aphasia: Theoretical considerations and nursing implications. *Journal of Neuroscience Nursing, 21,* 290–294.

Kelly-Hayes, M., Warf, P., Kannel, W., Sytkowski, P., D'Agostino, R., & Gresham, G. (1988). Factors influencing survival and need for institutionalization following stroke: The Framingham study. *Archives of Physical and Medical Rehabilitation, 69,* 415–418.

Kinsella, G. & Duffy, R. (1979). Psychosocial readjustment in the spouses of aphasic patients. *Scandinavian Journal of Rehabilitation Medicine, 11,* 129–132.

Krefting, L. & Krefting, D. (1991). Cultural influences on performance. In C. Christian & C. Baum (eds.), *Occupational therapy: Overcoming human performance deficits.* Thorofare, NJ: Slack.

Langenbrunner, J., Willis, P., Jencks, S., Dobson, A., & Lezzoni, L. (1989). Developing payment refinements and reforms under Medicare for excluded hospitals. *Health Care Financing Review, 10,* 91–107.

Lawton, M. (1970). Assessment, integration and environments for older people. *Gerontology, 10,* 38–46.

Lefebre, R. & Sanford, S. (1985). A multi-model questionnaire for stress. *Journal of Human Stress, 11,* 69–75.

Lin, N. (1986). Conceptualizing social support. In N. Lin, A. Dean, & W. Ensel (eds.), *Social support, life events, and depression* (pp. 17–30). New York: Academic Press.

Litman, T. (1962). Self-conception and physical rehabilitation. In A. Rose (ed.), *Human behavior and social processes.* Boston, MA: Houghton Mifflin.

Longerich, MC. (1986). *Helping the aphasic to recover his speech: A manual for the family.* Los Angeles, CA: LLU Press.

Lubinski, R. (1981). Environmental language intervention. In R. Chapey (ed.), *Language intervention strategies in adult aphasia.* Baltimore, MD: Williams & Wilkins.

Lubinski, R. (1988). A model for intervention: Communication skills, effectiveness and opportunity. In B. Shadden (ed.), *Behavior and aging: A sourcebook for clinicians.* Baltimore, MD: Williams & Wilkins.

Lubinski, R. (1991). Environmental considerations for elderly patients. In R. Lubinski (ed.), *Dementia and communication.* Philadelphia, PA: Decker.

Luterman, D. (1991). *Counseling the communicatively disordered and their families.* Austin, TX: Pro-Ed.

Lyon, J. (1992). Communication use and participation in life for adults with aphasia in natural settings: The scope of the problem. *American Journal of Speech-Language Pathology, 1,* 7–14.

Maitz, E. (1991). Family systems theory applied to head injury. In J. Williams & T. Kay (eds.), *Head injury and family matters.* Baltimore, MD: Paul Brookes.

Maslach, C. (1982). *Burnout: The cost of caring.* Englewood Cliffs, NJ: Prentice-Hall.

May, J. (1992). Working with diverse families: Building culturally competent systems of health care delivery. *Journal of Rheumatology, 19,* 46–48.

McCormick, G. & Williams, P. (1976). The Midwestern Pennsylvania Stroke Club: Conclusions following the first year's operation of a family centered program. In R. Brookshire (ed.), *Clinical aphasiology: Conference proceedings.* Minneapolis, MN: BRK.

McCubbin, H., Larsen, A., & Olson, D. (1981). *Family Crisis Oriented Personal Evaluation Scales (COPES).* St. Paul, MN: University of Minnesota.

McCubbin, H. & Patterson, J. (1983). The family stress process: A double ABCX model of adjustment and adaptation. In H. McCubbin, M. Sussman, & J. Patterson (eds.), *Advances and developments in family stress theory and research.* New York: Haworth Press.

McCubbin, H., Patterson, J., & Wilson, L. (1980). *Family Inventory of Life Events and Changes (FILE).* St. Paul, MN: University of Minnesota.

McGoldrick, M. & Carter, E. (1982). The family life cycle. In F. Walsh (ed.), *Normal family processes.* New York: Guilford Press.

McNeny, R. & Wilcox, P. (1991). Partners by choice: The family and the rehabilitation team. *Neurological Rehabilitation, 1,* 7–18.

Moos, R. (1976). *The human contest.* New York: John Wiley & Sons.

Norlin, P. (1986). Familiar faces, sudden strangers: Helping families cope with the crisis of aphasia. In R. Chapey (ed.), *Language intervention strategies in adult aphasia.* Baltimore, MD: Williams & Wilkins.

Olson, D., Portner, J., & Lavee, Y. (1985). *FACES III: Family social science.* Minneapolis MN: University of Minnesota.

Pasquarello, M. (1990). Developing, implementing, and evaluating a stroke recovery group. *Rehabilitation Nursing, 15,* 26–29.

Power, P. (1989). Working with families: An intervention model for rehabilitation nurses. *Rehabilitation Nursing, 14,* 73–76.

Rabinowitz, H. & Mitsos, S. (1964). Rehabilitation as planned social change: A conceptual framework. *Journal of Health and Human Behavior, 5,* 2–14.

Rau, M.T., Schulz, R., Tompkins, C., Rhyne, C., & Golper, L. (1986). The poststroke psychosocial environment of stroke patients and their partners: Some preliminary results of a longitudinal study. In R. Brookshire (ed.), *Clinical aphasiology.* Minneapolis, MN: BRK.

Rawlins, P., Rawlins, T., & Horner, M. (1990). Development of the family needs assessment tool. *Western Journal of Nursing Research, 12,* 201–214.

Robinson, R. & Benson, D.F. (1981). Depression in aphasia patients: Frequency, severity, and clinicopathological correlations. *Brain and Language, 14,* 282–291.

Rolland, J. (1988). A conceptual model of chronic and life-threatening illness and its impact on families. In C. Chilman, E. Nunnally, & F. Cox (eds.), *Chronic illness and disability,* Newbury Park, CA: Sage.

Rolland, J. (1990). Anticipatory loss: A family systems developmental framework. *Family Process, 29,* 229–243.

Rollin, W. (1987). *The psychology of communication disorders in individuals and their families.* Englewood Cliffs, NJ: Prentice-Hall.

Romano, M. (1989). The therapeutic milieu in the rehabilitation processes. In D. Krueger (ed.), *Rehabilitation psychology.* Rockville, MD: Aspen.

Rothenburger, R. (1990). Transcultural nursing overcoming obstacles to effective communication. *American Organization of Registered Nurses Journal, 51,* 1349–1363.

Safilios-Rothchild, C. (1970). *The sociology and social psychology of disability and rehabilitation.* New York: Random House.

Scheuerle, J. (1992). *Counseling in speech-language pathology and audiology.* New York: Merrill.

Shipley, K. (1992). *Interviewing and counseling in communicative disorders.* New York: Merrill.

Simon, A. & Agazarian, Y. (1967). *Sequential analysis of verbal interaction.* Philadelphia, PA: Research for Better Schools.

Starkstein, S. & Robinson, R. (1988). Aphasia and depression. *Aphasiology, 2,* 1–20.

Steger, H. (1976). Understanding the psychological factors in rehabilitation. *Geriatrics, 31,* 68–73.

Stern, R. & Bachman, D. (1991). Depressive symptoms following stroke. *American Journal of Psychiatry, 148,* 351–356.

Sue, D. & Sue D. (1990). *Counseling the culturally different: Theory and practice* (2nd ed.). New York: John Wiley & Sons.

Tanner, D. (1987). *The family's guide to stroke, head trauma, and speech disorders.* Tulsa, OK: Modern Education Corp.

Tanner, D. & Gerstenberger, R. (1988). The grief response in neuropathologies of speech and language. *Aphasiology, 2,* 79–84.

Tanner, D., Gerstenberger, D., & Keller, C. (1989). Guidelines for the treatment of chronic depression in the aphasia patient. *Rehabilitation Nursing, 14,* 77–80.

Taylor, M. (1958). *Understanding aphasia.* New York: Institute of Rehabilitation Medicine.

Trivette, C. & Dunst, C. (1988). Inventory of social support. In C. Dunst, C. Trivette, & C. Deal (eds.), *Empowering families: Principles and guidelines for practice.* Cambridge, MA: Brookline Book.

Turnbull, A. & Turnbull, H.R. (1991). Understanding families from a systems perspective. In J. Williams & T. Kay (eds.), *Head injury: A family matter.* Baltimore, MD: Paul Brookes.

Wahrborg, P. (1991). Assessment and management of emotional and psychological reactions to brain damage and aphasia. San Diego, CA: Singular Publishing Group.

Wallace, G. & Freeman, S. (1991). Adults with neurological impairment from multicultural populations. *Journal of the American Speech and Hearing Association, 33,* 58–62.

Watson, P. (1989). Indications of family capacity for participating in the rehabilitation process: Report of a preliminary investigation. *Rehabilitation Nursing, 14,* 318–322.

Watzlawick, P. & Coyne, J. (1980). Depression following strokes: Brief problem-focused family treatment. *Family Process, 19,* 13–18.

Wayne State University (1991). *Pathways.* Detroit, MI: Wayne State University Press.

Webster, E.J. & Newhoff, M.N. (1981). Intervention with families of communicatively impaired adults. In D.L. Beasley & G.A. Davis (eds.), *Aging communication processes and disorders*. New York: Grune & Stratton.

Wertz, R. (1983). Language intervention context and setting for the aphasic adult. In J. Miller, D. Yoder, & R. Schiefelbusch (eds.), *Contemporary issues in language intervention* (Report 12;1:116–220). Rockville, MD: ASHA.

West, J. (1981). Group treatment. In R. Brookshire (ed.), *Proceedings of the Clinical Aphasiology Conference* (pp. 149–152). Minneapolis, MN: BRK.

Westby, C. (1990). Ethnographic interviewing: Asking the right questions to the right people in the right ways. *Journal of Childhood Communication Disorders, 13*, 101–111.

Wilkerson, D., Batavia, A., & DeJong, G. (1992). Use of functional status measures for payment of medical rehabilitation services. *Archives of Physical and Medical Rehabilitation, 73*, 111–120.

Williams, J. (1991). Family reaction to head injury. In J. Williams & T. Kay (eds.), *Head injury: A family matter*. Baltimore, MD: Paul Brookes.

Ziolko, M. (1991). Counseling parents of children with disabilities: A review of the literature and implications for practice. *Journal of Rehabilitation, 57*, 29–34.

Chapter 13

Treating Life Consequences of Aphasia's Chronicity

Jon G. Lyon and Barbara B. Shadden

OBJECTIVES

This chapter will enable the reader to (1) assess the nature of interventions into aphasia's chronicity in terms of (a) their form, i.e., historically, currently, and potentially into the future; and (b) their intended purposes and treatment targets, which seemingly are most influential in living daily life effectively; (2) better understand the complexities of such interventions; and (3) cite possible treatment options.

INTRODUCTION

Aphasia's Chronicity: Its Effects on Daily Life

When one examines the literature pertaining to aphasia and its treatment, either historically or ontologically, a common theme prevails: this disorder usually arrives without warning and remains a permanent part of daily life thereafter. From descriptions of aphasiology's earliest roots (Schuell et al., 1964) to descriptions of its most recent developments (Davis, 2000; Worrall & Frattali, 2000), and from the perspectives of a wide variety of experts (people with aphasia [Newborn, 1998; Wulf, 1979], their family and friends [Labourel & Martin, 1993; Parr et al., 1997], clinicians [Lyon, 1998b; Pound, 1998], and researchers [LeDorze & Brassard, 1995; Wahrborg, 1991]) at any point in its evolution and treatment, the chronicity of aphasia remains a central issue of daily life.

For all the benefit that has accrued from what we have learned about aphasia, and all the good that has been derived from our treatments for people confronting aphasia, nothing "cures" its underlying pathology or its functional and psychosocial consequences, or eliminates the necessity of overhauling most of the primary domains of daily life (Sarno, 1991; Tanner & Gerstenberger, 1988). Furthermore, this perpetual state of interference in the living of life is not restricted to the person with aphasia, but rather affects the well-being of everyone who depended upon that person for their own daily sustenance, partnership, or companionship (Chwat & Gurland, 1981; Code et al., 1999).

As a result, the real-life consequences of aphasia are broader and deeper than first acknowledged by researchers and clinicians, or internalized by those confronting aphasia personally. In other words, social dysfunction in life extends well beyond the presenting symptom of an acquired disruption of language and communication (Darley, 1991; Simmons-Mackie, 2000). Not only do a host of ongoing "barriers" obstruct aspects of daily life such as maintaining a household, rearing a family, or working in a chosen job or profession, but more importantly, they often paralyze, undermine, and/or retard personal or intimate domains of life, such as sharing, discussing, wishing, and deciding jointly and mutually with key confidants, friends, and loved ones.

For many, this "interpersonal bond," entailing frequent access to and use of counsel, humor, support, comfort, respect, and love, significantly determines constancy and predictability in daily life, and ultimately defines wellness, both individually for the person with aphasia or significant other, and jointly for couples and dyads in which one partner has aphasia (Ryff & Singer, 2000; Ryff et al., in press). It is this massive and protracted disruption throughout 'life systems' that underscores what aphasia really is! The effects of the ongoing presence of permanent injury, herein referenced as "aphasia's chronicity," are what this chapter addresses. Without question, it is within the wide array of symptoms of lasting dysfunction that the most obstructive and detrimental forces to living a positive daily existence rest (Byng et al., in press; Life Participation Approach to Aphasia/LPAA, 2000).

Aphasia's Chronicity: Why Its Impact Is So Extensive

Aphasia's global effects on the living of ordinary life originate from its prime source of interference: the disruption of everyday communication. Unlike acquired and enduring injuries that primarily involve an isolated body part or an internal organ, the brain injury resulting in aphasia is not reducible to a circumscribed list of communicative losses or parts. In fact, if we attempt to isolate the effects of aphasia by removing everything else in life except these, we can only do so momentarily and artificially. We cannot consider aphasia in such a state of separation for long without seeing the resultant alterations to life itself.

The reason for the life-altering effect of aphasia is clear: the act of communicating serves no other purpose in daily life except as a *medium* or *conduit* through which people can consider, share, reflect, and decide about its form and possibilities. Thus, communication is not, in and of itself, a free-standing entity or 'thing.' It is, instead, as Kagan and Gailey (1993) have stated: "a currency" through which life is lived! As such, it allows personal and social entrance, acceptability, verification, and acclaim, while without it, one typically faces obstruction, disempowerment, and/or rejection. Again, the devastating effects of aphasia extend beyond the injured adult; they significantly impact partnerships and 'couples' of all kinds, most often couples in close relationships.

The citing of aphasia's broad impact on the living of life is not to imply that chronic physical injury (e.g., hemiparesis or hemiplegia) doesn't impact psychosocial wellness as well. In fact, depending on a person's image of self and daily reliance on refined or skilled motor movement, being rendered permanently disabled in arm or hand movements may be far more catastrophic to the professional athlete, for instance, than being speechless. When physical immobility occurs, however, it usually does not preclude entry and participation in other social realms of life.

People confronting the long-term effects of aphasia, however, do not share this ease of re-entry into an array of social options. Social participation in life rests with one's ability to engage others, interact, share, and maintain parity and acceptance within such exchanges. For people with aphasia, the degree of interference in such realms may vary from mild to severe, subtle to overt, understood to misunderstood. Even the 'mildest' forms of aphasia can render seismic and enduring consequences to daily life. For instance, Elman and Bernstein-Ellis (1995) have documented how lasting clinically 'minimal' disruptions in spoken communication can translate into job loss, lowered status, altered self-identity, and reduced well-being in professionals who relied on refined communication skills to do their work, e.g., trial attorneys, corporate executives, physicians, ministers, and actors/actresses.

Thus, protracted communication breakdown often penetrates to the core of self and daily life, not just within those tasks directly requiring communication, as if these alone constituted 'the broken parts.' The aftershocks of long-term language/communication dysfunction seep much deeper. This is the fact that defines and validates communication's true nature, an integral and inseparable conduit in the conducting, living, and experiencing of daily life.

Aphasia's Chronicity: Intervention

Aphasia's permanency requires that affected parties somehow and in some way confront, cope with, and ultimately decide how they wish to live with its chronic consequences. There are no longitudinal data that specifically tell us when survivors come to truly realize or know that aphasia will remain a part of daily life. What we do know descriptively about this process (Buck, 1968; Parr, 1994; Parr et al., 1999), though, suggests that somewhere near the end of the first year post-onset and then continuing over a period of months and sometimes years, affected parties slowly come to entertain that notion and integrate its reality into their daily lives.

Understandably, such a realization begins first with an insidious sense of entrapment by the void of what has not returned, rather than enlightenment over what might now be possible given this unwelcomed shift in life (Malone et al., 1970; Parr et al., 1997). It seems that coming to accept aphasia's permanence requires regular and substantial doses of 'living with it' daily, that is, experiential knowledge. Thus, learning to cope begins with an acknowledgment of permanency and continues to develop through observing, feeling, reacting, and modifying daily life first-hand. From this foundation, successful coping then develops from integrating alternative ways of making daily life feel, and hopefully work, harmoniously again (Luterman, 1996; Lyon, 1998a; Parr et al., 1999).

What emerges from the descriptive data of such life modifications is that change comes at differing rates and with differing implications. The varied pathways of adjustment differ for all affected parties (Parr et al., 1997). Although the recognition and acknowledgment of aphasia's chronicity is extremely important to subsequent healthy reordering of many of life's offerings, it still represents but the first step in reclaiming a meaningful and purposeful lifestyle. As affected parties naturally begin to turn their attention from restoration of deficited functions to finding improved ways to ensure harmony in life as is, a fundamental philosophical shift occurs. Instead of focusing simply on fixing what isn't working, participants begin looking for effective ways to incorporate what still works. When this shift occurs, one officially enters the realm of management of aphasia's chronicity.

To date, treatment of aphasia's chronicity has received little formal attention or just due in America. In fact, until the past decade, there were no well-documented methodologies or outcomes that directly targeted rejuvenation of life systems. We refer specifically to the lack of methods for lessening aphasia's enduring dominance over feeling 'able,' and over desiring or choosing to participate in daily life. This treatment void has existed even though these perceived barriers, frequently surrounded by fear and self-depreciation, often constitute the greatest challenge, far greater than language disability, per se, to restoring a sense of personal comfort and harmony in daily life.

A critical part of this treatment void has been the absence of a societally endorsed plan to pay for such services. Approximately two million individuals confront the daily dilemmas of how to live life purposefully and meaningfully with aphasia's ongoing presence constantly before them (National Aphasia Association Website/www.aphasia.com). Again, the importance of this number is not its size, although quite substantial, but the disproportionality of known or tried methods of intervention to the magnitude of daily disruption to life experienced by such individuals. Even partial removal of many of these chronic life barriers would stand to impact prime components of wellness (like purpose and direction in daily life and positive relationships with others) that Ryff and Singer (1998) have identified as essential to maintaining a 'positive contour of health.'

This chapter attempts to focus on remediation of the consequences of aphasia's chronicity, that is, how we might establish effective methods and procedures for restoring meaning, purpose, comfort, and pleasure to daily life, given life's vastly reconstituted form and its perpetual strengths and weaknesses. The form and content of this work originate purely from a 'hands-on' perspective, that is, what we've experienced, observed, internalized, and concluded as clinicians and clinical researchers in efforts to make the workings of daily life easier, more tolerable, and ultimately of greater choice and pleasure for those we treat. It begins with an overview of our therapeutic past in relationship to aphasia's chronicity; a summary of the elements from this past that may further the pursuit and development of effective methods of intervention; some theoretic and trial offerings to date; their current status as exemplified in two case scenarios; and finally, where we may wish to proceed in the years ahead.

TREATMENT OF APHASIA

Our Past

In the modern era (post World War II), aphasia treatment in America evolved out of a medical model of management (Eisenson, 1954; Wepman, 1951). In other words, it originated from a disease-identification/elimination perspective, where the therapeutic intent was to describe, diagnose, prescribe, and over time, prognosticate about which methods and with which people our interventions might yield optimal returns (Porch, 1967). Within such a model, it made sense to attack the injury's prime core of linguistic dysfunction. Inferentially, it then followed that if disordered daily functions could be restored to near-normal levels in clinical settings, then enduring benefits to daily life and reduced consequences of injury, might result.

Beginning in the late 1950s and extending through the 1960s and early 1970s, operantly driven stimulation packages dominated the aphasia treatment landscape (Schuell et al., 1964). As long as such methods could demonstrate sustained gains on standardized measures, involving the repair of basic listening, reading, speaking, and/or writing skills, their import or reimbursement was never questioned, either by providers or by payers.

Early in this era, a small contingent of clinical practitioners and researchers did treat aphasia's chronicity, although their efforts were known more as support than treatment. These clinicians and clinical researchers not only conceived of aphasia's deficit as extending well beyond language repair, but they specifically highlighted and targeted the need for and importance of assisting affected parties in their adjustment to altered perceptions of self and life systems, primarily through peer group interaction (Agranowitz et al., 1954; Backus, 1952; Bloom, 1962; Sarno, 1981). Through the use of long-term group therapy, both client and spouse/caregiver-oriented, they promoted free-flowing conversation, regardless of its linguistic form or accuracy, to further personal interaction and psychosocial adjustment to injury. At that time, the form and operation of such groups compared closely to the prime constructs that now define and govern group treatment in today's more progressive centers for the management of chronic aphasia (Elman, 1999). Nevertheless, the mainstream of treatment in America at that time focused primarily on isolating and fixing broken or disrupted language processes within the injured adult. This was considered the 'real' therapy.

By the late 1970s and early 1980s, pressure was increasing on clinical researchers to demonstrate that such linguistic repair not only aided clinical performance but transferred to untreated conditions in real life, a phenomenon termed "treatment generalization" (Kearns, 1989; Thompson, 1989). Although indirect, such attempts represented the first formal acknowledgment of aphasia's chronicity within a medical model of management. No longer was clinical restoration considered sufficient; this 'fixing' needed to lead toward accrued life benefits at home and in real life settings for its validity. In this formal broadening of the scope of aphasia management, treatment shifted, and instead of targeting just language repair, it began probing (1) the augmentation of verbal expression and (2) the definition of governing properties of dyadic conversation with a person having aphasia.

In the first instance, forms of circumventing limited oral-verbal communication, like AMERIND (Skelly, 1979; Duffy & Duffy, 1984), communication boards and spontaneous writing (Collins, 1986), as well as drawing (Lyon, 1989; Lyon, 1995a,b), were devised around a Davis/Wilcox 'PACE-like' premise (Davis & Wilcox, 1985) that permitted any workable expressive route or routes to drive everyday exchanges. There was a premium placed on the successful completion of the exchange of content, irrespective of its social acceptability normatively or personally.

In the second instance, clinical researchers began seriously investigating the nature of dyadic, open-ended conversations through "discourse methodology" (Bottenberg et al., 1987;

Nicholas & Brookshire, 1993). These investigations sought to broadly define the hows and whys of more natural interactions when coping with the residuals of linguistic injury. Again, while their prime intent was to understand and enhance real life use, these pioneering investigations focused primarily on augmenting communication within the person with aphasia rather than targeting the style of the normal interactant or of the dyad itself, and considered clinical rather than real-life settings.

By the late 1980s and early 1990s, clinical researchers had sufficient data to suspect that initial attempts at circumventing restricted verbal communication, although clearly an improvement over the use of highly restricted communicative forms, were still no better in terms of treatment generalization (Thompson, 1989). As a rule, little of what had been clinically trained appeared to transfer readily to everyday life and what did was often revised or personalized to meet the needs and wishes of individual interactants (Simmons, 1993). More importantly, when attempting to uncover probable cause for this sparse transfer of treatment effects, lack of use in real life did not necessarily relate directly to functional ability, that is, the inherent skill in using trained clinical strategies. In fact, individuals could often readily retrieve and/or demonstrate proficiency with clinically trained strategies when prompted, but still elected, of personal choice, not to use them in real life (Simmons, 1993).

Such lack of use seemingly was tied to other real life issues, some communicative in nature and some not. On the communication side (Simmons-Mackie & Damico, 1997), real life use seemed bound to being:

- highly automatic, or not arduous to call up or implement.
- socially driven and governed, and not just serving as an expedient means of exchanging basic "functional" needs/wants.
- acceptable and refined to the degree that its form 'fit' within the communicative styles and desires of all participants and not just the person with aphasia.

On the noncommunication side (Lyon, 1992; Sarno, 1993), real life use required numerous modifications within self-concept and image, such as

- Aphasic interactants knowing about, understanding, and compensating altered feelings and attitudes toward self, others, and their changed status in life.
- Others (those closely bound to the injured party…family, close friends, and relatives) equally compensating for their altered feelings and attitudes toward/about the disordered person.
- Others knowing how and willing to empower their aphasic partner to be 'more,' often requiring a delicate balance between dependency, independence, and interdependency.

Thus, adopting a communicative strategy in natural settings depends on more than supplementing the act of communication. It requires an awareness of how existing options may fit, work, and enhance personal and social processes and systems for all interactants in daily life (Lyon, 2000a; Simmons-Mackie, 2000).

A Current View

This expanded view of challenges to enablement reinforces what the World Health Organization (WHO, 1980) proclaimed over two decades ago when they categorized chronic states of dysfunction of impairment (the originating physical/psychological injury), disability (the functional consequences of such injury), and handicap (the personal and social consequences of such functional losses). Viewed this way, chronic dysfunction harbors a multitude of consequential sequelae that may not, in form, resemble original symptoms, but are every bit as influential in the obstructing and continuance of daily life. Because of this, these later acquired symptoms are as integral to defining the nature of the disorder as are its presenting symptoms. Of late, treatments have begun to emerge that target the broadness of dysfunction within a WHO framework (Elman & Bernstein-Ellis, 1999c; Kagan, 1998; Lyon, 2000a; Parr et al., in press; Simmons-Mackie, 2000; Worrall & Frattali, 2000).

Byng et al. (in press) have proposed a treatment grid that crosshatches life-related goals (enhancement of communication, adaptation of identity, access to auto- nomy and choice of lifestyle, identification of barriers to social participation, health, promotion/illness prevention, and healthy psychological states) across a variety of real-life contexts (the aphasic adult, immediate social environment, community, and society/citizenship). What is immediately apparent from their array of treatment targets is the broadening of venues toward the enhancement of life, and not just the repair of communication within the injured adult. As well, it is this basic tenet that underlies the Life Participation Approach to Aphasia (LPAA, 2000) that was reprinted in the opening chapter of this section.

Although LPAA targets chronicity, it does not restrict its treatment focus to a time well post-onset. Rather, it promotes a view of aphasia as a life-long predicament for all persons intimately involved, no matter at what stage post-onset individuals are referred. Because of this, treatment methods focus on different life themes depending on where, in form and time, individuals may be. Although the chronology of treatment differs for each set of individuals affected by aphasia, an LPAA treatment profile, based on individual needs, resources, and desires, might look at targets such as these: (1) lessening the emotional trauma and shock of injury for everyone during the initial days and weeks of treatment through frequent visits, encouragement, question-answering, introducing the topic of what has happened and what will likely follow; (2) providing specific information and restorative care between 2 and 4 weeks post-onset and establishing a collaborative means of identifying what is most needed at that time in daily life; and (3) starting to shift the emphasis toward encouraging and allowing the person with aphasia to perform more independently or interdependently at home (6 to 10 months post-onset) while concomitantly striving to lessen the load on the caregiver so he/she can return to work and not worry or feel guilty.

Accordingly, LPAA treatment targets are not bound or driven by repair of language/communication dysfunction, but rather, aim at minimizing the effects of life barriers for all persons closely connected to this ongoing shift in life. Treatment form and emphasis center around adjusting feelings/attitudes about self and others, strengthening intrapersonal and interpersonal communication and increasing participation in activities of choice. The model represents a step in a historical trend toward aphasia's management including more and more direct involvement in life functions and systems. Encouragingly, there seems to be growing evidence that aphasia's management may be moving more toward active inclusion of methods that speak to aphasia's influence on daily life.

COPING WITH APHASIA

In the past, concerns about normalizing life processes after the termination of formal treatment have fallen under the broad rubric of "coping." This literature is extensive and can be broadly subdivided into two broad emphases: (1) theorists/scientists studying the coping process itself (Kubler-Ross, 1969; Norlin, 1986; LaPointe, 1997), and (2) individual testimonials (Newborn, 1997; Wulf, 1979) and group testimonials (Chwat & Gurland, 1981; LeDorze & Brassard, 1995; Parr, 1994; Parr et al., 1997) from survivors themselves.

With respect to the theory of coping, two themes prevail: one that ascribes to an ascending progression of steps or stages in adjustment (Tanner & Gerstenberger, 1988; Wahrborg, 1991; LaPointe, 1997), and a second that stresses the importance of prior biases, strategies, and outcomes in confronting and resolving former crises in life (LaPointe, 1997).

Among personal accounts of the coping process, favorable outcomes appear bound to a variety of internal and external factors, like personality, the perceived severity of chronic injury on the living of life, and the ability to remain open to and focused on personal growth in spite of altered life forms and processes that often look and feel less than before onset (Newborn, 1997; Wulf, 1979). Equally apparent in positive accounts of coping is the importance of individuality. Collectively, people coping with aphasia share certain broad longitudinal milestones with others of a similar fate, but success seems more dependent on idiosyncratic or personalized forms, processes, and outcomes (Parr et al., 1997). Whereas a thorough review of the coping literature rests beyond our scope here, we continue with a condensed version, including

those aspects which may be most pertinent to successfully managing aphasia's chronicity.

Ascending a Series of Steps or Stages

This perspective of coping is rooted in Kubler-Ross's (1969) earlier works involving common reactions and adjustments, or 'coming to terms,' with terminal diseases. It is based on the presence of, and possible need to pass through a series of coping steps or stages (shock, denial, bargaining/compromise, anger, acceptance) before life can resume in a meaningful manner and direction. More specifically, when translated into coping with aphasia, there have been numerous parallel views or constructions. For example, Tanner and Gertenberger (1988) speak of a "grief response," which encompasses ascending steps similar to those described by Kubler-Ross, not around loss of life but with respect to loss of one's prior self. While such a view is common throughout the coping literature when physical or psychological injury involves permanent disability (Easton, 1999; Livneh & Antonak, 1990; Matson & Brooks, 1977), there is little evidence within the anecdotal aphasia literature for such a specific progression of coping steps, or the exclusivity of any single step at a particular point in time.

Parr et al. (1997) interviewed 50 dyads, each with a member 5 or more years post-onset, about their feelings and adjustments to the chronicity of aphasia. They found no standard progression of coping. Rather, their data revealed substantial idiosyncratic variability in the manner that dyads had come to resolve their issues of life adjustment. Each brought to this arena their own approaches, beliefs, strengths and weaknesses, and ultimate outcomes. There were, within these, anecdotal reports of identifiable portions of all of Kubler-Ross's steps or stages. These elements did not sequentially align with any particular order of occurrence, however, nor did they arrange themselves in any single pattern.

For example, one person with aphasia might be 'angry' over the inability to work, 'in denial' about returning to pre-stroke communication levels, and 'accepting' that conversation with family and friends was impractical at the moment. The spouse, on the other hand, might be 'accepting' that communication may never be the same (although unclear as to what this actually means) and 'in denial' over the impact of such a loss in daily life or to the daily dynamics that previously supported and defined their relationship. Also, the Parr et al. data suggest that working through a step like anger, denial, etc., did not preclude its subsequent re-emergence. Coming to realize and/or accept that speech was not going to fully return did not preclude cyclic bouts of frustration and/or anger over this issue, depending upon the circumstance and importance of the communiqué. Finally, such variability in coping was not restricted to the person with injury and the significant other, but was also found in other dyads involving family, friends, and others.

Thus, for a majority of Parr et al.'s subjects, there was no evidence of a set coping progression, although anger and denial were typically more prevalent at first, often giving way over time to some form of internal compromise and/or acceptance. More characteristic, though, was a continuous and overlapping ebb and flow of all of Kubler-Ross's stages, their appearance and reappearance depending on the personal and collective subtleties of those affected.

Factors Influencing Coping Outcomes

Another given in the aphasia literature dealing with coping is that favorable outcomes often depend on survivors' abilities to counteract the natural sequelae of permanent injury (depression, fatigue, and stimulus overload) while effectively calling upon and implementing pre-injury strategies, successful ways of resolving earlier crises or conflicts in life (LaPointe, 1997; LaPointe, 1999).

Depression

Avoiding or overcoming the darkness that may pervade daily life following brain injury with aphasia is not reducible to a list of behavioral traits or strategies that might foster understanding and acceptance of one's altered self and/or life processes. The data to date, instead, point to a complex interaction among physiological and psychological substrates that likely influence and govern emotional stability (Gainotti, 1997; Robinson et al., 1984). Code et al. (1999) maintain that this process likely involves a continuum, along which falls the interplay of severity, location of brain injury, and day-to-day fluctuations in mood. Early on, for example, structural neurobiochemical changes within the brain, depending on the size and location of lesion, may dominate emotional stability. Later on, when the biochemistry of the brain has either stabilized or been augmented through antidepressant medications, reactive 'blues' in response to lasting functional losses may emerge as more influential. Regardless of the individual composition of these forms of depression, both types may persist over long durations unless treated. Besides the use of antidepressants, behavioral interventions often aid, especially with reactive depression.

Fatigue and Stimulus Overload

Another area in which personal biases and strategies influence coping is fatigue and stimulus overload. Living with aphasia (whether one's own or that of a family member) is an exhausting process (Shadden,1999). The degree of exhaustion, and the unpredictable 'ups and downs' of the fatigue experience, are often underestimated by those outside of the situation. In responding to this fatigue, or to the "too much, too fast" experience of stimulus overload, individuals will bring premorbid emotional styles and coping strategies to the situation. One person may lash out in anger, another

may feel helpless to control the mental shutdown, a third may withdraw. Failure to acknowledge and work through these response patterns can result in a failure to manage aphasia consequences effectively.

Biases in Managing Prior Life Crises

LaPointe (1997) has detailed a list of pre-injury personality tendencies or biases that may influence the manner and outcomes of coping with aphasia. They include temperament, hardiness, introspection, dispositional optimism, locus of control, and closeness of family connections. A favorable portrait of each would include:

- temperament: stable activity, adaptability, engagement rather than withdrawal from new stimuli/challenges, attentiveness, pleasant and stable moods, persistence, and predictability.
- hardiness: resistance to stress.
- introspection: looking 'inward' and calling upon personal strengths and skills.
- dispositional optimism: viewing life's challenges in a favorable light, that is, a glass half full rather than half empty.
- locus of control: belief that life outcomes rest more in the hands of those affected than being preordained.
- family closeness: strong familial bonds.

Thus, it may well be that people's previous patterns of viewing and reacting to earlier crises in life may influence their coping strategies and outcomes with aphasia. What is less clear therapeutically is whether those who might operate at the opposite end of these spectra (displaying discouragement, a defeatist attitude, dispositional pessimism, a sense that life's outcomes rest outside their control, and possessing minimal social/familial support) can be significantly aided in changing, or acquiring better coping skills. If so, in what ways, when, and to what degree might they be assisted?

Personal Accounts of Individuals

The aphasia literature is replete with numerous and superb personal testimonials of what aphasia *is* and perhaps, more importantly, how it feels to live with aphasia, day-in-and-day-out:

I don't...I not...I can't–all no, not–what is it I can?
I miss the color of life!
They give me pills...so today, now, is okay...but what about the tomorrows?
I look, say, at the anger and think through it...same with frustration...because the frustration is always there. It's a part of everything, every few minutes of the day.

Such quotes are but a small sampling of the diverse personal commentaries on what aphasia brings to 'the living' of daily life (Bergquist et al., 1994; Knox, 1971; Newborn, 1997; Parr et al., 1997; Wulf, 1979). Noteworthy within these brief encapsulations are certain often-shared themes: an abrupt awareness and accentuation of one's own mortality; initial confusion and ignorance about what has happened; and fear about one's basic survival and being able to return to a productive role in society. Many who elect to speak or write about their personal experiences and challenges years later, detail a torturous remaking of self and daily life. Within these, there is often a theme of initial hopelessness slowly evolving toward affirmation of a new, often quite different, form of persona and daily life. And for a smaller number of people, there comes through this transformation, confirmation that the new form holds certain benefits that otherwise would never have been known or experienced had aphasia not been present.

For significant others, the onset of aphasia seems no less traumatic and often more so in terms of their sense of hopelessness to contribute anything meaningful to the restoration of life to its prior form. With time to adjust, they too report threats to their own self-preservation and well-being, not linked so much to self-esteem but to guilt (over what they perceive as neglect in preventing this occurrence); shame (over its lasting effects/consequences); embarrassment (over how others in society may perceive it and those affected); and fatigue (over added burdens and stresses of dealing with life). As well, the accounts of significant others often speak to having to assume unfamiliar roles while being held solely responsible for re-establishing and maintaining daily harmony and balance, their own as well as the couple's (Parr et al., 1997; Shadden, 1999).

Accounts of Couples and Groups

Group studies of coping with aphasia's chronicity support the individual trends cited above, yet reveal distinct discrepancies in perceptions and expectations across parties (persons with aphasia, significant others, family members, therapists, and employers). Discrepant perceptions pertain to the nature and severity of the problem, what is needed most, and what the future might bring. Clearly, if key players in the process of coping with aphasia do not concur fundamentally in their perceptions of current realities and future needs and possibilities, coming to successfully live with aphasia seems less probable (Kagan, 1995; Brumfitt, 1993).

With respect to "what's wrong," common discrepancies include the following:

- people with aphasia single out motor impairments as most troublesome, while family members (and therapists) are more likely to perceive cognitive and linguistic impairments as most challenging and burdensome (Hermann et al., 1993).
- cognitive impairment, in general, is associated with greater caregiver burden and reduced coping (Tower et al., 1997; Smerglia & Deimling, 1997; Noonan & Tennstedt, 1997).

- family members report more negative emotions in stroke patients than self-reported by patients themselves (Henry, 1984).
- although some studies suggest spouses' and children's perceptions of aphasic language deficits are congruent with language testing, other group data indicate that spouses overestimate the linguistic and communicative competence of the aphasic individual (Furbacher & Wertz, 1983; Chwat & Gurland, 1981; Flowers et al., 1979; Helmich et al., 1976).
- aphasic persons appear to show little concern about or awareness of caregiver depression, often describing the family unit as stable and emotionally supportive (Hermann et al., 1993). In contrast, family members report considerable depression and other negative emotions, often expressing concern about the integrity of the family unit.
- spousal perceptions of aphasic partners' attributes tend to be negative in general (Zraick & Boone, 1991); commonly selected descriptors include "demanding," "temperamental," "confused," and "immature."

Clearly, differences in perceptions of the fundamental nature of the problem can lead to a mismatch between what people with aphasia, significant others, and health professionals believe is needed. For instance:

- aphasic persons have a need to remain valued, interactive partners in close relationships, and social contexts. Family members, particularly spouses, may have the same need but can be devastated and sometimes immobilized by role changes, loss of intimacy, and disrupted communication.
- individuals with aphasia and significant others experience numerous role changes. Aphasic persons have a need to be autonomous, yet supported (assisted), in as many premorbid roles as possible. However, family member concerns about deficits and apparent dependencies may lead to a need to control, monitor, and otherwise limit the activities of the person with aphasia (Boisclair-Papillon, 1993).
- speech-language pathologists believe improved functional communication and relative communicative independence are major priorities. Family members may feel the effort needed to achieve these goals is too exhausting or overwhelming.
- both aphasic individuals and family members have a need to re-establish some new stability or family equilibrium.

However, perceptions of what may be needed to reach that stability may be quite different.

Lack of perceptual congruence is also obvious when expectations about future performance and behavioral change are compared across groups. The Code-Müller protocols (CMP) have been particularly useful in exploring these perceptions (Code et al., 1999; Hermann & Wallesch, 1989). In their work, speech-language pathologists were significantly more pessimistic than relatives and clients with respect to anticipating improvement in the ability to work, to communicate with strangers, and to form new relationships. Clients and relatives actually anticipated improvement in communication and in the ability to cope with embarrassment. Relatives further expected improvements in independence and the ability to deal with frustration. Different health care professionals demonstrated considerably different expectations about aspects of treatment and recovery.

Finally, expectations for recovery are also linked to other spousal variables, such as personality (Oranen et al., 1987; Batt-Leiba et al., 1998; Wahrborg & Borenstein, 1989). For example, premorbidly nurturant spouses reported higher levels of marital satisfaction and sharing. Also, greater spousal age is associated with lower optimism (Code et al., 1999).

What tendencies, then, might we find in the coping literature as it pertains to the treatment of aphasia's chronicity? We would suggest that these may be among them:

- coping, to be successful, involves more than adjustment by the person with aphasia; it must merge the life patterns and preferences of all closely involved parties.
- coping, to date, has been more of a self-determined and self-actualized process than clinically targeted and treated. Even for those who actively take part in peer support groups, 'hearing from others' often offers generic solutions rather than ones tailor-made to that person's personality, needs, or life contexts. Accordingly, survivors must search out their own paths, preferred strategies, and outcomes.
- coping, typically, does not follow a prescribed set of stages or steps, but rather involves a highly self-styled path that addresses idiosyncratic perceptions, needs, biases, strengths, and weaknesses.
- coping, to be successful, may mean that dyads not only understand and share perceptual congruence about the nature of restrictions to interpersonal communication (linguistic shortcomings, attentiveness, processing load, and problem-solving restrictions), but also remain close and intimate in an effort to (a) minimize natural consequences of injury (depression, fatigue, and overstimulation), and (b) maximize successful pre-injury strengths and strategies.
- to date, no clinical evidence exists, there is other than that derived from peer group support, to know whether treating the coping process, itself, might help.
- the process of successful coping with aphasia need not consume the remainder of life; with time, it, too, can be successfully placed in its rightful place of importance in terms of life's variables and priorities.

TREATMENT OF THE CHRONICITY OF APHASIA

If treatment of aphasia's chronicity is broadened to embrace its influences on life systems (Byng et al., in press; LPAA,

2000), and if successful coping is an integral part of achieving these ends, how might we best proceed?

Treatments for the consequences of aphasia's chronicity are only in their infancy, and are diverse in their form, purpose, setting, and type of participation. It seems likely that we will find that no single means of management (group, dyadic, or individual) or single participant (person with aphasia, significant other, family, friend, employer, or stranger) is sufficient to return disrupted life systems to preferred or optimal states of wellness. Depending upon the presenting needs and coping biases, both individually and collectively, a combination of methods, crafted idiosyncratically and hierarchically around existing life barriers, will likely represent the best intervention plan.

Group Interventions

Later in this text, Kearns and Elman detail the forms, purposes, and potential benefits of group therapy in aphasia. There is an existing, well-documented body of literature to support its treatment efficacy for people confronting the long-term effects of aphasia, both in terms of communicative and psychosocial gain (Elman & Bernstein-Ellis, 1999a,b). In fact, group methods may stand as the only known and well-established means of offsetting much of the chronic sequelae of aphasia.

As exemplified in the following true scenario, the benefits of such therapy are not always fully apparent, even at the time of intervention. In this instance, a group member, a stroke survivor's spouse, accidentally encountered the group leader at a local restaurant. Her husband, a stroke survivor of many years, had died months earlier following a protracted illness. Immediately upon seeing this friend and professional, she reached out, pulled her close, and began to cry. Interspersed in this emotional release were the words, "...without that stroke group, I would have quit years ago! I'd come to each meeting mad and depressed and leave feeling like I could make it for another month. I think it even helped me deal with his dying, because I felt I had been a decent wife to him when he was sick!" Such are the extensive and profound life benefits derived from such shared treatment forums.

The current authors, however, have been involved with another treatment form, direct intervention for minimizing idiosyncratic life barriers within relationships. The remainder of this chapter presents methods that focus on individualized real-life treatment strategies aimed at confronting and working with idiosyncratic life challenges, with the goal of restoring a greater sense of connection and harmony within relationships. While none of these methods precludes the concurrent value of group intervention, they offer individualized real-life treatment strategies which address the concerns of people confronting aphasia within their natural dyads and relationships, and in tailor-made ones.

Individualized Real-Life Interventions

It is not that providers haven't long known of the lasting consequences of aphasia; they have (Schuell et al., 1964). But until recently, these enduring aspects have been viewed primarily as inescapable residuals from permanent brain injury. That is, as therapists, we have been seen as justified in our individualized treatment plans that targeted functional loss, either by attempts to repair it or to circumvent it. However, what remained as the unremediable part of injury was left to survivors to learn to live with by themselves. Thus, there has been an absence of formal individualized treatment plans, both methodologically and reimbursably, that speak to the enhancement of daily life after formal restorative care ends.

Life Participation Approaches

Advocates for broadening the treatment of aphasia to include this larger domain view participation in life as more than the use of discreet communication skills (Byng et al., in press; LPAA, 2000). These clinicians and clinical researchers perceive such participation as linked to life factors, such as perception of self and others, being socially bonded or connected with those who matter most in life, and exercising control, autonomy, and choice over daily offerings. As a result, interventions have begun to arise that target participation in life as the prime focus, rather than as simply ancillary or addressed long post-onset (Kagan, 1998; Simmons-Mackie, 2000). Such interventions stem from the established connection that wellness in life relies heavily on personal worth, esteem, autonomy, choice, growth, and meaningful connections with others (Ryff & Singer, 1998).

In this life participation framework, Lyon (1997a,b, 1998, 2000a,b) has probed a number of therapeutic entry points that might enhance access, entrance, and daily involvement in preferred roles/activities in life. In each of these therapeutic probes, participants became active agents in determining their own direction and involvement in daily life, even if those forms of involvement differed substantially from pre-injury. Even when participation was in highly reformed or restricted activities, there was the assurance of personal determination, control, and immersion in real-life contexts and experiences involving selected people, settings, situations, and dilemmas. That is, the therapy focus was on personal engagement in real-life settings where participants could begin to evaluate and integrate existing levels of function. Over time and with sensitivity to equating challenge with skill, the therapy goal was for participants to come to acknowledge and better accept life differences 'with' aphasia, and perhaps even discover an unexpected value or merit in their altered forms.

It was hypothesized, as well, that becoming more engaged in chosen pursuits in life afforded other psychological and personal benefits. With more time involved in the 'doing' rather than in the 'thinking about' life, there might be a reduced tendency toward critical self-evaluation of one's needs, wants, and/or worth. Finding an alternative to an egocentric propensity necessitates looking beyond what is no longer possible to what still is. Also, by attempting to equate current skills with achievable outcomes, it opened the door to discovering self-driven/motivated participatory patterns to sustain participants out of choice. Due to commonly depreciated views of self, such undertakings involved successful management of the anxiety over failure to act in one's changed state of being (Csikzentimihalyi, 1990, 1993, 1997).

It was in this theoretic framework of intervention that "Communication Partners" emerged nearly a decade ago (Lyon, 1997; Lyon et al., 1997). This form of treatment links the person with aphasia with a novel, yet interested and motivated, life participant/facilitator/interactant. The purpose of this treatment was to reinstitute a basis for partaking in chosen activities of daily life by slowly and systematically exploring possible venues with a companion who did not have a prior (pre-onset) referent, and whose interest and role in therapy was simply to assist the person with aphasia to feel and experience success, comfort, and pleasure in re-engaging in daily life. Initially, the partner was shown and taught how to communicate with the adult with aphasia, that is, several weeks to a month of weekly or biweekly meetings led by the clinician. Thereafter, this dyad, again aided through planning and supervision from the clinician, set about exploring and establishing activities of the injured adult's choice in real-life settings. This latter treatment phase typically lasted 3 to 6 months with weekly meetings between participants to discuss what had happened the previous week and what of that needed to be expanded, revised, or redirected in the week ahead. All chosen activities were idiosyncratic, that is, specially crafted to the interests and needs of the person with aphasia. Examples included volunteering at a local food bank, visiting 'less fortunate' residents at a local nursing home who had no family or social ties, attending to the formal gardens surrounding a private country club, aiding a casino executive in ways of improving staff and gaming efficiency, and coming to feel 'able' and comfortable joining a local bowling league.

To assess the value a Communication Partner's treatment approach, 10 triads (person with aphasia, the community volunteer, and prime caregiver) were subjected to a multiple based, single-subject design (Lyon et al., 1997). Two informal probes were devised to assess anticipated changes to communication (that is, the person with aphasia's readiness and use of effective communicative strategies in daily life, the Communication Readiness and Use Index-CRUI) and psychosocial well-being (that is, direction, participation in life, and feelings about self and others, the Psychosocial Well-being Index-PWI). An appendix attached to the above publication contains both measures. Within this study, pre- and post-treatment comparisons yielded significant differences ($P < .05$) on both the CRUI and PWI. As important, activities of choice initiated in treatment frequently continued after partner support was withdrawn. As well, aphasic participants viewed such activities as far superior to sitting idly at home, that is, coming to take part in life rather than passively waiting to be acted upon.

Yet, although these re-engagement activities were therapeutically beneficial to the person with aphasia, that is, in promoting self-initiation, self-determination, and self-confirmation of value in his/her altered state of being, they often were not sufficient to counteract aphasia's apparent domination over much of the remainder of daily life. Beyond what was adequately addressed by the intervention was the realm of disappointments and dilemmas relating to important others in daily life. As a result, the following changes were made to treatment targets:

- enhancement of dyadic (spouse/client) communication in the home and everyday life.
- restructuring daily activities for all parties closely affected.

The form, manner of pursuit, and outcomes of these revised treatment targets have been detailed elsewhere (Lyon, 1998b; Lyon, 2000a,b). We highlight here just those findings that pertain directly to isolating more effective methods in the treatment of aphasia's chronicity.

Dyadic Communication Within the Home

From therapeutic attempts to improve dyadic communication between spouse/caregiver and the person with aphasia in the home, the following conclusions emerged from observational data (Lyon, 1998b):

- formal rehabilitation seldom addresses a form of dyadic communication in the home, either due to a perception of its appropriateness at that time in recovery or reimbursement constraints.
- if such communication repair is targeted, methods typically focus on enhancing the quantity, efficiency, and completeness of information exchanged (the transactional aspects of communicating), not how to keep interactants personally, socially, and comfortably connected in life (the interactional aspects of communicating).
- for dyadic interactions to occur with ongoing ease and frequency in real-life contexts, they must:
  —keep interactants bonded as people and interactants who care for each other, not just in that exchange but in other major realms of life as well.
  —come to occur naturally and automatically for everyone involved.
- with respect to the development and implementation of methods for enhancing interactional aspects of communication:
  —they typically require a different focus and set of communicative strategies from those used to foster transactional communication.

—their basic form and purpose are often easy to understand but less so to implement (that is, interactants, especially the uninjured/normal participant, tend to gravitate solely to how well and/or fully information is exchanged. In contrast, people with aphasia often know that communicative success is not always possible, and seek, instead, to develop ways that permit them to remain valued and connected with those people they care the most about).

—even when informed of and in agreement about interactional aspects of communicating, normal interactants often struggle at first to know what to do and when, and how to stay personally connected.

- with respect to the development and implementation of methods for enhancing transactional aspects of communication:
  —normal interactants are typically stymied over what is or isn't functional within the aphasic partner's communicative repertoire and how to best maneuver to keep their conversations productive and their outcomes meaningful.
  —when the person with aphasia is severely verbally restricted (nonverbal communicator), interactional gains are still possible, as well as the sharing of basic content. However, access or exchange of detailed information about daily life typically requires excessive amounts of time and effort on everyone's part to be maintained. Not surprisingly, couples quickly learned to avoid or ignore such conversational realms and/or topics.

Enhancing Participation in Life for All Affected Parties

To help determine what to treat within this broadened range of targets, we devised some informal measures that assessed:

- how much of daily life was viewed to be of choice by all people affected by the ongoing presence of aphasia.
- how current activities, measured as a ratio of free-time to obligated-time pursuits, compared with pre-injury/onset ratios (Lyon, 2000a,b).

In theory, our thinking was that greater mutual comfort, ease, and pleasure in life might follow from increasing the percentage of time all affected parties spent in daily activities of choice, and by having that time more closely correspond to the ratio of free and obligated-time experienced pre-onset. In this revised paradigm, the treatment participants were not just people with aphasia, but others (spouse, caregiver, family) who were in constant contact with the injured adult, and whose lives had been dramatically altered.

Within a brief period of time and over a limited number of treatment cases (Lyon, 2000a,b), the following trends have emerged:

- modifications of daily activities for spouse/caregiver were often much harder to carry out than were those of the person with aphasia due to real and perceived constraints in daily schedules. Although the spouse/caregiver may understand, and agree with, the therapeutic need to change current routines, their enactment required greater prompting, supervision, encouragement, and follow-up.

- such modifications in daily life were frequently viewed by the spouse/caregiver as a 'luxury,' and not an absolute necessity. As such, their implementation was often seen as 'selfish' rather than reasonable or justifiable, especially when enactment required time away from, or independent of, the person with aphasia.

- when changes were made by both the spouse/caregiver and the person with aphasia, there was greater perceived harmony and comfort in life, both individually and in jointly shared time.

- such changes further aided the normalization of daily life for all people involved. However, alone, they appeared once again to fall short of achieving sustainable levels of daily comfort.

- such changes addressed the outward, cosmetic shortcomings of daily life while minimally altering the inward ones of key relationships. That is, they peripherally aided in restructuring daily routines to assure some personal comfort for all, but they did not sufficiently address or compensate for altered personal feelings, connections, and attitudes about how members of the dyad viewed themselves and each other. To better clarify these latter points, we offer a couple of brief case examples.

Case Studies

Betty and Thomas

This first case stands out in that the caregiver/significant other (Betty) holds an advanced degree (PhD) in Speech-Language Pathology with clinical emphasis and expertise in aging and acquired neurogenic disorders in adults. In these ways, she not only is knowledgeable about aphasia, but has directed the teaching and training of graduate students entering the field of speech-language pathology for over 20 years. As well, she has overseen and continues to oversee the treatment of people confronting aphasia, both acutely and chronically. When involved in aphasia's chronicity, she has worked extensively with peer groups for both patients and caregivers. It is noteworthy, as well, that Betty's spouse, Thomas, was a mental health counselor who co-hosted peer support groups prior to his own stroke and aphasia.

Thomas's "brain attack" involved his right cerebral hemisphere and rendered him communicatively impaired with a moderate to severe fluent, Wernicke-like aphasia. Although it may be questioned whether 'all' of his subsequent communicative deficits were purely aphasic or a combination of right hemispheric involvement, his residual linguistic profile conformed more closely to that of an aphasic adult, suggesting either crossed or mixed cerebral dominance for language. Even today, nearing several years post-onset, Thomas still possesses fundamental deficits in linguistic processing and it is these communicative shortcomings and their effects on the living of daily life that are highlighted here.

In the beginning, Betty's thorough understanding and knowledge of the nature and chronicity of Thomas's aphasia permitted greater access and outward ease in adjusting to this life change. Being as informed as she was about such matters, she possessed a clearer sense of what to expect in terms of communicative return and use in the ensuing months and years. Accordingly, she quickly accepted that Thomas's and their communication would never be the same. Yet, she reasoned that if the basic elements of daily life could be successfully negotiated, then the lasting consequences of Thomas's injury would be tolerable and manageable.

Such a view proved beneficial at first, but what naturally evolved was a different story. Prior to his stroke, Thomas was quite adept as a communicator, both in his role as a mental health counselor and within other social settings where he often found himself 'on stage,' for example, telling stories and jokes at a local pub at the end of the day. Within his relationship with Betty at home, however, his communication was often more sparing, still bound to humor, but typically nonanalytical in style.

Upon returning home after a challenging day in academia, Betty's venting over work-related dilemmas often fell on deaf ears. Although Thomas would, indeed, hear and understand the intent of her messages, his natural inclination was seldom to comment, and if he did, it was simply an acknowledgment. Now, however, over a year post-onset, having regained sufficient use of language to qualify as a moderate/mild anomic-Wernicke aphasic, Thomas began 'to try' to listen closely to Betty's work-related concerns. Due to linguistic processing deficits, though, his responses suggested numerous auditory misperceptions or sequential omissions. Yet, unlike his prior communicative self, he now very much wanted to hear, understand, and assist her.

At first, Betty's approach was to respond with interest and to try to repair Thomas's misperceptions so that a more accurate portrayal of her topic could then be addressed. In attempting this, she realized that Thomas's previous habit of passively listening, paying attention yet not directly intervening, was far easier and preferable in many ways to attempting to treat his current linguistic and cognitive limitations. Had there been the tendency on his part prior to injury to delve into her dilemmas, that might have been encouraged. However, with Thomas's current language abilities, the interactive process was too demanding for Betty to sustain on any ongoing basis. Thus, she was faced with wanting to help her spouse and at the same time not wanting to be entrapped in a lengthy process that only added to, rather than served, her basic needs. As a result, she gradually began withdrawing from such communicative contexts and carefully guarded information about her day from her husband upon returning home from work. As well, she found herself beginning to avoid previously enjoyed social activities, because the effort to facilitate a verbal exchange between Thomas and others likewise was becoming more and more exhausting. More importantly, these subtle acts of communicative withdrawal were impacting the closeness of their relationship as a whole.

This brief account is but a small part of Betty and Thomas's total encounter with coming to terms with aphasia's chronicity. What it illustrates, though, is the subtle askewness that may permeate personal relationships, even when one of the participants is very knowledgeable about the nature and management of aphasia. More importantly, this case highlights how such 'less visible' features of personal relating/interacting, if not recognized and understood early on, may, over time, threaten or even erode intimacy within the relationship itself. Finally, Betty's unanticipated dilemma with her spouse came not from Thomas's inability or unwillingness to interact, but the complex requisites of what that task required. For Betty, it involved conflicting desires to aid Thomas on the one hand and to attend to her own physical, mental, and emotional needs and limitations on the other.

Ken and His Business Associates

Ken is a 64-year-old commercial real estate developer who had formed his own company a decade and a half prior to suffering a cerebral stroke (left cerebral artery occlusive event) that left him with a mild/moderate anomic aphasia. He was 1 year and 6 months post-onset when this treatment began. Prior to that, he had extensive speech/language rehabilitation in a more traditional sense. At the time of our treatment, there were no visible signs of hemiparesis, although he claimed that strength and muscle coordination (when playing tennis and golf) were noticeably less on the right side of the body. His speech and communication (including writing) were highly functional, although impaired if examined thoroughly. Having previously performed at extremely proficient levels of competency within his business, he was well aware of, and sensitive to, his multiple and enduring deficiencies (linguistic, cognitive, physical, and social) even though they would be classified as minor on a normative scale.

At our treatment's outset, Ken's anomia continued to be of prime concern to him, especially within social and business exchanges. He officially remained the president of his company although his two sons oversaw daily operations. These management roles were new for his sons who,

although knowledgeable of the business before Ken's stroke, had only been tangentially involved in its leadership. Given Ken's earlier devotion and commitment to work (16–18 hours daily, 5–6 days per week), he instinctively sought, and somewhat expected, similar performance standards from his sons now.

We began this treatment phase by asking Ken to make a list of those daily functions that he would choose to be more involved with, followed by a list of what currently stood in the way of such participation. Not too surprisingly, at the top of his list was the desire to be more active in his business, and what stood in the way were (a) his inability to succinctly and accurately communicate his views, and (b) what he perceived was his sons' lack of knowledge about and effectiveness in dealing with his communication. As well, Ken's desire to be more involved in the company did not include returning to his previous role as CEO. Rather, he wanted to confine his time and input to teaching and assisting his sons in the firm's strategic planning and management. He wanted to ensure that its operations were sound and pointed in the right direction, but as well, he wanted to turn over its operations thereafter to them.

We began treatment by asking Ken to enumerate the types and forms of business contexts and interactions that would be necessary to accomplish his desired ends. Next, we sat down with his sons in a couple of joint meetings to ascertain their perspectives of this process. In these meetings, we assessed their sense of Ken's communicative impairment, the extent to which it interfered with their interactions with him in the business, and their reaction to Ken's desire to be more present in the firm's strategic planning and management.

Both sons appeared reasonably knowledgeable of aphasia in general and of the prime communicative features influencing their father's effectiveness as a communicator in the business. They had devised their own set of compensatory strategies for interacting with him, many of which were functional and in daily use. They were open to learning and trying any other recommendations that might further their interactions with their father. They were agreeable, too, to looking into ways of fostering their father's input in the company.

As a starting point, all parties agreed to have Kevin begin attending weekly staff planning meetings, where company policy issues were presented and decided upon. A week later, we all convened at such a meeting. What was most noteworthy about that gathering was the absence of any significant miscommunication. That is, it was not Ken's word-finding failure or his inability to fully and expediently explain the particulars of a topic that stood in the way of his participation. True, certain communiqués were delivered in a piecemeal or telegraphic fashion, but within the shared context/referent of that group, his point and its implications were quickly and accurately understood. In fact, staff members often supplied missing content, acknowledged his concern, and openly stated their opinions, both in agreement and opposition. Thus, what had been perceived as the life barrier by Ken his inadequate communication skills, was less influential.

What was striking, however, was the fact that Ken and his sons had very distinct differences in personality and philosophy. These differences encompassed how, what, and when matters should be resolved in the running of the business, as well as the control over these issues. Prior to his injury, Ken would have simply countermanded his sons' opinions and objections, both verbally and through his seniority. Now, though, having lost and relinquished power in the conduct of the firm's daily business and lacking the verbal ease and agility to defend his personal preferences, he was in the novel position of feeling 'able' but subjugated to a lesser role and position of authority.

In treatment, then, the emphases shifted to ways of keeping father and sons united and strong in their business dealings through conversing in a manner and at a time that permitted optimal sharing of thought. Instead of Ken erupting in front of the entire staff over philosophical differences which undermined his sons' authority and ability to lead, we moved to weekly private meetings where they could more openly and freely discuss and resolve such differences.

Once again, much as in Betty's and Thomas's case, the true barrier in life was not at the surface level of communicative breakdown, but deeper, tied more to the underpinnings within communiqués: intent, philosophy, and personal power. It was not that Kevin's sons couldn't decode his verbal message; they could. But his style and potential volatility threatened their working relationship as well as their personal ties, if it was left unaddressed.

In conclusion, these two case presentations serve to highlight another complex level of communicative breakdown that may be more problematic than the basic repair of communicative forms/use. They suggest that the gravest threat to restoring quality to daily life may rest with disruptions to the intimacy of relationships with others. And unless we better understand, address, and incorporate these latter aspects in our thinking, our treatments of aphasia's chronicity may only skim the outer surface of what is most needed and necessary.

INTIMACY IN RELATIONSHIPS: THE CORNERSTONE TO WELLNESS

Ryff and Singer (2000) make the distinction that there is greater agreement among experts over what constitutes "sickness," than an interest or reliable sense of what constitutes "wellness." When researchers are pressed to supply their definitions, multiple views emerge of wellness, like "quality living, flourishing, and the good life, in both philosophical and social scientific accounts." These researchers have demarcated key psychosocial constructs that seemingly underlie wellness across life spans, differing cultures, and gender. When reduced to core components, they center around six separate, yet related constructs: purpose and direction in daily life, personal growth, self-acceptance, mastery of the environment, autonomy, and meaningful connections with others (Ryff & Singer, 1998).

Of these, they state:

"Central among the core criterial goods comprising optimal living is having quality ties to others. Across time and settings, people everywhere have subscribed to the view that close, meaningful ties to others is an essential feature of what it means to be fully human. Moreover, in philosophical accounts of the good life, notable prominence is given to mutual love, affection and empathy, deep personal relations, love's bond, intimacy, and parent/child connection. Zest in life, according to Bertrand Russell, comes, more than anything, from feeling loved and from giving love and affection." (in press)

Accordingly, Ryff and Singer (2000) have immersed themselves in research that may lead the way in helping us discern the effect of intimacy in close relationships to establishing and maintaining "wellness" in life. Although their work only tangentially relates to the prime theme here, that is, helping people remain intimately connected in life when aphasia persists, it serves to define how intimacy in relationships might be viewed and assessed in terms of overall physical and psychological wellness.

In this respect, Ryff et al. (in press) reviewed findings from a national survey study (MacArthur Research Network for Successful Midlife Development). A total of 1880 cases of normal adults from the lower 48 contiguous states were interviewed by phone to determine the quality of their relationships with spouse, other family members, and friends. These authors indicate that previous studies of relationship bonds to others often measured closeness in terms of size or proximity of one's social networks, that is, whether people were married, divorced, or single, and how many friends one had. In contrast, however, Ryff et al. reported that the approach in the MacArthur Research Study was to probe more emotionally binding features of relationships by asking questions like, "How often do you argue?" "How well are you understood?" and "How much do significant others in life appreciate you?" As well, such questions are important in assessing the intimacy of relationships with people confronting aphasia's chronicity. To complete this picture, it likely would necessitate plotting change over time, that is, pre-injury closeness (from the infancy of the relationship, midway in its existence, to a time just prior to injury), post-injury closeness (months post-onset, a year out, to the present moment) and projected closeness (anticipated levels in the next year and 5 years hence).

What emerged from the MacArthur Research Study was that strong social connections/bonds (that is, not arguing a lot and feeling understood and appreciated) highly correlated with a lower number of reported health symptoms and chronic health conditions, and overall subjectively assessed good health. The implication of these findings, according to Ryff and Singer, is that there is no artificial or real separation between psychosocial and physical health, especially when it entails this 'core' component of wellness in daily life. When unwellness was perpetuated, such disruptions not only exacerbated levels of daily stress and grief, they translated directly into physiological decline, that is, physiological signs that suggested 'wear and tear' on basic bodily functions. If sustained, this unwellness may contribute to premature morbidity and shortened life spans (Ryff et al., in press).

Based on this premise, these researchers recently compared three measures of personal intimacy to a physiological stress indicator termed "allostatic load" in a subsample of 106 normal adults (57 males; 49 females). The measures of intimacy included (1) parent/child bonding (Parental Bonding Scale: Parker et al., 1979), intimacy in current relationships (Personal Assessment of Intimacy Relationships/PAIR: Schaefer & Olsen, 1981), and social ties/bonds with others (a subsection of Ryff's Measure of Psychological Well Being, 1989).

In this latter study, the PAIR test of intimate relationships was subdivided into two broad categories: (1) emotional/sexual (E/S), the ease, form, and completeness of sharing feelings and physical closeness, and (2) intellectual/recreational (I/R), the scope of communication for sharing one's thinking, companionship, and mutually enjoyed experiences together. Two other test domains of the PAIR, social (that is, ties to people outside the relationship) and conventionality (that is, ability to make a good impression with/around others) were not tested.

"Allostasis" refers to the ability to remain stable through the process of change, "the dynamism of internal physiology and the fact that healthy functioning requires ongoing adjustments and adaptations of the internal physiologic milieu." In this study, allostatic load referred to the collective normalcy of nine physiologic stress/strain indicators, five of which were viewed as secondary sequelae of stressful challenge: blood pressure, waist-hip ratio, cholesterol to high-density lipoprotein ratio, total glycosylated hemoglobin level, and high-density lipoprotein level alone, and four of which were seen as mediators of physiological responses to adverse challenge: urinary cortisol level urinary norepinephrine level, urinary epinephrine level, and DHEA (Seeman, 1997). All allostatic load indicators were procurable through standard blood and urine samples.

Their findings were numerous, and too extensive to report in full here. But of particular interest to couples confronting aphasia may be their results pertaining to intimacy's form in highly bonded couples, and the relational importance of strong intimacy to lower allostatic loads.

From PAIR data, they found concurrently high E/S and I/R scores in highly bonded couples. That is, few instances occurred where intimacy scores were high on E/S and low on I/R or high on I/R and low on E/S. Although it is less apparent whether E/S prompts I/R or I/R prompts E/S, both appear integral to intimacy. With respect to social and communicative challenges that aphasia imposes on normal marital bonds, it would appear that it is NOT just one aspect of intimacy that may be important to preserve, but the need to assure that all domains are attended to (emotional, sexual, intellectual, and recreational)! Those PAIR domains not tested in this study, that is, social and conventionality, may prove influential with those confronting aphasia's permanency as well.

When intimacy and allostatic load data were compared in their study, in general, stronger parental/child and spousal ties yielded lower allostatic load scores (less physiological stress/strain) while weaker parental/child and spousal ties produced higher allostatic load scores. Recall from the earlier case scenarios, it was not the loss, per se, of the mechanics of communication that was most stressful and interfering to daily life; instead it was the camouflaged subtleties (involving differences in intent, personal desire/need, process, power, and control within interpersonal dynamics) underpinning those communiqués. For Betty and Thomas, it was how to remain closely aligned when communicative content and intent became confused and their ongoing repair was more taxing than productive for the couple. For Ken and his sons, it was how to stay professionally productive when feelings and personal investiture in management style, philosophy, and authority/power dominated.

Relative to Ryff et al.'s findings, wouldn't it be interesting to know some things about Betty and Thomas's and Ken and his sons' allostatic load levels? Specifically it might be useful to know the following:

- how current levels compare with pre-injury levels.
- how current levels compare with Ryff et al.'s norms.
- how these values correlate with current levels of personal intimacy and/or stress associated with coping with aphasia.
- what might be undertaken therapeutically to more normalize current levels.

SHIFTING TREATMENT PARADIGMS

We now turn to describing our attempts at normalizing aspects of personal intimacy in dyads dealing with aphasia. Within this chapter's main theme of trying to delineate the nature and treatment of aphasia's chronicity, two evolutionary processes emerge. These processes of change seem to create a 'full circle,' although they end up in a different place from where they began. Thus, they deserve comment as we shift to considering a treatment paradigm that includes not only general life participation, but intimate connections within relationships.

Evolutionary Process 1: From Repair of Linguistic Communication to Repair of 'Self' and Life Participation to Repair of Interpersonal/Social Communication

The first evolution involves the broadening of the concept of repair, that is, from one of dealing with communication in the brain-injured adult to one of confronting obstructed life systems for everyone closely involved. Although this expanded view compares closely with the earlier contributions of Byng et al. (in press), as well as the theoretical constructs of LPAA (the opening chapter of this section), it also suggests that close personal ties with others or intimacy in key relationships in life rests at 'the core' of many life challenges/stresses associated with aphasia's permanency.

The circular course of evolution into this expanded treatment framework began with us as therapists working in a more traditional manner, attempting to restore as much linguistic/communicative function as possible. Our traditional forms of restoration of basic language functions have been severely restricted in today's health care system. But even when speech-language pathologists had optimal fiscal support for traditional services, we knew that clinical improvement did not necessarily transfer directly or fully into real-life use. As a result, remedial efforts have gradually shifted toward methods of establishing real-life use, or increased 'functionality' (Worrall & Frattali, 2000). In this latter phase of intervention, the importance of enhancing self-chosen participation in daily life for all parties affected has become more central (Byng et al., in press; LPAA, 2000). Such interventions have not only given people cause for increased communication in real life, they have frequently bolstered self worth/confidence, autonomy, and purpose and direction in life.

Participation alone, however, appears insufficient to return the workings of daily life to sustainable and frequent periods of comfort, harmony, pleasure, and "flow." When we look for probable cause for this inadequacy, it would appear that disrupted communication still rests at the root of the matter. Yet, its form, nature, and method of intervention appear quite different from simply completeness or accuracy of message delivery. Rather, this communicative breakdown involves interpersonal/social connections with others, that is, maintaining the integrity and closeness of personal and social bonds with those in life who matter the most, successful personal intimacy in key relationships in life.

Evolutionary Pattern 2: From Physiological Reactivation of Brain Processes to Psychological Wellness to Physiological Wellness

The second evolution in treatment practices we have been exploring involves broadening targets to center on wellness in life (or as Ryff & Singer [1998] refer to it: "a positive health contour"), not confined to either linguistic repair or even psychosocial wellness.

At the beginning of this historical progression, traditional stimulation techniques once claimed to enhance renewed use of linguistic function through physiological modification of existing neural cortical pathways, that is, either the establishing of new networks around lesion sites or summoning support from previously uninvolved cortical areas in the brain (e.g., the right hemisphere). Yet, such neural repair failed to address the need and importance of psychological repair to offset the consequences of permanent physiological cortical injury. Over time, and more recently, interventions have arisen in an attempt to counteract the disruptions which have accrued within key life domains (personal, familial, and social/communal). As Ryff et al. (in press) are discovering, as crucial as achieving such psychosocial wellness may be to those impacted by aphasia's chronicity, it would now appear that such wellness is not, nor likely has it ever been, separate from overall physiological wellness.

Therapeutic Options: Old and New

In the modern era (post World War II), we began our treatment of aphasia by attempting to remediate a part of the communicative 'whole,' and in many ways, the more apparent part. It does not seem strange that to help our clients make their preferred workings of daily life sustainable and harmonious, we may need to hone and refine our treatment skills in still another communicative realm—helping people stay socially and personally connected with others when aphasia remains an integral and ongoing part of their lives. The necessity to allocate time and resources to such ends comes from other recent inquiries as well. Parr et al. (1998) sampled the opinions of 50 sets (the person with aphasia and his/her prime 'carer') of people coping with the long-term effects of aphasia as to what treatment strategies were most needed in daily life. Common themes among their respondents were (a) respect individual interpretations and beliefs, (b) acknowledge the complexity of aphasia and the multiple contexts in life that it influences, (c) ensure treatments to be sustained and its effects sustainable, (d) address life systems, as well as individual impairments, (e) educate and train others, (f) affirm individual, social, and collective identities, (g) promote social change, (h) provide relevant and accessible information, and (i) promote autonomy and self-help. Embedded in this diverse list of unmet needs is clearly the theme of making daily life better and such changes sustainable.

In this regard, it is not as if we are without effective long-term solutions for intervention at the moment. In America today, the National Aphasia Association lists over 200 long-term, peer support groups that meet regularly to inform and aid in the adjustment of living life with its many changed forms and stressors. In addition, the increasing numbers of innovative treatment centers in North America, specifically for the management of aphasia's chronicity, are producing documentable evidence of ongoing enhancement of communication and psychosocial well-being in daily life (Avent, 1997; Elman & Bernstein-Ellis, 1999c; Holland & Beeson, 1999; Kagan & Cohen-Schneider, 1999; Marshall, 1999; Walker-Batson et al., 1999). As well, in the United Kingdom, there is a network of self-empowerment groups that strives to place purpose/meaning, self-determination, and autonomy back into daily routines and schedules (Action for Dysphasic Adults [ADA]; Coles & Eales, 1999). Thus, such group venues constitute a significant 'handhold' in addressing aphasia's chronicity.

Yet, as good and as essential as group intervention may be, it may lack the necessary specificity or methodology to speak to or resolve the idiosyncratic needs of those involved. As a start, it is apparent that we need to supplement traditional language-based assessment tools. In addition to the use of standardized measures of language and communication, there is a need to move more toward interviews, group dialogues, questionnaires, rating scales, and other creative evaluation formats that probe functioning beyond standard speech and language use and repair. Equally clear, measures need to address the status of individuals with aphasia, family members, and the network of friends. Assessment domains must be broadened to include emotional state (mood, affect); quality of life, life satisfaction, and psychosocial well-being (and related constructs); coping, resources, and stress; interactional measures; caregiver burden and stress; and perceptions of disability and adaptation to illness and disability.

Also, with respect to defining a framework for treating intimacy in relationships, we need to know more about current states of interpersonal function:

- how do pre-injury levels compare to Ryff et al.'s normative data?
- how have levels varied over time post-onset?
- in what manner do they change?
- how extensively do they change?
- what means and strategies aid couples (when aphasia is notably present in daily life) in keeping personal intimacy present, strong, and healthy? As a part of this inquiry, it would be interesting and beneficial to know how certain couples may have increased their personal intimacy due to or around this complication in life, especially when communication is more severely compromised.
- among those who have experienced continued strong intimacy, what has proven challenging to their success?

From such inquiries, we might better fuse a set of rules and guidelines that might prompt new interventions, although they likely exist in some form elsewhere right now in treatment for addictions, abusive or self-destructing behaviors, and parent/child dysfunction.

Since interpersonal disruptions in life, secondary to aphasia, rest firmly within the scope of disordered communication, they are justifiably within our professional purview. However, devising the most effective ways of overcoming them, ones that not only impact social communication but the living and quality of daily life, requires a broadening of our own interactive and interpersonal skills. We refer here to a multidisciplinary approach, a blending of social, psychological, and rehabilitative experts/personnel. Such integrative intervention realms, though only partially understood may eventually bring us closer to managing the entirety and complexity of aphasia's chronicity.

KEY POINTS

1. Sustainable and effective treatment of aphasia requires MORE than remediation of acute impairment in language/communication systems; it requires conscious awareness of and inclusion of methods that offset chronic barriers to the living of daily life.
2. Remediation of aphasia's chronicity involves the inclusion of significant others in daily life as much as it does to the person with aphasia.
3. Although establishing effective strategies of communication are unquestionably a key ingredient to ensuring useful and enduring differences in daily life, they are but a starting point.
4. Comfortably and actively re-engaging in daily life involves a complex array of personal and social factors. Among these, keeping people closely and optimally linked in daily life (intimate) may be central to achieving long-term therapeutic success.

References

Agranowitz, A., Boone, D., Ruff, M., Seacat, G., & Terr, A. (1954). Group therapy as a method of retraining aphasics. *Quarterly Journal of Speech, 40,* 170–182.

Avent, J.R. (1997). *Manual of cooperative group treatment for aphasia.* Boston, MA: Butterworth-Heinemann.

Backus, O. (1952). The use of a group structure in speech therapy. *Journal of Speech and Hearing Disorders, 21,* 17, 116–122.

Batt-Leiba, M.I., Hills, G.A., Johnson, P.M., & Bloch, E. (1998). Implications of coping strategies for spousal caregivers of elders with dementia. *Topics in Geriatric Rehabilitation, 14,* 54–62.

Bergquist, W.H., McLean, R., & Kobylinski, B.A. (1994). *Stroke survivors.* San Francisco, CA: Jossey-Bass.

Bloom, L. (1962). A rationale for group treatment for aphasic patients. *Journal of Speech and Hearing Disorders, 27,* 11–16.

Boisclair-Papillon, R. (1993). The family of the person with aphasia. In R. Lafond, R. DeGiovani, Y. Joanette, J. Ponzio, & M.T. Sarno (eds.), *Living with aphasia: Psychosocial issues* (pp. 173–186), San Diego, CA: Singular Publishing Group.

Bottenberg, D., Lemme, M.L., & Hedberg, N.L. (1987). Effect of story content on narrative discourse of aphasic adults. In R.H. Brookshire (ed.), *Clinical aphasiology, Vol. 17* (pp. 202–209). Minneapolis, MN: BRK.

Brumfitt, S. (1993). Losing your sense of self: What aphasia can do. *Aphasiology, 7,* 569–575.

Buck, M. (1968). *Dysphasia: Professional guide for family and patients.* Englewood Cliffs, NJ: Prentice Hall.

Byng, S., Pound, C., & Parr, S. (in press). *Living with aphasia: A framework for therapy interventions.* London: Whurr.

Chwat, S. & Gurland, G.B. (1981). Comparative family perspectives on aphasia: Diagnostic, treatment, and counseling implications. In R.H. Brookshire (ed.), *Proceedings of clinical aphasiology conference* (pp. 212–225). Minneapolis, MN: BRK.

Code, C., Hemsley, G., & Herrmann, M. (1999). The emotional impact of aphasia. *Seminars in Speech and Language, 20,* 19–31.

Code, C., Müller, D.J., & Herrmann, M. (1999). Perceptions of psychosocial adjustment of aphasia: Application of the Code-Müller Protocols. *Seminars in Speech and Language, 20,* 51–63.

Coles, R. & Eales, C. (1999). The aphasia self-help movement in Britain: A challenge and an opportunity. In R. Elman (ed.), *Group treatment of neurogenic communication disorders: The expert clinician's approach* (pp. 107–114). Boston, MA: Butterworth-Heinemann.

Collins, M.J. (1986). *Diagnosis and treatment of global aphasia.* San Diego, CA: Singular Publishing Group.

Csikzentimihalyi, M. (1990). *Flow: The psychology of optimal experience.* New York: HarperCollins.

Csikzentimihalyi, M. (1993). *The evolving self.* New York: Harper-Collins.

Csikzentimihalyi, M. (1997). *Finding flow: The psychology of engagement with everyday life.* New York: HarperCollins.

Darley, F.A. (1991). I think it begins with an A. In T. Prescott (ed.), *Clinical aphasiology, Vol. 20* (pp. 9-20). Austin, TX: Pro-Ed.

Davis, G.A. (2000). *Aphasiology: Disorders and clinical practice.* Needham Heights, MA: Allyn and Bacon.

Davis, G.A. & Wilcox, M.J. (1985) *Adult aphasia rehabilitation: applied pragmatics.* San Diego, CA: College-Hill Press.

Duffy, R.J. & Duffy, J.R. (1984). *Assessment of nonverbal communication.* Tigard, OR: C.C. Publications.

Easton, K.L. (1999). The post-stroke journey: From agonizing to owning. *Geriatric Nursing, 20,* 70–76.

Eisenson, J. (1954). *Examining for aphasia.* New York: The Psychological Corporation.

Elman, R.J. (ed.) (1999). *Group treatment of neurogenic communication disorders: An expert clinician's approach.* Boston, MA: Butterworth-Heinemann.

Elman, R.J. & Bernstein-Ellis, E. (1995). What is functional? *American Journal of Speech-Language Pathology, 4,* 115–117.

Elman, R.J. & Berstein-Ellis, E. (1999a). Psychosocial aspects of group communication treatment. *Seminars in Speech and Language, 20,* 65–72.

Elman, R.J. & Berstein-Ellis, E. (1999b). The efficacy of group communication treatment in adults with chronic aphasia. *Journal of Speech-Language Hearing Research, 42,* 411–419.

Elman, R.J. & Berstein-Ellis, E. (1999c). Aphasia group communication treatment: The Aphasia Center of California approach. In R. Elman (ed.), *Group treatment of neurogenic communication disorders: The expert clinician's approach* (pp. 47–56). Boston, MA: Butterworth-Heinemann.

Furbacher, E. & Wertz, R.T. (1983). Simulation of aphasia by wives of aphasic patients. In R.H. Brookshire (ed.), *Clinical aphasiology conference proceedings* (pp. 227–232). Minneapolis, MN: BRK.

Flowers, C.R., Beukelman, D.R., Bottorf, L.E., & Kelley, R.A. (1979). Family members' predictions of aphasic test performance. *Aphasia, Apraxia, Agnosia, 1,* 18–26.

Gainotti, G. (1997). Emotional, psychological and psychosocial problems of aphasic patients: An introduction. *Aphasiology, 11,* 635–650.

Kagan A. (1995). Revealing the competence of aphasic adults through conversation: A challenge to health professionals. *Topics in Stroke Rehabilitation, 2(1),* 15–28.

Kagan A. (1998). Supported conversation for adults with aphasia: Methods and resources for training conversation partners. *Aphasiology, 12,* 816–830.

Kagan, A. & Cohen-Schneider, R. (1999). Groups in the introductory program at the Pat Arato Aphasia Centre. In R. Elman (ed.), *Group treatment of neurogenic communication disorders: The expert clinician's approach* (pp. 97–106). Boston, MA: Butterworth-Heinemann.

Kagan, A. & Gailey, G. (1993). Functional is not enough: Training conversational partners for aphasic adults. In A.L. Holland & M.M. Forbes (eds.), *Aphasia treatment: World perspectives.* San Diego, CA: Singular Publishing Group.

Kearns, K. (1989). Methodologies for studying generalization. In L.V. McReynolds & J. Spradlin (eds.), *Generalization strategies in the treatment of communication disorders* (pp. 13–30). Toronto: BC Decker.

Knox, D. (1971). *Portrait of aphasia.* Detroit, MI: Wayne State University Press.

Kubler-Ross, E. (1969). *On death and dying.* New York: Macmillan.

Labourel, D. & Martin, M.M. (1993). In D. Lafond, R. DeGiovani, Y. Joanette, J. Ponzio, & M.T. Sarno (eds.), *Living with aphasia: Psychological issues* (pp. 151–172). San Diego, CA: Singular Publishing Group.

LaPointe, L.L. (1997). Adaptation, accommodation, aristos. In L.L. LaPointe (ed.), *Aphasia and related nurogenic language disorders* (2nd ed.) (pp. 265–287). New York: Thieme.

LaPointe, L.L. (1999). Quality of life with aphasia. *Seminars in Speech and Language, 20,* 5–17.

LeDorze, G. & Brassard, C. (1995). A description of the consequences of aphasia on aphasic persons and their relative and families, based on the WHO model of chronic diseases. *Aphasiology, 9,* 239–255.

Livneh, H. & Antonak, R.F. (1990). Reactions to disability: An empirical investigation of their nature and structure. *Journal of Applied Rehabilitation Counseling, 2,* 12–21.

Life Participation Approach to Aphasia (LPAA) (2000). *ASHA Leader, 5(3),* 4–6.

Luterman, D.M. (1996). *Counseling persons with communication disorders and their families* (3rd ed.). Austin, TX: Pro-Ed.

Lyon, J.G. (1992). Communication use and participation in life for adults with aphasia in natural settings: The scope of the problem. *American Journal of Speech-Language Pathology, 1,* 7–14.

Lyon, J.G. (1995a). Drawing: Its value as a communication aid for adults with aphasia. *Aphasiology, 9,* 33–50.

Lyon, J.G. (1995b). Communicative drawing: An augmentative mode of interaction. *Aphasiology, 9,* 84–94.

Lyon, J.G. (1996). Optimizing communication and participation in life for aphasic adults and their prime caregivers in natural settings: A use model for treatment. In G. Wallace (ed.), *Adult aphasia rehabilitation* (pp. 137–160). Boston, MA: Butterworth-Heinemann.

Lyon, J.G. (1997). Volunteers and partners: Moving intervention outside the treatment room. In B. Shadden & M.T. Toner (eds.), *Communication and aging* (pp. 299–324). Austin, TX: Pro-Ed.

Lyon, J.G. (1998a). *Coping with aphasia.* San Diego, CA: Singular Publishing Group.

Lyon, J.G. (1998b). Treating real-life functionality in a couple coping with severe aphasia. In N. Helm-Estabrooks & A.L. Holland (eds.), *Approaches to the treatment of aphasia* (pp. 203–239). San Diego, CA: Singular Publishing Group.

Lyon, J.G. (2000a). Finding, defining, and refining functionality in real life for people confronting aphasia. In L. Worrall & C. Frattali (eds.), *Neurogenic communication disorders: A functional approach* (pp. 137–161). New York: Thieme.

Lyon, J.G. (2000b). Service delivery for people confronting aphasia: Some thoughts and practical suggestions in troubled times. *American Speech-Language-Hearing Association Special Interest Division 2, 9*(5), 18–22.

Lyon, J.G., Cariski D., Keisler, L., Rosenbek, J., Levine, R., Kumpula, J., Ryff, C., Coyne, S., & Blanc, M. (1997). Communication partners: Enhancing participation in life and communication for adults with aphasia in natural setting. *Aphasiology, 11,* 693–708.

Malone, R., Ptacek, P., & Malone, M. (1970). Attitudes expressed by families of aphasics. *British Journal of Communication Disorders, 5,* 174–179.

Marshall, R. (1999). A problem-focused group treatment program for clients with mild aphasia. In R. Elman (ed.), *Group treatment of neurogenic communication disorders: The expert clinician's approach* (pp. 57–66). Boston, MA: Butterworth-Heinemann.

Matson, D. & Brooks, L. (1977). Adjusting to multiple sclerosis: An explorative study. *Social Science and Medicine, 11,* 245–250.

Nicholas, L.E. & Brookshire, R.H. (1993). A system for quantifying the informativeness and efficiency of the connected speech of adults with aphasia. *Journal of Speech and Hearing Research, 36,* 338–350.

Newborn, B. (1997). *Return to Ithica.* Bergenfield, NJ: Penguin USA.

Norlin, P.F. (1986). Familiar faces, sudden strangers: Helping families cope with the crisis of aphasia. In R. Chapey (ed.), *Language intervention stragegies in adult aphasia* (2nd ed.) (pp. 174–186). Baltimore, MD: Williams & Wilkins.

Oranen, M., Sihvonen, R., Aysto, S., & Hagfors, C. (1987). Short Report. Different coping patterns in the families of aphasic people. *Aphasiology, 1,* 889–911.

Parker, G., Tupling, H., & Brown, L.B. (1979). A parental bonding instrument. *British Journal of medical Psychology, 52,* 1–10.

Parr, S. (1994). Coping with aphasia: Conversations with 20 aphasic people. *Aphasiology, 8,* 457–466.

Parr, S., Byng, S., Gilpin, S., & Ireland, C. (1997). *Talking about aphasia.* Philadelphia: Open University Press.

Parr, S., Byng, S., & Pound, C. (1998). *Perspectives, partnerships, practicalities and policies: Developing a sustainable service for people with aphasia.* Presentation at the Clinical Aphasiology Conference, Asheville, NC.

Parr, S., Pound, C., Byng, S., & Long, B. (1999). *The aphasia handbook.* Great Britain: Connect Press.

Porch, B.E. (1967). *Porch Index of Communicative Ability, Volume I: Theory and development.* Palo Alto, CA: Consulting Psychologists Press.

Pound, C. (1998). *Power, partnerships and perspectives: Social model approaches to long term aphasia therapy and support.* Presented at the 8th international aphasia rehabilitation conference, S. Africa.

Robinson, R.G., Kubos, K.L., Starr, L.B., Rao, K., & Price, T.R. (1984). Mood disorders in stroke patients: Importance of location of lesion. *Brain, 107,* 81–93.

Ryff, C.D. (1989). Happiness is everything, or is it? Explorations on the meaning of psychological well-being. *Journal of Personality and Social Psychology, 57,* 1069–1081.

Ryff, C.D. & Singer B. (1998). The contours of positive human health. *Psychological Inquiry, 9,* 1–28.

Ryff, C. & Singer, B. (2000). Interpersonal flourishing: A positive health agenda for the new millennium. *Personality and Social Psychology Review, 4,* 30–44.

Ryff, C., Singer, B., Wing, E., & Love, G.D. (in press). Elective affinities and uninvited agonies: Mapping emotion with significant others onto health. In C.D. Ryff & B.H. Singer (eds.), *Emotion, social relationships, and health.* New York: Oxford University Press.

Sarno, M.T. (1981). Recovery and rehabilitation in aphasia. In M.T. Sarno (ed.), *Acquired aphasia* (pp. 485–529). New York: Academic Press.

Sarno, M.T. (1986). *Understanding aphasia: A guide for family and friends* (3rd ed.). New York: New York University Medical Center.

Sarno, M.T. (1991). The psychological and social sequelae of aphasia. In M.R. Sarno (ed.), *Acquired aphasia* (2nd ed.) (pp. 499–515). New York: Academic Press.

Sarno, M.T. (1993). Aphasia rehabilitation: Psychosocial and ethical considerations. *Aphasiology, 7,* 321–334.

Schaefer, M.T. & Olsen, D.H. (1981). Assessing intimacy: The PAIR inventory. *Journal of Marital and Family Therapy, 9,* 47–60.

Schuell, H.M., Jenkins, J.J., & Jimenez-Pabon, E. (1964). *Aphasia in adults.* New York: Harper and Row.

Seeman, T.E., Singer, B., McEwen, B., Horwitz, R., & Rowe, J.W. (1997). The price of adapation: Allostatic load and its health consequences: MacArthur studies of successful aging. *Archives of Internal Medicine, 157,* 2259–2268.

Shadden, B. (1999). *Fatigue and stress: Impact on spouse interactions with an aphasic adult.* Presentation at American Speech-Language-Hearing Association Convention, San Francisco, CA.

Simmons, N. (1993). An ethnographic investigation of compensatory strategies in aphasia. University Microfilms International, Ann Arbor, Michigan.

Simmons-Mackie, N.N. (2000). Social approaches to the management of aphasia. In L. Worrall & C. Frattali (eds.), *Neurogenic communication disorders: A functional approach* (pp. 162–188). New York: Thieme.

Simmons-Mackie N.N. & Damico, J. (1997). Reformulating the definition of compensatory strategies in aphasia. *Aphasiology, 8,* 761–781.

Skelly, M. (1979). *Amer-Ind gestural code based on universal American Indian hand talk.* New York: Elsevier.

Smerglia, V.L. & Deimling, G.T. (1997). Care-related decision-making satisfaction and caregiver well-being in families caring for older members. *Gerontologist, 37,* 658–665.

Tanner, D.C. & Gerstenberger, D.I. (1988). The grief response in neuropathologies of speech and language. *Aphasiology, 2,* 97–84.

Thompson, C.K. (1989). Generalization research in aphasia: A review of the literature. In T. Prescott (ed.), *Clinical aphasiology, Vol. 18* (pp. 195–222). Boston, MA: College-Hill Press.

Tower, R.B., Kasl, S.V., & Moritz, D.J. (1997). The influence of spouse cognitive impairment on respondents' depressive symptoms: The moderating role of marital closeness. *Journal of Gerontology, 52B,* S270–S278.

Wahrborg, P. (1991). *Assessment and management of emotional and psychosocial reactions to brain damage and aphasia.* San Diego, CA: Singular Publishing Group.

Wahrborg, P. & Borenstein, P. (1989). Family therapy in families with an aphasic member. *Aphasiology, 3,* 93–98.

Walker-Batson, D., Curtis, S., Smith, P., & Ford, J. (1999). An alternative model for treatment of aphasia: The lifelink approach. In R. Elman (ed.), *Group treatment of neurogenic communication disorders: The expert clinician's approach* (pp. 67–76). Boston, MA: Butterworth-Heinemann.

Wepman, J.M. (1951). *Recovery from aphasia.* New York: Ronald Press.

World Health Organization (1980). *International Classification of Impairments, Disabilities, and Handicaps.* Geneva, Switzerland: WHO.

World Health Organization (1997). *International Classification of Impairments, Activities, and Participation (ICIDH-2).* Geneva, Switzerland: WHO.

Worrall, L. & Frattali, C. (eds.) (2000). *Neurogenic communication disorders: A functional approach.* New York: Thieme.

Wulf, H.H. (1979). *Aphasia, my world alone.* Detroit, MI: Wayne State University Press.

Zraick, R.I. & Boone, D.R. (1991). Spouse attitudes toward the person with aphasia. *Journal of Speech and Hearing Research, 34,* 123–128.

Chapter 14

Group Therapy for Aphasia: Theoretical and Practical Considerations

Kevin P. Kearns and Roberta J. Elman

Group therapy for aphasia evolved in the United States as a practical response to the large influx of head-injured veterans returning from World War II. At that time, relatively few professionals were specifically trained to provide clinical services for aphasic individuals, and burgeoning caseloads necessitated group treatment. Group therapy has remained a common method of treating aphasia in the United States and abroad (Fawcus, 1989; Pachalska, 1991a; Tsvetkova, 1980).

Ironically, changes in reimbursement and public policy (Frattali, 1992) and a renewed interest in psychosocial aspects of recovery from aphasia have stimulated a renewed interest in group treatment (Avent, 1997a,b; Borenstein et al., 1987; Brindel et al., 1989; Elman, 1999; Elman & Bernstein-Ellis, 1999a,b; Marshall, 1999a,b; Pachalska, 1991a,b; Radonjic and Rakuscek, 1991). Lyon (1992) argued that clinical aphasiologists broaden their clinical perspective by incorporating psychological as well as functional communicative goals into the endeavors, and they should use treatment plans that facilitate or encourage "participation in life." Similarly, Frattali has noted, "We must remember that human communication sciences and disorders is a discipline dedicated to improving the quality of life of persons with communication disorders" (p. 81).

Of course, interest in the broader aspects of recovery from aphasia are not new. Descriptive accounts of group therapy and its benefits abound in the aphasia literature (Agranowi, 1954; Aronson et al., 1956; Chenven, 1953; Gordon, 1976; Holland, 1970; Inskip & Burris, 1959; Nielson et al., 1948; Schlanger & Schlanger, 1970; Wepman, 1947). Advocates have claimed that group intervention results in widespread changes in speech and language skills and increased psychosocial adjustment to aphasia. Unfortunately, there have been few objective studies to support these claims, and the efficacy of group therapy for aphasia is just now being established. Although the results of recent investigations indicate that group therapy is an effective form of aphasia

management (Aten 1982; Avent, 1997a; Brindely et al., 1989; Elman & Bernstein-Ellis, 1999a,b; Radonjic & Rakuscek, 1991; Wertz et al., 1981) aphasiologists have only begun to give attention to this important area of clinical investigation. Renewed interest in group therapy for aphasia is reflected in recent publications that specifically address clinical goals and procedures for group intervention (Avent, 1997b; Elman, 1999; Marshall, 1999; Vickers, 1998). These texts are a welcome addition to the clinical armamentarium since most clinical aphasiology textbooks contain only brief descriptions of group treatment and minimal discussion of procedures employed in group therapy (Brookshire, 1992; Darley, 1982, 1992; Eisenson, 1973; Jenkins et al., 1981; Sarno, 1981). Prior to the recent publication of texts that focus on group treatment, few critical summaries of the group treatment literature were available (Fawcus, 1989; Marquardt et al., 1976).

While recognizing the need for empirically based group treatment procedures, recent interest in broader rehabilitation goals has occurred within a conceptual and methodological framework that heretofore had been lacking. From a conceptual perspective, clinical aphasiologists have begun to appreciate the complexities associated with facilitating generalized changes in our aphasic patients (Van Harskamp and Visch-Brink, 1991). More important, an ecological perspective on intervention, which considers the complexity of environmental, personal, social, emotional, and communicative factors on treatment, is finally evolving into specific, testable treatment suggestions for both individual and group therapy (Aten et al., 1982; Davis & Wilcox, 1981; Elman & Bernstein-Ellis, 1999a,b; LaPointe, 1989). Consistent with the trend toward a more ecological approach to intervention, a concomitant emphasis on methodological issues may provide a procedural framework for group therapy. For example, calls for reliable and appropriate functional (Frattali, 1992) and psychosocial assessment tools (Lyon, 1992) as well as the development of a generalization planning approach to intervention (Kearns, 1989; Thompson, 1989) have direct relevance to group intervention for aphasia.

OBJECTIVES

There is a continuing need to synthesize the group treatment literature, describe current clinical practice, and develop specific treatment approaches that can be clinically useful and experimentally validated. Therefore, the purpose of this chapter is to (a) critically review and summarize the aphasia group therapy literature and (b) present a perspective on group therapy for aphasia that is consistent with information in the literature on facilitating generalization. Suggestions will also be provided regarding the future role of speech-language pathologists in this area of rehabilitation.

The content and focus of group therapy for aphasia is predominately a function of the skills and biases of the group leader (Elman, 1999; Marquardt, 1982; Marquardt et al., 1976). In general, however, most aphasia groups focus on one or more of the following parameters: psychosocial adjustment, speech-language treatment, and/or counseling (Eisenson, 1973; Fawcus, 1989). This clinical taxonomy is, of course, somewhat arbitrary, since communication and psychosocial factors are intricately related and improvement of one factor may affect the other (Marquardt et al., 1976). Therefore, the interrelatedness and complexity of therapeutic goals in group treatment for aphasia should be kept in mind during the following discussion of group treatment approaches.

GROUP TREATMENT APPROACHES

Psychosocial Groups

Although psychotherapeutic and sociotherapeutic approaches to group management have been distinguished in the aphasia literature (Marquardt et al., 1976), these approaches share more similarities than differences. That is, despite differing descriptive labels, the purpose and procedures discussed in reports of sociotherapeutic and psychotherapeutic group therapy are often indistinguishable. Psychosocial groups provide a supportive atmosphere where aphasic individuals can ventilate feelings and learn to cope with the psychological impact of aphasia. In addition, the goals and procedures of these groups emphasize interpersonal relationships while providing social contacts with other persons "in the same boat." The primary purpose of psychosocial aphasia groups is to foster the development of emotional and psychological bonds that help group members cope with the consequences of aphasia (Ewing, 1999; Inskip & Burris, 1959; Luterman, 1996; Oradei & Waite, 1974; Redinger et al., 1971; Yalom, 1985).

Earliest reports of psychosocial group treatment gave minimal attention to subject description, procedural specification, or evaluation of treatment results (Backus &

Dunn, 1947, 1952; Blackman, 1950; Blackman & Tureen, 1948; Godfrey & Douglas, 1959). Aronson et al. (1956), however, provided a detailed description of a "social-psychotherapeutic" approach to group therapy and attempted to evaluate the effectiveness of their program. They developed a task continuum in an attempt to facilitate group discussion, provide an emotional outlet, and allow patients to develop interpersonal relationships. Tasks in the hierarchy ranged from nonverbal (e.g., music rhythm group) to solely verbal (e.g., group discussion), and they included (a) using rhythmic musical instruments, (b) participating in group singing, (c) listening to short stories read by a group leader, (d) participating in various speech games and discussion of proverbs, (e) taping and replaying speech samples, and (f) taking part in group-centered discussion. Activities from the hierarchy were introduced as needed to maintain motivation and facilitate group interaction whenever adequate group discussion could not be elicited.

The effectiveness of this approach was evaluated for 21 chronic and acute patients who attended an average of 14 hourly treatment sessions. Results of interviews and clinical ratings revealed that the patients and staff reacted quite favorably to the treatment program. The group leaders also observed a reduction in anxiety, increased intragroup support, and a heightened ability for constructive self-criticism among group members. Another early report of psychosocial group therapy notable for its attempt to outline specific group treatment procedures was provided by Schlanger and Schlanger (1970). They recommended the use of role playing as a method of reducing anxiety about communication and establishing spontaneous, functional discourse in the group setting. Their primary purpose was to "try to 'get something across' both inter- and intra-personally" (p. 230) through the use of (a) gesture and pantomime, (b) role playing one's self in realistic situations, (c) role playing other individuals, and (d) psychodrama.

Gestures and pantomime were employed to enhance the communication of chronic aphasic patients who had severely limited verbal abilities. Gestural and pantomime training included the use of descriptive gestures to transmit information about pictorial referents, pantomiming daily activities such as mailing a letter, and using "universal" iconic gestures.

Following gesture and pantomime training, the patients participated in role-playing activities involving nonstressful and stressful situations. Nonstressful situations included activities such as shopping or attending a picnic. Role playing in stressful situations involved having patients interact with a clinician in a "Candid Camera"–like situation. Unexpected events were blended into everyday experiences so that the patient had to problem solve and communicate in a natural situation.

Another aspect of this approach involved having the aphasic individuals role play other people during simulated situations. During this activity, patients used pantomime and verbal skills to depict people in contrived scenes from a bakery, a florist, and so on. A final aspect of the Schlanger and Schlanger (1970) group treatment program used psychodrama to act out the problems and frustrations of each group member. During this activity, patients assumed roles that allowed them to vent feelings and release hostility.

The aphasia group members gradually progressed through the four facets of training, and several benefits of the program were noted. Patients demonstrated an increased ability to cope with stressful situations, a reduction in anxiety concerning communication deficits, a feeling of accomplishment, loss of emotional inhibition, and better insight into feelings and problems. Schlanger and Schlanger (1970) concluded that role-playing activities provide an important means of adjusting to the psychosocial impact of aphasia.

More recent clinical reports have also targeted psychosocial goals within the aphasia group setting. Borenstein et al. (1987), for example, examined the psychological, linguistic, and neurological effects of a 5-day intensive residential treatment program for aphasic patients and their relatives. Eleven aphasic patients and seven family members attended the group. Sessions were conducted by a speech-language pathologist, a psychologist, and a neurologist, and formal assessments of family members' psychological adjustment and aphasic participants' language ability and neurological status were conducted. The content of the intervention program included family-centered therapy, social excursions that encouraged functional communication, and group discussions of everyday problems and adjustment strategies. Reevaluations of the participants conducted 1 year after the intensive treatment period revealed some improvements in psychological and interpersonal adjustment but not in neurological or communicative status. A 10-year follow-up was reported for eight of the original participants (Wahrborg et al., 1997). The improvements that had been achieved at the end of the course of treatment were diminished at the 10-year follow-up. All but one of the participants showed a more severe aphasia at the 10-year follow-up. However, seven of the eight participants reported that their quality of life was improved at 10 years post-treatment as compared with the end of the psychosocial group.

Johannsen-Horbach and colleagues (1993) reported on their aphasia groups which focused on aspects of coping with aphasia and its consequences. Two groups were described—one for younger participants (eight members, ages 26–51) and one for elderly participants (seven members, ages 60–80). Content of the group treatment included interactional and conversational exchange about psychosocial burden, communication strategies (e.g., PACE; Davis & Wilcox, 1985), role playing, and tasks from a verbal/visual memory training program. The groups, led by a psychologist and a speech-language pathologist, met once a week for 2 hours. The younger group met a total of 22 times and the elderly group met for a total of 16 times. The authors reported that participants had higher degrees of self-esteem following

participation in the group treatment and that participants were able to utilize "new behavioral strategies." The authors stated that younger participants had more difficulty accepting their deficits as compared with the elderly clients and that younger participants wanted to focus their efforts on communicative deficits. The authors concluded that their observations support the usefulness of psychosocial groups and reinforce their belief that separating participants by age was a useful clinical strategy.

Hoen et al. (1997) reported on psychosocial changes following participation in their community-based program offered to those with aphasia following stroke and head injury. Their study evaluated changes on a condensed form of Ryff's Psychological Well-Being Scale (1989). Thirty-five clients with aphasia received volunteer-run communication groups twice weekly for half-days. In addition, a social worker led caregiver support groups with 12 family members. Although improvement was measured over a 6-month time period, treatment time in the program prior to enrollment in the study was not controlled. In addition, total treatment time for each subject was not reported. Results indicated that clients with aphasia showed positive changes on the Ryff scales, which measure autonomy, environmental mastery, personal growth, purpose in life, and self-acceptance. The scale designed to assess positive relations with others did not show significant change. The results for family members were also encouraging. Family members showed significant change on all scales except for "environmental mastery." Despite these positive findings, the authors note that the design of this study is flawed and the study does not permit an objective assessment of the benefits of group intervention.

Penman and Pound developed a short-term self-advocacy group for people with aphasia at the City Dysphasic Group at City University in London, England (Pound, 1998; Penman, in press). The course ran for 10 weeks with 2-hour sessions. The focus of the group was twofold: (1) to identify disabling barriers in the environment; and (2) to develop a positive personal identity that was inclusive of aphasia and disability. Two people, a speech-language therapist and a person with aphasia, facilitated the groups. Eight individuals with chronic aphasia participated. Group discussion was used as the vehicle for working on many different issues including communication, self-esteem, autonomy, leisure life, and financial status.

The outcomes of the therapy were evaluated by examining personal interviews and personal portfolios that had been developed by each group member. Post-treatment evaluations suggested that group members felt more confident, had improved self-esteem, and were more positive about living with aphasia. Participants also reported feeling an increased sense of social participation and 'belonging.'

Useful supplements to the specific psychosocial treatment programs outlined above are provided by Ewing (1999) and Luterman (1996). These authors summarize information regarding group process, group dynamics, and other group considerations that speech-language pathologists must be aware of when facilitating treatment groups. Both authors emphasize group techniques that need adaptation when working with members who have neurogenic communication disorders.

Summary and Observations

There is a general consensus in the literature that psychosocial group therapy provides psychological, emotional, and social benefits for individuals with aphasia. Specific benefits that have been reported include an opportunity for increased socialization; a supportive atmosphere in which aphasic individuals can express anger, hostility, and other emotions; and the development of skills that allow patients to cope with emotional and lifestyle changes resulting from aphasia (Aronson et al., 1956; Backus & Dunn, 1947; Blackman, 1950; Blackman & Tureen, 1948; Byng et al., 1998; Eisenson, 1973; Friedman, 1961; Godfrey & Douglass, 1959; Hoen et al., 1997; Inskip & Burris, 1959; Johannsen-Horbach et al., 1993; Marquardt et al., 1976; Oradei & Waite, 1974; Penman, 1999; Redinger et al.,1971; Schlanger & Schlanger, 1970). Despite near-unanimous agreement regarding the benefits of psychosocial group treatment, it should be cautioned that the findings of the majority of reports in this area are based on subjective assessment and anecdotal observations. Data-based studies are practically nonexistent in the psychosocial group literature, and those that have been reported have not been rigorous (Aronson et al., 1956; Godfrey & Douglass, 1959; Oradei & Waite, 1974). Although the psychometric difficulties involved in measuring psychological and social parameters are substantial, there is a pressing need to begin evaluating the psychosocial impact of group treatment for aphasia.

Prerequisite to the establishment of a solid database for this approach to aphasia management is the development of specific replicable treatment procedures. Unfortunately, with few notable exceptions (Aronson et al., 1956; Schlanger & Schlanger, 1970), investigators have not delineated specific treatment principles or procedures for conducting psychosocial group therapy for aphasia. Descriptions in the literature do not provide the procedural detail necessary to translate them into clinical practice (e.g., Friedman, 1961; Oradei & Waite, 1974; Redinger et al., 1971), and psychosocial group therapy remains largely an undefined entity. Moreover, when attempts have been made to document the effectiveness of psychosocial treatment groups (e.g., Borenstein et al., 1987), failure to meet minimal psychometric standards limits the usefulness of these efforts.

Family Counseling and Support Groups

In addition to the psychosocial adjustment difficulties of aphasic individuals, the emotional, psychological, and lifestyle changes for family members of aphasic individuals have also been documented (Friedland & McColl, 1989; Johannsen-Horbach et al., 1993; Kinsella & Duffy, 1978, 1979; Lafond et al., 1993; Lyon, 1998; Malone, 1969; Parr et al., 1997; Rice et al., 1987). Over 30 years ago Malone (1969) observed that "in most cases the family as a closely knit unit no longer existed" (p. 147) once a family member was stricken by aphasia. He concluded that family counseling programs are needed to help spouses and family members learn about aphasia and cope with its devastating consequences. The group setting is frequently used for counseling and educating aphasic patients and their families.

Brookshire (1997) notes that the primary objective of family support or counseling groups is to educate aphasic patients and their families about the nature of aphasia and to explore the impact of aphasia on family dynamics. Counseling groups provide a medium for discussing physical, psychological, and social consequences of brain damage. They also serve as a forum for expressing feelings and learning to adjust to newly acquired family roles and lifestyle changes. Brookshire observed that patient-family and spouse support groups also function as a social or recreational outlet for aphasic individuals and their families.

Examples of family counseling groups abound in the aphasia literature (Bernstein, 1979; Davis, 1992; Derman & Manaster, 1967; Friedland & McColl, 1989; Gordon, 1976; Johannsen-Horbach et al., 1993; Kisley, 1973; Mogil et al., 1978; Newhoff & Davis, 1978; Porter & Dabul, 1977; Puts-Zwartes, 1973; Redinger et al., 1971). Turnblom and Myers (1952) provided one of the earliest examples of group counseling for families of aphasic individuals. Following this early report, there was a virtual neglect of this area of rehabilitation for approximately 20 years. Redinger et al. (1971) subsequently described a multidisciplinary discussion group for severely impaired aphasic patients and their spouses. The purpose of the group was to facilitate emotional adjustment and help the group members work through family and social issues through problem-oriented discussions. The group consisted of several co-leaders (a speech-language pathologist, a psychiatric nurse, and a psychiatrist), six aphasic patients, and four spouses who met on a weekly basis for 1 year. Participation of the spouses was viewed as a critical element in rehabilitation, since problems discussed in the group inevitably involved adjustment difficulties that were shared by the aphasic patients and their spouses.

Redinger and his colleagues (1971) observed that the group evolved through several stages during the course of therapy. Initially, there was a period of anxiety, and group members experienced difficulty communicating with one another. During the second stage, the members expressed regrets about their condition and complained about various factors associated with rehabilitation. Finally, during the third stage of treatment, the group evolved into a friendly, understanding, and supportive unit. As the group evolved through these stages, participants gradually became better adjusted to home and social environments, and they developed a more realistic view of family problems. In addition to these benefits, the counseling group also provided a social outlet for patients and spouses.

Many reports of spouse counseling groups highlight the importance of planning treatment to meet the specific needs of individual aphasic patients and their families. Gordon's (1976) spouse counseling group, for example, developed in response to the expressed needs of the wives of aphasic patients. The group provided an atmosphere in which spouses acquired a better understanding of aphasia, felt free to express feelings and share their reactions, and worked through problems that occurred as a result of their husband's aphasia. The ultimate goal of the group was to improve the interpersonal relationships of the aphasic individuals and their spouses.

A speech-language pathologist and a psychiatric social worker acted as co-leaders for the group. Meetings were held on a weekly basis, and attendance ranged from 4 to 10 spouses per session. The duration of individual spouse participation in the group varied from several months to 3 years. The co-leaders adopted a nondirective counseling approach in which wives increasingly assumed more responsibility for the content and direction of the group while the leaders provided information and guidance as needed. Psychosocial aspects of adjustment addressed by the social worker included feelings of resignation, guilt and loneliness, shifts in family roles, and the need to maintain interests outside of the home. The speech pathologist discussed the nature of aphasia, prognosis for recovery of language skills, and strategies for improving communication with their aphasic partners. Wives were encouraged not to demand verbal responses from their husbands, to accept nonverbal communication, and to modify their input to their aphasic partners.

Gordon (1976) concluded that wives' emotional problems hindered communication with their aphasic husbands prior to participation in the group. Relatedly, the group helped to alleviate many of the wives' emotional problems, and formal psychotherapy was seldom required. Gordon cautioned, however, that multiple repetitions were often needed before the wives comprehended group-counseling information. Some redundancy may, therefore, be necessary for spouses to receive maximum benefit from group treatment.

Bernstein (1979) also described a multidisciplinary spouse group that evolved out of concern for the emotional needs of family members. He stressed that interpersonal problems between aphasic patients and their wives may interfere with speech-language treatment attempts. More important, he believed that the family unit itself may be endangered if we ignore the emotional and psychological trauma suffered by spouses and other family members. He stressed that we cannot meet the complex emotional needs of spouses by simply providing a list of "do's and don'ts" and discussing them. Bernstein (1979) also indicated that the team leaders also

benefited from the group. He stated, "We are all better clinicians for the experience" (p. 35).

Recognizing the scarcity of studies in the aphasia counseling area, Newhoff and Davis (1978) reported their attempt to objectively plan and implement a spouse-intervention program. Four spouses, two male and two female, participated in this study. Spouses were individually interviewed to determine target areas for intervention, and a questionnaire was administered before and at the termination of the study to evaluate the effectiveness of the program.

The questionnaire examined seven areas: (a) communication strategies, (b) changes in lifestyle and social pursuits, (c) spouses' feelings regarding their partner's disability, (d) spouses' perception of how well they understood their partner's problems, (e) actual level of spouse understanding, (f) spouse-partner independence, and (g) advice sought by spouses. The items in the questionnaire were all "Do you. . ." questions. For example, one item asked, "Do you talk with your spouse as you did before the accident?" (Newhoff & Davis, 1978, p. 320). The spouses circled appropriate answers on a seven-point rating scale that ranged from "very often" to "never."

The spouse intervention group met for 50-minute sessions once a week for a period of 7 weeks. A speech-language pathologist served as group leader, but the spouses provided the direction for the group. The leader served as a catalyst for discussions and provided information as needed. The purpose of the group was to accomplish the following "counseling functions": (a) provide information to the spouses, (b) receive information from spouses that might be useful during their partner's rehabilitation, (c) facilitate the spouses' acceptance of their own feelings and help them accept and understand their aphasic partners, and (d) effect change in the spouses' behavior.

After 7 weeks of group counseling, the questionnaire was readministered to evaluate the effectiveness of the intervention. A comparison of responses to pre- and post-study questionnaires revealed considerable variability in the spouses' responding, and no discernible pattern of change was apparent. However, Newhoff and Davis (1978) concluded that they had accomplished their primary counseling objectives. They also concluded that, although the measurement problems involved in evaluating group counseling are difficult, they are not insurmountable.

Rice et al. (1987) also described their social support group for the spouses of 10 aphasic patients. The purpose of this 12-week group was to provide information and social support, enhance psychosocial adjustment, and facilitate communication between aphasic persons and their spouses. The authors reported significant improvement on scales of psychological adjustment for those individuals who consistently attended the group. No significant differences were found in post-treatment functional communication ability of aphasic patients whose spouses regularly attended versus those whose spouses did not regularly attend. Although this report is noteworthy for its attempt to evaluate the psychosocial effects of the spouse counseling group, results must be interpreted cautiously given the small number of participants included in the evaluation and the lack of appropriate experimental control. Friedland and McColl (1989) attempted to operationalize the definition of social support for their spouse program. Their model conceptualizes social support as having three dimensions: source of support, types of support, and how satisfied the patient is with the support received. Common sources of support may include personal, friend/family, community, and professional resources. Relatedly, the type of support received may include emotional and informational. Their parsing of social support has potential as a taxonomy for future studies of counseling and support groups.

Summary and Observations

Patient and family counseling groups have been widely advocated in the aphasia literature. The primary purpose of patient-family and spouse groups has been to provide educational information regarding aphasia and to provide emotional support for aphasic individuals and their families. Generally, speech pathologists and psychologists have acted as group co-leaders for aphasia counseling groups. Their primary function has been to lead topic-oriented discussions that center on communication and emotional adjustment issues. The emphasis in counseling groups for aphasic individuals and their relatives has been on "working through" the communication, emotional, and lifestyle changes that affect family dynamics.

The devastating effects of aphasia on interpersonal relationships and the family unit are well documented and the need for counseling aphasic persons and their families is unassailable. There is, however, little documentation as to the best format for accomplishing counseling objectives in the group setting. Although not specifically mentioned in most reports of group counseling, topic-oriented discussions should be accompanied by printed counseling information and/or appropriate audiovisual materials. Bevington (1985), for example, described an educational program that included the use of videotaped educational materials, lectures, and printed materials. The National Aphasia Association (NAA) is a nonprofit organization that promotes public education, research, rehabilitation, and support for people with aphasia and their families. The NAA website (www.aphasia.org) provides access to a variety of counseling and educational materials that can be used to support individual or group counseling efforts. Websites for other professional organizations, such as the National Stroke Association (www.stroke.org), also provide an invaluable resource for the clinical management and counseling of persons with aphasia.

Information provided in the counseling packets can be supplemented with counseling films. Printed information

provided in patient-family counseling can be supplemented with videotaped material such as: *Pathways: Moving Beyond Stroke and Aphasia* (Adair Ewing & Pfalzgraf, 1991) and *What Is Aphasia?* (Adair Ewing & Pfalzgraf, 1991).

Films and printed materials can be shared with aphasic individuals and/or spouses prior to their participation in counseling and support groups. This common information base allows new members to immediately interact with the other group members if they wished to do so. Clinical experience indicates that this approach alleviates some of the anxiety that may be present prior to entering the group. Discussions generated from the counseling materials may also help clinicians determine if a client or spouse might benefit from individual counseling. For example, spouses can be referred to a clinical psychologist for evaluation if they do not appear to be psychologically ready to share their feelings and emotions in the group setting. Similarly, spouses who discuss sensitive issues such as divorce or suicide may also be referred for individual counseling.

The invaluable contributions of professionals specifically trained in psychological assessment and counseling emphasize the importance of an interdisciplinary approach to family counseling for aphasia. Group counseling sessions are often very emotionally laden, and speech-language pathologists require specific training in order to manage the psychological and emotional impact of disability (Ewing, 1999; Kearns & Simmons, 1985; Luterman, 1996). Group counseling for aphasia may be best conducted within a multidisciplinary approach that recognizes and treats emotional and psychological difficulties that arise from disordered communication (Friedland & McColl, 1989; Pachalska, 1991a; Radonjic & Rakuscek, 1991).

Speech-Language Treatment Groups

Speech-language treatment of aphasic patients has been conducted in group settings for nearly half a century. Yet, despite its history of longevity, group therapy for aphasia remains a controversial area. Many authors have viewed group therapy as an "adjunct" to, or substitute for, individual therapy (Chenven, 1953; Eisenson, 1973; Marquardt et al., 1976; Makenzie, 1991; Schuell et al., 1964; Smith, 1972), but not a substitute for it. Schuell et al. (1964), for example, noted that "we are unable to have confidence in group therapy as a basic method of treatment for aphasia" (p. 343), since benefits derived from group treatment are likely to be emotional or social in nature. Similarly, although he acknowledges potential speech-language benefits, Eisenson (1973) states, "The first and most important (objective) is providing psychological support for individuals within the group" (p. 188). The prevalent attitude has been that group treatment methods may not facilitate speech-language recovery in aphasia, but they are not, at least, detrimental to recovery.

In opposition to the stance that group therapy for aphasia is merely palliative, a number of authors have indicated that group intervention is an effective means of treating speech-language deficits (Aten et al., l981, 1982; Avent, 1997a; Bloom, 1962; Elman & Bernstein-Ellis, 1999a,b; Fawcus, 1989; Garrett & Ellis, 1999; Graham, 1999; Holland & Beeson, 1999; Makenzie, 1991; Marshall, 1993, 1999a,b; Walker-Batson et al., 1999; Wertz et al., 1981). Although the data are not yet available to conclude that individual and group therapy for aphasia are equally effective, recent data and opinions that support this conclusion are stimulating investigative interest in the group treatment approach. In the sections that follow, we will examine the speech-language treatment group literature and explore emerging trends in this area.

Advocacy Reports

For our purposes the term "advocacy reports" is used to designate articles that advocate the use of group speech-language treatment for aphasia without clearly delineating treatment procedures or presenting data to support their position. Johnston and Pennypacker (1980) originally described an advocacy research style as one in which the experimenter's prejudices interfere with his or her objectivity. That is, the experimenter "has taken the role of an advocate who defends a cause, not a scientist who searches for understanding" (p. 424).

Advocacy reports may reflect, in part, a paucity of efficacy research, strong clinical bias toward unproven techniques, and a genuine interest in sharing clinical ideas. Clinicians are often more influenced by teachers, colleagues, and non-data-based presentations than they are by clinical research. This has often been the case in clinical aphasiology, where few data existed regarding the efficacy of group therapy approaches. Unfortunately, discussions of group therapy for aphasia continue to be based primarily on clinical experience and bias. Some descriptions of group therapy approaches have attempted to document change in psychosocial (Borenstein et al., 1987) and communication skills (Radonjic & Rakuscek, 1991) following intervention. However, few studies have incorporated appropriate experimental controls, such as the use of control groups and reliable measurement techniques. These limitations may negate the contributions of such efforts, making them comparable to earlier advocacy reports.

The current emphasis on intensive, multidisciplinary, functional aphasia treatment groups is reminiscent of approaches that have been advocated for decades (Borenstein, et al., 1987; Pachalska, l991a; Repo, 1991). Sheehan (1946) was among the earliest advocates of group speech-language treatment for aphasia. Her initial writings described "group speech classes" in which small groups of aphasic patients worked on everyday vocabulary. Five or six patients usually participated in the group at a given time. The specific content of "lessons" included greetings and farewells, personal identification information, money, calendar use, right-left orientation, and body part identification. As Sheehan (1946) noted, "The list is endless—a product of a little imagination and ingenuity and of observation of the things needed by the patients in their daily living" (p. 152). Sheehan (1948) was an early advocate of establishing individualized goals for each aphasic patient in treatment groups.

Wepman (1947) described a model program for inpatient rehabilitation of aphasic individuals. The program was carried out by a multidisciplinary team that included speech-language pathologists, psychologists, occupational and physical therapists, social workers, and special education teachers. Both individual and group speech therapy sessions were included in the program. The speech-language pathologist directed speech-related groups, and special educators taught writing, spelling, reading, and arithmetic in a group setting. Wepman outlined an intensive program that included 6 to 8 hours of treatment per day, 5 days per week. He concluded that an intensive, multidisciplinary approach is necessary if aphasic patients are to make maximum gains in therapy. A similar approach for patients with "motor aphasia" was outlined by Corbin (1951).

While the earliest writers in the area emphasized the importance of functional communication therapy in the group setting, the rationale for this approach was not fully developed for several years. Bloom (1962) was the first author to clearly articulate a pragmatic philosophy of group treatment for aphasia. Her rationale for group treatment combined an awareness of contextual influences on communication and meaning with an appreciation for the power of operant training techniques.

Although several treatment groups were conducted in her setting, Bloom emphasized the feasibility of group treatment for severely impaired patients. Aphasic individuals participating in her rehabilitation program attended one session of individual treatment, one session of auditory stimulation, and an hourly group session each day. The primary goal of group treatment was to improve functional communication abilities. All treatment activities were directed toward improving performance of "activities of daily living." Unlike many of the previous reports of group treatment, this approach did not segment sessions into classroom-like activities according to separate language modalities.

Bloom (1962) emphasized a situational group approach in which language stimulation was provided in meaningful contexts. Situations that occurred in daily experience were recreated in the naturalistic group environment, while role playing and rote memorization of scripts were avoided. Verbal tasks were used to practice greetings, directions, ordering from a menu, and handling money. In addition, auditory stimulation was also provided during group sessions.

Summary and Observations

To summarize, advocacy style treatment reports promoted the use of group therapy techniques as a primary method of intervention for aphasia. These reports described ongoing group treatment programs and presented a sampling of tasks employed in the group setting. There was consensus agreement that group speech-language treatment was efficacious, although data to support this claim were lacking.

Despite their shortcomings, advocacy reports of group treatment for aphasia were farsighted in several respects. They were, for example, ahead of their time in recommending a multidisciplinary treatment approach (Nielson et al., 1948; Sheehan, 1946; Wepman, 1947). Sheehan (1946) held regular team conferences that included speech-language pathologists, occupational therapists, and physical therapists. An effort was made to coordinate these services so that an overall plan of rehabilitation could be developed. Wepman (1947) also strongly advocated the multidisciplinary approach, and he indicated that "only by this overall cooperative approach can the maximum recovery level for the brain injured aphasic adult be achieved" (p. 409). Advocacy reports laid the historical foundation for current group therapy approaches that incorporate a multidisciplinary format (Pachalska, 1991a; Radonjic & Rakuscek, 1991; Walker-Batson et al., 1999).

In addition to establishing a multidisciplinary approach to aphasia management, early advocates of group therapy were nearly unanimous in their call for intensive therapy regimen (Corbin, 1951; Huber, 1946; Sheehan, 1948; Wepman, 1947). Wepman (1947) and his contemporaries suggested daily treatment, and many advocated several sessions per day. Huber (1946), for example, indicated that most aphasic patients could participate in 3 to 6 hours of therapy daily when appropriate rest periods were scheduled. Perhaps the most impressive aspect of the early group treatment literature is the consistent emphasis on functional, real-life treatment activities (Agranowitz et al., 1954; Bloom, 1962; Corbin, 1951; Huber, 1946; Sheehan, 1946, 1948). During the embryonic stages of group therapy for aphasia, clinicians developed treatment tasks that were based on the patients' communicative needs in the living environment. Treatment approaches included a consideration of contextual factors despite the lack of a supporting theoretical basis for "pragmatic" aspects of communication.

The previous examples of advocacy reports are primarily from the post–World War II era. However, recent reports reviewed below are also advocacy in nature (Borenstein et al., 1987; Friedland & McColl, 1989; Radonjic & Rakuscek, 1991; Rice et al., 1987). These authors present data obtained from uncontrolled group treatment studies to support the effectiveness of their approaches. Whereas earlier advocacy reports presented detailed clinical information and subjective clinical impressions, more recent descriptions of group therapy have included relatively less detailed information regarding clinical techniques and quasi-experimental results.

Taken together, early and more recent advocacy reports appear to have had a subtle and perhaps negative impact on the cumulative growth of objective information in this area. That is, the legacy of advocacy reports has been the tacit acceptance of the efficacy of group therapy for aphasia despite meager evidence to support this claim. Initial group therapy reports provided convincing, albeit unsubstantiated, testimonials as to the effectiveness of this method of patient management and more recent efforts have included clinical data that provide an appearance of scientific legitimacy. However, acceptance of subjective reports and uncontrolled treatment data as evidence for the efficacy of group treatment may have had the deleterious effect of retarding legitimate investigative efforts in this area. Over 20 years ago Gilbert et al. (1977) stated that "repeated weakly controlled trials are likely to agree and build up an illusion of strong evidence because of a large count of favorable studies. Not only does this mislead us into adopting and maintaining an unproven therapy, but it may make proper studies more difficult to mount" (p. 687). It seems that advocacy reports of group therapy have seduced clinicians and researchers alike into uncritically accepting this approach, and the cumulative effect of this literature has been an "illusion of strong evidence." Recent data-based clinical efforts represent a legitimate initial effort to examine treatment effectiveness, but these efforts must be followed up with more rigorous efficacy studies that examine specific treatment approaches for clearly defined groups of aphasic patients.

In the section that follows, we will examine contributions to the group treatment literature and explore the current status of research in this area. Five types of aphasia treatment groups—direct, indirect, sociolinguistic, transition, and maintenance groups—will be considered.

Direct Language Treatment Groups

Davis (1992) has distinguished "direct" from "indirect" treatment approaches. He states that:

Direct approaches focus the clinician-patient interaction on the exercising of specific language processes. They are referred to as stimulus-response training, in which the clinician elicits specific language responses from the patient. They are structured...so that the patient is using discrete functions such as auditory language comprehension or word retrieval (p. 241).

Brookshire (1997) was apparently referring to "direct" speech-language training groups when he noted that many aphasia treatment groups are didactic, relatively structured, and clinician directed. Tasks that are chosen for direct treatment groups of 10 mimic those used in individual treatment.

Holland (1970) provided an early example of the application of "stimulus-response training" in a direct group treatment program. She applied "shaping and reinforcement procedures to direct language work with aphasics in a group setting" (p. 385). Unlike previously discussed group treatment reports, she established specific treatment goals in an attempt to improve verbal categorization, naming, plurality, subject-verb agreement, and syntactic ordering abilities. Language tasks were arranged in hierarchies of difficulties so that patients of various severity levels could participate in the same group. Although Holland did not report objective data to support her exploratory approach, she indicated that she was able to arrange treatment so that individual patient needs were met. Additional examples of direct language treatment groups are available from studies of specific training techniques. Skelly et al. (1974), for example, combined group treatment with individual treatment in their study of the effects of Amer-Ind sign on patients' verbal production. They stated that the sign group was an integral part of their gestural program. Skelly et al. did not evaluate the contributions of group training to the acquisition of Amer-Ind signs. Relatedly, Sparks et al. (1974) used "less structured" Melodic Intonation Therapy (MIT) in direct group treatment for aphasia. Although not specifically evaluated in their study, they suggested that group MIT therapy may increase patients' ability to intone basic, purposeful utterances.

More often than not, group therapy is viewed as an adjunct to individual therapy (Davis, 2000). Makenzie (1991) recently examined the effectiveness of a combined regimen of direct individual and group intervention. The five subjects in this study had previously been dismissed from nonintensive speech therapy after having plateaued. All participants were at least 9 months post-onset of aphasia. The primary focus of this investigation was to examine the value of an intensive period of therapy.

The stated aim of the aphasia group was "information giving." All participants were encouraged to use an available modality to communicate effectively during discussions of daily topics. In addition, each individual participated in daily individual therapy in which two verbal goals were targeted for improvement. In total, subjects received approximately 85 hours of individual and group therapy during a 1-month period. A 1-month period of no treatment followed the period of intensive therapy. A screening battery for aphasia, a test of verbal naming ability, and a test of functional communication were among the measures used to evaluate treatment gains. The results of this clinical report indicate that all five patients improved on at least one clinical measure. Some decrease in performance was found following a period of no treatment.

Indirect Language Treatment Groups

Indirect treatment approaches are unstructured and may consist of general conversation, social groups, role playing, and field trips (Davis, 1992). Many of these approaches are purported to have therapeutic merit for improving deficient language skills despite the fact that they are largely undefined. Previously presented examples of psychosocial group therapy for aphasia, which used unspecified or poorly described techniques, differ from indirect treatment approaches primarily in the orientation and general goals of the group leaders. That is, whereas the general purpose of psychosocial groups has been to facilitate emotional and psychological adjustment to aphasia, the orientation of indirect language training groups has been to stimulate language recovery.

Despite the vague nature of indirect treatment groups, there is reason to believe that loosely defined language stimulation and group discussion are commonly applied treatment methods. In a survey of group therapy for aphasia in a Veterans Administration Medical Center, Kearns and Simmons (1985) asked clinicians to estimate the percentage of time spent on various clinical activities during a typical aphasia group treatment session. The respondents indicated that "general, topic oriented discussions" were the most prevalent (31%) activity engaged in during group treatment. Considerably less group treatment time was spent on "structured tasks" (word retrieval, etc. [22%]).

As in all areas of group treatment for aphasia, there are few data available regarding the effectiveness of indirect language treatment groups. The poorly defined nature of these treatment approaches severely limits investigators' ability to examine the usefulness of such approaches. However, a Veterans Administration cooperative study on aphasia compared the effectiveness of individual treatment and indirect group treatment (Wertz et al., 1981). A treatment protocol was developed to help ensure uniform training within both groups. Strict selection criteria were also used in this study, and only patients having a single, left-hemisphere, cerebrovascular accident were included.

Aphasic subjects in both treatment conditions received 8 hours of therapy a week for up to 44 weeks. Subjects in the group treatment condition received 4 hours of therapy in a social setting and 4 hours of recreational activities. Group treatment activities did not include direct manipulation of speech or language abilities. That is, no specific treatment tasks were presented to improve performance in verbal, auditory, visual, or graphic language modalities. Typical group tasks included participation in discussions of current events or other interesting topics. Subjects in the individual treatment condition received 4 hours of direct "stimulus-response" treatment of speech and language deficits. Specific tasks were presented for the various language modalities, and contingent feedback and reinforcement were provided by the clinician. In addition to individual treatment, subjects also received 4 hours per week of machine assisted treatment.

The results of this study revealed that subjects in the individual treatment condition improved significantly more than subjects in the indirect treatment group conditions on overall performance on the Porch Index of Communicative Ability

(PICA) (Porch, 1967). No significant differences were apparent on other language tests. Furthermore, subjects in both the individual and group treatment conditions made significant gains in their language test scores beyond the recognized period of spontaneous recovery. The authors concluded that there were relatively few differences in the amount or type of improvement exhibited by subjects in the two treatment conditions. Wertz et al. (1981) surmised that "individual and group treatment are efficacious means for managing aphasia" (p. 593).

Sociolinguistic Treatment Groups

Sociolinguistic treatment groups have evolved as a reaction to the highly structured treatment techniques employed in direct treatment approaches. Proponents of sociolinguistic treatment approaches have pointed out that direct treatment approaches may limit the types of communicative exchanges that occur between the clinician and the patient. Wilcox and Davis (1977), for example, found that clinicians primarily produced "questions" and "requests" during direct treatment sessions, and patients responded to the clinicians with assertions. A similar pattern of restricted responding was evident in a social group setting. Clinicians and patients produced a restricted number of "speech acts" in both settings. Wilcox and Davis concluded that individual and group treatment should be less didactic and permit the exchange of a wider variety of communicative interactions including advising, arguing, and congratulating.

Davis (1992) also advocates a sociolinguistic approach to group therapy for aphasia. Rather than drilling patients on specific treatment tasks that are adapted from individual treatment, he recommended that group sessions emphasize interaction among the patients while minimizing clinician directiveness. For example, principles of Promoting Aphasic's Communicative Effectiveness (PACE) therapy (Davis & Wilcox, 1981) can be incorporated into group treatment so that patients "take turns, convey new information, practice using multiple channels, and provide each other with feedback to overcome obstacles" (p. 263).

As a participant in the panel discussion of group therapy for aphasia conducted by Aten et al. (1981), Haire elaborated on Davis's principles of treatment. She defined the purpose of group treatment as an attempt to "maximize (the patients') communicative strengths in order to improve interpersonal communication" (Aten et al., 1981, p. 146). Her group treatment activities centered around a preplanned task or game, and PACE treatment principles were incorporated into the sessions. Aten et al. (1982) investigated a sociolinguistic treatment approach that was described as "group functional communication therapy." Seven chronic aphasic patients participated in this study. All subjects had suffered a single, left-hemisphere, cerebrovascular accident at least 9 months prior to the initiation of treatment. The subjects participated in

hourly group sessions twice weekly for a period of 12 weeks, and a total of 24 treatment sessions were administered.

The goal of treatment was to improve functional communication, and a variety of everyday communicative situations were selected for training from the Communicative Activities of Daily Living (CADL) (Holland; 1980). The "real-life" training situations included (a) shopping, (b) giving and following directions, (c) greetings, (d) giving personal information, (e) reading signs, and (f) gestural expression of ideas. Therapy activities included role playing and use of menus, grocery lists, and other materials from the patients' living environment. The results of training were evaluated by examining pre- and post-study performance on the PICA (Porch, 1967) and the CADL. Pre- and post-treatment PICA scores revealed nonsignificant differences, but statistically significant differences were apparent for pre- and post-treatment CADL scores. The authors concluded that group functional communication treatment is efficacious and that functional measures such as the CADL should be included in our clinical assessments.

A partial replication of the Aten et al. study was provided by Bollinger et al. (1993). In this study, group treatment was provided using a treatment/withdrawal design with "structured" treatment followed by a period of no treatment. Ten chronically aphasic individuals who were at least 18 months post-onset received 3 hours a week of group treatment for a total of 40 weeks. Treatment consisted of 10-week segments of "contemporary group treatment" and "structured television viewing group treatment" alternating with 10 weeks of no treatment. "Contemporary Group Treatment" consisted of greetings and socialization, a core activity focusing on a real-life activity, and specific communication-related activities such as group repetition of words and naming activities. "Structured Television Viewing Group Treatment" consisted of subjects watching specific television programs with later group discussion of specific communicative elements by group members. Bollinger et al. found significant improvement on both the CADL and the PICA but not on the third measure of language which tested auditory comprehension. Results did not demonstrate the superiority of either treatment.

Avent (1997a) described the use of cooperative learning methods with eight brain-injured individuals (seven post-CVA and one TBI). A single-subject multiple baseline across behaviors design was used to evaluate the effectiveness of cooperative group treatment on narrative and procedural discourse of participants. Each participant was paired with another into a total of 4 dyads. The speech-language pathologist's role was to provide guidance and structure to the treatment. Each participant with aphasia alternated in the role of "recaller" and "facilitator" of 10 narrative and 10 procedural stories having 100 to 120 words each. Initially, the therapist read the target story aloud with participants listing 8 to 10 key words and/or phrases from the story. Then the recaller retold the story. Each dyad's facilitator used the key words/phrases to cue his/her partner as needed. The therapist also prompted the facilitator to cue the reteller with the key words. Following a practice period, the reteller once again told the story followed by feedback from both the facilitator and the therapist. Five procedural stories and five narrative stories were used in treatment with the remaining stories used as generalization probes.

The outcome measure in this study was an analysis of content units (Nicholas & Brookshire, 1993). Results indicated that following 18 sessions of cooperative group treatment, three of the eight participants improved their narrative and procedural discourse in the treatment stories and the generalization probes. However, the remaining five participants showed either slight improvement or no change in performance. Avent concludes that participants who showed improvement were those with the mildest aphasia as measured pre-treatment by the Western Aphasia Battery and the content unit analysis (ie., 20% or higher content units per minute).

Graham (1999) describes the use of aphasia groups in subacute and skilled nursing facilities. Graham uses the ASHA FACS (1995) as a framework for planning and evaluating treatment in these groups. Following evaluation to determine communication strengths and weaknesses as well as the ability to use compensatory strategies, patients are enrolled into group treatment. Group members may also be enrolled in individual treatment sessions. Both individual and group treatment goals are selected from the ASHA FACS in combination with Hartley's (1995) functional communication goals. Treatment groups consist of two to six members which meet 5 days a week for 45-minute sessions. Treatment tasks focus on functional and "survival" skills and Graham describes how she uses videotape segments for viewing and discussion by group members.

Garrett and Ellis (1999) describe a group language intervention program developed in 1994 at the University of Nebraska-Lincoln's Speech Language and Hearing Clinic. The primary goal of this aphasia group program is to provide a vehicle for individuals with long-term aphasia to continue to improve their communication skills. In addition, the program provides learning opportunities for graduate students in speech-language pathology. The authors describe the Nebraska treatment program as combining principles of discourse, thematicity, contextual support, and functional use. A continuum of language activities, communication goals, and scaffolding strategies are incorporated into conversation, context building, language mediation, and discourse activities. The authors provide specific communication goals and explicit prompting information. Group sessions are 90 minutes in length with 6 to 10 people participating in each group. Garrett and Ellis report that group members frequently indicated that the groups helped them to become more competent communicators.

Additional data are needed to establish the validity of sociolinguistic group treatment for aphasia. For example, evaluation of the efficacy of discourse exercises (Osiejek, 1991) and other communication-based therapies in the group setting are warranted.

Transition Groups

In addition to the direct, indirect, and sociolinguistic treatment approaches described above, several authors have described transition or maintenance group treatment for aphasia. Brookshire (1997) indicates that transition groups, "...prepare patients for communication in daily life by giving them training and practice with strategies and problem solving skills that are useful in daily life" (p. 286). Tasks employed in these groups, such as role playing, are usually selected to help aphasic individuals adapt to communicative situations that occur in their living environment. Information may also be provided in transition groups regarding community services, such as adult day-care centers and home health services. Transition groups often meet one or more times weekly, and patients usually participate in these groups for a limited and specified period of time prior to discharge from treatment.

As a member of the group therapy panel conducted by Aten et al. (1981), West described her unique approach to transition groups. Three groups, a discharge-planning group, a community involvement group, and a stroke club group, were used to facilitate the transition between inpatient hospital services and release to the home environment. Patients in West's program participated in each of the groups in sequential order in an attempt to develop an increasing level of functional independence from the hospital staff.

The overall goals of the transition groups were (a) to help patients accept changes in physical and cognitive abilities, (b) to develop a realistic view of progress and altered ability, (c) to assist patients in finding an alternate lifestyle within available family and community resources, (d) to reinforce gains made in individual therapy, and (e) to help patients with community placement.

In addition to these general goals, each group had a specific purpose. For example, the main purpose of the discharge-planning group was to prepare patients for lifestyle changes that would occur on dismissal from the hospital. Practical difficulties encountered during home visitations were also discussed in this group.

Once patients were discharged from the hospital, they participated in the community involvement group in an attempt to facilitate emotional and psychological adjustment to their new environment. The emphasis in this group was on helping patients accept their new lifestyles and assist them in developing productive alternate lifestyles. The group also discussed emotional incidents that occurred in the home setting, and provided an opportunity for emotional venting by the group members. The community involvement group attempted to "confront reality without destroying hope" (Aten et al., 1981, p. 150).

The final stage in West's transition group program was participation in a monthly "stroke club." This group provided emotional support and education, and it helped patients maintain the level of communicative ability that had been reached following individual speech-language treatment. In general, West concluded that her three-group transition process was successful because it reduced dependency on the hospital staff and integrated patients into existing family and community structures.

Maintenance Groups

In the final analysis, West's "stroke club" group appears similar in function to a "maintenance group." Brookshire (1997) notes that maintenance groups provide regular stimulation so that patients' speech-language skills do not deteriorate once they are dismissed from intensive individual therapy. He indicates that maintenance group activities are frequently social in nature and may emphasize social interaction and communication in social contexts. Participation in maintenance groups may last from months to years, depending on the individual needs of the patient and his or her family. Brookshire observed that maintenance group meetings are seldom held more than once per week and may be held only once per month. Maintenance groups continue to be a medium for encouraging retention of therapeutic gains made during aphasia rehabilitation (Springer, 1991).

Hunt (1976) described a language maintenance group that provided support, information, and language stimulation for patients who had been dismissed from individual treatment. Eight to twelve patients participated in the groups, which met once a week for 2 hours. Family members were excluded from group participation.

The emphasis of this maintenance program was on stimulation of language in a social setting. Group activities were planned around the patients' interests and included movies, slide presentations, and guest speakers. These activities provided an opportunity for using residual language skills. Although specific language goals were not established, all attempts to communicate in the group setting were reinforced.

Hunt (1976) concluded that the social language group provided valuable language stimulation, practice of previously acquired abilities, social interaction, and entertainment. The maintenance group also acted as a source of information, support, and referral for the families of aphasic patients, and it provided a valuable training experience for student clinicians.

Coles and Eales (1999) describe Action for Dysphasic Adults (ADA), which provides self-help groups for individuals with aphasia in the United Kingdom. Speech-language therapists work for ADA as regional development advisers.

Each adviser supports a number of self-help groups and provides direction as each group is formed. The speech-language therapist also serves as the link to the national body. Ultimately, each group is run by its members with the speech-language therapist providing assistance only when requested. As different locales have varied interests and/or needs, each group identifies relevant goals and sets its own rules, including the number of members permitted in the group.

Multipurpose Groups

Taxonomies of group treatment procedures for aphasia are inherently flawed, since clinicians often identify several purposes for their groups. The results of Kearns and Simmons's (1985) survey of clinical practices indicate that 80% of the respondents listed multiple goals for their groups. As might be expected, language stimulation, often in combination with support or social goals, was the most frequent aim (84%) of aphasia groups. Following language stimulation, the next most frequently listed goals were emotional support (59%), carryover (47%), and socialization (45%). As previously indicated, attempts to classify types of aphasia group treatment approaches are generally for the sake of convenience alone, and they should not be construed as being a reflection of clinical reality. More often than not, group therapy is undertaken with several aims in mind even when a primary focus is evident. Most recent reports of group treatment for aphasia reveal that programs are typically multipurpose in nature, often combining psychosocial and speech-language goals into treatment.

Kagan et al. (1990, 1999) described a unique, community-based group treatment approach that is designed to facilitate functional communication, promote independence, and maintain gains made as a result of individual therapy. An important aspect of the program is the use of community volunteers who are trained and supervised by speech-language pathologists to work on communication goals with aphasic individuals in a group setting. A comparison of the results of pre- and post-testing for chronic aphasic patients who participated in the community group versus a group of untreated community-dwelling control subjects was reported. Results revealed significant improvement in the post-treatment performance of the group participants on a test of communicative effectiveness (CETI; Lomas et al., 1989 [see Chapter 6]) but not on traditional language testing. A significant between-group difference favoring the treated patients was also found on this measure.

Radonjic and Rakuscek (1991) described a multipurpose group that was established to decrease emotional tension; prevent social isolation; encourage the need for communication; encourage ability to search for, develop, and use communication in social situations; and develop confidence and self-respect. The group was developed by a clinical psychologist and a speech-language pathologist, and it generally ranged in size from 4 to 7 participants with a maximum of 10 group members. Group activities included such varied activities as "learning about each other, relaxation techniques, games to strengthen psycholinguistic ability, drawing, pantomime, and therapeutic techniques involving music" (p. 451).

A five-point scale of communication was administered at the beginning and end of each patient's participation in an attempt to examine the impact of intervention. A descriptive analysis of difference scores for 108 aphasic patients revealed improvements on patients' post-treatment communication ratings as compared with pre-treatment ratings. The authors concluded from their analysis that the best results were obtained for patients who participated in at least 10 treatment sessions in small groups having three to five members. Although intriguing, these clinical data must be replicated under more rigorous experimental conditions before they can be considered unassailable.

Pachalska (1991a) reviewed the group therapy literature and presented her treatment approach. Based on her review of the literature and her clinical experience, she suggests making groups as homogeneous as possible in terms of patient type and level of language involvement. Pachalska also recommends that the size of aphasia groups should not exceed four or five and that treatment sessions should last no more than an hour. A structured treatment approach is also advocated. Pachalska refers to a "holistic" method of treatment, which apparently refers to a multidisciplinary, multipurpose approach, such as her own Complex Aphasia Rehabilitation Model (CARM). Citing publications in her native language (Polish) she asserts that the holistic approach is "the most effective approach" (p. 547) to group treatment. CARM is described as having both individual and group treatment components, and group therapy is seen primarily as an adjunct to individual treatment. Group sessions are run by a multidisciplinary team of clinicians who provide cognitive physiotherapy, physical therapy, speech therapy, psychotherapy, and sociotherapy. Tasks are directed toward facilitating natural conversation. Pachalska (1991b) indicates that a goal of CARM is to stimulate transfer of information between the cerebral hemispheres; consequently, both linguistic and nonlinguistic stimuli are employed in treatment, and special emphasis is placed on "language-oriented art therapy." Linguistic materials used in therapy include popular poems and word games. In addition to the language emphasis, other aspects of rehabilitation such as physical therapy and group discussions with family members are also included. Social activities, such as "car rallies," are also considered as part of the rehabilitation process. Pachalska (1991a) makes the broad claim that "all abilities which underwent training in the programme significantly improved, and that the disturbances in the communicative, psychological and social domains were eliminated to a considerable degree; the reintegration was more complete" (p. 551).

The clinical forum that highlighted Pachalska's (1991a,b) work included commentaries by distinguished aphasiologists (Aten, 1991; Fawcus, 1991; Loverso, 1991; Repo, 1991; Springer, 1991). Fawcus (1991) emphasized that "the whole essence of group work is its flexibility and spontaneity" (p. 555) and cautioned against using overly structured approaches. Others agree that the mechanics of group therapy, such as group size and session length, cannot be dictated by prescription (Loverso, 1991; Springer, 1991). Our clinical experience is consistent with their suggestion that group sessions longer than 1 hour are possible and that larger groups are manageable and sometimes desirable. Larger, more heterogeneous groups may be particularly appropriate when the emphasis is not on direct communication or language training (Springer, 1991).

Another example of a multipurpose group is provided by Marshall's (1993, 1999b) description of problem-focused group therapy for mildly aphasic patients. The goals of this program are to provide a forum for discussing social, vocational, and recreational reintegration into society and assisting members in solving everyday communication problems. Examples of the problem-solving activities used during treatment include communicating in an emergency, meeting new people, and preparing for a physician's visit. Unique aspects of this program include the fact that it provides one of the few available descriptions of clinical management for mildly aphasic patients, and it provides a rationale for intervention that focuses on everyday problems and community reintegration. Clinical data are presented that show the range of post-treatment improvements on standardized language test scores for the 18 patients for whom pre- and post-treatment comparisons were available. Marshall recognizes the potential of functional communication assessments for evaluating progress in group therapy (Lomas et al., 1989), and he suggests that seldom-used formats, such as client self-report, may also provide a measure of clinical accountability. This issue is further considered in the sections that follow.

Walker-Batson and colleagues (1999) describe the Texas Women's University transdisciplinary Aphasia Center Lifelink© program, which uses theme-based activities to prepare clients for community re-entry. Lifelink© is a half-day university-based program with graduate students in speech-language pathology, physical therapy, and occupational therapy in addition to rehabilitation professionals providing services. Clients are assessed on a battery of measures to evaluate speech and language skills, participation in leisure activities, affect/mood, and quality of life. Speech-language treatment is determined by placement of each client on the "recovery-compensation continuum" (Elman, 1994). Intensity of intervention is based on the client's severity level as measured by the *Boston Diagnostic Aphasia Examination* (Goodglass & Kaplan, 1983). The most severe clients receive individual as well as group treatment; those with less severe aphasia are discharged from individual treatment with continuation in group therapy and community activities. The authors describe a "Visual Retrieval Language System" that provides theme-related vocabulary and structure for each client and is used in both individual and group treatment. Group size ranges from three to five members and groups are 75 minutes in length. Group sessions often focus on themes developed by the clinician; however, higher level groups may select their own topics.

Holland and Beeson (1999) describe the University of Arizona group treatment program. Treatment is focused on facilitating successful communication using any modality in addition to client specific communication strategies. Groups are 1 hour in length, include between five and seven members and are facilitated by faculty and graduate students. Holland and Beeson suggest that the Arizona treatment groups serve many purposes including direct and indirect language treatment, modeling of communication strategies, psychosocial support, and continuing education for group members, their families, and the student-clinicians. (Separate groups are conducted for family members.) Holland and Beeson report the Western Aphasia Battery (WAB) scores for 40 chronically aphasia individuals pre/post group participation. All had participated in the aphasia group for at least 1 calendar year. More than one-third of the group members showed a positive change of at least 5 points on the WAB. A regression analysis suggested that individuals who were younger and closer to onset improved more than those older and further from stroke onset.

Elman & Bernstein-Ellis (1999a) investigated the efficacy of group communication treatment on linguistic and communicative performance for 24 participants with chronic aphasia. Their research design utilized random assignment to immediate and deferred treatment groups. Groups were balanced for age, education level, and initial aphasia severity. While in the treatment condition, all participants received 5 hours of group treatment weekly provided by a speech-language pathologist for a total of 4 months. The focus of treatment was on increasing initiation of conversation and exchanging information using whatever means possible. Communicative topics were relatively unconstrained, with a wide variety of topics addressed, including psychosocial and post-stroke issues. Specific clinical procedures and content are described in detail in Bernstein-Ellis and Elman (1999). While awaiting group communication treatment, deferred treatment group participants engaged in activities such as support, performance, or movement groups in order to control for the effects of social contact.

Dependent measures included the Shortened Porch Index of Communicative Abilities (SPICA, Disimoni et al., 1980), the Western Aphasia Battery—Aphasia Quotient (WAB AQ: Kerstesz, 1982), and the Communicative Abilities in Daily Living (CADL: Holland, 1980). All participants received these tests at entry, after 2 and 4 months of treatment, and following 4 to 6 weeks of no treatment. In addition, deferred treatment group participants received an additional administration of the measures just before beginning treatment.

Results revealed that group communication treatment was efficacious. Participants receiving treatment had higher scores on the SPICA and WAB AQ compared with those not receiving treatment. In addition, those participants with moderate-to-severe aphasia who received treatment had higher scores on the CADL compared with those not receiving treatment. Significant improvement was observed after both 2 months and 4 months of treatment. No significant decline was observed at the time of follow-up. This study is the first to demonstrate that group communication treatment, and not social contact alone, is responsible for treatment gains.

Elman and Bernstein-Ellis (1999b) also report on the preliminary results from participant and caregiver interviews collected during and after group communication treatment. Semi-structured interviews were conducted with questions focusing on the positive and negative aspects of participation in the communication treatment groups. Interview transcripts were transcribed verbatim and a qualitative analysis (Miles & Huberman, 1994; Strauss & Corbin, 1990) applied. In this analysis, positive and negative aspects of group treatment were noted and then coded and grouped into common themes. Finally, all transcripts were reread multiple times to produce a limited number of themes that captured the information expressed in the interviews.

Interview data for 12 participants and their relatives/caregivers are reported. The positive psychosocial aspects of group communication treatment reported by participants with aphasia included: like being with others, like the support of others with aphasia, like making friends, like being able to help others, like seeing others improve, and feel more confident. The positive speech-language aspects included: enjoy conversations, improvement in talking, and improvement in reading/writing. The relatives/caregivers reported very similar positive psychosocial and speech-language aspects of their family member's/client's participation in group communication treatment. Psychosocial aspects included: more confident, more social, more independent, more motivated, like making friends, happier, and like helping others. Positive speech-language aspects included: improvement in talking and improvement in reading/writing. Negative aspects were rarely reported. It is important to note that many of these psychosocial behaviors were not directly treated during group communication treatment. Elman and Bernstein-Ellis posit that many of these changes are a result of increased confidence and motivation that participants gained from attending the groups. They suggest that the group environment can be an extremely powerful one for producing change.

Efficacy of Speech-Language and Multipurpose Treatment Groups

Examination of group treatment as a primary and independent form of patient management has only recently been undertaken (Aten et al., 1982; Avent, 1997a; Elman &

Bernstein-Ellis, 1999a,b; Radonjic and Rakuscek, 1991; Wertz et al., 1981). In addition, several studies have explored the value of combined individual and group treatment for aphasia (Chenven, 1953; Makenzie, 1991; Smith, 1972). Research evaluating the effectiveness of specific group speech-language treatment is growing, but the scientific basis of clinical aphasiology will not be sturdy unless this investigative effort continues.

Summary and Observations

Recent reports of group speech-language treatment for aphasia were reviewed, and five group therapy approaches were identified. These included (a) direct language treatment groups, (b) indirect language treatment groups, (c) sociolinguistic treatment groups, (d) transition groups, and (e) maintenance groups. Although each approach is unique, the common denominator among them is that their primary purpose is to facilitate recovery and/or maintenance of speech-language abilities. There is, however, considerable variability among group treatment approaches. Speech-language treatment groups range from structured, so-called "stimulus-response" approaches to essentially undefined, indirect treatment approaches. Group treatment tasks also show considerable variability and include specific techniques such as MIT (Sparks et al., 1974) as well as group discussions and recreational activities (Wertz et al., 1981). As previously noted, the variety of group treatment approaches probably reflects the training and biases of the clinicians who conduct group therapy (Elman, 1999; Marquardt et al., 1976).

There are, of course, obvious parallels between speech-language treatment group therapy and individual therapy for aphasia. Direct language treatment groups, for example, often employ tasks similar to those used in individual treatment sessions. Similarly, clinicians conducting sociolinguistic group therapy often adopt recently developed functional treatment approaches, such as PACE therapy (Davis & Wilcox, 1981), to the group format. Given these parallels between individual and group treatment, Holland's (1975) inquiry about the differences between these two approaches is poignant. If a group leader sequentially treats each individual in a group, and there is little interaction other than individual exchanges between the clinician and a given patient, the result may be inefficient individual treatment in a group setting. To avoid this possibility, group leaders must be aware of the strengths and communicative needs of individual group members. Ideally, tasks should be structured so that all group members can participate (Holland, 1970), but interactive aspects of communication should not be sacrificed (Davis, 1992; Ewing, 1999). Moreover, the objectivity of direct approaches should be combined with the common-sense rationales for sociolinguistic group therapy. The development of data-based, pragmatic treatment approaches will be challenging, but clinical aphasiologists have recently demonstrated

the feasibility of this approach to program development (Cochrane & Milton, 1984; Davis & Wilcox, 1985; Elman & Bernstein-Ellis, 1999a,b; Kearns, 1986; Osiejek, 1991).

Clinicians should eschew indirect treatment approaches that have no explicit communication goals and serve as a social outlet for their aphasic patients. While socialization can be a legitimate goal of group therapy for aphasia, clinicians should be leery of letting group treatment deteriorate into totally unstructured activities that neither facilitate nor support identified communication aims. Like individual therapy for aphasia, group intervention should be based on sound clinical logic, and it should be goal directed without being overly rigid (Fawcus, 1991).

CLINICAL ACCOUNTABILITY

Measurement problems encountered in group therapy are significant but not insurmountable, and proper attention must be given to assessing speech-language treatment gains in the group setting. To date, few authors of group therapy reports have attempted to measure treatment gains, and those who have examined the success of treatment have, for the most part, relied on standardized tests of aphasia (Aten et al., 1982; Wertz et al., 1981). Although tools designed to measure functional communication ability (Holland, 1980; Lomas et al., 1989) may be of particular value, standardized aphasia tests do not measure interactive aspects of communication, and the development and use of reliable supplemental measurement tools, in addition to qualitative methods of investigation, are sorely needed (Elman & Bernstein-Ellis, 1999b; Garrett, 1999).

The importance of measurement issues in group therapy for aphasia cannot be overestimated. Kearns and Simmons (1985) reported that 73% of survey respondents used periodic standardized testing to evaluate group members, and 33% employed standardized testing in combination with "behavioral ratings of task performance." Surprisingly, 20% of the clinicians indicated that patient performance was *not* routinely evaluated. A recurring problem for clinicians who run aphasia groups is the issue of clinical accountability; finding appropriate measures for assessing the effects of group therapy is problematic. As Aten (1991) pointed out in his commentary on Pachalska's work, treatment effectiveness will not be easily demonstrated until better assessments of psychosocial changes and conversational language are available. Similarly, Loverso (1991) addressed the need to develop and adopt tools that examine the roles of individuals within aphasia groups and the interaction of these roles during treatment. This novel suggestion is exemplified by the earlier work by Loverso et al. (1982), in which they demonstrated the reliability of a process evaluation form. Loverso et al. (1982) assessed the "roles" of individual group members and classified their interactions. They demonstrated that task (e.g., information giving and receiving), maintenance (e.g., encouraging following), and nonfunctional (e.g., disruptive) behaviors could be reliably rated in the small-group setting. Other novel, supplemental measures that may be employed in aphasia groups include the use of discourse analyses and interactive coding procedures (Cochrane & Milton, 1984).

Given the nature of the abilities targeted for intervention in group settings, clinicians often must devise their own clinical probes or "mini-tests" to sample skills such as turn-taking ability, initiation of interactions, and other skills, since standard assessments are not routinely available. Garrett (1999) describes numerous outcome measures that clinicians can use to assess basic communication skills, functional communication, quality of life, customer satisfaction, and overall cost-benefit ratios. Garrett states that most of these measures can be adapted for use in medical, outpatient, and/or community settings. Whatever the procedure or outcome measure chosen, it is important to evaluate the communicative abilities of aphasia group members routinely.

GUIDING PRINCIPLES

Thus far we have considered psychosocial, family counseling and support, and speech-language treatment groups for aphasia. Among the speech-language treatment reports, we distinguished early advocacy groups from more recent speech-language and multipurpose treatment groups. Our review of recent speech-language treatment group reports revealed a number of distinct approaches including direct language treatment groups; indirect language treatment groups; and sociolinguistic, transition, and maintenance groups. It should be apparent from this brief summary that no single therapeutic model can accommodate the variety of aphasia groups that have been reported in the literature. However, recent trends in the generalization literature may serve as a cornerstone for the development of eclectic, principled group treatment approaches.

The ultimate goal of aphasia therapy is to develop maximum communication ability in nontraining settings and situations. In essence, generalization of target behaviors across stimuli, settings, people, behavior, and time (i.e., maintenance) is the desired end product of therapy. Treatment effects are notoriously restrictive, and generalization is the exception rather than the rule in aphasia rehabilitation and other applied fields as well. There is, however, a growing generalization literature that provides suggestions regarding specific techniques that may facilitate carryover (Baer, 1981; Horner et al., 1988; Hughes, 1985; Kearns, 1989; McReynolds & Spradlin, 1989; Spradlin & Siegel, 1982; Warren & Rogers-Warren, 1985). A philosophy of group management that is geared toward facilitating generalization may provide an opportunity to empirically test our assumptions about generalization and allow us to examine the efficacy of group therapy for aphasia.

Reviews of the aphasia generalization literature also indicated that generalization of aphasia treatment effects is not an automatic by-product of intervention (Thompson, 1989). More often than not, clinical investigations of aphasia are what Stokes and Baer (1977) labeled "Train and Hope Studies." That is, investigators attempt to measure generalization of communicative improvements, but they seldom do anything to actively try and achieve generalized responding. Furthermore, when generalization does not occur following intervention, no additional follow-up steps are taken to obtain carryover. If the ultimate goal of aphasia therapy is to achieve maximum communicative functioning in settings and situations where patients live, work, and interact, then we have an obligation to do everything in our power to achieve functional carryover. As Horner et al. (1986) note, "[T]here is an ethical obligation, if not a responsibility, to make sure that generalization programming is incorporated into every program that endeavors to make important social and life-style changes for clients" (p. 16).

Generalization Planning

Clinical practice in speech-language pathology often includes four discrete and relatively independent sequential phases involving assessment, intervention, generalization, and maintenance. As is true of other clinical specialties in speech pathology, clinical aphasiologists have attended to the assessment and intervention phases of the clinical process while placing relatively little emphasis on generalization and maintenance. In contrast to the traditional approach to treatment planning, a generalization planning approach to the clinical process is conceptualized as a means of integrating the known clinical phases into a continuous loop that incorporates specific procedures to maximize the possibility of promoting generalization (Baer, 1981; Horner et al., 1988; Hughes, 1985; Warren & Rogers-Warren, 1985).

Kearns (1989) notes the following differences between a generalization planning approach to intervention and the traditional discrete phase approach. First, the separation of the clinical process into discrete phases encourages the establishment of clinical goals based on performance on clinical tasks within the treatment setting. Thus, within the traditional model, an aphasia test is given during the assessment phase, and the results of testing are used to establish clinical goals. When these goals are met, clinicians may then begin to examine aspects of generalization and maintenance. By contrast, a generalization planning approach to clinical management assumes that carryover of improvements in functional communicative abilities is the primary goal of intervention, and, as a result, assessment, goal setting, and intervention are all influenced by this assumption. The desire to facilitate generalization is foremost from the initial contact with the aphasic person and his or her family. Within a generalization planning framework, carryover of functional abilities is the clinical glue that bonds all aspects of patient management into an integrated whole. Thus, all steps in the process are woven together for the express purpose of effecting change in patients' ability to communicate in nonclinical settings, and with people and in situations that they experience in daily life. Whereas generalization and maintenance are too often a clinical afterthought with the discrete phase model of clinical practice, their attainment is the driving force behind generalization planning.

The distinction between traditional treatment planning and generalization planning is far more than philosophical. After all, most clinical aphasiologists would contend that carryover is a primary goal of group therapy. From a practical viewpoint, however, a generalization training approach is procedurally more complex and sometimes more time consuming than its traditional counterpart. For example, whereas the discrete phase approach to assessment of aphasic individuals may include standard and nonstandard tests of language and functional communication, the generalization planning approach expands the evaluation process to include gathering information directly relevant to maximizing the chances of obtaining carryover of treatment effects. Expansion of the traditional assessment may include, for example, naturalistic observations, interviewing significant others to determine communicative need, and recording and analyzing spontaneous interactions with familiar and unfamiliar partners. Baer (1981) suggests using every means available to make lists of all (communication) behaviors, settings, individuals, people, and actions of significant others that might affect generalization. These lists can then be narrowed down to a reasonable few and prioritized for the purposes of deciding what combination of client behaviors and environmental factors need to be altered to maximize the probability of obtaining generalization.

The primary outcome of an expanded, more ecologically valid assessment is to choose *generalization* goals. That is, based on the information gathered, the clinician attempts to determine the most critical factors that should be targeted for intervention if improved communicative ability is likely to carry over to real-life settings and conditions. Importantly, the clinician also sets a criterion for evaluating whether a sufficient level of generalization occurs. The clinician is also charged with the task of determining how best to measure progress toward generalization goals. Since there are rarely specific tests available to determine if generalization of specific target behaviors improves, clinicians must often develop their own means of assessing performance or adapt nontraditional measures (Garrett, 1999). These clinical probes (i.e., mini-tests) can be periodically given over time to evaluate progress toward generalization goals. This information can subsequently be graphed and used as a visual aid to monitor treatment effectiveness (Connell & McReynolds, 1988; Kearns, 1986a). In addition, ongoing assessment and visual-graphic data presentation also serve as a guide in making

treatment decisions. For example, clinical probe data can be examined to determine if generalization occurs to targeted people, settings, and conditions, and appropriate modifications can be made to intervention strategies as needed. Since it is clear that generalization of aphasia treatment effects does not automatically occur as a result of intervention, it is imperative that progress toward generalization goals be monitored so that appropriate clinical modifications can be initiated.

Kearns (1986a; Kearns & Scher, 1988; Kearns & Yedor, 1991), for example, reported a treatment approach, Response Elaboration Training (RET), which has been adopted clinically in group settings. The thrust of this approach is to use a forward chaining technique to lengthen patient-initiated utterances and encourage response variety. Novel appropriate utterances are encouraged and reinforced. That is, any patient-initiated response that was relevant for a given stimulus item is acceptable regardless of the form or content of the response. A unique aspect of this approach is that the patient directs the content of treatment. Once treatment stimuli are selected, patients' spontaneous utterances are used as building blocks for developing more elaborate responses. The clinician combines successive patient responses, models them for repetition by the patient, and then prompts him or her to provide additional information. Each novel elaboration is subsequently added to the chain until the patient's spontaneous responses are lengthened to preselected levels. Throughout RET an interactive, turn-taking format is maintained so that it can be readily adopted to group treatment. That is, each spontaneous conversational turn during group activities can serve as an opportunity for the clinician to prompt more elaborate verbal (and nonverbal) responses and to reinforce the use of novel but appropriate utterances.

Although the RET format has not been experimentally tested in the group setting, a series of studies has examined the efficacy and generalization of the approach for individual aphasic patients. Results to date indicate that generalized increases in verbal response length and variety have occurred following RET (Kearns, 1986; Kearns & Scher, 1989; Kearns & Yedor, 1991). In addition, this approach has also been successfully applied to facilitate improvements in nonverbal means of communication (Gaddie-Cariola et al., 1990) and communicative drawing (Kearns & Yedor, 1991).

RET and other "loose training" approaches to treatment are based, in part, on the rationale that loosening and diversifying treatment parameters may facilitate generalization (Baer, 1981; Horner et al., 1988; Hughes, 1985; Stokes & Baer, 1977; Stokes & Osnes, 1986). Attempts to target generalization directly as a goal of therapy by incorporating procedures that may facilitate carryover are an integral component of a generalization planning approach to intervention for aphasia. The group setting provides an environment for refining this clinical process, and it also provides a rich arena for future research and development of strategies that promote generalization.

By appropriately targeting generative responding in the group setting, we may increase the probability of obtaining carryover to the natural environment. Generalization training should, however, go beyond simply reinforcing selected responses when they occur. Task hierarchies should be developed to elicit responses under conditions that increasingly approximate the natural environment.

SUMMARY

In summary, a generalization planning approach has been reviewed and related to group therapy for aphasia. It was suggested that group therapy for aphasia may provide a means of incorporating generalization prompting techniques. The group setting provides an important link between individualized treatment and the natural environment. Only future research can determine the most effective means of using group treatment to facilitate generalization.

FUTURE TRENDS

Group therapy for aphasia is at a crossroads. We can fall back on the worn path of investigative complacency, or we can continue along a newer path of rigorous research in order to determine the efficacy of group aphasia treatment (Elman & Bernstein-Ellis, 1999). Although the choice may seem obvious, the road to group therapy research will continue to be challenging. We must begin by overcoming the assumption that we have developed efficacious already group treatment methods. Group therapy for aphasia has become strongly entrenched in our clinical repertoire because of historical precedent and practical clinical exigencies. There are, however, very few experimental studies of group treatment methods to guide our clinical practice. Intensive group treatment research will not be forthcoming unless we overcome the "illusion of strong evidence" (McPeek & Mostellar, 1977) that supports current clinical practices. The future direction of group therapy for aphasia depends on whether clinical aphasiologists will continue to research group treatment methods aggressively. The ultimate goal of research in this area should be to identify specific, replicable, and effective group treatment procedures. Ideally, it would be desirable to be able to predict with reasonable certainty which patients would benefit from which types of group treatment. Thus, future research should eventually compare the relative effectiveness of group treatment methods.

In addition to investigating treatment approaches, the future direction of group therapy for aphasia will bring an increased awareness of the training needs of group clinicians. It has already been suggested that not all clinicians are appropriately trained to conduct group therapy (Eisenson, 1973; Elman, 1999; Ewing, 1999; Sarno, 1981). We do not, however, have academic or training guidelines to evaluate the skill level of group leaders. Kearns and Simmons (1985) found that 74% of a large sample of clinicians who conduct group therapy for aphasia reported no additional training beyond their speech-language pathology coursework. Only 24% of the survey respondents indicated that they had taken coursework or training in group dynamics, counseling, or related areas. While it is not clear exactly what type of additional training is advisable for group clinicians, this issue must be addressed in the near future. Group therapy for aphasia presents additional challenges that are not encountered in individual sessions, and investigators and academicians alike need to consider clinical training factors relating to group intervention.

In addition to research and training, the future direction of group treatment will also be shaped by technological advances. The rapid development of computer technology, including the Internet, will, no doubt, have an impact on group treatment methods. Individualized treatment programs that are available may be expanded to allow patients to interact with one another and jointly solve communication problems. Similarly, treatment approaches may be enhanced by the expanding video technology, and taped or simulated communicative interactions may eventually replace static picture cards as the primary stimulus material used during group sessions. In the final analysis, the future direction of group therapy for aphasia will depend on people rather than technology. If researchers are firmly committed to this area of investigation and clinicians are willing to challenge traditional assumptions about the effectiveness of group approaches, then the benefits of group therapy for aphasia may eventually be fully realized.

KEY POINTS

Given the historical roots, it would be tempting to conclude that group therapy for aphasia is nothing more than, "old wine in a new bottle." It should be emphasized, however, that group therapy for aphasia, while in existence since the post–World War II era, has taken on a new and more important role in clinical practice.

1. The advent of managed care and the resultant decrease in services for aphasic individuals (Elman & Bernstein-Ellis, 1995; Frattali, 1998; Warren & Kearns, 2000) have forced clinicians and clinical researchers to reevaluate the efficiency and efficacy of their therapy techniques.
2. In the context of reductions in reimbursement for clinical services and less time to treat aphasic persons, it is clear that sound group therapy approaches are playing an increasingly significant role in patient management.

3. General trends in rehabilitation, including the emphasis on treating individuals at the level of handicap or well-being rather than treating their impairments per se also bode well for the future of group therapy for aphasia.

4. Multipurpose groups that attempt to address the needs of the "whole" patient are rapidly becoming the norm rather than the exception. Importantly, the resurgence of interest in group techniques is not simply a matter of necessity.

5. Clinical researchers have recently developed novel group treatment methods (Avent, 1997b; Bernstein-Ellis & Elman, 1999; Kagan et al., 1990) that incorporate clearly articulated treatment rationales and there is long overdue interest in issues relating to measuring client progress in treatment (Garrett, 1999).

6. Treatment efficacy is finally being put to the scientific test and data are accumulating to support the use of group treatment for aphasia (Elman & Bernstein-Ellis, 1999; Marshall, 1993).

7. Group therapy for aphasia should now be considered an essential component of our clinical armamentarium rather than a convenient supplement to individual treatment.

References

Adair Ewing, S. & Pfalzgraf, B. (1991). *Pathways: Moving beyond stroke and aphasia.* Detroit, MI: Wayne State University Producer.

Adair Ewing, S. & Pfalzgraf, B. (1991). *What is aphasia?* Detroit, MI: Wayne State University, Producer.

Agranowitz, A., Boone, D., Ruff, M., Seacat, G., & Terr, A. (1954). Group therapy as a method of retraining aphasics. *Quarterly Journal of Speech, 40,* 17–182.

Aronson, M., Shatin, L., & Cook, J.C. (1956). Sociopsychotherapeutic approach to the treatment of aphasic patients. *Journal of Speech and Hearing Disorders, 21,* 352–364.

Aten, J. (1991). Group therapy for aphasic patients: Let's show it works. *Aphasiology, 5,* 559–561.

Aten, J.L., Caligiuri, M.P., & Holland, A. (1982). The efficacy of functional communication therapy for chronic aphasic patients. *Journal of Speech and Hearing Disorders, 47,* 93–96.

Aten, J., Kushner-Vogel, D., Haire, A., West, J.F., O'Connor, S., & Bennett, L. (1981). Group treatment for aphasia panel discussion. In R.H. Brookshire (ed.), *Clinical aphasiology conference proceedings* (pp. 141–154). Minneapolis, MN: BRK.

Avent, J.R. (1997a). Group treatment in aphasia using cooperative learning methods. *Journal of Medical Speech-Language Pathology, 5*(1), 9–26.

Avent, J.R. (1997b). *Manual of cooperative group treatment for aphasia.* Boston, MA: Butterworth-Heinemann.

Backus, O. & Dunn, H. (1947). Intensive group therapy in speech rehabilitation. *Journal of Speech and Hearing Disorders, 12,* 39–60.

Backus, O. & Dunn, H. (1952). The use of a group structure in speech therapy. *Journal of Speech and Hearing Disorders, 17,* 116–122.

Baer, D.M. (1981). *How to plan for generalization.* Austin, TX: Pro-Ed.

Barlow, D.H., Hayes, S.C., & Nelson, R.O. (1984). *The scientist practitioner: Research and accountability in clinical and educational settings.* New York: Pergamon Press.

Bernstein, J. (1979). A supportive group for spouses of stroke patients. *Aphasia Apraxia Agnosia, 11,* 30–35.

Bernstein-Ellis, E. & Elman, R. (1999). Group communication treatment for individuals with aphasia: The Aphasia Center of California approach. In R. Elman (ed.), *Group treatment for neurogenic communication disorders: The expert clinician's approach* (pp. 47–56). Boston, MA: Butterworth-Heinemann.

Bevington, L.J. (1985). The effects of a structured educational programme on relatives' knowledge of communication with stroke. *Australian Journal of Communication Disorders, 13,* 117–121.

Blackman, N. (1950). Group psychotherapy with aphasics. *Journal of Nervous Mental Disorders, 111,* 154–163.

Blackman, N. & Tureen, L. (1948). Aphasia: A psychosomatic approach in rehabilitation. *Transactions of American Neurological Association, 73,* 1931–96.

Bloom, L.M. (1962). A rationale for group treatment of aphasic patients. *Journal of Speech and Hearing Disorders, 27,* 11–16.

Bollinger, R., Musson, N., & Holland, A. (1993). A study of group communication intervention with chronically aphasic persons. *Aphasiology, 7,* 301–313.

Borenstein, P., Linell, S., & Wahrborg, P. (1987). An innovative therapeutic program for aphasic patients and their relatives. *Scandinavian Journal of Rehabilitation Medicine, 19,* 51–56.

Brindely, P., Copeland, M., Demain, C., & Martyn, P. (1989). A comparison of the speech of ten chronic aphasics following intensive and no-intensive periods of therapy. *Aphasiology, 3,* 695–707.

Brookshire, R.H. (1997). *An introduction to neurogenic communication disorders* (5th ed.). Saint Louis, MO: Mosby Year Book.

Chenven, H. (1953). Effects of group therapy upon language recovery in predominantly expressive aphasic patients. Doctoral dissertation, New York University.

Cochrane, R. & Milton, S.B. (1984). Conversational prompting: A sentence building technique for severe aphasia. *Journal of Neurological Communication Disorders, 1,* 423.

Coelho, C.A. & Duffy, R. (1985). Communicative use of signs in aphasia: Is acquisition enough? *Clinical Aphasiology, 15,* 222–228.

Coles, R. & Eales, C. The aphasia self-help movement in Britain: A challenge and an opportunity. In R. Elman (ed.), *Group treatment for neurogenic communication disorders: The expert clinician's approach* (pp. 107–114). Woburn, MA: Butterworth-Heinemann.

Connell, P. & McReynolds, L.V. (1988). A clinical science approach to treatment. In L. McReynolds, N. Lass, & D. Yoder (eds.), *Handbook of speech-language pathology and audiology* (pp. 1058–1075). Toronto: BC Decker.

Corbin, M.L. (1951). Group speech therapy for motor aphasia and dysarthria. *Journal of Speech and Hearing Disorders, 16,* 21–34.

Darley, F.L. (1982). *Aphasia.* Philadelphia, PA: WB Saunders.

Davis, G.A. (2000). *Aphasiology disorders and clinical features*. Boston, MA: Allyn and Bacon.

Davis, G.A. (1992). *A survey of adult aphasia*. Englewood Cliffs, NJ: Prentice Hall.

Davis, G.A. & Wilcox, M.J. (1981). Incorporating parameters of natural conversation in aphasia treatment. In R. Chapey (ed.), *Language intervention strategies in adult aphasia*. Baltimore, MD: Williams & Wilkins.

Derman, S. & Manaster, H. (1967). Family counseling with relatives of aphasic patients at Schwab Rehabilitation Hospital. *ASHA, 9*, 175–177.

Disimoni, R., Keith, R., & Darley, R. (1980). Prediction of PICA overall score by short version of the test. *Journal of Speech and Hearing Research, 23*, 511–516.

Eisenson, J. (1973). *Adult aphasia*. New York: Appleton-Century-Crofts.

Elman, R.J. (1994, October). Aphasia treatment planning in an outpatient medical rehabilitation center: Where do we go from here? In C. Coelho (ed.), *Neurophysiology and neurogenic speech and language disorders special interest division 2 newsletter* (pp. 9–13). Rockville, MD: American Speech-Language-Hearing Association.

Elman, R. (ed.), (1999). *Group treatment of neurogenic communication disorders: The expert clinician's approach*. Woburn, MA: Butterworth-Heinemann.

Elman, R. & Bernstein-Ellis, E. (1995). What is functional? *American Journal of Speech and Language Pathology, 4*, 115–117.

Elman, R. & Bernstein-Ellis, E. (1999a). The efficacy of group communication treatment in adults with chronic aphasia. *Journal of Speech, Language, and Hearing Research, 42*, 411–419.

Elman, R. & Bernstein-Ellis, E. (1999b). Psychosocial aspects of group communication treatment: Preliminary findings. *Seminars in Speech & Language, 20*(1), 65–72.

Ewing, S. (1999). Group process, group dynamics, and group techniques with neurogenic communication disorders. In R. Elman (ed.), *Group treatment for neurogenic communication disorders: The expert clinician's approach* (pp. 9–16). Boston, MA: Butterworth-Heinemann.

Fawcus, M. (1989). Group therapy: A learning situation. In C. Code & D.J. Müller (eds.), *Aphasia therapy* (2nd ed.). London: Cole & Whurr.

Fawcus, M. (1991). Managing group therapy: Further considerations. *Aphasiology, 5–6*, 55–557

Frattali, C.M. (1998). *Measuring outcomes in speech-language pathology*. New York: Thieme.

Frattali, C.M. (1992). Functional assessment of communication: Merging public policy with clinical views. *Aphasiology, 6–I*, 630–683.

Friedland, J. & McColl, M. (1989). Social support for stroke survivors: Development and evaluation of an intervention program. *Physical and Occupational Therapy in Geriatrics, 7*, 55–69.

Friedman, M.H. (1961). On the nature of regression in aphasia. *Archives of General Psychiatry, 5*, 60–64.

Gaddie, A., Keams, K., & Yedor, K. (1989). A qualitative analysis of response elaboration training effects. *Clinical Aphasiology, 19*, 171–184.

Gaddie-Cariola, A., Kearns, K., & Defoor-Hill, L. (1990). Response elaboration training: Treatment effects using a visual

communication system. Paper presented at the annual meeting of the American Speech-Language-Hearing Association, Seattle, WA.

Garrett, K. (1999). Measuring outcomes of group therapy. In R. Elman (ed.), *Group treatment for neurogenic communication disorders: The expert clinician's approach* (pp. 17–30). Woburn, MA: Butterworth-Heinemann.

Garrett, K. & Ellis, G. (1999). Group communication therapy for people with long-term aphasia: Scaffolded thematic discourse activities. In R. Elman (ed.), *Group treatment for neurogenic communication disorders: The expert clinician's approach* (pp. 85–96). Woburn, MA: Butterworth-Heinemann.

Gilbert, T.P., Mcpeek, B., & Mosteller, F. (1977). Statistics and ethics in surgery and anesthesia. *Science, 198*, 684–699.

Godfrey, C.M. & Douglass, E. (1959). The recovery process in aphasia. *Canadian Medical Association Journal, 80*, 618–624.

Gordon, E. (1976). A bi-disciplinary approach to group therapy for wives of aphasics. Paper presented at the Annual Convention of the American Speech and Hearing Association, Houston, TX.

Goodglass, H.E. & Kaplan, E. (1983). *The assessment of aphasia and related disorders* (2nd ed.). Philadelphia, PA: Lea & Febiger.

Graham, M. (1999). Aphasia group therapy in a subacute setting: Using the American Speech-Language-Hearing Association Functional Assessment of Communication Skills. In R. Elman (ed.), *Group treatment for neurogenic communication disorders: The expert clinician's approach* (pp. 37–46). Woburn, MA: Butterworth-Heinemann.

Hoen, R., Thelander, M., & Worsley, J. (1997). Improvement in psychological well-being of people with aphasia and their families: Evaluation of a community-based programme. *Aphasiology, 11*(7), 681–691.

Holland, A.L. (1970). Case studies in aphasia rehabilitation using programmed instruction. *ASHA, 35*, 377–390.

Holland, A.L. (1975). The effectiveness of treatment in aphasia. In R.H. Brookshire (ed.), *Clinical aphasiology conference proceedings, 1972–1976* (pp. 145–159). Minneapolis. MN: BRK.

Holland, A.L. (1980). *Communicative abilities in daily living*. Baltimore, MD: University Park Press.

Holland, A.L. & Beeson, P. (1999). Aphasia groups: The Arizona experience. In R. Elman (ed.), *Group treatment for neurogenic communication disorders: The expert clinician's approach* (pp. 77–84). Woburn, MA: Butterworth-Heinemann.

Homer, R.H., Dunlap, G., & Koegel, R.L. (1988). *Generalization and maintenance: Lifestyle changes in applied settings*. Baltimore, MD: Paul H. Brookes.

Horwitz, B. (1977). An open letter to the family of an adult patient with aphasia. *The National Easter Seal Society for Crippled Children and Adults, 30*, Reprint A-186.

Huber, M. (1946). Linguistic problems of brain-injured servicemen. *Journal of Speech Disorders, II*. 143–147.

Hughes, D.L. (1985). *Language treatment and generalization: A clinician s handbook*. San Diego, CA: College Hill Press.

Hunt, M.I. (1976). Language maintenance group for aphasics. Paper presented at the Annual Convention of the American Speech and Hearing Association, Houston, TX.

Inskip, W.M. & Burris, G.A. (1959). Coordinated treatment program for the patient with language disability. *American Archives of Rehabilitation Therapy, 7*, 27–35.

Jenkins, J.J., Jimenez-Pabon, E., Shaw, R.E., & Sefer, J.W. (1981). *Schuell's aphasia in adults: Diagnosis prognosis and treatment* (2nd ed.). Hagerstown, MD: Harper & Row.

Johannsen-Horbach, H., Wenz, C., Funfgeld, M., Herrmann, M., & Wallesch, C. (1993). Psychosocial aspects in the treatment of adult aphasics and their families: A group approach. In A. Holland & M. Forbes (eds.), *Aphasia treatment: World perspectives.* San Diego, CA: Singular Publishing Group.

Johnston, J.M. & Pennypacker, H.S. (1980). *Strategies and tactics of human behavioral research.* Hillsdale, NJ: Lawrence Erlbaum.

Kagan, A., Cambell-Taylor, I., & Gailey, G. (1990). A unique community based programme for adults with chronic aphasia. Paper presented at the Fourth International Aphasia Rehabilitation Congress, Edinburgh.

Kagan, A. & Cohen-Schneider, R. (1999). Groups in the introductory program at the Pat Arato Aphasia Centre. In R. Elman (ed.), *Group treatment for neurogenic communication disorders: The expert clinician's approach* (pp. 97–106). Woburn, MA: Butterworth-Heinemann.

Kearns, K.P. (1986a). Flexibility of single-subject experimental designs II: Design selection and arrangement of experimental phases. *Journal of Speech and Hearing Disorders, 51,* 204–214.

Kearns, K.P. (1986b). Systematic programming of verbal elaboration skills in chronic Broca's aphasia. In R.C. Marshall (ed.), *Case studies in aphasia rehabilitation* (pp. 225–244). Austin, TX: Pro-Ed.

Kearns, K.P. (1989). Methodologies for studying generalization. In L.V. McReynolds & J. Spradlin (eds.), *Generalization strategies in the treatment of communication disorders* (pp. 13–30). Toronto: BC Decker.

Kearns, K.P. & Scher, G. (1988). The generalization of response elaboration training effects. *Clinical Aphasiology, 18,* 223–242.

Kearns, K.P. & Simmons, N.N. (1985). Group therapy for aphasia: A survey of Veterans Administration Medical Centers. In R.H. Brookshire (ed.), *Clinical aphasiology conference proceedings* (pp. 176–183). Minneapolis, MN: BRK.

Kearns, K.P. & Yedor, K. (1991). An alternating treatments comparison of loose training and a convergent treatment strategy. *Clinical Aphasiology, 20,* 223–238.

Kearns, K.P. & Yedor, K. (1992). Artistic activation therapy: Drawing conclusions. Paper presented at the Clinical Aphasiology Conference, Durango, CO.

Kertesz, A. (1982). *Western Aphasia Battery.* New York: Grune & Stratton.

Kinsella, G. & Duffy, F.D. (1978). The spouse of the aphasic patient. In Y. Lebrun & R. Hoops (eds.), *The management of aphasia.* Amsterdam: Swets-Zeitlinger.

Kinsella, G. & Duffy, F.D. (1979). Psycho-social readjustments in the spouses of aphasic patients. *Scandinavian Journal of Rehabilitation Medicine, 11,* 129–132.

Kisley, C.A. (1973). Striking back at stroke. *Hospitals, 47,* 4–72.

Lafond, D., Joanette, Y., Ponzio, J., Degiovani, R., & Sarno, M. (eds.) (1993). *Living with aphasia: Psychosocial issues.* San Diego: Singular Publishing Group.

LaPointe, L.L. (1989). An ecological perspective on assessment and treatment of aphasia. *Clinical Aphasiology, 18,* 1–4.

Lomas, J., Pickard, L., Bester, S., Elbard, H., Finlayson, A., & Zoghab, C. (1989). The Communicative Effectiveness Index: Development and psychometric evaluation of a functional communication measure for adult aphasia. *Journal of Speech and Hearing Disorders, 54,* 113–124.

Loverso, F.L. (1991). Aphasia group treatment, a commentary. *Aphasiology, 5,* 567–569.

Loverso, F.L., Young-Charles, H., & Tonkovich, J.D. (1982) . The application of a process evaluation form for aphasic individuals in a small group setting. In R.H. Brookshire (ed.), *Clinical aphasiology conference proceedings* (pp. 1–17). Minneapolis, MN: BRK.

Luterman, D. (1996). *Counseling persons with communication disorders and their families* (3rd ed). Austin, TX: Pro-Ed.

Lyon, J.G. (1992). Communication use and participation in life for adults with aphasia in natural settings: The scope of the problem. *American Journal of Speech-Language Pathology, 1–3,* 7–14.

Lyon, J. (1997). *Coping with aphasia.* San Diego: CA: Singular.

Makenzie, C. (1991). Four weeks of intensive therapy followed by four weeks of no treatment. *Aphasiology, 5* (4–5), 435–437.

Malone, R.L. (1969). Expressed attitudes of families of aphasics. *Journal of Speech and Hearing Disorders, 34,* 146–151.

Marquardt, T.P. (1982). *Acquired neurogenic disorders.* Englewood Cliffs, NJ: Prentice-Hall.

Marquardt, T.P., Tonkovich, J.D., & Devault, S.M. (1976). Group therapy and stroke club programs for aphasic adults. *Journal of the Tennessee Speech-Hearing Association, 20,* 2–20.

Marshall, R.C. (1993). Problem focused group therapy for mildly aphasic clients. *American Journal of Speech-Language Pathology, 2*(2), 31–37.

Marshall, R.C. (1999). *Introduction to group treatment for aphasia: Design and management.* Woburn, MA: Butterworth-Heinemann.

Marshall, R.C. (1999b). A problem-focused group treatment program for clients with mild aphasia. In R. Elman (ed.), *Group treatment for neurogenic communication disorders: The expert clinician's approach* (pp. 57–65). Woburn, MA: Butterworth-Heinemann.

McReynolds, L.V. & Spradlin, J. (1989). *Generalization strategies in the treatment of communication disorders.* Toronto: BC Decker.

Miles, M. & Huberman, A. (1994). *Qualitative data analysis* (2nd ed.). Thousand Oaks, CA: Sage.

Mogil, S., Bloom, D., Gray, L., & Lefkowitz, N. (1978). A unique method for the follow-up of aphasic patients. In R.H. Brookshire (ed.), *Clinical aphasiology conference proceedings* (pp. 314–317). Minneapolis, MN: BRK.

Newhoff, M.N. & Davis, G.A. (1978). A spouse intervention program: Planning, implementation and problems of evaluation. In R.H. Brooksbire (ed.), *Clinical aphasiology conference proceedings* (pp. 318–326). Minneapolis, MN: BRK.

Nicholas, L. & Brookshire, R. (1993). A system for quantifying the informativeness and efficiency of the connected speech of adults with aphasia. *Journal of Speech and Hearing Research, 36,* 338–350.

Nielson, J.M., Schultz, D.A., Corbin, M.A., & Crittsinger, B.A. (1948). The treatment of traumatic aphasics of World War II at Birmingham. General Veterans Administration Hospital, Van Nuys, California. *Military Surgery, 102,* 351.

Oradei, D.M. & Waite, J.S. (1974). Group psychotherapy with stroke patients during the immediate recovery phase. *American Journal of Orthopsychiatry, 44,* 386–395.

Osiejek, E. (1991). Discourse exercises in aphasia therapy. *Aphasiology, 5*(45), 443.

Pachalska, M. (1991a). Group therapy for aphasia. *Aphasiology, 5*(6), 541–554.

Pachalska, M. (1991b). Group therapy: A way of integrating patients with aphasia. *Aphasiology, 5*(6), 573–577.

Penman, T. (1999). Breaking down the barriers. *Bulletin of the College of Speech and Language Therapists*, August, 14–15.

Porch, B. (1967). *The Porch Index of Communicative Ability*. Palo Alto, CA: Consulting Psychologists Press.

Porter, I.L. & Dabul, B. (1977). The application of transactional analysis to therapy with wives of adult aphasic patients. *ASHA, 19*, 24.

Pound, C. (1998). Power, partnerships and practicalities: Developing cost-effective support services for living with aphasia. Paper presented at the Clinical Aphasiology Conference, Asheville, NC.

Puts-Zwartes, R.A. (1973). Group therapy for the husbands and wives of aphasics. *Logopaed, Fomiatr, 45*, 93–97.

Radonjic, V. & Rakuscek, N. (1991). Group therapy to encourage communication ability in aphasic patients. *Aphasiology, 5*(4–5), 451–455.

Rao, P. (1986). The use of Amer-Ind code with aphasic adults. In R. Chapey (ed.), *Language intervention strategies in aphasia* (2nd ed.) (pp. 360–369). Baltimore, MD: Williams & Wilkins.

Redinger, R.A., Forster, S., Dolpbin, M.K., Godduhn, J., & Wersinger, J. (1971). Group therapy in the rehabilitation of the severely aphasic and hemiplegic in later stages. *Scandinavian Journal of Rehabilitation Medicine, 3*, 89–91.

Repo, M. (1991). The holistic approach to rehabilitation: A commentary. *Aphasiology, 5*, 571–572.

Rice, B., Paul, A., & Müller, D. (1987). An evaluation of a social support group for spouses of aphasic partners. *Aphasiology, I*, 247–256.

Sarno, M.T. (1981). Recovery and rehabilitation in aphasia. In M.T. Sarno (ed.), *Acquired aphasia*. New York: Academic Press.

Schlanger, P.H. & Schlanger, B.B. (1970). Adapting role-playing activities with aphasic patients. *Journal of Speech and Hearing Disorders, 35*, 229.

Schuell, H., Jenkins, J.J., & Jimenez-Pabon, E. (1964). *Aphasia in adults*. New York: Harper and Row.

Sheehan, V.M. (1946). Rehabilitation of aphasics in an army hospital. *Journal of Speech and Hearing Disorders, 2*, 149–157.

Sheehan, V.M. (1948). Techniques in the management of aphasics. *Journal of Speech and Hearing Disorders, 13*, 241–246.

Skelly, M., Schinsky, L., Smith, R.W., & Fust, R.S. (1974). American Indian Sign (AMERIND) as a facilitator of verbalization for the oral verbal apraxic. *Journal of Speech and Hearing Disorders, 39*, 445.

Smith, A. (1972). *Diagnosis, intelligence, and rehabilitation of chronic aphasics: Final report*. Ann Arbor, MI: University of Michigan.

Sparks, R., Helm, N., & Albert, N. (1974). Aphasia rehabilitation resulting from melodic intonation therapy. *Corte, 10*, 303–316.

Spradlin, J.E. & Siegel, G.M. (1982): Language training in natural and clinician environments. *Journal of Speech and Hearing Disorders, 47*, 2.

Springer, L. (1991). Facilitating group rehabilitation. *Aphasiology, 6*, 563–565.

Stokes, T.F. & Baer, D.M. (1977). An implicit technology of generalization. *Journal of Applied Behavior Analysis, 10*, 349–367.

Stokes, T. & Osnes, P.P. (1986). Programming generalization of children's social behavior. In P.S. Strain, M. Guralnick, & H. Walker (eds.), *Children's social behavior: Development, assessment, and modification* (pp. 407–443). Orlando, FL: Academic Press.

Strauss, A. & Corbin, J. (1990). *Basics of qualitative research: Grounded theory procedures and techniques*. Thousand Oaks, CA: Sage.

Thompson, C.K. (1989). Generalization in the treatment of aphasia. In L.V. McReynolds & J. Spradlin (eds.), *Generalization strategies in the treatment of communication disorders* (pp. 82–115). Toronto: BC Decker.

Thompson, C.K. & Kearns, K.P. (1991). Analytical and technical directions in applied aphasia research: The Midas touch. *Clinical Aphasiology, 19*, 41–54.

Tsvetkova, L.S. (1980). Some ways of optimizing aphasic rehabilitation. *International Journal of Rehabilitation Research, 3*, 183–190.

Turnblom, M. & Myers, J.S. (1952). A group discussion program with the families of aphasic patients. *Journal of Speech and Hearing Disorders, 17*, 383–396.

Van Harskamp, F. & Visch-Brink, F.E.G. (1991). Goal recognition in aphasia therapy. *Aphasiology, 5–6*, 529–535.

Veterans Administration (1983). *A stroke: Recovering together*. St. Louis: V.A. Regional Learning Resources.

Vickers, C. (1998). *Communication recovery: Group conversation activities for adults*. San Antonio, TX: Communication Skill Builders.

Wahrborg, P., Borenstein, P., Linell, S., Hedber-Borenstein, E., & Asking, M. (1997). Ten-year follow-up of young aphasic participants in a 34-week course at Folk High School. *Aphasiology, 11*(7), 709–715.

Walker-Batson, D., Curtis, S., Smith, P., & Ford, J. (1999). An alternative model for the treatment of aphasia: The Lifelink© approach. In R. Elman (ed.), *Group treatment for neurogenic communication disorders: The expert clinician's approach* (pp. 67–75). Woburn, MA: Butterworth-Heinemann.

Warren, R.L. & Kearns, K.P. (2000). The influence of capitation on rehabilitation and clinical aphasiology. Paper presented at the Clinical Aphasiology Conference, Waikola, HI.

Warren, S.F. & Rogers-Warren, A.K. (eds.) (1985). *Teaching functional language*. Austin, TX: Pro-Ed.

Wepman, J.M. (1947). The organization of therapy for aphasia: 1. The inpatient treatment center. *Journal of Speech and Hearing Disorders, 12*, 405–409.

Wertz, R.T., Collins, M.H., Weiss, D., Kurtzke, J.F., Friden, T., Porch, B.E., West, J.A., Davis, L., Matovitch, V., Morley, G.K., & Resurreccion, E. (1981). Veterans Administration cooperative study on aphasia: A comparison of individual and group treatment. *Journal of Speech and Hearing Research, 24*, 580–594.

Wilcox, M.H. & Davis, G. (1977). Speech act analysis of aphasic communication in individual and group settings. In R.H. Brookshire (ed.), *Clinical aphasiology conference proceedings* (pp. 166–174). Minneapolis, MN: BRK.

Section IV

Traditional Approaches to Language Intervention

Chapter 15

Schuell's Stimulation Approach to Rehabilitation

Joseph R. Duffy and Carl A. Coelho

OBJECTIVES

The objectives of this chapter are to familiarize the reader with Schuell's definition, theory, and classifications of aphasia; describe the principles, rationale, goals, procedures, and techniques associated with Schuell's stimulation approach to aphasia rehabilitation; and provide an overview of the literature on stimulus variables that may affect aphasic patient performance.

This chapter deals with an approach to the treatment of aphasia which places its primary emphasis on the stimulation presented to the aphasic person. Hildred Schuell was among the most lucid, scientific-minded, and insightful clinicians to propose and offer support for this approach. Because of her major role in its development, the approach described in this chapter is often referred to as "Schuell's aphasia therapy" or "Schuell's stimulation approach."

The work of Hildred Schuell in aphasiology spanned two decades and included significant contributions in the areas of diagnostic testing, classification of aphasic patients, and theory development regarding the underlying nature of aphasia. It was probably this sound foundation in theory, evaluation, and methods of observing and categorizing behavior that helped develop the compelling rationale for the stimulation approach. Its sound foundation also helps to explain why the stimulation approach represents one of the main schools of thought in aphasia therapy and has been one of the most widely used treatment approaches for aphasia employed in this country for a number of years (Darley, 1975; Davis, 1993; Sarno, 1981). In this chapter, Schuell's definition, theory, and classifications of aphasia will be reviewed briefly as prerequisites for understanding the stimulation approach. The remainder of the chapter will emphasize the principles, rationale, and specific goals, procedures, and techniques associated with the stimulation approach to aphasia rehabilitation.

Before proceeding, it is necessary to delimit further the territory to be covered in this chapter. First, it is recognized that virtually all approaches used by speech-language pathologists for the treatment of aphasia necessarily must involve stimulation of some kind (Wepman, 1953); for that reason, the stimulation approach may be thought to encompass all approaches to aphasia rehabilitation. The presence of numerous other chapters in this book, however, makes it clear that this is not intended to be the case. The material presented here is conceptually related to Schuell's specific approach to treatment, and it is her name which serves to signal the scope of this chapter and distinguish it from other treatment approaches which use stimulation in more broadly or more narrowly defined ways.

The second point is intended to qualify the narrowed scope described in the previous paragraph. Although Schuell was a "prime mover" in the development of the stimulation approach, many other clinicians and investigators have contributed to the development or refinement of its rationale, principles, design, and techniques. Wepman's (1951) contribution, for example, is particularly noteworthy, as it was the first complete elaboration of the approach (Darley, 1972). Therefore, while all current approaches to treating aphasia will not be discussed, attention will be given to the contributions of many individuals in addition to Hildred Schuell. Receiving special emphasis will be those investigations which continuously help to refine the approach by identifying stimulus factors which influence the adequacy of language performance in aphasic persons.

PREREQUISITES TO UNDERSTANDING THE STIMULATION APPROACH

Definition and Primary Symptoms of Aphasia

Systematic observation and testing of over a thousand aphasic patients led Schuell and her colleagues to define aphasia as "a general language deficit that crosses all language modalities and may or may not be complicated by other sequelae of brain damage" (Schuell et al., 1964, p. 113). The language modalities referred to in the definition include comprehension of spoken language, speech, reading, and writing. The "other sequelae"—nonphasic disturbances—most often would include modality-specific perceptual disturbances, dysarthrias, and sensorimotor deficits (including apraxia of speech). Also, other complications and secondary symptoms, such as a reduction of communication generated by depression or an altered attitude toward communication, may occur as a reaction to the primary symptoms of aphasia (Jenkins et al., 1975).

Schuell consistently viewed a reduction of available vocabulary, linguistic rules, and verbal retention span, as well as impaired comprehension and production of messages, as the primary characteristics of aphasia (Schuell, 1969, 1974a; Schuell & Jenkins, 1961a; Schuell et al., 1964). In addition, her observations indicate that not only does the impaired ability to retrieve and use the language code cross all modalities, it tends to be evident in all modalities in a similar manner. Finally, "the impairment is regular and orderly, and operates in a manner that is lawfully related to known language phenomena" (Schuell et al., 1964, p. 104). The occurrence of similar deficits across modalities within patients, as well as the predictable nature of those deficits, are important additional characteristics and they figure strongly in the rationale and procedures used in the stimulation approach.

Underlying Nature of Aphasia

In most scientific clinical endeavors it is preferable that the rationale for using a particular method precede the application of the method. This is particularly important in clinical aphasiology because we cannot always confidently, though superficially, say, "I use this approach because it works!" Until the efficacy of any approach to the rehabilitation of aphasia is unequivocally demonstrated, what we do at least must be defensible on theoretical grounds. Schuell (1974b) supported such a notion with her belief that "what you do about aphasia depends on what you think aphasia is" (p. 138). Therefore, it is important that our method(s) of treatment be linked to our beliefs about the organization of language in the brain and the nature of language breakdown which occurs when the brain is damaged. The adoption of such beliefs, however, is complicated by an abundance of choices. In fact, the existence of numerous beliefs about the underlying nature of aphasia has as one of its primary symptoms the existence of numerous approaches to treatment. Since treatment is subject to such beliefs, it is essential that we have some understanding of the model of language and beliefs about the nature of aphasia which specifically underlie the stimulation approach. If such a model and beliefs are palatable, procedures and techniques become logical extensions of the underlying rationale.

Schuell's beliefs about the organization of language and the nature of language breakdown in aphasia can be summarized as follows:

1. Language cannot be thought of as a simple sensorimotor dichotomy or a three-system cortical relay involving reception, transmission, and execution (Schuell et al., 1964). Such classical models were rejected because they ignore the complexity of perceptual and motor processes and view language as an activity bound to sensation and movement. They also allow aphasia to be thought of in terms of isolated, pure disorders reflecting disturbances at different stages of the dichotomy or relay system (for example, receptive or Wernicke's aphasia, conduction aphasia, expressive or Broca's aphasia). To many investigators, including Schuell, such notions do not correspond to modern concepts of neurophysiology and, more important, to the clinical behavior of most aphasic patients.

2. Neurophysiologically, language is the result of the dynamic interaction of complex cerebral and subcortical activities. Such complex interactions preclude the existence of simply segregated sensory and motor divisions and, in effect, place the existence of isolated sensory or motor deficits outside the realm of aphasia. Likewise, the various elements of language cannot be separated neurophysiologically. For example, the relationship between the semantic and syntactic aspects of language is so strong that their separation at the physiological level is arbitrary at best (Schuell et al., 1964).

3. The language mechanism contains a system of stored, learned elements and rules whose use and maintenance require discrimination, organization, storage, comparison, retrieval, transmission, and feedback control. Like Wepman et al. (1960), Schuell viewed language as an integrative activity that is linked to sensory and motor modalities, but not bound to them. That is, the stored elements and rules are common (central) to all input and output modalities—speech, verbal comprehension, reading, and writing "... involve the same referents and the same categorizations of individual and collective experience" (Schuell et al., 1964, p. 104). In the adult, therefore, language can exist unimpaired even in the presence of severe sensory and/or motor deficits, although it might be difficult to receive or express language through an impaired modality. Conversely, the language mechanism can be impaired in the absence of sensory or motor deficits, although in such instances the disturbance will be reflected in all modalities because the same language system is utilized by (or linked to) all input and output modalities through which language is channeled. Consequently, aphasia is viewed as a multimodality disturbance which is unidimensional in nature. That is, not only do all modalities tend to be impaired in aphasia, they also tend to be impaired in the same manner and to about the same degree.

4. It is important to recognize that Schuell's unidimensional, multimodality concept of aphasia does not require that aphasic patients vary only along a severity continuum. Schuell and Jenkins (1961b) wrote that

among aphasic patients "...many dimensions of impairment resulting from language deficit are identifiable, and need to be studied, in addition to the common or general dimension of language deficit" (p. 299). They also stated that "...at a given level of language deficit, language tests may be arranged in subgroups which show systematic regularities in aphasic performance in various modalities as well as systematic differences in the performance of various segments of aphasic populations." The point here is that Schuell did not believe that all aphasic patients were alike. However, based on her clinical observations and objective analyses of data, she chose to emphasize the apparent universal feature of the disorder—a general disturbance of language which is reflected in a similar manner in all modalities.

5. In aphasia, the problems of most patients appear more related to performance factors than to competence factors (Schuell, 1969). That is, it appears that linguistic elements and rules are not lost or destroyed but that the language system is working with reduced efficiency or is "...swamped in noise, due to faulty connections, disturbed internal signal sources, defective speech analyzers, and the general asynchronous chaos of processes whose mass action can no longer be properly coordinated" (Jenkins et al., 1975, p. 59). Schuell's belief that language is not lost or destroyed in aphasia is an important factor in determining that the stimulation approach is not one which involves the "teaching" or "reteaching" of language.

6. Although the language mechanism can exist separately from input and output modalities, our primary language processes are acquired and organized through complex, interacting sensory systems and sensorimotor processes. Notably, auditory processes are at the apex of those interacting systems which aid in the acquisition, processing, and control of language (Schuell et al., 1964). The importance of auditory processes for language and in the stimulation approach to language remediation will be discussed in more detail later.

Classification of Aphasia

Schuell's classification system for aphasia is unique when compared with most other popular systems. Her view of aphasia as a multimodality, unidimensional impairment clearly precluded categorizing patients according to modality of impairment (expressive, receptive, agraphia, alexia, etc.) or the element of language involved (semantic, syntactic, anomic, etc.). Instead, her classification system aimed at descriptive and predictive utility by classifying patients according to severity of language impairment, the presence or absence of related sensory or motor deficits, and prognosis. Originally, Schuell's system contained five categories and two minor syndromes. Later (Jenkins et al., 1975), the

minor syndromes were treated as major categories. The seven categories can be summarized as follows:

Simple Aphasia

Relatively mild multimodality language impairment with no specific perceptual, sensorimotor, or dysarthric components. Prognosis for recovery is excellent.

Aphasia with Visual Involvement

Mild aphasia complicated by central impairment of visual discrimination, recognition, and recall. Prognosis for language recovery is excellent but reading and writing recover more slowly.

Aphasia with Persisting Dysfluency

Mild aphasia with associated verbal dysfluency as an apparent result of proprioceptive disturbance (Jenkins et al., 1975). Prognosis for recovery from aphasia is excellent but continued conscious control over speech execution remains necessary.

Aphasia with Scattered Findings

Moderate aphasia with a variety of problems compatible with generalized brain injury (e.g., dysarthria, visual involvement, emotional lability). Although potential for functional language exists, prognosis is limited by the concomitant physiological and psychological problems.

Aphasia with Sensorimotor Involvement

Severe language impairment with impaired perception and production of phonemic patterns. Prognosis is for limited but functional recovery of language with persisting signs of sensorimotor impairment.

Aphasia with Intermittent Auditory Imperception

Usually severe aphasic impairment with severe involvement of auditory processes. Recovery of some language may occur but normalcy is not achieved.

Irreversible Aphasia Syndrome

Nearly complete multimodality loss of functional language skills. Prognosis for recovery of functional language is poor.

The above classifications are useful in planning treatment with the stimulation approach in two ways. First, the various categories indicate severity of language impairment and, therefore, give some indication of the level at which stimulation should be directed. Second, the identification of associated nonaphasic deficits indicates those input avenues with the least intact access to the language system, and those output avenues through which evidence of language processing is least likely to be valid or interpretable. Such input and output problems signal a possible need to modify stimuli or restructure response demands. They also identify nonlinguistic disturbances which also may require remediation.

APPROACH—GENERAL DESCRIPTION

Definition and Rationale

The stimulation approach can be defined as that approach to treatment which employs strong, controlled, and intensive auditory stimulation of the impaired symbol system as the primary tool to facilitate and maximize the patient's reorganization and recovery of language. It is an approach which recognizes that stimuli to which an intact language system can respond may be inadequate for eliciting responses from an impaired system. Because "sensory stimulation is the only method we have for making complex events happen in the brain" (Schuell et al., 1964, p. 338), the approach employs the manipulation and control of stimulus dimensions to aid the patient in making maximal responses.

Although numerous input modalities may be used, the auditory modality is at the foundation of the stimulation approach. The use of intensive, controlled auditory stimulation is supported by the following:

1. Sensory stimulation affects brain activity. For example, sensory input alters the electrical activity of the brain; increasing stimulus strength increases the frequency of firing of neurons and the number of fibers activated; the threshold of response can be altered by repetitive stimulation (Eccles, 1973; Thompson, 1967); animals maintained in enriched environments show positive changes in brain structure and function when compared with animals in standard or deprived environments (Ansell, 1991); structural changes in the brains of experimental animals occur in cortical areas presumably related to the behaviors they learn in response to specific stimuli (Ansell, 1991). Thus, at the neurophysiological level stimulation can and does influence brain structure and function.

2. Many lines of research indicate that repeated sensory stimulation is essential for the acquisition, organization, storage, and retrieval of patterns in the brain. Language "patterns" appear to be no exception because language proficiency is largely the result of linguistic stimulation and experience. In addition, it is likely that language retrieval works through patterns of excitation laid down during original learning, and that appropriate stimuli are required for adequate retrieval (Schuell et al., 1964).

3. The auditory system is of prime importance in the acquisition of language, and ongoing functional language is dependent on the auditory system for processed information and control through feedback loops (Schuell et al., 1964).

4. Numerous studies indicate that nearly all aphasic people exhibit deficits in the auditory modality (Duffy & Ulrich, 1976; Schuell, 1953b; Schuell et al., 1964; Smith, 1971). It has been suggested that many of the multimodality impairments which aphasic patients experience stem from these auditory deficits (Schuell, 1953b), and that recovery of auditory functions, for many patients, is a prerequisite to recovery of other speech and language abilities (Brookshire, 1976a; Holland & Sonderman, 1974). Finally, the clinical observations of Schuell et al. (1955, 1964) and Schuell (1953a, 1969) suggest that the use of intensive, controlled auditory stimulation results in multimodality improvement which is greater than when treatment focuses on movement patterns or on each modality separately. Schuell (1974c) considered the notion of intensive auditory stimulation to be "the most important clinical discovery that we ever made" (p. 112).

5. The use of intensive auditory stimulation is consistent with the definition of aphasia as a multimodality deficit due to an underlying disturbance of language. That is, if the patient's problems in each modality are a reflection of a common underlying language disturbance, then it makes sense to channel treatment through the auditory modality because of its crucial link to language processes. In doing so, we should expect that gains made through the auditory modality will extend to all other input and output language channels.

A caveat regarding the primacy of the auditory modality in treatment is in order. Experience tells us there are some patients for whom the auditory channel is not the most appropriate avenue for stimulation. For example, there are those with disproportionately severe impairment of auditory processes who, on baseline testing, respond more favorably to written or gestural input. For such individuals the primary stimulus channel in therapy may be visual instead of auditory. The use of intensive auditory stimulation in the stimulation approach should therefore be viewed as a rule for which there are important-to-recognize exceptions.

What the Stimulation Approach is Not

The stimulation approach can be further understood by identifying some things which it is not. Wepman (1953, 1968) argued that aphasic patients do not recover because they are taught to speak. He indicated that the purpose of stimulation is not to convey new learning but rather to focus on "old learning" and stimulate the patient to produce new integrations for language. Schuell et al. (1955, 1964) emphasized that aphasia clinicians are not teachers; their role is to stimulate the adequate functioning of disrupted processes. Martin (1975), viewing the stimulation approach as conceptually related to cognitive theories of learning, indicated that the approach is an attempt ". . . to reorganize a system already reorganized by brain damage" (p. 73). He pointed out that because the approach is based on a model which views aphasia as an interference with (not a loss of) language processes, therapy does not emphasize memory or the reproduction of stimuli as stimulus-response (S-R) learning approaches do. Instead, the approach emphasizes the action elicited within the patient by the stimuli presented. Such an approach treats the patient as an active participant in the reorganization of language, and gears stimulation to maximize the ability of the patient to participate in the process.

Finally, what Taylor (1964) has called nonspecific stimulation, or the spontaneous recovery approach, is not part of the approach being discussed here. Nonspecific stimulation would include merely talking to the patient as much as possible, working to establish rapport, socialization, or interest, and reducing anxiety. Clearly, such approaches to treatment should be distinguished from the more carefully planned and controlled approach which is the focus of this chapter.

Individuals for Whom the Approach is Appropriate

Relative to Severity

The rationale and general goals of the stimulation approach do not preclude its use with particular degrees of language impairment. However, the approach is not invariant along the severity continuum. The severity of aphasia should and does influence the nature of stimulation, specific treatment goals and procedures, and the frequency and duration of treatment. For example, severe aphasia (Schuell's irreversible aphasia syndrome) may sharply limit the use of the stimulation approach, and reduce treatment to a short-term program aimed at improving comprehension, counseling of the patient and family, and the prevention of withdrawal and depression (Schuell, 1969). Variations of the approach as a function of severity will be discussed in more detail later.

Relative to Associated but Nonaphasic Communicative Deficits

The stimulation approach attempts to improve language or reduce the functional handicap imposed by disruption of language processes. It is not intended to remediate problems which often coexist with aphasia, such as perceptual deficits, apraxia of speech, or dysarthrias; such deficits may interfere with communication but do not disturb language per se. When present, they require treatment which differs significantly from the stimulation approach used for the treatment of the aphasia. The treatment of concomitant nonaphasic deficits may be secondary to, take precedence over, or coincide with aphasia therapy. Although the presence of nonaphasic deficits often places limits on the application of the stimulation approach and the expected outcome of aphasia therapy, their presence does not necessarily preclude the use of the stimulation approach to treat the aphasia; nor does the presence of aphasia and the use of the stimulation approach to treat it necessarily preclude the use of other approaches to treat the nonaphasic deficits.

Philosophical Underpinnings

Before discussing the general principles and design of intervention, a brief summary of the general philosophy underlying the stimulation approach is in order. This philosophy should temper any desire on the part of the reader for a rigid, universal approach to treatment.

First, Schuell et al. (1964) stated: "We believe in a general philosophy of treatment, but not an arbitrary method. There is no room for rigidity in clinical practice . . . If the method leaves the patient behind, or if a patient outstrips the method, the method must be altered" (p. 332). Schuell believed that the main objective of treatment is to increase communication and that techniques merely assist in achieving that end. Therefore, methods should be flexible enough to be discarded if they are not working.

Second, diagnosis is a crucial part of the therapeutic process. That is, treatment must not proceed without some knowledge of the patient's assets and liabilities in each modality and some information about why performance breaks down when it does. Only with such information do we know what to work on and where to begin.

Third, treatment must be relevant. The neurological, linguistic, and social needs and interests of the patient need to be considered and utilized (Schuell et al., 1964; Wepman, 1953, 1968). Not only do such considerations reflect the clinician's personal sensitivity, they also help identify motivating material and pinpoint stimuli which may have very strong associational linkages in the patient's brain.

Finally, as stated earlier, treatment should be logically related to beliefs about the nature of aphasia. With the stimulation approach, there is no material to be taught, and no student to learn a lost language. There is a person whose communication ability may be improved with appropriate stimulation. Such a philosophy significantly affects the principles and conduct of therapy.

GENERAL PRINCIPLES OF REMEDIATION

The design of intervention used in the stimulation approach is based on a number of general principles, many of which were articulated by Schuell et al. (1964). A number of additional, very practical principles which also apply to the stimulation approach have been presented by Brookshire (1997). It should be noted that several of these principles are indigenous to good clinical practice, regardless of the specific approach used. They are addressed here because they have grown out of observations of patients treated with a general stimulation approach. Information pertinent to the validity of the applied principles will be presented when the design of intervention is discussed. The general principles derived from those discussed by Schuell and/or Brookshire are:

1. Intensive auditory stimulation should be used. As noted earlier, this is the framework of the stimulation approach, and is based on the primacy of the auditory modality in language processes and the notion that the auditory modality represents a key area of deficit in aphasia. The auditory modality need not be used exclusively. One modality may be used to reinforce another, and combined auditory and visual stimulation may be especially appropriate.

2. The stimulus must be adequate—it must get into the brain. Therefore, it needs to be controlled, perhaps along a number of dimensions. The application of this principle may be highly dependent upon baseline data, and may involve considerable individualized pretreatment planning. Brookshire (1997) states that tasks should be at a level of difficulty where "patients are working at or just below their maximum performance level (i.e., approximately 60% to 80% immediate and correct responses and to increase task difficulty when immediate correct responses exceed 90% to 95%)" (p. 225).

3. Repetitive sensory stimulation should be used. Auditory material which is ineffective as a single stimulus may become effective after it is repeated a number of times before the patient responds.

4. Each stimulus should elicit a response. This is the only way we can assess the adequacy of stimulation, and it provides important feedback which the patient and clinician may use to modify future stimuli and responses.

5. Responses should be elicited, not forced or corrected. If a stimulus is adequate, there will be a response. If a response is not elicited, the stimulus was not adequate. What the patient needs in such cases is more stimulation, not correction or information about why a response was inadequate.

6. A maximum number of responses should be elicited. A large number of adequate responses indicates that a large number of adequate stimuli have been presented. Numerous responses also provide frequent feedback and reinforcement of language, and help increase confidence and language attempts outside the treatment setting.

7. Feedback about response accuracy should be provided when such feedback appears beneficial, and patients should be shown their progress. The necessity for feedback may vary from patient to patient but it generally is advisable. Showing patients their progress may be motivating, reinforcing, and extremely helpful in "proving" that progress is taking place, or that different approaches or termination of treatment should be considered.

8. The clinician should work systematically and intensively. Treatment requires a sequenced plan of action. It should be implemented often enough to meet the patients' needs, taking into account their overall condition and prognosis for recovery.

9. Sessions should begin with relatively easy, familiar tasks. This allows for adjustment and "warm-up" time and enables the patient to proceed to more difficult activities after experiencing success.

10. Abundant and varied materials (Schuell et al., 1955) that are simple and relevant to the patient's deficits should be used. Treatment does not involve the learning of vocabulary or rules so content need not be limited to "items-to-be-learned." As Wepman (1953) indicated, the specific content of treatment is not as important as the manner in which it is conducted. A variety of material also reduces the frustration often induced by drilling on a small amount of material.

11. New materials and procedures should be extensions of familiar materials and procedures. This allows the patient to concentrate on language processing and minimizes the possible disruptive effects of new material and response demands.

DESIGN OF INTERVENTION

In this section, those factors which must be considered in developing a treatment program will be considered. Since, by definition, the most important component of the stimulation approach is the stimulation provided to the patient, those variables which are potentially most important to structuring stimulation will receive primary emphasis. Response demands, feedback, and the sequencing of treatment steps also will be discussed. The reader is cautioned that the recommendations offered here for implementing the stimulation approach are based on rather broad generalizations derived from a potpourri of research and observation of heterogeneous groups and individual patients. Consequently, few, if any, of the recommendations can be assumed to apply effectively to all aphasia patients.

Structure of Stimulation

A great deal of information has been acquired about stimulus variables which may affect aphasic patient performance. Such data are largely the result of basic clinical and experimental research and are not primarily derived from specific treatment studies. The data are, nonetheless, invaluable to the clinician who must decide how to make stimulation adequate and effective during treatment. As Holland (1975) and Tikofsky (1968) have suggested, one strategy for designing treatment is to follow leads provided by research by turning the experimental techniques designed to isolate a particular problem into potential treatment tasks. Nowhere in the aphasiology literature are there so many "leads" as in the area related to stimulus variables that affect performance.

These leads have at least three practical applications to patient management. First, knowledge about stimulus manipulations that may maximize performance can be used to ensure that a patient is working at a level where "failure" is minimized. Second, and conversely, knowledge about stimulus manipulations can be applied in the opposite direction to challenge mildly impaired patients or those who respond without difficulty to tasks designed to maximize performance. Third, many of the factors to be discussed may be useful when counseling people in the patient's environment who need information about how best to communicate with the patient in everyday interactions. The following represents a review of the variables most relevant to the structuring of stimulation.

Auditory Perceptual Clarity (Volume and Noise)

Although Schuell et al. (1964) suggested that most patients prefer to hear speech at conversational levels, they indicated that an increase in volume (not shouting!) is sometimes desirable. Only a few controlled studies have been conducted to evaluate the effects of increasing volume on auditory comprehension.

Glaser et al. (1974) found that auditory comprehension of aphasic persons under sound field conditions at conversational level was superior to comprehension under earphones (binaurally and monaurally) at 25 dB above conversational level. Because of the interaction between volume level and earphone/sound field methods of presentation, the results are difficult to interpret, but they do suggest that increasing volume above normal levels does not facilitate comprehension.

McNeil et al. (1979a) found no significant improvement in a group of 10 aphasic patients on a word discrimination and word sequencing task or on portions of the Revised Token Test (McNeil & Prescott, 1978) when stimuli were presented under earphones at 75, 85, and 100 dB SPL (Sound Pressure Level). Group data were representative of individual performance. The authors concluded that simple increases in stimulus intensity do not improve aphasic patients' auditory comprehension.

Although there is little evidence to support increasing the volume of auditory stimulation, it does appear that reducing noise or increasing the signal/noise ratio is beneficial. Aphasic patients often complain about the negative effects of noise on performance (Rolnick & Hoops, 1969; Skelly, 1975). Although Birch and Lee (1955) found that a binaural masking tone improved aphasic patients' naming and reading performance, other investigators have not concurred. Weinstein (1959), Wertz and Porch (1970), Schuell et al. (1964), and Siegenthaler and Goldstein (1967) found either no difference in performance accuracy in quiet versus noise or found noise to have a detrimental effect on performance on language tasks. Darley (1976) concluded from a review of

such studies that "background noise apparently reduces the efficiency of the patient's performance" (p. 4).

These studies suggest that reducing noise or working in quiet generally facilitates language performance. Simply increasing loudness, on the other hand, does not appear useful, although it may enhance performance in isolated cases. Many clinicians feel confident in advising patients' families that verbal comprehension is typically better in quiet than in the presence of a variety of distracting or competing auditory stimuli (TV, radio, background conversation, etc.).

Nonlinguistic Visual-Perceptual Clarity (Dimensionality, Size, Color, Context, Ambiguity, and Operativity)

Visual materials are often used as an integral part of the stimuli to which patients are asked to respond. The importance of visual stimulation, in fact, led Eisenson (1973, p. 162) to call Schuell's stimulation approach to treatment a "visual-auditory" approach. Clinical observations suggest that the properties of visual stimuli may influence responses, and the importance of the visual modality to language behavior in general has led to the investigation of visual redundancy as a potential factor influencing linguistic processing in aphasia.

In a study of 21 patients with severe verbal comprehension deficits, Helm-Estabrooks (1981) compared performance on a single-word comprehension task in which stimulus conditions consisted of line drawings, each on individual cards arranged in rows; smaller line drawings of items, all on a single page; and real objects around the room. For the group as a whole, picture-pointing was superior to identification of objects around the room, but there were no differences between the two picture conditions; however, not all patients followed the group pattern. Helm-Estabrooks concluded that auditory comprehension can be influenced by variables extrinsic to central auditory processing, such as visual search skills.

Bisiach (1966) compared the naming performance of nine aphasic subjects in response to pictures of realistic colored objects, line drawings of the same objects, and the same line drawings with superimposed curved or jagged lines. Although there were no differences among stimulus conditions for object recognition, subjects' naming of the realistic colored pictures was 15 to 18% more accurate than their naming of line drawings and distorted line drawings. The visual redundancy of the realistic colored drawings was felt to facilitate naming.

Benton et al. (1972) examined the naming performance of 18 aphasic persons in response to real objects, large line drawings, and small line drawings. Accuracy of real object naming was superior to that for small line drawings; accuracy for large line drawings fell in-between. The redundancy provided by three-dimensionality was felt to enhance the conceptual associations underlying word retrieval. Because of the relatively small differences between conditions, however, the authors questioned the clinical significance of their results. The possible insignificance of three-dimensionality was supported by Corlew and Nation (1975), who found no differences in the performance of 14 aphasic persons when they named the 10 common real objects used in the Porch Index of Communicative Ability (PICA) (Porch, 1967) than when they named reduced-size line drawings of the same objects.

In a theoretically interesting study, Whitehouse and Caramazza (1978) compared the ability of 10 aphasic persons to identify line drawings of three objects (cup, bowl, glass) varying in physical features such as height and width. Stimuli consisted of prototypes (unambiguous representations) of the three objects as well as drawings in which the height-width dimensions were varied in order to make the perceptual distinction among the objects "fuzzy." In addition, some of the drawings had a handle, some did not. Context (functional information) was also varied by presenting stimuli alone or in context with a coffee pot, cereal box, or water pitcher. Subjects "named" the pictures by selecting from multiple choice presentations of the names of the three objects. Results were not uniform across subjects. Those with a diagnosis of Broca's aphasia performed similarly to normal control subjects in their use of context and in their ability to deal with fuzzy perceptual boundaries. Patients with a diagnosis of anomic aphasia, however, had difficulty integrating and using perceptual and functional cues (dimension and context). These findings and those of Caramazza et al. (1982) have led to the conclusion that, for some patients, naming difficulty is related to an inability to organize adequately the concepts underlying word meaning in terms of functional and perceptual information, as opposed to difficulty with retrieval of an adequately perceived/conceived lexical item. Although the implications of these findings for clinical practice are neither clear-cut nor universal, it appears that the perceptual characteristics of visual stimuli should be as unambiguous as possible for all patients. Placing a target object in a redundant conceptual setting (pairing a cup with a coffee pot) may enhance word retrieval when the target is perceptually ambiguous. When pairing a target stimulus with other visual stimuli, the additional stimuli should never introduce ambiguity about the nature of the target.

Finally, the findings of Gardner (1973) suggest that the number of modalities in which associations may be evoked should be considered when selecting visual materials for treatment. He compared naming of pictures of "operative" objects (discrete, firm to the touch, and available to several modalities—for example, "rock") to that for "figurative" objects (not operative—for example, "cloud"), while accounting for the effects of picturability and word frequency. Most aphasic patients performed more accurately in response to the operative items and the effects of operativity were most pronounced for patients with difficulty initiating speech. Gardner argued that operative items were superior because they aroused associations in several modalities, whereas the

figurative items were limited to visual associations. This perspective is supported by the findings of Nickels and Howard (1995), who noted that operativity and imageability (i.e., how easy it is to create a visual or auditory image of the referent) were predictive of naming performance for some aphasic individuals. The implication for treatment, therefore, is that visual stimuli which also may trigger auditory, tactile, kinesthetic, or olfactory associations are potentially more effective in aiding word retrieval than stimuli which trigger only visual associations.

To summarize, although some data suggest that some properties of visual stimuli are relatively unimportant to aphasic performance it does seem that the clarity and redundancy of visual stimuli can influence linguistic processing (Cararnazza & Berndt, 1978). Darley (1976) recommends that we "play safe" and use the redundant and realistic stimuli in treatment. The most potent visual stimuli appear to be characterized by three-dimensionality, color, redundant physical properties, operativity, and a lack of ambiguity in perceptual characteristics and context.

Linguistic Visual Perceptual Clarity (Size and Form)

There are few data to suggest that the size or form of reading material affects comprehension, but a few clinical observations are relevant. Rolnick and Hoops (1969) reported that aphasic patients complain about small print for word and sentence stimuli and prefer large print, even when visual field deficits are not present. McDearmon and Potter (1975) observed varying preferences for upper case, lower case, or script stimuli. Schuell et al. (1955) recommended upper case print for patients with visual impairments and felt that script should not be introduced until the reading rate for printed material is normal.

Boone and Friedman (1976) examined 30 aphasic patients' single word reading comprehension in response to cursive versus manuscript stimuli, and Williams (1984) investigated the same factors' influence on the word and sentence comprehension of 20 patients. Neither study found significant differences between the two written forms. Williams, however, observed that 2 of her patients reliably responded better to one form than the other.

There is no compelling evidence to suggest that the size and form of written input are powerful stimulus factors affecting reading comprehension. When providing reading material for patients, however, the clinician should be aware of a general preference for large print, and potential idiosyncratic preferences for upper case, lower case, cursive, or manuscript format.

Method of Delivery of Auditory Stimulation

Many clinicians have speculated about ways to improve the delivery of auditory stimuli to patients. For example, can live-voice, binaural, free-field stimulation be improved upon?

The use of earphones is intuitively attractive because of its potential for reducing extraneous noise and focusing attention. Schuell et al. (1964), however, observed that patients usually prefer direct presentation to earphones because they rely on more than auditory cues and perhaps because earphones produce distortions to which they are sensitive. The preference for free-field presentation is supported by the previously mentioned study by Glaser et al. (1974). They found that the comprehension under free-field conditions was superior to binaural and right and left ear monaural presentations through earphones. The superiority of the free-field condition was maintained even when the intensity of the earphone conditions was 25 dB greater than in the free-field.

It has been suggested that selective left ear/right hemisphere presentation of auditory stimuli may improve comprehension. Such speculation is based on the results of dichotic listening studies which have found a left ear advantage for aphasic patients (e.g., Johnson et al., 1977; Sparks et al., 1970). LaPointe et al. (1977) examined aphasic patients' responses to portions of the Token Test (DeRenzi & Vignolo, 1962) when presented to the right ear, left ear, or binaurally, and found no significant differences among the three conditions. They concluded that selective monaural presentation of auditory stimuli is not a useful procedure. McNeil et al. (1979b) examined the effects of selective binaural SPL variations in which stimuli were presented at 85 or 100 dB SPL to one ear while stimuli to the other ear were presented at 70 dB SPL. Although a trend toward better comprehension on some tasks was noted when the left ear was more intensely stimulated, their general conclusion was that unilateral intensity increase is not a potent mechanism for improving auditory comprehension.

The data to date indicate that response adequacy to free-field presentation is not exceeded when earphones are used, and that selective stimulation of one ear/hemisphere does not surpass binaural stimulation. It should also be noted that the findings of Green and Boller (1974) and Boller et al. (1979) suggest that live-voice presentation is superior to taped presentation of stimuli. Therefore, there are no compelling reasons for us not to continue to present auditory stimuli directly with live voice, binaurally, and in the free-field.

Discriminability (Semantic, Auditory, Visual)

Verbal responses of aphasic patients are often characterized by errors associated in meaning or experience. Such errors (e.g., "table" for "chair") are, in fact, the "best" errors a patient can make (Schuell & Jenkins, 1961a; Schuell et al., 1964). These characteristics suggest that response alternatives provided to patients should not promote semantic errors. This is particularly relevant for comprehension tasks which require the patient to choose from among a set of alternatives (e.g., responding to a verbally and/or visually presented word or sentence by pointing to one of several choices). Assuring that response choices are unrelated semantically often will facilitate speed and accuracy of performance. Conversely, tasks can remain unchanged in nature but often can be made more difficult by introducing semantically related response choices (Duffy & Watkins, 1984; Pizzamiglio & Appicciafuoco, 1971).

Semantic discriminability among response choices is more important than visual perceptual discriminability. This is illustrated by the findings of Chieffi et al. (1989). Their aphasic patients made more errors on a single word comprehension task when response choices were semantically related (e.g., banana, apple, grapes) than when they were visually related (e.g., wheel, button, lifebelt). Performance on a task in which response choices were both semantically and visually related (e.g., chair, bench, stool) was poorer than in the semantically related condition, suggesting that semantic and perceptual effects may be cumulative, although the authors argued that the semantic demands of the combined semantic and visual task were more potent than the visual ones.

Difficulty discriminating between words with minimal phonemic differences (e.g., cake/take, horse/house) is an important aspect of auditory impairment in some patients (Schuell, 1973). In addition, aphasic patients may confuse letters or words with similar visual configurations (e.g., E/F; p/b; store/stone).

An investigation by Linebaugh (1986) sheds some light on the importance of semantic, auditory, and visual discriminability in single word reading comprehension tasks. He presented a picture-to-written word matching task to 25 aphasic patients under two conditions. In one, all three response foils (written words) were either semantically, auditorily, or visually related to the target response. In the other, the three foils consisted of one semantically, one auditorily, and one visually related word. When all foils were of the same type, error rates were higher with visually than with auditorily related foils, with no differences among other foil comparisons. When foils contained one of each foil type, both semantic and visual errors were more frequent than with auditory, with no differences between semantic and visual errors. There was considerable variability among subjects in their patterns and degree of susceptibility to the semantic, visual, and auditory influences, with a minority of subjects making more than 50% of their errors in one category and only 2 subjects doing so in both experimental conditions. These findings suggest that semantic and visual discriminability, on average, are more potent than auditory discriminability in single word reading tasks, but the power of each factor is seldom overwhelming in individual patients.

The discriminability factor apparently is also relevant to word retrieval tasks. The findings of Mills et al. (1979), for example, have implications for the semantic distinctiveness of visual stimuli used in naming tasks. (They also are relevant to the information discussed under nonlinguistic visual perceptual clarity.) They examined the effects of "uncertainty" on the naming performance of 10 aphasic patients, with uncertainty defined as "the number of equally probable binary choice decisions necessary to achieve a final name selection from one or several correct names available in the lexicon" (p. 75). For example, shown a picture of a cup, most control subjects respond "cup"; there are few alternative correct responses (little uncertainty). On the other hand, a picture of a country home in winter generates considerable uncertainty because "winter....country," "cabin....house," and other words would be reasonable responses, thus requiring a greater number of word retrieval decisions. The aphasic patients made significantly more errors and had greater response latencies in response to high uncertainty pictures than in response to low uncertainty pictures, leading the authors to conclude that uncertainty affects aphasic naming performance. Their findings suggest that another way to simplify word retrieval on picture naming tasks is to select stimuli to which there are only a few alternative responses. Similarly, reducing the number of response alternatives reduces error probability on point-to comprehension tasks.

In summary, there are compelling data to suggest that verbal comprehension tasks in which several response choices are offered can maximize performance if alternatives are semantically unrelated to the target response. The auditory and visual perceptual "distinctiveness" of the target from response alternatives may also be important, with visual similarity generally being more important than auditory similarity on written word comprehension tasks. Although there is considerable variability among patients in their responsiveness to these semantic, auditory, and visual influences, reducing the number of response choices on point-to tasks will usually lead to improved performance.

Combining Sensory Modalities

Although the auditory modality is paramount in the stimulation approach, the use of several modalities in combination is often recommended. Schuell (1974b) indicated that various modalities should be used to reinforce one another and, in fact, felt that patients often do better when auditory and visual stimuli are combined. Schuell and Jenkins (1961a) reported that patients do better on single word comprehension tasks when written and auditory stimuli are used instead of auditory stimuli alone.

Goodglass et al. (1968) examined the naming performance of 27 patients in response to auditory (characteristic sound associated with the target item), tactile, olfactory, and picture stimuli. They found a uniformity in performance across all modalities for the great majority of patients, although reaction times were fastest to visual stimuli. By extension, the work of Mills (1977) and Smithpeter (1976) suggest that combining some of those stimuli may enhance performance. Mills found that pairing an environmental sound (e.g., whinny)

with a picture to be named (e.g., horse) facilitated naming performance over time, generalized to nondrilled words, and resulted in post-therapy improvement in naming without the auditory stimulus. Smithpeter reported that olfaction was effective in stimulating accurate language responses in some aphasic patients when it preceded or accompanied other stimuli.

Caramazza and Berndt (1978) cite the work of North (1971) who found that aphasic patients' word recall improved when information was available through several sense modalities. North argued that various senses may contribute additively to word recall. Gardner's (1973) previously discussed findings regarding operativity suggest that such additivity of multisensory stimulation need not be overt. That is, performance may be enhanced if visual stimuli, for example, are capable of "arousing" multisensory associations.

Combining the auditory and visual modalities is the most widely used form of multisensory stimulation, and a number of studies support the practice, although with some qualifications. Gardner and Brookshire (1972) found naming and single word reading performance of eight aphasic patients to be better during combined auditory and visual stimulation than during auditory or visual stimulation alone. By varying the order in which the stimulus conditions were presented, they also determined that combined stimulation facilitated performance during subsequent unisensory stimulus conditions. While analysis of single subject profiles indicated that combined stimulation may not be best for all patients, their results generally supported the conclusion that combined stimulation is better than unisensory. They also suggest that combined auditory-visual stimulation should generally precede auditory or visual stimulation alone, at least on treatment tasks requiring naming responses. Halpern (1965a,b), reporting similar results, supported the concept of multisensory stimulation, but noted that a multisensory approach sometimes can be distracting. Additional evidence related to multisensory stimulation may be derived from the study of electrophysiological activity in the brain during various stimulation activities. Moore (1996) investigated the hemispheric alpha asymmetries (through the use of EEG) of normal males and females and aphasic males during recall and recognition of high and low imagery words presented auditorily, visually, and in a multimodality (combined auditory and visual) condition. Results indicated that the aphasic subjects demonstrated higher mean scores on the recall and recognition tasks during the multimodality condition than during either the visual or auditory alone conditions. Further, for the aphasic subjects the multimodality stimulation appeared to activate the left hemisphere to a greater degree than either auditory or visual stimulation alone. Moore comments "the multimodality stimulation appears to have facilitated the left hemisphere's participation in language processing, which may have contributed to increased language performance" (p. 683).

Auditory stimulation often involves some potentially useful visual input as well; for example, the patient's visual contact with the examiner may provide a number of facilitory verbal or paralinguistic cues. Green and Boller (1974) found that the comprehension of severely impaired aphasic patients was not as accurate or appropriate when stimuli were presented by tape or with the examiner behind the patient as when stimuli were presented face-to-face. Boller et al. (1979) confirmed the superiority of face-to-face presentation over the use of taped stimuli, and Lambrecht and Marshall (1983) showed that the comprehension of severely impaired patients was better when they looked and listened than when stimuli were just heard. Whether the performance differences in these studies were due to situational, extralinguistic cues, or additional visual verbal input through lip-reading is not clear. Such an interpretation is supported by recent studies of the contribution of visual sources of contextual information to speech perception. Records (1994) reported that as auditory information became more ambiguous, aphasic individuals with poor language comprehension made greater use of accompanying referential gestures to facilitate their understanding of verbal messages. Similarly, the successful application of therapy focused on auditory discrimination of minimal pairs at the phonemic level, utilizing lip reading, has also been reported (Morris et al., 1996). Regardless, it seems that having the visual and auditory attention of the patient during the presentation of verbal material is important. Other combinations of sensory input have been noted to be facilitative as well. For example, Lott et al. (1994) successfully paired tactile-kinesthetic cues (i.e., tracing letters on the palm of the hand) with visual cues to improve reading skills of an aphasic individual with alexia.

To summarize, providing multimodality stimulation can improve response adequacy for many aphasic patients, and combining auditory and visual stimulation may be the best and most practical way of doing so. Combined auditory-visual stimulation may facilitate responses to subsequent unisensory stimuli and, therefore, may be employed first when responses to unisensory stimulation are deficient to a significant degree. Other modalities, such as the tactile, also may be helpful. It seems that the effectiveness of multimodality stimulation stems from the redundancy of information it provides and the additional associations that it may help to trigger. This appears desirable for many patients, although the clinician needs to be sure that such multiple inputs improve performance and that they do not somehow overload or exceed the capacity of the patient to use them effectively.

Stimulus Repetition

Repetitive sensory stimulation is a principle of treatment espoused by Schuell et al. (1964). They recommended, for example, that on word recognition or repetition tasks as many as 20 repetitions of a stimulus word might be appropriate/necessary before eliciting a response. Few studies, however, have directly examined the effects of repetitive stimulation on language comprehension or expression in aphasic patients.

Helmick and Wipplinger (1975) examined naming behavior in one aphasic patient under a nontreatment and two treatment conditions, each condition containing different target words. In a minimal stimulus condition, six "stimulations" (including verbal identification, contextual cue, picture identification/discrimination, tracing and copying) were provided before eliciting a naming response. In the maximum stimulus condition, the six stimulations were repeated four times for each word. Both conditions were more effective than the nontreatment condition, but there were no differences between the results obtained from minimum and maximum stimulation. The authors concluded that a relatively small amount of stimulation can be as effective as a great deal of stimulation.

LaPointe et al. (1978) evaluated the effects of two methods of repetition of Token Test commands on the auditory comprehension of 12 aphasic patients. In one condition, stimulus repetitions of commands preceded responses. In the other, repetition occurred only following incorrect responses. When items were repeated following failure (to a ceiling of four repetitions of the original stimulus), significant improvement occurred in response to the first and second repetitions; further but nonsignificant gains were noted for the third and fourth repetitions. In numeric terms, while accuracy was 24% without repetition, it rose to 58% after repetition to ceiling level. Degree of language impairment was negatively correlated with gains from repetition. In contrast, when items were presented twice or four times prior to a response, no significant group gains over the no-repetition condition were noted. However, there were some individual subject differences—one subject did "remarkably poorer" when commands were repeated prior to responses and another apparently benefited from the preresponse repetition.

Considering the lack of experimental support, the use of numerous repetitions prior to eliciting a response cannot be considered a verified, generally applicable principle of aphasia treatment. Some individuals may respond differently to preresponse repetitive stimulation, however, with some benefiting and others deteriorating. In contrast, repetition of stimuli subsequent to errors generally does appear to increase adequate responses, with maximum benefits derived from the first or second repetition.

Rate and Pause

It has been suggested that slowing speech rate may aid auditory comprehension (Schuell et al., 1964) and this is something experienced clinicians apparently are aware of subconsciously. Salvatore et al. (1978) reported that experienced clinicians give Token Test commands more slowly than do their inexperienced colleagues by inserting more pause time within commands. They also found that experienced clinicians tend to slow their presentation rate when repeating commands that previously had generated error responses. Such clinician behavior obviously is not desirable during standardized diagnostic testing and some baseline procedures, but it does offer indirect support for the facilitating effect of rate reduction on verbal comprehension.

Gardner et al. (1975) examined sentence comprehension in 46 aphasic patients with comprehension problems ranging from mild to severe. They reported improvement in comprehension—independent of form of aphasia—when sentences were spoken at a rate of one word per second. They recommended that, when proceeding from single word to sentence stimuli, words initially should be "slowly enunciated."

Weidner and Lasky (1976) found improved performance in a group of 20 aphasic patients on four measures of auditory comprehension when presentation rate was reduced from 150 words per minute (wpm) to 110 wpm. Differences between the two rate conditions were greatest for patients scoring above the 50th percentile on the PICA. Similarly, Poeck and Pietron (1981) induced an 11 to 12% improvement in Token Test scores of a group of 42 aphasic patients by electronically expanding speech rate by 25%. Pashek and Brookshire (1982) extended these findings by showing that reducing rate from 150 wpm to 120 wpm facilitated paragraph comprehension in a group of 20 patients; performance was facilitated in those with poor as well as those with good sentence level comprehension.

The facilitative effect of reduced rate also has been demonstrated for a patient with aphasia and severe auditory imperception (Albert & Bear, 1974). The authors found that their patient's comprehension improved dramatically when rate was slowed to "one-third or less of normal."

Liles and Brookshire (1975) examined the comprehension of 20 patients when 5-second pauses were inserted into various portions of Token Test commands. The insertion of pauses facilitated comprehension for many of their patients. Patterns of patient performance led them to hypothesize that the pauses aided the processing of strings of lexical items but not the processing of syntactic components. In contrast, Hageman and Lewis (1983) inserted 2-second pauses at major within-sentence breaks of the Revised Token Test and failed to find qualitative or quantitative performance differences when compared to a no-pause condition. They suggested that a 2-second pause may not be long enough to facilitate performance.

Salvatore (1976) reported facilitation of comprehension for an aphasic patient when 4-second pauses were inserted into Token Test commands. By gradually fading pause duration it was also possible to maintain improved comprehension

with 2- and sometimes only 1-second pauses. Although there was no generalization to nonpause stimulation, the results do suggest that pause time can be faded, to some degree, while maintaining high levels of comprehension.

Are the effects of rate reduction and pause insertion cumulative? Lasky et al. (1976) examined the effects of rate reduction (120 vs. 150 wpm) and the insertion of 1-second interphrase pauses on the sentence comprehension of 15 aphasic persons. Comprehension improved when rate was slowed or when pauses were inserted, and combining reduced rate and interphrase pauses resulted in the best performance.

In an effort to examine how slowing rate facilitates comprehension, Blumstein et al. (1985) compared aphasic patients' comprehension of sentences spoken at normal rates to (1) a vowel condition, in which vowel duration in each word was increased (140 wpm), (2) a word condition, in which silences were added between words (110 wpm), (3) a syntactic condition, in which silences were added at constituent phrase boundaries (90 wpm), and (4) a natural condition, in which sentences were read at a naturally slowed rate (110 wpm). In general, reducing rate had a relatively small facilitory effect and was significant only for the syntactic condition and only for patients with Wernicke's aphasia. The authors concluded that it may not be slowed rate per se that facilitated comprehension but rather the effect of a syntactically well-placed pause on the processing of preceding syntactic and semantic elements. Although this may be the case, the fact that the rate of the syntactic condition (90 wpm) was slower than any other slowed condition confounds the interpretation and leaves open the possibility that slowing rate to a comparable degree in other ways might also facilitate comprehension.

The positive effects of slowed rate may not be as robust for narrative discourse. Nicholas and Brookshire (1986a) examined narrative comprehension across two test sessions in aphasic patients with relatively good and relatively poor comprehension; narratives were spoken at fast (190–210 wpm) versus slow (110–130 wpm) rates. Only the group with relatively poor comprehension benefited from rate reduction and this held only for the first of the two test sessions. In addition, the facilitory effect of slow rate was not present for all patients in the poor comprehension group. The authors concluded that the effect of slow rate was undependable and transitory, and they noted that variables with strong effects on comprehension at the sentence level may have only weak effects at the level of discourse.

To summarize, it appears that slowing rate and lengthening pauses at phrase boundaries can have a facilitory effect on sentence comprehension. This effect is neither always present nor generally dramatic, and there are no consistent indications across studies that the ability to benefit from rate and pause modifications is tied to either type or severity of aphasia. The positive effects of slowing rate may be less consistent and pervasive at the level of discourse than at the sentence level. From a practical standpoint, however, it is reasonable to accept Nicholas and Brookshire's (1986a) advice that "... it seems reasonable to counsel those who speak with brain-damaged listeners to speak slowly, because slow speech rate does not affect most brain-damaged listeners negatively, and for some it may be beneficial, at least on some occasions" (p. 469).

Length and Redundancy

As previously stated, Schuell felt that reduced verbal retention span is a near universal feature of aphasia. Although pervasive, she reported that retention deficits are highly reversible with the use of carefully controlled intensive auditory stimulation characterized by gradual increases in stimulus length (Schuell, 1953a; Schuell et al., 1955).

The importance of stimulus length receives additional support from a number of sources, including patients themselves. Rolnick and Hoops (1969), in interviews with several mild aphasic patients, found numerous complaints about the processing and retention demands imposed by lengthy messages. Patients felt that reduced message length facilitated comprehension and retention.

In addition, numerous studies have demonstrated that, with other factors held constant, sentence comprehension tends to decrease as length increases (e.g., Curtiss et al., 1986; Shewan & Canter, 1971; Weidner & Lasky, 1976).

Although Goodglass et al. (1970) found that 52 patients with different classical forms of aphasia had varying degrees of success on a verbally presented retention span test, all were deficient to some degree. Albert (1976) examined the ability of 28 aphasic patients on a short-term memory task in which they pointed to objects named serially by the examiner. They were inferior to control subjects and nonaphasic brain-injured patients on total item retention and in retention of the accurate sequence of presentation. Response patterns indicated that sequencing problems increased as information load increased. Information load and sequencing deficits were both present regardless of clinical type of aphasia. The findings of Martin and Feher (1990) suggest that degree of short-term memory limitation in aphasia affects semantic processing (i.e., sentences with a large number of content words) but is not strongly related to processing of syntactic complexity. Finally, Gardner et al. (1975) found poorer comprehension when length increased from single words to nonredundant sentences containing the same single words.

Length appears to be an important factor in the visual as well as the auditory modality. Siegel's (1959) 31 aphasic patients had more difficulty reading words of two or more syllables (six or more letters) than they did single-syllable words of less than five letters. Halpern (1965a,b) compared verbal responses of 33 patients on tasks involving single word repetition, reading single words, and reading single words with simultaneous auditory and visual stimulation. Stimuli in each task were either long (two or more syllables or six letters) or short (one syllable or less than four letters), and also varied as a function of abstraction level and part of speech. Results showed that long words resulted in more verbal errors, including preservation, than did short words, regardless of modality of presentation. Differences between errors on long and short words were greatest for the visual modality. On the basis of his findings, Halpern recommended that, for such tasks, auditory or auditory/visual stimulation usually should precede visual stimulation alone.

Going beyond the word level, Webb and Love (1983) examined the reading abilities of 35 aphasic patients and found more errors on sentence recognition than on letter or word recognition; more errors on oral reading of sentences and paragraphs than on letters or words; and more errors on paragraph comprehension than on sentence comprehension.

Friederici et al. (1981) have shown that word length also influences writing. In their group of 12 aphasic patients, written accuracy was reduced by more than 50% as word length increased from one to three syllables. Increased word length (i.e., number of phonemes in the spoken word) has also been shown to negatively influence naming performance in some individuals with aphasia (Nickels & Howard, 1995).

Wepman and Jones (1961) found that verbal responses to words are easier than verbal responses to sentences whether stimuli are presented auditorily or visually. At the word level, verbal responses to written stimuli were better for one-syllable than two-syllable words. On the other hand, verbal responses to auditorily presented words did not differ between one- and two-syllable words. In contrast to Halpern's (1965a,b) findings, they indicated that the length factor for sentence material is most pronounced for the auditory, not the visual, modality. It is possible that the different results are due to the fact that Halpern dealt with variations of length within single words while Wepman and Jones were referring to differences between words and sentences. If so, this highlights the fact that differences in the processing and/or retention of words between modalities are not identical to differences in the processing and/or retention of sentences (and discourse) between modalities.

It is important to note that the detrimental effects of increasing message length may vary as a function of message redundancy. For example, the findings of Gardner et al. (1975) support the notion that aphasic patients comprehend redundant sentences better than nonredundant sentences of equal length. Clark and Flowers (1987) demonstrated that increasing sentence redundancy facilitated comprehension even when redundant sentences were longer and syntactically more complex than nonredundant ones (e.g., sentences like "Which one is the book you read?" were easier than "Which one is the book?"). Also, the remarkable sensitivity of the Token Test to subtle comprehension deficits is at least partially due to the nonredundant properties of its verbal stimuli. Clearly, the potent effect of length strongly interacts with redundancy; the two factors can seldom, if ever, be considered separately. Further discussion of this interaction can be found in the section on grammar and syntax.

To summarize, there can be little doubt that controlling length at the word and sentence level is a potent stimulus factor for most or all aphasic patients, and most clinicians discuss this factor when counseling families about their verbal input to the aphasic person. Length is an influential factor regardless of whether stimuli are auditory, visual, or auditory/visual. In the visual modality, reducing length at both the word and sentence level can be expected to facilitate comprehension. For auditory input, length may be relatively unimportant at the word level, but it becomes highly important when proceeding from the word to phrase to sentence level. When controlling length, it seems that nonredundant components are the most crucial elements to control, since increases in message redundancy may limit or even overcome the generally negative effects of increases in message length. This may be particularly true at the paragraph and narrative discourse levels (to be discussed in the section on context).

Cues, Prompts, and Prestimulation

It is well recognized that, under the right circumstances, the skillful clinician can employ a variety of techniques—often referred to as cues, prompts, or prestimulation—which will facilitate patients' word retrieval or comprehension. Such techniques are often used following an inadequate response to a less powerful stimulus. However, when less powerful stimuli consistently are incapable of generating a high proportion of adequate responses, the cue (prompt or prestimulus) may become a distinct treatment condition to which acceptable responses must be generated prior to proceeding to the less powerful stimuli. In this section, a number of potentially useful cues that have not been identified already under other headings will be discussed.

McDearmon and Potter (1975) offered a number of suggestions regarding representational prompts, which they defined as symbolic or realistic cues which directly suggest the concept referred to in a response; prompts are strongly related to the concepts of stimulus redundancy and multimodality stimulation. They suggest that more than one representation of the response be presented and that one representation—the prompt—gradually be faded. For example, on naming tasks, pictures and their written names may be presented with resultant adequate responses; the written prompts may then be faded gradually by blocking out increasing portions of the word until it is entirely eliminated. Some other suggested prompts, not already implied under other headings, include tracing letters to facilitate letter

recognition, writing words to aid word retrieval, pantomime or Amerind sign to facilitate word retrieval, and using pictures in conjunction with corresponding written words to facilitate reading.

Barton et al. (1969) examined word retrieval of 36 patients under three conditions: picture naming, sentence completion (e.g., "you clean teeth with a _____") and object description. In order, the most powerful cues were sentence completion, picture naming, and object description. It is important to note, however, that 44% of the subjects in their study did not follow the group's ordering of responses to the three naming conditions. This highlights the importance of examining the individual patient's responsiveness to stimulus cues; a powerful cue for one patient may not be powerful for another. Along these lines, Marshall and Tompkins (1982) and Golper and Rau (1983) point out that careful analysis of individual patient strategies may provide clues about the best cues for the clinician to provide during therapy; such information may also be used to increase the patient's own use of successful cues.

Freed et al. (1995) examined two cuing techniques with 30 moderately aphasic individuals in associative learning tasks. Real English words were paired with black-and-white abstract symbols and subjects were required to label each symbol. During the task subjects were given either their own previously elicited associations for the word-symbol pairs (personalized cues) or associations developed by the examiner (provided cues). Results indicated that both cuing techniques were equal in terms of yielding correct responses. The authors observed that in the "provided cue" condition subjects were given complete rationales for why the cues were used; thus, the provided cues may have inadvertently become similar to personalized cues. Freed et al. concluded that both the provided and personalized cues contained components that might be beneficial to include in a treatment protocol for word retrieval deficits.

Linebaugh and Lehner (1977) have described a cuing program for word retrieval that is based on two principles: (1) that recovery is best served by eliciting the desired response with a minimal cue, and (2) that when a cue is successful, continued elicitation of the appropriate response with less powerful cues is reinforcing and conducive to stimulating the processes underlying word retrieval. When a patient is unable to name a pictured object, the following cues, in order, are given until an adequate response is elicited: directions to state the object's function, clinician states the function, clinician states and demonstrates function, sentence completion, sentence completion plus the silently articulated first phoneme of the response, sentence completion plus the vocalized first sound, sentence completion plus the first two phonemes vocalized, and, finally, word repetition. When an adequate response is elicited, the order of cues is reversed until the patient names the picture without a cue. Linebaugh and Lehner presented data for several patients which demonstrate improved word retrieval and generalization to nontreatment words. Importantly, they indicate that cuing hierarchies must be individually determined.

A facilitative effect of semantic cues also seems to exist for on-line tasks (tasks in which the cues are not necessarily obvious to the patient). Chenery et al. (1990) studied patients' ability to recognize whether the second word in a pair of verbally presented words was real or nonsense when the first word was functionally related to the target (e.g., eat-knife), superordinally associated (e.g., cutlery-knife), unrelated (door-knife), or nonsense (e.g., lamiel-knife). Subjects were told to ignore the first word. All aphasic subjects, including a subgroup with severe comprehension and naming deficits, more accurately identified words as real in response to the functional and superordinate semantic primes than in the other priming conditions. This led to a conclusion that information is preserved in semantic memory in aphasia. (This on-line facilitation of semantic processing may partially explain why redundancy can facilitate sentence comprehension.) In a related study, Leonard and Baum (1997) noted faster responses to words preceded by primes that were both phonologically and orthographically related to the target word (e.g., words which shared both spelling and sound syllable rhyme, "blood-flood") than those that were unrelated (e.g., "dish-room"). Phonologically related primes (i.e., word pairs shared syllable rhymes but were orthographically unrelated, e.g., "seed-bead") alone did not facilitate reaction times, and responses were also slower relative to the primes that were orthographically but not phonologically related (i.e., word pairs shared rhyme spelling but were pronounced differently, e.g., "tough-cough").

Podraza and Darley (1977) investigated the effects of three types of prestimulation on picture naming in five aphasic patients. The prestimulus conditions (cues presented prior to picture presentation) included the first phoneme of the target word; an open-ended sentence; three words, one of which was the target word; and three semantically related words. Naming was generally facilitated by the phoneme, open-ended sentences, and three-words-containing-the-target-word cues, while performance decrements occurred for the three semantically related words cues. The facilitative failure of the semantically related word cues is in disagreement with Weigl's (1968) and Blumstein et al.'s (1982) findings that such cues may serve a "deblocking function" and facilitate retrieval. Podraza and Darley suggest that their own patients may already have been operating in the appropriate "semantic field" (Goodglass & Baker, 1976) and that additional stimuli in that field may have served to confuse the selection of an appropriate response. Similarly, patients with Wernicke's aphasia, who frequently make phonemic errors, benefit less from phonemic cues than do patients with other types of aphasia (Kohn & Goodglass, 1985).

Breen and Warrington (1994) have also compared a variety of cues in an individual with severe anomia. Phonologic and semantic cues were noted to be far less facilitative, in a naming task, than were sentence frames (i.e., sentence completion). Further, neither picture frames, associated verbs, or syntactically correct but semantically meaningless sentence frames were effective cues. The authors suggest that there may be two modes of name retrieval, one that utilizes a nominative system and a second that employs an on-line language processor involved in propositional speech production. It is the latter system that may account for the preservation of fluent speech in individuals with severe anomia. Similarly, sentence completion cues containing a semantically related word were noted to be more effective than semantically empty sentence frames (e.g., "This is a _____") or semantic information alone (i.e., associated verbs) in facilitating naming performance in eight aphasic subjects (McCall et al., 1997). These findings were felt to support the notion that naming is enhanced most by a combination of syntactic and semantic variables.

Stimley and Noll (1991) examined naming accuracy in a group of aphasic patients when pictures were accompanied by a semantic cue (e.g., this is something you wear on your foot, for "sock") or a phonemic cue (e.g., this is something that starts with /S/, for "sock"). Compared with a no-cue condition, the semantic and phonemic cues both facilitated naming, although the average effect was only in the order of 9 to 10%; the authors felt the small effect may have been because cues were presented for all items, not just following failure to name without a cue. They also observed (as have others) that semantic errors were more frequent in the semantic cue condition and that phonemic errors were more frequent in the phonemic cue condition (Li & Canter [1991] have made similar observations). Thus, while semantic and phonemic cues are generally facilitative, they also tend to "move" errors toward the cuing category.

Other recent investigations have examined the effects of only semantic cues on naming performance. Semantic feature analysis (SFA) is an elaborate cuing technique in which the client is encouraged to produce words semantically related to the target. For example, for the target word "pan" the cues might involve questions related to its use (cooking), its properties (metal, copper, wooden handle), where it might be used (kitchen), what group it belongs to (cookware), and what might be associated with it (stove, spoons, ladles, pots). Semantic feature analysis is thought to improve retrieval of conceptual information by accessing semantic networks (Massaro & Tompkins, 1992). By activating the semantic network surrounding the target, the target itself should be activated above its "threshold" level, thus increasing the likelihood that its name can be retrieved. Results have consistently documented improved confrontational naming scores with the SFA technique for treated pictures as well as generalization to untreated pictures (Boyle & Coelho, 1995; Coelho et al., 2000; Lowell et al., 1995). However, generalization to connected speech has either been quite modest

(Coelho et al., 2000) or not observed at all (Boyle & Coelho, 1995).

Whether or not a semantic cue should be accompanied by the referent word has also been investigated (LeDorze et al., 1994). Using a comprehension task format, two types of semantic cues were compared. In the first, the aphasic individuals were to point to a picture (in a field of three pictures) of the referent word presented, next to match the written word to the corresponding picture, and then to answer a question about the referent word (e.g., for the word "organ," "Does an organ have just one keyboard?"). The other cuing procedure also involved three steps; in the first the aphasic individuals were to point to a picture of the referent word identified by a definition, next to match a written definition to the corresponding picture, and finally, answer a yes-no question related to the referent word (e.g., for the word "lobster," "Does this mollusk have pincers?"). Results indicated that naming improved significantly when the semantic cues were accompanied by the referent word. The authors speculate that naming was facilitated because both word form and word semantics were activated.

Some recent efforts have attempted to tailor the type of cue to the level at which naming tends to break down. Thompson et al. (1991) examined the effects of a phonemic cuing treatment program on two patients with Broca's aphasia whose naming deficits appeared related to phonological breakdowns (e.g., they had naming difficulties in spite of being able to match spoken words to pictures and perform conceptual matching tasks; in other words, they appeared to have access to word meaning but not the phonological form of words). The program consisted primarily of providing a rhyming cue (e.g., "it sounds like mat" for the target "bat") or, if that failed, the first phoneme, whenever the patient failed to name without a cue. Both subjects improved in oral naming and there was some generalization to untrained items and to oral reading tasks. Li and Williams (1989) examined the effect of semantic and phonemic cues on noun and verb naming after failure to name on picture confrontation. Patients with Broca's and conduction aphasia responded better to phonemic than semantic cues and the opposite pattern occurred for patients with anomic aphasia. In general, phonemic cues were more effective than semantic cues for nouns, and the two cue types did not differ for verbs. This suggests that cue type effectiveness may vary both as a function of the source of naming failure (semantic versus phonologic, presumably related to aphasia type) and word category (nouns versus verbs).

Are cues presented in combination more effective than single cues? Weidner and Jinks' (1983) findings say yes. They examined the naming performance of 24 patients who were presented with single cues (e.g., sentence completion, written words, first phoneme) or cues in combination. Combined cues were more facilitative than were single cues or single cues presented in succession. They suggest that if one cue fails, a combination of cues may help.

Finally, cuing also may facilitate sentence production. Roberts and Wertz (1986) used a contrastive task paradigm to facilitate sentence production in two chronic aphasic patients. After demonstrating comprehension of sentence meaning, patients imitated the clinician's production of a sentence (e.g., "the bed is made") and then spontaneously produced a minimally contrasting sentence in response to a picture stimulus (e.g., "the bed is not made"). Imitation was then faded over additional steps to a point where the patient had to produce on their own both contrasting sentences in response to picture stimuli. Both patients' sentence production improved and there was evidence of some carryover to spontaneous sentence production.

It is reasonable to conclude that there are a large number of cues, prompts, and preparatory stimuli which may facilitate language processing in aphasia. Care must be taken to demonstrate the utility of cues in each case because even the most widely used facilitators may not be effective for every patient. Careful analysis of the level at which language tends to break down (e.g., semantic versus phonologic) and the types of successful cues that patients adopt spontaneously can help identify the type of cuing likely to be most successful.

Frequency and Meaningfulness

It has been established repeatedly that the reduction of available vocabulary in aphasia is related to the frequency of occurrence of words in the language. Schuell (1969, 1974d) also predicted a reduction of available linguistic rules and a hierarchy for their recovery, and speculated that the hierarchy is related to the frequency of occurrence of those structures in general or individual language usage.

Schuell et al. (1961) tested the auditory comprehension of 48 aphasic patients in response to four word lists varying in frequency of occurrence. Decrements in performance as a function of decreasing word frequency were found, supporting the conclusion that word frequency is an important factor in comprehension. They also reported that single word comprehension improves in an orderly and predictable manner that is strongly related to word frequency. Relatedly, Gerratt and Jones (1987), in a reaction time task, have shown that aphasic, like nonaphasic individuals, recognize words as real (versus nonsense) more rapidly when they have multiple meanings and high frequency of occurrence than when they have few meanings and low frequency of occurrence.

Word frequency remains a factor at the sentence level. Shewan and Canter (1971) found that increasing vocabulary difficulty (reducing word frequency) reduced the accuracy and promptness of sentence comprehension in aphasic patients. In addition, frequency of occurrence also applies to phrases and sentences as they occur as familiar units. For example, Van Lancker and Kempler (1987) have shown that aphasic patients comprehend familiar phrases (idiomatic expressions such as "while the cat's away the mice will play") more readily than novel sentences matched for word frequency, length, and structure.

Word frequency effects are also apparent in verbal output, reading, and writing. For example, Schuell et al. (1964), Gardner (1973), and Williams and Canter (1982) have reported negative correlations between errors on naming tests and frequency of occurrence; Siegel (1959) found that less frequently occurring words were more difficult to read than frequently occurring words; Bricker et al. (1964) reported that word frequency (and length) accounted for almost all aphasic spelling errors; and Santo Pietro and Rigrodsky (1982) found that verbal perseveration on naming and reading tasks increased as word frequency decreases.

In contrast to the notion that word frequency is an important factor in verbal expression, Nickels and Howard (1995) found small effects of word frequency on naming performance. In a series of experiments with two groups of aphasic individuals, the authors investigated eight variables on naming: word age-of-acquisition, operativity (i.e., figurative versus operative), frequency, familiarity (i.e., based on a rating of how often one might see, hear, or use referent word), imageability (i.e., ease of creating visual or auditory image of referent), concreteness (i.e., how accessible to sensory experience subjects rated referent word), length (i.e., number of phonemes in spoken word), and visual complexity (i.e., complex versus simple based on number of elements in stimulus picture). The first group consisted of six fluent and six nonfluent individuals, and the second group consisted of three nonfluent, two nonfluent with apraxia of speech, two with primarily apraxia of speech, and eight with fluent aphasia. Results indicated a far less marked effect of frequency on naming when the effects of the other variables had been accounted for (i.e., by means of simultaneous multiple regression or discriminate analysis procedures). Further, because of intercorrelations between variables and the wide range of variables which have been found to affect naming performance in aphasic individuals findings must be interpreted cautiously. The authors concluded that previously the effects of frequency on naming have been overstated due to the confounding effect of other variables such as length and imageability. Finally, the two groups of aphasic individuals studied showed quite different patterns of predictor variables for naming performance and the variables which affected individuals' performances was often different from those of the group, calling into question the applicability of conclusions drawn from group studies (Nickels & Howard, 1995).

Although word frequency is certainly positively correlated among speakers of the language, we need to bear in mind that word frequency for individuals is determined by their unique experiences, needs, occupation, culture, and numerous other factors (the word "aphasia" is certainly more available to the speech-language pathologist than it is to the political scientist!). Although word lists such as Thorndike and Lorge's (1944) are useful in selecting stimulus material, it is also important that we identify verbal stimuli that are meaningful, relevant, and personally significant to the individual (Schuell, 1969; Schuell et al., 1955; Wepman, 1953).

The importance of this was demonstrated by Wallace and Canter (1985), who examined severely impaired aphasic patients' responses to personally relevant versus nonpersonal stimuli on verbal and reading comprehension tasks (e.g., "Is your birthday in _____" versus "Is Christmas in February?"), repetition tasks (e.g., patient repeats his or her name versus another name), and naming tasks (e.g., television versus giraffe). Performance was better in response to personally relevant materials on all tasks, although the authors pointed out that personally relevant stimuli had a generally higher frequency of occurrence than nonpersonal material. Relatedly, Correia et al. (1989) asked if gender bias in pictures used to elicit narrative responses from male aphasic patients affects what they say about them. After having nonaphasic subjects identify picture stimuli as male or female biased (e.g., men working out in a gym versus women in a beauty salon), they used the stimuli to obtain narratives from aphasic and non-brain-damaged subjects. Subjects produced more words in response to male-biased stimuli, but there were no differences in measures of efficiency or amount of information conveyed. The authors concluded that gender bias in picture stimuli is not of great concern (at least for males) unless the number of words in responses is important. Thus, some dimensions of personal relevance may or may not affect all dimensions of performance to the same or to an important degree.

The concept of meaningfulness is also tied to emotion and expectations. Reuterskiöld (1991) has demonstrated that patients with significant verbal comprehension deficits perform more adequately on single word comprehension tasks when stimuli consist of objects and actions with emotional connotations (e.g., casket, kissing) than when they have no obvious emotional connotations (e.g., paper, typing). Graham et al. (1987) examined aphasic patients' comprehension in response to contextually relevant commands (e.g., ring the bell), contextually neutral commands (e.g., touch the bell), and contextually inappropriate commands (e.g., roll the bell). Contextually related tasks were easier than neutral or inappropriate ones, leading the authors to state that "if we pair objects with actions that are most expected both in terms of meaning and structure, we facilitate comprehension" (p. 183). Finally, Deloche and Seron (1981) and Kudo (1984) have established that comprehension is better when sentence meaning does not violate our knowledge of the world (e.g., "the policeman arrests the thief") than when meaning is implausible or unlikely (e.g., "the thief arrests the policeman").

Abstractness

It has been suggested that aphasic individuals have more difficulty with abstract than with concrete words (Goldstein, 1948) and that they categorize words in a relatively concrete emotional manner when compared with nonaphasic individuals (Zurif et al., 1974).

Two problems present themselves when the concept of abstractness arises. First, abstractness is strongly tied to—and difficult to separate from—frequency of occurrence (concrete words occur more frequently than abstract words). Spreen (1968), however, has pointed out that words scaled as abstract are not perceived or recalled as readily as words scaled as concrete even when frequency of occurrence is controlled. Halpern (1965a), controlling for frequency of occurrence, found that aphasic patients made more verbal errors in response to written words of high or medium abstractness than in response to words of low abstractness. Abstractness did not play a role in repetition of verbally presented stimuli, however.

The second problem is more relevant to stimulus selection and is related to the fact that abstractness is a difficult concept to define. Words, however, are scalable on an abstractness dimension (Darley et al., 1959), and Spreen (1968) has suggested that degree of abstractness can be related tangibly to sense experience ("book" is more concrete than "hope" because it presumably generates more multimodality associations).

The performance of aphasic patients suggests that we should be aware of the abstractness factor when selecting and ordering stimulus material. Problems related to isolating and defining abstractness, however, present practical clinical problems. Fortunately, we probably account for most of the effects of abstractness when we account for the more easily defined concepts of word frequency and intersensory redundancy or operativity.

Part of Speech and Semantic Word Category

When word retrieval and comprehension abilities are examined or treated at the single word level, there is a tendency for clinicians to focus on nouns, particularly object-nouns. However, evidence makes it clear that all parts of speech and word categories are typically affected in aphasia. This speaks against an object-noun orientation to treatment.

Because different parts of speech (e.g., nouns versus verbs) serve different linguistic functions, it seems possible that, for some patients or under some circumstances, they may present differing levels of difficulty. Consistent with this notion, recent research has demonstrated selective impairments in nouns versus verbs in some aphasic individuals. For example, verb production has been noted to be more difficult than nouns for agrammatic aphasic individuals, while nouns appear to be more problematic than verbs for some individuals with anomic aphasia (Marshall et al., 1988; Miceli et al., 1988;

Miceli et al., 1984; Orpwood & Warrington, 1995; Saffran et al., 1989; Thompson et al., 1994; Williams & Canter, 1987; Zingeser & Berndt, 1990). In addition, when there is a discrepancy between nouns and verbs on synonym generating and sentence generation tasks, the difference favors nouns over verbs (Kohn et al., 1989). Finally, that the processing of nouns versus verbs can differ is also supported by the finding of Li and Canter (1991) that aphasic patients responded better to phonemic than semantic cues for noun naming but that there was no difference between the cue types for verb naming; the authors felt that the greater concreteness, static nature, and imagability of nouns than verbs might explain some of the differences between them.

The observation that the naming may be differentially impaired across semantic categories has led investigators to question whether verb production might also be differentially affected; that is, that certain types of verbs may be more difficult than others for some individuals. According to Thompson et al. (1997) an important distinction among verbs pertains to their syntactic properties, such as the number and type of arguments or participant roles required by certain verbs. Like other classes of words, verbs are acquired and stored in memory on the basis of their phonological form and lexical category. However, verbs are also represented in the lexicon by virtue of the sentence structures in which they occur. For example, the verb "wash" must always be followed by a noun phrase and by a prepositional phrase. These phrase structure rules are referred to as strict subcategorization and are related to but separate from argument structure. Argument structure pertains to meaning relations between the verb and constituents within a sentence, or to the number of participant or thematic roles described by a verb. For example, the verb "wash" has two participant roles: an Agent (someone doing the washing) and a Theme (the thing being washed). The verb "put" has three roles: an Agent (someone doing the putting), a Theme (thing that is put), and a Location (place where the thing is put). For certain verbs all participant roles must be specified in sentence production for the sentence to be grammatical. Returning to the example of the verb "put," it is obligatory that all three of its arguments be represented when it is used, whereas for other verbs some arguments are optional and do not need to be specified in the syntax. This is the case for the verb "eat," which can be produced with an Agent only, as in "Tom ate," or with both its arguments, as in "Tom ate the corn." The critical issue is that the verb's lexical representation includes information about its argument structure and that the grammaticality of sentences and syntax is determined by these argument structures and their representation in the sentence (Thompson et al., 1997).

To investigate the type of verb deficits in aphasic individuals, Thompson et al. (1997) examined verb and verb argument structure production in 10 agrammatic aphasic and 10 nonbrain-damaged individuals. Production of six types of verbs: obligatory one-place (verbs with only one external argument—e.g., "The boy smiles"), obligatory two-place (verbs requiring both arguments—e.g., "The boy catches the ball"), obligatory three-place (verbs that require three arguments—e.g., The girl gives the bone to the dog"), optional two-place (verbs that require one external argument and a second optional argument—e.g., "The woman eats" and "The woman eats spaghetti"), optional three-place (verbs that require an Agent and Theme, but a third argument is optional—e.g., "The woman throws the stick" and "The woman throws the stick to the dog"), and complement verbs (verbs that require external and internal arguments—e.g., "the girl knows the answer" and "The girl knows the cat is in the tree") in confrontation and elicited labeling conditions. Results indicated the aphasic individuals produced obligatory one-place verbs correctly significantly more often than the three-place verbs. In addition, a consistent hierarchy of verb difficulty was found in both the confrontation and elicited conditions. Data indicated that argument structure properties of verbs are important dimensions of lexical organization which influence verb retrieval.

Differences may also exist for other word categories and tasks. Halpern (1965a) found that aphasic patients made more errors when repeating or reading adjectives and verbs as opposed to nouns. Siegel (1959) and Marshall and Newcombe (1966) reported similar findings for reading tasks. In contrast, Noll and Hoops (1967) did not find selective spelling difficulty among nouns, verbs, adjectives, and adverbs for a group of 25 patients, but did find that pronouns, prepositions, and conjunctions were more difficult than other parts of speech. Finally, Goodglass et al. (1970) found different comprehension patterns among Broca's, Wernicke's, and anomic patients across measures of receptive vocabulary (nouns and verbs) and measures of comprehension of directional and grammatical prepositions.

Stimulus selection should consider possible differences among substantive word categories—such as nouns, verbs, and adjectives—with nouns likely to be easiest when word frequency is controlled. In general, the literature suggests that grammatical words—such as prepositions, conjunctions, and articles—are more difficult to comprehend for aphasic patients than are substantive words (Lesser, 1978). The above findings suggest that both semantic categories and grammatical class are critical aspects of lexical organization. Such differences should be considered in stimulus selection.

The possibility that specific semantic word categories may be selectively impaired in aphasia is a matter of debate (see Lesser [1978], pp. 97–107), but some studies suggest that semantic word categories should be considered for some patients. For example, Goodglass et al. (1966) assessed the naming and comprehension of objects, actions, letters, numbers, and colors in aphasic patients. Objects and actions were the easiest to comprehend, and

letters the most difficult—but objects were the most difficult to name and letters the easiest. This not only suggests differences among word categories but also implies that the difficulty of a particular category may vary between input and output tasks.

Although many investigators and clinicians argue convincingly against common or marked differences among semantic word categories, it does appear that stimuli restricted to a single semantic category (e.g., objects) occasionally may yield misleading diagnostic and treatment results. Thus, consideration of semantic category may lead to the identification of treatment stimuli with varying degrees of difficulty.

Grammar and Syntax

As noted earlier, Schuell hypothesized that there is a hierarchically based reduction of available linguistic rules in aphasia. Although her idea that such a hierarchy is based on the frequency of occurrence of grammatical structures in general language usage is untested and perhaps overly simplistic in light of current linguistic theory, there is ample evidence that grammatical complexity is an important factor in language activities. In other words, as is true for intact language users, there is a grammatical hierarchy of difficulty for aphasic patients; some grammatical structures are more difficult to comprehend and produce than others. Grammar and syntax, therefore, are important variables to consider when devising language stimuli. Following is a sampling of the numerous studies that have examined the relationship between grammatical variations and performance in aphasia. For more information on these factors, see Chapter 24 in this volume.

The importance of grammar is illustrated by the fact that, even when lexical comprehension is quite good, sentence interpretation may be impaired because of grammatical processing deficits. Caramazza and Zurif (1976), for example, have shown that some patients have problems when sentence comprehension is dependent upon syntax rather than on the logical relations expressed by individual semantic elements. To illustrate, the meaning of the semantically constrained sentence, "The apple that the boy is eating is red," can be derived from an understanding of the meaning of its critical elements and the limited logical relationships that exist among them. That is, our knowledge of the world tells us it must be the boy who is eating and not the apple, and it must be the apple that is red. On the other hand, consider the requirements for accurate comprehension of the reversible sentence, "The girl that the boy is hitting is tall." Here, either the boy or the girl logically can do the hitting and either can be tall. Correct interpretation requires the appropriate pairing of boy with hitting and girl with tall, an interpretation arrived at only through adequate syntactic processing. Several studies have found that some patients have considerably more difficulty comprehending reversible sentences than they do semantically constrained ones, implying the presence of significant deficits in grammatical processing (Caramazza & Zurif, 1976; Kolk & Friederici, 1985; Sherman & Schweikert, 1989; Wulfeck, 1988).

There is ample additional evidence that sentences requiring structural-syntactic analysis are generally difficult for aphasic patients (usually regardless of aphasia type), and that sentence comprehension probably is maximized when interpretation can be based on world knowledge and the understanding of critical individual elements (e.g., see Ansell & Flowers, 1982a,b; Blumstein et al., 1983; Caplan & Evans, 1990; Curtiss et al., 1986; Friederici, 1983; Gallaher, 1981; Gallaher & Canter, 1982; Mack, 1982; Parisi & Pizzaniiglio, 1970; Peach et al., 1988). Constructing sentence stimuli with this in mind is of practical import for another reason; Gallaher and Canter (1982) suggest that the syntactic impact on comprehension in *real life* may be minimal because much of what is said in everyday communication can be interpreted on the basis of real-world knowledge and comprehension of lexical items, with grammar and syntax providing largely redundant information.

Demands for processing of grammar and syntax should not and cannot be avoided entirely. There are a number of studies that provide very useful information about the relative processing ease or difficulty of a variety of grammatical and syntactic devices for aphasic patients. The following represent a sampling of these findings:

1. Present tense sentences are easier than past or future tense sentences (Naeser et al., 1987; Parisi & Pizzamiglio, 1970; Pierce, 1981). When tense changes, the use of an additional tense marker tends to facilitate tense comprehension (e.g., "the man has caught the ball" should be easier than "the man caught the ball"; "the man has already combed his hair" should be easier than "the man has combed his hair"). Words like "yesterday" and "tomorrow" also help to mark tense (Ansell & Flowers, 1982b; Pierce, 1981, 1982, 1983).

   The distinction discussed in the preceding paragraph is one example of what seems to be a fairly consistent hierarchy of syntactic difficulty that can affect comprehension. For example, gender, negative/affirmative, and singular/plural distinctions tend to be easier than past/present, subject/object, and past/future/present distinctions. Within distinctions, the marked features tend to be more difficult; for example, negative is more difficult than affirmative, plural more difficult than singular, and future and past more difficult than present tense (Lesser, 1974; Naeser et al., 1987; Parisi & Pizzamiglio, 1970).

2. Other morphologic distinctions can also affect comprehension. For example, Goodglass and Hunt (1958) examined the ability of aphasic patients to comprehend and express noun plurals and possessives which are represented by identical phonological forms (e.g., horses-horse's). Expressively, patients made many more errors on possessive endings than on plurals. Receptively, the same pattern was noted with the additional observation that third person singular verbs also generated more errors than plurals. Goodglass and Berko (1960) have reported similar error patterns. Goodglass (1968) indicated that such patterns of deficit are independent of form of aphasia (nonfluent versus fluent) and, therefore, are not just specific to patients who are labeled "agrammatic." At the same time, it is important to keep in mind that syntactic deficits in aphasia are not an all-or-none phenomenon. In addition, the source of agrammatic production errors appears to be independent of comprehension errors (Goodglass et al., 1993). The deficits typically encountered are relative, not absolute, and aphasic patients (even "agrammatic" ones) are often able to process a good deal of syntactic information (Baum, 1989).

3. Aphasic patients tend to use an active subject-verb-object (SVO) strategy for processing sentences and find active sentences easier to comprehend than other forms. In general, this means that sentences in which the order of mention reflects the agent-action-object relationship ("the mother kissed the baby") are easier than when word order does not reflect that relationship ("the policeman was punched by the robber") (Ansell & Flowers, 1982b; Brookshire & Nicholas, 1980, 1981; Friederici & Graetz, 1987; Grossman & Haberman, 1982; Hickok & Avrutin, 1995; Hickok et al., 1993; Laskey et al., 1976; Pierce, 1983; Shewan & Canter, 1971). As mentioned above, SVO sentences that are nonreversible are easier than reversible sentences.

4. Aphasic patients tend to have more difficulty processing grammatically encoded (compact) sentences (e.g., "the man greeted by his wife was smoking a pipe" or "the woman was taller than the man") than sentences which are simplified syntactically by expansion into a series of propositions ("the man was greeted by his wife and he was smoking a pipe" or "the woman was tall and the man was short") (Goodglass et al., 1970; Nicholas & Brookshire, 1983). Similarly, individuals with aphasia have more difficulty processing object-gap relative clauses (e.g., "It was the farmer that the robber chased") than subject-gap relative clauses (e.g., "It was the farmer that chased the robber") (Hickok & Avrutin, 1995). These findings demonstrate that sentence comprehension is not simply a function of amount of information and length, because compact and expanded sentences can contain the same amount of information and easier-to-comprehend sentences can be longer than compact ones. Results like these also highlight the complexity of the interactions among stimulus factors and show that maximizing the facilitative effect of one factor may increase the difficulty

imposed by another; for example, the generally desirable strategy of reducing sentence length may necessitate a generally undesirable increase in syntactic complexity. In addition, it has become evident that factors influencing sentence comprehension do not have the same effects on discourse comprehension and that performance on sentence level material does not always predict discourse comprehension (Brookshire & Nicholas, 1984) (for further discussion, see section on Context).

5. Syntactic context, or the form in which sentence level tasks are expressed, can influence response appropriateness, if not accuracy. For example, Green and Boller (1974) evaluated auditory comprehension in severe aphasia by testing differences in response to commands, yes/no questions, and information questions when such tasks were directly worded (e.g., "point to the ceiling"), indirectly worded (e.g., "I would like you to point to the ceiling"), or directly worded but preceded by an introductory sentence (e.g., "Here's something. Point to the ceiling"). Commands constituted the easiest task, followed by yes/no questions and the information questions. The various syntactic contexts did not affect response accuracy but directly worded items were associated with a greater number of appropriate (relevant, although incorrect) responses than were indirectly worded items. Directly worded items preceded by an introductory sentence were easier than indirectly worded items.

6. As discussed in the previous section, verb argument structure properties are important influences of lexical organization for verb retrieval. They are also important factors in sentence production in agrammatic aphasic individuals. Previous research has indicated that agrammatic aphasic subjects do not produce all argument structures required by the verb in their sentence productions (Caplan & Hanna, 1996; Thompson et al., 1994; 1995). Thompson et al. (1997) have also investigated the effects of these structures on sentence production in agrammatic aphasic individuals during narrative tasks. The aphasic subjects produced fewer verbs than the normal subjects. In addition, the aphasic individuals showed a preference for producing simple one- and two-place verbs (i.e., verbs with the fewest participant roles) and rarely produced three-place or complement verbs (i.e., the most complex verbs). When complex verbs were produced by the aphasic subjects, they were produced in their simplest argument structure forms. These results indicated that sentence production was also influenced by the number of arguments or participant roles as well as by the type of arguments required by the verb. The complexity of the verb (i.e., the number of possible argument structure configurations) influenced sentence production, with simple verbs produced correctly with their arguments more often than complex ones. Finally,

obligatory arguments were produced correctly more often than optional ones, even when production of optional arguments was requested.

A number of syntactic and grammatical factors may influence comprehension, repetition, and verbal formulation performance. It also appears that the hierarchy of difficulty for a number of syntactic and grammatical tasks may be differentially influenced by nature of aphasia. Because variations in the grammatical and syntactic complexity of language have such effects, they should be accounted for when structuring stimulation for treatment purposes.

Context

In recent years, there has been a surge of interest in aphasic patients' discourse comprehension and expression, the factors that influence discourse comprehension and expression, and the relationship of discourse to word and sentence level abilities. Findings indicate that word and sentence comprehension do not predict very well the comprehension of discourse (Brookshire & Nicholas, 1984; Hough, 1990; Hough et al., 1989; Pashek & Brookshire, 1982; Stachowiak et al., 1977; Waller & Darley, 1978) and that discourse comprehension is often better than single-sentence comprehension. Brookshire (1997) points out that because communication in daily life usually occurs more in the form of connected speech than as single sentences, it may be that measures of sentence comprehension underestimate daily life comprehension competence.

Context, redundancy, predictability, and extralinguistic cues within discourse and conversation facilitate communication for aphasic patients. The following summary represents a sampling of findings from studies of aphasic patients' comprehension and expression of language in discourse or natural communicative contexts. They provide clues for the design of intervention tasks that, for some patients, may be easier than shorter and apparently simpler word and single-sentence level activities:

1. Comprehension of syntactically complex sentences (e.g., reversible passive sentences) is facilitated when preceded or followed by contextually relevant sentences containing semantic or syntactic information that predicts the relationship expressed in the target sentence (Boyle & Canter, 1986; Cannito et al., 1989; Pierce, 1988; Waller & Darley, 1978). (An example of a prior facilitative context task is: "The girl is on the ground. The girl was tripped by the boy. Who was tripped?" An example of a subsequent facilitative context task is: "The woman went to the library. She returned a book. Where did the woman go?" [Pierce, 1988]). Some studies also show that the context that precedes or follows a target sentence may not have to predict specific information as long as it facilitates the processing of the target information by, for example, identifying the topic, setting, or

theme (Cannito et al., 1986; Hough et al., 1989); however, nonpredictive context has also been noted not to facilitate comprehension of target sentences (Cannito et al., 1989; Cannito et al., 1996). Contextual facilitation for both types of paragraphs has been reported to increase as a positive function of stage of recovery from aphasia (Cannito et al., 1996). Aphasic individuals in the early stage of recovery (<1 month) demonstrated no advantage for predictive or nonpredictive narratives; aphasic individuals in the intermediate stage (1–6 months) demonstrated an advantage only for predictive narratives and chronic aphasic individuals (>6 months) exhibited facilitative effects of both predictive and nonpredictive narrative contexts. Finally, extralinguistic context, in the form of a picture depicting target sentence information, also facilitates comprehension (Pierce & Beekman, 1985), although Waller and Darley (1978) found that the facilitative effect of a contextual picture was less powerful than verbal context. Pierce (1991) has pointed out that these facilitative effects are most apparent for patients with relatively poor comprehension. The benefits of this kind of contextual cue seem to derive from redundancy or the fact that certain events or relationships are made more plausible than others.

2. Predictability provided by discourse may explain why it is comprehended better than sentences. Armus et al. (1989) found that mild-moderate aphasic patients' knowledge of scripts is not significantly compromised (scripts are used to organize common situations; for example, after repeatedly eating in restaurants we "know" the events that usually occur). Thus, if a patient has an internalized script for a discourse event it may allow him or her to predict what will happen next, infer what is not stated, and organize it for recall. The authors suggest that scripts may be used in treatment to facilitate comprehension, with fading of the degree to which discourse follows a script when comprehension improves.

3. Aphasic patients comprehend implied meanings quite well, especially in situations aided by extralinguistic context. In fact, Foldi (1987) reported that aphasic, like non-brain-injured people, tend to prefer the pragmatic interpretation of indirect requests over the literal interpretation. Wilcox et al. (1978) presented videotaped "natural" situations to patients in which the correct interpretation of an utterance was the meaning conveyed by the request in a particular context; for example, while the literal interpretation of "Can you move the table?" simply requires a yes-no response, the indirect, conveyed/contextual meaning is a request that the table be moved. Aphasic patients generally performed similarly to normal controls in their ability to use extralinguistic cues to comprehend the intent conveyed in many indirect requests. These results suggest that the use of natural communicative contexts in treatment may raise communicative performance over and above that derived from more traditional, relatively pure linguistic tasks, which often intentionally minimize extralinguistic cues. Linguistic information may help some patients appreciate the meaning of extralinguistic information. For example, Tompkins (1991) found that increased semantic redundancy facilitated the interpretation of emotions that were conveyed linguistically or prosodically to aphasic patients.

4. Aphasic patients have been shown to comprehend main ideas expressed in discourse—the most salient information—better than details, and information that is expressed directly better than information that must be inferred (Katsuki-Nakamura et al., 1988; Nicholas & Brookshire, 1986a). Of interest, increasing directness and salience (through repetition or elaboration) seems to be a more reliable way to improve discourse comprehension than is decreasing speech rate. Nicholas and Brookshire (1986b) have also shown that the advantage of directly expressed information over that requiring inference is maintained in multiple sentence reading tests.

5. Context can facilitate performance in certain word retrieval tasks. Hough (1989) and Hough and Pierce (1989) have shown this effect for tasks requiring generation of words in ad hoc categories, categories that are constructed for use in specialized contexts (e.g., things not to eat on a diet). Significantly, more items were generated when contextual vignettes preceded ad hoc category tasks (e.g., before listing things to take on a picnic, the patient heard "Sam wanted to spend time outdoors. It was a beautiful day so he packed up some items and went to a nearby park.") than when they did not. The facilitative effect of context was not found for common categories (e.g., foods). Hough and Pierce suggest that ad hoc category tasks may be useful for aphasic patients because they are more divergent in nature and allow reliance on experience and world knowledge to a greater extent than do common category tasks.

6. Methods used to elicit narrative discourse from aphasic patients have variable effects. For example, picture sequences representing stories generally lead to a greater number of words in narratives than do single pictured scenes, but the two types of stimuli generally do not affect other measures of production differently (Bottenberg et al., 1987). Gender-bias of pictures (e.g., men in a gym versus women in a beauty salon) may result in differences in number of words and information but does not affect wpm or efficiency, at least in males (Correia et al., 1990).

7. Main ideas are expressed to a proportionately greater degree than are details when stories are retold (Ernest-Baron et al., 1987). This may explain why patients get along reasonably well in daily life; it is usually main ideas that must be recalled rather than details.

8. Situational context may affect the manner in which aphasic patients respond. Glosser et al. (1988) reported that, in spite of their linguistic deficits, aphasic patients showed appropriate and predictable changes in response to nonlinguistic social contextual variables (e.g., face-to-face conversation versus telephone versus conversation over video monitors). In contrast, Brenneise-Sarshad et al. (1991) found few meaningful differences in the verbal output of aphasic patients when they narrated a sequenced picture story for a listener known to them who looked at the pictures as the story was being told versus a newly introduced person who could not see the picture stimuli. The authors felt that it may not be important to create treatment situations in which the patient believes the listener is naive to the information in order to obtain valid measures of communicative effectiveness.

In summary, the contextual information provided within discourse and natural communicative contexts can exert significant facilitative effects on language and communication for patients with aphasia. These effects occur not only for the processing of the main ideas and intents expressed in discourse but also extend "backward" to the comprehension and expression of semantic and syntactic relationships expressed within the context of discourse. It is clear that discourse tasks, particularly comprehension tasks, need not await recovery of word and sentence comprehension ability to become a focus of treatment. In fact, in some instances it appears that discourse should precede word and sentence level tasks in the treatment hierarchy.

Stress

Despite evidence that aphasic patients may be deficient in their ability to derive meaning from information provided by vocal stress (Baum et al., 1982) or that stress representation may be selectively impaired after brain damage (Cappa et al., 1997), it appears that stress can influence response adequacy in a positive way. For example, Swinney et al. (1980) have shown that aphasic patients respond more rapidly to stressed as opposed to unstressed words. More important, Pashek and Brookshire (1982) and Kimelman and McNeil (1987) found improved paragraph comprehension when exaggerated stress on critical words was employed. Pashek and Brookshire observed that improved comprehension in response to exaggerated stress was independent of improvement induced by slow rate, suggesting that slowed rate and exaggerated stress may be additive facilitators of auditory comprehension. More recently, Kimelman and McNeil (1989) showed that aphasic patients' comprehension of normally stressed target words in paragraphs is better when preceded by stressed as opposed to normally stressed context. The magnitude of the facilitative effect was greater for more severely impaired patients, those individuals most likely to need extralinguistic

cues for comprehension. Finally, Kimelman (1991) has presented data that suggest that the facilitative effect of stressing target words may actually derive from changes in duration and fundamental frequency in the context preceding the target word. Thus, it may be contextual stress modifications that alert the listener to the salience of the target word.

Eliminating consideration of information strongly associated with Melodic Intonation Therapy (MIT), the most representative study on stress and speech output in aphasia has been conducted by Goodglass et al. (1967). They found that fluent and nonfluent patients omitted initial unstressed function words much more frequently than initial stressed words in a sentence repetition task. The omission of unstressed words occurred more frequently for nonfluent patients. They also found that the stress pattern /-/, was easier to repeat than any other three-word pattern tested, when a function word was in the first or second position. Moreover, the facilitating effect of this stress pattern seemed to override grammatical complexity. For example, the negative interrogative "Can't you swim?" (/-/), was easier to repeat than the grammatically simpler "Can you swim?" (-//). The authors felt that nonfluent (and, therefore, usually apraxic) patients, in particular, may depend on stress features in order to initiate and maintain a flow of speech. Goodglass (1968) interpreted these and similar findings as supportive of the importance of "saliency" in the initiation of speech. That is, for many patients there is a need for a salient word in order to initiate speech—saliency being characterized by stress and phonological prominence, as well as other factors, already discussed, such as informational and personal significance.

The clinical implications of these findings are obvious. The selection of sentence and paragraph material for comprehension and repetition tasks should consider stress-saliency as a variable capable of affecting the verbal comprehension and verbal production of aphasic patients.

Order of Difficulty

Within a given treatment task, stimuli probably should be ordered so that more difficult items are presented last. This recommendation is based on evidence which suggests that success tends to breed success and failure breeds failure for patients with aphasia.

Brookshire (1972) studied the effects of task difficulty on naming behavior in nine patients. A group of easy-to-name and a group of hard-to-name pictures were derived from baseline measures for each patient and were subsequently presented in different orders. When easy pictures preceded hard pictures, responses to hard pictures were better than predicted by baseline measures. When easy pictures followed hard pictures, performance on easy pictures was poorer than expected on the basis of baseline measures. Brookshire speculated that when a patient experiences a high proportion of failures, emotional responses may be generated which disrupt subsequent responses. Although such negative effects tended to decay over time, he suggested that treatment should keep error rates low and that easy items should precede difficult ones. Brookshire (1976b) subsequently demonstrated very similar task difficulty effects for a sentence comprehension task in a group of 22 patients. The results differed from the study on naming only in that easy items facilitated comprehension on subsequent hard items for only a small number of patients.

Support for an order effect can be found in several other studies. Gardner and Brookshire (1972) found that naming performance under unisensory conditions often is facilitated when preceded by a generally easier auditory-visual stimulus condition, and that responses to auditory-visual stimuli are reduced when preceded by a generally more difficult visual stimulus condition. Similarly, Brookshire (1971b) found that forcing subjects to respond at rapid rates depresses performance on subsequent items in which they are given more time to respond. Finally, Brookshire and Lommel (1974) reported on the disruptive effects of failure on aphasic and nonaphasic brain injured subjects' performance on a nonverbal sequencing task.

Dumond et al. (1978) questioned (or qualified) the significance of the order effect. They readministered the PICA to 20 patients in split-half form, with the 18 subtests rearranged in two orders of difficulty—one ascending and one descending. No performance differences were found between the two orders of difficulty. In contrasting their results with those of Brookshire (1972), they pointed out that he examined a single task containing items of varying difficulty, while they examined differences across tasks containing items of equal difficulty. They also indicated that "the changes in difficulty level between subtests were apparently less extensive than the changes in difficulty level within Brookshire's experiment" (p. 358) and that this may have reduced subjects' perception of their performance adequacy. They concluded that presenting PICA-like tasks in order of increasing difficulty is not likely to adversely affect performance on nonevaluative tasks whose difficulty levels do not vary extensively.

The available data appear to warrant the following generalizations regarding order of presentation during treatment: error rates should be kept low; stimulus presentation generally should proceed from easiest to hardest, particularly within a given task and on tasks in which the patient is likely to be most sensitive to performance inadequacies; and if error rates are kept low, potential across-task order effects should be minimized. (In line with these generalizations, Crosky & Adams [1969] present some practical procedures for selecting and ordering vocabulary stimulus materials for individual patients.) Finally, it is reasonable to follow Brookshire's (1997) suggestion that sessions begin with familiar, easy tasks, proceed to less familiar and more difficult ones, and end with tasks that result in a great deal of success.

Psychological and Physical Factors

In addition to stimuli which are directly intended to stimulate language, factors which affect the psychological and physical "set" of patients can influence response adequacy.

Skelly's (1975) interviews with aphasic patients indicate that even relatively subtle signs of disinterest or impatience on the part of the clinician "bothers" patients. Stoicheff (1960) found that the overt attitudes expressed during instructions to patients can significantly affect responses. Using three groups of aphasic patients, she examined the effects of encouraging, discouraging, and neutral instructions and comments during performance on naming, reading, and self-evaluation tasks. After 3 days of exposure to one of the conditions, the self-evaluation, naming, and reading performance of the group receiving the discouraging instructions was lower than the performance of the groups receiving neutral or encouraging instructions. No differences were found between the encouraging and neutral conditions. Obviously, the performance differences were attributed to the negative effects of discouraging instructions. Finally, the previously discussed findings of Brookshire and his colleagues on the effects of order of stimulus difficulty suggest that failure, or stress induced by failure, may produce emotional responses that disrupt subsequent responses. It seems, therefore, that disruptive psychological effects may result from negative attitudes expressed by the clinician during instructions and performance, or from the failures the patient may experience during the course of a treatment session.

The effects of physical fatigue on language performance have been examined by Marshall and King (1973). Subjects were given the PICA following a period of isokinetic exercise and, on another day, following rest. PICA scores were significantly lower following exercise than following rest for Verbal, Graphic, and Overall PICA measures. Fatigue had its most pronounced effect on speaking and writing tasks. The authors suggested that language therapy be scheduled prior to physical exertion, such as physical or occupational therapy. In another study that probably reflects the cumulative effects of fatigue over the course of a day, Marshall et al. (1980) found that aphasic patients did better on assessment measures administered in the morning as opposed to the afternoon.

Psychological and physical factors may facilitate performance best when treatment is conducted in a positive, encouraging, success-producing milieu and at a time when the patient's physical status during the treatment day is optimal.

Pattern of Auditory Deficit

Auditory impairments are not uniform and may reflect a number of different underlying problems. As a result, to ignore differences in the auditory deficits of aphasic patients is to ignore a factor which may bear on the way we structure auditory stimulation in treatment. Consideration of such differences may help identify stimulus factors which are especially important for a given patient and, in some cases, may serve to qualify or alter the generalizations and recommendations that have been made about those factors thus far.

Brookshire (1974) summarized and discussed five kinds of auditory deficits whose characteristics may have an important bearing on treatment planning. They reflect the need to avoid considering auditory deficits in aphasia as a unitary problem. These deficits and implications for stimulus selection are the following.

Slow Rise Time

Patients whose auditory systems are characterized by slow rise time tend to miss the initial portion of incoming messages. They may be able to repeat or comprehend only the last part of sentences, may miss short messages entirely, or may do better on the final items of a subtest or treatment activity than on initial items. Brookshire suggests that the use of warning signals prior to presenting auditory stimuli may facilitate processing for these patients. Loverso and Prescott (1981) provide some indirect support for this. They found response times of aphasic subjects on a same-different visual judgment task to be reduced when the visual stimuli were preceded by a half-second warning tone; maximum benefit was derived when the tone preceded the stimulus by 1.5 sec. Presenting items with gradually increasing intervals between successive items may also help the patient keep his/her "processor" active over longer intervals or help activate the processor more quickly.

Patients with slow rise time illustrate the fact that generalizations about a number of stimulus factors do not always hold. For example, contrary to "average" performance, the patient with slow rise time may respond better to redundant sentences than to single words, or may respond more appropriately to directly worded input preceded by an introductory sentence than to a directly worded sentence alone.

Noise Buildup

Patients with noise buildup tend to respond more accurately to the initial portion of auditory messages than to following portions. More complex material tends to produce noise more rapidly than less complex material. Such patients may not be able to repeat or comprehend the final portion of sentences, may make more errors on complex than simple materials, and may deteriorate progressively across items on a particular task. Brookshire suggests that they may benefit from a program with messages of gradually increasing length and complexity, with gradually decreasing silent intervals between successive items.

Retention Deficit

Patients with retention deficits also deteriorate as length increases, but they are not as susceptible to complexity factors as are those with noise buildup. Performance breakdown tends to occur at the same point in all messages regardless of complexity. The important treatment consideration here is to gradually increase message length.

Information Capacity Deficit

Patients with information capacity deficit do not seem able to receive and process information at the same time (see Wepman, [1972] for a discussion of the "shutter principle"). In such cases, performance may be alternately good or poor within a message—good for information which is received and can be acted upon—poor for information directed at the system while processing of prior stimuli is taking place. Such patients may, for example, be able to repeat the beginning and end of a sequence of words, but not the middle elements. Brookshire suggests that these patients may benefit from the insertion of pauses within messages. Such pauses may initially be frequent and of relatively long duration, with fading of their frequency and duration as processing ability improves.

Intermittent Auditory Imperception

Patients with this problem constitute a separate category in Schuell's system of classification. Their auditory processing ability appears to fade in and out, randomly leading to sporadic and unpredictable performance. Because we do not understand the controlling factors in such a problem, Brookshire recommends that treatment be directed to other areas of deficit.

Brookshire points out that the above categories may be simplistic and incomplete, although the existence of several of them appears to have been verified by other investigators (McNeil & Hageman, 1979; Porch, 1967; Schuell et al., 1964). It is quite probable, however, that they exist in varying combinations within many patients, and are seen atypically in pure form. Regardless, the ability to recognize them when they occur has direct implications for the selection of potent stimulus factors when planning treatment.

Resource Allocation Model for Aphasia

The resource allocation model for aphasia proposed by McNeil and colleagues (McNeil & Kimelman, 1986; McNeil et al., 1990) has important implications for the application of the stimulation approach to aphasia. Essentially, what resource allocation models suggest is that all humans have a limited amount of cognitive resources for conducting mental or cognitive processes involved with perception, comprehension, memory, and response formulation. The mental energy or fuel required for carrying out these processes is referred to as processing resources and is contained in a central pool.

With the activation of any process, resources must be transferred from the pool to the process. The number of cognitive processes that are called upon simultaneously as well as the complexity of a given process determines how much fuel is drawn from the central resource pool. If the demands of the cognitive processes exceed the resources within the pool, the cognitive process(es) will not be provided with adequate resources and performance will be negatively affected. If on the other hand the resource demands for a given process are low the finite resources in the pool will not be exceeded and performance will be normal. The issue of whether brain damage reduces the amount of resources within the central pool or hinders access to the pool is unclear. However, in either case the allocation of suitable resources is insufficient for the task at hand and consequently the brain-damaged individual's performance on a given task is at a level below that of a non-brain-damaged person. Performance will vary depending on the number and complexity of cognitive processes called upon.

Brookshire (1997) notes that if elements of treatment tasks are simplified, the demands on the resource pool will be decreased, thus improving the aphasic individual's performance. For example, an aphasic individual with a visuoperceptual impairment is engaged in an auditory comprehension task involving pointing to black and white line drawings named by function ("point to the one used for…"). After ten trials he has made eight errors. The patient comments that he cannot see what the pictures represent so the clinician substitutes colored pictures for the line drawings. After ten more trials only three errors are noted. Although the targeted process was an aspect of auditory comprehension this task required the aphasic individual to call upon processes involved in visual perception that were impaired; consequently, the available resources were exceeded. By modifying the visual characteristics of the stimuli the visual perceptual demands of the task were decreased, freeing up cognitive resources, and performance on the auditory comprehension aspects of the task improved. As Brookshire notes "… clinicians can focus treatment on a targeted process by controlling the processing load associated with incidental task variables that are not related to the treatment objectives." (p. 217). The primary manner in which clinicians can manipulate the processing load is through manipulation of the task stimuli. Stimulus manipulations involve adjusting the factors that have just been discussed, such as visual perceptual clarity, length and redundancy, frequency and meaningfulness, grammar and syntax, etc. This gets to the heart of the stimulation approach; that is, the stimulus must be adequate—it must get into the brain.

Response Considerations

Although the emphasis of the stimulation approach is on input to the patient, it is obvious that the effectiveness of such stimulation can be assessed only if responses are elicited.

Regardless of the form of response, three of the general principles of remediation stated earlier are relevant to response considerations: (1) there should be a response to each stimulus, (2) responses should not be forced, and (3) a maximum number of responses should be elicited. To those we can add one additional principle—response demands generally should proceed from short to long. Just as length is a potent stimulus factor, it is also a potent response factor for most patients, with short responses nearly always easier than long ones. In addition to these principles, certain other response considerations must be addressed when planning treatment.

Response Mode

Decisions regarding the mode of response are based upon specific goals and baseline data. For example, if we wish to improve auditory comprehension or retention, we should place minimal demands on output and let baseline data aid us in selecting the most intact mode of response. If the goal is to improve spoken language ability, then the response mode has already been determined by the chosen goal.

Sometimes response adequacy in a particular modality can be facilitated by a simultaneous response in another modality. For example, Hanlon et al. (1990) found that patients with anterior lesions, hemiparesis, and Broca's aphasia named pictures more adequately when they simultaneously attempted to point to the picture with their hemiparetic right arm. (Note that this may represent facilitation of problems more related to apraxia of speech than to language per se.)

Output modes usually include pointing, nodding, object or picture manipulation, pantomime, other gestures, speech, and writing. "Point-to" tasks are used frequently when treatment focuses on auditory processes because the motor control of simple pointing responses usually is unimpaired. However, Brookshire (1997) observes that such tasks can be relatively difficult for some patients. Such observations reinforce the need for letting the individual patient's abilities determine the mode of response.

Temporal Relationship

The temporal relationship between stimulus and response should be considered. Responses may be elicited in unison with a stimulus, immediately following a stimulus, or after a delay. Patients also may be asked to repeat a response consecutively.

Unison responses may be especially appropriate for severely impaired patients because they give simultaneous auditory and visual feedback and are a step down the response hierarchy from repetition (Schuell et al., 1955; Wertz, 1978). Although immediate responses represent the most frequent and desirable temporal relationship, they may impose unreasonable demands on some patients; requiring rapid responses may depress performance adequacy for some patients. In such cases, allowing a delay for processing may be very useful. Marshall (1976), for example, found that delay was the most effective response "strategy" employed by aphasic patients for word retrieval.

How much delay? Schuell et al. (1964) suggested 60 seconds for some tasks. Brookshire (1971b) found that 30 seconds were better than 0, 5, or 10 seconds on an object naming task but noted that when patients were able to name objects they usually did so within 10 seconds. It seems that delays allowed for processing rarely should have to exceed 30 seconds, and probably should not, considering the principle that treatment should elicit a large number of responses.

On comprehension tasks the effect of imposing delays between stimulus and response may not be predictable. Schulte (1986) examined 10 aphasic patients' comprehension on a token test type of task in which 0, 5-, 10-, and 20-second delays were imposed before patients were allowed to look at response choices and respond. No consistent effects on comprehension were found among the delay conditions for the group as a whole, but performance within subjects varied by nearly 20% between some conditions and a few of the more severely impaired patients benefited from brief delays in some conditions. Schulte suggested that, for some patients, imposed delay may facilitate full processing before a response but that it may be detrimental for others because of poor rehearsal mechanisms or reduced retention capacity. It therefore appears that imposing a delay between stimulus presentation and response has no generally predictable influence on sentence comprehension accuracy, but that it may be a useful response parameter if its effects are predictable for individual patients.

In addition to using delay as an aid to comprehension or formulation, imposing delays before allowing the patient to respond may be a useful strategy for improving retention span. Imposing a delay between a patient's response and the next stimulus also may be an effective strategy for reducing perseveration in some patients. Santo Pietro and Rigrodsky (1982) found that the frequency of perseveration on sentence completion, naming, and reading tasks decreased as the time between a response and subsequent stimulus increased from 1 to 10 seconds.

Delay sometimes can be used actively by patients to improve response adequacy (this point could also be considered under the section dealing with consequences/feedback). Berstein-Ellis et al. (1987) instructed a mildly impaired aphasic patient with reduced conversational fluency (because of hesitation, revisions, and paraphasias) in the use of a pacing board (Helm, 1979) to slow speech rate. This reduced syntactic and paraphasic errors and permitted the same or more information to be conveyed with fewer verbalizations. Whitney and Goldstein (1989) used a different technique and achieved the same result for three mildly aphasic patients whose discourse was dysfluent because of revisions, repetitions, and audible pauses. After learning to recognize and identify their dysfluencies from audiorecorded samples of their speech, the patients were trained to monitor/identify their dysfluencies during picture description tasks. This resulted in reduced speech rate, a dramatic reduction of dysfluencies, and increased efficiency in the form of increased length of uninterrupted utterances.

Finally, there are some subtle uses of temporal relationships in stimulus presentation that may influence processing demands and response adequacy. Brookshire and Nicholas (1980) have shown that aphasic patients tend to use a find-and-compare strategy on sentence verification tasks in which the truth value of a sentence is based on a comparison with a simultaneously presented picture stimulus; that is, instead of processing the full meaning of the sentence, they may simply match key words to elements in the picture. To force the patient to deal with the fuller meaning of the sentence, they suggest that the spoken sentence and the picture stimulus presentations be staggered (e.g., present sentence, then present picture) rather than simultaneous. It is quite possible that this more challenging approach to stimulus presentation in a verification task would also apply to point-to comprehension tasks (that is, present sentence and then present picture choices).

Response Characteristics

Although accuracy is certainly the most commonly expected response characteristic, it is not the only relevant one. Green and Boller (1974) found that severely impaired patients, unable to respond very accurately to auditory tasks, often are able to respond appropriately; that is, they show signs of rudimentary comprehension by, for example, looking around the room when asked to point to the door, or nodding when asked yes/no questions. In such cases, appropriateness of response may be the most appropriate initial response expectation. At the other end of the continuum, when a patient can respond with a relatively high degree of accuracy, it may be appropriate to expect a reduction of self-corrections, or incomplete, delayed, or distorted responses. (Such response characteristics are reflected in Porch's multidimensional scoring scale.) The important point is that response expectations need not be geared solely to accuracy. For some patients, a high degree of accuracy may not be possible and expectations may have to be lowered; for others, a high proportion of accurate responses may still leave considerable room for response refinement along a number of other response dimensions.

Consequences (Feedback)

The stimulation approach presumes that the stimulus (antecedent event) is that part of the treatment sequence which facilitates, or is largely responsible for, the ability of the patient to respond adequately. This is in contrast to operant approaches, in which increased adequacy of responses is attributed primarily to the controlling influence of consequences on subsequent behavior. Because antecedents are theoretically the crucial modifier of language processing in the stimulation approach, however, does not mean that we should not respond to patient behavior.

Feedback about response accuracy and appropriateness should be given when appropriate. Boone (1967) suggests that any specific response-contingent feedback may be trivial or unnecessary when patients are motivated (as is usually the case), know the target response, and can assess their response in relation to the target. Support for this comes from the finding that mild to moderately impaired aphasic patients modify their picture descriptions in response to failure in a referential communication task in the same way nonaphasic speakers do. In the relatively rare case where a patient is not motivated, response contingent rewards or punishment may be necessary; but, in general, reinforcement or punishment have little effect on speech and language performance in aphasia (Brookshire, 1977). When patients are motivated but give deficient responses, it may be most appropriate to confirm response adequacy or give information about the closeness of a response to the target. Whether feedback is in the form of reward, punishment, confirmation, or information, Brookshire's (1971a) finding that markedly to severely impaired patients were sensitive to the effects of short delays between responses and their consequences on a nonlanguage learning task implies that feedback, when appropriate, should be immediate.

What information should be given to patients when their responses are inadequate? First, in most instances, such information should not be negative. Stoicheff's (1960) findings suggest that discouraging comments during performance, such as "that's wrong," at least when combined with discouraging instructions, have a detrimental effect on performance. Second, Schuell et al. (1964) felt that one of the most common errors made by clinicians was overcorrection or overexplanation of errors, and that the proper contingency for an inadequate response is usually more stimulation. In support of this, Holland and Sonderman (1974), in their evaluation of an auditory comprehension program, felt that explaining errors to patients confused rather than aided subsequent performance. Brookshire and Nicholas' (1978) analysis of clinical interactions in aphasia treatment indicated that patients tend to make errors following corrective explanations of previous errors. It seems that confirmation of adequate performance may be helpful and encouraging, and generally represents good clinical practice. Explanation and correction, on the other hand, should be carefully controlled and concise, bearing in mind that such feedback may be of little value, may waste time, and may be counterproductive.

In addition to considering response-dependent feedback, general encouragement and reassurance during a treatment session is always desirable. Brookshire (1997) supports the value of showing patients their progress over time, with graphs often being an effective format for doing so. Such feedback—aside from being information the patient has a right to know about—has motivational and reinforcement functions, and provides a framework for discussing and/or supporting the continuation, alteration, or termination of certain treatment activities.

Sequencing Steps in the Treatment Program

Where to Start

Schuell et al. (1964) indicated that treatment should begin where language breaks down and should proceed through gradually increasing levels of difficulty. Bollinger and Stout (1976), arguing for the critical importance of stimulation in treatment, suggested that treatment should progress from highly clinician-cued antecedent events to low-cued events in which the patient carries most of the processing load. Brookshire (1997) offers more specific suggestions regarding starting points which can be summarized as follows:

1. Treatment should begin at levels where slight deficiencies exist and never where performance is completely inadequate. This assures that patients are not pushed beyond their capacity but forces them to work near capacity.
2. Tasks where 60 to 80% of responses are correct and immediate represent good starting points. That is, not more than 20 to 40% of responses should be self-corrected or delayed.
3. Tasks should not be too easy. Difficulty should be increased when 90% or more of responses are completely adequate in the dimensions that are the focus of treatment.

The selection of appropriate starting points should be based on adequate baseline data, for without such information treatment begins without knowing if tasks or stimuli are appropriate. Baseline data may be established through standardized tests, systematic sampling of patients' responses to their environment (this is critical for the establishment of relevant practical tasks and stimuli) or selected stimuli, or probing of variations in stimuli to see how changes influence speech and language behavior (Hendrick et al., 1973). For example, standardized testing may indicate that the ability to identify objects named from among 10 choices is very adequate (e.g., 90% immediate, accurate responses), but that identifying object-by-function from among 10 choices is below the level at which treatment would be appropriate (e.g., 50% inaccurate responses). Subsequent assessment of responses to functional items might confirm standardized results, but probing might establish that identifying those same objects-by-function from among only four choices generates response characteristics at a level appropriate for treatment (e.g., 80% accurate with 20% delayed or self-corrected responses). Such baseline data identify a starting point for stimulating auditory abilities, specify the stimulus conditions and response expectations to be employed during treatment, and give direction about the organization of succeeding steps. No less important is the fact that baseline data provide a pretreatment measure of ability against which the results of treatment can be compared.

Criteria for Determining Success

Once tasks and stimuli have been established and target behaviors or response characteristics have been identified, we must determine a criterion for acceptable performance. When this criterion is reached, it is assumed that the specific task is no longer necessary and that the patient is ready to move on to tasks with greater demands. Experienced clinicians agree that a target behavior criterion of 90% is generally appropriate (Brookshire, 1997; LaPointe, 1977). LaPointe also suggests that the criterion be maintained for three consecutive sessions before terminating the task to ensure that the behavior is stable. When a patient's performance plateaus at a level below the criterion for a number of sessions, he suggests that the task be terminated or modified to make it slightly easier.

Compatibility of the Stimulation Approach and Programming

The discussion of the design of intervention has included information about stimulus and response considerations, contingencies, the selection of starting points, and progression of activities. The acquisition of baseline data and the setting of criterion levels also have been highlighted. All of these considerations can be strongly associated with programmed approaches to treatment. This may be somewhat surprising because the appearance of information about the stimulation approach and programmed approach to treatment in the same discussion has been typically in the form of contrast (e.g., see Darley, 1975; and Sarno, 1974). Although operant-programmed approaches are dissimilar to the stimulation approach because of their emphasis on consequences as the primary modifiers of behavior, it is inappropriate to consider the stimulation approach and the application of general programming principles as mutually exclusive treatment strategies (LaPointe, 1978b). A careful reading of Schuell's work shows that her principles and suggestions regarding treatment are compatible with the rigor and systematic nature of programming. Her admonitions to choose realistic goals, know where performance breaks down, elicit large numbers of responses, work systematically, and discard techniques when they aren't working are things that a systematic, behavioral approach—programming—is highly capable of assisting. It seems most appropriate, in this context, to consider programming as a tool for systematically implementing the stimulation approach. Programming is particularly desirable because of its commitment to accountability and its capacity for making treatment replicable and accessible to analysis

(Holland, 1975; LaPointe, 1983). LaPointe's (1977) "Base-10 Programmed Stimulation" and Bollinger and Stout's (1976) "Response-Contingent Small-Step Treatment" are excellent, clinically applicable examples of the compatibility of the stimulation approach and structured behavioral methods.

EXAMPLES OF THERAPY TASKS

The preceding discussion of the design of intervention included numerous implied suggestions about tasks and techniques that may be appropriate for therapy. In this section a number of specific tasks will be listed. They are offered as examples of activities that are considered appropriate for aphasic patients and have enjoyed varying or undefined degrees of success. They are not offered as prescriptions or even as recommendations, for given our current state of knowledge we have no way of predicting reliably which tasks and techniques work best with individual patients.

The focus of the examples will be on tasks that emphasize auditory processes, because that is consistent with the stimulation approach. A number of examples of tasks requiring verbal output, many of which also involve auditory input, also will be given. It should be understood that nearly all auditory and verbal tasks are readily adaptable to the reading and writing modes. However, a few examples of tasks unique to reading and writing also will be given.

The examples offered here cover a range of difficulty so as to include suggestions which are appropriate for mildly to severely impaired patients. The tasks are ordered from the anticipated easiest to hardest, but the reader is cautioned that the order provided is not empirically derived, and probably cannot be, because of patient variability. It is also important to note that difficulty level can be altered, not only by switching tasks, but also by altering certain stimulus factors or stimulus-response relationships associated with a given task. For example, increasing the number of response choices in a point-to auditory comprehension task may significantly increase task difficulty.

Many of the examples given below have been derived from suggestions offered in the following sources: Schuell et al. (1955, 1964); Schuell (1953a); Brookshire (1997); Kearns and Hubbard (1977); LaPointe (1978a); Darley (1982); and Rosenbek et al. (1989). Many other examples are of such universal, longstanding use that they defy or make trivial accurate referencing.

Tasks Emphasizing Auditory Abilities

Point-to Tasks

These activities involve the presentation of information auditorily and require a simple identification-by-pointing response. The ease of the motor response allows patients to focus primarily on the reception, processing, and retention of the auditory message. Difficulty level on these and many other auditory tasks can be altered by variations of many of the stimulus factors discussed earlier in the chapter (rate, pause, stress, similarity and number of response choices, visual cues, syntactic complexity, etc.). Many of these tasks can be employed as speech activities by requiring verbal instead of gestural responses. Some examples follow:

1. Point to an item (picture or object) named.
2. Point to an item described by function ("Point to the one used for writing").
3. Point to an item in order to complete a sentence ("Please pass the bread and _____").
4. Point to an item in response to questions ("What do you find in the kitchen?"—stove). A more complex but analogous task might involve responses to questions based on preceding sentence or paragraph material.
5. Point to two (or more) items named ("Point to the book and point to the pen" or "Point to book; comb").
6. Point to two (or more) items described by function.
7. Point to an item best described by a sentence ("Those people are very busy"—represented by people building a house).
8. Point to an item whose name is spelled.
9. Point to an item described by a varying number of descriptors ("Point to the large white circle," "Point to the one that is long, silver, and sharp"—knife).

Following Directions

These tasks allow for greater flexibility and complexity in the auditory demands placed upon the patient.

1. Follow one-verb instructions ("Pick up the pen").
2. Follow two-object location instructions ("Put the pencil in front of the cup").
3. Follow two-verb instructions ("Point to the cup. Pick up the eraser").
4. Follow two-verb instructions with time constraint ("Before touching the penny, pick up the spoon").

Yes-No Questions and Sentence Verification

These formats also increase flexibility, can reduce the possible effects of visual deficits on performance, and often allow for the extension of stimulus material beyond the immediate environment. Only a simple verbal or nonverbal response is required.

1. Questions dealing with general information ("Was Kennedy President in 1861?")
2. Questions requiring phonemic discrimination ("Do people wear shoes and blocks on their feet?")
3. Questions requiring semantic discrimination ("Do you start a car with a tire?")

4. Questions about picture material ("Is the boy wailing?"—picture of boy running).
5. Questions involving verbal retention ("Are cows, horses, dogs, trees, and lions all animals?")
6. Questions about preceding sentences or paragraph material ("I like to swim, play tennis, and go to the ballpark. Did I say I like to play football?")
7. The above question examples may be converted to sentence or paragraph verifications tasks, in which the patient is asked to verify the truth of various statements ("Kennedy was President in 1861. . . . Cows, horses, dogs, trees, and lions are all animals," etc.).

Response Switching

These tasks require the patient to switch responses from item to item and, therefore, require close attention to the nature of the task on each trial. Such activities may simply combine the auditory tasks previously discussed or also may include items requiring speech, reading, or writing abilities. For example, a response switching activity might include the following successive items:

1. Point to the door.
2. Give me the cup.
3. Is the floor lower than the ceiling?
4. Spell your name.
5. How are you feeling today?
6. Have I asked you to give me the cup?
7. Read this and do what it says to do.

Tasks Emphasizing Verbal and Auditory Abilities

Repetition Tasks

These require reception and retention of auditory information and the ability to repeat the information verbally. Auditory comprehension is not necessary, although it may facilitate performance. Minimal demands are placed on word retrieval.

1. Repeat spoken words.
2. Repeat phrases ("in the house"; "on the beach"; "to the store"; "black and white"; "shoes and socks").
3. Repeat series of items ("book-table"; "penny-key-knife"; "long-under-baby-pencil").
4. Repeat stereotyped or functional phrases ("where are you going?"; "what time is it?"; "please pass the salt"; "how are you?").
5. Repeat sentences with or without corresponding picture stimuli ("the girl is chasing the boy"; "the cat is up in the tree").

Sentence or Phrase Completion

These tasks typically place more demand on auditory comprehension and word retrieval processes, and less demand on auditory retention than do repetition tasks. For most patients, they are more difficult than single-word repetition tasks but less difficult than single-word recall tasks without auditory input.

1. Complete sentences with nouns with varying degrees of predictability ("Please pass the salt and _____"; "Throw me the _____"; "Read a _____"; "Buy me some _____").
2. Complete sentences with verbs ("I use a fork for _____"; "I use a paint brush for _____").
3. Complete paired-associates ("Black and _____"; "Hot and _____"; "Salt and _____").

Verbal Association

These tasks require verbal comprehension but minimal retention. Verbal retrieval processes are taxed.

1. Oral opposites (hot-cold; night-day; early-late).
2. Rhyming—clinician says word and patient rhymes (hot-pot).
3. Word fluency/rapid word retrieval—clinician provides a letter of the alphabet, a common category (e.g., clothes, sports), or a concept (e.g., things to do on vacation, things that can roll), and patient generates as many words, categories, or concepts as possible.
4. Synonyms—"think of a word that means the same as 'car'."

Answering Wh-questions

These tasks always place some demand on auditory comprehension and may require significant retention as well. Word retrieval and sentence formulation may be taxed to varying degrees.

1. Answer questions after imitative cues and a question prompt (clinician—"Answer the phone"-patient imitates-clinician—"What should I do?"; patient—"Answer the phone").
2. Answer questions after a model (clinician—"The boy went to the movies. What did the boy do?").
3. Answer familiar conversational questions ("How old are you?"; "How do you feel?").
4. Answer questions about preceding sentence or paragraph material (e.g., "John was on the ground. John was tripped by Mary. Who was on the ground?").
5. Answer general questions ("What do you do when you're hungry?"; "Who is the President of the U.S.A.?"; "How did you get here today?"). High-level patients may be asked questions requiring lengthy responses ("How do you change a flat tire?"; "Exactly how do you get from here to _____?").

Connected Utterances in Response to Single Words

Minimal demands are placed on auditory input processes. Maximal demands are on word retrieval and sentence formulation.

1. Use selected words of varying parts of speech, word class, tense, etc., in sentences (put-how; television; red; running; bigger; given).
2. Define words.
3. Use sentences beginning (or ending) with selected words or phrases (I eat; when; if, she).

Retelling

These tasks can place relatively heavy demands on comprehension and retention and always tax word retrieval and sentence formulation.

1. Listen to paragraph material and retell.
2. Listen to radio or television broadcast and retell.
3. Retell a familiar story.

"Self-Initiated" or Conversational Verbal Tasks

These tasks are not dependent upon pre-selected auditory input to the patient, with the exception of directions about the general nature of the task. Other stimuli may be used to focus content and aid retrieval, but the primary demands are placed on the patient's verbal retrieval and formulation abilities, and often on the ability to follow naturally occurring auditory and situational cues.

1. Name pictures.
2. Describe the function of objects.
3. Describe activities in pictures.
4. Tell everything possible about pictured objects or activities (urge patient to describe all possible uses of objects, objects' physical properties, associated situations, people, etc.).
5. Describe activity of the clinician (clinician points to two pictures—patient describes; clinician touches an object, places another object near it, and then places an object on top of another—patient describes the activity when completed).
6. General conversation about a selected topic with one or more individuals.
7. Open-ended conversation on unrestricted topics with one or more individuals.

Tasks Involving Reading and Writing Abilities

Reading

Nearly all of the tasks previously described involving auditory input can be adapted easily for reading tasks simply by using written input. Following are some additional tasks which are associated more uniquely with reading:

1. Match written words, phrases, or sentences to pictures (gradually reducing stimulus exposure time may be employed in an effort to increase reading rate).
2. Identify letters named by the clinician among a number of written choices.

3. Name letters.
4. Read in unison with the clinician with gradual increase in rate and/or fading of the clinician's input.
5. Fill in missing words in sentences from among written choices ("They went to the movies last [day, night, show, fight]"-"John is [to, went, going, come] in a little while").
6. Read sentences or paragraphs silently, followed by questions about content.
7. Read aloud a paragraph or story and then retell.

Writing

Most of the examples offered under the sections dealing with auditory and verbal activities also can be adapted readily to the writing mode merely by requiring written instead of gestural or verbal responses. Following are some additional tasks that are associated more uniquely with writing modality activities:

1. Copy forms, letters, and words.
2. Write letters to dictation.
3. Write words dictated letter-by-letter.
4. Write overlearned materials such as name, the alphabet, numbers 1–10, etc.
5. Fill in missing letters or words in written stimuli, with or without associated picture stimuli ("He is reading a book _____"; "He is reading a _____ b-ok").
6. Clinician reads paragraph material and the patient writes down the essential facts. Have the patient rewrite the paragraph based on those notes.

EFFICACY OF THE STIMULATION APPROACH

It is impossible to make a single empirically based statement about the efficacy of the stimulation approach. Nor would it be appropriate or particularly enlightening, within the context of this chapter, to review all of the group and single-subject studies which might bear on the issue of treatment efficacy (the reader is referred to Darley's [1972, 1975, 1982], Rosenbek et al.'s [1989], and Holland et al.'s [1996] comprehensive reviews of such studies and issues related to assessing the effectiveness of treatment). However, a number of general statements about the effectiveness of treatment, particularly the stimulation approach, may help put the current state of the art in perspective.

While no single study can conclusively "prove" the efficacy of treatment (Holland, 1975), reviews and observations by well-respected, active clinical aphasiologists and some neurologists generally have yielded cautious-to-confident conclusions that therapy helps aphasic patients (see, for example, Darley, 1977, 1979, 1882; Benson, 1979; Wertz, 1983, 1991; and Helm-Estabrooks, 1984). Today, the evidence accumulated from many group and single-subject treatment studies, including at least one well-designed randomized controlled clinical trial (Wertz et al., 1986), at the least, justifies a general conclusion that "... there is ample evidence that what we do for some aphasic patients does some good" (Wertz, 1991, p. 318). These general conclusions are well supported by the results of meta-analysis of both group and single-subject treatment studies (Robey, 1994, 1998; Robey & Schultz, 1998; Robey et al., 1999).

Do we know something about the effectiveness of the stimulation approach that we do not know about therapy for aphasia in general? We do know that Schuell and her colleagues believed in and reported observations of the effectiveness of the stimulation approach, excluding patients with an irreversible (severe) aphasic syndrome. Many other users of the approach also report measurable progress (for relatively recent, relatively unambiguous examples of studies supporting the efficacy of the stimulation approach, see Basso et al., 1979; Shewan & Kertesz, 1984; Marshall et al., 1989; Poeck et al., 1989; Wertz et al., 1981; and Wertz et al., 1986). Because of the widespread use of the stimulation approach, it probably has been studied more extensively than any other approach to treatment (although the interpretation of most efficacy studies requires this conclusion to be inferred since treatment approaches rarely have been well specified). Therefore, conclusions that therapy is generally effective are based on studies that have utilized, or probably have utilized, a stimulation approach. More pessimistically, we can say that much of our inconclusive evidence about treatment efficacy is derived from studies of the stimulation approach. However, it is very possible that such inconclusiveness is due more to the study of the treatment than to the treatment itself. Taken as a whole, treatment studies employing the stimulation approach are more conclusive than inconclusive, and the conclusion they generate is that it has a significant positive effect on the communication ability of many patients with aphasia.

FUTURE TRENDS

What does the future hold for the stimulation approach? Answering this question is risky business, subject to the predictor's biases and misconceptions, new fads and fashions, major advances in other therapy approaches, altered availability of funding for continued investigation, etc. With these pitfalls in mind, we can address three questions about the future: (1) Will we increase our understanding of the efficacy and dynamics of the stimulation approach? (2) Is the approach likely to change? (3) How will we understand and use it in relation to other therapy approaches?

Will we increase our understanding of the efficacy of the stimulation approach and the dynamics that explain its success? There are a number of reasons to anticipate that this will happen. First, clinical aphasiologists have made a commitment to accountability—a commitment to providing "proof" of the effectiveness, or lack thereof, of treatment for aphasia. Second, we have identified many of the flaws in our previous attempts, as well as those variables which must be accounted for in any study of treatment efficacy. Third, our measuring instruments have become more sensitive and reliable (e.g., the PICA). Fourth, we have begun to specify and study the dynamics of treatment more precisely (especially in single-subject studies) so that we know better what is effective and under what circumstances. Fifth, although we have acquired a substantial body of data about stimulus factors that affect the performance of aphasic patients in nontreatment conditions, we know very little about the specific effects of using such stimulus manipulation in ongoing treatment. That is, the simple observation of improved performance under a certain stimulus condition in a single-trial nontreatment study does not constitute proof that use of that stimulus factor in treatment will be responsible for short- or long-term language gains within or beyond the specific language task. This gap in our knowledge is true for many of the stimulus factors reviewed in this chapter and it is close to the heart of questions about whether stimulation in general and/or specific stimulation is important to inducing language gains with the stimulation approach. We are in position to test the effects of many stimulus factors in treatment, and it is likely that this will be pursued in the future. Finally, the effect of stimulus factors and other variables that affect communication in discourse, conversation, and natural communicative settings are receiving increased attention. These efforts should help identify the components of stimulation likely to have the greatest impact on communication in daily life and, thus, stimulus factors that are most meaningful to the patients we treat (i.e., social validation of the stimulation approach).

Is the stimulation approach likely to change? Probably not in any fundamental way. Major change is unlikely because the stimulation approach is an old and established one whose major principles and techniques have been reasonably well articulated and, in principle, consistently employed. It is likely that any major departures from the basic approach will be considered new approaches, given new names, and studied and employed separately. Several chapters in this volume reflect this trend and demonstrate divergence from the stimulation approach along many different lines.

The change that can be expected for the stimulation approach is refinement of our understanding of stimulus factors that do and do not influence performance and, as mentioned previously, an increase in our ability to selectively and effectively employ that knowledge in treatment. Hopefully, these changes will be rapid and numerous and significantly improve overall treatment efficacy. Probably they will be slow and painstakingly acquired. Certainly, they will require the efforts of many investigators who are interested in the increased understanding of the essence of aphasia as well as its effective management.

Finally, how will we understand and use the stimulation approach in relation to other therapy approaches? There is no way to answer this because so little has been done to compare the effects of different treatment approaches. This is at least partly due to the enormous past efforts expended to establish that treatment, in general, is effective, and to develop new approaches and preliminary efficacy data for them. Another reason, really not to be confronted until more comparative studies are attempted, has been perceived by Sarno (1981). She said: "It is probably appropriate that there have been few studies comparing treatment methods in view of the seemingly insurmountable methodological problems associated with such research and our present state of knowledge" (p. 512). Despite these past priorities and ever-present methodologic challenges, it can be argued that unless comparative studies are done, we will not learn what works best and with whom, and we will either become complacent in our use of a single "old and familiar" approach or will move randomly from one approach to another. There are numerous comparative questions that should be addressed. Among them: How do various treatment approaches differ in terms of ultimate level of recovery, time demands, cost-effectiveness, professional and family requirements, etc.? What is the best approach to use for patients with particular severity levels and forms of aphasia? Are some approaches more effective early post-onset, late post-onset? Is there a best sequence of approaches to use over the course of treatment? Is language recovery enhanced if certain approaches are used in combination? Do some approaches have to be used in isolation for them to be effective?

Some of the aforementioned questions will probably be addressed in the next 5 to 10 years. The number of approaches now in use make this increasingly necessary for rational, data-based clinical decision making. In addition, because more is known about the efficacy of the stimulation approach than almost any other, it will frequently be among the approaches compared. In fact, we might anticipate that it will be the standard against which the effectiveness of other approaches will be measured.

KEY POINTS

1. Schuell and colleagues defined aphasia as a generalized language deficit crossing all language modalities (i.e., comprehension of spoken language, oral-verbal expression, reading, and writing) that may or may not be complicated by other nonaphasic disturbances (i.e., perceptual disturbances, dysarthrias, and apraxia of speech).
2. It is important that an approach to the treatment of aphasia be linked to our belief about the organization of language in the brain and the nature of language breakdown after brain damage.

3. Schuell's beliefs regarding the organization of language and the nature of language breakdown in aphasia may be summarized as follows:
   a) Language is not a simple sensorimotor dichotomy or a three-system cortical relay involving reception, transmission, and execution.
   b) Neurophysiologically, language is the result of a dynamic interaction of complex cerebral and subcortical activities.
   c) In adults language can exist unimpaired in the presence of sensory and/or motor deficits. Conversely, language can be impaired in the absence of sensory or motor deficits. Consequently, aphasia is viewed as a multimodality disturbance which is unidimensional in nature.
   d) Individuals with aphasia demonstrate problems that appear to be more related to performance factors than to competence factors.
   e) Auditory processes are at the apex of those interacting systems which aid in the acquisition, processing, and control of language.

4. Schuell's classification system of aphasia aimed at descriptive and predictive utility by classifying patients according to severity of language impairment, presence or absence of related sensory or motor deficits, and prognosis. The system consists of seven categories:
   a) simple aphasia
   b) aphasia with visual involvement
   c) aphasia with persisting dysfluency
   d) aphasia with scattered findings
   e) aphasia with sensorimotor involvement
   f) aphasia with intermittent auditory imperception
   g) irreversible aphasia syndrome

5. The stimulation approach for rehabilitation of aphasia can be defined as that approach to treatment which employs strong, controlled, and intensive auditory stimulation of the impaired symbol system as the primary tool to facilitate and maximize the patient's reorganization and recovery of language.

6. The use of intensive, controlled auditory stimulation is at the foundation of Schuell's stimulation approach. The use of intensive, controlled auditory stimulation is supported by the following:
   a) Sensory stimulation affects brain activity.
   b) Repeated sensory stimulation is essential for acquisition, organization, storage, and retrieval of patterns in the brain.
   c) The auditory system is of prime importance in the acquisition of language, and ongoing functional language is dependent on the auditory system for processed information and control through feedback loops.

   d) Nearly all individuals with aphasia exhibit deficits in the auditory modality.
   e) Use of intensive auditory stimulation is consistent with the definition of aphasia as a multimodality deficit due to an underlying disturbance of language.

7. The design of intervention used in the stimulation approach is based on a number of general principles:
   a) Intensive auditory stimulation should be used.
   b) The stimulus must be adequate—it must get into the brain. Therefore, it needs to be controlled along a number of dimensions.
   c) Repetitive sensory stimulation should be used.
   d) Each stimulus should elicit a response.
   e) Responses should be elicited, not forced or corrected.
   f) A maximum number of responses should be elicited.
   g) Feedback about response accuracy should be provided.
   h) The clinician should work systematically and intensively.
   i) Sessions should begin with relatively easy, familiar tasks.
   j) Abundant and varied materials that are simple and relevant to the patient's deficits should be used.
   k) New materials and procedures should be extensions of familiar materials and procedures.

8. There is a great deal of information in the aphasiology literature related to stimulus variables that affect performance. Knowledge about stimulus manipulations that may maximize performance can be used to ensure that a patient is working at a level where "failure" is minimized. Such manipulations may also be used to challenge mildly impaired patients, and for counseling individuals in the aphasic patient's environment on how to best communicate with the patient in everyday interactions.

9. Nineteen stimulus variables have been identified and reviewed which may affect performance of aphasic individuals.

10. Resource allocation models suggest that humans have a limited amount of cognitive resources for conducting mental or cognitive operations. If elements of treatment tasks are simplified, demands of the resource pool will be decreased, thus improving the aphasic individual's performance. The primary manner in which clinicians can manipulate the processing load is through manipulation of the task stimuli.

11. Although the emphasis of the stimulation approach is on input to the patient, effectiveness of each stimulation can be assessed only if responses are elicited.

12. Treatment should begin where language breaks down and should proceed through gradually increasing levels of difficulty.

13. Conclusions that aphasia therapy is generally effective are based on studies that have utilized, or probably have utilized, a stimulation approach.

References

Albert, M.L. (1976). Short-term memory and aphasia. *Brain and Language, 3,* 28–33.

Albert, M.L. & Bear, D. (1974). Time to understand: A case study of word deafness with reference to the role of time in auditory comprehension. *Brain, 97,* 373–384.

Ansell, B.J. (1991). Slow-to-recover brain-injured patients: Rationale for treatment. *Journal of Speech and Hearing Research, 34,* 1017–1022.

Ansell, B.J. & Flowers, C.R. (1982a). Aphasic adults' understanding of complex adverbial sentences. *Brain and Language, 15,* 82–91.

Ansell, B.J. & Flowers, C.R. (1982b). Aphasic adults' use of heuristic and structural linguistic cues for sentence analysis. *Brain and Language, 16,* 61–72.

Armus, S.R., Brookshire, R.H., & Nicholas, L.E. (1989). Aphasic and nonbrain-damaged adults' knowledge of scripts for common situations. *Brain and Language, 36,* 518–528.

Barton, M., Maruszewski, M., & Urrea, D. (1969). Variation of stimulus context and its effect on word finding ability in aphasics. *Cortex, 5,* 351–365.

Basso, A., Capitani, E., & Vignolo, L.A. (1979). Influence of rehabilitation on language skills in aphasic patients: A controlled study. *Archives of Neurology, 36,* 190–196.

Baum, S.R. (1989). On-line sensitivity to local and long-distance syntactic dependencies in Broca's aphasia. *Brain and Language, 37,* 327–338.

Baum, S.R., Daniloff, J.K., Daniloff, R., & Lewis, J. (1982). Sentence comprehension by Broca's aphasics: Effects of some suprasegmental variables. *Brain and Language, 17,* 261–271.

Benson, D.F. (1979). Aphasia rehabilitation (editorial). *Archives of Neurology, 36,* 187–189.

Benton, A.L., Smith, K.C., & Lang, M. (1972). Stimulus characteristics and object naming in aphasic patients. *Journal of Communication Disorders, 5,* 19–24.

Berstein-Ellis, E., Wertz, R.T., & Shubitowski, Y. (1987). More pace, less fillers: A verbal strategy for a high-level aphasic patient. In R.H. Brookshire (ed.), *Clinical Aphasiology, Vol. 17* (pp. 12–22). Minneapolis, MN: BRK.

Birch, H.G. & Lee, M. (1955). Cortical inhibition in expressive aphasia. *A.M.A. Archives of Neurology and Psychiatry, 74,* 514–517.

Bisiach, E. (1966). Perceptual factors in the pathogenesis of anomia. *Cortex, 2,* 90–95.

Blumstein, S.E., Katz, B., Goodglass, H., Shrier, R., & Dworetsky, B. (1985). The effects of slowed speech on auditory comprehension in aphasia. *Brain and Language, 24,* 246–265.

Blumstein, S.E., Goodglass, H., Statlender, S., & Biber, C. (1983). Comprehension strategies determining reference in aphasia: a study of reflexivization. *Brain and Language, 18,* 115–127.

Blumstein, S.E., Milberg, W., & Shrier, R. (1982). Semantic processing in aphasia: Evidence from an auditory lexical decision task. *Brain and Language, 17,* 301–315.

Boller, F., Vrtunski, B., Patterson, M., & Kim, Y. (1979). Paralinguistic aspects of auditory comprehension in aphasia. *Brain and Language, 7,* 164–174.

Bollinger, R.L. & Stout, C.E. (1976). Response-contingent small-step treatment: Performance-based communication intervention. *Journal of Speech and Hearing Disorders, 41,* 40–51.

Boone, D.R. (1967). A plan for the rehabilitation of aphasic patients. *Archives of Physical Medicine and Rehabilitation, 48,* 410–414.

Boone, D.R. & Friedman, H.M. (1976). Writing in aphasia rehabilitation: Cursive vs. manuscript. *Journal of Speech and Hearing Disorders, 41,* 523–529.

Bottenberg, D., Lemme, M., & Hedberg, N. (1987). Effect of story on narrative discourse of aphasic adults. In R.H. Brookshire (ed.), *Clinical Aphasiology, Vol. 17* (pp. 202–209). Minneapolis, MN: BRK.

Boyle, M. & Canter, G.J. (1986). Verbal context and comprehension of difficult sentences by aphasic adults: A methodological problem. In R.H. Brookshire (ed.), *Clinical Aphasiology, Vol. 16* (pp. 38–44). Minneapolis, MN: BRK.

Boyle, M. & Coelho, C.A. (1995). Application of semantic feature analysis as a treatment for aphasic dysnomia. *American Journal of Speech-Language Pathology, 4,* 94–98.

Breen, K. & Warrington, E.K. (1994). A study of anomia: Evidence for a distinction between nominal and propositional language. *Cortex, 30,* 231–245.

Brenneise-Sarshad, R., Nicholas, L., & Brookshire, R.H. (1991). Effects of apparent listener knowledge and picture stimuli on aphasic and nonbrain-damaged speakers' narrative discourse. *Journal of Speech and Hearing Research, 34,* 168–176.

Bricker, A.L., Schuell, H., & Jenkins, J.J. (1964). Effect of word frequency and word length on aphasic spelling errors. *Journal of Speech and Hearing Research, 7,* 183–192.

Brookshire, R.H. (1997). An *introduction to neurogenic communication disorders* (5th ed.). St. Louis, MO: Mosby Year Book.

Brookshire, R.H. (1971a). Effects of delay of reinforcement on probability learning by aphasic subjects. *Journal of Speech and Hearing Research, 14,* 92–105.

Brookshire, R.H. (1971b). Effects of trial time and inter-trial interval on naming by aphasic subjects. *Journal of Communication Disorders, 3,* 289–301.

Brookshire, R.H. (1972). Effects of task difficulty on the naming performance of aphasic subjects. *Journal of Speech and Hearing Research, 15,* 551–558.

Brookshire, R.H. (1974). Differences in responding to auditory materials among aphasic patients. *Acta Symbolica, 5,* 1–18.

Brookshire, R.H. (1976a). The role of auditory functions in rehabilitation of aphasic individuals. In R.T. Wertz & M. Collins (eds.), *Clinical aphasiology conference proceedings 1972.* Madison, WI: Clinical Aphasiology Conference.

Brookshire, R.H. (1976b). Effects of task difficulty on sentence comprehension performance of aphasic subjects. *Journal of Communication Disorders, 9,* 167–173.

Brookshire, R.H. (1977). A system for coding and recording events in patient-clinician interactions during aphasia treatment sessions. In M. Sullivan & M.S. Kommers (eds.), *Rationale for adult aphasia therapy*. Omaha, University of Nebraska Medical Center.

Brookshire, R.H. & Lommel, M. (1974). Perception of sequences of visual temporal and auditory spatial stimuli by aphasic, right hemisphere damaged, and non-brain-damaged subjects. *Journal of Communication Disorders, 7*, 155–169.

Brookshire, R.H. & Nicholas, L.S. (1978). Effects of clinician request and feedback behavior on responses of aphasic individuals in speech and language treatment sessions. In R.H. Brookshire (ed.), *Clinical aphasiology conference proceedings*. Minneapolis, MN: BRK.

Brookshire, R.H. & Nicholas, L.E. (1980). Sentence verification and language comprehension of aphasic persons. In R.H. Brookshire (ed.), *Clinical aphasiology conference proceedings*, Minneapolis, MN: BRK.

Brookshire, R.H. & Nicholas, L.E. (1981). Verification of active and passive sentences by aphasic and monoaphasic subjects. *Journal of Speech and Hearing Disorders, 23*, 878–893.

Brookshire, R.H. & Nicholas, L.E. (1984). Comprehension of directly and indirectly stated ideas and details in discourse by brain-damaged and non-brain-damaged listeners. *Brain and Language, 21*, 21–36.

Cannito, M.P., Hough, M., Vogel, D., & Pierce, R.S. (1996). Contextual influences on auditory comprehension of reversible passive sentences in aphasia. *Aphasiology, 10*, 235–252.

Cannito, M.P., Jarecki, J.M., & Pierce, R.S. (1986). Effects of thematic structure on syntactic comprehension in aphasia. *Brain and Language, 27*, 38–49.

Cannito, M.P., Vogel, D., & Pierce, R.S. (1989). Sentence comprehension in context: Influence of proper visual stimulation? In T.E. Prescott (ed.), *Clinical aphasiology, Vol. 18* (pp. 433–446). Boston, MA: Little, Brown.

Caplan, D. & Evans, K.L. (1990). The effects of syntactic structure on discourse comprehension in patients with parsing impairments. *Brain and Language, 39*, 206–234.

Caplan, D. & Hanna, J.E. (1996). Sentence production by aphasic patients in a contained task. *Brain and Language, 63*, 184–218.

Cappa, S.F., Nespor, M., Ielasi, W., & Miozza, A. (1997). The representation of stress: Evidence from an aphasic patient. *Cognition, 65*, 1–13.

Caramazza, A. & Berndt, R.S. (1978). Semantic and syntactic processes in aphasia: A review of the literature. *Psychological Review, 85*, 898–918.

Caramazza, A., Berndt, R.S., & Brownell, H.H. (1982). The semantic deficit hypothesis: Perceptual parsing and object classification by aphasic patients. *Brain and Language, 15*, 161–189.

Caramazza, A. & Zurif, E.B. (1976). Dissociation of algorithmic and heuristic processes in language comprehension: Evidence from aphasia. *Brain and Language, 3*, 572–582.

Chenery, H.J., Ingram, J.C.L., & Murdoch, B.E. (1990). Automatic and volitional semantic processing in aphasia. *Brain and Language, 38*, 215–232.

Chieffi, S., Carlomagno, S., Silveri, M.C., & Gainotti, G. (1989). The influence of semantic and perceptual factors on lexical comprehension in aphasic and right brain-damaged patients. *Cortex, 25*, 592–598.

Clark, A.E. & Flowers, C.R. (1987). The effect of semantic

redundancy on auditory comprehension in aphasia. In R.H. Brookshire (ed.), *Clinical aphasiology, Vol. 17* (pp. 174–179). Minneapolis, MN: BRK.

Coelho, C.A., McHugh, R.E., & Boyle, M. (2000). Application of semantic feature analysis as a treatment for aphasic dysnomia: A replication. *Aphasiology, 14*, 133–142.

Corlew, M.M. & Nation, J.E. (1975). Characteristics of visual stimuli and naming performance in aphasic adults. *Cortex, 11*, 186–191.

Correia, L., Brookshire, R.H., & Nicholas, L.E. (1989). The effects of picture content on descriptions by aphasic and non-brain-damaged speakers. In R.H. Brookshire (ed.), *Clinical aphasiology, Vol. 18* (pp. 447–462). Boston, MA: Little, Brown.

Correia, L., Brookshire, R.H., & Nicholas, L.E. (1990). Aphasic and nonbrain-damaged adults' descriptions of aphasia test pictures and genderbased pictures. *Journal of Speech and Hearing Disorders, 55*, 713–720.

Crosky, C.S. & Adams, M.R. (1969). A rationale and clinical methodology for selecting vocabulary stimulus material for individual aphasic patients. *Journal of Communication Disorders, 2*, 340–343.

Curtiss, S., Jackson, C.A., Kempler, D., Hanson, W.R., & Metter, E.J. (1986). Length vs. structural complexity in sentence comprehension in aphasia. In R.H. Brookshire (ed.), *Clinical aphasiology, Vol. 16* (pp. 45–53). Minneapolis, MN: BRK.

Darley, F.L. (1972). The efficacy of language rehabilitation in aphasia. *Journal of Speech and Hearing Disorders, 37*, 3–21.

Darley, F.L. (1975). Treatment of acquired aphasia. In W.J. Friedlander (ed.), *Advances in neurology, Vol. 7*, New York: Raven Press.

Darley, F.L. (1976). Maximizing input to the aphasic patient. In R.H. Brookshire (ed.), *Clinical aphasiology conference proceedings*. Minneapolis, MN: BRK.

Darley, F.L. (1977). A retrospective view: Aphasia. *Journal of Speech and Hearing Disorders, 42*, 161–169.

Darley, F.L. (1979). Treat or neglect. *ASHA, 21*, 628–631.

Darley, F.L. (1982). *Aphasia*. Philadelphia: WB Saunders.

Darley, F.L., Sherman, D., & Siegal, G.M. (1959). Scaling of abstraction level of single words. *Journal of Speech and Hearing Disorders, 2*, 161–167.

Davis, G.A. (1993). *A survey of adult aphasia and related language disorders* (2nd ed.). Englewood Cliffs, NJ: Prentice-Hall.

Deloche, G. & Seron, X. (1981). Sentence understanding and knowledge of the world: Evidence from a sentence-picture matching task performed by aphasic patients. *Brain and Language, 14*, 57–69.

DeRenzi, E. & Vignolo, L.A. (1962). The Token Test: A sensitive test to detect receptive disturbances in aphasics. *Brain, 85*, 665–678.

Duffy, J.R. & Watkins, L.B. (1984). The effect of response choice relatedness on pantomime and verbal recognition ability in aphasic patients. *Brain and Language, 21*, 291–306.

Duffy, R.J. & Ulrich, S.R. (1976). A comparison of impairments in verbal comprehension, speech, reading, and writing in adult aphasics. *Journal of Speech and Hearing Disorders, 41*, 110–119.

Dumond, D.L., Hardy, J.C., & Van Demark, A.A. (1978). Presentation by order of difficulty of test tasks to persons with aphasia. *Journal of Speech and Hearing Research, 21*, 350–360.

Eccles, J.C. (1973). *The understanding of the brain*. New York: McGraw-Hill.

Eisenson, J. (1973). *Adult aphasia: Assessment and treatment*. Englewood Cliffs, NJ: Prentice-Hall.

Ernest-Baron, C.R., Brookshire, R.H., & Nicholas, L.E. (1987). Story structure and retelling of narratives by aphasic and non-brain-damaged adults. *Journal of Speech and Hearing Research, 30*, 44–49.

Foldi, N.S. (1987). Appreciation of pragmatic interpretations of indirect commands: Comparison of right and left hemisphere brain-damaged patients. *Brain and Language, 31*, 88–108.

Freed, D.B., Marshall, R.C., & Nippold, M.A. (1995). Comparison of personalized cuing on the facilitation of verbal labeling by aphasic subjects. *Journal of Speech and Hearing Research, 38*, 1081–1090.

Friederici, A.D. (1983). Aphasics' perception of words in sentential context: Some real time processing evidence. *Neuropsychologia, 21*, 351–358.

Friederici, A.D. & Graetz, P.A.M. (1987). Processing passive sentences in aphasia: Deficits and strategies. *Brain and Language, 30*, 93–105.

Friederici, A.D., Schoenle, P.W., & Goodglass, H. (1981). Mechanisms underlying writing and speech in aphasia. *Brain and Language, 13*, 212–222.

Gallaher, A.J. (1981). Syntactic versus semantic performances of agrammatic Broca's aphasics on tests of constituent-element-ordering. *Journal of Speech and Hearing Research, 2*, 217–223.

Gallaher, A.J. & Canter, G.J. (1982). Reading and lexical comprehension in Broca's aphasia: Lexical versus syntactical errors. *Brain and Language, 17*, 183–192.

Gardner, B. & Brookshire, R.H. (1972). Effects of unisensory and multisensory presentation of stimuli upon naming by aphasic patients. *Language and Speech, 15*, 342–357.

Gardner, H. (1973). The contribution of operativity to naming capacity in aphasic patients. *Neuropsychologia, 11*, 213–220.

Gardner, H., Albert, M.L., & Weintraub, S. (1975). Comprehending a word: The influence of speed and redundance on auditory comprehension in aphasia. *Cortex, 11*, 155–162.

Gerratt, B.R. & Jones, D. (1987). Aphasic performance on a lexical decision task: Multiple meanings and word frequency. *Brain and Language, 30*, 106–115.

Glaser, R., Stoioff, M., & Weidner, W.E. (1974). The effect of controlled auditory stimulation on the auditory recognition of adult aphasic subjects. *Acta Symbolica, 5*, 57–68.

Glosser, G., Wiener, M., & Kaplan, E. (1988). Variations in aphasic language behaviors. *Journal of Speech and Hearing Disorders, 53*, 115–124.

Goldstein, K. (1948). *Language and language disturbances*. New York: Grune & Stratton.

Golper, L. & Rau, M.T. (1983). Systematic analysis of cuing strategies in aphasia: Taking your "cue" from the patient. In R.H. Brookshire (ed.), *Clinical aphasiology conference proceedings*. Minneapolis, MN: BRK.

Goodglass, H. (1968). Studies on the grammar of aphasics. In S. Rosenberg & J. Koplin (eds.), *Developments in applied psycholinguistic research*. New York: Macmillan.

Goodglass, H. & Baker, E. (1976). Semantic field, naming, and auditory comprehension in aphasia. *Brain and Language, 3*, 359–374.

Goodglass, H., Barton, M.I., & Kaplan, E.F. (1968). Sensory modality and object naming in aphasia. *Journal of Speech and Hearing Research, 11*, 488–496.

Goodglass, H. & Berko, J. (1960). Agrammatism and inflectional morphology in English. *Journal of Speech and Hearing Research, 3*, 257–267.

Goodglass, H., Christiansen, J.A., & Gallagher, R. (1993). Comparison of morphology and syntax in free narrative and structured tests: Fluent vs. nonfluent aphasics. *Cortex, 29*, 377–407.

Goodglass, H., Fodor, I.G., & Schuloff, C. (1967). Prosodic factors in grammar: Evidence from aphasia. *Journal of Speech and Hearing Research, 10*, 5–20.

Goodglass, H., Gleason, J.B., & Hyde, M.R. (1970). Some dimensions of auditory language comprehension in aphasia. *Journal of Speech and Hearing Research, 13*, 595–606.

Goodglass, H. & Hunt, J. (1958). Grammatical complexity and aphasic speech. *Word, 14*, 197–207.

Goodglass, H., Klein, B., Carey, P.W., & Jones, K.J. (1966). Specific semantic word categories in aphasia. *Cortex, 2*, 74–89.

Graham, L.F., Holtzapple, P., & LaPointe, L.L. (1987). Does contextually related action facilitate auditory comprehension? Performance across three conditions by high and low comprehenders. In R.H. Brookshire (ed.), *Clinical aphasiology, Vol. 17* (pp. 180–187). Minneapolis, MN: BRK.

Green, E. & Boller, F. (1974). Features of auditory comprehension in severely impaired aphasics. *Cortex, 10*, 133–145.

Grossman, M. & Haberman, S. (1982). Aphasics' selected deficits in appreciating grammatical agreements. *Brain and Language, 16*, 109–120.

Hageman, C.F. & Lewis, D.L. (1983). The effects of intrastimulus pause on the quality of auditory comprehension in aphasia. In R.H. Brookshire (ed.), *Clinical aphasiology conference proceedings*. Minneapolis, MN: BRK.

Halpern, H. (1965a). Effect of stimulus variables on dysphasic verbal errors. *Perceptual and Motor Skills, 21*, 291–298.

Halpern, H. (1965b). Effect of stimulus variables on verbal perseveration of dysphasic subjects. *Perceptual and Motor Skills, 20*, 421–429.

Hanlon, R.E., Brown, J.W., & Gerstman, L.J. (1990). Enhancement of naming in nonfluent aphasia through gesture. *Brain and Language, 38*, 298–314.

Helm, N. (1979). Management of palilalia with a pacing board. *Journal of Speech & Hearing Disorders, 44*, 350–353.

Helm-Estabrooks, N. (1981). "Show me the . . . whatever": Some variables affecting auditory comprehension scores of aphasic patients. In R.H. Brookshire (ed.), *Clinical aphasiology conference proceedings*, Minneapolis, MN: BRK.

Helm-Estabrooks, N. (1984). Treatment of the aphasias. *Seminars in Neurology, 4*, 196–202.

Helmick, J.W. & Wipplinger, M. (1975). Effects of stimulus repetition on the naming behavior of an aphasic adult: A clinical report. *Journal of Communication Disorders, 8*, 23–29.

Hendrick, D.L., Christman, M.A., & Augustine, L. (1973). Programming for the antecedent event in therapy. *Journal of Speech and Hearing Disorders, 38*, 339–344.

Hickok, G. & Avrutin, S. (1995). Representation, referentiality, and processing in agrammatic comprehension: Two case studies. *Brain and Language, 50*, 10–26.

Hickok, G., Zurif, E.B., & Canseco-Gonzalez, E. (1993). Traces in the explanation of comprehension of Broca's aphasia. *Brain and Language, 45*, 371–395.

Holland, A.L. (1975). The effectiveness of treatment in aphasia. In R.H. Brookshire (ed.), *Clinical aphasiology conference proceedings*, Minneapolis, MN: BRK.

Holland, A.L., Fromm, D.S., DeRuyter, F., & Stein, M. (1996). Treatment efficacy: Aphasia. *Journal of Speech and Hearing Research, 39*, S27–S36.

Holland, A.L. & Sonderman, J.C. (1974). Effects of a program based on the Token Test for teaching comprehension skills to aphasics. *Journal of Speech and Hearing Research, 17*, 589–598.

Hough, M.S. (1989). Category concept generation in aphasia: The influence of context. *Aphasiology, 3*, 553–568.

Hough, M.S. (1990). Narrative comprehension in adults with right and left hemisphere brain-damage: Theme organization. *Brain and Language, 38*, 253–277.

Hough, M.S. & Pierce, R.S. (1989). Contextual influences on category concept generation in aphasia. In T.E. Prescott (ed.), *Clinical aphasiology, Vol. 18* (pp. 507–519). Boston, MA: Little, Brown.

Hough, M.S., Pierce, R.S., & Cannito, M.D. (1989). Contextual influences in aphasia: Effects of predictive versus nonpredictive narratives. *Brain and Language, 36*, 325–334.

Jenkins, J., Jiménez-Pabón, E., Shaw, R., & Sefer, J. (1975). *Schuell's aphasia in adults* (2nd ed.). New York: Harper & Row.

Johnson, J., Sommers, R., & Weidner, W. (1977). Dichotic ear preference in aphasia. *Journal of Speech and Hearing Research, 20*, 116–129.

Katsuki-Nakamura, J., Brookshire, R.H., & Nicholas, L.E. (1988). Comprehension of monologues and dialogues by aphasic listeners. *Journal of Speech and Hearing Disorders, 53*, 408–415.

Kearns, K. & Hubbard, D.J. (1977). A comparison of auditory comprehension tasks in aphasia. In R.H. Brookshire (ed.), *Clinical aphasiology conference proceedings*. Minneapolis, MN: BRK.

Kimelman, M.D.Z. (1991). The role of target word stress in auditory comprehension by aphasic listeners. *Journal of Speech and Hearing Research, 34*, 334–339.

Kimelman, M.D.Z. & McNeil, M.R. (1987). Emphatic stress comprehension on adult aphasia: A successful constructive replication. *Journal of Speech and Hearing Research, 30*, 295–300.

Kimelman, M.D.Z. & McNeil, M.R. (1989). Contextual influences on the audio comprehension of normally stressed targets by aphasic listeners. in T.E. Prescott (ed.), *Clinical aphasiology, Vol. 18* (pp. 407–420). Boston, MA: Little, Brown.

Kohn, S.E. & Goodglass, H. (1985). Picture-naming in aphasia. *Brain and Language, 24*, 266–283.

Kohn, S.E., Lorch, M.P., & Pearson, D.M. (1989). Verb finding in aphasia. *Cortex, 25*, 57–69.

Kolk, H.H.J. & Friederici, A.D. (1985). Strategy and impairment in sentence understanding by Broca's and Wernicke's aphasics. *Cortex, 21*, 47–67.

Kudo, T. (1984). The effect of semantic plausibility on sentence comprehension in aphasia. *Brain and Language, 21*, 208–218.

Lambrecht, K.J. & Marshall, R.C. (1983). Comprehension in severe aphasia: A second look. In R.H. Brookshire (ed.), *Clinical aphasiology conference proceedings*. Minneapolis, MN: BRK.

LaPointe, L.L. (1977). Base-10 programmed stimulation: Task specification, scoring, and plotting performance in aphasia therapy. *Journal of Speech and Hearing Disorders, 42*, 90–105.

LaPointe, L.L. (1978a). Aphasia therapy: Some principles and strategies for treatment. In D.F. Johns (ed.), *Clinical management of neurogenic communicative disorders*. Boston, MA: Little, Brown.

LaPointe, L.L. (1978b). Multiple baseline designs. In R.H. Brookshire (ed.), *Clinical aphasiology conference proceedings*. Minneapolis, MN: BRK.

LaPointe, L.L. (1983). Aphasic intervention in adults: historical, present, and future approaches. In J. Miller, D.E. Yoder, & R. Schiefelbusch (eds.), *Contemporary issues in language intervention* (ASHA Reports No. 12). Rockville, MD: American Speech-Language-Hearing Association.

LaPointe, L.L., Horner, J., & Lieberman, R. (1977). Effects of ear presentation and delayed response on the processing of Token Test commands. In R.H. Brookshire (ed.), *Clinical aphasiology conference proceedings*. Minneapolis, MN: BRK.

Lapointe, L.L., Rothi, L.J., & Campanella, D.J. (1978). The effects of repetition of Token Test commands on auditory comprehension. In R.H. Brookshire (ed.), *Clinical aphasiology conference proceedings*. Minneapolis, MN: BRK.

Lasky, E.Z., Weidner, W.E., & Johnson, J.P. (1976). Influence of linguistic complexity, rate of presentation, and interphrase pause time on auditory verbal comprehension of adult aphasic patients. *Brain and Language, 3*, 386–396.

Le Dorze, G., Boulay, N., Gaudreau, & Brassard, C. (1994). The contrasting effects of a semantic versus formal-semantic technique for the facilitation of naming in a case of anomia. *Aphasiology, 8*, 127–142.

Leonard, C.L. & Baum, S.R. (1997). The influence of phonological and orthographic information on auditory lexical access in brain-damaged patients: A preliminary investigation. *Aphasiology, 11*, 1031–1042.

Lesser, R. (1978). *Linguistic investigations of aphasia*. New York: Elsevier.

Lesser, R. (1974). Verbal comprehension in aphasia: An English version of three Italian tests. *Cortex, 10*, 247–263.

Li, E.C. & Canter, G.J. (1991). Varieties of errors produced by aphasic patients in phonemic cuing. *Aphasiology, 5*, 51–61.

Li, E.C. & Williams, S.E. (1989). The efficacy of two types of cues in aphasic patients. *Aphasiology, 3*(7), 619–626.

Li, E.C. & Williams, S.E. (1990). The effects of grammatic class and cue type on cuing responsiveness in aphasia. *Brain and Language, 38*, 48–60.

Liles, B.Z. & Brookshire, R.H. (1975). The effects of pause time on auditory comprehension of aphasic subjects. *Journal of Communication Disorders, 8*, 221–235.

Linebaugh, C.W. (1986). Variability of error patterns on two formats of picture-to-word matching. In R.H. Brookshire (ed.), *Clinical aphasiology, Vol. 16* (pp. 181–189). Minneapolis, MN: BRK.

Linebaugh, C. & Lehner, L. (1977). Cuing hierarchies and word retrieval: A therapy program. In R.H. Brookshire (ed.), *Clinical aphasiology conference proceedings*, Minneapolis, MN: BRK.

Lott, S.N., Friedman, R.B., & Linebaugh, G.W. (1994). Rationale and efficacy of a tactile-kinesthetic treatment for alexia. *Aphasiology, 8,* 181–196.

Loverso, F.L. & Prescott, T.E. (1981). The effect of alerting signals on left brain damaged (aphasic) and normal subjects' accuracy and response time to visual stimuli. In R.H. Brookshire (ed.), *Clinical aphasiology conference proceedings.* Minneapolis, MN: BRK.

Lowell, S., Beeson, P.M., & Holland, A.L. (1995). The efficacy of a semantic cuing procedure on naming performance of adults with aphasia. *American Journal of Speech-Language Pathology, 4,* 109–114.

Mack, J.L. (1982). The comprehension of locative prepositions in nonfluent and fluent aphasia. *Brain and Language, 14,* 18–92.

Marshall, J.C. & Newcombe, F. (1966). Syntactic and semantic errors in paralexia. *Neuropsychologia, 4,* 169–176.

Marshall, J., Pring, T., & Chiat, S. (1998). Verb retrieval and sentence production in aphasia. *Brain and Language, 63,* 159–183.

Marshall, R.C. (1976). Word retrieval behavior of aphasic adults. *Journal of Speech and Hearing Disorders, 41,* 444–451.

Marshall, R.C. & King, P.S. (1973). Effects of fatigue produced by isokinetic exercise on the communication ability of aphasic adults. *Journal of Speech and Hearing Research, 16,* 222–230.

Marshall, R.C. & Tompkins, C.A. (1982). Verbal self-correction behaviors of fluent and nonfluent aphasic subjects. *Brain and Language, 15,* 292–306.

Marshall, R.C., Tompkins, C.A., & Phillips, D.S. (1980). Effects of scheduling on the communication assessment of aphasic patients. *Journal of Communication Disorders, 13,* 105–114.

Marshall, R.C., Wertz, R.T., Weiss, D.G., Aten, J.L., Brookshire, R.H., Garcia-Bunuel, L., Holland, W.L., Kurtzke, J.F., LaPointe, L.L., Milianti, F.J., Brannegan, R., Greenbaum, H., Voge, D., Carter, J., Barnes, N.S., & Goodman, R. (1989). Home treatment for aphasia patients by trained nonprofessionals. *Journal of Speech and Hearing Disorders, 54,* 462–470.

Martin, A.D. (1975). A critical evaluation of therapeutic approaches to aphasia. In R.H. Brookshire (ed.), *Clinical aphasiology conference proceedings.* Minneapolis, MN: BRK.

Martin, R.C. & Feher, E. (1990). The consequences of reduced memory span for the comprehension of semantic versus syntactic information. *Brain and Language, 38,* 1–20.

Massaro, M.E. & Tompkins, C.A. (1992). Feature analysis for treatment of communication disorders in traumatically brain-injured patients: An efficacy study. *Clinical Aphasiology, 22,* 245–256.

McCall, D., Cox, D.M., Shelton, J.R., & Weinrich, M. (1997). The influence of syntactic and semantic information on picture-naming performance in aphasic patients. *Aphasiology, 11,* 581–600.

McDearmon, J.R. & Potter, R.E. (1975). The use of representational prompts in aphasia therapy. *Journal of Communication Disorders, 8,* 199–206.

McNeil, M., Darley, F.L., Rose, D.E., & Olsen, W.O. (1979a, June). Effects of diotic intensity increments on auditory processing deficits in aphasia. Paper presented to the Ninth Annual Clinical Aphasiology Conference, Phoenix, AZ.

McNeil, M., Darley, F.L., Rose, D.E., & Olsen, W.O. (1979b, June). Effects of selective binaural intensity variations on auditory processing in aphasia. Paper presented to the Ninth Annual Clinical Aphasiology Conference, Phoenix, AZ.

McNeil, M. & Hageman, C. (1979). Prediction and pattern of auditory processing deficits on the Revised Token Test. In R.H. Brookshire (ed.), *Clinical aphasiology conference proceedings.* Minneapolis, MN: BRK.

McNeil, M.R. & Kimelman, M.D.Z. (1986). Toward an integrative information-processing structure of auditory comprehension and processing in adult aphasia. *Seminars in Speech and Language, 7,* 123–146.

McNeil, M.R., Odell, K., & Tseng, C.H. (1990). Toward the integration of resource allocation into a general model of aphasia. In T. Prescott (ed.), *Clinical aphasiology, Vol. 20* (pp. 21–39). Austin, TX: Pro-Ed.

McNeil, M. & Prescott, T.E. (1978). *Revised token test.* Baltimore: University Park Press.

Miceli, G., Silveri, M.C., Nocentini, U., & Caramaza, A. (1988). Patterns of dissociation in comprehension and production of nouns and verbs. *Aphasiology, 2,* 207–220.

Miceli, G., Silveri, M.C., Villi, G., & Caramaza, A. (1984). On the basis for the agrammatic's difficulty in producing main verbs. *Cortex, 20,* 207–220.

Mills, R. (1977). The effects of environmental sound on the naming performance of aphasic subjects. In R.H. Brookshire (ed.), *Clinical aphasiology conference proceedings.* Minneapolis, MN: BRK.

Mills, R.H., Knox, A.W., Juola, J.F., & Salmon, S.J. (1979). Cognitive loci of impairments in picture naming by aphasic subjects. *Journal of Speech and Hearing Research, 22,* 73–87.

Moore, W.H. (1996). The effects of multimodality stimulation on hemispheric alpha asymmetries of aphasic and normal subjects. *Aphasiology, 10,* 671–686.

Morris, J., Franklin, S., Ellis, A.W., Turner, J.E., & Bailey, P.J. (1996). Remediating a speech perception deficit in an aphasic patient. *Aphasiology, 10,* 137–158.

Naeser, M.A., Mazurskil, P., Goodglass, H., Peraino, M., Laughlin, S., & Leaper, W.C. (1987). Auditory syntactic comprehension in nine aphasia groups (with CT scans) and children: Differences in degree but not order of difficulty observed. *Cortex, 23,* 359–380.

Nicholas, L.E. & Brookshire, R.H. (1986a). Consistency of the effects of rate of speech on brain-damaged adults' comprehension of narrative discourse. *Journal of Speech and Hearing Research, 29,* 462–470.

Nicholas, L.E. & Brookshire, R.H. (1986b). Types of errors in multiple sentence reading comprehension of aphasic adults. In R.H. Brookshire (ed.), *Clinical aphasiology, Vol. 16* (pp. 190–195). Minneapolis, MN: BRK.

Nicholas, L. & Brookshire, R.H. (1983). Syntactic simplification and context: Effects on sentence comprehension by aphasic adults. In R.H. Brookshire (ed.), *Clinical aphasiology conference proceedings.* Minneapolis, MN: BRK.

Nickels, L. & Howard, D. (1995). Aphasic naming: What matters? *Neuropsychologia, 33,* 1281–1303.

Noll, J.D. & Hoops, H.R. (1967). Aphasic grammatical involvement as indicated by spelling ability. *Cortex, 3,* 419–432.

North, B. (1971). Effects of stimulus redundancy on naming disorders in aphasia. Unpublished doctoral dissertation, Boston University.

Orpwood, L. & Warrington, E.K. (1995). Word specific impairments in naming and spelling but not reading. *Cortex, 31,* 239–265.

Parisi, D. & Pizzamiglio, L. (1970). Syntactic comprehension in aphasia. *Cortex, 6,* 204–215.

Pashek, G.V. & Brookshire, R.H. (1982). Effect of rate and stress on auditory paragraph comprehension in aphasic individuals. *Journal of Speech and Hearing Research, 25,* 377–383.

Peach, R.K., Canter, G.J., & Gallaher, A.J. (1988). Comprehension of sentence structure in anomic and conduction aphasia. *Brain and Language, 35,* 119–137.

Pierce, R.S. (1981). Facilitating the comprehension of tense related sentences in aphasia. *Journal of Speech and Hearing Disorders, 46,* 364–368.

Pierce, R.S. (1982). Facilitating the comprehension of syntax in aphasia. *Journal of Speech and Hearing Research, 25,* 408–413.

Pierce, R.S. (1983). Decoding syntax during reading in aphasia. *Journal of Communication Disorders, 16,* 181–188.

Pierce, R.S. (1988). Influence of prior and subsequent context on comprehension in aphasia. *Aphasiology, 2,* 577–582.

Pierce, R.S. (1991). Short Report: Contextual influences during comprehension in aphasia. *Aphasiology, 5,* 379–381.

Pierce, R.S. & Beekman, L.A. (1985). Effects of linguistic and extralinguistic context on semantic and syntactic processing in aphasia. *Journal of Speech and Hearing Research, 28,* 250–254.

Pizzamiglio, L. & Appicciafuoco, A. (1971). Semantic comprehension in aphasia. *Journal of Communication Disorders, 3,* 280–288.

Podraza, B.L. & Darley, F.L. (1977). Effect of auditory prestimulation on naming in aphasia. *Journal of Speech and Hearing Research, 20,* 669–683.

Poeck, K., Huber, W., & Willmes, K. (1989). Outcome of intensive language treatment in aphasia. *Journal of Speech and Hearing Disorders, 54,* 471–479.

Poeck, K. & Pietron, H. (1981). The influence of stretched speech presentation on Token Test performance of aphasic and right brain damaged patients. *Neuropsychologia, 19,* 135–136.

Porch, B.E. (1967). *Porch index of communicative ability.* Palo Alto, CA: Consulting Psychologists Press.

Records, N.L. (1994). A measure of the contribution of a gesture to the perception of speech in listeners with aphasia. *Journal of Speech and Hearing Research, 37,* 1086–1099.

Reuterskiöld, C. (1991). The effects of emotionality on auditory comprehension in aphasia. *Cortex, 27,* 595–604.

Roberts, J.A. & Wertz, R.T. (1986). TACS: A contrastic-language treatment for aphasic adults. In R.H. Brookshire (ed.), *Clinical aphasiology, Vol. 16* (pp. 207–212). Minneapolis, MN: BRK.

Robey, R.R. (1994). The efficacy of treatment for aphasic persons: A meta-analysis. *Brain and Language, 47,* 585–608.

Robey, R.R. (1998). A meta-analysis of clinical outcomes in the treatment of aphasia. *Journal of Speech, Language and Hearing Research, 41,* 172–187.

Robey, R.R. & Schultz, M.C. (1998). A model for conducting clinical outcome research: An adaptation of the standard protocol for use in aphasiology. *Aphasiology, 12,* 787–810.

Robey, R.R., Schultz, M.C., Crawford, A.B., & Sinner, C.A. (1999). Single-subject clinical-outcome research: Designs, data, effect sizes, and analyses. *Aphasiology, 6,* 445–474.

Rolnick, M. & Hoops, H.R. (1969). Aphasia as seen by the aphasic. *Journal of Speech and Hearing Disorders, 34,* 48–53.

Rosenbek, J., LaPointe, L.L., & Wertz, R.T. (1989). *Aphasia: A clinical approach.* Boston, MA: College-Hill.

Saffran, E., M., Berndt, R.S., & Schwartz, M.F. (1989). The quantitative analysis of agrammatic production: Procedure and data. *Brain and Language, 37,* 440–479.

Salvatore, A.P. (1976). Training an aphasic adult to respond appropriately to spoken commands by fading pause duration within commands. In R.H. Brookshire (ed.), *Clinical aphasiology conference proceedings,* Minneapolis, MN: BRK.

Salvatore, A.P., Strait, M., & Brookshire, R.H. (1978). Effects of patient characteristics on delivery of Token Test commands by experienced and inexperienced examiners. *Journal of Communication Disorders, 11,* 325–333.

Santo Pietro, M.J. & Rigrodsky, S. (1982). The effects of temporal and semantic conditions of the occurrence of the error response of perseveration in adult aphasics. *Journal of Speech and Hearing Research, 25,* 184–192.

Sarno, M.T. (1974). Aphasia rehabilitation. In S. Dickson (ed.), *Communication disorders: Remedial principles and practices.* Glenview, IL: Scott Foresman.

Sarno, M.T. (1981). Recovery and rehabilitation in aphasia. In M.T. Sarno (ed.), *Acquired aphasia.* New York: Academic Press.

Schuell, H. (1953a). Auditory impairment in aphasia: Significance and retraining techniques. *Journal of Speech and Hearing Disorders, 18,* 14–21.

Schuell, H. (1953b). Aphasic difficulties understanding spoken language. *Neurology, 3,* 176–184.

Schuell, H. (1969). *Aphasia in adults* (NINDS, Monograph No. 10). *Human communication and its disorders.* Washington, DC: Department of Health, Education and Welfare, National Institutes of Health.

Schuell, H. (1973). (Revised by J.W. Sefer). *Differential diagnosis of aphasia with the Minnesota test.* Minneapolis, MN: University of Minnesota Press.

Schuell, H. (1974a). Clinical symptoms of aphasia. In L.F. Sies (ed.), *Aphasia theory and therapy: Selected lectures and papers of Hildred Schuell.* Baltimore: University Park Press.

Schuell, H. (1974b). The treatment of aphasia. In L.F. Sies (ed.), *Aphasia theory and therapy: Selected lectures and papers of Hildred Schuell.* Baltimore: University Park Press.

Schuell, H. (1974c). The development of a research program in aphasia. In L.F. Sies (ed.), *Aphasia theory and therapy: Selected lectures and papers of Hildred Schuell.* Baltimore: University Park Press.

Schuell, H. (1974d). A theoretical framework for aphasia. In L.F. Sies (ed.), *Aphasia theory and therapy: Selected lectures and papers of Hildred Schuell.* Baltimore: University Park Press.

Schuell, H., Carroll, V., & Street, B. (1955). Clinical treatment of aphasia. *Journal of Speech and Hearing Disorders, 20,* 43–53.

Schuell, H. & Jenkins, J.J. (1961a). Reduction of vocabulary in aphasia. *Brain, 84,* 243–261.

Schuell, H. & Jenkins, J.J. (1961b). Comment on "dimensions of language performance in aphasia." *Journal of Speech and Hearing Research, 4,* 295–299.

Schuell, H., Jenkins, J.J., & Jiménez-Pabón, E. (1964). *Aphasia in adults.* New York: Harper & Row.

Schuell, H., Jenkins, J.J., & Landis, L. (1961). Relationship between auditory comprehension and word frequency in aphasia. *Journal of Speech and Hearing Research, 4*, 30–36.

Schulte, E. (1986). Effects of imposed delay of response and item complexity on auditory comprehension by aphasics. *Brain and Language, 29*, 358–371.

Sherman, J.C. & Schweickert, J. (1989). Syntactic and semantic contributions to sentence comprehension in agrammatism. *Brain and Language, 37*, 419–439.

Shewan, C.M. & Canter, G.J. (1971). Effects of vocabulary, syntax, and sentence length on auditory comprehension in aphasic adults. *Cortex, 7*, 209–226.

Shewan, C.M. & Kertesz, A. (1984). Effects of speech and language treatment on recovery from aphasia. *Brain and Language, 23*, 272–299.

Siegel, G.M. (1959). Dysphasic speech responses to visual word stimuli. *Journal of Speech and Hearing Research, 2*, 152–167.

Siegenthaler, B.M. & Goldstein, J. (1967). Auditory and visual figure-background perception by adult aphasics. *Journal of Communication Disorders, 1*, 152–158.

Skelly, M. (1975). Aphasic patients talk back. *American Journal of Nursing, 75*, 1140–1142.

Smith, A. (1971). Objective indices of severity of chronic aphasia in stroke patients. *Journal of Speech and Hearing Disorders, 36*, 167–207.

Smithpeter, J.V. (1976). A clinical study of responses to olfactory stimuli in aphasic adults. In R.H. Brookshire (ed.), *Clinical aphasiology conference proceedings*. Minneapolis, MN: BRK.

Sparks, R., Goodglass, H., & Nickel, D. (1970). Ipsilateral versus contralateral extinction in dichotic listening resulting from hemisphere lesions. *Cortex, 8*, 249–260 (1970).

Spreen, O. (1968). Psycholinguistic aspects of aphasia. *Journal of Speech and Hearing Research, 11*, 467–480.

Stachowiak, F.K., Huber, W., Poeck, K., & Kerschensteiner, M. (1977). Text comprehension in aphasia. *Brain and Language, 4*, 177–195.

Stimley, M.A. & Noll, J.D. (1991). The effects of semantic and phonemic prestimulation cues on picture naming in aphasia. *Brain and Language, 41*, 496–509.

Stoicheff, M.L. (1960). Motivating instructions and language performance of dysphasic subjects. *Journal of Speech and Hearing Research, 3*, 75–85.

Swinney, D.A., Zurif, E.B., & Cutler, A. (1980). Effects of sentential stress and word class upon comprehension in Broca's aphasics. *Brain and Language, 10*, 132–144.

Taylor, M.T. (1964). Language therapy. In H.G. Burr (ed.), *The aphasic adult: Evaluation and rehabilitation*. Charlottesville, VA: Wayside Press.

Thompson, C.K., Lange, K.L., Schneider, S.L., & Shapiro, L.P. (1997). Agrammatic and non-brain-damaged subjects' verb and verb argument structure production. *Aphasiology, 11*, 473–490.

Thompson, C.K., Raymer, A., & le Grand, H. (1991). Effects of phonologically based treatment on aphasic naming deficits: A model-driven approach. In T.E. Prescott (ed.), *Clinical aphasiology, Vol. 20* (pp. 239–261). Austin, TX: Pro-Ed.

Thompson, C.K., Shapiro, L.P., Li, L., & Schendel, L. (1994). Analysis of verbs and verb-argument structure: A method for quan-

tification of aphasic language production. In P. Lemme (ed.), *Clinical aphasiology, Vol. 23* (pp. 121–140). Austin, TX: Pro-Ed.

Thompson, C.K., Shapiro, L.P., Tait, M.E., Jacobs, B., Schneider, S., & Ballard, K. (1995). A system for the linguistic analysis of agrammatic language production (Abstract). *Brain and Language, 51*, 124–127.

Thompson, R.F. (1967). *Foundations of physiological psychology*. New York: Harper & Row.

Thorndike, E.L. & Lorge, I. (1944). *The teacher's word book of 30,000 words*. New York: Columbia University.

Tikofsky, R. (1968). Basic research in aphasic behavior: Could it and should it contribute to rehabilitation. In J. Black & E. Jancosek (eds.), *Proceedings of the conference on language retraining for aphasics*. Washington, DC: Social and Rehabilitation Service, Department of Health, Education, and Welfare.

Tompkins, C.A. (1991). Redundancy enhances emotional inferencing by right- and left-hemisphere-damaged adults. *Journal of Speech and Hearing Research, 34*, 1142–1149.

Van Lancker, D.R. & Kempler, D. (1987). Comprehension of familiar phrases by left- but not by right-hemisphere damaged patients. *Brain and Language, 32*, 265–277.

Wallace, G.L. & Canter, G.J. (1985). Effects of personally relevant language materials on the performance of severely aphasic individuals. *Journal of Speech and Hearing Research, 50*, 385–390.

Waller, M.R. & Darley, F.L. (1978). The influence of context on the auditory comprehension of paragraphs by aphasic subjects. *Journal of Speech and Hearing Research, 21*, 732–745.

Webb, W.G. & Love, R.J. (1983). Reading problems in chronic aphasia. *Journal of Speech and Hearing Disorders, 48*, 164–171.

Weidner, W.E. & Jinks, A.F.G. (1983). The effects of single versus combined cue presentations on picture naming by aphasic adults. *Journal of Communication Disorders, 16*, 111–121.

Weidner, W.E. & Lasky, E.Z. (1976). The interaction of rate and complexity of stimulus on the performance of adult aphasic subjects. *Brain and Language, 3*, 34–40.

Weigl, E. (1968). On the problem of cortical syndromes: Experimental studies. In M.L. Simmel (ed.), *The reach of the mind: Essays in memory of Kurt Goldstein*. New York: Springer.

Weinstein, S. (1959). Experimental analysis of an attempt to improve speech in cases of expressive aphasia. *Neurology, 9*, 632–635.

Wepman, J.M. (1951). *Recovery from aphasia*. New York: Ronald Press.

Wepman, J.M. (1953). A conceptual model for the process involved in recovery from aphasia. *Journal of Speech and Hearing Disorders, 18*, 4–13.

Wepman, J.M. (1968). Aphasia therapy: Some relative comments and some purely personal prejudices. In J. Black & E. Jancosek (eds.), *Proceedings of the conference on language retraining for aphasics*. Washington, DC: Social and Rehabilitation Service, Department of Health, Education and Welfare.

Wepman, J.M. (1972). Aphasia therapy: A new look. *Journal of Speech and Hearing Disorders, 37*, 203–214.

Wepman, J.M. & Jones, L.V. (1961). *Studies in aphasia: An approach to testing*. Chicago: University of Chicago Education Industry Service.

Wepman, J.M., Jones, L.V., Bock, R.D., & Van Pelt, D. (1960).

Studies in aphasia: Background and theoretical formulations. *Journal of Speech and Hearing Disorders, 25,* 323–332.

Wertz, R.T. (1978). Neuropathologies of speech and language: An introduction to patient management. In D.F. Johns (ed.), *Clinical management of neurogenic communicative disorders.* Boston: Little, Brown.

Wertz, R.T. (1983). Language intervention context and setting for the aphasic adult: When? In J. Miller, D.E. Yoder, & R. Schiefelbusch (eds.), *Contemporary issues in language intervention* (ASHA Reports No. 12). Rockville, MD: American Speech-Language-Hearing Association.

Wertz, R.T. (1991). Keynote paper: Aphasiology 1990: A view from the colonies. *Aphasiology, 5,* 311–322.

Wertz, R.T., Collins, M.J., Weiss, D., Kurtzke, J.F., Friden, T., Brookshire, R.H., Pierce, J., Holtzapple, P., Hubbard, D.J., Porch, B.E., West, J.A., Davis, L., Matovitch, V., Morley, G.K., & Ressureccion, E. (1981). Veterans Administration cooperative study on aphasia: *Journal of Speech and Hearing Research, 24,* 580–594.

Wertz, R.T. & Porch, B.E. (1970). Effects of masking noise on the verbal performance of adult aphasics. *Cortex, 6,* 399–409.

Wertz, R.T., Weiss, D.G., Aten, J.L., Brookshire, R.H., Garcia-Bunuel, L., Holland, A.L., Kurtzke, J.F., LaPointe, L.L., Milianti, F.J., Brannegan, R., Greenbaum, H., Marshall, R.C., Vogel, D., Carter, J., Barnes, N.S., & Goodman, R. (1986). Comparison of clinic, home, and deferred language treatment for aphasia: A Veterans Administration cooperative study. *Archives of Neurology, 43,* 653–658.

Whitehouse, P. & Caramazza, A. (1978). Naming in aphasia: Interacting effects of form and function. *Brain and Language, 6,* 63–74.

Whitney, J.L. & Goldstein, H. (1989). Using self-monitoring to reduce dysfluencies in speakers with mild aphasia. *Journal of Speech and Hearing Disorders, 54,* 576–586.

Wilcox, J.M., Davis, G.A., & Leonard, L.B. (1978). Aphasics' comprehension of contextually conveyed meaning. *Brain and Language, 6,* 362–377.

Williams, S.E. (1984). Influence of written form on reading comprehension in aphasia. *Journal of Communication Disorders, 17,* 165–174.

Williams, S.E. & Canter, G.J. (1982). The influence of situational context on naming performance in aphasic syndromes. *Brain and Language, 17,* 92–106.

Williams, S.E. & Canter, G.J. (1987). Action-naming performance in four syndromes of aphasia. *Brain and Language, 32,* 124–136.

Wulfeck, B.B. (1988). Grammaticality judgments and sentence comprehension in agrammatic aphasia. *Journal of Speech and Hearing Research, 31,* 72–81.

Zingeser, L.B. & Berndt, R.S. (1990). Retrieval of nouns and verbs in agrammatism and anomia. *Brain and Language, 39,* 14–32.

Zurif, E.B., Caramazza, A., Myerson, R., & Calvin, J. (1974). Semantic feature representation for normal and aphasic language. *Brain and Language, 1,* 167–187.

Zurif, E., Swinney, D., Prather, P., Soloman, J., & Bushell, C. (1993). An on-line analysis of syntactic processing in Broca's and Wernicke's aphasia. *Brain and Language, 45,* 448–464.

Chapter 16

Thematic Language Stimulation Therapy

Shirley Morganstein and Marilyn Certner Smith

OBJECTIVES

Our objectives in this chapter are to provide a theoretical background for *Thematic Language Stimulation*, an intervention technique for aphasia; explain the rationale for *TLS* and delineate its various components; provide suggestions for clinical and functional communication analysis as a precursor to the use of *TLS*; and provide a template for replication of *TLS* modules and directives for implementation in aphasia therapy.

INTRODUCTION

In the preceding chapter, Duffy and Coelho present Schuell's approach to aphasia rehabilitation. Her model remains one of the major approaches to intervention even as we begin the new millennium. The current approach is based on her model. Indeed, as a graduate student in the 1960s, the senior author was privileged to have studied with Schuell during her tenure at the University of Minnesota and the Minneapolis VA Hospital. This work formed the basis of *Thematic Language Stimulation*. While some approaches to aphasia management are based on abstract or theoretical models of language, some, like Schuell's, were conceived as a result of focused clinical observation and interaction with large numbers of patients. Recently, a variety of approaches have developed in response to changes in the way we perceive aphasia and/or the demands of the new therapy milieu. Specifically, the profession of speech-language pathology is looking more closely at the *person with aphasia* and how he or she functions, rather than *the disorder of aphasia*, as did Schuell. This is not to say that Schuell did not consider the interpersonal aspects of communication—quite the contrary. However, she focused on the devastating effect of impaired communication on the psychosocial functioning of the person with aphasia, rather than an interactive analysis of the dyadic exchange.

This current focus on function has led to some specific conversational intervention techniques emphasizing the training of interaction strategies rather than the language stimulation techniques derived from Schuell's model (Aten, 1994; Cochrane & Milton, 1984). Such social, environmental, and competence approaches to aphasia intervention (Simons-Mackie, 1997; Lubinski, 1994; Kagan, 1995; Boles, 1998) emphasize the communicative dyad, rather than underlying processes. Additionally, there are group interventions (Kearns, 1994; Avent, 1997) and educational approaches (Wertz, 1986) that are designed to assist in recovery from aphasia. Selecting the right approach for *a particular* patient at *a particular* time remains a challenge for the practicing aphasia therapist (Wertz, 1991). This is due, in part, to the absence of a significant body of research that might help us reliably identify specific candidates for specific techniques.

The present *Thematic Language Stimulation (TLS)* attempts to bridge the restorative and functional approaches by combining aspects of both. In its original form, *TLS* (Morganstein & Certner-Smith, 1982) strictly adhered to the principles of therapy specified by Schuell. More recently, however, the authors have expanded the approach to emphasize more its functional and educational potential. Despite the fact that it requires a good deal of time to create, adapt, and use properly, we have found *TLS* to be a helpful tool in the education and training of therapists as well as caregivers who must continue with the management of aphasia after we are no longer able to do so.

DEFINITION

Thematic Language Stimulation (TLS) is an organized program of aphasia therapy that uses thematically related vocabulary in multimodality stimulation to improve language processing and functional communication in adults. Specifically, it begins with a select group of words related in meaning, places them in particular linguistic contexts, uses them in tasks that employ both input and output modes, and targets improvement of underlying language processes to impact on conversational success. Thus, *TLS* extends concepts originally presented by Schuell et al. (1964) and Wepman (1953, 1972). In addition, the authors have recently been influenced by the work of Edith Kaplan (1989) and Nancy Helm-Estabrooks (1991) who emphasize the *process approach* in evaluation and treatment: understanding the *why* as well as the *what* about aphasia.

Like all stimulation approaches, *TLS* places the burden of success upon the therapist, since it is she or he who provides a possible neurobiological link between what the patient *knows* and what he or she can *produce*. Theoretically, restoration of language proficiency comes about by means of carefully controlled stimulation. Stimulation targets overall improved understanding, speaking, reading, and writing. Observation of the patient's behavior during stimulation reveals information about underlying processes. Awareness of these processes has value in the development of strategies for success in conversation. Ultimately, functional communication training utilizes inferences about underlying language processes to enhance the sending and receiving of information (Wertz, 1998).

TLS THEORY

Organizing Content and Delivery

The organization of the language used for stimulation is central to *TLS*. This is accomplished in two ways: first, in establishing a relevant, thematic "core vocabulary," and second, in creating predictable, systematic linguistic stimuli for each presented task.

Thematic Content

Wepman (1972), in his *content-centered treatment approach*, believes treatment should focus on ideas. He advocates for stimulation of thought to enhance verbal production during conversation. In contrast, *TLS* requires more stringent control of content and its manipulation within the session. Such content themes heighten the saliency of the therapy, and provide a context for language stimulation and subsequent conversation.

Most aphasiologists agree that treatment content should be *personally relevant* (Schuell, 1964; Wepman, 1972). At the most basic level, people tend to have more to talk about when the subject is connected to them (Wallace & Canter, 1985). Additionally, Marshall (1994) noted that for fluent aphasic patients, personally relevant material is "comforting and helps to break the garbage in-garbage out cycle." Human beings are simply more at ease and better equipped to talk about topics that interest them most. Therefore, in choosing a *TLS* topic relevant to the person with aphasia, we establish a heightened performance "edge" for therapy, as well as a shared referent for subsequent exchanges. Most important, it reassures the individual that we know more of who he or she is than he or she may be able to tell us. This helps to

create an atmosphere of respect that affirms his or her present value in therapeutic partnership.

TLS themes may be fairly universal, such as "cooking" or "sports." However, the authors commonly create units based upon the unique interests of specific patients. For example, we once used a family interview and a few trade magazines to construct a *TLS* unit on the garbage industry for a particular patient, and it proved a great success. Sometimes, the same units can be used with other individuals who display similar interests.

A *TLS* unit usually consists of eight to ten vocabulary words, primarily nouns and verbs which are highly related to a topic. From this pool of core vocabulary, a variety of language activities, all linked to the theme, are developed for language practice. (The reader is referred to Appendix 16-1 for an example of one such unit.) Subsequently, the functional communication segment uses extensions and elaborations on this theme.

Stimulation Delivery in *TLS*

For an excellent, comprehensive discussion of Schuell's stimulation therapy principles, the reader is referred to Duffy and Coelho's chapter in this text. Several of these principles are very important in the development and execution of *TLS* units and therefore warrant further elaboration here:

1. Stimulus Adequacy
   The adequate stimulus, by definition, is one which has an intended result. Therefore, stimuli must be sufficiently intense, focused, and redundant to create a neurobiological effect. In *TLS*, such stimulus adequacy is assured in several ways. First, the high degree of functionality and relevance of content ensures saliency. Second, redundancy is ensured by the repeated semantic and syntactic elements, and the use of multiple input and output channels in stimulus/response tasks. Third, the hierarchical development of task sequences builds and extends stimuli in familiar but varied contexts.
2. Maximal Patient Response
   TLS supports this principle by providing many opportunities for the patient to respond in all modalities. In every theme, the patient is bombarded linguistically. That is, between 10 and 15 different exercises are presented for each vocabulary item. Additionally, therapists are encouraged to repeat tasks with minor adaptations from session to session.
3. Extension of Materials and Language
   Using a variety of tasks that can be rearranged and adapted for use over a period of several sessions, therapists can broaden the stimulation base without shifting out of the theme. In addition, language can be extended further by utilizing environmental materials and objects such as a real restaurant menu for the restaurant unit, or a trade magazine for a specific chosen topic.

4. Systematic and Intense Presentation

TLS activities are composed and delivered systematically in order to obtain the greatest number of accurate responses. The progression is from introductory topical conversational material, to identification of theme vocabulary, to manipulation of language in carefully adapted and sequenced multimodality tasks, and a return to conversational format, all within one session. The degree to which patients achieve high numbers of "correct" responses in therapy is dependent on patient ability to respond and on the intensity of language stimulation delivered.

Functional Communication

The stimulation-facilitation component of *TLS* therapy is not its only benefit; it is equally important for the clinician to transition to a functional context. The desire for functional change is a powerful one, shared by clinician, patient, family members, and sources of funding.

Intervention in the functional domain has become central in several models of aphasia therapy. These social and ecological models propose that the effectiveness of intervention be measured by functional communication success in natural environments, and that therapeutic interventions employ analysis and problem solving in that milieu (Boles, 1998). In contrast, more clinically based stimulation approaches still need to transition to functional communication.

In many effective therapy models, treatment includes a problem-solving component in which the clinician tries various combinations of cues and strategies to facilitate improved language function (Chapey, 1994; Holland, 1998; Kaplan, 1989; Wepman, 1972; Wertz, 1998; Tompkins, 1994). This process draws upon the very essence of our practice as speech-language pathologists: the ability to observe symptoms and behavior and apply interventions that help. In *TLS*, because we are keeping the treatment structure consistent, the process itself becomes more of a focus. Freed of the necessity of constantly learning new directions and rules of therapy for new tasks, the patient engages more easily in problem-solving activity and can concentrate more on his or her own performance issues. This consistent structure helps both the clinician and patient to develop insights that assist in facilitating functional communication behaviors.

The present authors believe that *TLS* may provide a link from clinical to functional language stimulation by manipulation of the theme. The daily segue from clinical task to relevant, theme-based conversation moves the clinician and patient back and forth between both environments. Capitalizing on what may be improved access primed in the stimulation mode, the therapist skillfully shifts the environment of practice to functional conversation. Once there, clinician and patient continue the problem-solving process, exploring successful strategies, heightening awareness, and developing insight into what is really happening at this level.

ASSESSMENT FOR *TLS*

Regardless of the theoretical basis for provision of language treatment, clinicians need specific information about language function in order to develop a program. Schuell (cited in Byng et al., 1990) proposed that treatment planning requires knowledge of which cerebral processes are impaired, the level at which performance breaks down in each modality, and the reason that performance breaks down when it does. For the present authors, this is a prescription for a process-oriented examination of both functional performance and behaviors more typically elicited in a formal test milieu. While formal aphasia tests can provide some information, clinicians would do well to heed the warning inherent in Edith Kaplan's comment that "batteries are for cars, not for people" (1991).

Assessing aphasia is one of the most complex requirements of speech-language pathologists. Competent evaluation requires astute observation of language behavior, combined with a thorough knowledge of the range of possible symptoms and how they influence communication. The speech-language pathologist must also have the knowledge and skill to manipulate the environment and explore all possible avenues of success. Thus, proper aphasia assessment bridges both domains of science and art. When the therapist has a thorough understanding of the patient's clinical and functional picture, he or she can create an effective therapeutic milieu; specifically, he or she can choose a particular approach or environment suited to the information provided by the evaluation. Moreover, endpoint recommendations are more individualized and helpful for communicative partners.

Establishing Baseline Functional Conversation

At the onset of treatment, a baseline of functional communication is obtained. Although we have used some formal instruments to measure functional communication in research or for other purposes (Yorkston & Beukelman, 1980; Taylor, 1969), our approach for *TLS* is usually more informal. That is, we believe that the experienced clinician can usually answer questions about functional communication after a relatively short period of interaction with the patient. Therefore, we provide the following guided questions for beginning clinicians:

How well does the patient initiate and sustain conversation?

Assessment of the patient's overall level of participation in a conversational exchange establishes a baseline for measuring progress and helps the clinician develop initial ideas about intervention. Therefore, the relative burden of information exchange as well as the degree to which information must be inferred needs to be determined.

How well does the patient express himself or herself verbally and nonverbally?

Assessment focuses on content. Observations address the patient's relative use of alternatives to speech when they appear in the natural course of an exchange. This information about preferred modes and relative ease of success in any mode will assist in decisions about *TLS* activity selection and order. It will also guide the way in which we introduce options for enhanced communication and how we train the communicative partner.

How well does the patient follow conversation and directions? How complex can auditory demands be before performance breaks down?

Information about comprehension informs decisions about task selection and presentation and also about adjustments that need to be made in the therapist's verbal behavior when introducing tasks, counseling the patient, and in conversation. Skilled clinicians can derive a good deal of information during conversational exchange about the intermittency of auditory processing, whether the patient is aware of a loss in understanding, and how well he or she comprehends subtleties, humor, and/or sublinguistic information.

Assessing Clinical Performance on Tasks

TLS is strongly dependent on a process approach. Therefore, we continually ask "why?" when symptoms are revealed. It is only by understanding the "why" that we can answer "what" can be done about it in treatment. Standard aphasia tests tell some of the "what" that is important, but none of the "why." In comparing the various standard aphasia instruments, a core group of subtests occur repeatedly: repetition, naming, answering yes/no to questions, etc. The value of these subtests is that they assist the clinician in differential diagnosis of aphasia. However, they do not explain what to do with people once aphasia is confirmed. Therefore, the clinician must engage in further analysis, adding probes to explore cognition, behavior, and therapeutic style in order to determine "what to do" and "where to begin" in therapy.

Formal Testing

1. Repetition
   Some people with aphasia can repeat well, and some cannot. Since *TLS* relies completely upon the objective of "language in, language out," therapists must know whether or not repetition will be a primary stimulation task, one to avoid completely, or one that will need to be adapted but can still be used successfully. Any formal test of repetition can provide the level of breakdown with respect to length and complexity of units, but further observations are required to assist in therapy decision-making. For example, if repetition is better than

spontaneous speech, the clinician has discovered a key aural-oral connection to modify speech output. If it is worse, the clinician must look elsewhere for primary input, most likely the visual modality. In addition, for many individuals with aphasia, repetition is not a "can do/can't do" phenomenon. Many "can do" once some structural stimulation requirements are met, such as slowing the rate of presentation, or face-to-face delivery, particularly for the patient with apraxia. Such observations are critical to *TLS* planning and the success that can be achieved using this approach.

2. Sentence Construction
   Most formal aphasia batteries assess the ability of the patient to create sentences given a one-, two- or three-word stimulus. Creation or expansion of verbal utterances that are substantive and grammatically correct is an objective of many treatment approaches. The clinician learns more about how best to facilitate this for a particular patient when he or she knows (a) the required length and grammatical composition of stimuli, (b) the effect of vocabulary complexity, and (c) how much and what type of verbal or visual cues are needed to facilitate performance.

3. Automatic Language
   For some patients, automatic language is far more preserved than propositional language and should be facilitated first if it will create a base of success for the patient. Knowing the ease with which automatic language can be facilitated will help with therapy task selection and sequencing. For example, fill-in tasks with multiple choice response requirements are rich in predictability, and might be considered a natural extension of automatic language material.

4. Picture Description
   A pictorial cue can be powerful for some patients in eliciting a flow of ideas. When aural-oral presentation and response is tenuous, it can provide a starting point for therapy. In addition, the contrast between narrative and spontaneous expression can be explored with respect to the complexity of ideas and vocabulary generated, and the degree of clinician-initiated cuing necessary for a response.

5. Following Instructions
   While it is desirable to minimize task instructions to the patient at each session, it is important to determine each particular patient's needs for such repetition of procedures. When we apply process parameters to listening, the logical questions to be asked are (a) how complex and lengthy can directions be? (b) will a visual cue be needed to support the verbal request? (c) how does the rate of presentation affect comprehension? and (d) is the auditory mode a strong or weak one for the patient?

6. Yes/No Reliability
   For the more severely impaired patient, ability to respond readily and consistently in a yes/no question

format is an essential skill. Indeed, for all patients, it is a valuable task for auditory, verbal, and visual stimulation. In addition, prior to construction of a *TLS* unit, the parameters of length, complexity, ease, and facilitation requirements should be noted via descriptive comments.

7. Reading Comprehension

For many individuals with aphasia, reading comprehension is a valid alternative to auditory comprehension. In this instance, treatment will first emphasize presentation of information via the visual modality rather than the more traditional auditory mode. The comparison of results on subtests that tap auditory processing of directions and commands with those that examine silent reading of sentences and paragraphs allows the clinician to decide on a preferred input mode. It is also important to compare scores obtained during testing as well as the overall ease of performance in both modalities, since this information sometimes provides a clue about a patient's "hard wiring" for processing language. For example, if visual-graphic expression is more preserved and preferred to the aural-oral system, that will be the road we follow. Additionally, for some individuals, silent reading prior to verbal performance has a priming effect. It is only when a detailed process approach is applied to tasks that such important pieces of information are learned. This information can then be applied not only to task and cue selection, but can also be shared with the person with aphasia and his or her communicative partner. Thus, treatment decisions are made based on a balancing of the patient's strengths and weaknesses (Holland, 1998).

8. Oral Reading

Oral reading is another avenue that provides an opportunity to get language in and out. Therefore, the clinician needs to know if oral reading is more preserved than speaking, and whether or not the patient can correct errors that occur in this format. For some patients, visual stimuli are more salient. In addition, when the patient and clinician share visual reference in the same context, this may reveal specific symptoms and procedures for modification.

9. Graphic Expression

Writing adds to the sources of linguistic bombardment necessary to reach a threshold for response. Integrated into the therapy program, it comes to be thought of as a welcome addition, adding to the patient's repertoire of success. For the higher-level patient, one needs to know how much and what kind of assistance is needed for the production of words, phrases, sentences, or narratives, and whether or not a self-initiated written cue aids verbal performance. Therefore, clinical and functional graphic abilities are explored fully. The therapist investigates writing and drawing not only as an augmentative communication tool, but also as a source of stimulation itself. By integrating writing at an early stage of treatment, the clinician stimulates the patient's language system in

yet another way. Many individuals with global aphasia can copy neatly and accurately. In addition, after several such trials are combined with repetition, they may even produce the target word verbally without struggle.

Formal test probes represent our minimal set of evaluative exploration in both clinical and functional domains. In addition, observation of the patient provides useful clinical insight into performance including other aspects influencing performance.

Cognitive and Behavioral Considerations

There are several non-language behaviors that have impact upon the treatment planning process. Additional knowledge about the patient's cognitive and behavioral strengths and weaknesses will influence the treatment model or approach chosen. In the case of *TLS*, such an analysis is necessary to customize both the content and delivery of therapy materials. As in the language analysis, certain behaviors are observed, described, and noted for future reference.

Patient Involvement

For some patients, the purpose of therapy is obvious, and they "get with the program" immediately, respond well to the treatment materials, and provide the clinician with evidence that she or he is on the right track. For other patients, however, lack of insight is as much an obstacle to recovery as are their symptoms. *TLS* naturally works best with insightful, motivated patients who "get it." Therefore, very early in the period of evaluation and initial phases of therapy, we note the patient's ability to connect with the disorder, comment on his or her own internal processes or performance for such behavior on task, and other types of metacognitive analyses. However, because of the way it is structured, it is also a treatment approach which can facilitate improved insight and understanding about therapeutic process. Even at the lowest level of function for this type of reflection, we offer many opportunities and indicate to the patient that such concerns are not only worthwhile but essential to recovery. We share our observations with the patient and encourage him or her to do the same. This process is important because recovery does not happen via neurobiological stimulation alone, but via the insights patients derive from their own process. Therefore, we continually ask "why" of our patients, and sometimes, they can give us an answer.

Specific Symptom Awareness

Patients are asked to modify their symptoms as part of their therapeutic process. Some modifications result from the clinician's direct intervention; others result from patients' insight into a specific symptom and their resultant focused response to it. Naturally, patients with specific symptom awareness achieve greater progress. This is a natural extension of their symptom awareness or "getting it." Indeed, such awareness has a significant impact upon how we structure material in tasks and how we cue or strategize for success. We all have memories of such moments in our therapy sessions. For example, one author recalls a former patient with conduction aphasia who taught us the value of graphomotor association by producing a dictionary of words beginning with target sounds, and using that list to aid his pronunciation of words in general.

Task Orientation and Retention

When patients have good task orientation and retention of treatment set, directions need not be repeated from day to day. Subsequently, there is a natural flow from one task to the next, and one day to the next. In addition, because of its organization, *TLS* can assist even the low-level patient to prepare himself or herself cognitively for the tasks at hand. This, in turn, sometimes engenders feelings of competence in the "knowing" of what to do. Therefore, there is value in keeping structure constant and changing the items within.

Perseveration

For some patients, perseveration is a highly problematic and unwelcome intrusion in their communication. For these patients, the semantic relatedness of *TLS* can make perseveration even worse. Typically, this tendency is discovered once treatment is underway and the clinician observes that the patient's responses, rather than demonstrating the advances in vocabulary retrieval and sentence use, contain recycled errors in word choice which are not evolving into something better. *TLS* is not an appropriate treatment approach for such an individual.

Visual Perception

Because *TLS* relies heavily on multimodality stimulation, any visual problems that affect task presentation, such as the presence of hemianopsia or the need for altered print size, should be known in advance. For some patients, it may simply be a matter of modifying the aural/oral elements and adapting visual materials. For others with severe accompanying visual impairments, *TLS* may not be effective.

TREATMENT DELIVERY

Once the clinician has completed an assessment of conversational proficiency, language, and cognitive/behavioral status, she or he is ready to incorporate this information into an organized treatment delivery plan. However, one more set of questions needs to be answered before therapy can begin:

1. *Is this person a good candidate for TLS?*
   Candidacy for *TLS* is best determined in one or two sessions of trial therapy. However, certain rules of thumb seem to be of help in deciding which patients may potentially succeed. Good candidates are generally those with no marked perseveration or semantic confusion in task performance, with good ability to understand the purpose of therapy, stable emotional status, and some amount of visual language preservation. Severity level may vary, but patients with moderate to severe difficulties appear to profit best. Although preliminary research findings suggest otherwise, we feel the technique is of value to people with either fluent or nonfluent aphasia.

2. *How should tasks be chosen and sequenced?*
   Our analysis during assessment has told us very specifically which modalities and tasks are the strongest and weakest. Therefore, in order to adhere to the principle of stimulus adequacy, we begin there. In addition, since it will prime the session for all subsequent task presentations and adaptations, the first task should be one that provides a high probability of success. If it is known, for example, that the patient does not repeat well, but that he or she can read words and phrases both silently and orally with good success, then the *TLS* exercises chosen first will require him or her to do just that. Since treatment is multimodal, the next task might begin to include aural-oral requirements, such as answering questions using the same material just practiced visually. This might be followed by a writing task at a level compatible with demonstrated skills in this modality. For example, the patient might be able to copy or write the target words as the clinician dictates them.

3. *What cues are most beneficial to achieve maximal success in treatment?*
   Since successful language stimulation should neither involve too much struggle nor be so "easy" that it does not provide a neurobiological effect, an 80% success rate is targeted in *TLS* therapy. To achieve this level of success, considerable experimentation regarding facilitatory cuing takes place. However, our assessment analysis has provided clues about the likelihood they will or won't succeed. Therefore, the clinician answers questions such as: Are visual cues more powerful than auditory ones? How much spontaneous writing is possible with and without input from dictation? When can I fade out a verbal, auditory, or visual cue and still maintain an accurate response? When we determine cuing that works at baseline, we are also determining the beginning of a cuing hierarchy. These hierarchies are individualized and will change over time as the patient progresses and needs to be challenged further. However, maintaining a high level of success throughout treatment should be a constant goal.

4. *How do I select theme and vocabulary?*
   As mentioned earlier, theme selection is based upon each patient's interests; personal relevance generates ideas and themes that provide a shared reference point for all subsequent interaction. The inclusion of material based upon the patient's input reflects respect for his or her

personal contribution to the decision about treatment needs. Themes that are more concrete or even able to be pictured are easier for patients to conceptualize. However, it is entirely possible to select complex themes and create vocabulary and tasks that can be modified to levels consistent with normal language complexity. A minimum of six and maximum of ten words are recommended.

A closed set of core vocabulary permits manipulations that fulfill some of the content and delivery principles described earlier: redundancy, multimodality presentation, and predictable task inventory. The majority of words are nouns; however, an occasional verb or adjective is also desirable. For example, if the theme were "restaurant," appropriate vocabulary words might be *waitress, tip, table, menu, appetizer, water, check, chef, and order.*

The actual tasks that we have employed in our *TLS* work are familiar to any experienced aphasia clinician. What is different is the constancy of theme that connects them all, and the systematic way in which they are employed. A complete *TLS* unit on Industry is provided as an example for your review and personal use in Appendix 16.1.

PRELIMINARY RESEARCH WITH *TLS*

According to Darley (1972, as cited in Howard, 1986) "if speech pathologists are to have a role in the management of aphasic patients, it must depend not on wishful thinking, but on unequivocal demonstration of effectiveness in significantly altering, in a favourable way, the course of recovery." Therefore, after more than 10 years of clinical exploration with *TLS*, the authors embarked on a pilot research study to explore its efficacy.

In the 1980s, it was becoming more obvious that problems in the use of large group studies were clouding our ability to judge the value of aphasia therapy. The randomized controlled trials approach in England uniformly negated any treatment effects on aphasia; in the U.S., results were only somewhat better (Whurr et al., 1992) and difficult to evaluate because of the high dropout rate resulting in small numbers, a lack of homogeneity with respect to subject groupings, and a similar lack of uniformity in the therapy approaches employed across studies (Howard, 1986). Researchers increasingly began to turn to the use of single-subject designs (McReynolds & Thompson, 1986) because of their distinct advantages: simplicity of construction, relatively short duration, the use of the subject as his or her own control, the propensity for detailed descriptions of intervention techniques, and the ability to replicate procedures more readily from patient to patient (Morganstein & Certner-Smith, 1993). In a clinical milieu such studies are also more easily accomplished than are other designs. However, Siegel and Spradlin (1985, 1987) noted that therapists often find it difficult to integrate them into a typical service delivery model. In 1993, circumstances permitted the authors of this chapter some protected time for a pilot investigation into *TLS* efficacy.

Defining Success

In the early stages of our clinical work with *TLS*, we were relatively comfortable with clinical evidence that the approach was making language more available during the execution of tasks. As sessions progressed, performance seemed better during each session and from session to session. But if *TLS*, or for that matter any restorative technique, is to be judged efficacious, it must be held to the ultimate standard: improvement in conversational speech. We found immediate difficulties in selecting functional conversation as the improvement measure, since there were few quantifiable options from which to choose, and those available seemed insensitive to discriminating what would undoubtedly be very small changes. For that reason, we rejected the *CADL* (Holland, 1980), the *CETI* (Lomas et al., 1989), and the *FCP* (Taylor, 1969). We found support, however in our frustration:

"Clinicians and investigators who wish to quantify changes in the informativeness of the connected speech of adults with aphasia in response to manipulation of experimental variables have been hampered by the scarcity of standard measures for characterizing this aspect of connected speech"

(Nicholas & Brookshire, 1993).

At the time we embarked on our study, the only published system for measuring small improvements in discourse appeared to be that proposed by Yorkston and Beukelman in 1980. In their system, the individual's response to the cookie theft picture from the *Boston Diagnostic Aphasia Examination* (Goodglass & Kaplan, 1983) is analyzed for the number of *content units* produced and for a measure of communicative efficiency which is determined by the ratio of content units per minute of discourse. Content units (CUs), or groupings of information expressed by normal speakers in response to the cookie theft picture, are finite and offer a clear index of relative performance in response to this specific picture stimulus. While there remained concerns regarding the differences between connected speech elicited in this manner and that elicited in a conversational exchange, a content unit analysis seemed our best method of defining success: communication of information in discourse.

Design Choice

In general, single-subject studies investigating the efficacy of a particular approach to aphasia intervention employ either a reversal/withdrawal or multiple-baseline design (Pring, 1986). Our desire was to determine whether or not *TLS* was more effective than a "traditional" approach, and we therefore chose a reversal design in which *TLS* and non-*TLS* modules would alternate with each other for 3 weeks after a baseline determination of communicative efficiency. Modules 1 and 2 (*TLS*, non-*TLS*) were ordered such that subjects would receive either one first for a 3-week period. This served to control for the number of times each was received. The same CU analysis obtained at baseline was performed between each of the modules.

The decision regarding the content of the non-*TLS* module was of great concern because there are many differing approaches to aphasia therapy. Our personal journey involved exploration of many of these approaches, and we would and will employ many of them therapeutically when we feel it is an appropriate choice for a specific individual. However, our choice of non-*TLS* therapy for Module 2 was one derived from what seemed "the norm" for many speech-language pathologists: a "general language stimulation" approach employing a variety of exercises for word retrieval, comprehension, reading, and writing, but *without* controlled content and delivery around thematic structure and Schuellian principles.

Therefore, Module 2 employed activities from the many easily accessible aphasia workbooks frequently used by clinicians. These activities were administered by the authors subsequent to completion of the same evaluative procedures described above. In other words, we attempted to treat the patient with traditional speech and language tasks selected for the individual's level of performance in each modality but without regard to semantic uniformity across modalities. We did not hesitate to assist patients in achieving success on these tasks within the session, and provided whatever degree of stimulation and support was required for specific activities. However, we avoided any linking of materials with conversational topics. It may be argued that we did not provide the best possible non-*TLS* modules because of our bias. However, we are accustomed to delivering other kinds of therapy for those for whom *TLS* is not appropriate and we attempted to do that for this study. Our hope is that in future studies we will be able to employ other therapists so as to eliminate any possible bias in this regard.

Subject Selection

In attempting to balance limitations existing in our practice with our research desires, we chose individuals who were able to complete a 3-week course of treatment without regard to age, type of aphasia, etiology, duration of symptoms, or any other particular characteristic. All were screened for adequate vision and hearing, and received traditional aphasia testing prior to inclusion in the study. As required under the guidelines of ethical research, all participants were aware of the nature of the study.

Procedures

Prior to beginning the first module, in between modules, and again at the end of the last module, the responses of each patient to the cookie theft picture were audiotaped and videotaped. Written transcripts of these descriptions were

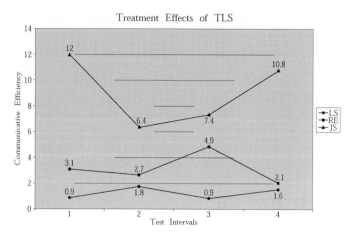

Figure 16–1.

obtained and analyzed according to the Yorkston and Beukelman procedure (1980). Each therapy session was also videotaped. All subjects received $^1/_2$ hour sessions of therapy 5 days per week for each of the 3 consecutive weeks.

Results

Pring (1986) offers some encouragement for the analysis of data in a visual rather than statistical manner when changes are likely to be small. Thus, as can be seen in Figure16–1, two of the three patients, both fluent aphasics, demonstrated treatment effects with *TLS*. That is, the communicative efficiency score (number of CUs divided by rate) increased after *TLS* modules and decreased after non-*TLS* modules, relative to baseline. There was no treatment effect for patient JS; in fact, his scores appear to be poorer with both treatment approaches than that achieved at baseline.

Discussion

Because of the very small number of patients in our study, there is little that can be confirmed about the efficacy of *TLS*. Certainly, we would need to test many more individuals before drawing any conclusions. What seems safe to assume, however, is that the use of a content unit analysis as a measure of discourse for revealing small, quantifiable changes in performance is a good idea. However, we found it interesting that our best results were obtained in treating fluent, rather than nonfluent aphasia, given our clinical impression that nonfluents respond quite well. We encourage anyone with interest to pursue such studies, and will attempt to do so ourselves with larger numbers of people and more varied diagnostic categories.

FUTURE TRENDS

During this decade we are changing models of service delivery faster than we had imagined possible in order to redefine our roles as experts and keep ourselves viable in the eye of the third party payer. What is it that the future holds for us in the way of an ethical, functional, and truly efficacious approach to aphasia recovery? Our best guess is that it will not be yet another technique but a change in how we use what we know about aphasia to enable the patient and his or her partners in life to have a better chance for success in communicating.

One positive change in aphasia therapy derived from our evolving health care system has been the rapid inclusion of the communication partner in the process of therapy. It has propelled us into a more realistic evaluation of the functional relevance of our approaches. At the same time, our expertise has shifted from only being a remediator to including being an educator for patient and family. In this role, we are teaching more about the disorder, its expected recovery course, and what each individual can do to help communicative success. The focus on process which is so essential to *TLS* assists in this regard.

Although communicative partners cannot generally provide *TLS* therapy, by observing sessions and talking with us they learn about how the person with aphasia organizes his or her language, employs appropriate strategies, and what he or she requires in the way of priming input in order to do his or her best. These are lessons that can be learned from many different approaches; *TLS*, because of its strong dependence upon structure, may simply be a more organized observational environment for shared insights. We hope to expand upon this aspect in future years by providing communicative partners with more formalized instruction in maximizing stimulation and materials.

KEY POINTS

1. *Thematic Language Stimulation* therapy may be seen as an extension of Schuellian stimulation principles; a core vocabulary of topically related words is used to generate language activities in multimodality stimulus/response formats.
2. *TLS* links functional communication ability and functional language performance.
3. *TLS* requires focused evaluation of language and behavioral processes.
4. The structure inherent in *TLS* preparation and delivery is useful in developing guidelines for family conversation training.

References

Aten, J.L. (1994). Functional communication treatment. In R. Chapey (ed.), *Language intervention strategies in adult aphasia* (pp. 292–303). Baltimore, MD: Williams & Wilkins.

Avent, J.R. (1997). Group treatment in aphasia using cooperative learning methods. *Journal of Medical Speech-Language Pathology*, 5(1), 9–26.

Boles, L. (1998). Conducting conversation: A case study using the spouse in aphasia treatment. *Neurophysiology and Neurogenic Speech and Language Disorders, a publication of ASHA SID 2, 19*(3), 24–31.

Byng, S., Kay, J., Edmundson, A., & Scott, C. (1990). Aphasia tests reconsidered. *Aphasiology, 4*(1), 24–31.

Chapey, R. (1994). Introduction to language intervention strategies in adult aphasia. In R. Chapey (ed.), *Language intervention strategies in adult aphasia* (pp. 2–26). Baltimore, MD: Williams & Wilkins.

Chapey R. (1994). Cognitive intervention: Stimulation of cognition, memory, convergent thinking, divergent thinking, and evaluative thinking. In R. Chapey (ed.), *Language intervention strategies in adult aphasia* (pp. 220–245). Baltimore, MD: Williams & Wilkins.

Cochrane, R. & Milton, S. (1984). Conversational prompting: A sentence-building technique for severe aphasia. *Journal of Neurology Communication Disorders, 1*, 4–23.

Duffy, J.R. & Coelho, C. (2000). Schuell's stimulation approach to rehabilitation. In R. Chapey (ed.), *Language intervention strategies in adult aphasia*. Baltimore, MD: Williams & Wilkins.

Goodglass, H. & Kaplan, E. (1983). *The Boston diagnostic aphasia examination*. Philadelphia, PA: Lea & Febiger.

Helm-Estabrooks, N. & Albert, M.L. (1991). *Manual of aphasia therapy*. Austin, TX: Pro-Ed.

Holland, A. (1980). *Communicative abilities in daily living*. Baltimore, MD: University Park Press.

Holland, A. (1995). Aphasia treatment: Clinical effectiveness in the new health care environment. Paper presented at a conference at JFK Johnson Rehabilitation Institute, Edison, NJ.

Holland, A. (1998). A strategy for improving oral naming in an individual with a phonological access impairment. In N. Helm-Estabrooks & A. Holland (eds.), *Approaches to the treatment of aphasia* (pp. 39–67). San Diego, CA: Singular Publishing Group.

Horner, J., Loverso, F.L., & Gonzalez Rothi, L. (1994). Models of aphasia treatment. In R. Chapey (ed.), *Language intervention strategies in adult aphasia* (pp. 135–145). Baltimore, MD: Williams & Wilkins.

Howard, D. (1986). Beyond randomised controlled trials: The case for effective case studies of the effects of treatment in aphasia. *British Journal of Disorders of Communication, 21*, 89–102.

Kagan, A. (1995). Revealing the competence of aphasic adults through conversation: A challenge to health professionals. *Topics in Stroke Rehabilitation, 2*(1), 15–28.

Kaplan, E. (1989). A process approach to neuropsychological assessment. In T. Boll (ed.), *Clinical neuropsychology and brain function: Research, measurement, and practice*. Washington, DC: APA.

Kaplan, E. (1991). Neuropsychological assessment & language treatment: A process-based approach. Seminar June 7–8 in Alexandria, VA, sponsored by Education Resources, Inc, Medfield MA and the Boston Neurobehavioral Institute, Boston, MA.

Lomas, J., Pickard, L., Bester, S., Elbard, H., Finlayson, A., & Zoghaib, C. (1989). The communicative effectiveness index: Development and psychometric evaluation of a functional communication measure for adult aphasia. *Journal of Speech and Hearing Disorders, 54*, 113–124.

Lubinski, R. (1994). Environmental systems approach to adult aphasia. In R. Chapey (ed.), *Language intervention strategies in adult aphasia* (pp. 269–291). Baltimore, MD: Williams & Wilkins.

Marshall, R.C. (1994). Management of fluent aphasic clients. In R. Chapey (ed.), *Language intervention strategies in adult aphasia* (pp. 389–406). Baltimore, MD: Williams & Wilkins.

McReynolds, L. & Thompson, C. (1986). Single-subject experimental designs. *Journal of Speech and Hearing Disorders, 51*, 306–312.

Morganstein, S. & Certner-Smith, M. (1982). *Thematic language stimulation.* Tucson, AZ: Communication Skill Builders.

Morganstein, S. & Certner-Smith, M. (1993). Aphasia and right-hemisphere disorders. In W. Gordon (ed.), *Advances in stroke rehabilitation* (pp. 103–133). Boston, MA: Andover Medical Publishers.

Nicholas, L.E. & Brookshire, R.H. (1992). A system for scoring main concepts in the discourse of non-brain-damaged and aphasic speakers. *Clinical Aphasiology, 21*, 87–99.

Pring, T.R. (1986). Evaluating the effects of speech therapy for aphasics: Developing the single case methodology. *British Journal of Disorders of Communication, 21*, 103–115.

Sarno, M.T. (ed.) (1981). *Acquired aphasia.* New York: Academic Press.

Schoonen, R. (1991). The internal validity of efficacy studies: Design and statistical power in studies of language therapy for aphasics. *Brain and Language 1991, 41*, 446–464.

Schuell, H., Jenkins, J.J., & Jimenez-Pabon, E. (1964). *Aphasia in adults: Diagnosis, prognosis and treatment.* New York: Harper & Row.

Siegel, G.M. (1987). The limits of science in communication disorders. *Journal of Speech and Hearing Disorders, 52*, 306–312.

Seigel, G.M. & Spradlin, J.E. (1985). Therapy and research. *Journal of Speech and Hearing Disorders, 50*, 226–230.

Simons-Mackie, N. (1997). Aphasia therapy: A functional social approach. Course presented at Kessler Institute for Rehabilitation, West Orange, NJ.

Taylor, M.L. (1969). *The functional communication profile.* New York: New York University Medical Center.

Wallace, G.L. & Canter, G.J. (1985). Effects of personally relevant language materials on the performance of severely aphasic individuals. *Journal of Speech and Hearing Disorders, 50*, 385–390.

Wepman, J.M. (1953). A conceptual model for the processes involved in recovery from aphasia. *Journal of Speech and Hearing Disorders, 18*, 4–13.

Wepman, J.M. (1972). Aphasia therapy: A new look. *Journal of Speech and Hearing Disorders, 37*, 201–214.

Wertz, R.T. (1986). Comparison of clinic, home, and deferred language treatment for aphasia. *Archives of Neurology, 43*, 653–658.

Wertz, R.T. (1991). Aphasiology 1990: A view from the colonies. *Aphasiology, 5*, (4–5), 311–322.

Whurr, R., Perlman Lorch, M., & Nye, C. (1992). A meta-analysis of studies carried out between 1946 and 1988 concerned with the efficacy of speech and language therapy treatment for aphasic patients. *European Journal of Disorders of Communication, 27*, 1–17.

Yorkston, K.M. & Beukelman, D.R. (1980). An analysis of connected speech samples of aphasic and normal speakers. *Journal of Speech and Hearing Disorders, 45*, 27–36.

APPENDIX 16-1
Thematic Language Stimulation (TLS) Unit on Industry with Instructions for Creating *TLS* Units.

How to create a *TLS* unit

Select between eight and ten words that have a close association to your chosen theme. These words will become your **core vocabulary,** used in each exercise. Use nouns primarily, but verbs and adjectives are fine as well.

Thirteen Exercises

Exercise 1. Repetition

This is controlled repetition practice, in which the stimuli gradually increase in length and complexity. Use each core vocabulary item and create a phrase and sentence sequence for them in which the target word is in the final position whenever reasonable.

Exercise 2. Speech Stimulation/Production

This is a grouping of four statements and one question which evolve for each core vocabulary item from repetition, to open-ended fill-ins, to generation of novel utterances. Begin with a statement for the patient to repeat in which the core vocabulary item is the last word. Create the next statement using the exact language as the first, but with the last word as a fill-in. Change the content of the next statement but retain the last word as fill-in. Create a question requiring the target word as an answer. End with a question relevant to the content just practiced, but designed to elicit a novel response.

Exercise 3. Categorization, Inclusion

This task is for identification of the core vocabulary in a list of words which vary in their semantic closeness to the target items. First, randomize core vocabulary items in a list of roughly twice its size. Use foils (other words) which are varied in the degree to which they may be related, visually or semantically, to the targets. The semantic closeness of the foils will determine the difficulty of the task.

Exercise 4. Categorization, Exclusion

This task requires elimination of one word in a set of four or five, which does not relate to the others, in order to create a convergent set. Then, the patient must supply an additional item which is within the category. Present at least four words as a group for comparison. Include space for the patient to write-in a novel word belonging to the class.

Exercise 5. Matching Related Words

This task involves matching synonyms and related words. Create two columns with core vocabulary on the left and words of high association or example on the right. The task is to connect the two.

Exercise 6. Sentence Fill-Ins, Multiple Choice

These are fill-in sentences for which the target word is one of the choices. For each fill-in sentence, three choices are offered. Semantic closeness of the foils determines complexity.

Exercise 7. Yes/No Questions

Questions are formulated with target vocabulary and the task is to provide a yes or no response.

Exercise 8. Simple Questions, Multiple Choice

Questions are developed for which correct answers are randomly ordered in a vocabulary grouping. Create three or four columns at the top of the page and list the core vocabulary. Below, create questions designed to elicit the core vocabulary in answer.

Exercise 9. Definitions, Multiple Choice

This task employs words or phrases which define the core vocabulary in a matching task. Using a two-column multiple choice format, list target vocabulary on the left and definitions on the right.

Exercise 10. Sentence Construction

Pairs of words are provided with which to create sentences. Create two columns. On the left list the core vocabulary first followed by a verb. In the next column, list a noun phrase.

Exercise 11. Sentence Arrangement

The patient is provided with a scrambled sentence for each core vocabulary item. Create out-of-order sentences of varied complexity, but within the mild to moderate range for each vocabulary item.

Exercise 12. Sentence Correction

The patient is provided with sentences containing two errors of either word choice, grammar, or spelling, which he or she must identify and correct.

Exercise 13. Simple Paragraphs, Multiple Choice Questions

A paragraph is created in which all or most of the vocabulary has been used. The patient must then answer some multiple-choice questions about the paragraph. When possible, use humor or idiomatic expressions to improve processing. Create three or four questions with multiple choice answers for practice in processing factual and implied information.

Vocabulary Unit: Industry
Exercise 1. **Repetition**

Directions: Repeat these words, phrases, and sentences.

union	management
to a union	good management
I belong to a union.	We must have good management.
employee	strike
an employee	a strike
He is an employee.	Will there be a strike?
benefits	wages
for benefits	her wages

We now pay for benefits.
corporation
large corporation
We work for a large corporation.
mining
coal mining
He works in coal mining.

Will they pay her wages?
farming
organic farming
Their family is in organic farming.

Vocabulary Unit: Industry
Exercise 2. **Speech Stimulation/Production**

Directions: Listen, fill in, and answer the questions.

1. I belong to a union.
   I belong to a _____.
   What do I belong to? _____
   What is the AFL-CIO? _____
   What do you think about unions?

2. Business must have good management.
   Business must have good _____.
   What must business have? _____
   What does the boss represent? _____
   What does management do?

3. He is an employee.
   He is an _____.
   What is he? _____
   What do you call a worker? _____
   How do you get to be an employee?

4. There may be a strike.
   There may be a _____.
   What may there be? _____
   What does the union threaten to do? _____
   When do you last remember a strike?

5. We have many company benefits.
   We have many company _____.
   What do we have at the company? _____
   What do we call an annual vacation with pay? _____
   What are some important benefits?

6. She earns high wages.
   She earns high _____.
   What does she earn? _____
   What is another word for salary? _____
   When are wages usually paid? _____

7. A major industry in Arizona is copper mining.
   A major industry in Arizona is copper _____.
   What is a major industry in Arizona? _____

How is copper found? _____

What other metals are mined? _____

8. His business is farming.

His business is _____.

What is his business? _____

If you study agriculture, what business are you in? _____

What crops can farmers grow? _____

9. We work for a large corporation.

We work for a large _____.

What do we work for? _____

What is General Motors? _____

Name some other corporations.

Vocabulary Unit: Industry
Exercise 3. Word Categorization, Inclusion

Directions: Circle the words that belong in the category, "Industry."

slap	respond
corporation	management
baseball	certainty
strike	benefits
army	outlaw
pears	triumphant
wages	farming
employer	union
teach	mining

Vocabulary Unit: Industry
Exercise 4. Word Categorization, Exclusion

Directions: 1. Cross out the word on each line that does not belong.
2. Write in a new word that does belong.

1. union   insect   labor   employee

   _____

2. farming   manufacturing   mining   seeking

   _____

3. benefits   wages   zebras   job

   _____

4. employer   management   corps   corporation

   _____

5. union   picket   pickax   strike

   _____

Vocabulary Unit: Industry
Exercise 5. Matching Related Words

Directions: Draw a line from each word in the left-hand column to the related word or phrase in the right-hand column.

union   chairman of the board
employee   precious metal

benefits	boss
mining	Local 82
management	worker
strike	thresher
wages	walk-out
farming	salary
corporation	401K

Vocabulary Unit: Industry
Exercise 6. Sentence Fill-Ins, Multiple Choice

Directions: Read the sentence, circle the correct word, and write it.

                         onion   union   united
1. The AFL-CIO is a strong _____.

                    employee   trooper   laughter
2. He works as my _____.

                         sweeps   many   benefits
3. Insurance is one of our company _____.

                         mining   feet   ashes
4. Pennsylvania is known for coal _____.

                    corporation   pizza   officer
5. General Foods is a large _____.

                         plan   strike   limb
6. The workers are going out on _____.

                    wages   clothes   types
7. He earns very high _____.

                         art   sailing   farming
8. In rural areas, the main industry is _____.

                    fuel   management   workers
9. Labor is sometimes in conflict with _____.

Vocabulary Unit: Industry
Exercise 7. Yes/No Questions

Directions: Read each question and mark "yes" or "no".

	YES	NO
1. Are unions organized?	____	____
2. Do employees work?	____	____
3. Are benefits bad?	____	____
4. Are energy sources found by mining?	____	____
5. Do some corporations go bankrupt?	____	____
6. Does management always win?	____	____
7. Can dogs earn wages?	____	____
8. Is farming a fuel?	____	____
9. Do workers sometimes go on strike?	____	____

Vocabulary Unit: Industry
Exercise 8. **Simple Questions, Multiple Choice**

Directions: Answer each question, using one of the words below:

union	employee	benefits
mining	corporations	management
strike	wages	farming

1. What is a rural industry? _____.
2. With whom does labor negotiate? _____.
3. What do workers earn? _____.
4. What are Xerox, 3M, and General Foods? _____.
5. In what industry are copper and gold found? _____.
6. What is another name for a walk-out? _____.
7. What do organized workers belong to? _____.
8. Who is someone hired? _____.
9. Besides pay, what "extras" do workers receive? _____.

Vocabulary Unit: Industry
Exercise 9. **Definitions, Multiple Choice**

Directions: Write the letter of each word next to its definition.

a. union   _____ salary
b. employee   _____ owner, supervisor
c. benefits   _____ organization of workers
d. mining   _____ agriculture
e. corporation   _____ worker
f. management   _____ business organization
g. strike   _____ dental plan, expense account
h. wages   _____ walk-out
i. farming   _____ energy sources

Vocabulary Unit: Industry
Exercise 10. **Sentence Construction**

Directions: Create sentences for these words and phrases.

union-join	strong union
employee-works	responsible employee
benefits-receive	fringe benefits
mining-dangerous	copper mining
management-supervises	good management
strike-go out	wildcat strike
wages-earn	low wages
farm-harvest	produce farming
corporation-form	large corporation

Vocabulary Unit: Industry
Exercise 11. **Sentence Arrangement**

Directions: Rearrange these words to form correct sentences.

1. a   union   I   to   belong

_____.

2. my   employee   he   is

_____.

3. company   has   my   many   benefits   fringe

_____.

4. he   mining   in   works   the   industry

_____.

5. management   disagree   sometimes   and   labor

_____.

6. Tuesday   will   they   go   strike   on

_____.

7. earns   higher   she   wages   I   than   do

_____.

8. work   hard   farming   is

_____.

9. large   is   Xerox   a   corporation

_____.

Vocabulary Unit: Industry
Exercise 12. **Sentence Correction**

Directions: Find and correct the errors in the sentences below.

1. The minor's onion is very strong.

_____.

2. He in a trusted employ.

_____.

3. When are my bennifits?

_____.

4. Mineing is an major industry.

_____.

5. Managment is always write.

_____.

6. They wore on strike for 12 day.

_____.

7. Wayges are paid on Firday.

_____.

8. Me uncle has bin in the farming business.

_____.

9. The formed a corpation.

_____.

Vocabulary Unit: Industry

Exercise 13. **Simple Paragraphs, Multiple Choice Questions**

Directions: Read the paragraphs. Then answer the questions.

Local 32 of the Restaurant Employee's Union went out on strike because management refused to grant the fringe benefits they asked for. Workers for the corporation said that wages were not the main issue. "If we don't get these benefits," said one union member, "I will go into coal mining or farming. At least then I will be able to heat my home and feed my family."

1. Which union went on strike?
   a. coal miners   c. farmers
   b. restaurant workers   d. corporation

2. What was not the main issue?
   a. benefits   c. farming
   b. wages   d. management

3. What did management refuse?
   a. a pay cut   c. membership
   b. farming rights   d. fringe benefits

Chapter 17

Cognitive Stimulation: Stimulation of Recognition/Comprehension, Memory, and Convergent, Divergent, and Evaluative Thinking

Roberta Chapey

OBJECTIVES

The objectives of this chapter are to define communication as a problem-solving, decision-making task; review the stimulation approaches to aphasia intervention; discuss the Guilford Structure-of-Intellect model; define cognition, intelligence, language, problem solving, decision making, learning, information processing, and composite abilities within the context of the Guilford model; discuss assessment within a cognitive stimulation approach to aphasia management; explain the general and specific objectives of cognitive stimulation therapy and suggest possible tasks and materials for such therapy; and discuss the relationship between cognitive stimulation therapy and Wepman's Thought Process Therapy, Kearns' Response Elaboration Training, and the Life Participation Approach to Aphasia.

I served as a speech pathologist for a 6-week summer program in the NYC Board of Education that included a group of 5-year-old nonverbal, language-impaired children. Each day I used subsequent activities and lessons from the *Peabody Language Development Kit* (1965), based on the Guilford Structure-of-Intellect model—specifically on divergent thinking, convergent thinking, and associative thinking. The results amazed me: the children gained a large amount of language in a very short time—so much so that they were not recommended for therapy that September. I became fascinated with the results, the kit, and the Guilford model, and did my doctoral dissertation on the application of part of the model to adults with aphasia: "Divergent Semantic Behavior In Adult Aphasia." The kit has subsequently been expanded to include multiple levels and is still used throughout the world.

COMMUNICATION: A PROBLEM—SOLVING/ DECISION—MAKING TASK

Communication is a problem-solving/decision-making task. One possible model of problem solving and decision making may be the Guilford Structure-of-Intellect model (see Figure 17–1). There are four reasons why this model may be appealing. First, it appears to have ecological and communicative validity. That is, communication usually involves deciding who can say what, to whom, in what way, where, and when (Prutting, 1979). It is a constant attempt to decide what is the message of best fit for this partner in this situation. It is the back and forth—the give and take—of ideas for a specific purpose or problem. During such communication, when we comprehend a literal or implied message (such as 'what time is it?' perhaps meaning 'you are late'), or comprehend that a problem exists, we use the mental operation of recognition/comprehension. When we comprehend a joke or double meaning of a word (such as 'If the #2 pencil is the most popular, why is it still #2' or 'Why is the time of day with the slowest traffic called rush hour?')—we use recognition/comprehension of systems. When we remember what was said, we use memory; when we ask ourselves, 'what are all the possible reasons that I can use to explain the fact that I'm late?' we use divergent thinking. (Divergent thinking is also called brainstorming or creativity.) When we think of relevant contingent and/or adjacent utterances we often use divergent thinking. When we decide between 'my car broke down,' 'I overslept,' and 'the dog turned off my alarm clock,' we use the mental operation of judgment.

When individuals have a communicative (or other) problem to solve or a decision to make they make use of whatever *content* (figural, symbolic, semantic, and/or behavioral), *mental operation* (recognition/understanding, memory, convergent thinking, divergent thinking, and/or evaluative thinking), and/or *product* (*or association*) (units, classes, relations, systems, and transformations)—or combination of

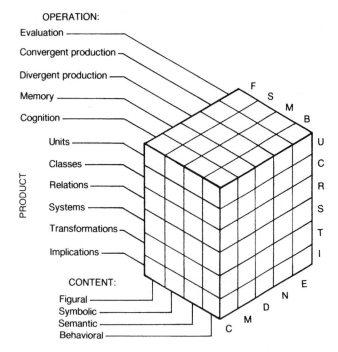

OPERATION:

Evaluation
Convergent production
Divergent production
Memory
Cognition

PRODUCT

Units
Classes
Relations
Systems
Transformations
Implications

CONTENT:

Figural
Symbolic
Semantic
Behavioral

F S M B U C R S T I N E D M C

Figure 17–1. Guilford's Structure of Intellect model.

them—that is/are called for by the specific communication (or other) problem or decision at hand.

STIMULATION APPROACHES TO LANGUAGE INTERVENTION IN APHASIA

The stimulation approaches to therapy form the cornerstone of language intervention strategies used with adult aphasic patients (Chapey, 1981a). None of these approaches attempts to teach naming or other specific responses to particular stimuli. Rather, each emphasizes the reorganization of language through stimulation or increased cortical activity through problem solving (Duffy & Coelho, 2001). The stimulation approach first articulated and later developed and refined by Schuell et al. (1955, 1964) places its **primary emphasis on the stimulation presented** to the aphasic individual. The stimulation approach is grounded in the observation that the patient has not lost linguistic elements or rules but, rather, that the language system is working with reduced efficiency. This approach, therefore, employs **strong, controlled**, and **intensive auditory stimuli** as the primary tool to facilitate and **maximize** the patient's **reorganization and recovery** of language. It emphasizes the **action elicited within the patient by the stimuli presented**, since "sensory stimulation is the only method we have for making complex events happen in the brain" (Schuell et al., 1964, p. 338). Some proponents of the stimulation approach encourage us to stimulate patient ability to solve problems (Jennings & Lubinski, 1981; Zachman et al., 1982), to predict outcomes, to determine causes of events (Zachman et al., 1982), and to think (Chapey,

1977a, 1981b; Chapey & Lubinski, 1979; Chapey et al., 1976, 1977).

In light of the current emphasis on cognition, one might ask what are the types of cortical activity that are increased through problem solving, predicting outcomes, and/or determining causes of events? **What complex events happen in the brain** when one stimulates a patient? What are cognition, intelligence, and information processing, and how do they relate to these complex events in the brain? Are problem solving and decision making unitary or composite abilities? What is the difference between cognitive processes and products? What language-based cognitive abilities elicit action within the patient and make complex events happen in the brain in order to stimulate the comprehension and production of language? Answers to these questions and operational definitions of these abilities are crucial if we are to develop a coherent and generative rationale for intervention, as opposed to the listing of tasks that should be presented to patients. We need a better understanding and specification of the processes we are stimulating in the brain, and an operational definition of the action elicited within the patient and the complex events that happen in the brain. We need to concretize the cognitive processes and the processes involved in problem solving and decision making. Specification of the underlying targets of our stimulation therapy may increase the effectiveness of our intervention efforts.

The following discussion represents one possible way to answer the above questions.

DEFINITIONS OF COGNITION IN THE PSYCHOLOGY LITERATURE

The study of cognition represents the work of numerous psychologists with a variety of related approaches. Thus, there is no single comprehensive theory of cognition. Rather, cognitive psychologists are viewed as "information-processing" theorists who seek to determine what "functional mental events transpire while a person actually behaves" (Rosenthal & Zimmerman, 1978). Their focus is not on observable behavior but, rather, on examining the characteristics of internal, central brain processing or mental events such as perception, recognition, reasoning, thinking, evaluation, concept formation, abstraction, generalization, decision making, and problem solving.

Cognition, then, is a **generic term for any process whereby an organism becomes aware of or obtains knowledge of an object** (English & English, 1958). It "refers to **all the processes** by which **sensory input is transformed, reduced, elaborated, stored, recovered, and used**" (Neisser, 1967, p. 4). It is a group of processes by which we achieve knowledge and command of our world, that is, a method of processing information. It is "the **activity of knowing**; the **acquisition, organization, and use** of knowledge" (Neisser, 1967, p. 1)—knowledge that will, in turn, influence or instigate and guide subsequent and more overt behavior (Rosenthal & Zimmerman, 1978). It should be noted that cognitive psychologists do not interpret the above mental processes as occurring in stages or in isolation but, rather, they are seen as dynamic and interacting variables.

HOW THE MIND WORKS

In his book "How the Mind Works," Steven Pinker (1997) presents a computational theory of the mind and suggests that the mind is not the brain but what the brain does. The brain's special status comes from what the brain does: information processing or computation. Thus, "beliefs and desires are *information*, incarnated as configurations of symbols" (p. 25). Computation "allows meaning to cause and be caused" (p. 25) by allowing patterns of connections and patterns of activity among the neurons (p. 25). The "content of brain activity lies in the patterns of connections and patterns of activity among the neurons" (p. 25). "Only when the program is run does the coherence become evident" (p. 25). It is the arrangement of neurons that matters. Programs are assemblies of simple information processing units (which are functionally specialized) which must assemble themselves. "A program is an intricate recipe of logical and statistical operations directed by comparisons, tests, branches, loops, and subroutines embedded in subroutines" (p. 27).

According to Pinker (1997), evolution equipped us with a neural computer that often supplies missing information and makes good guesses. It contains modules which are "defined by the special things they do with the information available to them, not necessarily by the kinds of information they have available" (p. 31). Pinker suggests that we need ideas "that capture the ways a complex device can tune itself to unpredictable aspects of the world and take in the kinds of data it needs to function" (p. 33). Intelligence, he says, "is the ability to attain goals in the face of obstacles by means of decisions based on rational (truth-obeying) rules" (p. 62).

INTELLIGENCE AS DEFINED IN THE PSYCHOLOGY LITERATURE

The most widely accepted definition of intelligence is that "intelligence is what the intelligence tests test." Another definition is the Structure-of-Intellect model (Figure 17–1), which was developed by J.P. Guilford (1967) during his 20 years as the director of the Aptitudes Research Project at the University of Southern California from 1949 to 1969. His project, funded by the Personnel and Training Branch of the Psychological Sciences Division of the U.S. Office of Naval Research, was designed to define various intellectual abilities in order to match the native skills of navy personnel to specific job requirements. For example, he sought to determine which subjects were best suited for officer status, for pilot training, and so on.

In an attempt to define the numerous intellectual abilities available to individuals and, thereby, achieve a **taxonomy of intellectual functioning**, Guilford and his colleagues (1967, 1971) developed numerous tests, each of which was thought to tap a specific intellectual ability. The validity of each test and ability was then assessed by performing numerous-factor analytic studies of responses to the tests and determining which tests loaded on specific statistical factors. Results of this research suggest that there are 120 factors in humans (Figure 17–1). These 120 factors are divided into three parameters: mental operations, contents, and products.

THE GUILFORD MODEL

There are five mental operations, four content areas, and six products of the Guilford model ($5 \times 4 \times 6 = 120$). An ability is a combination of one kind of operation, one kind of content, and one kind of product (e.g., convergent symbolic units, divergent semantic classes). Each operation is a computation.

Mental Operations

The five mental operations are cognition, memory, convergent thinking, divergent thinking, and evaluative thinking or judgment.

Cognition

The mental operation of cognition is basic to all other operations, hence, it is first. "If no cognition, no memory; if no memory, no production, for the things produced come largely from memory storage. If neither cognition nor production, then no evaluation" (Guilford, 1967, p. 63).

Cognition involves **knowing, awareness, attention, immediate discovery** (or rediscovery), and **recognition** of information in various forms (**comprehension** or understanding). Recognition involves acknowledgment that something has been seen or perceived previously. For example, cognition of semantic material might be tested by using a multiple-choice vocabulary test in which the correct alternative is a synonym of the word to be defined and the others are not. Tests of cognition determine how much the examinee knows or can readily discover on the basis of what is known. (The term "cognition" has been used to refer to all mental activity or operations by most cognitive psychologists. However, Guilford used the term to refer to one specific mental operation: recognition/comprehension, which can be confusing).

Memory

Memory is the power, act, or process of fixing newly gained information in storage. It involves the ability to insert new information into memory and to retain the new information. According to Guilford (1967), good memory tests require that subjects essentially have a full comprehension of the studied information. Therefore, test material is not difficult. Otherwise, tests may load on cognition, convergent thinking, and/or divergent thinking. The operation of memory, then, is the **fixation and retention** of new information.

Convergent Thinking

Convergent thinking is the generation of **logical conclusions** from given information, where emphasis is on achieving conventionally best outcomes. Usually, the information given fully determines the outcome, as in mathematics and logic. In accordance with the information given them, examinees must converge on the one right answer (Guilford, 1967; Guilford & Hoepfner, 1971).

Convergent production is in the area of **logical deductions** or **compelling inferences**. It involves the generation of **logical necessities**. An example of a convergent semantic test would be verbal analogies completion, in which the subject has to supply his or her own answers, or picture group naming, in which the individual writes a class name for each group of five pictured objects.

Divergent Thinking

Divergent production involves the generation of **logical alternatives** from given information, where emphasis is on **variety, quantity,** and **relevance** of output from the same source. It is concerned with the generation of logical possibilities, with the **ready flow of ideas** and with the **readiness to change the direction** of one's responses (Guilford, 1967). It involves providing ideas in situations where a proliferation of ideas on a specific topic is required. Such behavior necessitates the use of a **broad search of memory storage**, and the production of **multiple possible solutions** to a problem. It is the ability to **extend previous experience** and knowledge or to **widen existing concepts** (Cropley, 1967). Divergent behavior is directed toward **new responses**—new in the sense that the thinker was not aware of the response before beginning the particular line of thought (Gowan et al., 1967).

Divergent questions are open-ended and do not have a single correct answer. For example, the individual might be asked to list numerous things that are soft and fluffy, to think of problems that anyone might have in eating lunch, or to list what might happen if people no longer needed or wanted sleep. Responses can be grouped according to the number of ideas produced (**fluency**) and the variety of ideas suggested (**flexibility**). If an individual is asked to list objects that can roll, and responds with, "a baseball, a football, a basketball, a nickel, a dime, a quarter, a car, and a truck," this person would receive a fluency score of eight and a flexibility score of three (balls, money, transportation). Guilford also uses originality and elaboration scores to measure divergent ability.

Originality relates to the unusualness of the response. **Elaboration** is the ability to specify numerous critical details in planning an event or making a decision. Responses are also evaluated for relevance. Answers that are not relevant to the specific questions are not scored. Thus, if the above individual had responded, "Isn't that an interesting question?" or "I like to eat lunch," these responses would not be scored because they do not answer the question.

Evaluative Thinking or Judgment

According to Guilford (1967), judgment involves the ability of the individual to use knowledge to make **appraisals** or **comparisons**, or to formulate **evaluations** in terms of **known** specifications or **criteria**, such as correctness, completeness, identity, relevance, adequacy, utility, safety, consistency, logical feasibility, practical feasibility, or social custom. Although judgment behavior is based on the individual's previous experience and knowledge of the subject involved, it is always an **extension** of what is known. It is an appraisal or evaluation based on knowledge.

Guilford (1967) developed a number of tests to study judgment or evaluation skills. These tests require that the individual keep specific criteria in mind and select one best answer or solution from among several alternatives. In one test, for example, the individual chooses the best word for the sentence, "A sandwich always has (a) bread, (b) butter, (c) lettuce, (d) meat. Which one must it have in order to be a sandwich?" In another, the subject must judge whether a sentence expresses a complete thought. For example, "Is 'Milk comes from' a sentence?" In yet another test, the individual is given specific classifications and asked to determine if new information can be assigned to the previously established class. For example, "Should the word chair be put with the words cow and horse or with the words table and lamp?" Each judgment task has a predetermined best response or solution (Chapey & Lubinski, 1979).

Content

There are four broad, substantive, basic kinds (or areas) of information, material, or content that the organism discriminates. They are figural, symbolic, semantic, and behavioral.

Figural

Figural content pertains to "information in concrete form, as perceived or as recalled in the form of images." The term "figural" minimally implies figure-ground perceptual organization" (Guilford & Hoepfner, 1971).

Symbolic

Symbolic content pertains to "information in the form of **denotative signs having no significance** in and of themselves, such as letters, numbers, musical notations (and) codes" (Guilford & Hoepfner, 1971).

Semantic

Semantic content pertains to "information in the form of **conceptions** or **mental constructs** to which words are often applied. Therefore, it involves thinking and verbal communication. However, it need **not necessarily be dependent on words**. For example, meaningful pictures also convey semantic information" (Guilford & Hoepfner, 1971).

Behavioral

Behavioral content pertains to **psychological** information—that is, to essentially nonfigural and nonverbal aspects of human interactions, where the **attitudes, needs, desires, moods, intentions, perceptions,** and **thoughts** of others and of ourselves are involved. Some of the cues that the human organism obtains about **the attention, perception, thinking, feeling, emotions,** and **intentions** of others come indirectly through nonverbal means such as "body language." For example, this might involve matching two faces that are similar in terms of the mental state conveyed. Such ability enables us to keep aware of what behavior is going on and enables us to interpret it. It is important for coping with other individuals in face-to-face encounters, in solving interpersonal problems, in detecting and analyzing problems, and in generating information that is needed toward solutions. This type of content is sometimes called social intelligence (Guilford & Hoepfner, 1971).

Products

The six types of products are units, classes, relations, systems, transformations, and implications. They represent the **way that things are associated** in the mind—such that each level enters into the next level—producing a larger and larger number of **associations between and among items of information**. Thus, units enter into classes, classess into relations, relations into systems, etc. Therefore, products represent a possible continuum from simple (units) to complex (implications) (Chapey, 1994).

Units

Units are things to which nouns are often applied. They are relatively **segregated** or circumscribed items or "chunks" of information having "**thing**" character (Guilford & Hoepfner, 1971) and often refer to one item such as a cup or a chair. Units may be synonymous with Gestalt psychology "figure-on-ground." An example of a semantic units test might be a multiple-choice vocabulary test in which the correct alternative is a synonym of the word to be defined, and the others are not. Semantic units are **meanings, ideas,** or **thoughts**

in the form of a particular **whole**. Of the products, units are regarded as basic; hence they appear at the top (Guilford, 1967).

Classes

Units enter into classes or "**conceptions underlying sets of items** of information grouped by virtue of their common properties" (Guilford & Hoepfner, 1971). They involve common properties within sets—such as dishes or furniture. Such semantic classes involve **class ideas** or **concepts** or choosing the class name that best describes a given set of words or objects.

Relations

Relations are **meaningful connections** between items of information based upon variables or points of contact that apply to them (Guilford & Hoepfner, 1971). For example, a test of semantic relations can be the logical relations of a **syllogism** in which two premises and four alternative conclusions are presented, only one of which is correct. It might also involve an **analogy** task, in which case the individual must grasp the relations between the initial pair of words and apply it to the second—such as "soup is hot, ice cream is _____."

Systems

Relations enter into systems or **organized patterns** or items of information; they are complexes of interrelated or interacting parts (Guilford & Hoepfner, 1971). For example, a semantic system can be a "sentence—**a complex of relationships among ideas**, an organized thought—a sequence of events, or a common situation" (Guilford & Hoepfner, 1971). It might involve double meanings, puns, homonyms, and redefinitions or shifts in meaning.

Transformations

Systems enter into transformations or **changes** of various kinds such as **redefinitions, shifts, transitions,** or **modifications** in existing information.

Implications

Transformations enter into implications or **circumstantial connections** between items of information such as connections by virtue of contiguity, or any condition that promotes "belongingness" (Guilford & Hoepfner, 1971). Implications involve information **expected, anticipated, suggested,** or **predicted** by other information. For example, a semantic implication can be sensitivity to problems such as stating two things seen wrong with a common appliance or problems that might arise in the use of a given specific object.

Composite Abilities

According to Guilford and Hoepfner (1971):

It must not be supposed that, although the abilities are separate and distinct logically and they can be segregated by factor analysis, they function in isolation in mental activities of the individual. Two or more of the abilities are ordinarily involved in solving the same problem. The fact that they **habitually operate together in various mixtures** in ordinary mental functioning has been the reason for the difficulty of recognizing them by direct observation or even by ordinary laboratory procedures (pp. 19–20).

Indeed, it was largely through the construction of special tests, each one aimed at a specific ability, and the sensitive and searching procedures of factor analysis where Guilford and his colleagues clearly demonstrated the separateness of the various mental operations, contents, and products.

The following sections will explore the composite or unified notions of problem solving, decision making, and information processing.

PROBLEM SOLVING

According to Guilford and Hoepfner (1971), problem solving is a **complex composite ability**. A problem is presented whenever a situation calls for the individual doing anything novel in order to cope with something that is different from past behavior. Problem solving involves the use of all five mental operations, all types of content or information, and any kind of product, depending on the problem presented, the context in which the problem arises, and the kinds of products required in order to reach a solution.

Initially, the individual must become **aware** that a problem exists. This is a matter of cognition, often involving implications. Next, the problem must be **analyzed** or **structured**, which usually involves cognition of systems. After the problem is structured:

[the] individual generates a variety of alternative solutions, which is divergent production. If sufficient basis for a solution is cognized and then produced, there is convergent production (Guilford & Hoepfner, 1971, p. 31).

At each stage in the problem-solving process there is evaluation:

in the form of accepting or rejecting cognitions of the problem and generated solutions. At any step what happens may become fixated and retained for possible later use, so that memory is involved. When evaluation leads to rejections, there may be new starts, with revised cognitions and productions (Guilford & Hoepfner, 1971, p. 31).

Thus, problem solving can be said to have five steps: **preparation** (recognition of a problem, cognition); **analysis** (cognition); **production** (divergent and convergent); **verification** (evaluation); and **reapplication**.

The problem-solving factors found by Guilford and his colleagues using factor analyses are as follows:

Cognition	CMU		
	CMC		
	CMR		
	CMS	Inductive	Therefore, there are
	CMI[a]		8 factors involved
Divergent	DMU		in reasoning
	DMR		(5 cognition, 3
	DMT		convergent)
Convergent	NMC		
	NMR	Deductive	
	MNI		
Evaluation	EMI		

[a] sensitivity to problems = CMI, EMI.

DECISION MAKING

Decision making and planning ability both belong in the category of problem solving and usually entail all of the steps described above. Guilford (1967) notes that the more a problem, decision, or plan involves the generation of numerous responses or novelty, or the more creative the solution to the problem, the more it involves divergent production abilities—especially divergent transformation abilities—or possibly all transformation abilities.

INFORMATION PROCESSING

The present writer suggests that Guilford's (1967) Structure-of-Intellect (SOI) model can also be viewed as an information-processing model (Figure 17–2). Within this information-processing model, incoming sensory information is figural, symbolic, semantic, and/or behavioral. An attention mechanism selects a small portion of sensory information to be held for several seconds for further processing. This further processing takes place in the central processing unit. The processes of this **central processing unit** are **cognition, memory, convergent thinking, divergent thinking,** and **evaluative thinking** or **judgment**. It is suggested that these are the **functional mental events that transpire while a person actually behaves**. These are the **mental events** or **processes by which sensory information is transformed, reduced, elaborated, stored, recovered, and used**. This is the group of mental processes that are used to acquire, organize, store, and use knowledge, the processes whereby an organism becomes aware of or obtains knowledge of an object, event, or relationship.

Within this information-processing model, then, incoming figural, symbolic, semantic, and/or behavioral sensory

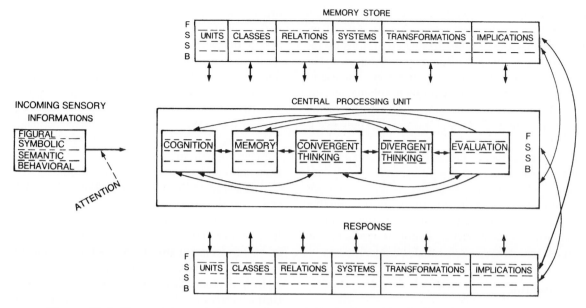

Figure 17–2. Human information processing model based upon the Guilford Structure of Intellect model (Chapey, 1994).

information is attended to and processed in the central processing unit by one or more of the five SOI mental operations. If the information is immediately recognized, known, comprehended, or understood, then the mental operation of cognition has occurred. When situations call for the individual to generate logical conclusions from given information, where emphasis is on achieving conventionally best outcomes, convergent thinking occurs. When a novel response is required, the divergent operation is generated. Inserting newly gained information into storage involves memory. Judging the appropriateness, acceptability, relevance, and/or correctness of information requires evaluation.

When the mental operations are used and **new** information or **knowledge is produced**, these **new discriminations** come about **in the form of new products**: units, classes, relations, systems, transformations, and implications. Products are the basic forms that figural, symbolic, semantic, and behavioral information take as a result of being processed by one or all of the organism's mental operations. These new associations are usually produced as responses and/or may also be processed by the mental operation of memory and inserted into memory storage.

Memory

It is important to differentiate between memory as an operation or short-term memory (STM) and long-term memory or memory storage. The operation of memory (or STM) is the act or process of **fixing** newly gained information in storage. In contrast, long-term memory is a storage area that contains everything that is **retained** for more than a few minutes, such as all learned experience, including language and the rules of language. It retains the products generated by the various mental operations as they process or act on experience. Thus, each individual has his or her own summary of past experiences, or a memory structure of the world in long-term memory. It has been shown that the capacity of this storage is not static or fixed; it is dynamic. Indeed, "the more you know, the more you can know, the more you remember, the more you can remember" (Muma, 1978). This "theory of the world in our heads serves as the foundation for learning." Indeed, what we know makes our experience meaningful.

One of the characteristics of long-term memory is that what is recalled is often not simply what was seen or heard but a modification of the original learning. That is, external stimuli cannot enter the organism. Rather, organisms do not react directly to representations of the world, but to information that they themselves construct (Guilford, 1967). An individual's representation of reality as internal symbols and the interrelations among these symbols are what is called "information." When the amount of memory we need to process is large, the operation of memory is capable of collapsing the data it receives (or "chunking" it) in more efficient ways and treating it in groups, such as classes. Through chunking, we can successfully deal with larger amounts of information with minimal difficulty in storage and retrieval. Chunking provides a way of representing information so that it conforms to one's conceptual organization (Muma, 1978), that is, one's previously stored associations or products.

When the individual is faced with a meaningful problem and uses all of the cognitive processes to solve a problem, the results of this information processing are frequently inserted into long-term memory. Rote memory, on the other hand, uses only one mental operation: memory. The use of more numerous operations during problem solving and the establishment of numerous associations, or products, during the process may be one reason why meaningful memory is longer lasting.

All of the mental operations depend on memory storage since all operations retrieve information from this store (Figure 17–2). That is, all of the mental operations search long-term memory in order to recall information that has been stored. Thus, there is cognitive retrieval, memory retrieval, convergent retrieval, divergent retrieval, and evaluative retrieval.

Perception/Attention

Where, one may ask, is perception in all this? In the literature, perception is defined as knowing and comprehending the nature of the stimulus (Muma, 1978). To perceive is to know. Attention is part of this process. Therefore, within this model, both perception and attention are viewed as part of cognition.

LEARNING

According to cognitive psychologists, learning is an active process of problem solving (Lazerson, 1975). A learning situation arises whenever our present cognitive structures prove inadequate for making sense of the world, when something in our experience is unfamiliar or unpredictable (Smith, 1975). Thus, learning is an interaction between the world around us and the theory of the world in our heads. In this view, the learner is seen as a scientist who constructs theories or forms hypotheses about the world and conducts experiments to test these hypotheses.

A distinguishing feature of the "cognitive" approach to learning is the assumption that what is learned are concepts or schema and conceptual associations about the relationships between and among objects, events, and relationships. This process of concept formation involves identifying common features and grouping together all things that have a common feature (i.e., forming classes). Concept learning involves the acquisition of a common response to dissimilar stimuli (Saltz, 1971). It is regarded as the process of making differentiations and discriminations, a process of recognizing similarities and differences or reorganizing material into new patterns or products. It involves the generation of lists of specific characteristics to differentiate membership into particular categories.

Concept formation enables us to transform the world of infinite appearances into finite essences (Saltz, 1971) and to organize past learning in such a way that it is no longer bound to the specific situation in which the learning occurred. Thus, instead of having to react to each object as something unique, we learn to make generalized responses to classes of objects. The generalized responses function as principles or laws. When we learn something in this type of generic manner, we are able to benefit from analogy when we deal with a new problem. When this occurs, one of the major objectives of learning has been accomplished. We are able to adapt to our environment in more satisfactory ways, and we are saved from subsequent learning (Bruner, 1968).

According to Bruner (1968), all of human beings' interactions with the world involve classifying input in relation to classes or categories that they have already established. It is Bruner's (1968) contention that to perceive is to categorize; to conceptualize is to categorize; to learn is to form categories; to make decisions is to categorize.

In SOI theory, learning is "the **acquisition of information** which comes about in the form of **new discriminations** in terms of **new products**" (Guilford & Hoepfner, 1971, p. 30). Learning and **concept formation employ the five operations** of the SOI theory. According to Guilford and Hoepfner (1971):

> . . . (no) item of information has been learned until it has been cognized. That which is learned cannot have any future effects unless it is fixated and retained (memory). Items of information produced (divergent and convergent) in response to new cues may also be fixated and remembered. In attempting to learn, the individual makes errors and he must discriminate between errors and correct information. This involves evaluation. Evaluation is conceived as playing an important role in reinforcement (p. 30).

Concept formations, the largest product of cognitive processing, are products of SOI operations and are called units, classes, relations, systems, transformations, and implications. Thus, the SOI model is also a model of learning.

Results of factor analyses led Guilford and his colleagues (1967, 1971) to redefine some of the terminology traditionally used in reference to learning. For example:

Serial learning is essentially dealing with systems, since learned order is a system.

Reasoning, redefined as relational thinking, involves mostly cognition and convergent production—but especially cognition of semantic systems (CMS).

Induction is thought to be in the area of cognition because of its discovery properties.

Deduction is primarily in the area of convergent production because it has to do with drawing firm conclusions.

Classifying objects involves cognition of semantic classes.

Sensitivity to problems is primarily cognition of meaningful implications.

Analysis and synthesis are not coherent SOI factors.

Abstraction, Generalization, and Transfer

Abstraction occurs when the person selectively picks "abstract dimensions of the object" and reacts to those dimensions and no others. With transfer, "he is obviously adding some personal component to his original learning experience. Thus, more than the literal, external properties of stimuli guide the individual's behavior" (Rosenthal & Zimmerman, 1978). Abstraction is apparent during concept development: "Concepts are developed by abstracting the common stimulus elements in a series of stimulus objects" (Staats, 1968). After having experience with the common stimulus elements of the concept, the individual will then be able to pick this common component from a new set containing the same element.

Abstraction and transfer are apparent during rule learning.

By a rule, we mean that two or more objects or events are related to one another in a systematic way. For example, we learn that a flashing red light signifies stopping before crossing an intersection. Later, we exhibit transfer of this rule by stopping when we unexpectedly see a flashing red light beside a stalled car on the highway (Rosenthal & Zimmerman, 1978).

Abstraction and transfer are involved in a judgment of class inclusion. For example, a baby concludes that certain objects are movable. Understanding the "abstract dimension" of moveability the child transfers this by adding some personal component to his or her original learning experience: The child knows that one way of moving something is to pull it; another way is to kick it; and yet another is to get a parent to pull it (Boden, 1980). This is analogous to the child who knows that the class of beads includes the subclass of green beads (Boden, 1980).

The transfer of learning to new stimuli means that the individual will add quite dissimilar response elements that were not directly related to his or her original learning (Rosenthal & Zimmerman, 1978). Transfer is an additional concept used in problem solving. It is when an individual uses something he or she learned previously and transfers it to a new situation. Positive transfer is when what was learned for one situation helps solve a problem in a new situation. Negative transfer is when what was learned for one situation makes it harder to solve a problem in a new situation. When an individual is continuously exposed to similar sorts of problems he or she learns strategies for solving them. A skill that can be transferred to solve problems in new situations is a strategy. Harry Harlow (1949) calls this "learning to learn."

Strategies can be transferred from one situation to another. A strategy can also be divided into its components, and then the components can be recombined in new ways (transformations). A transfer in which the components are recombined to 'suddenly' solve a problem is called insight. It is when a problem is solved with 'aha! Reaction' (Lazerson, 1975).

The intellectual ability to generalize is a significant component of the definition of "cognition." To incorporate specific knowledge and generalize it into everyday experiences is "cognition" well defined and developed (Scott et al., 1979).

Why We Solve Problems or Learn

According to cognitive psychologists, the mind possesses an innate order-generating capacity—a built-in drive to learn. We carry out that drive by acting on our environment. Thus, the individual must act on and interact with the physical, emotional, social, language, and thinking world in order for cognitive processing to occur. When something is unfamiliar or unpredictable, or when we do not understand, we are motivated to learn (Smith, 1975). According to Smith (1975):

We learn because we do not understand, cannot relate, cannot predict. Everything we know, then, is a consequence of all our previous attempts to make sense of the world. Our present knowledge arises out of a history of problem solving or of predicting the consequences of potential actions (p. 161).

We learn by relating new information to previous information and by seeing relationships among various bits of information.

For cognitive psychologists, learning is an active process that is significantly influenced by motivation, especially intrinsic motivation (Bruner, 1968), and by curiosity (Yardley, 1974). Bruner (1968) explains this intrinsic motivation in terms of curiosity drive, a drive to achieve competence, and a need to work cooperatively with others, which he termed reciprocity.

Leon Festinger (Lefrancois, 1982) conceived of cognitive dissonance, the motivating effect of possessing simultaneously compatible items of information. "It is assumed that dissonance leads to behavior designed to reduce conflict" (Lefrancois, 1982, p. 71). An individual remembers more distinctly and for longer periods of time material that is somewhat different from what is already known. If it is completely new and unrelated to anything in his or her cognitive structure, according to Ausubel (Lefrancois, 1982, p. 225), rote learning rather than meaningful learning will occur. If it is too similar, it is rapidly forgotten.

Other variables that intervene between the stimuli and the response are the individual learner's purpose, aspirations, beliefs, and ideals (Marx, 1970). In addition, the learning potential of an individual includes the requisite intellectual capacities, the ideational context, and the existing store of knowledge as it is currently organized (Ausubel, 1965). It is on this basis that the potential meaningfulness of learning material varies with factors such as age, intelligence, occupation, and cultural membership.

Two people, therefore, are likely to respond differently to the very same stimuli because of what they have already learned, what they feel they are capable of achieving, differences in the ways their minds work, or other differences that distinguish one person from another (Dember & Jenkins, 1979). Smith (1975) observes there are two other crucial conditions for the individual to exercise a capacity to learn. One is that the individual have the expectation that there is something to learn; second, the learner must have some reasonable expectation of a positive outcome.

COGNITION

Cognition, then, can be operationally defined as the **use of the five mental operations**: cognition (recognition/ understanding/comprehension), memory, convergent thinking, divergent thinking, and evaluative thinking or judgment. These are the mental events or processes by which we learn or obtain knowledge of our world, by which we organize, store, recover, and use that knowledge. Knowledge is a product of cognition and is associated or organized into units, classes, relations, systems, transformations, and implications.

LANGUAGE DEFINED

Psycholinguistics is the study of the mental processes underlying the acquisition and use of language (Slobin, 1971). Within the context of the Guilford model, incoming information or **language experience** is **semantic and behavioral** (Figure 17–3). This information is then **processed by** one or more of the **five cognitive operations**: cognition, memory, convergent thinking, divergent thinking, and evaluative thinking. These are **the mental processes underlying the acquisition and use of language**.

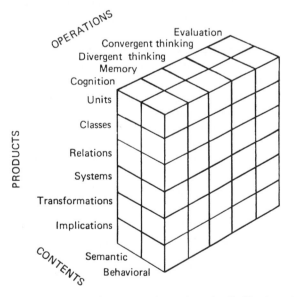

Figure 17–3. Model of language based on the Guilford model (Chapey, 1994).

Language is something we know (Slobin, 1971). It is a body of knowledge represented in the brains of speakers of a language, whose content is inferred from overt behavior (Slobin, 1971). According to Bloom and Lahey (1978), language can be defined as "a knowledge of a code for representing ideas about the world through a conventional system of arbitrary signals for communication" (p. 23). Specifically, there are **three types of language knowledge**: content, form, and use. Thus, "language consists of some aspect of content or meaning that is coded or represented by linguistic form for some purpose or use in a particular context" (p. 23). These three types of language knowledge come together in both understanding and saying messages and indeed linguistic competence can be defined as the interaction of content, form, and use (Bloom and Lahey, 1978; Lahey, 1988).

Content: Language Represents Ideas About the World

Psycholinguistic research suggests that our

... code or means of representing information can operate only in relation to what (we) the speaker and hearer of the language know about objects and events in the world. Speakers of a language need to know about objects and actions in order to know the names for objects and actions. (O)ne cannot know about sentences and the relations between the parts of a sentence unless one also knows about relations between persons and objects in different kinds of events ... It is the knowledge that individuals have about objects, events and relations in the world that is coded by language—ideas about events are coded, not events themselves (Bloom & Lahey, 1978, p. 5).

It is this knowledge, these **ideas**, that are the **meaning, topic,** or **subject** matter involved in conversation. For example, an individual might comment about a specific **object**, such as a pipe, a particular **action**, such as eating lunch, or a specific **relation**, such as between Harry and his pipe. Or, meaning could relate to a **content category** such as possession, or having or owning an object, quality, or ability; recurrence, or the reappearance of an object or event; or rejection, the opposition to an action or object.

An individual learns to understand and use language in relation to the ideas or mental concepts that have been formed through experience (Bloom & Lahey, 1978). The experience of many different objects—some of which are more alike than others—is "an active process whereby persons perceive patterns of structure and invariance in the environment" (Bloom & Lahey, 1978, p. 7), such as similarities among different chairs and the mobility of certain objects and not others. The ability to perceive the similarities in repeated encounters with physical and social events involves the ability to process and analyze experience using the five cognitive processes. Words and categories represent regularities that the individual notes in his or her environment. Individuals learn new words and categories gradually, by testing hypotheses of what a word means in different situations in which they think one or another word might fit (Bloom & Lahey, 1978; Lahey, 1988). This results in the organization or association of information—or the formation of schema into **units** (or chunks of information having 'thing' character; things to which words are often applied; meaning, ideas, or thoughts in the form of particular wholes—such as a cookie); **classes** (or conceptions underlying sets of items such as cookies); **relations** (or meaningful connections between items of information—such as all desserts); **systems** (or complexes of interrelated or interacting relationships among objects, ideas and events; double meanings, puns, homonyms, and redefinitions or shifts in meaning—such as "This is what I call cheesecake"); **transformations** (or various types of changes such as redefinitions, shifts, transitions, or modifications in existing information—such as when baking a cake, if a recipe calls for two eggs and there is only one, one might open one egg, put it into a measuring cup, and then double the volume by adding water or milk); and **implications** (or the formation of hypotheses of what is expected, anticipated, suggested, or predicted by other information—such as "Desserts are sweet, fattening, and taste good; are sold in a bakery; are frequently chocolate; can often become stale or spoil" and so forth).

New experiences may cause the brain to place the experience into an existing unit or class; to create a new concept; to reprocess existing information and reformulate the structure of individual units or to group units together into classes, systems, and/or relations; to transform the information; and/or to see the implications of such information.

Language content is developed and used within the context of the speech act. Communication, which is a problem-solving task, is usually initiated and/or maintained in order to convey meaning about certain topics or ideas or to convey an intent. For example, during communication, an individual may become aware that it is necessary to describe something (an intent) that he or she knows (cognition). The individual may sort through all the possible ways to express this intent (divergent thinking) and may make a judgment, based on past experience, that certain content would be inappropriate (evaluation) for his or her purpose, intent, or listener. The individual therefore comes to a logical conclusion about the conventionally best content for his or her intent (convergent thinking), and then conveys the content to the listener.

Form: Language Is a System

The **rules** of language specify **how to arrange symbols to express ideas** (McCormick & Schiefelbush, 1984). Specifically, a system of rules determines the "ways in which sounds combine to form words and words combine to form sentences for representing knowledge" (Bloom & Lahey, 1978, p. 7). For words, a limited number of rules specify which sounds can and cannot combine. For sentences, a limited number of rules specify how linguistic elements (words

and morphemes) are combined to code meaning (Bloom & Lahey, 1978; Lahey, 1988). According to Slobin (1971), syntax is a device that relates sound and meaning. Thus, the form of language or system of rules "is the means for connecting sounds or signs with meaning" (Bloom & Lahey, 1978, p. 15). Linguistic competence is a system of rules that relates semantic interpretations of a sentence to their acoustic phonetic representations (Slobin, 1971). It is a set or system of rules for processing utterances (Slobin, 1971).

Two rule systems in English are **word order** and **markers**. Word order tells us about the subject-object relationship. There are two types of markers: function words ('the', 'a', 'with') and suffixes ('-s', '-ing'). The markers do such things as identify classes (for example, 'the' identifies a noun), specify relations ('with' relates 'girl' to 'eyes'), or signal meanings ('-ing' signals ongoing activity, '-s' signals plurality), and so on (Slobin, 1971, p. 2).

Chomsky (1957) postulated that there are **two basic sorts of rules or two levels of sentence interpretation**. **Phrase structure rules** generate **deep structures**, which are directly related to the meaning of the sentence. The semantic component of grammar "relates deep structures to meanings" (Slobin, 1971, p. 19). Transformational rules convert deep structures into surface structures. The surface level of a sentence is directly related to the sentence as it is heard. The phonological component of grammar "converts surface structures into sound patterns of spoken utterances" (Slobin, 1971, p. 19).

According to Chomsky (1972), the surface structure is often misleading and uninformative: "Our knowledge of language involves properties of a much more abstract nature, not directly in the surface structure" (p. 32). Since the meaning is not always directly expressed in the sounds we hear, we must have rich inner mental structures that make it possible to utter and comprehend sentences (Slobin, 1971). We cannot explain language learning on the basis of observable "stimuli" and "responses" alone, because all of the information for the processing of speech is not present in observable behavior" (Slobin, 1971, p. 19). Rather, the individual is biologically predisposed to learn a set or system of rules for processing utterances.

Grammar then is:

> . . . a device for pairing phonetically represented signals [into a] system of abstract structures generated by the syntactic component. Thus, the syntactic component must provide for each sentence (actually for each interpretation of each sentence), a semantically interpretable deep structure and a phonetically interpretable surface structure, and in the event that these are distinct, a statement of the relation between these structures (Chomsky, 1964, p. 52).

Abstract structural patterns underlie grammatical sentences. Understanding a sentence is based on knowledge of this structure. Indeed, "you can only make sense of the string of words you hear if you "know . . . the grammar of your language" (Slobin, 1971). This syntactic knowledge or finite system of rules makes it possible for us to comprehend and generate an infinite number of sentences and connect sounds or signs with meaning.

These rules of language that allow us to process and/or generate utterances and connect sounds or signs with meaning are learned by "listening to the language of the environment and abstracting from it the rules that are used to generate it" (Naremore, 1980). Individuals do not learn language form and then apply it to meaning. Rather, they focus on what they see and hear and "use their conceptual capacity for linguistic inductions" (Bloom & Lahey, 1978, p. 72) to develop a knowledge of language content, form, and use in order to communicate meaning. Meaning is the essence of language (Goodman, 1971).

Developing a language system is a problem-solving task. It involves, among other things, hypothesis formation, abstraction, transfer, judgment of class inclusion, and generalization. As individuals process and use semantic and behavioral information, they become aware that the system of rules they now possess is not adequate for expressing meaning or what they would like to say. Becoming aware that a problem exists is a matter of cognition, often involving implications. Next, the problem in the rule system is analyzed or structured, which usually involves cognition of systems. After the problem is structured, the individual generates a variety of possible ways to code what he or she wishes, which is divergent production. If sufficient basis for a solution to the rule system is cognized and then produced, there is convergent production. At each stage in the process, there is evaluation or judgment in the form of accepting or rejecting cognitions of the problem and generated solutions. At any step, what happens may become fixated and retained for possible later use, so that memory is involved. When evaluation leads to rejections, there may be new starts, with revised cognitions and productions.

Thus, we learn new forms of language when our present system of rules proves inadequate for expressing meaning. The acquisition of new rules comes about in the form of new discriminations in terms of new products. Individuals learn rules gradually by testing hypotheses of what a form can express in different situations where they think the rule might be appropriate for the expression of meaning.

Use: Language Is Used for Communication

Communication is an assertive act of coping—an active problem-solving task. It is a constant attempt to vary the content, form, and acceptability of a message; to switch or shift sets of reference as topics change (Muma, 1975); and to be sensitive to the influence of one's communicative partner and the physical context in which communication occurs (Prutting & Kirchner, 1983) in order to achieve a message

of best fit and thus effective and efficient communication (Muma, 1975).

Therefore, **communicative competence** implies knowledge of how to converse with different partners and in different contexts (Craig, 1983) and knowledge of the rights, obligations, and expectations underlying the maintenance of discourse (Ochs & Schieffelin, 1979). It is a knowledge of who can say what to whom, in what way, where and when, and by what means (Prutting, 1979).

Pragmatics involves the acquisition and use of such conversational knowledge and of the semantic rules necessary to communicate an intent in order to affect the hearer's attitudes, beliefs, or behaviors (Lucas, 1980). Such semantic knowledge develops and is "used within the context of a **speech act**, a theoretical unit of communication between a speaker and a hearer" (Lucas, 1980). According to Searle (1969), the speech act includes "what the speaker means, what the sentence (or other linguistic elements) uttered means, what the speaker intends, what the hearer intends, what the hearer understands, and what the rules governing linguistic utterances are" (p. 12). Speech acts include making promises, statements, requests, assertions, and so on (Table 17–1). In Searle's (1969) theory, the proposition is the words or sentences produced, and the elocutionary force of this proposition is the speaker's intent in producing the utterance.

Thus, pragmatics involves the interactional aspects of communication including sensitivity to various aspects of

---

TABLE 17–1

Discourse Structures

1. Physical context variables
2. Communicative partner variables
3. Communication of intent

Label	Greeting	Attention
Response	Repeating	Protesting (Dore, 1974)
Request	Description	
Request	Order	Warn (Searle, 1969)
Assert	Argue	
Question	Advise	

4. Turn taking
   A. Initiation of speech act
   B. Maintenance of communication
      (i) Role switching/turn taking
      (ii) Sustaining a topic
         a. Contingent utterances
         b. Adjacent utterances
         c. Feedback to speaker
         d. Repair/revision
         e. Code switching

social contexts (Prutting & Kirchner, 1983). It is an analysis of the use of language for communication. The emphasis is not on sentence structure but on how meaning is communicated—how units of language function in discourse (Prutting & Kirchner, 1983).

Pragmatics is inextricably related to cognition, and indeed the conversational knowledge or discourse structures that are derived by an individual are the products of one or all of the five SOI cognitive processes or operations. The incoming semantic and/or behavioral information is processed by cognition, memory, convergent thinking, divergent thinking, and/or evaluative thinking in order to generate pragmatic (semantic and/or behavioral) units, classes, relations, systems, transformations, and implications. Communication, and therefore pragmatics or language use, is an active process of problem solving. We learn new pragmatic rules when our present pragmatic knowledge proves inadequate for a situation or when something in our experience is unfamiliar or unpredictable. The acquisition of new pragmatic information comes about in the form of new discourse structures, as a result of the use of one or all of the five mental operations of the SOI model.

Discourse Structures

A number of cognitive/pragmatic products or discourse structures are discussed in the literature. They relate to physical context variables, communicative partner variables, communication of intent, and turn-taking rules (including topic selections, maintenance and change, code switching, and referential skills) (Table 17–1).

Physical Context Variables

A pragmatic view of language assumes that language will vary with each context, that contexts are dynamic, and that any language sample will therefore be the interactive product of contextual variables and the individual's structural linguistic knowledge (Gallagher, 1983). Various conversational settings may affect the number and variety of utterances produced by a speaker (Gallagher, 1983). For example, one may have a rule that says, "Don't talk in church"; one that says, "Don't talk loudly in an elegant restaurant"; and yet another that says, "Cheer loudly for your team at a football game."

As individuals encounter various contexts or settings, they categorize or classify these contexts and simultaneously or subsequently develop rules for interacting in specific types of contexts. The individual tries to determine if he or she knows or recognizes the context; may perhaps try to think of all of the other possible responses or behaviors that might be appropriate to this context; may make judgments about certain variables within the context; may try to hypothesize what is expected, anticipated, or suggested for this or for analogous situations; and so on.

Communicative Partner Variables

Specific communicative partners may affect the length, complexity, redundancy, fluency, and responsiveness (such as elaborations of comments), semantic relatedness of comments, and the amount of eye contact during an utterance (Gallagher, 1983). Indeed, partner characteristics such as **age, sex, familiarity,** and **status** frequently affect communication. Again, the individual categorizes and classifies partners and develops rules for interacting with specific partners, types of partners, and groups of partners.

When a person first encounters a potential communicative partner, he may determine if he knows or recognizes the partner or type of partner. He may sort through all the possible topics or intents that would be appropriate for this partner and subsequently judges or evaluates the form, reference, and acceptability of various possible communications and the implications of such communication.

Communication of Intent

Language is used to communicate a variety of intentions. For example, Dore (1974) specified the following intents: **to label, to respond, to request, to greet, to protest, to repeat, to describe,** and **to call attention** to something. The intents specified by Searle (1969) are **to request, to assert, to question, to order, to argue, to advise,** and **to warn.**

Language intent may be communicated and comprehended through semantic-syntactic utterances and/or by previous or subsequent utterances. In addition, intent may be expressed (and comprehended) through facial expression or accompanying actions, gestures, or tone of voice. What is not said may also communicate intent. One can also say one thing and mean another. Individuals frequently use their knowledge of the physical context variables and the communication partner to help them decipher between what is said and what is meant. Thus, the communication of intent involves the use of semantic content (what is said) as well as behavioral content, or the nonfigural and nonverbal information that communicates the **attitudes, needs, desires, moods, intentions, perceptions,** and **thoughts** of others and ourselves. It may even involve the use of symbolic content when symbolic gestures are used.

Individual intents are semantic and/or behavioral units—that is, items or "chunks" of information. These units are developed when the brain processes semantic and behavioral experiences using the five cognitive operations. New experiences may cause the brain to place the experience into an existing unit or class; to create a new concept; to reprocess existing information and reformulate the structure of individual units or to group units together into classes, systems, and/or relations; and/or to see implications of such information. The way in which the individual chooses to communicate an intent at any particular point will reflect his or her knowledge of physical context variables and his or her communicative partner(s). Thus, the individual evaluates group membership, ability of the listener to interpret the various levels of complexity, receptiveness to various intents, and so on. Comprehension of the intent will be based on the units, classes, systems, relations, transformations, and implications that the listener has already established, as well as the information, associations, or products that he or she has constructed with respect to this specific partner or class of partner, this type of context, and this type of topic. According to Haviland and Clark (1974), comprehension of an utterance in context also involves relating new information to assumed information. Thus, the individual makes a judgment based on past experience, as to what is new information and what he or she can assume this particular partner knows.

Turn Taking Rules

The reciprocal nature of communication involves a number of aspects, including the **initiation of the speech act** and the maintenance of communication. Initiation of the speech act (as speaker) includes topic selection and introduction and/or change of topic. Usually, the communicative act should contain **new, relevant**, and what is judged to be sincerely **wanted** information. It is important to evaluate the implicitly shared information aspect of the communication act. Thus, **topical or referential identification** involves searching one's long-term memory for information that is judged to be relevant to this partner, wanted by this partner, and perhaps interesting.

Maintenance of communication involves a number of variables. First, **role taking** involves the establishment and variation of roles with respect to the speaker and the listener and the reciprocal roles of speaker-initiator and listener-respondent.

The **listener's** role is to comprehend the **speaker's** message, which involves cognition. He maintains his role with nonverbal (behavioral) responses that are "characterized by visual orientation rather than gaze avoidance" (Davis & Wilcox, 1981, p. 172), a head nod, or leaning forward. He may also respond with a short and usually affirmative verbal response such as "yes."

Feedback to the speaker is also essential. This involves the listener's ability to monitor and evaluate the speaker's message and ability/willingness to indicate whether he or she believes it is effective and acceptable. Listener feedback will depend on the listener's previously established concepts of effectiveness and acceptability in general and his or her concepts relevant to this speaker and this context. Occasionally, the listener will assist the speaker in conveying the message, which involves cognition, judgment, and possibly convergent and divergent thinking.

Role switching may occur as the result of the speaker's desire to relinquish the role. It can be communicated and/or comprehended semantically and/or behaviorally. In many instances, nonverbal (behavioral) cues are used by partners to signal a wish to maintain or change roles (Harrison, 1974; Rosenfeld, 1978). The speaker usually retains his or her role by gaze avoidance and a hand gesture that is not maintained or not returned to a resting state through a phonetic clause juncture (Rosenfeld, 1978). When a speaker wants a listener's reaction, he or she signals "with a pause between clauses" or "with a rising or falling pitch at the end of a phonemic clause" (Davis & Wilcox, 1981, p. 171). Thus, the listener needs to use knowledge of such cues as well as the cues themselves in order to formulate a judgment concerning the speaker's willingness to switch roles. However, when role switching occurs in the absence of the speaker's readiness to switch, it may be accompanied by overloudness and a shift of the head away from the speaker (Davis & Wilcox, 1981), which would be behavioral content.

Maintenance of communication may also involve a response that **sustains a topic** (the listener becomes the speaker)—one that involves a specific response to the speech act. For example, **contingent utterances** are utterances that share the same topic with the preceding utterance and that add information to the prior communication act. A contingent utterance is an elaboration of the speaker's topic. Production of contingent utterances would usually involve semantic and behavioral cognition in order to understand or comprehend an utterance and its intent; convergent production, or a logical and sequentially ordered response; and divergent thinking, or an elaboration of a topic and judgment as to the relevance, accuracy, and appropriateness of a response in this context to this communicative partner.

Maintenance of communication also involves a **sequential organization of topics**. Thus, **adjacent utterances** are also used. These are utterances that occur immediately after a partner's utterance but are not related to the speaker's topic. Such utterances are considered logical or possible elaborations of communication and therefore involve convergent and divergent semantic thinking.

Repair and **revision** are also part of discourse maintenance and regulation. This involves the speaker's sensitivity to cues provided by the listener, which involves semantic and behavioral cognition and judgment, and the ability to respond to such cues by repeating and/or modifying the message when necessary. It involves the speaker's use of convergent production, divergent production, and judgment. Moves by the speaker and the listener to repair sequences and respond to such regulatory devices as requests for clarification are essential to the maintenance of communication (Fey & Leonard, 1983).

Code switching is the degree to which the individual can produce stylistic variations in the form or frequency of specific acts to meet situational requirements (Fey & Leonard, 1983), such as the ability to role play. Judgment is essential.

In an article written in 1975, John Muma addressed the issue of role/code switching. In this article, he differentiated between two different variations in one's method of communication. One he called "dump" and the other "play." **Dumping** pertains to the issuance of a coded message. **Play** involves ascertaining needed changes for appropriate recoding of a message and making necessary adjustments in order to achieve the message of best fit. According to Muma (1975), role-taking attitudes involve the active resolution of communicative obstacles of form, reference, and acceptability in an effort to achieve the message of best fit for a particular situation and listener. It is the ability to issue a "message in the most appropriate form for conveying intended meanings to a particular person for particular efforts" (p. 299). In role taking, "both speaker and listener are active participants in formulating, perceiving and revising messages until necessary adjustments are made in form, reference or psychological distance, and acceptability in order to convey intended meanings" (p. 299). The objective of true communication is aimed at ascertaining or judging the message most suited to achieve effective and efficient communication.

Content, Form, and Use

Language learning and use, then, are problem-solving tasks. A problem is presented whenever a situation calls for the individual doing anything novel in order to cope with something that is different from his or her past behavior. A problem is a question or a proposition that necessitates consideration and a solution (Webster, 1977). Problem solving involves the use of all five mental operations, all types of content or information, and any kind of product, depending on the context in which the problem arises and the kinds of products required in order to reach a solution.

If the information is immediately recognized, known, comprehended, or understood, the mental operation of cognition has occurred. When situations call for the individual to generate logical conclusions from given information where emphasis is on achieving conventionally best outcomes, convergent thinking occurs. When a novel response is required, the divergent operation is generated. Inserting newly gained information into storage involves the operation of memory. Judging the appropriateness, acceptability, relevance, and/or correctness of information requires evaluation.

The three **types of language knowledge** that develop and are used (**content, form,** and **use**) **are products of these five mental operations**. Normal language functioning, then, requires the efficient action and interaction of all five cognitive processes in order for effective decoding (cognition, memory) and encoding (convergent thinking, divergent thinking, evaluative thinking) to occur.

ASSESSMENT OF COGNITIVE OPERATIONS

Guilford and Hoepfner (1971) developed a number of tests to assess each of the five mental operations. A list of some of these tests follows.

Semantic Awareness/Recognition Tests

Verbal Comprehension. Choose a word that means about the same as the given word.

Reading Comprehension. Answer questions about a short passage.

Verbal Opposites. Give a word that is opposite in meaning to the given word.

Sentence Synthesis. Rearrange scrambled words to make a meaningful sentence.

Vocabulary. Choose the alternative word that has the same meaning as a word that completes a sentence.

Semantic Memory Tests

Picture Memory. Recall names of common objects pictured on a previously studied page.

Recalled Words. Recall words presented on a study page.

Word Recognition. Recognize whether given words were on a previously studied page.

Memory for Facts. Answer questions regarding information previously given in two sentences.

Convergent Semantic Tests

Picture Group Naming. Write a class name for each group of five pictured objects.

Associations. Write a word that is associated with each of two given words.

Largest Class. Form the largest class possible from a given list of words so that the remaining words also make a class.

Attribute Listing. List attributes of objects needed to serve a specific function.

Divergent Semantic Tests

Common Situations. List problems that are inherent in a common situation.

Brick Uses. List many different uses for a common object.

Product Improvement. Suggest ways to improve a particular object.

Consequences. List the effect of a new and unusual event.

Object Naming. List objects that belong to a broad class of objects.

Differences. Suggest ways in which two objects are different.

Similarities. Produce ways in which two objects are alike.

Word Fluency. List words that contain a specified word or letter.

Planning Elaboration. List many detailed steps needed to make a briefly outlined plan work.

Semantic Evaluation Tests

Word Checking. Choose one of four words that fits a single criterion.

Double Descriptions. Select the one object of four that best fits two given descriptions or adjectives.

Class Name Selection. Select a class name that most precisely fits a group of four given words.

Commonsense Judgment. Select the two best of five given reasons why a briefly described plan is faulty.

Behavioral Tests

Alternate Expressional Groups. Group pictured expressions in different ways so that each group expresses a common thought, feeling, or intention.

Cartoon Predictions. Choose one of three alternative cartoon frames that can be most reasonably predicted from the given frame.

Expression Grouping. Choose one of four expressions that belongs with a given group by virtue of common psychological dispositions.

Expressions. Choose one of four expressions that indicates the same psychological state as another given expression.

In addition, Torrance (1966) adapted Guilford and Hoepfner's (1971) work on divergent thinking and developed the *Torrance Test of Creative Thinking* (Torrance, 1966). (Norms are available only for children.) Parts of this test along with other tests from Guilford and Hoepfner (1971) have been used with aphasic, right-brain-damaged, closed-head-injured, and elderly individuals (Braverman, 1990; Chapey, 1974, 1983; Chapey & Lubinski, 1979; Chapey et al., 1976, 1977; Diggs & Basili, 1987; Law & Newton, 1991; Schwartz-Crowley & Gruen, 1986), in order to assess abilities and impairments of specific mental operations in these groups. The *Test of Problem Solving* (Zachman et al., 1983), developed to measure reasoning abilities in children, can also be used with adults to assess specific cognitive semantic abilities such as explaining inferences, determining causes, answering negative 'wh' questions, determining solutions, and avoiding problems.

Other techniques for assessing cognitive semantic abilities can be obtained through the Educational Testing Services' Test Collection Department which has a number of unpublished research instruments measuring aptitude and cognition. Several of these measures target Guilford and Hoepfner's (1971) mental operations.

Clinicians who use the cognitive semantic approach to intervention may also evaluate the specific language assets and liabilities of each patient so that the therapeutic effort is individualized to fit the needs, interests, and abilities of each person who receives such therapy. For example, clinicians may want to explore the nature of each patient's language impairment—including performance on appropriate tasks, types(s) of errors made, and the manner in which each patient goes about tasks (Byng et al., 1990).

Clinicians may also need to break tasks (such as comprehending sentences, reading aloud single words, gesturing,

hailing a bus, filling in a check, turn taking) down into their component processes and examine the functioning of each of those processes in detail (Byng et al., 1990, p. 82) in order to derive hypotheses about the nature of the underlying processing problems in the language deficits in specific patients. A more in-depth discussion of assessment techniques can be found in Chapter 4.

INTERVENTION

The present writer agrees with Martin (1979):

Normal functioning is the "efficient action and interaction of the cognitive processes which support language behavior within and by the organism." The disorder is "(a) reduction of the efficiency of action and interaction of the cognitive processes which support language behavior."

Therapy is "the attempt to manipulate and to excite the action and interaction of the cognitive processes which support language behavior within and by the organism so as to maximize their effective usage . . . Therapy [is] directed toward the subsystems which process language" (pp. 157–158).

Within the context of the present chapter, **the cognitive processes** or **subsystems that process language are cognition, memory, convergent thinking, divergent thinking,** and **evaluation.** Aphasia is a reduction in the efficient action and interaction of these processes. Therapy is an attempt to manipulate and excite the action and interaction of these processes. We employ strong, controlled, and intensive figural, symbolic, semantic, and behavioral stimuli—most frequently, semantic stimuli—in order to elicit the action of cognition, memory, convergent thinking, divergent thinking, and evaluation. These are the cognitive processes or the complex events that happen in the brain.

What is happening between the stimulus and the response is that the individual is using one or all of his or her mental operations. **Task input** is defined as figural, symbolic, semantic, and/or behavioral. **Processing** occurs through the use of cognition, memory, convergent thinking, divergent thinking, and evaluative thinking. **Output** is generated in units, classes (or categories), relations, transformations, systems, and implications. This holds true for problem-solving, decision-making, learning, and language tasks.

Rationale

A cognitive approach to therapy is based on the belief that **propositional** language (H. Jackson, cited in Head, 1915) or **functional communication is an active problem-solving task** that **necessitates the use of all five cognitive processes.** These operations are the intervening mediating variables or constructs responsible for language comprehension and production. Thus, cognitive semantic therapy advocates the stimulation of all five mental operations, since this type of processing is required for the comprehension and production of spontaneous language. Indeed, most definitions of language and communication have components that are highly suggestive of all five operations. For example, Hughy and Johnson (1975) state that language is used primarily for information getting and giving, problem solving, and persuasion. Another definition, that proposed by Muma (1975), notes that communication entails the ability to switch or shift sets of reference as topics change, to initiate such shifts, and to overcome obstacles to communication flow. Both definitions reflect the fact that language and communication require the use of all five cognitive processes.

Ability to produce functional communication or spontaneous speech also involves what Noam Chomsky (1957, 1964) refers to as deep structure and surface structure. **Deep structure** specifies the **basic relationship** being expressed—who did what to whom. It tells the meaning relationship. The surface structure is the actual sentences that are spoken and written. **Meaning is often not audible or visible**. Rather, the listener or reader must identify the relationships of the concepts to the events being communicated or described. Understanding a message depends on the memory structure of the people involved in the communication. The entire structure is not communicated if the receiver of the information can already be assumed to understand certain basic concepts. That is, some relations are assumed to be known or to be relatively easy to discover and therefore not necessary to mention.

According to Chomsky (1957, 1964), not everything we know about a sentence is revealed in the superficial string of words. That is, all information for processing speech is not present in observable behavior. Meaning is not directly expressed in the sounds we hear and the words we read. Our capacity to interpret sentences depends on our knowledge of deep structure. We don't learn a set of utterances (surface structures). Rather, we learn methods of processing utterances. We have rich cognitive structures that make it possible to utter and comprehend sentences.

In everyday communication, surface structure is frequently deficient, misleading, and uninformative. For example, there are extensive deletions, extensive use of pronouns, and ambiguous referents. But meaning structure may be communicated nevertheless. Therefore, language is an aid to communication. Production of spontaneous, functional language and therefore deep and surface structure requires the use of all five mental operations. These are the methods for processing utterances. These are the rich cognitive structures that make it possible to comprehend and produce sentences. Cognitive therapy therefore targets all five mental operations for the production of meaningful ideas and the elaboration of those ideas.

A third rationale is based on the observation that aphasic patients are unable to produce the highest-level central nervous system integrations (Wepman, 1951). Research by Bolwinick (1967) indicates that the **highest-level** cognitive integrations are **thinking**—such as convergent thinking, divergent thinking, and evaluative thinking; **problem solving**—all five cognitive operations are viewed as essential components of problem solving; and **creativity**—divergent thinking is used as a synonym for creativity. Tasks using all five mental operations will focus on the essence of the aphasic impairment: inability to produce the higher-level cognitive integrations.

Cognitive therapy is also rooted in the observation that aphasia is a problem in language **retrieval** (Schuell et al., 1964), or in the searching and scanning mechanism that selects among many possibilities. Schuell and coworkers (1964) noted that the search mechanism is controlled by instructions, directing it to go to a specific address and bring out information. They suggest that appropriate stimuli are required to activate or reactivate patterns. The information-processing model presented in this chapter hypothesizes that divergent production and evaluative production involve the use of a broad search of memory storage, while cognition and convergent production involve a narrow search of long-term memory. Tasks that stimulate retrieval under a variety of cognitive operations appear to facilitate the patient's reorganization and retrieval of language. Specifically, the stimuli presented foster the action of a broad and narrow search of memory within the individual. The clinician attempts to manipulate the patient's retrieval strategy in order to aid the patient in making maximal responses.

Another appeal of the Guilford model is that it is a **model of learning** (Chapey, 1994) and, indeed, the acquisition and use of knowledge may involve the use of the five mental operations in the model: recognition/comprehension, and convergent, divergent, and/or evaluative thinking (Chapey, 1994).

In addition, the Guilford **SOI model has statistical validity**. That is, the entire model has been proven to exist in "normal" individuals (Guilford, 1967; Guilford & Hoepfner, 1971) and the mental operations have been proven to exist in individuals with aphasia (Chapey, 1974, 1977a, 1983, 1988, 1992, 1994; Chapey & Lubinski, 1979). The fourth appeal of the model is that some individuals may solve problems and make decisions more effectively and efficiently when they use a structured problem-solving, decision-making model.

Accountability

Despite the **wide acceptance of the cognitive and pragmatic approaches** to therapy in our literature, and the acceptance of the **distinction between deep structure and surface structure**, many intervention agencies and many government agencies mandate that each therapy session have an operationally written, behavioral goal. Many clinicians also use such goals. For example, the audience (ASHA certified speech-language pathologists) at a workshop were asked to write short-term goals for a moderately language-impaired patient. More than half wrote goals such as "By the end of this session, X will say the name of five common objects."

Behavioral, operationally written objectives are counterproductive to the development of language. They are unacceptable within both a cognitive model and a pragmatic model of intervention. Behavioral objectives target surface structures. Cognitive and pragmatic intervention focus on meaning or deep structure. In cognitive-pragmatic intervention, we attempt to increase the patient's viability as a communicative partner (Lubinski, 1986).

Behavioral, operationally written objectives are inappropriate because they ignore the fact that **meaning is the essence of language** and that meaning is **not an observable behavior**. They ignore the fact that a conversation is like a game. It involves a series of moves by participants. Every conversation is altogether new for the participants. Therefore, we continually communicate creativity (Lindfors, 1980). (Lindfors's text concerns language intervention in children.)

Behavioral, operationally written objectives ignore the **fact that content and form are developed and used within the context of a speech act.** The individual develops communicative competence "through discerning rules underlying the diverse interaction contexts which she observes and in which she participates" (Lindfors, 1980, p. 311).

Behavioral, operationally written objectives ignore the fact that the **speaker's intent** in producing an utterance and a **hearer's intent** in hearing an utterance **are the essence of communication and meaning. The intent of the message is the reason we communicate.** The intent is the function that language serves. We use verbal utterances to express an intention or function. We use language to question, to request, and to inform. Our attention as speakers and listeners is on the meaning, the intention of what someone is trying to say (Cazden, 1976). Language forms are heard through the meaning intended (Cazden, 1976). Thus, **communication is idea oriented**, not word oriented. Language is rooted in meaning, not in surface structures. Language is used for communication. It is a tool, not an end in itself. **Language is an aid to communication.**

Clinical aphasiologists may wish to encourage regulating agencies to realize that language is facilitated by an environment that focuses on meaning rather than on form. Getting the message across is more important for individuals than the form they use to do so.

These agencies should realize that "language is not labeling or matching pictures to words or repeating what someone else said" (Holland, 1975, p. 518). (Holland's article concerns language intervention in children.) Instead, **language is "an active, dynamic interpersonal interchange"** (Holland, 1975, p. 518). If we focus on tasks like labeling, matching pictures to words, or repeating what someone else said, "we run the risk of inadvertently teaching the erroneous principle that language is a skill on the order of playing

the piano. This helps the (individual)... miss the point of communicating" (Holland, 1975, p. 518).

Language training must be to some very significant extent concerned with helping (the individual)... discover his potential as a verbal communicator. Without this discovery, language will remain something akin to a well practiced talent, a recital, not a...part of him (p. 519).

Verbalizations must not replace language. Drill is not language. According to Lindfors (1987), "there is no language apart from meaning" (p. 217). Language "is communicating—the back and forth, the give and take of ideas, not... the mindless parroting of rigid, fixed forms" (Lindfors, 1980, p. 218). Where in a language drill is the meaning that we know to be the very base of language (Lindfors, 1980)? Where is the creativity, the novel expression, that is the core of language? Where is the communicating—the interacting with someone, about something, for some reason (Lindfors, 1987)?

Drill is opposed to language in its meaninglessness, in its rigidity, in its purposelessness (Lindfors, 1987). Drill may make clients very good at doing drills but not at using language and communication. Indeed, according to Lindfors, drill may adversely affect language growth and retrieval. She maintains that **problem solving, planning, discussing ideas, brainstorming, recording ideas, presenting ideas,** and **selecting the best ideas** involve **listening, speaking, reading,** and **writing with a purpose.** The real question is: Is the individual a more effective user of language after completing an exercise or drill? The answer is no. We become more effective communicators as a result of using language in communication with others. According to Lindfors (1980):

labeling syntactic (or semantic) items simply makes you a better "syntactic item labeler" (at least for a few days). Talking about forms doesn't help you express meaning more effectively (p. 220).

Lindfors apparently believes that it is inappropriate to structure a simple-to-complex sequence of forms. Rather, the communication itself will determine the language forms the individual uses and responds to. She believes that we need **to focus on language use for effective communication.** When we do so, our clients may then use the language forms that help them accomplish effective communication.

Individuals, Lindfors (1987) claims, become effective interactants as they have more **opportunities to interact.** Language intervention should **reflect** the individual's **interests, goals, activities, concerns,** and **life participation.** Natural shaping of semantics and syntax happens not through sequenced curriculum but through feedback as to whether one has been understood and whether one has achieved the purpose of the communication.

New meanings find expression as individuals **wonder, question, inform, argue,** and **reason** through language in real-life situations rather than contrived situations (Lindfors, 1987). Language lives in **shared experience, in decision making,** and **in planning**. Language is stimulated and facilitated by an environment rich in diverse verbal and nonverbal experiences. Language lives and grows **in rich experiences**.

As human beings, we develop a theory of the world in our head (Smith, 1975). Our theory shapes the way we look at past experience (recall and interpret it), and the way we look at new experience. We comprehend or interpret the world by relating new experience to the already known—by placing new experiences in our existing cognitive structure or "theory" (Smith, 1975). To learn is to alter our existing cognitive structure when experience does not conform to our theory (Lindfors, 1987).

Language helps us to comprehend and learn—especially as language is used in **questioning** (curiosity and procedural or social-interactional questioning), **focusing attention, making understandings more precise, making understandings more retrievable, reinterpreting past experience,** and **going beyond present personal experiences** (Lindfors, 1987). Interaction is essential to both comprehension and learning. In real gut-level, meaningful learning, what is to be learned cannot be specified in advance. Such learning is characterized by **curiosity, exploration, problem solving, planning, decision making, discussion of ideas, brainstorming,** and **evaluative thinking** (Chapey, 1988, 1992; Guilford, 1967; Lindfors, 1980, 1987).

The present pressure to establish accountability has actively discouraged exploration, curiosity, and problem solving. Skills, drills, rules, and facts become ends in themselves (Lindfors, 1987). We have packaged clinical programs with a renewed emphasis on memorizing words, on defining words, on identifying parts of speech in sentences that no one ever said or ever will say, so that individuals can get higher standardized test scores and move on to the next highest level of memorization, definition, and identification (Lindfors, 1987).

As a profession, we are first and foremost concerned that our clients become competent communicators (Frattali, 1992). Emphasis on learning rote skills and specified sets of behaviors means increased emphasis on the use of lower-level cognitive processes (Lindfors, 1987). **Lower-level** cognitive behavior means that clients can **give back** the same information they received (recalling, memorization), but to display **higher-level** cognitive behavior, they must **go beyond** the given information some way—**relating it** to something else, **reorganizing** it, **inferring** from it, and **using** it as a springboard for creatively solving new problems. It involves **applying, analyzing, synthesizing,** and **evaluating**. **Questioning** is the individual's most important tool for learning—especially curiosity questioning (Lindfors, 1987). **Conversation** should be the locus, process, and goal of

language intervention (Warren & Rogers-Warren, 1985). **Content-centered discussion therapy** and **embellishment of ideas** within a topic (Wepman, 1972, 1976) should be our focus.

THERAPY OBJECTIVES

Therefore, the objective of a cognitive approach to rehabilitation is to stimulate the five cognitive processes—cognition (awareness/attention, immediate discovery, recognition, comprehension), memory, convergent thinking, divergent thinking, and evaluative thinking—in order to improve overall functional communication. Whenever possible, the focus should be on the stimulation of these abilities within the context of conversational discourse. That is, conventional discourse is seen as the procedural plan for intervention. Whenever possible, turn taking, cuing, modeling, and reinforcement are essential components of therapy.

General Objectives

The general objectives are:

1. To stimulate ability to recognize and comprehend language
2. To stimulate ability to fix new information in memory in order to improve communication
3. To stimulate ability to generate logical information or conclusions during communication
4. To stimulate ability to generate logical alternatives to given information, to produce a quantity and variety of responses during communication, and to be able to elaborate on ideas and plans during communication
5. To stimulate ability to make judgments or appraisals or to formulate evaluations in terms of criteria such as correctness, completeness, identity, relevance, adequacy, utility, safety, consistency, feasibility, social custom, and so forth in order to communicate more effectively and efficiently
6. To stimulate the integration of all cognitive operations through the use of problem-solving, decision-making, and planning tasks and through conversational discourse in order to communicate more effectively and efficiently.

There are four levels of specific objectives within this approach. However, this model of therapy suggests that, regardless of the level at which the patient is functioning, the initial stage of intervention should focus on language-related cognition: knowing, awareness, immediate discovery, recognition, comprehension, and understanding. This suggestion is based on the rationale that individuals with aphasia should be provided with an opportunity to hear and grasp the language behavior of others over and over again. That is, auditory stimulation is seen as an essential component of language retrieval in aphasic patients (Schuell et al., 1955). Thus, for example, the clinician might videotape a group of normal adults responding to a divergent task such as: "Can you think of a problem that anyone might have in eating lunch?" Concomitantly, the patient could be reinforced for all listening and attending behavior. Specifically, movements of the eye that result in a better visual stimulus for the patient or movements of the ear that result in a better auditory stimulus (Staats, 1968) of the videotape would be reinforced. Although no verbal responses would be required during this phase of therapy, all verbal responses that relate to the task at hand could be highly reinforced.

Exposure to the videotaped responses of others may prove to be a vicarious learning experience (Bandura & Walters, 1963; Harris & Evans, 1974) for the individual with aphasia. This suggestion appears to be in consonance with Cooper and Rigrodsky's (1979) finding that persons with aphasia are able to model the verbal behavior of normal subjects and improve their explanations of material that is presented. If modeling is to occur, however, it may be helpful to consider several facts. First, it may be beneficial if the subjects on the videotape are of comparable age and sex as the individual with aphasia, so that the patient will identify with the person who is producing the divergent responses. Second, the clinician could attempt to choose tasks that are interesting and relevant to the particular subject. Third, since Pieres and Morgan (1973) empirically determined that a relaxed, receptive, and uncritical environment increased the divergent behavior of normal subjects, it may be important to provide this type of climate for persons with aphasia. This exposure to the divergent semantic behavior of others, perhaps filed in competitive "game show" style (Torrance, 1974), can continue to be a component of the intervention strategy throughout the process of therapy.

Principles

Intervention should be oriented toward the following traditional therapeutic principles:

1. Begin with the tangible (here and now) and move toward the representational.
2. Begin with the concrete and move toward the abstract.
3. Begin with the simple and move toward the complex.
4. Begin with the real and move toward the complex.
5. Begin with actions on objects and move toward verbalizations concerning these actions.
6. Begin with simple classifications and move toward reclassifications and multiple classifications.
7. Begin with exaggerated sensory stimulation—for example, talking through a microphone or using a variety of inflectional patterns (McConnell et al., 1974)—and gradually decrease this exaggeration.
8. Begin with short stimuli/responses and move toward longer stimuli/responses.

9. Begin with continuous reinforcement and move toward intermittent reinforcement (Grant et al., 1951; Jensen & Cotton, 1960).
10. Begin with clinician reinforcement and move toward self-reinforcement (Staats, 1968).

During the course of both diagnosis and therapy, the aphasiologist will attempt to isolate specific conditions under which language retrieval is maximized and to increase the number and variety of these conditions. That is, with whom and under what conditions does language behavior increase? The clinician may wish to manipulate some of the following variables and observe their effect on patient behavior: the listener, referent, intent, situation, cuing devices, repetition and reauditorization, intonation, level of abstraction, cognitive complexity, linguistic complexity, length of stimuli, and frequency of occurrence of word stimuli. The conditions that augment semantic retrieval for each cognitive operation should become an integral component of all subsequent sessions. Examples of specific objectives at each of the four levels of therapy are presented below.

Level I. Specific Objectives

To stimulate ability

Cognition

To be aware of time/space/speech/emotional voice tone
To recognize stimulus equivalence such as matching letters/matching objects to objects/matching objects to pictures/matching words to pictures/matching words to objects
To recognize very high-frequency, concrete objects/events/relationships named
To recognize own name/family names
To follow one-part, simple commands
To understand simple greetings/requests/questions.

Memory

To remember one to two letters/words/pictures
To remember one to two high-frequency, concrete objects/events named.

Convergent Thinking

To repeat one-syllable, high-frequency objects/events/relationships
To produce automatic language
To complete high-probability closure tasks.

Level II. Specific Objectives

To stimulate ability

Cognition

To recognize concrete, high-frequency, familiar objects/events/relationships

To recognize family names/body parts/community helper occupations

To recognize high-frequency objects given their function

To recognize high-frequency events described

To recognize concrete, brief ideas

To comprehend simple conversation with one person

To understand concrete, high-frequency statements about objects such as existence/nonexistence /recurrence /rejection/denial/possession/food/clothing/personal care objects

To understand concrete, high-frequency, brief statements about events such as playing/eating/activities of daily living

To comprehend concrete agent-action and action-object constructions

To comprehend concrete yes/no questions

To comprehend concrete active and negative phrases/sentences

To comprehend articles

To comprehend morphological inflections such as plural /s/, /z/, possessive /s/, /z/, past /t/, /ed/

To comprehend concrete noun phrases and verb phrases

To recognize forms/letters/pictures

To recognize high-frequency printed words and pictures

To match high-frequency printed words to spoken words

To recognize printed letters.

Memory

To remember one to three concrete, high-frequency objects/events/relationships, serially

To execute one- to two-step commands, serially

To remember one to four pictures, serially

To group items to facilitate ability to recall.

Convergent Thinking

To produce automatic language

To complete high-probability phrases/closure tasks

To name high-frequency objects/events/relationships

To comment on objects noting their existence, nonexistence, recurrence, location, possession, and so forth

To talk about common objects such as food, clothing, furniture, transportation

To comment on events such as cooking, eating, activities of daily living

To produce agent-action and action-object constructions

To produce concrete speech acts such as requesting, informing, greeting, questioning

To name members of categories

To list many words that start with a specific letter

To generate numerous and varied objects within a class

To list numerous possible topics of conversation.

Level III. Specific Objectives

To stimulate ability

Cognition

To recognize high- and low-frequency objects/events/relationships

To recognize high- and low-frequency objects/events/relationships described by function

To recognize letter/color/form/number names, and rhyme words

To recognize phonetically similar words

To recognize categories

To comprehend concrete ideas/sentences

To understand relationships between words

To understand statements about objects such as existence/nonexistence/recurrence/rejection/denial/possession/attribution/food/furniture/clothes/personal care objects/health/kitchen utensils, family/other people/places/locations

To understand statements about events such as play/entertainment/eating/activities of daily living/cooking/feelings/sports/school/work/travel/time/news

To understand concrete speech acts such as requesting/ordering/advising/warning/questioning/describing/greeting/repeating/protesting

To hold the thread of discussion in mind, identifying main ideas

To distinguish between relevant and irrelevant information

To understand television/movies

To comprehend inferences

To comprehend short paragraphs

To recognize the existence of problems

To recognize own errors and errors of others

To comprehend simple, concrete analogies

To comprehend active and negative sentences

To comprehend pronouns such as personal, reflexive, indefinite, demonstrative, interrogative, negative

To comprehend adjectives such as color, size, shape, length, height, width, age, taste, temperature, speed, distance, comparative, superlative

To comprehend adverbs with -ly

To comprehend conjunctions

To comprehend prepositions such as locative/temporal/directional

To read concrete, high-frequency and low-frequency sentences

To read and comprehend sequences of material

To read and comprehend short paragraphs

To read and identify main ideas

To read and obtain facts
To read and locate answers
To read and draw conclusions
To read and grasp relationships
To read and grasp inferences
To read street signs
To read newspaper headlines/newspaper stories/newspaper ads.

Memory

To identify one to five names serially
To follow one- to five-part directions and commands
To remember one to five ideas/facts just presented
To group items to facilitate recall
To remember meaning in sentences/short paragraphs/ stories/songs.

Convergent Thinking

To answer questions about self, family, everyday life
To name high- and low-frequency objects/events/relation- ships
To name categories
To name objects/events/relationships within categories
To describe objects/events/relationships
To tell the function of objects, the purpose of events
To define words
To judge the suitability of class inclusion
To judge the similarity of relationships
To judge the suitability of class properties
To identify absurdities
To evaluate implications
To express simple ideas with specificity
To sequentially order ideas or topics toward a purpose
To retell stories—both the literal (who, when, what, where) details and the inferential implications
To describe procedures
To state the relationship between objects/events such as sim- ilarities/differences
To predict possible outcomes
To make inferences and draw conclusions
To answer true/false, yes/no, and wh-questions
To write letters and numbers
To write own name and address
To write sentences with high-frequency, concrete words.

Divergent Thinking

To produce numerous logical possibilities/perspectives/ideas where appropriate
To provide a variety of ideas where appropriate
To change the direction of one's responses
To generate categories of objects/events/relationships/ideas
To predict many different possible outcomes of situations

To generate many different solutions to problems
To list many different problems inherent in situations
To generate numerous steps in a plan
To elaborate on a topic.

Evaluative Thinking

To judge the correctness, completeness, identity, relevance, adequacy, utility, safety, consistency, logical feasibility, and social acceptability of facts
To judge the suitability of words to a topic.

Level IV. Specific Objectives

To stimulate ability

Cognition

To comprehend high- and low-frequency objects/events/ relationships
To recognize concrete and more abstract classes/concepts
To understand relationships among objects/events/ideas
To comprehend analogies
To recognize problems
To recognize own errors and errors of others
To comprehend concrete and more abstract speech acts in conversation with one to five partners
To follow changes in the topic of conversation
To hold the thread of discussion in mind and identify main ideas
To understand changes in interpretation
To comprehend TV/movies
To comprehend more rapid, complex conversations
To comprehend longer sentences/directions/commands
To comprehend more complex/abstract relationships such as comparative, possessive, spatial, temporal, inferential, familial, part-whole, object-action, action-object, cause- effect, sequential, degree, and antonym and synonym relationships
To comprehend negative, passive, and question transforma- tions
To read both short, concrete, and longer, more abstract sen- tences/paragraphs
To read and identify main ideas
To read and obtain facts
To read and locate answers
To read and draw conclusions
To read and grasp relationships
To read and draw inferences
To comprehend newspaper stories/ads
To comprehend catalog/mail order forms
To comprehend a menu
To comprehend a table of contents/index
To use a dictionary/telephone directory.

Memory

To remember one to nine high- and low-frequency objects/events/relationships/categories

To remember facts and commands of increasing length and complexity

To remember meaning in sentences and paragraphs

To use hierarchical organization to facilitate recall

To cluster information to facilitate recall.

Convergent Thinking

To describe high- and low-frequency objects/events/relationships

To indicate the function of high- and low-frequency objects/events/relationships

To specify attributes of objects

To specify the defining attributes of concepts

To define words

To express ideas clearly and with variety

To use language to communicate specific ideas

To use language to elicit specific responses

To express relationships between and among objects/events/relationships and ideas such as similarities and differences

To produce analogies

To sequentially order ideas toward a purpose

To use language to request, inform, explain, question, greet, advise, thank, order, negotiate

To keep meaning going in conversation

To produce class names for groups of words/pictures

To logically deduce the most predictable outcome of a set of facts

To tell the literal (who, what, when, where) details of a story

To make inferences and draw conclusions

To write high- and low-frequency words, sentences, and paragraphs.

Divergent Thinking

To produce numerous logical possibilities and perspectives where appropriate

To provide a variety of ideas where appropriate

To change the direction of one's responses

To stimulate ability to generate many different uses for common and uncommon objects

To predict many possible outcomes of a situation

To list many different problems inherent in a common situation

To think of many different ways to initiate a conversation

To think of many different ways to maintain a conversation

To define many possible rules for communicative partners and communicative contexts

To think of many different ways to repair conversation

To elaborate on topics

To elaborate on or list many different steps needed to do a particular task.

Evaluative Thinking

To make appraisals, comparisons, and formulate evaluations regarding correctness, completeness, relevance, adequacy, utility, safety, consistency, logical feasibility, and social acceptability

To judge the intent of messages

To judge the coherence of a conversation

To judge what can and cannot be said in different contexts, to different partners

To use context and partner variables to decipher between what is said and what is meant

To determine the meaning of proverbs

To judge a situation in which a proverb could be used

To select the word that best fits a single criterion

To select the best of given reasons why a briefly described plan is faulty.

Integration of the Five Cognitive Processes

Within the present therapeutic approach, all five mental operations are integrated in therapy by requiring responses that involve composite abilities. **Problem solving, planning, decision-making tasks,** and **conversational interaction** are excellent for this purpose, since they are composite operations or processes depending on the content of the problem, decision, or conversation and on how the problem/decision/conversation is worded or phrased. Thus, while conversational interaction such as the use of speech acts is sometimes convergent in nature, it will also often involve the use of other mental operations and become problem solving, planning, and decision making in nature depending on the listener, the context, and the intent. Individuals can be stimulated to use language **to question, to request, to inform, to wonder, to argue, to reason,** and **to comprehend** such speech acts.

In addition, formulating solutions to problems posed in the "Dear Abby," or "Dear Meg," column in the local newspaper can be used to stimulate all five cognitive operations. If carefully chosen, such tasks reflect "real-life" situations that patients face—or can allow them to increase their self-concept, since their opinion is being sought and valued. The use of such tasks is conversational in nature and frequently allows for reciprocal role reversal. These tasks can therefore be used to stimulate **brainstorming, discussing, recording and presenting ideas,** and **selecting best outcomes**. They can also be used to stimulate individuals **to question** (curiosity, procedural, and social-interactional), **to focus attention, to make understanding more precise, to reinterpret past experience**, and **to go beyond** present personal experience. Conversational management, conversational **turn taking, topic manipulation,** and **conversational repair** management can also be targeted using these tasks.

Thus, whenever possible, intervention should involve the stimulation of two or three or more mental operations. For example, the clinician might begin a session by asking the client, "Can you list all of the things that can be folded?" After the patient has produced some responses, the clinician summarizes these responses and asks, "Can you think of anymore?" (Table 17–2). When the client has finished responding, the clinician then uses convergent techniques such as those described by Aurelia (1974), Butfield and Zangwill (1946), Goldstein (1948), Keenan (1975), Sarno et al. (1970), Schuell et al. (1955), Vignolo (1964), and Wepman (1953) to stimulate retrieval of appropriate and desired responses that the patient had not produced. Such techniques might involve confrontation naming, recognition naming, oral spelling, reading, categorizing similar responses, creating sentences with a word, and so forth (Table 17–2). In an attempt to develop each patient's ability to correct his or her own errors, the clinician may use cuing techniques such as those suggested by Berman and Peelle (1967). For example, the initial letter of a word could be used as a cue technique. Alternative stimuli for self-cuing might include (a) the first phoneme of a word; (b) the association of a word with a gesture; or (c) the use of an incorrect associational response to cue the correct verbal response. Subsequently, the aphasiologist attempts to transfer the semantic material retrieved in the convergent context and integrate this information into a divergent one. For example, the clinician might ask another divergent question that would call for some of the responses that the patient has been able to retrieve, such as, "Can you think of all of the things that we could pull over our heads?" (Table 17–2). Progress is evaluated by keeping a record of the number and variety of responses produced by the patient (Table 17–2).

Spontaneous language tasks that have divergent, convergent, and/or evaluative components are also used in therapy. For example, the clinician might present a picture description task such as the 'Cookie Thief' picture from the Boston Diagnostic Aphasia Examination (Goodglass & Kaplan, 1972), and encourage the client to produce as many responses as possible (see Yorkston & Beukelman [1977]). Clients can also be encouraged to produce functional spontaneous communication related to a specific theme (Wepman, 1976), such as food, nutrition, food service, restaurants, great parks, interesting sights, vacation destinations, health and diet, sexual issues, social security, legal and money issues, current events, and pharmaceutical issues (AARP's Modern Maturity magazine provides interesting and timely topics for the 50+ audience). In each instance, the clinician records the number and variety of ideas produced by the client.

Levels III and IV. Specific Objectives to Stimulate Use of Composite Abilities

To stimulate ability

To use language to explain, request, correct information, report, advise, question, greet, thank, argue, negotiate

To comprehend speech acts produced by another

To overcome obstacles in communication

To keep meaning going in conversation

To role play (especially to take the viewpoint of someone else) during communication

To select, introduce, maintain, and change the topic of conversation

To initiate and maintain conversation

To use language to discuss objects, events, relationships

To use language to communicate specific ideas

To use language to elicit specific responses

To use language to verbalize a variety of possibilities and perspectives such as the pros and cons of ideas and issues, the advantages and disadvantages of certain actions, ideas

To vary language depending on the context

To vary language depending on the partner

To comprehend various speech acts and intents in relationship to various partners and contexts

To produce stylistic variations to meet situational requirements

To overcome obstacles in communication

To repair and revise communication

To use cues as a signal to repeat or modify messages

To provide feedback to the speaker, as listener, such as requesting message clarification/repetition/restatement, requesting that the message slow down, requesting the message in alternate form, indicating agreement/disagreement with message

To define the problems and solutions inherent in certain objects, events, and relationships

To use a telephone

To use a telephone directory, a dictionary, and a television schedule

To use street and store signs and maps.

THERAPY TASKS AND MATERIALS

Guilford and Hoepfner (1971) developed a number of tasks for each of the five mental operations. Some of these tests have been listed previously under "Assessment." All of these tasks can be readily used to stimulate specific mental (cognitive) operations during therapy. Most traditional workbooks in the field of aphasia have presented tasks that stimulate cognition (recognition/comprehension) and convergent thinking. However, within the last few years, a number of workbooks have been published that focus on the stimulation of divergent thinking, evaluative thinking, problem solving, and decision making.

TABLE 17–2

Sample Therapy Plan That Includes Both Divergent and Convergent Tasks

Objective	Tasks[a]	Cue	Evaluation
General—to stimulate the communication of ideas *Specific*—to stimulate language related to a holiday, Christmas, through divergent and convergent thinking	Greeting *Divergent Tasks* 1. We're coming close to Christmas. What are all of the things that you think of when you think of Christmas?	After 2 minutes summarize responses given and ask, "Can you think of anymore?"	1. (a) List responses: _____ _____ Total fluency: _____ 1. (b) List categories: _____ _____ Total flexibility: _____
	2. Someone mentioned that Santa carries a sack. Can you think of all of the things that could fit into Santa's sack?	Same as above	2. Score as in number one
	3. What are all of the things we might get for Christmas that: could be folded? couldn't be folded? might break if they were dropped? wouldn't break if they were dropped? we could wash? could be hauled in a truck? we could pull over our head? might have buttons? could be worn in summer (winter)? could be made of paper? could come in a box? could be round (square)? are made of glass (plastic, rubber)? someone could drink? someone could eat? has handles? has a neck? moves?	Same as above	3. Score as in number one
	4. List all of the things that you could possibly use a Christmas box for (or bells, string, ribbon).	Same as above	4. Score as in number one
	5. How could you improve a___so that it would be more useful (better, more fun)?	Same as above	5. Score as in number one
	6. If Santa didn't have a sack, he could use___. If Santa lost his belt, he could use___.	Same as above	6. Score as in number one
	7. Imagine you are in a department store (church, living room) at Christmas time. What are all of the things that you might possibly see?	Same as above	7. Score as in number one

continued

continued

Objective	Tasks[a]	Cue	Evaluation
	8. Let's make up a story about Christmas.	Same as above	8. Score as in number one
	9. The word *Christmas* begins with the sound "k." What other words can you think of that start with "k"? The word bell begins with the sound "b." What other words can you think of that start with "b"?	Same as above	9. Score as in number one
	10. What are all of the possible questions that you could ask about this Christmas picture?	Same as above	10. Score as in number one
	11. List all of the different parts of Santa's suit. How could we change each one to make it better?	Same as above	11. Score as in number one
	12. Suppose that we did not celebrate Christmas anymore. What do you think might happen? Can you guess?	Same as above	12. Score as in number one
	13. List all of the problems that someone might have in shopping for a Christmas present.	Same as above	13. Score as in number one
	14. Someone mentioned a cymbal and a drum. They make noise. Can you list all of the things that could be used to make noise?	Same as above	14. Score as in number one
	15. Santa's suit is red. What are all of the other things that could be red?	Same as above	15. Score as in number one
	16. Tomorrow we will have a Christmas party. What are all the different things we'll need to do before the party? *Convergent Tasks* Present responses given to question number one. Oral and/or visual representation of responses can be used. (Later, responses to question two, then three, etc., can be presented.)	Same as above	16. Score as in number one
	Responses that might be appropriate to this question but that were not given by the patient are now presented.	Give first sound of a word	Use Porch's (1971) multidimensional scoring system to evaluate responses
	Convergent techniques that might be used to stimulate retrieval of items not produced are as follows: a) confrontation naming b) definition naming c) closure naming d) recognition naming e) repetition naming f) following oral and/or printed directions or commands g) yes/no comprehension h) word associations: antonyms, synonyms i) rhyming j) description	Give first letter of a word Give semantic association	

continued

continued

Objective	Tasks[a]	Cue	Evaluation
	k) recognition spelling		
	l) oral spelling		
	m) analogies		
	n) recognition of categories		
	o) spontaneous generation of categories		
	p) concept learning		
	q) reading		
	r) writing		
	s) copying		
	t) creating sentences with words		
	u) creating sentences telling the function of an object		
	v) memory tasks		
	w) read a story—ask questions		
	x) read a story and retell a story		
	y) role play		

[a] Turn taking, cuing, modeling, and reinforcement are essential components of therapy.

RELATIONSHIP OF COGNITIVE INTERVENTION TO WEPMAN THOUGHT PROCESS THERAPY

Wepman (1972) notes that the aphasic patient frequently **substitutes** a word that is associated with a word he or she is attempting to produce, and that the remainder of the individual's communicative effort often relates to the approximated rather than to the intended word. In addition, the aphasic person's inaccurate verbal formulation may feed back an altered message to the thought process and change the thought process so that it is in consonance with the utterance. For example, if the patient is trying to say "circle" and instead utters "square," his or concept of circle may change so that it agrees with the utterance, and the patient will begin to think of a circle as a square. Wepman (1972) suggested that aphasia may be a thought process disorder in which **impairment of semantic expression is the result of an impairment of thought processes** that "serve as the catalyst for verbal expression" (p. 207).

Individuals who cannot retrieve the most appropriate lexical symbol for a context are impaired in their ability to communicate a number and variety of specific propositional ideas. When the remainder of the aphasic's communication relates to the approximated rather than the intended word, spontaneous language will be even more impaired, since, in this instance, the aphasic patient becomes incapable of using the learned code to communicate his or her true feelings and thoughts.

For Wepman (1972, 1976), the **first** stage of therapy **is content-centered, discussion therapy** in which the patient is stimulated to remain on a topic. Similarly, cognitive therapy is content centered and idea oriented; the individual is encouraged to generate functional communication and to produce a variety of ideas related to topics.

During Wepman's (1972, 1976) **second** stage of therapy, individuals are encouraged to **elaborate** on various topics. The ability to elaborate on a topic is a divergent ability. Thus, Wepman's thought process therapy involves stimulating convergent, divergent, and evaluative thinking as well as recognition/comprehension and memory.

RELATIONSHIP OF COGNITIVE INTERVENTION TO RESPONSE ELABORATION TRAINING

Response elaboration training (RET) is a program developed by Kearns (1985, 1990; Gaddie et al., 1991; Kearns & Potechin, 1988; Kearns & Yedor, 1991) to **increase the length and information content** of verbal responses of nonfluent aphasic patients. RET is a "loose training" program that attempts to loosen control over stimuli and response during therapy by using client-initiated responses as the primary content of therapy. The emphasis is on **shaping and chaining** client-initiated responses. Patients are encouraged to **elaborate** (think divergently) on "whatever they are reminded of" when they are responding to picture stimuli of everyday activities and sports. Naming and describing are discouraged. Informational content rather than linguistic form is reinforced.

Specifically, according to Kearns (1990),

The basic RET sequence entails (1) eliciting spontaneous responses to minimally contextual picture stimuli, (2) modeling and reinforcing initial responses, (3) providing "wh" cues to prompt clients to elaborate on their initial responses, (4) reinforcing attempted elaborations and then modeling sentences that combine initial and all subsequent responses to a given stimulus picture, (5) providing a second model of sentences that combine previous responses and then requesting a repetition of the sentence, (6) reinforcing repetitions of combined sentences and providing a final model of the sentence. Throughout this sequence clients' responses are not directly corrected by the clinician. Instead, naturalistic feedback is provided during the structured interactions through conversational modeling.

Progress during RET is measured by counting the number of content words per stimulus picture (**fluency**) and the variety of responses to the same stimulus picture (**flexibility**). Novel and varied responses are encouraged. Thus, RET stimulates fluency, flexibility, originality, and elaboration—or divergent semantic thinking as well as functional spontaneous speech, which necessitates all five mental operations.

Kearns' (1990) data demonstrate that RET procedures facilitate an increase in the amount of information (i.e., number of content words) generated by aphasic individuals. Further, a moderate degree of generalization across stimuli, people, and settings was reported.

RELATIONSHIP OF COGNITIVE INTERVENTION TO LPAA

Communication creates and is created by life participation. Therefore, the LPAA model directs our choice of **goals, priorities, activities, strategies** used in intervention to the **purpose, direction, meaning, comfort, pleasure, needs, life participation decisions and problems** of each individual affected by aphasia. Such life participation necessitates the use of effective and efficient problem-solving and decision-making skills (see Tables 17–3 and 17–4). In addition, various life span theorists emphasize the **importance of social integration** and participation **for the physical and emotional health and well-being** of all individuals. Indeed, such participation in mundane yet meaningful, valued activities of everyday life provide the structure and meaning for living life (Duchan, 1999).

Case Study

P is a 67-year-old mild to moderately impaired male with aphasia, 3 months post-stroke, with a left CVA and right hemiplegia who lives with his wife, T. Before the stroke, both were active in the local church, but they hadn't returned since P's stroke. Both reported feeling isolated and cut off from life and wanted to go to an upcoming church-sponsored event—a trip to Atlantic City, NJ (famous for its gambling casinos, reasonable meals, Atlantic Ocean beaches, and shopping). Both had reservations about how practical and advisable their involvement might be and about the reaction they might receive from others.

Goals

Life-enhanced participation governed management from day one (see Tables 17–1 and 17–2). The main goal was

to restore purpose, direction, meaning, comfort, and pleasure in the daily lives of P and T by facilitating their access to communication partners and events of their choice and to train caregivers, family, friends, and neighbors to communicate more effectively with both individuals. Therefore, the initial GOALS were:

To determine the extent to which P and T and persons associated with them are able to partake and achieve life participation goals.

To determine the extent to which P and T and persons associated with them are being hindered in the attainment of such goals.

To identify and increase personal and environmental factors which facilitate harmony, comfort, purpose, and participation in life.

To identify and decrease personal and environmental obstacles which disrupt harmony, comfort, purpose, and life participation.

To identify and facilitate attainment of the needs and goals of all individuals in the environment.

To increase/maximize P's ability to initiate and direct conversation/discussions, convey a number and variety of ideas across (with or without prompts, props, and cues), convey a message using whatever strategy is useful (e.g., to encourage use of graphic and drawing representations, use of natural gesture, pictures, travel brochures, menus, books, etc.), and practice conversational skills within the context of conversational exchanges.

To focus on conversation as a collaborative achievement, to provide communication/conversational support, and when appropriate and necessary, to train partners/communities in these techniques to use volunteers as conversational partners.

To provide and demonstrate a problem-solving, decision-making approach model for P and T and to encourage them to structure theme-oriented, problem-solving, decision-making, conversationally based interactions using the five mental operations.

Goals were constantly assessed, weighed, and prioritized to determine which personal and environmental factors should be targets of intervention and how best to provide freer, easier, and more autonomous access to activities and social connections. Every attempt was made to have consumer-based/self-generated rather than clinician-generated goals and activities and to provide autonomous choice whenever possible.

Methods

The upcoming trip to Atlantic City appeared an attractive initial target of intervention since it meant so much to P and T and since it focused on doing things which result in communication as participation—rather than on communication itself. Therefore, intervention focused on developing strategies and skills to increase the possibility of success directly related to re-engagement in/participation in the upcoming event. Most therapy tasks were problem-solving, decision-making, role-playing tasks focused on the five mental operations. However, where appropriate, therapy also made use of Wepman's (1972; 1976) content-centered discussion therapy (see above); Conversational Prompting (Cochrane & Milton, 1984); Conversational Coaching (Holland, 1991); training of conversation partners (Kagan & Gailey's, 1993); Response Elaboration Training (Kearns, 1985) (see above, Chapter 1, and Chapter 14); PACE therapy techniques (Davis & Wilcox, 1981); and for restorative, impairment-centered, skill-level work: Stimulation Therapy (see Chapter 15 by Duffy & Coelho), and Thematic Stimulation Therapy (see Chapter 16 by Morganstein & Certner-Smith, this edition).

Education

The church social committee, several participants of the up-coming trip, and the home care nurse attended two meetings in which they viewed the video, "What is aphasia?" and discussed the language, psychological, and social consequences of aphasia. Sample tasks under the five mental operations included:

Divergent Thinking

What are all the possible environmental barriers that will make functioning (including communication) in a bus difficult?

What are all of the possible ways that can limit their impact or change the environment to make communication more successful?

What are all the environmental factors that will make functioning (including communication) in the casino difficult?

What are all the things we can do to increase the chances of communication success in this environment?

What are all the environmental barriers that make group communication more difficult than individual communication?

What are all the things we can do to decrease the level of this difficulty?

What are all the things that we can do to increase our (our partner's) communication success/failure?

What are all the things that communication partners can do to help someone to be more successful in getting his or her ideas across?

In addition, the therapist led the group in a discussion and modeled strategies for facilitating communication—such

as those suggested by Simmons-Mackie (see Chapter 11, Appendix 11-1, this edition); interactive drawing (Lyon, 1994, 1995); alerting to topic initiation and change; cuing/retrieval feature analysis, suggested by Boyle and Coelho (1995); and communication consequences, developed by Norris and Hoffman (1990).

For example, the communication consequences discussed by Norris and Hoffman (1990) include (1) acknowledgments or **confirming the truth value** of an utterance; (2) using very **specific language**; (3) **extensions** or adding new ideas within the same topic; (4) **nonverbal** responses; (5) verbatim **repetitions**; (6) restating or **rewording** what was said; (7) **summarizing** and **integrating**; (8) **negation** or indicating how and why what was said is untrue or unclear; (9) **self-talk**; (10) **parallel-talk**; (11) **semantically contingent remarks**; (12) sharing **personal reactions**; (13) **questions and comments**; (14) **predictions and projections**; (15) requests for **repair or clarification**; (16) requests for **repetition**; (17) **concept formation**.

Interaction with Patient and Spouse

During intervention, both partners discussed some of the same questions as above. In addition, other tasks such as those discussed below were used with the partners.

Comprehension and Memory

The POSSE strategy suggested by Englert and Mariage (1991) was used to facilitate comprehension of and memory for content for stories. P = **PREDICT** what ideas may be in the story; O = **ORGANIZE** your thoughts (What happens? Where is it? What does it look like? Main idea?); S = **SEARCH the STRUCTURE** (draw the structure out schematically); S = **SUMMARIZE** the main idea; E = **EVALUATE**, compare, clarify, predict. For example, the patient and spouse were asked to predict what the article "STAY BUSY, LIVE LONGER, EXPERTS SUGGEST" (*NY TIMES*, 8/24/99, p. F8), might be about and what the author might possibly mean by the word busy.

Later, the patient and spouse were asked to draw a picture of the information in the article by putting the main idea in the middle of the page (stay busy = live longer) (+sense of purpose = live longer) and other ideas around it (Physical Activity; Social Activity; Productive Activity: Cooking, Shopping, Volunteering, Gardening).

Divergent Thinking

What are all the things that people can possibly do to live longer?

What are all the ways that you could possibly apply this information to your everyday lives?

TABLE 17–3

Pre- and Post-Therapy Questionnaire for Life Participation/ Communication: For the Person with Aphasia and Significant Others. Both Observational and Self-Reported—With and Without Support

Identity
Autonomy of life participation
   In social context
   In family
   In medical context
Degree of life participation
   In life events
   With other people
Relationships
   Value as participant
   Role
Count of number of people seen
   Of places
   Of activities
Environmental barriers (and changes)
Changes in social connection

Communication function (Simmons, 1993)
   Interactional (sharing ideas, thoughts, and opinions)
      Verbal, gestural, cued
   Transactional (transfer of information)
      Verbal, gestural, cued
Ability to communicate independently
Personal competence revealed
Impairment (and changes in)
Ability to cope with impairment

Degree of comfort
   Function
   Involvement
   Pleasure
   Success
   Quality of daily life
Feelings of self-esteem
Feeling of being in control of one's life
Level of flow in one's life

Analysis of specific life events (Duchan, 1999)
   Participants: Who is participating?
   Goal: Why are they participating?
   Type of interaction: What is the type of social interaction required?
   Part of activity: What part of the activity are they engaged in?
   Attitudes: What are the attitudes of the participants:
      Toward activity?
      Toward their partners?
      Toward goals?
   Expectations: (e.g., for social connection; general improvement in sense of well-being)

Perception of (and changes in perception)
   Health care worker
   Family
   Significant others

TABLE 17–4

Reengagement, Enhancement/Inclusion Strategies to Facilitate Meaningful, Functional, Optimal Access to Participation in Life, Well-Being, Wellness, and Quality of Life: A Plan for Action

Goals	Outcomes
Foster optimal meaningful, purposeful life participation, autonomy, and choice of lifestyle and activities	Increased meaningful ties to others
Facilitate optimal inclusion in and meaningful, purposeful connection to social and community activities/life	
Encourage strong social connections with people that matter, such as spouse, caregiver, family, close friends	
Facilitate the restoration of function, purpose, direction, pleasure, comfort, and sense of well-being in daily life	Mastery of environment
Encourage optimal mastery of daily life events	
Encourage and facilitate support from significant others to optimize meaningful, purposeful life participation	Purpose/direction
Encourage and facilitate support for significant others to optimize meaningful, purposeful life participation	Self-acceptance
Recognize and remove environmental, structural, attitudinal, and informational barriers that limit or prevent participation in normal social and community life	Harmony
Increase community resources that support life participation	Well-being
Work to build protected communities where individuals are valued participants	Wellness
Enhance psychological adjustment, promote health and wellness, and foster a healthy sense of identity through life participation	Quality of life Communication effectiveness
Reflect the fact that adaptation to the changes brought about by stroke is a complex, dynamic process that requires time and skill	Consumer satisfaction
Recognize and recalibrate the psychological effects that aphasia has on personal, social, and collective identities, self-esteem, relationships, and role definitions	
Promote healthy psychological adjustment to grief and stress associated with the changes imposed by aphasia	
Facilitate the development of self-actualization, self-assertiveness, and self-advocacy skills	
Recognize and reduce negative internal barriers that decrease or prevent individuals from actively participating in life	
Reflect the curative factors in group work and the healing power of intimacy	
Increase feelings of harmony/well-being and quality of life	
Reflect the fact that communication is a medium through which humans share life's experiences, happenings, and outcomes as well as ideas and feelings about them	
that communication is inseparably bound to people, places, and purposes for its use	
that communication creates and is created by participation in life	
that communication is flexible and dynamic	
Focus on conversation—and conversation as a collaborative achievement	
Foster reasons to communicate	
Strive to enhance level of participation in conversation	
Promote abilities/opportunities	
to communicate to maintain social relationships	
to communicate in natural, authentic contexts and social units or dyads	
to communicate to transmit information	
to communicate basic needs	
Empower individuals to demonstrate or reveal communicative competence and acknowledge such competence	
Work to increase ability to communicate independently	
Provide communication/conversational support, when appropriate and necessary, and train partners and communities in these techniques	

continued

continued

> Work to reduce impairments while focusing on revealing competence/function
> Work to reduce impairments in the context of reducing barriers to life participation
> Relate functional communication to environmental factors as well as impairment
> Increase continuity and access to intervention

Intervention is a consumer-driven, dynamic, assistive, advising, empowering, interactive, collaborative process that responds to the significant, immediate and long-term consequences that aphasia imposes on the flow of daily living and recognizes that **communication is inseparably bound to people, places, and purposes for its use** and that **communication creates and is created by participation in life**. All intervention goals reflect the complexity of aphasia and the multiple contexts that it affects. Such goals are established collaboratively and are constantly assessed, weighed, prioritized, and renegotiated in order to decrease the devastating negative consequences of aphasia, foster adaptation to change, and increase meaningful social participation, purpose, harmony, and well-being in the lives of all those affected by aphasia. It is a process that evolves and changes over time, increasingly empowering those who receive it to be responsible for their own care. Outcomes are measured qualitatively and quantitatively.

What are all the personal and environmental factors that can increase (and decrease) life participation for individuals with aphasia, their families, and their communities?

What are all the things that add purpose, direction, and meaning to our daily lives?

What are all the things that can possibly lead to comfort and pleasure in our lives?

What are all the things we can do to restore the purpose, direction, and meaning in P and T's life?

What are all the ways that the trip to Atlantic City relates to this article?

What other things can you think of that relate to this article?

PRE TRIP questions included:

Who are the possible participants in the group?

What are all the things we could possibly think of to plan a trip to Atlantic City?

What are all the things we could possibly need to consider in planning a bus trip?

What are all the things you can think of about Atlantic City?

What are all the things you can think of about the Jersey Shore?

What are all the things you might possibly see in Atlantic City?

What are all the possible things that someone might bring with him or her on a trip to Atlantic City?

What are all the possible things that someone might do (participate in) in Atlantic City (go to the beach, nightclubs, restaurants, go shopping, walk on the boardwalk, swim, sightsee, etc.)?

What are all the possible things we need to take care of before we go to Atlantic City (personal care, banking, medical, etc.)?

What are all the safety rules we might possibly follow on a trip (to Atlantic City)?

What are all the topics someone could possibly talk about on a trip?

What are all the possible ways that someone can be a good conversational partner?

What are all the things a good citizen should do when he or she goes to a new place?

What are all the things we could possibly change that could increase our ability to go on these trips?

What are all of your strengths that will make this a successful trip?

What are all the possible things that someone can do to make a trip successful?

What are our weaknesses that could possibly hinder you from having a successful trip?

What are all the possible community resources that someone could possibly be able to use in preparing for a trip?

Who are all the possible people who might be able to help us make a trip more successful?

What are all the things that could possibly restrict your access to a trip to Atlantic City?

What are all the possible problems we might have in going to Atlantic City with a church group (getting to the bus, on the bus, in the casinos, in the restaurants, at the beach/boardwalk, in the shops, on the way home, etc.)?

What are all of the possible environmental/structural, attitudinal, informational obstacles that limit or prevent participation in a trip to Atlantic City?

What are all the possible things we might be able to do to avoid these problems?

What are all the possible ways we could solve each of these problems?

What are all the possible ways to cope when we have a problem?

What are all the things we can possibly eat in Atlantic City?

What are all the possible foods that someone can eat in a restaurant?

What are all the things we should eat in order to be healthy?

What are all the things we shouldn't eat in order to stay healthy?

What are all the things that we can bring to Atlantic City that can be folded? Can't be folded? That someone could drink? That someone could eat?

What are all the ways that someone can get to Atlantic City?

What are all the things that could fit into a bus?

What are all the possible places that someone can go by bus?

What are all the possible activities that we can attend through the church?

POST TRIP: Consumer Satisfaction Questionnaire

What were all of the possible benefits of going on the trip?

What were all the possible benefits of being members of the group?

What are all the feelings that you have about the trip?

What are all of the positive things that happened on the trip?

What were all of the problems that occurred that we did/didn't anticipate?

What are all of the ways we could possibly have anticipated them?

What are all of the ways we could possibly have solved them or coped with them?

What are all of the ways we (or others) could have been better conversational partners?

What are all of the things that we did before the trip that made the trip more successful?

What are all the things that we did that gave us a feeling of connection with others? A feeling of comfort and harmony?

What are all of the things that we could have done to have made the trip more successful?

Memory

To facilitate P's memory several strategies were used. First, the **scaffolding** techniques or prompts suggested by Norris and Hoffman (1990) were used. These included various prompts to cue P for more information. They included:

Relational Prompts.

Additive (and . . .)

Temporal (and then; first; after; next; and when; while)

Causal (because; so; since; so that's; in order to . . .)

Adversative (but; except; however; except that . . .)

Conditional (of; unless; if—then; in case; or . . .)

Spatial (in; next to; until he got to; which was on . . .)

Contingent Queries or Wh questions to prompt for agents, actions, objects, locations, or relational information.

Summarization or **Evaluation** gives the individual a second opportunity to communicate.

Binary Choices offer alternative utterances.

Phonemic Cues offer the initial sound or syllable of a target word.

In addition, the semantic feature analysis developed by Boyle and Coelho (1995) was used. This technique prompts the individual to identify the specific features of target pictures that they find hard to retrieve or name. For example, for "a quarter" P needed to identify the **GROUP:** money, coin; **USE:** buy things; **ACTION:** give, get, spend; **PROPERTIES:** round, shiny, large; **LOCATION,** in a pocket, at a bank, in the casino; **ASSOCIATION:** spending, getting things.

Cognition

Recognition/comprehension tasks included:

Reading and following signs, directories, menus, travel brochures from the chamber of commerce, the casinos, and the AAA.

Comprehending the video "What is Aphasia?"

Comprehending the video "Casino."

Comprehending other videotaped material.

Comprehending newspaper stories (e.g., "Ruling in California Crimps Indian Plans for a Casino Empire" by Todd Purdum, *NY Times*, 8/24/99, pp. A1 and A11; "Little Tribe, Casino Threatened, Battles U.S.," *NY Times*, 8/28/99, p. A7; and "Stay Busy, Live Longer, Experts Suggest," *NY Times*, 8/24/99, p. F8).

Reading short stories about gambling, Atlantic City, and the Jersey Shore.

Skill-building, impairment-level recognition and understanding tasks included:

Matching Related Words (e.g., Draw a line from each word in the left-hand column to the related word in the right-hand column.)

Word Categorization Tasks (Circle the words that belong in the category "Atlantic City.")

Word Categorization Exclusion (e.g., Cross out the word on each line that does not belong). **Write in a new word that does belong.**

Yes/No Questions (e.g., Read each question and mark "yes" or "no.")

Sentence Arrangement of scrambled sentences for targeted core vocabulary items (e.g., Rearrange these words to form correct sentences:

Atlantic City are we to going.)

Convergent Tasks

Answering Wh-questions.

What can I do when someone doesn't understand me?

What can I do when I don't understand someone else?

What can I do to get my partner to help me when I can't get my idea across?

What can I do to help my partner to get his idea across when I can't understand him?

Using social greetings.

Object manipulation and description—such as a slot machine

Acting out and describing sequences with props—such as using the slot machines or ordering lunch

Picture description—such as—describe this picture of "Taj Mahal Casino" or "Caesar's Palace Casino"

Event description—such as describe roulette

Discussing videotaped material

Structured answers—such as What does the dealer deal? How many cards are in a deck?

Identifying places and activities

Answering questions about reading material or videos.

Barrier tasks

Skill/impairment level convergent tasks included:

Repetition of Core Vocabulary (e.g., Atlantic City—To Atlantic City—We're going to Atlantic City)

Closure tasks (e.g., We're going to Atlantic City. We're going to _____.)

Naming tasks (e.g., What do we swim in?)

Category naming

Defining core vocabulary

Using core vocabulary words

Giving directions

Creating sentences for target core vocabulary items (e.g., Create sentences for these words and phrases. Game—play)

Multiple choice questions relating to core vocabulary

Evaluative thinking or judgment tasks included:

Which activity should we work on first? Atlantic City or the Garden Club lecture?

Which trip means more to you: the trip to Atlantic City or the lecture on roses?

Which game is easier to play: the slot machines or poker?

Since the trip is in August, which would be more useful to have with us: a bathing suit or gloves?

A beach towel or a coat?

Sun tan lotion or a lamp?

I can't read the menu. Should I ask the waitress to tell me the choices or just point to anything?

Which is more important for a pay phone call: a quarter or a five dollar bill?

Which is closer to New York: Atlantic City or Florida?

Which is faster: a plane or a bus?

I don't know how to play a game. Which should I do first: watch others play or start to play myself?

The sign says "Wet floor." Should I walk across it or wait until it is dry?

Integrative tasks included:

Conversation

Procedural discourse

Narrative discourse

Unstructured discussions—such as the pros and cons of gambling, of a group trip, of going to the beach, etc.

Role playing talking to fellow travelers on the bus

Role playing being in the casino

Role playing ordering in a restaurant

Role playing shopping in a store

Role playing being at the beach

Watching video tapes about Atlantic City and discussing them.

Reading stories about the New Jersey shore and Atlantic City and discussing them.

CONCLUSION

In summary, the model of problem solving and decision making presented here appears to be applicable to the LPAA approach because of its relevance to everyday life participation through its very specific structure or strategy for solving problems and the proven validity of the five mental operations in "normals" and individuals with aphasia. It is hoped that use of this model, especially when used in conjunction with other models such as those cited in this chapter, will help those who use it to become more active, accurate, thorough, and effective problem solvers and decision makers. Making it possible to achieve workable and effective solutions, resolutions, and adaptations to changing opportunities for participation in contexts that really matter, thereby facilitating optimum social, vocational, and recreational activity and reintegration.

However, most of the literature on cognition specifies what is learned, or the products of cognition. Similarly, the literature in language intervention specifies therapy objectives or what is to be learned. Therapy objectives emphasize the types of tasks used. The goal of therapy is the appropriate accomplishment of these tasks. The criterion of success is based on the percentage of appropriate versus inappropriate responses.

Today, however, speech-language pathologists are shifting from an orientation of simplistic listing of tasks used in therapy, which define them as technicians, to a comprehensive understanding of the rationale behind the selection of these tasks and a description of why these tasks stimulate complex events to happen in the brain; this defines them as true clinicians.

An attempt to separate tasks into input, processing, and output components and, more important, the identification of the subsystems whose interaction is necessary for processing and specification of the complex events that happen in the brain, may save us from performing therapy tasks backward. That is, we recognize that what we are attempting to stimulate in therapy is the patient's mental operations or processes, since these appear to be the complex events that happen in the brain. We also stimulate these mental operations because functional language requires the use of these mental processes. Thus, language therapy must reflect the fact that language is communicating—that it is the give and take of ideas. It must reflect the belief that meaning is the essence of language; that communication is idea oriented, not word oriented; that it is purpose/intent oriented. It must be recognized that the speech act involves creativity and novelty of expression. This is the core of language. Language is an aid to communication.

There are several other advantages to applying the Guilford model to adult aphasia. Most importantly, it enables us to identify and operationally define the action elicited within the patient by the stimuli presented, the complex events that happen in the brain, and/or the cognitive processes that are used in generating language products, such as words, classes, rules of languages, and semantic implications. It enables us to make use of an empirical statistically documented model or taxonomy of behaviors, in order to give the concepts of cognition, information processing, and problem solving a firm, comprehensive, and systematic theoretical and yet operationally defined foundation. Guilford supported the separate and distinct existence of each of the 120 abilities in normal individuals through the use of repeated research studies using factor analysis. Some of these abilities, such as memory, divergent thinking, convergent thinking, evaluative thinking or judgment, and semantic and behavioral content, have also been documented in persons with adult aphasia, right brain damage, closed-head injuries and aged (Braverman, 1990; Chapey, 1977b; Chapey & Lubinski, 1979; Chapey et al., 1976; Diggs & Basili, 1987; Law & Newton, 1991; Lubinski & Chapey, 1978; Schwartz-Crowley & Gruen, 1986). In addition, this model provides a set of tests whose validity and reliability have been established. These tests can be used in therapy to stimulate specific parameters of the model and also to assess, evaluate, and describe patient behavior. Use of these tests may help us to someday make a statement about the efficacy of treatment based on this model.

FUTURE TRENDS IN COGNITIVE SEMANTIC INTERVENTION

Recovery today is very documentation oriented—very focused on cost containment. This orientation generates a "pricing by activity" mentality in which government and insurance agencies emphasize unimportant but measurable goals, activities, and abilities. Many of these do not help the patient to regain as much functional, meaningful propositional language as possible or to increase his or her ability to become better adept at the back and forth—the give and take of ideas.

The current emphasis on measurable, operationally written behavioral goals should be reconsidered. In the future, we need therapy goals and procedures that are based on rich and shared experiences that encourage individuals to apply, analyze, synthesize, and evaluate such real-life experience; relate it to something else; reorganize it; infer from it; and use it as a springboard to solve new problems creatively. A cognitive approach to recovery appears to meet this need. In addition, it has the added advantage that stimulating thinking and cognitive processing may facilitate the aphasic individuals' natural acquisition ability, or their ability to acquire language independently.

A cognitive approach may also stimulate generalization. Therefore, there is a strong need to develop additional therapy materials appropriate for this approach. In addition, there is a strong need to develop assessment protocols that will measure these cognitive-semantic processes separately and within the context of functional, meaningful communication. Such a measure may help clinicians to assess progress in therapy and generalization and therefore sharpen our quality assurance systems.

KEY POINTS

1. The Guilford Structure-of-Intellect model contains four types of content, five mental operations, and six types of products or associations.
2. **Intelligence** can be defined within this model in terms of 120 abilities (content × operation × product). Therefore, we can assess the individual's intelligence for each ability.
3. **Cognition** can be operationally defined by the use of one or more of the five mental operations in the Guilford model: recognition/understanding, memory, convergent thinking, divergent thinking, and evaluative thinking.
4. **Communication** is a problem-solving, decision-making task that usually involves the back and forth, give and take of ideas between partners in a specific context. This usually involves the use of one or all five mental operations or cognitive processes.
5. **Language** involves the use of three types of knowledge: content, form, and use or function. Each of these can be defined within the context of the Guilford model as semantic and behavioral information processed by one or more of the five mental processes and resulting in one or more associations or products.
6. Spontaneous speech, communication, problem solving, decision making, learning, and information processing are **composite abilities** often requiring several abilities to function together in order to achieve a desired goal.
7. The objective of cognitive stimulation therapy is to stimulate the five mental operations at various levels of complexity and in composite abilities such as spontaneous speech in order to increase ability to participate in meaningful and personally relevant activities and life goals.

References

Aurelia, J. (1974). *Aphasia therapy manual.* Danville, IL: Interstate.
Ausubel, D. (1965). Introduction. In R. Anderson & D. Ausubel (eds.), *Readings in the psychology of cognition.* New York: Holt, Rinehart & Winston.

Bandura, A. & Walters, R. (1963). *Social learning and personality development.* New York: Holt, Rinehart & Winston.

Berman, M. & Peelle, L. (1967). Self-generated cues: A method for aiding aphasic and apractic patients. *Journal of Speech and Hearing Disorders, 32,* 372–376.

Bloom, L. & Lahey, M. (1978). Language development and language disorders. New York: John Wiley & Sons.

Boden, M. (1980). *Jean Piaget.* New York: Viking Press.

Bolwinick, J. (1967). *Cognitive processes in maturity and old age.* New York: Springer.

Boyle, M. & Coelho, C. (1995). Application of semantic feature analysis as a treatment for aphasic dysnomia. *American Journal of Speech-Language Pathology, 4,* 4, 11, 94–98.

Braverman, K.M. (1990). Divergent semantic and behavioral production skills in aphasia and right-hemisphere communication impairment. Unpublished doctoral dissertation. University of Cincinnati, Cincinnati, OH.

Bruner, J. (1968). *Processes of cognitive growth: Infancy.* Worcester, MA: Clark University Press.

Butfield, E. & Zangwill, O. (1946). Reeducation in aphasia: A review of 70 cases. *Journal of Neurology, Neurosurgery and Psychiatry, 9,* 75–79.

Byng, S., Kay, J., Edmundson, A., & Scott, C. (1990). Aphasia tests reconsidered. *Aphasiology, 4*(1), 67–92.

Cazden, C.B. (1976). How knowledge about language helps the classroom teacher-or does it? A personal account. *Urban Review, 9,* 74–91.

Cantor, N. & Sanderson, C.A. (1999). Life task participation and well-being: The importance of taking part in daily life. In D. Kahneman, E. Diener, & N. Schwarz (eds.) (1999). *Well-being: The foundations of hedonic psychology* (prepublication copy). New York: Russell Sage Foundation.

Carver, C.S. & Scheier, M.F. (1982). Control theory: A useful conceptual framework for personality-social, clinical, and health psychology. *Psychological Bulletin, 92,* 111–35.

Chapey, R. (1974). Divergent semantic behavior in aphasia. Unpublished doctoral dissertation. Columbia University, New York.

Chapey, R. (1977a). A divergent semantic model of intervention in adult aphasia. In R. Brookshire (ed.), *Clinical aphasiology: Conference proceedings.* Minneapolis, MN: BRK.

Chapey, R. (1977b). The relationship between divergent and convergent semantic behavior in adult aphasia. *Archives of Physical Medicine and Rehabilitation, 58,* 357–362.

Chapey, R. (ed.) (1981a). *Language intervention strategies in adult aphasia.* Baltimore, MD: Williams & Wilkins.

Chapey, R. (1981b). Divergent semantic intervention. In R. Chapey (ed.), *Language intervention strategies in adult aphasia.* Baltimore, MD: Williams & Wilkins.

Chapey, R. (1983). Language-based cognitive abilities in adult aphasia: Rationale for intervention. *Journal of Communication Disorders, 16,* 405–424.

Chapey, R. (1988). Aphasia therapy: Why do we say one thing and do another? In S. Gerber & G. Mencher (eds.), *International perspectives on communication disorders.* Washington, DC: Gallaudet University.

Chapey, R. (1992). Functional communication assessment and intervention: Some thoughts on the state of the art. *Aphasiology, 6*(1), 85–93.

Chapey, R. (1994). Cognitive intervention. In R. Chapey (ed),

Language intervention strategies in adult aphasia. Baltimore, MD: Williams & Wilkins.

Chapey, R., Duchan, J., Elman, R., Garcia, L., Kagan, A., Lyon, J., & Simmons-Mackie, N.: the LPAA group (2000). Life Participation Approach to Aphasia: A statement of values. *The ASHA Leader, 5*(3), Feb. 15, 4–6.

Chapey, R. & Lubinski, R. (1979). Semantic judgment ability in adult aphasia. *Cortex, 14,* 247–255.

Chapey, R., Rigrodsky, S., & Morrison, E. (1976). The measurement of divergent semantic behavior in aphasia. *Journal of Speech and Hearing Research, 19,* 664–677.

Chapey, R., Rigrodsky, S., & Morrison, E. (1977). Aphasia: A divergent semantic interpretation. *Journal of Speech and Hearing Disorders, 42,* 287–295.

Chomsky, N. (1957). *Syntactic structures.* The Hague: Mouton.

Chomsky, N. (1964). *Current issues in linguistic theory.* The Hague: Mouton.

Chomsky, N. (1972). *Language and mind.* New York: Harcourt, Brace & Jovanovich.

Cochrane, R. & Milton, S. (1984). Conversational prompting: A sentence building technique for severe aphasia. *Journal of Neurological Communication Disorders, 1,* 4–23.

Cooper, L. & Rigrodsky, S. (1979). Verbal training to improve explanations of conservation with aphasic adults. *Journal of Speech and Hearing Research, 33,* 818–828.

Craig, H. (1983). Application of pragmatic language models for intervention. In T.M. Gallagher & C.A. Prutting (eds.), *Pragmatic assessment and intervention issues in language.* San Diego, CA: College Hill Press.

Cropley, A. (1967). *Creativity.* London: Longman.

Davis, G.A. (1983). *A survey of adult aphasia.* Englewood Cliffs, NJ: Prentice-Hall.

Davis, G.A. & Wilcox, M.J. (1981). Incorporating parameters of natural conversation in aphasia treatment. In R. Chapey (ed.), *Language intervention strategies in adult aphasia.* Baltimore, MD: Williams & Wilkins.

Dember, W. & Jenkins, J. (1979). *General psychology: Modeling behavior and experience.* Englewood Cliffs, NJ: Prentice-Hall.

Diggs, C. & Basili, A. (1987). Verbal expression of right cerebrovascular accident patients: Convergent and divergent language. *Brain and Language, 30,* 130–146.

Dore, J. (1974). A pragmatic description of early language development. *Journal of Psycholinguistic Research, 3,* 343–350.

Duchan, J. (April, 1999). Personal communication on LPAA.

Duffy, J.R. & Coelho, C. (2001). Schuell's stimulation approach to rehabilitation. In R. Chapey (ed.), *Language intervention strategies in adult aphasia.* Baltimore, MD: Lippincott Williams & Wilkins.

Englert, C.S. & Mariage, T.V. (1991). Making student partners in the comprehension process: Organizing the Reading 'POSSE.' *Learning Disability Quarterly, 14,* 129.

English, H.B. & English, A.C. (1958). *A comprehensive dictionary of psychological and psychoanalytic terms.* New York: McKay.

Fey, M. & Leonard, L.B. (1983). Pragmatic skills of children with specific language impairments. In T. Gallagher & C.A. Prutting (eds.), *Pragmatic assessment and intervention issues in language.* San Diego, CA: College Hill Press.

Frattali, C. (1992). Functional assessment of communication: Merging public policy with clinical view. *Aphasiology, 6*(1), 63–63.

Gaddie, A., Kearns, K., & Yedor, K. (1991). A qualitative analysis of response elaboration training effects. In T. Prescott (ed.), *Clinical aphasiology: Conference proceedings, 21*, 171–184.

Gallagher, T. (1983). Pre-assessment: A procedure for accommodating language use variability. In T. Gallagher & C. A. Prutting (eds.), *Pragmatic assessment and intervention issues in language*. San Diego, CA: College Hill Press.

Goldstein, K. (1948). *Language and language disturbances*. New York: Grune & Stratton.

Goodglass, H. & Kaplan, E. (1972). *The assessment of aphasia and related disorders*. Philadelphia, PA: Lea & Febiger.

Goodman, P. (1971). *Speaking and language: Defense of poetry*. New York: Random House.

Gowan, J., Demos, G., & Torrance, E. (1967). *Creativity: Its educational implications*. New York: John Wiley & Sons.

Grant, D., Hake, H., & Hornseth, J. (1951). Acquisition and extinction of verbally conditioned response with different percentages of reinforcement. *Journal of Experimental Psychology, 42*, 1–5.

Guilford, J.P. (1967). *The nature of human intelligence*. New York: McGraw-Hill.

Guilford, J.P. & Hoepfner, R. (1971). *The analysis of intelligence*. New York: McGraw-Hill.

Harlow, H. (1949). The formation of learning sets. *Psychological Review, 56*, 51–56.

Harris, M. & Evans, R. (1974). The effects of modeling and instruction on creative responses. *Journal of Psychology, 86*, 123–130.

Harrison, R.P. (1974). *Beyond words: An introduction to nonverbal communication*. Englewood Cliffs, NJ: Prentice-Hall.

Haviland, S.E. & Clark, H.H. (1974). What' new? Acquiring new information as a process in comprehension. *Journal of Verbal Learning and Verbal Behavior, 13*, 512–21.

Head, H. (1915). Hughlings Jackson on aphasia and kindred affections of speech. *Brain, 38*, 1–7.

Herzog, A.R., Rogers, W.L., & Woodworth, J. (1982). *Subjective well-being among different age groups*. Ann Arbor: University of Michigan, Survey Research Center.

Holland, A. (1991). Pragmatic aspects of interaction in aphasia. *Journal of Neurolinguistics, 6*, 197–211.

Holland, A. (1975). Language therapy for children: Some thoughts on context and content. *Journal of Speech and Hearing Disorders, 40*, 514–23.

Hughy, J. & Johnson, A. (1975). *Speech communication: Foundations and challenges*. New York: Macmillan.

Jennings, E. & Lubinski, R. (1981). Strategies for improving productive thinking in the language impaired adult. *Journal of Communication Disorders, 14*, 255–71.

Jensen, G. & Cotton, J. (1960). Successive acquisitions and extinctions as related to differing percentages of reinforcement. *Journal of Experimental Psychology, 60*, 41–49.

Kagan, A. (1998). Philosophical, practical and evaluative issues associated with "Supported Conversations with Adults with Aphasia": A reply. *Aphasiology, 12*(9), 851–864.

Kagan, A. & Gailey, G. (1993). Functional is not enough: Training conversation partners for aphasic adults. In A. Holland & M. Forbes (eds.), *Aphasia treatment: World perspectives*. San Diego, CA: Singular Publishing Group.

Kahneman, D., Diener, E., & Schwarz, N. (eds.) (1999). *Well-being: The foundations of hedonic psychology* (prepublication copy). New York: Russell Sage Foundation.

Kearns, K. (1985). Response elaboration training for patient initiated utterances. *Clinical Aphasiology, 15*, 196–204.

Kearns, K.P. (1985). Response elaboration training for patient initiated utterances. In R. Brookshire (ed.), *Clinical aphasiology: Conference proceedings* (pp. 196–204). Minneapolis, MN: BRK.

Kearns, K.P. (1990). Broca's aphasia. In L. LaPointe (ed.), *Aphasia and related neurogenic language disorders*. New York: Thieme.

Kearns, K.P. & Potechin, G. (1988). The generalization of response elaboration training effects. In T. Prescott (ed.), *Clinical aphasiology*. Boston, MA: College Hill Press.

Kearns, K. & Yedor, K. (1991). An alternating treatments comparison of loose training and a convergent treatment strategy. In T. Prescott (ed.), *Clinical aphasiology, 20*, 223–238.

Keenan, J.A. (1975). *A procedure manual in speech pathology with brain-damaged adults*. Danville, IL: Interstate.

Kuypers, J. & Bengtson, V.L. (1990). Toward understanding health in older families impacted by catastrophic illness. In T.H. Brubaker (ed.), *Family relationships in later life* (2nd ed.) (pp. 245–266). Newbury Park, CA: Sage.

Lahey, M. (1988). *Language disorders and language development*. New York: Macmillan.

Law, P. & Newton, M. (1991). Divergent semantic behavior in aged persons. Atlanta, GA: American Speech-Language-Hearing Association Convention.

Lazerson, A. (ed.). (1975). *Psychology today*. New York: Random House.

Lefrancois, G. (1982). *Psychological theories of human learning* (2nd ed.). Belmont, CA: Brooks-Cole.

Lindfors, J.W. (1980; rev. 1987). *Children's language and learning*. Englewood Cliffs, NJ: Prentice-Hall.

Lubinski, R. (1986). A social communication approach to treatment in aphasia in an institutional setting. In R. Marshall (ed.), *Case studies in aphasia rehabilitation*. Austin, TX: Pro-Ed.

Lubinski, R. & Chapey, R. (1978). Constructive recall strategies in adult aphasia. In R. Brookshire (ed.), *Clinical aphasiology: Conference proceedings*. Minneapolis, MN: BRK.

Lucas, E. (1980). *Semantic and pragmatic language disorders: Assessment and remediation*. Rockville, MD: Aspen.

Lyon, J. (1995). Drawing: Its value as a communication aid for adults with aphasia. *Aphasiology, 9*(1), 33–94.

Lyon, J. (1994). Drawing: Its value as an aid for adults with aphasia. *Aphasiology, 8*.

Martin, A.D. (1979). A critical evaluation of therapeutic approaches to aphasia. In R. Brookshire (ed.), *Clinical aphasiology: Conference proceedings*. Minneapolis, MN: BRK.

Marshall, R. (1999). A problem-focused group treatment program for clients with mild aphasia. In R. Ellman (ed.), *Group treatment of neurogenic communication disorders: The expert clinician's approach* (pp. 57–65). Woburn, MA: Butterworth-Heinemann.

Marx, M. (1970). *Learning theories*. London: Macmillan.

McConnell, F., Love, R., & Smith, B. (1974). Language remediation in children. In S. Dickson (ed.), *Communication disorders: Remedial principles and practices*. Glenview, IL: Scott Foresman.

McCormick, L. & Schiefelbush, R. (1984). *Early language intervention: An introduction*. Columbus, OH: Charles E. Merrill.

Morganstein, S. & Certner-Smith, M. (1982). *Thematic language stimulation*. Tucson, AZ: Communication Skill Builders.

Morganstein, S. & Certner-Smith, M. (2001). Thematic language stimulation therapy. In R. Chapey (ed.), *language intervention strategies in adult aphasia*. Baltimore, MD: Lippincott, Williams & Wilkins.

Muma, J. (1975). The communication game: Dump and play. *Journal of Speech and Hearing Disorders, 40,* 296.

Muma, J.R. (1978). *Language handbook: Concepts, assessment and intervention.* Englewood Cliffs, NJ: Prentice-Hall.

Naremore, R. (1980). Language disorders in children. In T. Hixon, L. Shriberg, & J. Saxman (eds.), *Introduction to communication disorders.* Englewood Cliffs, NJ: Prentice-Hall.

Neisser, U. (1967). *Cognitive psychology.* New York: Appleton-Century-Crofts.

Norris, J. & Hoffman, P. (1990). Language intervention within naturalistic environments. *Language, Speech and Hearing Services in the Schools, 21,* 72–84.

Ochs, E. & Schieffelin, B. (eds.) (1979). *Developmental pragmatics.* New York: Academic Press.

Peabody Language Development Kit. Level One (1965). Circle Pines, MN: American Guidance Service.

Pieres, E. & Morgan, F. (1973). Effects of free associative training on children's ideational fluency. *Journal of Personality, 41,* 42–49.

Pinker, S. (1997). How the mind works.

Porch, B. (1971). Multidimensional scoring in aphasia testing. *Journal of Speech and Hearing Research, 14,* 776–792.

Prutting, C. (1979). Process/pra/ses/n: The action of moving forward progressively from one point to another on the way to completion. *Journal of Speech and Hearing Disorders, 44,* 3–10.

Prutting, C. & Kirchner, D. (1983). Applied pragmatics. In R.M. Gallagher & C.A. Prutting (eds.), *Pragmatic assessment and intervention issues in language.* San Diego, CA: College Hill Press.

Rosenfeld, N.M. (1978). Conversational control function of nonverbal behavior. In A.W. Siegman & S. Felstein (eds.), *Nonverbal behavior and communication.* Hillsdale, NJ: Lawrence Erlbaum.

Rosenthal, T. & Zimmerman, B. (1978). *Social learning and cognition.* New York: Academic Press.

Ryff, C.D. (1989). Happiness is everything, or is it? Explorations on the meaning of psychological well-being. *Journal of Personality and Social Psychology, 57,* 1069–81.

Saltz, E. (1971). *The cognitive bases of human learning.* Homewood, IL: Dorsey Press.

Sarno, M., Silverman, M., & Sands, E. (1970). Speech therapy and language recovery in severe aphasia. *Journal of Speech and Hearing Research, 13,* 607–623.

Schuell, H., Carroll, V., & Street, B. (1955). Clinical treatment of aphasia. *Journal of Speech and Hearing Disorders, 20,* 43–53.

Schuell, H., Jenkins, J., & Jiminez-Pabon, E. (1964). *Aphasia in adults.* New York: Harper & Row.

Schwartz-Crowley, R. & Gruen, A. (1986). Rehabilitation assessment of communicative, cognitive-linguistic, and swallowing functions. *Trauma Quarterly, 3*(1), 63–65.

Scott, W., Osgood, W., & Peterson, C. (1979). *Cognitive structure, theory and measurement of individual differences.* New York: Halstead Press.

Searle, J. (1969). *Speech acts.* London: Cambridge University Press.

Simmons, N. (1993). An ethnographic investigation of compensatory strategies in aphasia. Dissertation. Louisiana State University and Agricultural and Mechanical College.

Simmons-Mackie, N. (1996). CVA and related communication disorders: Assessment and treatment of aphasia. NJ: Presentation. December 6.

Simmons-Mackie, N. (in press). Social approaches to the management of aphasia. In L. Worrall & C. Frattali (eds.), *Neurogenic communication disorders: A functional approach.*

Simmons-Mackie, N., Damico, J., & Damico, H. (1999). A qualitative study of feedback in aphasia treatment. *American Journal of Speech-Language Pathology, 8,* 218–230.

Slobin, D. (1971). *Psycholinguistics.* Glenview, IL: Scott Foresman.

Smith, F. (1975). *Comprehension and learning.* New York: Holt, Rinehart & Winston.

Staats, A. (1968). *Learning, language and cognition.* New York: Holt, Rinehart & Winston.

Torrance, E.P. (1966). *Torrance Test of Creative Thinking.* Princeton, NJ: Personnel Press.

Torrance, E.P. (1974). Interscholastic brainstorming and creative problem solving competition for creatively gifted. *Gifted Child Quarterly, 18,* 3–7.

Vignolo, L. (1964). Evolution of aphasia and language rehabilitation: Retrospective exploratory study. *Cortex, 1,* 344–367.

Warren, S. & Rogers-Warren, A.K. (eds.). (1985). *Teaching functional language.* Austin, TX: Pro-Ed.

Webster's new collegiate dictionary (1977). Springfield, MA: G. & C. Merriam.

Wepman, J. (1951). *Recovery from aphasia.* New York: Ronald Press.

Wepman, J. (1953). A conceptual model for the processes involved in recovery from aphasia. *Journal of Speech and Hearing Disorders, 18,* 4–13.

Wepman, J. (1972). Aphasia therapy: A new look. *Journal of Speech and Hearing Disorders, 37,* 203–214.

Wepman, J. (1976). Aphasia: Language without thought or thought without language. *ASHA, 18,* 131–136.

Wepman, J.M., Jones, L.U., Bock, R.D., & Van Pelt, D. (1960). Studies in aphasia: Background and theoretical formulations. *Journal of Speech and Hearing Disorders, 25,* 323–332.

Yardley, A. (1974). *Structure in early learning.* New York: Citation Press.

Yorkston, K. & Beukelman, D. (1977). A system for quantifying verbal output of high level aphasia patients. In R. Brookshire (ed.), *Clinical aphasiology: Conference proceedings.* Minneapolis, MN: BRK.

Zachman, Jorensen, C. & Barrett, M., et al. (1983). Manual of exercises for expressive reasoning. Mouline, IIL: LinguiSystems.

Zukav, G. (1989). *The seat of the soul.* New York: A Fireside Book. Simon & Schuster.

Chapter 18

Management of Wernicke's Aphasia: A Context-Based Approach

Robert C. Marshall

OBJECTIVES

Clinicians who like order, control, and certainty tend to "shy away" from the patient with Wernicke's aphasia. Beginning clinicians may struggle to keep the patient from "taking over" the treatment session. I hope that this chapter will lead those who are ambivalent or fearful about treating Wernicke's aphasia to increased levels of competence and "comfort" planning and providing interventions for these patients. Specific chapter goals are (1) to provide a rationale for the context-based approach to management of Wernicke's aphasia; (2) to apply information from the aphasia literature to context-based management; and (3) to show how context-based intervention can be used to promote functional communication in daily communicative contexts for patients with Wernicke's aphasia.

Personal Interests

Patients with Wernicke's aphasia have held my interest for 35 years. Writing and talking about these patients has made me more aware of the unique combinations of skills needed to manage these patients (Marshall, 2000; Marshall, 1981, 1982, 1983, 1986, 1987a, 1987b; Marshall et al., 1985; Marshall & Tompkins, 1982; Starch et al., 1986; Marshall et al., 1991; Sullivan et al., 1986). These patients fail to match our behavioral expectations for those we want to help. They are difficult to test, sometimes uncontrollable, and may not always say "Thank you." Perhaps this is because few guidelines exist for planning interventions for patients with Wernicke's aphasia (Marshall, 1994). Treating these clients requires a combination of science, art, and common sense. Science comes from knowing what the literature tells about people with aphasia. Good clinical decision making constitutes the art.

Common sense comes from being aware of what is important for communication in those contexts in which the patient communicates daily.

Patients with Wernicke's aphasia surprise us with what they can and cannot do. For example, GW was unable to repeat words, but when given the word "screw," made an appropriate gesture and said "I'd like to." MA, seen in an extended care facility (ECF), performed poorly on the Porch Index of Communicative Ability (PICA, Porch, 1967), but expressed clearly a need to go home. She convinced the physician she could manage her affairs and he sent her home rather than keep her in the ECF. Recently, I met BC, a 70-year-old man with chronic Wernicke's aphasia. BC was unable to do the easiest tasks (e.g., repetition, matching) of the *Boston Diagnostic Aphasia Examination* (BDAE, Goodglass & Kaplan, 1983), but we have great conversations about the Boston Red Sox.

Wernicke's Aphasia: A Description

Classical descriptions of Wernicke's aphasia exist (Goodglass & Kaplan, 1983; Kertesz, 1979). These describe patients with disproportionately impaired auditory comprehension in relation to fluent speech. The fluent speech is contaminated with semantic and literal paraphasic errors and in severe cases, neologistic jargon. These deficits result from a lesion in the posterior branches of the left middle cerebral artery: the primary auditory cortex (Areas 41 and 42), Wernicke's area (Area 22), and portions of the second temporal and angular gyri, with possible white matter extension (Bachman & Albert, 1990). Because these areas are the crossroads for all incoming auditory and visual information, reading, writing, repetition, and other language functions are also severely impaired. In comparison to the other fluent aphasia syndromes (anomic, transcortical sensory, conduction), Wernicke's aphasia is the most severe and has the poorest prognosis (Brookshire, 1997). Improvement follows a fluent route with the endpoint usually being anomic aphasia (Kertesz, 1984; Pashek & Holland, 1988).

RATIONALE FOR CONTEXT-BASED INTERVENTION

The topics covered in this book suggest (1) that there are many ways to treat aphasia and (2) that clinical management of this complex problem must take into consideration a multitude of problems—linguistic, cognitive, behavioral, social, and familial (Rosenbek et al., 1989). Why is a context-based approach advocated for patients with Wernicke's aphasia? For one thing, it seems that a patient might be more interested in working on his or her communication problems in a contextual situation. It became apparent to me long ago when speech-language pathologists were still called "speech correctionists." At a staff inservice, a veteran clinician showed how "to correct in a context." Her treatment materials were two "sow bugs" that she used when working with two children with frontal lisps. The opportunities for eliciting productions of /s/ and /z/ in this contextual situation are obvious, and the children were far more excited working on correcting their lisps in this situation than by drilling on words.

Many Aphasic Clients Communicate Better in a Context

It is surprising when the patient with fluent aphasia cannot point to the "cigarette" on the PICA, but responds enthusiastically to "Have you got a cigarette?" or "Don't you know smoking is bad for you?" Several studies show that persons with aphasia perform better when personally relevant materials are used (Busch & Brookshire, 1982; Gray et al., 1977; Van Lancker & Klein, 1990; Van Lancker & Nicklay, 1992; Wallace & Canter, 1985). If provided a script, some patients comprehend and speak better than in noncontextual situations (Brookshire, 1992). Differences between aphasic patients' understanding of noncontextual and contextual material suggests that "establishing a context" may aid comprehension for patients (Meyers & Linebaugh, 1981; Stachowiak et al., 1977; Wilcox et al., 1978) and performance in a context is at variance with noncontextual situations.

Allows Intervention to Target Functional Communication Sooner

The communication deficits associated with Wernicke's aphasia and the rapid movement by this type of patient through the health care system requires that work on exchanging messages begin sooner, not later. If not, Wernicke's aphasia could be mistaken for another problem. For example, VL was hospitalized following a left-hemisphere stroke. He tried to tell his physician that his wife had a "drinking problem" and without supervision might use up all of their savings. He became so angry when his disrupted communications could not be understood that he was restrained, sedated, and sent to an ECF without being referred to the speech-language pathologist. He underwent an expensive psychiatric evaluation and spent 2 months in the ECF before starting rehabilitation. Had some time been taken to communicate with VL in this context to solve the problem, this unfortunate event might not have happened.

Helps the Patient Cope with Problems at Home

The causative lesions in Wernicke's aphasia spare the primary motor cortex. These patients have few rehabilitation needs other than speech and language therapy and are discharged early. Therefore, context-based intervention is well-suited for coping with these early transitions from hospital to home. Focusing on the immediate communication need can prevent making ill-advised decisions about what patients can and cannot do. JZ was a 57 year-old man with a resolving Wernicke's aphasia who owned an auto shop. He had no physical problems and was scheduled for immediate discharge. Frustrated by his pervasive word-finding difficulties, JZ vowed to sell his business. His brief inpatient treatment, instead of targeting word-finding problems, focused on convincing him that accurate naming was not necessary to be a mechanic. JZ discovered that he would be better off working than going on disability and he resumed his responsibilities without difficulty.

Compensates for Limited Rehabilitation Services

Within the context-based approach there is a substantial amount of counseling, education, and general guidance. This is vital because patients with Wernicke's aphasia receive fewer rehabilitation services than do their nonfluent counterparts. In inpatient rehabilitation, a team of professionals supports the nonfluent client and his family. Discharge plans are made. Counseling and information about stroke is provided. Going from the supportive, structured rehabilitation setting to home is smoother because preparations can be made. These luxuries are not always available for patients who have speech and language treatment as their primary rehabilitation need. Nevertheless, Wernicke's aphasia has serious disabling consequences for day-to-day communications and the patient is not always ready for what he or she will face at home. Because communication at home occurs in a context, the approach described herein is useful in helping the patient solve immediate problems vital to his or her well-being and to that of the family.

Enhances Participation in Life

Physical handicaps do not limit the Wernicke's patient from participating in activities, but speech and language deficits make him/her fearful to resume former activities. While halting speech and hemiparesis "signals" the nonfluent patient's partners that something is wrong, the Wernicke's patient "looks fine" and may be treated rudely. BH needed specific parts for his car. He went to the auto parts store, but when he got to the window he could not remember the part numbers. The clerk was impatient. BH was embarrassed and he said "the hell with it." In a context-based treatment this scenario was role played by BH and his clinician. Alternatives to not communicating were explored. BH felt that better preparation was required. He agreed to have his wife help him make a list of the parts and their numbers in the future. This strategy would allow him to continue doing something important to him. These and other similar problems can be addressed in a context-based approach in a constructive way.

APPLICATIONS

Context-Based Intervention and Functional Treatment Tasks

Lyon (1998) suggests that if patients are to get where they want to go in the rehabilitation journey (1) skills that are not working must work better, and (2) skills that are working must be made to work more completely and functionally. Functional needs change throughout rehabilitation. Immediately after a stroke, the speech-language pathologist may work with the patient to help him or her follow a medication schedule. In the rehabilitation setting, treatment stresses skills (e.g., ordering food in a restaurant) and sub-skills (reading and producing single words) used in communicative activities of daily living. When the aphasia is chronic, interventions seek to reduce handicaps by increasing participation in activities that were formerly enjoyed (e.g., returning to church).

Context-Based Treatment and Group Treatment

Group treatment is making a comeback as a primary method for treating patients with aphasia (Marshall, 1998a). The context-based approach is extremely useful in group treatments that stress problem solving, mutual cooperation, and other methods intended to reduce disability (Avent, 1997; Elman, 1998; Marshall, 1998b). The benefits of group treatment have been demonstrated in several studies (Aten et al., 1982; Bollinger et al., 1993; Elman & Burnstein-Ellis, 1999; Marshall, 1993; Wertz et al., 1981). It is anticipated that group treatment approaches will continue to flourish as long as funding for aphasia treatment is limited.

SPECIFIC DEFICITS

Auditory Comprehension

Impaired auditory comprehension is a hallmark of Wernicke's aphasia, especially in the early post-onset period. Comprehension improves for some, but not all patients. The context-based approach stresses (1) clinician manipulation

of linguistic and timing variables (e.g., rate, pause, and stress manipulation) in a contextual communication setting to maximize comprehension for the patient, and (2) teaching caregivers how to do the same thing through demonstration and modeling. For this reason, a brief review of the effects of linguistic and timing variables on comprehension of aphasic persons is necessary, but it should be pointed out that the research cited here was not specifically confined to comprehension performance of patients with Wernicke's aphasia.

Linguistic Variables

Normal individuals alter linguistic content of their speech according to whom they are speaking. For example, I make adjustments in what I say to my 93-year-old father when I call him on the phone or speak to him in person. Linguistic features discussed here include message length, syntactic complexity, reversibility and plausibility, vocabulary level, and redundancy. These features can be discussed at the word, sentence, and discourse levels.

Message Length

Comprehension of patients with aphasia is affected by a reduced auditory-verbal retention span (Schuell et al., 1965; Darley, 1982). Typically, aphasic patients retain shorter messages better than longer messages and this is usually the case whether those messages are sequences (e.g., words, numbers), sentences, or spoken discourse (paragraphs and stories).

Syntactic Complexity

Syntactic complexity influences sentence and discourse comprehension. Aphasic patients understand affirmative statements (e.g., John is running), better than negative statements (John is not running), and active declarative sentences (The boy is running), better than passive sentences (The boy ran). Message comprehension in aphasia is enhanced by reducing the syntactic complexity of spoken messages.

Reversibility and Plausibility

Reversible sentences (e.g., The boy is chasing the girl) have a subject and an object that can be transposed without creating an implausible sentence. They are more difficult to comprehend than nonreversible sentences (e.g., The boy is eating cake) (Caramazza et al., 1978). Verb markers may compensate for reversibility. Pierce (1981, 1982) found that marked reversible sentences (The girl was *being* hit by the boy) were understood better than unmarked reversible sentences (The girl was hit by the boy). In addition, the "plausibility" of the reversible sentence affects comprehension. For example, the construction: "The nurse helps the doctor" may be easier for a patient with aphasia to comprehend than the sentence:

"The girls charm the soldier" (Deloche & Seron, 1981; Kudo, 1984).

Vocabulary Level

Reduced available vocabulary is a cardinal feature of aphasia, and its effects on auditory comprehension are noticeable at word, sentence, and discourse levels (Schuell & Jenkins, 1961).

Single Word Comprehension

Aphasic individuals comprehend some single words better than others. Words that are frequently used in their native language (e.g., dog) are easier to understand than less common words (e.g., Basenji). Short words (e.g., bat) are easier than longer ones (e.g., banana). Personally relevant words (e.g., "plaintiff" for a lawyer) may be comprehended better than impersonal words. Verbs that can be pictured (e.g., kicking) may be easier to understand than verbs that are difficult to picture (e.g., curtail) (Brookshire & Nicholas, 1982). If the patient must select among words in a set of semantically related items (e.g., orange, apple, banana), he or she will have greater difficulty than when the set of words is semantically dissimilar (Goodglass & Baker, 1976; Marshall & Brown, 1974).

Sentence Comprehension

Semantic relatedness also affects sentence comprehension. For example, the question: "Was Abraham Lincoln the first president of the United States?" may stump the patient, because it is semantically falsified (Brookshire, 1997), but, "Is Abraham Lincoln the president now?" might prompt a correct response. Personal relevance and word frequency also influence sentence comprehension. Two studies have shown that personally relevant yes-no questions (Is your name John?) are more apt to be answered correctly by aphasic patients than questions about the immediate environment (Are you in the intensive care ward?). Questions about the environment, however, are easier than those containing impersonal information (Do apples grow on trees?) (Busch & Brookshire, 1982; Gray et al., 1977). Further, both yes-no questions and those requiring longer responses are problematic for aphasic patients when higher-level reasoning and the making of inferences are required (Brookshire, 1997). Thus, the patient with aphasia may be stumped by the question: "Does everyone put money in the bank?" Sentences that require comparisons (e.g., Is one pound of flour heavier than two?) are also more difficult for aphasic patients. Nicholas and Brookshire (1981) found this tended to occur if the comparative sentence contained "surprising" information (e.g., A brick is harder than a diamond), instead of anticipated information (e.g., A brick is harder than a pillow). Finally, aphasic patients respond better to directly worded sentences and commands (Open the door) than to those which are indirectly worded (Now I would like you to open the door).

Discourse Comprehension

Discourse comprehension (e.g., understanding stories, conversation, narratives, etc.), is affected by many of the factors discussed previously. Brookshire and co-workers have illustrated that discourse comprehension is improved when the main ideas of the narrative are highlighted in relation to the less important details of the passage (Brookshire & Nicholas, 1982, 1984, 1993; Wegner et al., 1984). Informational discourse that is directly stated is more apt to be comprehended by a patient with aphasia than discourse that requires the patient to make assumptions and use inference on the basis of implied information (Nicholas & Brookshire, 1995; Katsuki-Nakamura et al., 1988). Discourse comprehension is facilitated if the speaker uses cohesive ties to link the information together (Halliday & Hasan, 1976). For example, lexical ties repeat words and appropriate synonyms (e.g., *Susan & Andy got out of the car.* **Susan** *wore a blue dress.* **Andy** *wore a black tuxedo*) to accomplish these linkages. Discourse that is coherent is also easier to comprehend. Brookshire (1997) suggests that coherence relates to the overall unity of the discourse and that multiple variables contribute to this feature. This may be similar to listening to a lecture where the speaker follows a carefully constructed outline to support the central premise of the talk rather than skipping haphazardly from point to point.

Redundancy

To increase message redundancy speakers repeat, paraphrase, and augment so as to highlight important information of the utterance. Aphasic listeners benefit from message redundancy. Gardner and colleagues (Gardner et al., 1975) found that semantically redundant sentences (e.g., The cat is furry), were better understood than sentences with semantic distracters (e.g., The cat is sour) and neutral sentences (The cat is nice). West and Kaufman (1972) noted aphasic patients to respond better to Token Test commands where information was repeated (e.g., *Show me the* **green** *circle and the* **green** *square*), than when it was not (e.g., *Show me the green circle and the red square*). At the discourse level, Gravel and LaPointe (1983) noted rehabilitation team members varied the number of repetitions and revisions in communicating with aphasic patients of different severity levels.

Timing Variables

Aphasic listeners often accuse the speaking partner of talking too fast (Skelly, 1975). Those who treat aphasic patients regularly have a "knack" for adjusting the timing of their message when talking to some aphasic patients. This was seen in a novel experiment (Salvatore et al., 1975) that compared the speech rates of experienced and inexperienced clinicians in giving Token Test commands to low- and high-level aphasic patients. The experienced clinicians slowed rate of speech (by using pauses) for the low-level patients, but not the high-level patients. These differential adjustments were not observed for the inexperienced clinicians. Results suggest that clinicians "naturally" do what is necessary to facilitate comprehension by adjusting timing variables.

Rate

Aphasic patients comprehend spoken material better at slightly slower than normal rates. This is true for single words (number sequences) (Cermak & Moreines, 1976), sentences (Weidner & Lasky, 1976; Lasky et al., 1976), and paragraph-length material (Pashek & Brookshire, 1982). Slowing rate by using pauses gives the patient time to "catch up" and/or process information in meaningful "chunks" and has a positive effect on comprehension.

Pause Types

Three forms of pauses have been employed to enhance the comprehension of aphasic subjects: within-sentence, inter-stimulus, and imposed.

Within-Sentence Pauses

Within-sentence pauses occur at syntactical boundaries within sentences (e.g., *The little girl/is pushing/the big boy*). In spoken discourse, these pauses may be placed at syntactical boundaries or between sentences themselves. Pauses group the information in meaningful units called "chunks" for the listener. This facilitates storage and processing, and aids comprehension. Just how long within-sentence pauses should be appears to vary from patient to patient (Fehst & Brookshire, 1980; Salvatore, 1979), but the recommended length is about 3 seconds (Salvatore, 1979).

Interstimulus Pauses

Interstimulus pauses are brief silent intervals between stimulus presentations. These stimuli might be commands, yes-no statements, or informational questions. This type of pause is beneficial for the aphasic patient who accumulates "noise" in his auditory system and tends to perform increasingly poorly across a series of messages (Brookshire, 1974). Brief, quiet interstimulus pauses permits the noise to dissipate.

Imposed Pauses

Imposed pauses are intended to reduce impulsivity. Impulsive responders act before they have processed the information completely. An imposed pause forces the patient to "wait" before responding. In some instances, imposed pauses have been shown to prevent anticipatory response errors (Yorkston et al., 1977), but this finding is not universal (Toppin & Brookshire, 1978).

Alerting Signals

Deficits in attention may cause the patient to miss initial portions of messages or fail to comprehend short messages entirely. Not picking up a topic may also be the result of inattention. Sometimes patients have problems moving from an inactive to an active processing mode, a problem Brookshire (1974) calls "slow rise time." Alerting signals prepare the patient for an incoming message and may help him or her reallocate his or her attention and thus improve comprehension (Cambell & McNeil, 1983). Examples of alerting signals would be phrases (e.g., *Get ready; Here's the next one*), tones (Marshall & Thistlethwaite, 1977), and visual signals (Loverso & Prescott, 1981). A semantic prime might also function as an alerting signal. An example would be presenting the patient with the word "vehicle" before asking questions about driving or about favorite cars.

Stress

Aphasic patients are more responsive to the stressed than the unstressed words of sentences and paragraphs (Kimelman & McNeil, 1987; Pashek & Brookshire, 1982; Swinney et al., 1980). Stress is accomplished by giving added prosodic emphasis to important words in the message. Another way to do this is to put the important words in a prominent location, preferably the beginning or the end of the utterance (Darley, 1976). These manipulations, coupled with wording statements, directly heighten stimulus saliency. Saliency, as defined by Goodglass (1973), is "the psychological resultant of the stress, the informational significance, the phonological prominence, and the affective value of a word." Saliency is an important concept in addressing the auditory comprehension problems of the Wernicke's patient.

USING THE CONTEXT-BASED APPROACH

Use of the context-based approach requires a clinician who is not technique bound. The context-based approach relies on clinician flexibility and a willingness to experiment. It focuses more on successful communication and less on what the patient says and how. Flexibility indicates a willingness to switch, to deviate from a plan, and to make on-line decisions to enhance communication. Experimentation involves balancing clinical science, art, and the all important common sense mentioned earlier. It is important that the clinician be "free" of the tethers of having to elicit a specific number of "pre-selected" responses and try different strategies and strategy combinations to improve message comprehension and message exchange.

Intervention is presented in two stages, early and late. Early interventions begin in the acute care hospital and, depending on the patient's participatory status, extend into inpatient rehabilitation. Later interventions occur in outpatient settings and the patient must cope with the permanent residuals of aphasia, and when aphasia is interfering with the activities of daily living. In both stages, assessment, support, and guidance, as well as intervention tactics will be emphasized.

Early Context-Based Intervention

The patient with Wernicke's aphasia needs immediate attention from the speech pathologist because of his or her severe comprehension and expressive deficits. Many are unaware that they do not understand or are not understood. Some appear confused and/or agitated. If the factors responsible for these behaviors are not identified and dealt with appropriately by the speech-language pathologist, the patient's behavior could be misinterpreted. LB's fluent, neologistic speech and lack of comprehension was seen as "drunk and disorderly conduct" by the police because his stroke occurred in a bar. Instead of a hospital, LB was taken to detox. In their efforts to help, family and medical staff may make similar mistakes or become frustrated with the mismatches among their questions and the patient's answers. Contributing further to the patient's chaos is the fact that neurologists and medical students find Wernicke's patients "interesting" from a diagnostic standpoint. Hence, the entire "medical food chain" from senior physician to first-year medical student badger the patient with requests such as repeating "No ifs ands or buts."

In the early intervention period, the clinician assumes the role of "behavioral engineer" with patients like LB. His or her job is to get communication "on the right track." This is a time when (1) the patient is changing physically, cognitively, and in other ways; and (2) when he or she is moving through the health care system rapidly. The clinician must change speeds, tracks, and heed important signals that suggest what to do. Not only does he or she guide the patient, but also the family and treatment team as the patient increases his or her ability to participate in treatment. To plan this trip and make it as "smooth" as possible, the clinician needs information from "special" assessment procedures.

Assessment

The word "special" is used for good reason. Few patients with Wernicke's aphasia can be assessed formally in the early post-onset period. They are befuddled by the easiest tasks of a standardized aphasia test battery (e.g., naming, repetition, sentence completion, matching). Moreover, their performance on these tasks yields little useful information. Early assessment in Wernicke's aphasia should rely on parastandardized testing, observation, and personal information about the patient.

Parastandardized Assessment

Spark's (1978) paper *Parastandardized Examination Guidelines for Adult Aphasia* (PSE) is always assigned to students in my aphasia class. It offers a systematic format to obtain the information needed to get communication on the right track in the early post-onset period until formal evaluation can be attempted. The PSE is flexible. Its results provide information that is immediately useful in determining what facilitates and what hinders comprehension and expression. PSE information can be used to plan early interventions. Spark's guidelines cover several content areas, most of which are applicable to the patient with Wernicke's. The guidelines, with some modifications (of my own) are summarized in Table 18–1. Results of the PSE give a quick picture of the patient's strengths and weaknesses, and more specifically, what variables the clinician can manipulate to aid comprehension and information exchange. Experienced clinicians can conduct the PSE without using many notes, but beginning clinicians may want to record their interactions with the patient and/or use material provided in Table 18–1 to develop a form to follow when examining the patient. When possible, the PSE should be carried out in a reasonably quiet room, free from distractions of the hospital ward and its interruptions.

An important supplement to the PSE are the clinician's observations of the patient. Holland (1982, 1983) suggests that aphasic people be observed communicating in other environments and with different partners. Possible situations in which the patient might be observed include watching television, using the phone, writing, reading, eating, and making purchases in the gift shop. Interactive situations in which similar observations might be made include talking with a caregiver (e.g., Dr., nurse, OT), talking with a family member, talking with another patient, and talking with a stranger. If the patient is able to go home for weekend passes or short visits and if the family has a video camera, a tape might be made for the clinician to review.

A third component of early assessment involves gathering personal information about the patient's history, background, and pre-morbid communication status. Today's clinicians are pressed for time and lengthy patient-family interviews may not be conducted. Several alternatives are available. One is to have a significant other (SO) develop a short biography about the patient, providing information about work, friends, hobbies, interests, likes, dislikes, accomplishments, education, and the like. Autobiographical information can be supplemented with photographs and other suitable materials. Questionnaires for this purpose have been developed in several aphasia centers and these are reviewed in a recent text on group treatment (Marshall, 1978). Green (1984)

TABLE 18–1

Modified Parastandardized Examination Guidelines for Patients with Fluent Aphasia.

Feature 1. Therapeutic Set		
Area of Concern	**Negative Signs/Behaviors**	**Positive Signs/Behaviors**
Ease or difficulty establishing and maintaining a therapeutic set	Hostility towards examiner; distractibility due to ambient noise	Accepts the therapist in the situation, displays a realistic appraisal of situation, and acknowledges clinician is there to help
Presence of rigidity or perseveration	Continuing to produce a response without regard to change in stimulus; difficulty switching tasks	Recognizing task switches; awareness of errors and effort to correct them
Behavioral rigidity	Ego-minded responses—e.g., when asked "What do you wear on your head?" says "I don't ever wear hats."	Ability to role play and pretend

Feature 2. Pragmatics		
Area of Concern	**Negative Signs/Behaviors**	**Positive Signs/Behaviors**
Follows conversation rules	Limited turn taking; not aware when to terminate a conversation; violates social conventions	Obeys conversational conventions
Realizes the reasons for language processing deficit	Blames problems on outside forces, e.g., missing dentures, people talking too fast, no glasses	Understands that he or she has had a stroke
Initiates communication	Initiates few communication interactions; only responds when asked to	Initiates communication to make needs known
Persistence in face of failure	Gives up when communication snag occurs	Persists until he or she has communicated his or her thought

Feature 3. Auditory Comprehension		
Area of Concern	**Negative Signs/Behaviors**	**Positive Signs/Behaviors**
Peripheral hearing loss	Asks for repeats; phonemic confusions, e.g., rake/lake; history of working in noise	Examiner judges hearing acuity to be within normal limits
Understanding a conversation	Looking confused or perplexed; difficulty following conversation containing personally relevant material	Responds more enthusiastically to conversation about personal interests, e.g., sports, family, work
Comprehension in structured auditory comprehension tasks	Difficulty pointing to objects, body parts, following simple commands	Once oriented to task points to objects, body parts, and follows simple commands
Responses to different methods of presentation	Not helped by slower rate; alerting phrases; shorter, simplified messages; orientation to topic	Comprehension of conversation and structured material when clinician uses different methods of presenting material
Comprehension when verbal output is restricted	Examiner is unable to halt "press of speech" or patient's comprehension does not improve when speech is restricted	Comprehension in conversation and on structured tasks improves when patient is asked to "listen" rather than talk
Intrapersonal monitoring	Does not ask for repeats or verify what is said	Asks for repetitions; verifies what has been said

Continued

Continued

Comprehension when treatment materials are thematically organized	Comprehension does not improve when questions flow from mutually known topic, e.g., family	Comprehension improves when task is organized, e.g., I want to know about your family. Are you married? Do you have any children? Are the children still at home?
Effect of visual supplementation	No improvement when provided a visual cue (e.g., written word "Military")	Comprehension improves with visual cue in form of written word: e.g., Were you in the service? What branch of the military were you in?
Self-criticism	No awareness of errors in speech output	Aware of errors and possibly upset by them

Feature 4. Verbal Expression

Area of Concern	Negative Signs/Behaviors	Positive Signs/Behaviors
Accuracy and use of substantive words	Not aware when correct target has been produced; empty speech; rejects target word when it is provided; errors do not resemble target word	Aware that speech lacks content words; recognizes target word when provided; errors are variable and sometimes approximate the target word
Quantity of speech	Unrestricted verbal output with no awareness of its content	Fluent speech that sometimes becomes less fluent as the patient evidences concern for his or her errors
Grammatical structure	High number of paragrammatic errors (e.g., he/she, from/for, they/we) and lack of awareness of them	Speech reflects full range of grammatical constructions with few paragrammatic errors
Degree to which paraphasic errors approximate target word	Errors bear no resemblance to target word (e.g., pillow): "grabbitz, rafunta."	Errors contain some of the constituents of the target word: pister, pillar and may "in the ball park."
Self-correction accuracy and effort	No awareness of errors; makes no effort to correct errors; overcorrects a response when its meaning has been conveyed	Recognizes most errors; makes efforts to correct errors and sometimes succeeds
Stimulability	No improvement when errors are pointed out and model provided; response does not improve with semantic or phonetic cue	May improve production when model provided; responds to semantic or phonetic cues
Response to restriction in verbal output	Brief responses continue to be in error	Verbal expression is improved when shorter responses are elicited
Verbal compensations	Unable to find alternative means of verbal expression to convey intended word (zebra)	Conveys meaning of target word through description (black and white horse thing) or other means
Compensations in other modalities	Uses only speech to express thoughts	Uses alternative modalities, e.g., writing, gesturing

Author's Modifications Based on the Work of Sparks, R. (1978). *British Journal of Disorders of Communication, 13*, 135–146

has described an interview format for obtaining a detailed communication history on patients with aphasia. Swindell and colleagues (Swindell et al., 1982) have also developed a questionnaire for surveying personal and communication styles of persons with aphasia.

PSE results, observational data, and personal knowledge about the patient are integral to planning and implementing context-based interventions. Information of this nature is more than sufficient to allow the clinician to (1) return the consult to the physician; and (2) begin an early intervention program to bridge the gap to more structured treatment.

Goals of Early Context-Based Intervention

Goals of early intervention are to (1) establish a therapeutic set; (2) create different contexts for communication; (3) heighten auditory comprehension in established contexts;

TABLE 18–2

Examples of How a Communicative Context Might be Established for a Patient with Fluent Aphasia in the Early Intervention Period.

Strategy	Stimulus	Clinician Comment	Patient Response
Use of humor	Five men doing a paint job one could handle	"Wow! That's a heck of a way to spend the taxpayer's money."	"Just terrible. Oh God."
Shared knowledge	Clinician discovers she and patient live in the same part of town.	"I understand you live in Soho." "Me too." "Do you ever eat at Galluchi's?"	"Yeah." "Oh really?" "Expensive, but good, good, good."
Prop	Road Atlas on table	"I understand you are from the west coast."	"Right." (reaches for Atlas and points out California)
Emotion	Patient eating at bedside	"Are you really going to eat that crap?"	"Oh yeah. I gotta."
		"I bet you would prefer a steak."	"Right rare" (gestures thickness of steak)
Environmental feature	Patient's ring from Stanford	"Good looking ring on your finger. Does Stanford have a good team this year?"	"I think all the way."

and (4) maintain the flow of communication in information exchanges with partners, again in established contexts.

Therapeutic Set

Sparks (1978) uses the term therapeutic set to describe the patient's attitude towards the therapeutic environment. Sometimes, patients are changing so rapidly they feel no need for treatment. Once sent home, they may disconnect from the treatment setting and "fall through the cracks." For these patients, it is important to ensure that the patient and the family know that "the door is open" for further evaluation and treatment on an outpatient basis. For the Wernicke's patient who is not improving so rapidly, establishing a therapeutic set can be problematic. One reason is that the patient may not grasp what is wrong. Another is that the useful "get started tasks" that help "engage" nonfluent aphasic clients in treatment (e.g., counting, sentence completion) make little sense to a patient with Wernicke's aphasia. Nevertheless, it is necessary to establish a therapeutic set so the patient will know help is available. One approach is for the clinician to show the patient that his or her skills may help the patient get his or her message across to the family and the treatment care team. Mr. W., a 47-year-old man with severe Wernicke's, provides an example. When evaluated, he was anxious to tell the clinician something important. While the clinician needed information about Mr. W.'s language processing abilities, it was helpful to "trouble shoot" the situation. Using yes-no questions, trial and error, and lots of guessing, the clinician learned Mr. W. was worried about his dog because no was home to care for the animal when Mr. W. came to the hospital. The clinician dealt with the situation and this communication success helped establish a therapeutic set.

Creating a Context

To create a context, it is necessary to communicate with the patient about something that is important. These are issues he or she is concerned about (e.g., going home, work, family, health, money, living situation), rather than something out of a box (e.g., a picture card). A context creates expectations for the patient about what will be said and engages a "top-down" processing system, which is often better preserved than the "bottom-up" processing system. Top-down models of auditory comprehension emphasize listeners' general knowledge of the world and information that is mutually known by speaker and listener (Brookshire, 1992). Sometimes, this prompts better comprehension and verbal expression for the Wernicke's patient.

Information used to create a context can come from several sources: background information from the significant other, the medical chart, and the patient's autobiography. Certain props (e.g., maps, pictures) can also be used to create a context. Table 18–2 provides some representative examples. When a communicative context has been established, the clinician works to maximize comprehension within that context by selectively manipulating linguistic and timing variables. The analogy "finding a hole in the screen" will be used to demonstrate this process.

Finding a Hole in the Screen. Visualize looking at a large meshed screen that someone has thrown mud at. Some of the squares are plugged with mud; others are open.

The partner is seated on one side of the screen and the patient on the other. Successful comprehension involves getting the message through "an open square." Failure results when the message cannot get through a "plugged" square. Patients with severe comprehension deficits have many holes plugged; as comprehension improves, more squares in the screen open. The clinician's job is to find a way to get the message through an "open hole." Establishment of a communication context "primes the patient" for this to happen by laying down a template. Successes occur as the clinician manipulates linguistic and timing variables accordingly. This is illustrated in the following example:

Clinician: I would like to talk to you about your family. (Establish context)

Patient: Oh boy.

Clinician: I know you have a *large* family (presents written word "FAMILY" (**Stress, visual supplement**)

Patient: Oh, my family, well it's a big one.

Clinician: I understand you have quite a few children. How many do you have? (**Increased redundancy**)

Patient: Let me see, Tony, Markee, Martee, Muckee—Oh no.

Clinician: That's a hard word to say, but I'm interested in HOW MANY (stresses this word): four, five, six (gestures higher) (**Re-direct to topic, stress, gestural supplement**)

Patient: No more than that. (Holds up 10 fingers).

Clinician: Wow, ten kids. That must keep you busy. All boys? (**Humor, syntactic simplification**)

Patient: No way, no way. Lots of girls. Holds up seven fingers.

Clinician: Seven girls. That means you have three boys (holds up three fingers) (**Verify, gestural supplementation**)

Patient: Yep, three of them.

Clinician: I understand one of your *boys* is quite *famous*. (**Stress key words; put words at the end of the sentence**)

Patient: Huh? (looking quizzical). What did you say?

Clinician: I'm glad you asked me to repeat that question. Any time. I was asking about your FAMOUS son. (**Reinforce for asking for repeat; stress word famous; redundancy**)

Patient: Oh, you mean Buddig, Bodie, Booby.

Clinician: Right, Buddy. I understand he's a rather good football player? (Buddy is really a baseball player) (**Give false information to help patient integrate and consolidate response**)

Patient: Not that one, the other one.

Clinician: Sorry, wrong sport. You mean golf? (**Humor, again give information to integrate and consolidate response**)

Patient: Nope.

Clinician: Tennis? (**Humor, continue to consolidate and integrate**)

Patient: Get out of here.

Clinician: Baseball? (**Syntactic simplification; one word; salient word**)

Patient: That would be the one. He's a (gestures pitching motion) you know.

Clinician: A pitcher? Wow. Is he right or left handed? (**Emotion and facial expression; redundancy**)

Patient: One of these (gestures with his left hand).

In the forgoing example, a communicative context informs the patient that the conversation was to be about his family. Then the clinician selectively manipulates linguistic and timing variables (see boldfaced text), in this context to work on comprehension. Limited attention was given to the patient's production errors and the clinician required only short verbal responses from the patient. In such situations, the clinician notes those manipulations that are helpful in getting messages "through the open holes of the screen" and makes adjustments accordingly. In the early post-onset period, much of the work done to maximize comprehension in contexts is trial and error. The most successful clinicians constantly "experiment" to keep the patient on track. Some of the specific tactics that help are (1) using visual supplements (e.g., gesture, written words); (2) using humor and descriptive language; (3) alerting the patient to topic changes; (4) reinforcing and encouraging the patient to ask for repeats; (5) maximizing redundancy with semantic support; (6) providing the patient paralinguistic cues (tone of voice, facial expression, emphasizing or stressing certain words) to heighten meaning; (7) structuring requests for information such that the patient can respond with short answers (e.g., yes or no, select from a choice of two words); and (8) filling in the word for the patient if that is necessary to keep him or her focused on the comprehension exercise. As the patient improves, some strategies are abandoned and others retained and expanded upon.

Speech Flow

Speech flow in patients with Wernicke's aphasia may be unchecked (excessive) or restricted. The former results when comprehension is severely disrupted and talking is less punitive than listening. The term "press of speech" has been applied to patients who cannot inhibit their speech output. If this output is markedly defective a situation is created where the "defective utterances" are fed back to an impaired auditory system, a condition called "the garbage out-garbage-in cycle (Marshall, 1994). Conversely, as the patient with Wernicke's aphasia improves his or her auditory comprehension, speech flow may be restricted. The reason for this is that the patient is starting to recognize errors and to notice how others respond to these errors. Speech flow can be reduced by excessive and nonproductive self-correction efforts, circumlocution, and fruitless word search. These behaviors are, in some cases, desirable. However, when they disrupt communications with friends, family, and the treatment team in the early post-onset period, intervention is necessary.

TABLE 18–3

Examples of Word Search Behavior in Communicative Interactions That Require Clinical Decision Making. Target Word is Shown in Brackets

Scenario 1 (cigarette)

Patient PJ: "You smoke a cig, a sigg, oh what is it? I want one now. Smittring, ciggerthing, almost, what is it called? You put in your mouth and smuch it. Smucher, smuch, smukker, chitter, No."

Scenario 2 (Alaska)

Patient HB: "I always wanted to go to Alasta, where its cold, Alasta, Alaskan, Alasker (pause). Clinician signals to go on. HB: "Alaska.""

Scenario 3 (coffee)

Patient BB: "Well since my heart went bad, my Dr. said no more cokkee, I mean coffee. It's not good for my blood pressure."

Scenario 4 (bathroom)

Patient SA: Approaches nurse grimacing and saying "Oh, oh, oh gotta go, gotta go. Ok please?" Nurse: "Say bathroom."

Scenario 5 (hospital)

Patient RG: "They took me right to the hottle, hopil, hosital, for the sick people, lots of doctors, you know, hostile, hosital, where you work of course. I just can't get it today. Maybe tomorrow."

Excessive Flow. The garbage-out and garbage-in cycle can be interrupted with a stop strategy. This involves directing the patient to listen to himself or herself and to stop when he or she hears an error. The clinician can signal the occurrence of an error, but the goal is to have clients identify and correct their errors, first in treatment, and then outside the clinic. At times, merely stopping the patient from talking so much, encouraging shorter replies, and framing questions so that answers are within his or her capabilities will suffice.

Some patients with copious speech output cannot use a stop strategy because comprehension and self-monitoring skills are too impaired. Martin (1981a) offers an alternative. Instead of stopping the patient and correcting his or her errors, Martin suggests that clinicians become better interpreters and translators of the patient's defective utterances. By paraphrasing the patient's utterances, modeling, and reinforcing the patient for communicative adequacy (getting the message across), the clinician is able to break the garbage-out and garbage-in cycle. An example follows:

Patient: (Waving an issue of the *American Kennel Club Magazine*). "Here's the one smasher, master boy, oh nuts! It's there, where is it? My caster, the ones out there where I live. I know it. What's wrong with me? (Pause). Smash. M-A-T-T-E-R. Matteree. Oh God."

Clinician: "I understand you are a dog breeder. What types of dogs do you raise?"

Patient: (opening the magazine) "Well they're not in here but they are big and mean." (Opens the page to show Bulldogs) "Almost like this, but bigger. Smasbees, masters, mastees, oh nuts. Why can't I say it?" (Now frustrated)

Clinician: "Do you mean Bull Mastiffs? They are big fellows?"

Patient: "Bull Mastiffs, Bull Mastiffs, that's it. You got it. Those are my boys." (Now enthusiastic)

Clinician: "Very protective animals?"

Patient: "Oh you bet, they'll bite your head off if you mess with me."

In this scenario, the AKC magazine was the prompt that established the communicative context. The clinician's knowledge of the situation and the patient's interests in dogs allowed him to interpret the patient's defective utterances and to break the cycle.

Restricted Flow. If a patient struggles excessively and that struggle interferes with communication of basic needs, the clinician needs to consider strategies to maintain speech flow and exchange of information What is needed here is on-line clinical decision making. Some of the things to try when the patient's flow is so restricted that communication is affected follow.

Fill In. When struggle is excessive and it is apparent that the client will not "hit the target" word, the clinician may choose to fill in the missing word. Scenario one in Table 18–3 shows a portion of PJ's 3-minute effort to produce the word "cigarette." The best decision is for the clinician to supply the word or write the missing word for PJ and move on.

Keep Trying. Sometimes the patient gets so close to the target, it is tempting to supply the missing word. If the target word is truly "on the tip of the patient's tongue," reflected in Scenario 2 in Table 18–3, the patient might be encouraged to keep trying with a phrase like "Tell me more" or "You're almost there." Simple hand signals to keep trying may be employed similarly. These tactics allay the patient's fear that he or she will be interrupted and prompt him or her to continue the communicative effort.

Accept the Effort. In Scenario 3 in Table 18–3, the client clearly communicates the essence of what he wants to say, namely that he does not drink coffee because of a heart condition. Here, the clinician should acknowledge that the message has been understood. The clinician would do this by providing feedback based on communicative adequacy in a statement like "Oh yes, I drink too much coffee myself."

Reward Persistence. When the patient tries to work through a communication snag, acknowledge the effort so as to minimize the effects of failure. Comments that might fit the behavior exhibited in Scenario 4 in Table 18–3 might be "I like the way you stuck with that," "You really worked hard on that word," or "That word is tough today." Rewarding persistence is more important at the "thought level" than the word level. For example, for the patient who struggled with the word such as "cigarette" in Scenario 1, supplying the missing word to "fill the gap" and maintain communication flow may help. However, when the patient is showing persistence in sharing "new information" (e.g., His daughter is getting married August 6), encourage persistence and reinforce it.

Variability. One patient called his wife "Mildred" on one day and "Bernice" (his ex-wife's name), the next. This upset the patient and he usually hit his head saying "Mildred, Mildred, Mildred—stupid." In situations such as seen in Scenario 5, it is important to help the patient understand the day-to-day fluctuations in word retrieval efforts. Encourage them that this variability is a product of the stroke and not because they are stupid or crazy. Sometimes a visual aid or material from the National Aphasia Association may be useful here.

Support and Guidance

Treatment hours in the early post-onset period with the Wernicke's aphasic patient are limited. Clinicians need allies. The primary allies are the patient's caregivers. Support and guidance are those things the speech-language pathologist does to educate all other communicative partners of the patient on how they can communicate with the patient. Caregivers need to know how to heighten comprehension when speaking to the patient. They also need to know how to restrict and promote speech flow. The more support and guidance the better, as hospital staff and family members usually welcome the chance to be of assistance. The major benefit of support and guidance is that these activities create more communication opportunities for the patient.

Assistance from a caregiver is best gained by using a demonstration rather than a lecture. For example, Czvik

(1977) noted that family members disagreed with the speech-language pathologist's test results on patients' auditory comprehension deficits, and tended to view aphasia as "an expressive problem" only. Demonstrations that illustrate how comprehension is aided by the use of repetition, speaking at a slower rate, and how techniques to encourage communication flow help facilitate information exchange may yield better results than sharing the results of the Token Test.

Observation of the patient and the caregiver communicating with each other may give the clinician valuable information on who is and who is not coachable. Sometimes, caregivers do naturally what aphasia clinicians would like them to do when talking to the aphasic client. We can learn from these individuals. Some caregivers, however, talk too rapidly, do not talk at all, fail to listen, and change topics abruptly. They may be so overwhelmed by the impact of a stroke on the family that they are unable to think about maximizing comprehension and promoting speech flow. They need our support and guidance. Unfortunately, there are also the lost causes. These are caregivers with the responsibility of caring for an aphasic partner who has been in a troubled relationship. They may be angry and not interested in helping. They also need support and guidance, but from a psychologist.

Later Treatment

Later intervention begins about 4 to 8 weeks post-onset. By this time the clinician using the context-based approach is adept at communicating with the patient. The patient with Wernicke's aphasia has probably improved his or her comprehension status, but still has specific problems. These can now be addressed, but also within a context-based approach. The patient will also have pronounced word-finding difficulties or have evolved to become an anomic aphasic, as suggested by many authors (Kertesz & McCabe, 1977; Pashek & Holland, 1988). There are many model-based and other programs for treating word-finding problems of patients with aphasia. These are covered in detail in other chapters and will not be dealt with here. Because most of these programs focus on single words and are essentially acontextual, word-finding problems of patients with Wernicke's aphasia will continue to be addressed within the context-based approach stressed in this chapter.

Assessment

When the patient is seen in the outpatient setting, he or she will be able to participate in formal testing. Ideally, assessment will include the administration of a comprehensive battery such as the BDAE, WAB, PICA, or MTDDA. When necessary, free-standing tests that further probe the patient's comprehension, naming, reading, writing, and other functions may be used. Some form of functional assessment

TABLE 18–4

Examples of Functional Tasks to Improve Auditory Retention.

Retention Task Item	Example
Phone number	874–2384
Person's name	Joe Blackstone
Recipe step	two tablespoons sugar
Items from grocery	eggs, milk, juice, cereal
Directions	Go two blocks, turn left
License plate	ARQ 349
ATM code	2953
Important date	February 12, 1999

such as the *Communication Activities of Daily Living* (CADL, Holland, 1980), the *Everyday Language Test* (ANELT, Blomert, 1990), or *ASHA FACS* (Frattali et al., 1995), may be useful. The clinician may ask a family member to complete any one of a number of scales, rating measures, or forms to provide an index of social validation of the disabling and handicapping aspects of the aphasia. For more complete information on assessment the reader is referred to Chapter 4 of the text.

Specific Auditory Comprehension Problems

Attention Deficits

Attention deficits cause patients to miss beginning portions of messages and to miss short messages entirely (Brookshire, 1974; Loverso & Prescott, 1981). It helps to alert the patient that a message is coming with a verbal ("Listen to me!") or nonverbal (cup hand to ear) signal. Attention problems may result in a patient not picking up a topic change. Again, an alerting phrase such as "Let's talk about something else," or supplying the patient with a written cue identifying the new topic may help. Attention deficits can also be addressed directly in treatment sessions. One means of doing this is through the use of a rapid alternating question technique. Here, the clinician mixes up asking yes-no and information questions, as well as simple commands, as depicted in Table 18–4. To use this technique, the patient must be able to give short answers. To do this he or she must attend carefully to each stimulus.

Understanding Single Words

Certain Wernicke's patients do not attach meaning to single words. Some reflect distinct dissociations between spoken and written words (Franklin, 1989). There are two behavioral indicators of this problem. One is more difficulty identifying objects or pictures (e.g., knife) by name

than by function (Which one is for cutting meat?). A second is a monotone-like repetition of the word and a perceived "insensitivity" to its meaning or if the patient looks "perplexed." For example, patient CR when told "Point to your cheek," replied "Cheek, cheek, cheek (flat voice). There's no such thing as cheek." When single word insensitivity interferes with communication, the clinician may want to provide contextual support and increase redundancy. For the aforementioned example with patient CR, contextual support might involve presenting the sentence, "Children have rosy cheeks."

Perseveration

Perseveration involves repetition of a response after the stimulus has changed and that response is no longer appropriate. These responses may occur if a topic shift is not picked up (e.g., the patient continues to respond as though the conversation was about his family when work is the topic), or if the patient remains "stuck" processing the former stimulus when a new stimulus is presented. In the above example, RC understood the word "cheek" when provided contextual support, but for the next command "Show me your knee," pointed to his cheek and said "cheek." Wepman (1972) regarded perseveration as a byproduct of not giving the patient enough time to "integrate" and "consolidate" responses. He theorized that the mind functions similarly to a camera shutter. When the shutter is open, stimulation is possible. If the shutter is closed, new information cannot be processed and perseveration occurs. To aid the patient in integrating and consolidating responses, the clinician gives extra time and energy to that response. The following sequence provides an example:

> Clinician: "How many cheeks do you have?"
> Patient: "Two." Puff out your cheeks!
> Clinician: "Say the word cheek."
> Patient: "Cheek."
> Clinician: "Write the word cheek."
> Patient: (Writes word.)
> Clinician: "Do you put rouge on your cheeks?"
> Patient: "No, the wife."

The Treatment of Aphasic Perseveration program (TAP, Helm-Estabrooks et al., 1987) is another way to reduce perseveration. Rather than focus on correcting the patient's perseverative errors that occur in response to a new stimulus, TAP highlights that a new response is called for. Some mechanisms for accomplishing this are (1) to explain why the patient is in the TAP program for and to encourage him or her to ask for help; (2) to establish new stimulus sets before introducing new material; (3) and to "sensitize" the patient to perseverative errors. Sometimes this is done in a "dramatic fashion." For example, for patient RC (perseverating on cheek), the clinician could write the word "cheek" on a piece of paper, and then tear it in half and throw it in the wastebasket. This would shift his attention to a new stimulus.

Retention Problems

Aphasic patients have short-term memory limitations. These restrict comprehension of sentences, paragraphs, and conversation both in contextual situations (e.g., conversation), and when performing "off-line" tasks (e.g., repeating digits, following two-part commands). Not surprisingly, those who treat aphasia have an endless variety of workbooks and other materials to treat retention deficits. Most of these materials are noncontextual. Non-brain-damaged individuals use strategies to help them remember important information (e.g., phone numbers, ATM pin numbers, people's names). These strategies are applied in a context, and important information that aphasic people need to remember can be handled similarly. Table 18–4 provides examples of tasks that can be used to address retention problems in the context-based approach.

Retention Strategies. A retention strategy is something that "helps one remember to remember." These strategies are both behavioral and compensatory.

Asking for a Repetition. The patient can ask for assistance. He or she might be coached to say, "Hey, I did not get all of that," or "Could you run that by me again?" He or she could be encouraged to verify what was said by re-stating the "gist" of the message. A less obvious tactic for getting the partner to repeat might be to give him or her "a questioning look." This might be appropriate in certain social situations when directly asking one to repeat would be awkward.

Chunking. The patient could ask the partner to provide the information to be retained in small chunks. For example, a phone number might be presented as 975-40-22. Different ways of chunking information can be experimented in the treatment session to identify what works best with whom.

Rehearsal. The patient may benefit from using a rehearsal strategy. For example, he or she might repeat a telephone number three or four times to himself or herself before attempting to write the number on the note pad. When given directions such as: "Go two blocks north and turn left," he or she might again repeat the directions a time or two before getting back on the road.

Personalized Cuing. The use of personalized cues to aid later recall of information has been shown to be beneficial for patients with aphasia (Freed & Marshall, 1995; Starch et al., 1986). Personalized cuing involves linking the to-be-remembered piece of information (e.g., ATM pin number = 2946) with personally relevant cue (e.g., Year of the stock market crash = 29; year discharged from the Army = 46).

Memory Aids. One technological advance useful in compensating for retention problems is the message answering machine. The patient can play the message back several times before returning the call to make sure he or she has comprehended the message. Another might be to simply write down the message to be retained using a "post-it" or note pad or request that the speaker write down what he or she has instructed the patient to remember (e.g., grocery items, directions from the Dr.).

Increasing Complexity of Retention Tasks. The clinician has options for increasing the complexity of the retention tasks worked on in treatment. The most obvious is increasing the length of the message the patient needs to remember. Another is to have the patient wait for a brief period of time before responding. A third is to inject new material between the delivery of the message to be retained and the patient's response. Another may be to work on retention under conditions of competing noise (in a cafeteria), or under threat of interruption (a phone ringing). Treatment aimed at improving the patient's retention skills can also go hand in hand with treatment of syntactic deficits.

Treating Syntactic Comprehension Deficits

Information summarized earlier in the chapter stressed that certain syntactic constructions were more difficult for aphasic persons to comprehend than others. It appears that syntactic constructions that "surprise" the patient with their implausibility, reversibility, or complex wording are difficult to comprehend. While it is important to simplify the syntactic complexity of messages when talking to the Wernicke's patient, there are some treatment tasks that can be used to improve syntactic comprehension using personally relevant materials within the framework of the context-based approach. Specific examples include sentence verification, comprehension of yes-no questions of increasing difficulty, and the use of rapid alternating questions, presented earlier. Table 18–5 shows how these procedures can be used to work on syntactic comprehension problems in the context-based approach.

Sentence Verification. In sentence verification tasks, the patient sees a picture or hears a spoken message. He or she then verifies if the message is true of false. This activity can also be carried out using written stimuli. The clinician counts the number of correct responses and may also want to measure how long it takes the patient to make a decision. Table 18–5 provides an example of the procedure.

Yes-No Questions. Earlier in the chapter, the point was made that all yes-no questions are not equal. Some are easy to comprehend. Some are difficult because they require interpretation and reasoning. Syntactic comprehension can also be worked on using these types of questions, again within a personalized context. See Table 18–5 for an example.

TABLE 18–5

Context-Based Syntactic Processing Activities for Sentence Verification, Yes-No, and Rapid Alternating Question Tasks.

Sentence Verification

[A family portrait including the patient (John), his wife (Emma), his children (Bob, Peter, Emily, Karen, Heather), his parents (John Sr., Martha), and the family dog (Emerson)]

Clinician Activity	Correct Answer
Point to a girl older than Bob.	Points to Heather
Show me Martha's husband.	Points to John Sr.
Where is Emerson's mother?	"No way."
Who is Bob's little sister?	"Emily's one."
Who are you the son of?	"Her and him." (points to parents)
The two olders kids are. . .	"Bobby and Peter."

Yes-No

[Jerry, the patient, sells cars at a local dealership. The clinician has researched this topic carefully]

Do you sell clothes?	No
Are cars expensive to make?	Yes
Do customers sell cars to salesman?	No
Do you sell cars?	Yes
Do salesmen sell cars to customers?	Yes
Are automobiles cheap?	No

Alternating Questions

[Same portrait as sentence verification exercise. Clinician points to appropriate item when giving stimulus to verify]

Clinician Activity	Correct Answer
She is older than Bob.	No
This is Martha's husband.	Yes
He gets more attention than you do (dog).	Yes
This is Bob's little sister.	Yes
You are our son.	Yes
These two are oldest.	Yes

Information on which the Activity is Based on is Provided in Brackets.

Rapid Alternating Questions. The rapidly alternating questions procedure described earlier also lends itself to working on syntactic comprehension. See Table 18–5 for an example.

Discourse Comprehension

The patient with Wernicke's aphasia, like other brain-injured individuals, is limited in the neural resources he/she can devote to a language-processing task (Murray, 1999; McNeil et al., 1991). Hence, patients have problems "doing two things at once" (e.g., listening to a conversation if the television is playing). Background noise and competing noises may also have a negative influence on comprehension (LaPointe & Erickson, 1991). Improving discourse comprehension within the context-based approach will depend greatly on the patient's needs and severity level. Each patient brings to the clinic personal preferences in the form of social activity (e.g., understanding conversation at a party), passive listening needs (understanding lectures plays, movies, television programs), and interactive listening needs (following a conversation with the wife). Earlier, the importance of

making information within spoken narratives "salient" was emphasized. Some treatment strategies for doing this within the context-based approach and improving discourse comprehension follow

Withdraw. Patients comprehend better if they are rested. Taking a nap before an event where lots of listening is required or before the spouse comes home from work may aid comprehension. When auditory overload occurs, the patient may recover from the competitive listening situation by "taking a break." Some need counseling that it is permitted to "be prepared" to listen and that it is not "unmanly" to take some time off when rest helps.

Prestimulation. If the patient knows what to listen for, better comprehension may result. The patient can be "prestimulated" for attending a movie, play, or watching a television show by reading or being read a synopsis of the program beforehand. The partner might take a few moments to summarize what has gone on in the play or the movie during intermission. Similarly, the television can be muted during the commercial break and the partner can again summarize what has happened so far.

Supplementary Input. Having a closed caption option on the television may aid comprehension of news and other programs. Other forms of providing supplementary input may be used to ready the patient for a particular event. For example, patient BR was worried about how he would get along at a large family reunion. Since the last reunion, 5 years ago, BR had suffered his stroke. Supplementary information involved reviewing photographs from the prior reunion. BR talked about the people, their interests, and who was and was not still living. Essentially, he prepared to become an active listener and a participant in the reunion. The review and priming of BR with supplementary information also had some psychological value because he could discuss how he would deal with the subject of his stroke with the attendees.

Cooperative Group Treatment. Avent's (1997) cooperative group treatment provides an excellent strategy for facilitating discourse comprehension. Here, group members listen to a narrative and determine mutually what salient features of the narrative are important to remember in the retelling of the narrative. One person is selected as the recaller and the other group members act as facilitators. The recaller summarizes the narrative. The facilitators provide him or her cues and prompts to aid recall. The recaller provides feedback to the facilitators on the effectiveness of their coaching. In this situation, there are many opportunities to enhance discourse comprehension. For example, the patient can follow the story, underlining important phrases and words, or write these down—if able—as the narrative is told.

Treatment of Production Deficits in the Context-Based Approach

The Wernicke's patient is impaired on many metalinguistic tasks: naming, sentence production, repetition, sentence completion, and others. Face-to-face communication, however, involves much more than successful performance on these specific skills. Treatment to improve the aforementioned specific skills is covered in other sections of this text. In addition, the text contains a significant amount of information on treatment of naming problems using model-based and other methods. For the most part, these treatments focus on single words. Because the context-based approach is primarily interactive, and because single word treatments are presented in detail elsewhere, they will not be discussed here. Patient VL provides a starting point for talking about treatment of production deficits in Wernicke's aphasia using a context-based approach.

VL had severe Wernicke's aphasia. On the PICA, he could not name objects (knife), complete sentences (You cut meat with a___), or repeat. His overall PICA mean of 9.62 placed him "at the 41st percentile in a large random sample of left-hemisphere damaged adults. Nevertheless, VL and I could talk about anything. One day we had the following conversation:

> RCM: "How's it going?"
> VL: "Not so good these days."
> RCM: "What's the trouble?"
> VL: "Well we've got these—I can't say it, but I can show you."
> RCM: "OK."
> VL: "Well, it's this (points to his ear) and it's this (points to his head which is bald).
> RCM: "Something about your ear and your head?"
> VL: "The first part is right. It's this (again points to head) but I don't have any. If I wanted some, I could get some. You know. Then I wouldn't have this anymore. I'd put it on every day. Maybe a black one like you."
> RCM: "Your hair? You mean a wig?"
> VL: "That's it. They're all over the place. We had to have the pests in. (holds nose) What a deal?"
> RCM: "You have earwigs?"
> VL: "All over the place."

My direct attempts to get VL to produce the word "earwig" were fruitless, but after we had talked about his pest control problems, he produced a reasonable approximation of the word later in the session. It appears when patients with Wernicke's aphasia are "pinned down" to producing a single word, they often fail. The context-based approach provides the patient some flexibility in his responses rather than forcing a pre-selected response. Once the patient has produced a response in a context and that response has been integrated and consolidated, it may be possible to work directly on producing that response, be it a word or phrase.

Thought-Centered Therapy

Wepman's thought-centered approach serves as the foundation for the approach to word-finding problems stressed in this chapter (Martin, 1981b; Wepman, 1972). Wepman stressed that "speech should be the handmaiden of thought"—not visa versa. Treatment materials were contextual (e.g., topics of pre-stroke interests), and were introduced for the patient to respond to verbally. Like Martin's (1981a) approach to the treatment of jargonaphasia (a severe form of Wernicke's aphasia), thought-centered treatment does not focus on correcting the patient's verbal efforts, but on the clinician keeping communication "on track" by reflecting back the client's intended thoughts and paraphrasing when word-finding problems interfere. Wepman stressed using thought therapy with those he described as pragmatic aphasics, or "the talking aphasics." Clinicians who read accounts of thought-centered therapy, however, are apt to find it a bit "loose." And because some structure in treatment is needed, particularly in order to be able to account for what we do, we need to examine other approaches that fit within the context-based method.

PACE. *Promoting Aphasic Communicative Effectiveness* (PACE, Davis & Wilcox, 1985; Davis, 1980) was developed to make treatment situations more like natural communicative interactions. PACE stresses the use of new information, equal participation for both speaker and listener, freedom of communication channel selection (patient can gesture, write, draw, point, or speak), and the use of feedback based on communicative adequacy, not production accuracy. There are no reports of PACE treatment with Wernicke's aphasia specifically. However, PACE seems appropriate for these clients. These patients follow turn-taking rules in conversation (Ferguson, 1998; Scheinberg & Holland, 1980). While the patient with Wernicke's aphasia is highly verbal and may not use alternate modes of communication (Marshall et al., 1997), this is not always the case. Some patients use gestures to supplement their defective verbal output and communicate specific information (Ahlsen, 1991; Simmons & Zorthian, 1979). Drawing provides another option for some patients (Lyon & Helm-Estabrooks, 1987; Lyon & Sims, 1989). For example, CB, a severe Wernicke's aphasic, markedly increased the amount and the accuracy of his communications after drawing a floor plan of his house.

Basic PACE intervention involves clinician and client alternately describing pictures unknown to each other. Conventional PACE treatment has been found to improve the verbal expression of aphasic patients, but these studies have not been restricted to those with Wernicke's aphasia (Glindemann et al., 1991; Li et al., 1988; Springer et al., 1991). PACE need not be limited to the use of pictures, however. Pulvermuller and Roth (1991) offer extensions that are applicable to the context-based intervention approach. These stress different speech acts such as requesting, bargaining, and tasks demanding sequential actions (planning a vacation) that parallel those of actual communication situations. Picture description tasks, cartoon sequences, and conversations about famous people are other PACE adaptations that fit within a context-based approach (Carlomagno et al., 1991). Many of the suggestions offered by Harris in the use of reminiscence therapy as a language intervention (Harris, 1997) also can be adapted to a PACE format. For example, patients often respond robustly to queries about events such as buying their first car, where they met their wife, what they were doing when JFK was assassinated.

Game Therapy. Games provide an excellent resource for working on communication in a context. These might include "twenty one," poker, checkers, monopoly, and other similar games. McDonald and Pearce (1995) have described how the "dice" game can be used to assess pragmatic language skills in patients with closed-head injuries. With their appropriate pragmatic and turn-taking skills, patients with Wernicke's aphasia can work on communicating in a context using such games. An example was patient PN, a young man with resolving Wernicke's aphasia. He was a single parent and one of his immediate needs was to improve his use of numbers. PN was an avid "crap shooter." He was able to work on processing and production of numbers when allowed to show the clinician how to shoot craps.

Loose Training Methods. Loose training methods are another vehicle for working on communication in a context while still providing an amount of structure for the treatment session. Response Elaboration Training (RET, Kearns, 1986; Kearns & Scher, 1989; Kearns & Yedor, 1991) emphasizes the shaping and chaining of patient-initiated rather than clinician-selected responses. The goal of RET is to facilitate generalized improvement of the patient's ability to elaborate on conversational topics and share communicative burden. Table 18–6 shows how RET was used with a patient with Wernicke's aphasia in talking about a baseball game.

Partner Training. The patient will have many more communicative interactions with partners other than the clinician. Partners are co-workers. Throughout this chapter, family education and guidance through demonstration, modeling, and the use of constructive feedback has been stressed. Essentially, partners need to be as good at heightening comprehension and "keeping the conversation on track" with the Wernicke's patient as speech-language clinicians. Partner training, which can be carried out in a variety of ways, is the mechanism for doing this. For example, Simmons and colleagues (Simmons et al., 1987) used videotaped conversational samples between spouse and aphasic partner to train the spouse to minimize interruptive behaviors and to replace these with open-ended questions. Videotape instruction has also been used to teach comprehension-enhancing strategies (Linebaugh et al., 1984). Lyon and others (Lyon et al., 1997) use a "treatment triad" consisting of community volunteer, spouse, and aphasic patient. Phase one of the program establishes functional, reliable bonds and trust between the aphasic person and the partners and stresses the use of strategies to optimize effective exchange of information using a PACE-like format. In the second phase, the aphasic person plans and carries out activities of choice with the partner in naturalistic settings. These activities involve idiosyncratic wants and desires such as visiting a friend, getting a haircut, or planting flowers. The potential for working on communication in a context is obvious.

TABLE 18–6

Response Elaboration Training (RET) With a Fluent Aphasic Patient.

Step 1
Verbal Instruction and Stimulus Presentation

Clinician: "Tell me about this picture, as completely as you can."
Patient: "He took it right to that sucker. To the hole, to the hole."

Step 2
Elaboration, Model, Reinforce

Clinician: "Bill Walton dunks the ball over Kareem—Good."
Patient: No response

Step 3
"Wh Cue"

Clinician: "What is going on here?"
Patient: "Playing in the Western Conference finals. Wowie. Gonna beat the Lakers four straight. Wait and see."

Step 4
Combine Patient Responses, Model, Reinforce

Clinician: "Bill Walton dunks the ball over Kareem in the Western Conference finals against the Lakers—Great."
Patient: No response

Step 5
Request Repetition and Model

Clinician: "You try and say the whole thing. Bill Walton dunks the ball over Kareem in the Western Conference finals against the Lakers.
Patient: "Walton dunks on Kareem in the finals with the Lakers."

Step 6
Reinforce, Model

Clinician: "Good work. Bill Walton dunks the ball over Kareem in the Western Conference against the Lakers."

Group Treatment: Long-Term Support and Guidance.
As mentioned earlier, group treatment is re-surfacing as a method of providing treatment for patients with aphasia. Groups provide an excellent method of addressing the long-term consequences of Wernicke's aphasia and for continuing to work on communication in a context as long as the patient feels he or she can benefit from attendance. Recently, several books have been written on this subject (Avent, 1997; Elman, 1998; Marshall, 1998a). The chapter by Kearns and Elman in this text provides a comprehensive review of group treatment. I mention two programs here as examples of how group treatment might be used with patients with Wernicke's aphasia. The first is a recreationally focused therapy which seems most applicable to patients with severe Wernicke's aphasia (Fox, 1990). Here, the goal is to expand clients' recreational options and to increase their participation in recreational pursuits formerly enjoyed, but abandoned since the stroke. Group members (1) select an activity (e.g., bowling); (2) plan the activity; (3) identify barriers that need to be overcome to do the activity; (4) assign suitable roles for performing the activity (e.g., finding out the cost of going bowling); and (5) perform the activity. Subsequent treatment sessions are used to discuss the activity and determine what went well, poorly, and how to improve participation in the future.

Marshall's problem-focused approach offers a method for providing long-term support and guidance to less severe Wernicke's patients, particularly those who have evolved to an anomic stage (Marshall, 1993, 1998). The group focuses on solving problems that come up in their lives. Group interactions emphasize solutions and alternatives for handling specific problems. For example, patient RA was distraught because he needed extra time to disassemble and re-assemble his furnace. It was a task he had always done quickly and without difficulty. The group brainstormed solutions. RA learned that he might improve his performance by being more organized. Another client, CM, was overwhelmed with credit card offers. Unable to read the "fine print" she overextended herself to where her income did not cover the interest payments. Group discussions prompted her to (1) seek individual treatment to learn how interest works; (2) to seek consumer credit counseling to develop a plan to regain financial solvency; and (3) to tear up her credit cards.

FUTURE TRENDS

Holland (1995) suggests that the crystal ball is "cloudy" for specialists in neurogenic language disorders. There is a degree of anxiety as the profession seeks to cope with and adjust to changes in health care delivery. These changes will potentially affect patient care, student training, and professional autonomy. One change on the horizon is that clinicians will need to be more innovative in delivering treatment. Communication opportunities for the patient will need to be expanded beyond the confines of the therapy room. Paramount among these efforts to expand services to include the environment are partner training, group treatment options, and support groups for both patients and families. Another service delivery trend for the future is to provide better education about stroke and its consequences, where to go for services, and what to expect from providers. Organizations such as the National Aphasia Association, American Heart Association, and the Academy of Neurological Communication Disorders and Sciences are taking the lead in this regard.

Student training and exposure to difficult clients like those with Wernicke's aphasia warrants scrutiny. Few students know how to talk to any patient with aphasia, let alone a patient with a problem as complex as Wernicke's aphasia. Student training in settings outside of the university is becoming scarce as clinicians adjust to health care changes. Quantity and quality of student training, however, is vital to the profession's survival and sacrifices will need to be made.

Ultimately, aphasia treatment's future will be decided by its consumers: the patient and the family, the payer (insurance companies and Medicare), and by peers (physicians who refer patients for evaluation and treatment). All seek answers to the same question. What does speech and language treatment do to improve the patient's day-to-day functioning and quality of life? Since communication occurs in a context, it is how the patient with Wernicke's aphasia gets along in life's contextual situations that treatment efficiency will be judged. One certain trend of the future will be that of putting more importance on outcome measurement systems that document treatment's effects in day-to-day activities.

Most aphasic persons want one thing more than any other: to be able to do the things that nonaphasic people do. If improving naming accuracy or sentence production does this, well and good. However, communication-focused treatments delivered in a context will receive much attention from clinical aphasiologists in the future. There are plenty of signals that this movement is already under way.

I am optimistic that the "meat axe" approach to curbing health care costs will be abandoned and the pendulum of change will swing back to midline. Wernicke's patients like PN have convinced me that treatment helps. When asked how he felt treatment had helped, PN said:

"When I had a stroke, I though everything would be as it was before. When I found out that I was going to have problems I was afraid. I was afraid I couldn't pay my bills or write checks. Because I didn't talk so good, I was afraid they would take my house. I was afraid I would lose my son. I still don't talk as good. I have a lot of work to do. But after being in therapy, I'm not afraid anymore." PN was fortunate to have received both individual and group treatment.

Wernicke's aphasia that evolved to a later-stage anomic deficit was addressed by helping him do what was needed to be an effective single parent: drive, pay bills, communicate with his son, talk to his physician, and deal with his former wife's lawyer. Improved communication in these contexts enabled PN to work on specific deficits such as repetition and word retrieval later on his own using home programs and the computer. Ultimately, he decided when he had had enough treatment. It happened when PN started to think less about being aphasic and more about participating in life. Bringing about this attitudinal change in aphasic persons may be the most important trend for the future and the consummate challenge for all who treat aphasic people, regardless of type or severity.

References

Ahlsen, E. (1991). Body communication as compensation for speech in a Wernicke's aphasic—a longitudinal study. *Journal of Communication Disorders, 24,* 1–12.

Aten, J., Caliguiri, M., & Holland, A.L. (1982). The efficacy of functional communication therapy for chronic aphasic patients. *Journal of Speech and Hearing Disorders, 47,* 93–96.

Avent, J. (1997). *Manual of cooperative group treatment for aphasia.* Boston: Butterworth-Heinemann.

Bachman, D.L. & Albert, M. (1990). Auditory comprehension in aphasia. In H. Goodglass (ed.), *Handbook of neuropsychology* (pp. 281–306). New York: Elsevier.

Benson, D.F. (1967). Fluency in aphasia: Correlation with radioactive scan localization. *Cortex, 1,* 373–392.

Blomert, L. (1990). What functional assessment can contribute to setting goals in aphasia therapy. *Aphasiology, 4,* 307–320.

Bollinger, R., Musson, N., & Holland, A.L. (1993). A study of group communication intervention with chronically aphasic persons. *Aphasiology, 7,* 301–313.

Brookshire, R.H. (1974). Differences in responding to auditory-verbal materials among aphasic patients. *Acta Symbolica, 1,* 1–18.

Brookshire, R.H. (1997). *Introduction to neurogenic communication disorders* (5th ed.). St Louis: Mosby.

Brookshire, R.H. (1992). *Introduction to neurogenic communication disorders* (4th ed.). St Louis: Mosby Yearbook.

Brookshire, R.H. & Nicholas, L.E. (1982). Comprehension of directly and indirectly pictured verbs by aphasic and nonaphasic listeners. In R.H. Brookshire (ed.), *Clinical aphasiology conference proceedings* (pp. 200–206). Minneapolis, MN: BRK.

Brookshire, R.H. & Nicholas, L.E. (1984). Comprehension of directly and indirectly stated main ideas and details in the discourse of brain-damaged and non-brain-damaged listeners. *Brain and Language, 21,* 21–36.

Brookshire, R.H. & Nicholas, L.E. (1993). *The Discourse Comprehension Test,* Minneapolis, MN: BRK.

Busch, C. & Brookshire, R.H. (1982). Aphasic adults' comprehension of yes-no questions. Unpublished manuscript.

Campbell, T.F. & McNeil, M.R. (1983). Effects of presentation rate and divided attention on auditory comprehension in acquired childhood aphasia. Abstract. In R.H. Brookshire (ed.),

Clinical aphasiology conference proceedings (pp. 193–194). Minneapolis, MN: BRK.

Caramazza, A., Zurif, E.B., & Gardner, H. (1978). Sentence memory in aphasia. *Neuropsychologia, 16*, 661–669.

Carlomagno, S., Losanno, N., Emanuelli, S., & Casadio, P. (1991). Expressive language recovery or improved communication skills: Effects of PACE therapy on aphasics' referential communication and story telling. *Aphasiology, 5*, 419–424.

Cermak, L. & Moreines, J. (1976). Verbal retention deficits in aphasic and amnesic patients. *Brain and Language, 3*, 16–27.

Czvik, P. (1977). Assessment of family attitudes towards aphasic patients with severe auditory processing disorders. In R.H. Brookshire (ed.), *Clinical aphasiology conference proceedings* (pp. 160–164). Minneapolis, MN: BRK.

Darley, F.L. (1976). Maximizing input to the aphasic patient. In R.H. Brookshire (ed.), *Clinical aphasiology conference proceedings* (pp. 1–21). Minneapolis, MN: BRK.

Darley, F.L. (1982). *Aphasia*. Philadelphia: WB Saunders.

Davis, A.G. (1980). A critical look at PACE therapy. In R.H. Brookshire (ed.), *Clinical aphasiology conference proceedings* (pp. 248–257). Minneapolis, MN: BRK.

Davis, A.G. & Wilcox, M.J. (1985). *Adult aphasia: Applied pragmatics*. San Diego, CA: College Hill Press.

Deloche, G. & Seron, X. (1981). Sentence understanding and knowledge of the world: Evidences for a sentence-picture matching task performed by aphasic patients. *Brain and Language, 14*, 57–69.

Elman, R.J. (1998). *Group treatment of neurogenic communication disorders: The expert clinician's approach*. Boston: Butterworth-Heinemann.

Elman, R. & Burnstein-Ellis, E. (1995). What is functional? *American Journal of Speech-Language Pathology, 4*, 115–117.

Elman, R. & Burnstein-Ellis, E. (1999). The efficacy of group communication treatment in adults with chronic aphasia. *Journal of Speech, Language, and Hearing Research, 42*, 411–419.

Fehst, C.A. & Brookshire, R.H. (1980). Aphasic subjects' use of within-sentence pause time in a sentence comprehension task. Abstract. In R.H. Brookshire (ed.), *Clinical aphasiology conference proceedings* (pp. 66–67). Minneapolis, MN: BRK.

Ferguson, A. (1998). Conversational turn-taking and repair in fluent aphasia. *Aphasiology, 12*, 1007–1031.

Fox, L. (1990). Recreation focused treatment for generalization of language skills in aphasic patients. Paper presented at American Speech-Language-Hearing Association, Seattle, WA. (November).

Franklin, S. (1989). Disassociations in auditory word comprehension: Evidence from nine fluent aphasic patients. *Aphasiology, 3*, 189–208.

Frattali, C., Thompson, C., Holland, A., Wohl, C., & Ferketic, M. (1995). *Functional assessment of communication skills for adults*. Rockville, MD: American Speech-Language-Hearing Association.

Freed, D.B. & Marshall, R.C. (1995). The effects of personalized cueing on the long term naming of realistic visual stimuli. *American Journal of Speech-Language Pathology, 4*(4), 105–108.

Gardner, H., Albert, M.L., & Weintraub, S. (1975). Comprehending a word: The influence of speed and redundancy on auditory comprehension in aphasia. *Cortex, 11*, 155–162.

Glindemann, R., Willmes, K., Huber, W., & Springer, L. (1991). The efficacy of modeling in PACE-therapy. *Aphasiology, 5*, 425–429.

Goodglass, H. (1973). Studies on the grammar of aphasics. In H. Goodglass & S. Blumstein (eds.), *Psycholinguistics and Aphasia* (pp. 183–215). Baltimore: Johns Hopkins Press.

Goodglass, H. (1981). The syndromes of aphasia: Similarities and differences in neurolinguistic features. *Topics in Language Disorders, 1*:1–12.

Goodglass, H. & Baker, E. (1976). Semantic field naming, and auditory comprehension in aphasia. *Brain and Language, 3*, 339–374.

Goodglass, H. & Kaplan, E. (1983). *The assessment of aphasia and related disorders* (2nd ed.). Philadelphia: Lea & Febiger.

Gravel, J. & LaPointe, L.L. (1983). Length and redundancy in health care providers' speech during interactions with aphasic and nonaphasic listeners. In R.H. Brookshire (ed.), *Clinical aphasiology conference proceedings* (pp. 211–217). Minneapolis, MN: BRK.

Gray, L., Hoyt, P., Mogil, S., & Lefkowitz, N. (1977). A comparison of clinical tests of yes/no questions in aphasia. In R.H. Brookshire (ed.), *Clinical aphasiology conference proceedings* (pp. 265–268). Minneapolis, MN: BRK.

Green, G. (1984). Communication in aphasia therapy: Some of the procedures and issues involved. *British Journal of Disorders of Communication, 19*, 35–46.

Halliday, M. & Hasan, R. (1976). *Cohesion in English*. New York: Longman.

Harris, J.L. (1997). Reminiscence: A culturally and developmentally appropriate language intervention for older adults. *American Journal of Speech-Language Pathology, 6*, 19–26.

Helm-Estabrooks, N, Emery, P., & Albert, M. (1987). Treatment of aphasic perseveration (TAP) program. *Archives of Neurology, 44*, 1253–1255.

Henderson, A., Goldman-Eisler, F., & Skarbek, A. (1966). Sequential temporal patterns in spontaneous speech. *Language and Speech, 9*, 207–216.

Holland, A.L. (1995). A look into a cloudy crystal ball for specialists in neurogenic language disorders. *American Journal of Speech-Language Pathology, 3*, 34–36.

Holland, A.L. (1980). *Communicative Activities of Daily Living*. Baltimore, MD: University Park Press.

Holland, A.L. (1983) Remarks on observing aphasic people. In R.H. Brookshire (ed.), *Clinical aphasiology conference proceedings* (pp. 345–349). Minneapolis, MN: BRK.

Holland, A.L. (1982). Observing functional communication in aphasic adults. *Journal of Speech and Hearing Research, 47*, 50–56.

Katsuki-Nakamura, J., Brookshire, R.H., & Nicholas, L.E. (1988). Comprehension of monologues and dialogues by aphasic listeners. *Journal of Speech and Hearing Research, 53*, 408–415.

Kearns, K.P. (1986). Systematic programming of verbal elaboration skills in chronic Broca's aphasia. In R.C. Marshall (ed.), *Case studies in aphasia rehabilitation* (pp. 225–244). Austin, TX: Pro-Ed.

Kearns, K.P. & Scher, G.P. (1989). The generalization of response elaboration training effects. *Clinical Aphasiology, 18*, 223–242.

Kearns, K.P. & Yedor, K. (1991). Alternating treatments comparison of loose training and a convergent treatment strategy. *Clinical Aphasiology, 20*, 223–238.

Kertesz, A. (1979). *Aphasia and associated disorders*. New York: Grune & Stratton.

Kertesz, A. (1984). Neurobiological aspects of recovery from aphasia in stroke. *International Rehabilitative Medicine, 6*, 122–127.

Kertesz, A. & McCabe, P. (1977). Recovery patterns and recovery in aphasia. *Brain, 100*, 1–18.

Kimelman, M.Z. & McNeil, M.R. (1987). An investigation of emphatic stress comprehension in aphasia: A replication. *Journal of Speech and Hearing Research, 30*, 295–300.

Kudo, T. (1984). The effect of semantic plausibility on sentence comprehension in aphasia. *Brain and Language, 21*, 208–218.

LaPointe, L.L. & Erickson, R.J. (1991). Auditory vigilance during divided task attention in aphasia. *Aphasiology, 5*, 511–520.

Lasky, E.Z., Weidner, W.E., & Johnson, J.P. (1976). Influence of linguistic complexity, rate of presentation, and interphrase pause time on auditory-verbal comprehension of adult aphasic patients. *Brain and Language, 3*, 386–395.

Li, E.C., Kitselman, K., Dusatko, D., & Spinelli, C. (1988). The efficacy of PACE in the remediation of naming deficits. *Journal of Communication Disorders, 21*, 491–503.

Linebaugh, C., Margulies, C.P., & Mackisack-Morin, L.E. (1984). The effectiveness of comprehension-enhancing strategies employed by spouses of aphasic patients. In R.H. Brookshire (ed.), *Clinical aphasiology conference proceedings* (pp. 188–197). Minneapolis, MN: BRK.

Loverso, F.L. & Prescott, T.E. (1981). The effects of alerting signals on left brain damaged (aphasic) and normal subjects' accuracy and response time to visual stimuli. In R.H. Brookshire (ed.), *Clinical aphasiology conference proceedings* (pp. 55–67). Minneapolis, MN: BRK.

Lyon, J. (1998). *Coping with aphasia*. San Diego, CA: Singular.

Lyon, J.G., Cariski, D., Keisler, L., Rosenbek, J., Levine, R., Kumpula, J., Ryff, C., Coyne, S., & Blanc, M. (1997). Communication partners: Enhancing participation in life and communication for adults with aphasia in natural language settings. *Aphasiology, 11*, 693–708.

Lyon, J.G. & Helm-Estabrooks, N. (1987). Drawing: Its communicative significance for expressively restricted aphasic adults. *Topics in Language Disorders, 8*, 61–71.

Lyon, J. & Sims, E. (1989). Drawing: Its use as a communicative aid with aphasic and normal adults. *Clinical Aphasiology, 18*, 339–351.

Marshall, R.C. (1978). *Clinician controlled auditory stimulation for aphasic adults*. Tigard, OR: CC Publications.

Marshall, R.C. (1981). Heightening auditory comprehension for aphasic patients. In R. Chapey (ed.), *Language intervention strategies in adult aphasia* (pp. 297–324). Baltimore: Williams & Wilkins.

Marshall, R.C. (1982). Management of Wernicke's aphasia. *AAO Exchange, 2*, 3–7.

Marshall, R.C. (1983). Communication styles of fluent aphasic clients. In H. Winitz (ed.), *Treating language disorders* (pp. 163–180). Baltimore: University Park Press.

Marshall, R.C. (1986). Treatment of auditory comprehension deficits. In R. Chapey (ed.), *Language intervention strategies in adult aphasia* (2nd ed.). (pp. 370–393). Baltimore: Williams & Wilkins.

Marshall, R.C. (1987a). The fluent aphasias: Strategies for management. Short Course presented at the annual convention of the American Speech-Language-Hearing Association, New Orleans (November).

Marshall, R.C. (1987b). Management of fluent aphasias: Evaluation, treatment, counseling. Purdue University Interactive Television Series. West Layfayette, IN (April).

Marshall, R.C. (1993). Problem-focused group treatment for clients with mild aphasia. *American Journal of Speech-Language Pathology, 2*, 31–37.

Marshall, R.C. (1998). A problem focused group program for clients with mild aphasia. In R. Elman (ed.), *Group treatment of neruogenic communication disorders: The expert clinician's approach* (pp. 57–66). Boston: Butterworth-Heinemann.

Marshall, R.C. (1994). Management of fluent aphasic clients. In R. Chapey (ed.), *Language intervention strategies for adult aphasia* (pp. 390–406). Baltimore: Williams & Wilkins.

Marshall, R.C. (1998). *Introduction to group treatment for aphasia: Design and management*. Boston: Butterworth-Heinemann.

Marshall, R.C. (2000). Speech fluency and aphasia. In H. Riggenbach (ed.), *Perspectives on fluency*. Ann Arbor, MI: University of Michigan Press.

Marshall, R.C. & Brown, L.J. (1974). The effects of semantic relatedness upon the verbal retention of aphasic adults. In B. Porch (ed.), *Clinical aphasiology conference proceedings* (pp. 3–13).

Marshall, R.C., Freed, D.B., & Phillips, D.S. (1997). Communicative efficiency in severe aphasia. *Aphasiology, 11*, 373–384.

Marshall, R.C., Neuburger, S.I., & Phillips, D.S. (1991). Sentence comprehension and repetition in conduction aphasia. *Clinical Aphasiology, 19*, 151–162.

Marshall, R.C. & Thistlethwaite, N. (1977). Verbal and nonverbal alerters: Effects on auditory comprehension of aphasic subjects Unpublished manuscript.

Marshall, R.C., Rappaport, B.Z., & Garcia-Bunuel, L. (1985). Self-monitoring behavior in a case of severe auditory agnosia with aphasia. *Brain and Language, 24*, 297–313.

Marshall, R.C. & Tompkins, C.A. (1982). Verbal self-correction behaviors of fluent and nonfluent aphasic subjects. *Brain and Language, 15*, 292–306.

Martin, A.D. (1981a). Therapy with the jargonaphasic. In J. Brown (ed.), *Jargonaphasia* (pp. 305–326). New York: Academic Press.

Martin A.D. (1981b). An examination of Wepman's thought centered therapy. In R. Chapey (ed.), *Language intervention strategies in adult aphasia* (pp. 141–154). Baltimore, MD: Williams & Wilkins.

McDonald, S. & Pearce, S. (1995). The 'dice' game: A new test of pragmatic language skills after closed head injury. *Brain Injury, 9*, 255–271.

McNeil, M., O'Dell, K., & Tseng, C. (1991). Toward the integration of resource allocation into a general theory of aphasia. *Clinical Aphasiology, 20*, 21–40.

Meyers, P. & Linebaugh, C. (1981). Comprehension of idiomatic expressions by right-hemisphere damaged adults. In R.H. Brookshire (ed.), *Clinical aphasiology conference proceedings* (pp. 254–261). Minneapolis, MN: BRK.

Murray, L.I. (1999). Attention and aphasia: Theory, research, and clinical implications. *Aphasiology, 13*, 91–112.

Nicholas, L.E. & Brookshire, R.H. (1981). Effects of pictures and picturability on sentence verification by aphasic and nonaphasic subjects. *Journal of Speech and Hearing Research, 24*, 292–298.

Nicholas, L.E. & Brookshire, R.H. (1995). Comprehension of spoken narrative discourse by adults with aphasia, right hemisphere brain damage, or traumatic brain injury. *American Journal of Speech-Language Pathology, 4*, 69–81.

Pashek, G.V. & Brookshire, R.H. (1982). Effects of rate of speech and linguistic stress on auditory paragraph comprehension of aphasic individuals. *Journal of Speech and Hearing Research, 25*, 377–383.

Pashek, G. & Holland, A.L. (1988). Evolution of aphasia in the first year post-onset. *Cortex, 24*, 411–423.

Pierce, R.S. (1981). Facilitating the comprehension of tense related sentences in aphasia. *Journal of Speech and Hearing Research, 24*, 364–368.

Pierce, R.S. (1982). Facilitating the comprehension of syntax in aphasia. *Journal of Speech and Hearing Research, 25*, 408–413.

Porch, B.E. (1967). *Porch Index of Communicative Ability.* Palo Alto, CA: Consulting Psychologists.

Pulvermuller, F. & Roth, V.M. (1991). Communicative aphasia treatment as a further development of PACE therapy. *Aphasiology, 5*, 39–50.

Rosenbek, J.C., LaPointe, L.L., & Wertz, R.T. (1989). *Aphasia: A clinical approach.* Boston: Little, Brown.

Salvatore, A. (1979). Clinical treatment of auditory comprehension deficits in acute and chronic aphasic adults: An experimental analysis of within-message pause duration. In R.H. Brookshire (ed.), *Clinical aphasiology conference proceedings* (pp. 203–212). Minneapolis, MN: BRK.

Salvatore, A., Strait, M., & Brookshire, R.H. (1975). Effects of patient characteristics on the delivery of Token Test commands by experienced and inexperienced examiners. In R.H. Brookshire (ed.), *Clinical aphasiology conference proceedings* (pp. 103–112). Minneapolis, MN: BRK.

Schienberg, S. & Holland, A. (1980). Conversational turn-taking in Wernicke's aphasia. In R.H. Brookshire (ed.), *Clinical aphasiology conference proceedings* (pp. 106–110). Minneapolis, MN: BRK.

Schuell, H. & Jenkins, J.J. (1961). Reduction of vocabulary in aphasia. *Brain, 84*, 243–261.

Schuell, H., Jenkins, J.J., & Jiminez-Pabon, E. (1965). *Aphasia in adults: Diagnosis, prognosis, and treatment.* New York: Harper & Row.

Simmons, N.N., Kearns, K.P., & Potechin, G. (1987). Treatment of aphasia through family member training. In R.H. Brookshire (ed.), *Clinical aphasiology conference proceedings* (pp. 106–116). Minneapolis, MN: BRK.

Simmons, N. & Zorthian A. (1979). Use of symbolic gestures in a case of fluent aphasia. In R.H. Brookshire (ed.), *Clinical aphasiology conference proceedings* (pp. 278–285). Minneapolis, MN: BRK.

Skelly, M. (1975). Aphasic patients talk back. *American Journal of Nursing, 75*, 1140–1142.

Sparks, R. (1978). Parastandardized examination guidelines for adult aphasia. *British Journal of Disorders of Communication, 13*, 135–146.

Springer, L., Glendemann, R., Huber, W., & Willmes, K. (1991). How efficacious is PACE-therapy when 'Language Systematic Training' is incorporated? *Aphasiology, 5*, 391–399.

Stachowiak, F.J., Huber, W., Poeck, K., & Kerchensteiner, W.

(1977). Text comprehension in aphasia. *Brain and Language, 4*, 177–195.

Starch, S.A., Marshall, R.C., & Neuburger, S.I. (1986). Who's on first? A treatment approach for name recall with aphasics. In R.H. Brookshire (ed.), *Clinical aphasiology conference proceedings* (p. 73). Minneapolis, MN: BRK.

Sullivan, M.P., Fisher, B., & Marshall, R.C. (1986). Treating the repetition deficit in conduction aphasia. In R. Brookshire (ed.), *Clinical aphasiology conference proceedings* (pp. 172–180). Minneapolis, MN: BRK.

Swindell, C., Pashek, G., & Holland, A. (1982). A questionnaire for surveying persons and communicative style. In R.H. Brookshire (ed.), *Clinical aphasiology conference proceedings* (pp. 50–63). Minneapolis, MN: BRK.

Swinney, D., Zurif, E.B., & Cutler, A. (1980). Effects of sentential stress and word class upon comprehension in Broca's aphasics. *Brain and Language, 10*, 132–144.

Toppin, C.J. & Brookshire, R.H. (1978). Effects of response delay and token relocation on Token Test performance of aphasic subjects. *Journal of Communication Disorders, 11*, 65–78.

Van Lancker, D. & Klein, K. (1990). Preserved recognition of familiar personal names in global aphasia. *Brain and Language, 39*, 511–529.

Van Lancker, D. & Nicklay, C.K. (1992). Comprehension of personally relevant (PERL) versus novel language in two globally aphasic patients. *Aphasiology, 6*, 37–62.

Wallace, G.J. & Canter, G. (1985). Effects of personally relevant language materials on the performance of severely aphasic individuals. *Journal of Speech and Hearing Disorders, 50*, 385–390.

Wegner, M.L., Brookshire, R.H., & Nicholas, L.E. (1984). Comprehension of main ideas and details in coherent and noncoherent discourse by aphasic and nonaphasic listeners. *Brain and Language, 21*, 37–51.

Weidner, W.E. & Lasky, E.Z. (1976). The interaction of rate and complexity of stimulus on the performance of adult aphasic subjects. *Brain and Language, 3*, 34–40.

Wepman, J.M. (1972). Aphasia therapy: A new look. *Journal of Speech and Hearing Disorders, 37*, 203–214.

Wertz, R.T. (1986). Response to treatment: A case of chronic aphasia. In R.C. Marshall (ed.), *Case studies in aphasia rehabilitation* (pp. 59–73). Austin, TX: Pro-Ed.

Wertz, R.T., Collins, M.J., Weiss, D., Kurtzke, J.F., Friden, T., Brookshire, R.H., Pierce, J., Holtzapple, P., Hubbard, D.J., Porch, B.E., West, J.A., Davis, L., Matovich, V., Morley, G.K., & Resurreccion, E. (1981). Veterans Administration Cooperative Study on Aphasia: A comparison of individual and group treatment. *Journal of Speech and Hearing Research, 21*, 580–594.

West, J.F. & Kaufman, M. (1972). Some effects of redundancy on the auditory comprehension of adult aphasics. Paper presented at the annual convention of the American Speech-Language-Hearing Association, San Francisco (November).

Wilcox, M.J., Davis, A.G., & Leonard, L.B. (1978). Aphasics' comprehension of contextually conveyed meaning. *Brain and Language, 3*, 362–377.

Yorkston, K.M., Marshall, R.C., & Butler, M. (1977). Imposed delay of response: Effects on aphasics' auditory comprehension of visually and non-visually cued material. *Perceptual and Motor Skills, 44*, 647–655.

Chapter 19

Rehabilitation of Subcortical Aphasia

Stephen E. Nadeau and
Leslie J. Gonzalez Rothi

OBJECTIVES

The objectives of this chapter are to elucidate features and mechanisms of thalamic and nonthalamic subcortical aphasias; to analyze these aphasias in terms of the impairment they reflect in the neural networks supporting language function; to analyze these networks from the perspective of parallel distributed processing models of neural function in order to define the implications of network dysfunction for rehabilitation strategy and outcome; and to review behavioral consequences of subcortical lesions associated with aphasia that may seriously interfere with the rehabilitation process.

INTRODUCTION

Subcortical aphasia is defined as a language disorder associated with damage to subcortical brain structures such as the basal ganglia, the thalamus, or white matter pathways in the general vicinity of these structures. Usually it is caused by ischemic strokes, less often by intracerebral hemorrhages. When these disorders were first described, it was assumed that the aphasia was a direct consequence of the damage to subcortical structures that was revealed by structural imaging studies, such as computed tomographic (CT) scans and magnetic resonance images (MRI). Further research has shown this assumption to be substantially incorrect (see Nadeau & Crosson, 1997, for a more extensive analysis). Aphasia is actually an indirect consequence of subcortical lesions. In the case of subcortical aphasias stemming from thalamic lesions, the language disorders appear to result from the impact of thalamic dysfunction on cerebral cortical function (i.e., a neural systems disorder). In the case of subcortical aphasias stemming from lesions outside the thalamus, the language disorders reflect either the invisible cortical damage associated with the vascular event that caused the visible subcortical

lesion (i.e., a pathological correlate), or they reflect the impact of the subcortical lesion on pathways between the thalamus and language cortex (i.e., a neural systems disorder similar to that in thalamic aphasia).

We will begin this chapter by enlarging on the neural mechanism of thalamic aphasias and the pathogenesis of nonthalamic subcortical aphasias. In the course of this, we will also review the linguistic features of these disorders with a particular emphasis on the dysfunction of underlying neural systems that they reflect. We know of no adequately controlled scientific studies of the efficacy of therapy for subcortical aphasias. Therefore, we will proceed on the assumption that for therapy to be effective, it must be specific to the impaired systems. We will seek to understand the nature of the neural system impairment in these aphasias from the perspective of parallel distributed processing (PDP) (also known as connectionist) models of neural network function. As we hope to show, a PDP conceptualization has some very specific implications for the types of therapeutic approaches likely to be effective under various circumstances. We will conclude with a consideration of nonlinguistic behavioral disorders that are frequently present in patients with subcortical aphasia, and which may have a major impact on prognosis.

THALAMIC APHASIAS

The thalamus is located at the very center of the cerebrum at its junction with the midbrain (Figure 19–1). Although its function is by no means simple, it is far simpler and far better understood than that of any other cerebral structure. In essence, it functions as a *relay device*. Specific groups of neurons within the thalamus (nuclei) relay sensory information from more peripheral neural waystations to the cerebral cortex. For example, visual information is transmitted from the retinas via a specific thalamic nucleus, the lateral geniculate body (LGB), to the primary visual cortex (calcarine cortex) in the occipital lobes. Auditory information is relayed through a chain of nuclei within the brainstem to another thalamic nucleus, the medial geniculate body, from whence it is transmitted to primary auditory cortex (Heschl's gyrus) on the dorsal surface of the temporal lobe deep within the Sylvian or lateral fissure of the brain. Somatosensory information is relayed by

457

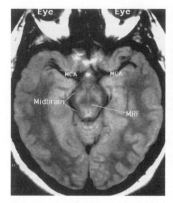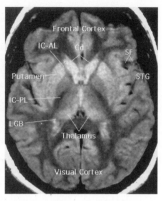

Figure 19–1. Major cerebral structures and landmarks relevant to the problem of subcortical aphasia: midbrain reticular formation (MRF), middle cerebral artery (MCA), head of the caudate nucleus (Cd), anterior limb of internal capsule (IC-AL), posterior limb of internal capsule (IC-PL), lateral geniculate body (LGB), Sylvian fissure (SF), superior temporal gyrus (STG). The image on the left is 2 cm below the image on the right. Heschl's gyrus lies on the medial aspect of the superior temporal gyrus. Wernicke's area is located somewhat more posteriorly on the dominant superior temporal gyrus; because the brain is sliced obliquely in this MRI (as in most), it is visible only on the next higher slice.

two major pathways within the spinal cord and brainstem to two specific thalamic nuclei, ventral posteromedial (subserving the face), and ventral posterolateral (subserving the body), from which it is then relayed to the somatosensory cortex on the surface of the cerebral hemispheres. Thus, these three pairs of nuclei relay information derived from sensory organs outside the brain to the cerebral cortex. The remainder of the thalamic nuclei relay information from one part of the brain to another. For example, neural transmission from motor areas of the cerebrum to the cerebellum and the basal ganglia is relayed back to separate portions of the ventrolateral nucleus of the thalamus, thence back to motor areas of the cortex. For all of these nuclei, as indeed for every nuclear group in the thalamus, the cortical connections are two way; that is, the projections from the cortex back to the thalamus are just as extensive as the projections from the thalamus to the cortex.

Of particular interest with respect to language and language-related processes are two other nuclear groups: the dorsomedial nucleus and the pulvinar-lateral posterior (LP) complex. They resemble the ventrolateral nucleus in that they relay information originally derived from cerebral cortex back to the cerebral cortex. However, the dorsomedial nucleus relays information from the prefrontal cortex (those portions of the frontal lobes implicated in executive functions and goal-oriented behavior), as well as several subcortical structures, back to the prefrontal cortex. The pulvinar/LP complex relays projections from the frontal, temporal, and parietal cortices (including those portions of the dominant

hemisphere directly implicated in language function) back to these same cortices. As we shall see below, there appears to be a logical relationship between dysfunction in these two nuclear groups and particular features of thalamic aphasias.

At this point, we must add a complicating feature to our original, oversimplistic conceptualization of the thalamus as a relay device: the thalamus is actually a regulated or *gated relay device*. This gating feature helps to address two questions. First, alert readers of the foregoing discussion will undoubtedly have asked what could conceivably be the purpose of long connections descending from, for example, the temporoparietal cortex to the pulvinar/LP complex, only to be sent right back to the very same cortex. The answer appears to be that the purpose for passing cortical information through the thalamus is to subject that information (and by implication, the originating cortex) to the regulatory mechanism provided by the thalamic gate. Second, it turns out that strokes involving either the dorsomedial nucleus or the pulvinar/LP complex (the thalamic regions most directly linked to language cortex) are extremely rare. Thus, if we are going to explain thalamic aphasia in terms of dysfunction of these two regions, we must look for another cause of dysfunction than direct damage. It appears that thalamic strokes producing aphasia, even though they almost invariably spare these nuclear groups, nevertheless damage key aspects of the thalamic gating mechanism. At this point we must address four questions: (1) how does the thalamic gating mechanism work? (2) how do strokes impair its function? (3) what purpose could such a gating mechanism serve? and (4) what is likely to be the specific impact of disorders of the gating mechanism on the function of overlying cortex, most specifically, language cortex? The neuroscientific data needed to answer these questions are very limited, so our answers necessarily involve considerable inference and speculation.

(1) How Does the Thalamic Gating Mechanism Work?

Nearly the entire thalamus is enveloped by a paper-thin layer of cells comprising the thalamic reticular nucleus (NR, Figure 19–2). The cells of this nucleus, unlike those in the remainder of the thalamus, send their projections (axons) back into the thalamus, where they synapse both on thalamic relay neurons and on inhibitory thalamic interneurons. These cells employ an inhibitor neurotransmitter (gamma-aminobutyric acid, or GABA). They are thus admirably suited to potentiating thalamic transmission to the cortex (by inhibiting the interneurons), or to blocking thalamic transmission to the cortex (by disinhibiting the interneurons and thus inhibiting relay neurons).

The neurons of the thalamic reticular nucleus are in turn regulated by a host of brain systems. We will focus on the two systems that appear to be most important. The *first* is the midbrain reticular formation (MRF), a complex and poorly understood network of neurons within the core of the

FRONTAL CORTEX

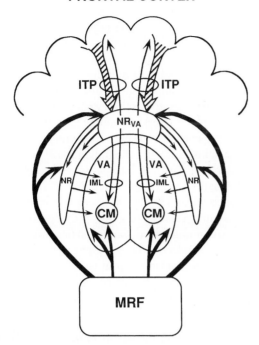

Figure 19–2. Schematic diagram of essential relationships involved in the regulation of the thalamic gating mechanism. See text for details. ITP, inferior thalamic peduncle; NR, nucleus reticularis; NR$_{VA}$, the portion of NR immediately anterior to ventral anterior nucleus (VA) that receives input both from the midbrain reticular formation (MRF) and the prefrontal cortex via the ITP; CM, center median nucleus; IML, internal medullary lamina, the white matter fascicle separating the medial from the lateral thalamus and containing the connections between prefrontal cortex and CM.

midbrain immediately below the thalamus. The midbrain reticular formation defines our level of wakefulness or arousal. With very high levels of arousal, the midbrain reticular formation strongly excites the thalamic reticular nucleus, causing it to inhibit thalamic inhibitory interneurons, thereby allowing all neural transmission to pass readily through the thalamus in an essentially unregulated fashion (i.e., it is transmitted by thalamocortical relay neurons without restraint). With low levels of arousal, as in deep sleep or coma, the thalamic reticular nucleus is relatively inactive, allowing generalized inhibition of thalamic transmission by thalamic inhibitory interneurons. Thus, in this circumstance, all neural transmission through the thalamus is blocked. In this way, the impact of the midbrain reticular formation on thalamic transmission is *global and nonselective*.

The *second* major regulatory system is provided by projections from the cerebral cortex, particularly the prefrontal cortex, to the thalamic reticular nucleus, via the inferior thalamic peduncle (ITP). These projections provide a mechanism by which thalamic transmission from specific regions

of specific nuclei can be selectively gated to the cortex. Thus, this system is *local and selective*.

(2) How Do Strokes Impair the Function of the Thalamic Gate?

The projections from both the midbrain reticular formation and the prefrontal cortex link to the thalamic reticular nucleus in a dense neural complex near the anterior pole of the thalamus (NR$_{VA}$), immediately adjacent to the ventral anterior (VA) nucleus of the thalamus. The mechanism by which the prefrontal cortex regulates the thalamic gate also appears to require the participation of a nucleus buried deep within posterior portions of the thalamus called the center median nucleus (CM). Fibers from the prefrontal cortex to and from the center median nucleus pass within the thalamus in a neural fascicle called the internal medullary lamina (IML). Immediately in front of the thalamus, these fibers pass through a white matter bundle called the inferior thalamic peduncle (ITP), which is continuous with the anterior limb of the internal capsule and the deep frontal lobe white matter (Figures 19–1 and 19–2). Although the means we use to localize strokes within the thalamus are prone to error, it appears that all the thalamic strokes that have been reported to result in aphasia have involved either the ventral anterior nucleus at the nexus of the connections between the prefrontal cortex (the ITP), the midbrain reticular formation, and the thalamic reticular nucleus; the internal medullary lamina carrying connections from the prefrontal cortex to the center median nucleus; or the center median nucleus itself. Thus, it appears that all strokes causing thalamic aphasia damage the regulatory system for the thalamic gate for the entire hemi-thalamus. This would implicate transmission from all thalamic nuclei, including the pulvinar/LP complex, which is heavily connected to language cortices. Thalamic strokes that are not associated with aphasia appear to spare this set of structures. Thus, the small subcortical strokes causing thalamic aphasia appear to impair the function of the thalamic gate by damaging the regulatory mechanism of the frontal lobe's center median for that gate.

(3) What Purpose Could Such a Gating Mechanism Serve?

The brain contains approximately 100 billion neurons organized into hundreds of systems, each of which is nearly infinitely malleable. Given this situation, it appears logical that there must be some systems whose function is simultaneously to maintain order and to optimize the resources that are brought to bear on a particular problem. As we have begun to understand the nature of neural network processing (see PDP, below), it has become apparent that individual neural networks are intrinsically self-optimizing. That is, they function automatically, without supervision, to provide the best available information despite noisy or incomplete input or the presence of network damage. However, there is still the problem of how to allocate processing demands among a multitude of different systems or within the parts of single systems. A number of different lines of research have begun to delineate the executive systems that subserve this purpose.

Fifteen years ago, Moran and Desimone (1985) performed a clever experiment that provides particular insight into the fundamental nature of this process. They were recording the activity of single neurons in inferior temporal cortex (visual association cortex) of macaque monkeys. In one study, they identified a neuron that was sensitive only to red light. If the monkey had been trained to pull a lever in order to receive a reward of a squirt of apple juice whenever a red light came on, this neuron fired vigorously in response to the red light. However, if the monkey had been trained to be rewarded for a lever pull in response to a green light, this neuron failed to fire in response to a red light. In other words, this neuron required two inputs to fire, one from visual cortex signaling the presence of red, and one from elsewhere in the brain, presumably the frontal lobes, signaling that red was behaviorally important because it indicated an opportunity to get a reward. During the red-light rewarded condition, input from the frontal lobes preferentially sensitized red-sensitive neural systems. This corresponded to particular attention by the monkey to red lights. The process exhibited by the monkeys in the experiment of Moran and Desimone can be termed *intentional attention* because it constitutes a deliberate allocation of sensory (visual) resources in order to achieve a particular end (get a juice reward).

Attention may also be reactive. We will, for example, orient to a brilliant flash of light because of the intrinsic value the brain assigns to this particular type of stimulus. A precise but flexible balance must be maintained between intentional and reactive attentional systems. For example, a rat must engage intentional attention to search for edible material, but must simultaneously maintain reactive attention in order to detect approaching predators.

The attentional phenomena we have been discussing so far involve the selection of particular neural networks or fragments of networks in cerebral association cortices in the service of focusing sensory organs at some particular locus in the environment (i.e., orienting). There is now abundant reason to believe that precisely analogous processes occur in polymodal or supramodal cerebral cortices, such as those supporting language function, that correspond to thinking and the formulation of behaviors other than orienting. These processes have been the focus of considerable study over the past 20 years (Fuster, 1991; Goldman-Rakic, 1990). The term "working memory" is often used to refer to the information maintained by the selected neural network (e.g., memory that the color red is important, in the Moran and Desimone experiment), although we prefer the more neutral term *selective*

engagement. In this conceptualization, attentional processes represent a subtype of selective engagement.

Nonhuman primate research suggests that, at this stage in the evolution of the brain, the thalamus is no longer involved in gated relay (selective engagement) of visual or auditory information, and probably only minimally involved in regulating the relay of somatosensory information that is processed at the level of *primary* sensory cortices. That is, attentional mechanisms in these modalities have been subsumed by the cerebral cortex. However, thalamic nuclei such as the dorsomedial nucleus and the pulvinar/LP complex have evolved in tandem with the burgeoning of cerebral cortex in higher primates, indirect evidence that their function has not been superceded. The development of cortical dysfunction after thalamic lesions in humans provides further, more direct evidence of ongoing thalamic participation in at least certain aspects of selective engagement. Thus, in humans, thalamic gating mechanisms appear to be most important in regulating selective engagement of *association* cortices supporting higher neural functions such as language.

(4) What is Likely to be the Specific Impact of Disorders of the Thalamic Gating Mechanism on the Function of Overlying Cortex, Most Specifically, Language Cortex?

The neuroscience of thalamocortical interaction has not advanced to the point of providing an answer to this question and we are primarily dependent upon human data in the inferences we draw on this subject. Thalamic aphasia is characterized by anomia in spontaneous language (at times of very severe degree), some impairment in naming to confrontation, normal grammar, normal articulation, and flawless repetition. In the worst cases, modest impairment in comprehension may be noted. Some patients make semantic paraphasic errors and rare patients, primarily those with thalamic hemorrhages, transiently produce neologisms. Can we relate this pattern of deficits to any fundamental functional attributes of the cerebral cortices involved? We have proposed that linguistic deficits wrought of thalamic dysfunction reflect selective functional impairment of cortices supporting declarative memories with sparing of cortices supporting procedural memories (Nadeau & Crosson, 1997).

Declarative or explicit memory consists of knowledge of facts and events and is ordinarily available to conscious recollection. It is represented in association cortices throughout the brain. New declarative memories are encoded by a system comprised of the hippocampus, cortices overlying the hippocampus, several structures in the limbic system (which presumably help to define which facts are worth remembering), and the dorsomedial nucleus and anterior nuclear group of the thalamus (Squire, 1987, 1992).

Nondeclarative memory consists of a heterogeneous collection of abilities including skills and habits, implicit memory, and some forms of classical conditioning. Nondeclarative memory is reflected only in behavioral change, as when one's tennis game improves with practice, or as when an experimental subject demonstrates an autonomic response or a correct decision when re-exposed to a stimulus previously presented too briefly to provide even a sense of familiarity, let alone a basis for conscious recognition. Skills, habits, and some forms of classical conditioning are represented in motor and premotor cortex, cerebellum, and possibly the basal ganglia. Unlike declarative memory, nondeclarative memory does not appear to require a special auxiliary processing mechanism like the hippocampal system to be instantiated. Patients with impaired declarative memory generally have preserved nondeclarative memory.

The principal linguistic deficit exhibited by patients with thalamic aphasia is in lexical-semantic access (Nadeau & Crosson, 1997), a process that clearly depends on declarative memories. In contrast, linguistic processes involving phonological processing and grammar are spared. Although we have declarative knowledge of the spelling of words, we rely on entirely automatic processes not available to conscious recollection in the actual production of spoken words. Although we have declarative knowledge of the concepts about which we plan to speak, the process of translating concepts into clause sequences and appropriate phrase structures is also an automatic one, unavailable to conscious recollection. Thus, the sparing of phonological and grammatical processes in thalamic aphasia appears to indicate sparing of procedural memory systems.

We have concluded that aphasia caused by thalamic strokes reflects a disorder of some type of selective engagement that impairs the function of language cortices connected to the thalamus (primarily the pulvinar/LP complex) that support declarative knowledge. The linguistic properties of thalamic aphasia favor rehabilitation strategies focused on impaired lexical-semantic function. Our conclusions about the neural basis of thalamic aphasia favor rehabilitation strategies directed at dysfunctional declarative memory systems.

NONTHALAMIC SUBCORTICAL APHASIA

Whereas the development of aphasia after thalamic lesions is a natural consequence of disruption of the function of neural systems implicated in language processing, the development of aphasia after nonthalamic subcortical lesions appears to be largely a consequence of direct damage to language cortices that is not visible on imaging studies, reflecting mechanisms of stroke pathogenesis. That is, nonthalamic subcortical aphasias are not fundamentally different in character or pathogenesis from cortical aphasias.

At first the problem of nonthalamic subcortical aphasia seems formidable, given the enormous variety in size and location of lesions and the spectrum of linguistic disorders observed. In our approach to this problem, we chose to simplify

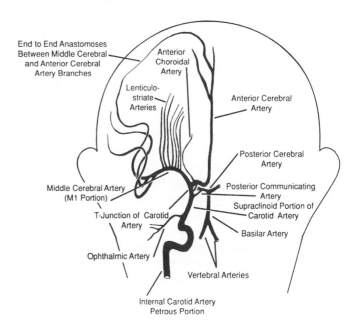

Figure 19–3. Anterior-posterior view of cerebral vascular anatomy relevant to the problem of nonthalamic subcortical aphasia.

by focusing on one single type of subcortical lesion producing aphasia, the striatocapsular infarct (Nadeau & Crosson, 1997). We did so for two reasons. First, this is a relatively common lesion that is typically fairly stereotyped in size and configuration. Second, because this infarct is apparently confined to structures that appear to have nothing to do with language (the head of the caudate nucleus, the anterior half of the putamen, and the interleaved anterior limb of the internal capsule), the very existence of aphasia in patients with this lesion provided compelling evidence of either an unrecognized neural mechanism or a completely non-neural mechanism. The latter proved to be the case.

The striatocapsular infarct is caused by the propagation of thrombus or the embolization of blood clot into the proximal (M1) portion of the middle cerebral artery (Figure 19–3). There, the clot occludes the lenticulostriate arteries supplying the head of the caudate nucleus, the anterior limb of the internal capsule, and much of the putamen, causing essentially complete infarction (death) of these structures. However, it should be noted that this same clot also severely reduces the flow of blood to middle cerebral artery branches supplying the overlying cerebral cortex. This cortex becomes entirely dependent upon blood flowing backward into middle cerebral branches from their connections (anastomoses) with branches of the anterior cerebral artery and the posterior cerebral artery. If these anastomoses are abundant and large, the cortex will be relatively spared. If they are sparse and small, a massive stroke will occur. It might be objected that if there is ischemia sufficient to cause aphasia, the damaged tissue should be apparent on imaging studies, but this clearly is not the case. However, cerebral blood flow studies in patients with striatocapsular infarcts and otherwise normal structural images have shown dramatic reductions in cortical blood flow in precisely the regions that would be expected from the character of the aphasia (e.g., hypoperfusion in the posterior perisylvian temporal region in patients with features of Wernicke's aphasia). Furthermore, although the cortex in such patients initially appears to be normal, a year later, repeat studies demonstrate hemispheric cortical atrophy, unequivocal evidence of earlier cortical damage (Weiller et al., 1993).

If reduced or absent blood flow in the middle cerebral artery is indeed the mechanism of nonthalamic subcortical aphasia, one would predict that cortical damage could occur anywhere within the cortex supplied by the middle cerebral artery, delimited only by the pattern and adequacy of arterial anastomoses. One would then expect aphasias of all types with striatocapsular infarcts or any other subcortical infarct reflecting proximal middle artery occlusion. This turns out to be the case. In addition, some subcortical infarcts, as well as hemorrhages into the putamen, disrupt the connections between language cortex and the thalamus. Thus, they are likely to add features of thalamic aphasia to whatever language disorder results directly from the cortical damage. Striatocapsular infarcts may also disrupt frontothalamic projections traversing the anterior limb of the internal capsule.

One can immediately conclude from the foregoing discussion that nonthalamic subcortical aphasias are not likely to be fundamentally different, either in character of pathogenesis, from cortical aphasias, and that they should be treated in the same way. Furthermore, unlike aphasias due to thalamic lesions, which appear to be intrinsically limited to impairment in declarative memory systems, cortical aphasias may implicate both declarative and procedural systems. Thus, nonthalamic subcortical aphasias are as varied as cortical aphasias and they may include impairment in grammatical and phonological function as well as lexical-semantic function.

PARALLEL DISTRIBUTED PROCESSING MODELS OF LANGUAGE FUNCTION

Essential Attributes and Implications for Generalization

Because thalamic aphasias are associated with lexical-semantic deficits implicating declarative memory systems and nonthalamic subcortical aphasias may involve, in addition, grammatical and phonological deficits implicating procedural memory systems, we will turn in this section to the neural network structures underlying these different memory systems in an effort to determine what implications the attributes of these structures have for rehabilitation strategies. Specifically, we will focus on parallel distributed processing (PDP) systems, which appear to constitute fundamentally valid models of neural network structure and function.

PDP models are comprised of large numbers of very simple processing units, each of which is connected to many, if not most, of the other units in the model. They have great practical appeal because they can be built on computers and tested in simulations for their ability to account for observed behavior. They also have great theoretical appeal. Although current PDP models are in many ways simplistic, they capture the essence of neural network architecture. Studies of animals as diverse as cockroaches, leeches, lampreys, and monkeys have demonstrated neural system after neural system that operates according to PDP principles. Finally, the ability of PDP models of human brain systems to recapitulate both normal and pathological function provides a great deal of confidence in their fundamental validity even while we recognize flaws in their details.

In any PDP model, the information is stored (as in the brain) as the pattern of connection strengths between units (neurons in the brain). Learning constitutes alteration of the connection strength patterns (neural synaptic strengths). We will focus on two particular PDP models, the "rooms-in-a-house" model of Rumelhart and colleagues (Rumelhart et al., 1986) and the connectionist model of reading developed by Plaut and colleagues (Plaut et al., 1996). The rooms-in-a-house model, an auto-associator model, has the organizational structure of a declarative memory system. Lexical-semantic deficits (whether in thalamic, nonthalamic subcortical, or cortical aphasia) reflect a deficit in this system or its links to pattern associators. The reading model, a pattern associator, has the organizational structure of a procedural memory system. Grammatical and phonological deficits (whether cortical or subcortical in origin) reflect defects in pattern associator networks.

The "Rooms-in-a-House" Model

The "rooms in a house" model is comprised of 40 "feature" units, each corresponding to an article typically found in particular rooms or an aspect of particular rooms. Each unit is connected with all the other units in the network—an attribute that defines the model as an *auto-associator network* (Rumelhart et al., 1986). Connection strengths capture the likelihood that any two features will appear in conjunction in a typical house. When one or more units is clamped into the on state (as if the network had been shown these particular features or articles), activation spreads throughout the model and the model eventually settles into a steady state that implicitly defines a particular room in a house. Thus, clamping "oven" ultimately results in activation of all the items one would expect to find in a kitchen and thereby *implicitly* defines, via a *distributed representation*, the concept of a kitchen (Figure 19–4). No kitchen unit *per se* is turned on. Rather, kitchen is defined by the pattern of feature units that are activated. The 40-unit model has the capability of generating distributed representations of a number of different rooms

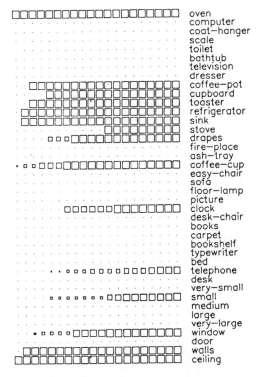

oven
computer
coat–hanger
scale
toilet
bathtub
television
dresser
coffee–pot
cupboard
toaster
refrigerator
sink
stove
drapes
fire–place
ash–tray
coffee–cup
easy–chair
sofa
floor–lamp
picture
clock
desk–chair
books
carpet
bookshelf
typewriter
bed
telephone
desk
very–small
small
medium
large
very–large
window
door
walls
ceiling

Figure 19–4. Evolution of the pattern of activation in the "rooms-in-a-house" model when the units "ceiling" and "oven" are clamped in the "on" position. Time elapses from left to right. The size of each square indicates the degree of activation of that particular feature unit. (From Rumelhart, D.E., Smolensky, P., McClelland, J.L., Hinton, G.E. [1986]. Schemata and sequential thought processes in PDP models. In J.L. McClelland, D.E. Rumelhart, PDP Research Group [eds.], *Parallel distributed processing, Vol. 2* [pp. 7–57]. Cambridge, MA: MIT Press.)

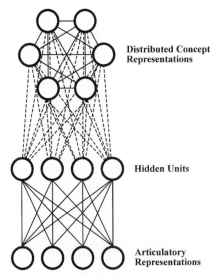

Distributed Concept Representations

Hidden Units

Articulatory Representations

Figure 19–5. Hypothetical structure of the linkage of an auto-associator network to a pattern associator network that would be capable of translating a pattern of activity in the auto-associator network corresponding to the distributed representation of a concept into the pattern of activity across motor units corresponding to the distributed representation that would produce the appropriate motoric output.

in a house (e.g., bathroom, bedroom, living room, study), subcomponents of rooms (e.g., easy chair and floor lamp, desk and desk-chair, window and drapes) and blends of rooms that were not anticipated in the programming of the model (e.g., clamping both bed and sofa leads to a distributed representation of a large, fancy bedroom replete with a fireplace, television, and sofa).

This auto-associator model, simple though it is, has the essential attributes of a network that might be capable of generating the distributed representations of meaning underlying lexical-semantic function. The brain's lexical semantic auto-associator must be comprised of vastly more that 40 features, enabling an enormous repertoire of distributed representations corresponding to the vast number of concepts we are capable of representing. In order for the distributed representations defining concepts to be translated into words, they must be linked via a pattern associator network to neural networks underlying articulatory representations (Figure 19–5). The singular attribute of this particular pattern associator is that the relationships between distributed representations

of meaning and distributed representations of articulatory word forms are almost completely arbitrary. That is, there is generally no relationship between the form of a word and its meaning. Thus, in general, learning of the relationship between meaning and articulatory word form that enables us to say one word will provide no assistance in the production of other words. It seems that learning in this system cannot generalize.

In fact, as David Plaut (1996) has shown in a reading model, the situation is not quite this simple or the implications for rehabilitation quite so dire. First, it needs to be recognized that a damaged network still contains a great deal of the knowledge originally stored in it, and that this residual knowledge spans the entire domain of the original knowledge. Thus, although network damage may result in rather severe anomia, rather modest adjustments in connection strengths may be adequate to bring elicited articulatory patterns above the minimum threshold needed for word production to succeed. Second, although the relationship between articulatory word form and word meaning is almost completely arbitrary, this arbitrariness largely applies to the pattern of connections between hidden units and articulatory units in Figure 19–5. In contrast, the pattern of connections between semantic units and hidden units captures some of the structure latent in the semantic domain, defined by the degree to which different concepts share attributes. Thus, as demonstrated by Plaut in computer simulations, retraining a network wherein the damage is nearer semantic representations may be associated with significant generalization to concepts that share semantic features with the members of the training set. Optimizing strengths of connections to semantic features of trained items can enhance production of untrained items to the extent that they share these same features. On the other hand, if the network damage is nearer articulatory representations, the generalization will tend to be minimal. Variations in lesion locus may thus explain a substantial portion of the variability in generalization observed in rehabilitation studies (reviewed by Plaut). If the principles of generalization elucidated here prove neurologically valid, then one would predict that retraining of a patient with lexical-semantic impairment due to either thalamic or posterior nonthalamic subcortical aphasia (anomic, transcortical sensory, Wernicke's, conduction) should be associated with some generalization, whereas retraining of patients with lexical-semantic impairment associated with anterior nonthalamic subcortical aphasias (e.g., transcortical motor aphasias as described by Lichtheim, 1885, and McCarthy & Warrington, 1984) should be associated with little if any generalization.

Plaut (1996) has also made the provocative suggestion, again supported by the results of computer simulations, that training with modestly atypical exemplars of semantic categories (e.g., penguin as opposed to sparrow) may produce better generalization than training with typical exemplars. This is because atypical words provide better information about semantic dimensions on which category members may vary, and thus support generalization to other atypical words. Furthermore, atypical words in aggregate can provide a good approximation of the central tendency of a semantic category. Training with typical words, in contrast, can facilitate the production of other typical words but will often fail to amend connections supporting semantic features underlying atypical words; therefore, generalization to atypical words will not tend to occur.

The Reading Model

The pattern associator model of single-syllable word reading developed by Plaut and colleagues (Plaut et al., 1996) (Figure 19–6) was comprised of three layers: (1) an input layer of 105 grapheme units grouped into clusters, the first cluster comprised of all possibilities for the one or more consonants of the onset, the second cluster comprised of all the possible vowels in the nucleus, and the third cluster comprised of all possibilities for the one or more consonants in the coda; (2) a hidden unit layer of 100 units; and (3) an output layer of 61 phoneme units grouped into clusters comprised of all the possibilities for onset, nucleus, and coda, respectively (as for the graphemes). Local representations were used for the graphemes and phonemes. There were one-way connections from each of the grapheme input units to each of the hidden units, and two-way connections between each of the hidden

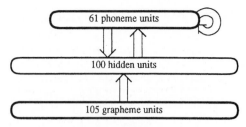

Figure 19–6. One version of the PDP reading model developed by Plaut et al. (From Plaut, D.C., McClelland, J.L., Seidenberg, M.S., Patterson, K. [1996]. Understanding normal and impaired word reading: Computational principles in quasi-regular domains. *Psychological Review, 103*, 56–115.)

units and each of the phoneme output units. Every output unit was connected to every other output unit, providing the network the capability for "settling into" the best solution (as opposed to its own approximate solution). The model was trained by successively presenting, in pairs, the orthographic representation of every English single-syllable word (in excess of 2000), and the desired phonologic output. The model was equipped with a learning device such that, to the extent that the actual output deviated from the target output, the strengths of connections throughout the model were slightly adjusted to reduce the discrepancy. Ultimately, the model learned to produce the correct pronunciation of all the words. One of the most striking things about the trained model is that it was able to produce correct pronunciations of plausible English nonwords (i.e., orthographic sequences it had never encountered before). How was this possible?

One might have inferred that the model was simply learning the pronunciation of all the words by rote. If this had been the case, however, the model would have been incapable of applying what it had learned to novel words. In fact, what the model learned was the relationships between *sequences* of graphemes and *sequences* of phonemes that are characteristic of the English language. To the extent that there is a limited repertoire of such sequences, the model was able to learn it and then apply that knowledge to novel forms that incorporated some of the sequential relationships in this repertoire. The information the model acquired through its long experience with English orthographic-phonologic sequential relationships went considerably beyond this, however. Certain sequences, those most commonly found in English single-syllable words, were more thoroughly etched in network connectivity. Such sequences included the most commonly used rhyme constituents. The model encountered difficulty (reflected in prolonged reading latency) only to the extent that it incorporated different, competing pronunciations of the same orthographic sequence. Thus, it was slow to read "pint," because in every case but "pint," the sequence "int" is pronounced /Int/ (e.g., mint, tint, flint, lint). It was also slow, though not quite so slow, to read words like "shown" because there are two equally frequent alternatives to the pronunciation of "own" (gown, down, town versus shown, blown, flown). This behavior precisely recapitulates the behavior of normal human subjects given reading tasks.

The capacity of the model to read nonwords reflects its ability to capture patterns in the sequential relationship between orthographic and articulatory word forms and to apply this knowledge to novel word forms. Thus, the model is intrinsically generalizing. Training with a limited corpus that nevertheless captures the preponderant sequential relationships should be adequate. Procedural knowledge in general is intrinsically generalizing. Thus, acquiring skill in playing tennis confers ability to hit the ball in almost any situation, even when that situation has never been precisely encountered before.

The procedural knowledge we access when speaking involves the acoustic-articulatory sequential relationships underlying phonologic processing and several types of sequence knowledge underlying grammatical function, including word class sequence knowledge captured by phrase structure rules, and implicit sequential relationships between concepts expressed in clause organization and verb predicate argument structure. Like other procedural knowledge, highly repeated practice of a representative corpus of skills by aphasic patients (cortical or nonthalamic subcortical) in these different domains should generalize. Knowledge acquisition will be implicit and subconscious. The extent to which metalinguistic knowledge (e.g., explicit knowledge of grammatical rules) can aid this process is unclear and represents a complex issue beyond the scope of this discussion.

Summary

In this section we have attempted to lay the groundwork for discussion of PDP models. Specifically, we have focused on the fundamental differences between auto-associator networks (the likely basis for semantic knowledge) and pattern associator networks (the likely basis for lexical-semantic knowledge, and for phonological and grammatical knowledge). We have considered the way in which the architecture of an auto-associator model and the knowledge implicitly incorporated therein might support distributed representations of concepts, and the way in which the architecture of pattern associators can implicitly support sequence knowledge. We have concluded with inferences on generalization during rehabilitation that follow from the essential structure of these neural network models, namely, that auto-associator models, in their connections with the pattern associator networks that enable input and output, have modest capabilities for generalization, whereas pattern associators supporting knowledge of relationships between two classes of sequences, are intrinsically generalizing (e.g., as in grammatical and phonological function).

Other Inferences From PDP Models Regarding Rehabilitation

We offer here a number of logical arguments pertinent to language rehabilitation that derive from a PDP conceptualization of neural architecture. All are testable hypotheses.

Implications of Hebbian Learning

We have noted that in PDP models, the information lies in the strengths of connections between units. The concept that this might be true in the brain was first proposed independently by Ramón y Cajal (1923) and Tanzi (1893), but it was really developed by Donald Hebb (1949). Hebb proposed that connection strengths develop to the degree that there is simultaneous activation of two connected units. Training of PDP models is extremely important—simply because the heuristic learning devices that have been employed are by far the most efficient means of setting connection strengths in models incorporating hundreds of thousands if not millions of connections.[1] PDP studies using brain-like (Hebbian) learning principles are being done. However, progress has been limited by the paucity of our knowledge about how the brain actually does learn (adjust its connection strengths). Nevertheless, neuroscientific studies of species ranging from primitive mollusks (*Aplysia*) to higher primates suggest that learning in the brain does incorporate some variation of the Hebbian principle.

What implications does the Hebbian principle have for rehabilitation? In most patients with aphasia (as opposed to those with dementia), we can generally assume that the cerebral representation of concepts is substantially intact.[2] Language rehabilitation in these patients therefore consists predominantly of training one or more pattern associator networks, e.g., the pattern associator linking distributed concept representations with articulatory representations in the anomic patient, or the pattern associator linking orthographic sequence representations to articulatory sequence representations in the patient with acquired phonological dyslexia. In some disorders associated with aphasia, the cerebral representations of concepts are degraded. This is true both in disorders with diffuse damage to association cortices (e.g., Alzheimer's disease) and in disorders associated

---

[1] A two layer model with 400 units in each layer, each unit in one layer connected to every unit in the other layer, would contain 160,000 connections.

[2] This is true to the extent that concepts are instantiated as distributed representations involving association cortices throughout the brain—and are therefore substantially impervious to the effects of a single focal lesion. It is not true to the extent that there is some cerebral geographic specificity to the representation of a particular concept. For example, patients who have recovered from herpes simplex encephalitis often have extensive damage to the inferior surfaces of the temporal lobes, most of which comprise visual association cortex. These patients may have severely depleted representations of concepts that are predominantly visual, e.g., living things. Thus, these patents exhibit a category-specific naming defect for living things. Patients with more dorsal (and unilateral, dominant hemisphere) temporoparietal lesions (at times associated with aphasia) may exhibit a category-specific naming deficit for tools because of associated damage to cerebral representations of movement knowledge about objects.

with diffuse dysfunction of histologically intact association areas (e.g., thalamic aphasia). In these disorders, rehabilitation consists substantially of training the auto-associator networks supporting meaning such that links between semantic feature representations are reinstated, thus enabling the generation of distributed concept representations.

To maximize the efficiency of Hebbian learning, the input and desired output patterns need to be as clear and explicit as possible. Thus, treating anomia or alexia using an algorithm that relies primarily on acoustic feedback is less likely to be effective than one that relies on articulatory motor feedback, particularly if the brain links between acoustic and articulatory representations are damaged as they are in all the perisylvian aphasias (Broca's, Wernicke's, conduction, and global) and in many patients with nonthalamic subcortical aphasia. After all, the point of the treatment is to facilitate articulatory production. Even normal subjects will tend to hear the phonemic sequence they see being mouthed, even when the actual acoustic stimulus corresponds to a slightly different phonemic sequence—the McGurk effect (McGurk & MacDonald, 1976). At the least, clinicians can provide articulatory motor feedback simply by having patients view their faces as they provide feedback. There is evidence that treatment algorithms employing intensive and explicit means of providing articulatory motor feedback may be highly successful (Conway et al., 1998). In patients with dysfunction of association cortices supporting distributed concept representations (semantics), the links between associated semantic features need to be made as clear and explicit as possible.

The Hebbian principle also makes signal delay potentially relevant. Focal cerebral activation will be maximal at time of stimulus onset and will remain high only to the extent that working memory is normal in the particular modalities involved. Given the often-disseminated damage associated with strokes, working memory may not be normal and focal activation patterns may rapidly decay with time. This suggests that feedback regarding the correct response should occur either simultaneously with or very shortly after stimulus presentation.

Implications of Associative Properties of PDP Networks

The Need For Rich and Converging Inputs

In PDP networks, activation flows freely from one part of a network to another and from network to network, constrained only by the strengths of the network connections and the activity of selective engagement systems. Thus, multiple sources of input that converge to establish a given distributed representation increase the probability that the desired distributed representation will be generated and that variously related competing distributed representations will not. The implication of this principle for rehabilitation is that stimuli should be as rich and polymodal as possible. High-quality color graphics or real objects, which enable visual, tactile, and even olfactory input, are likely to be more effective than black and white line drawings.

Multiple Parallel Pathways

There is accumulating evidence that many if not all language functions in the brain are subserved by two, perhaps more parallel pathways. The most clearly explicated process is reading, wherein grapheme to phoneme, lexical, and semantic routes have been posited (Coltheart et al., 1993). PDP models incorporating two routes, a grapheme sequence–phoneme sequence route and a grapheme cluster–semantic distributed representation–phoneme cluster route, can adequately account for all the observed behavior (Plaut et al., 1996). There is corresponding evidence of two routes involved in writing (Roeltgen & Heilman, 1984).

The mechanisms underlying the syndrome of optic aphasia are controversial, but one major hypothesis is that there are two routes to object naming, one involving a pattern associator network that links visual representations directly to articulatory representations (enabling us to learn and remember the name of an utterly meaningless symbol or drawing, for example), and a second route linking visual representations to semantic representations, thence to articulatory representations (Shuren & Heilman, 1993). In this conceptualization, optic aphasia occurs because a damaged visual-articulatory route generates incorrect patterns of activation in articulatory cortex that compete with correct distributed representations generated via the semantic route. This renders the patient incapable of output, i.e., anomic, when naming to confrontation, but fluent when speaking spontaneously, in which there is not competition from the corrupted visual-articulatory route.

Spontaneous language production has not been recognized as a two-route process. However, there is compelling evidence that it is (see Figure 19–7). The linkage of acoustic to articulatory representations incorporates sequence knowledge, in exactly the same fashion as in the reading model of Plaut et al. (1996). This sequence knowledge provides the basis for the existence of joint phonemes, rhymes, syllables, root forms, suffixes, and closed class words as relatively preserved entities in aphasic patients. When this route is damaged, as in conduction aphasia, patients make phonemic and syllabic substitution errors during repetition. The linkage from semantic to articulatory representations incorporates sequences at the articulatory end, but because these are not linked to sequences at the semantic end, the network connections (incorporating the hidden units) in the semantic-articulatory linkage do not incorporate knowledge about prevalent sequential patterns (as did the network in the reading model of Plaut et al., 1996). In short, this is a "whole word" route that incorporates no sublexical knowledge except at the movement level. Thus, errors in

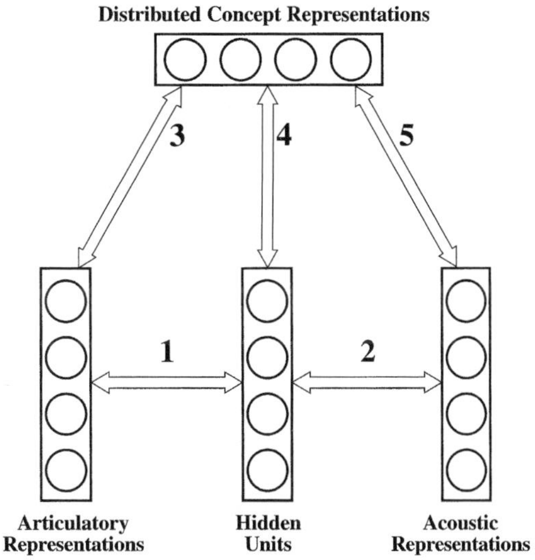

Distributed Concept Representations

Figure 19–7. Pools of neurons supporting distributed representations are depicted as sets of 4 circles, and the massive interconnectivity between the pools (probably two-way) as open arrows. The core of the language processor, which supports word and nonword repetition, and is located predominantly in dominant perisylvian cortex, consists of the articulatory representations, acoustic representations, and their interposed hidden units and connecting links 1 and 2. This core supports the knowledge of the relationship between sound sequences and articulatory motor sequences characteristic of the language spoken. This is not an acoustic element to phoneme transcoder. Rather, it is a transcoder of acoustic sequences to articulatory sequences. Connecting links 3, 4, and 5 represent connections between cortex supporting semantic distributed representations and the core phonologic processor. Additional pools of intermediate hidden units are left out for purposes of clarity. Two output links are posited (3 and 4) because patients with conduction aphasia routinely demonstrate sublexical paraphasias (e.g., phonemic paraphasias) in spontaneous language at the same time that there may be dramatic dissociations in these patients between the frequency of sublexical paraphasias in spontaneous language and in repetition. These observations suggest that there must be semantic-articulatory links that are whole word based (pathway 3) and that incorporate knowledge of phonologic sequences (pathway 4). It should be stressed that pathway 3 does not instantiate sublexical knowledge except at the movement level. This conceptualization parallels that thought to underlie reading, in which there is unequivocal evidence of lexical-semantic and phonologic pathways (Plaut et al., 1996). Pathways 1, 3, and 4 and the units they link comprise the basis for the phonologic output lexicon. The effortful, often unsuccessful production of single words in spontaneous speech with relatively spared naming to confrontation observed in some patients with transcortical motor aphasia could be explained by damage to pathway 3, leading to verbal paraphasic interference with articulatory representations generated by pathway 4. The essentials of this idea were first proposed by Lichtheim (1885) and later, Goldstein (1948). In some cases, there may also be damage to pathway 4, leading to phonemic paraphasias in spontaneous language (McCarthy & Warrington, 1984).

naming (or the spontaneous production of major lexical items) stemming from damage to this route will not result in phonemic paraphasias or neologisms. The patient will either be anomic or will make semantic paraphasic (whole word) errors. However, we know that most patients with aphasia due to perisylvian lesions (especially Wernicke's and conduction aphasias, sometimes Broca's aphasia), and some patients with nonthalamic subcortical aphasia, make literal paraphasic errors in spontaneous language and during naming. Some of these might occur because of phonemic distinctive feature substitutions due to damage to articulatory representations themselves, but this is unlikely to be the case with more posterior lesions and certainly cannot account for the joint phoneme and syllabic selection errors commonly seen in patients with Wernicke's or conduction aphasia. This means that semantic representations must have access to the sequence knowledge (hence, sublexical knowledge)

that has been acquired by the acoustic-articulatory system (Figure 19–7). Interestingly, there has been some debate in the literature about how essential repetition impairment is to the diagnosis of conduction aphasia. Some have tended to view it as a *sine qua non*, while others have pointed out that some patients with conduction aphasia actually make more phonemic paraphasic errors and neologisms during spontaneous language production and naming than during repetition. Positing a two-route model for spontaneous language production resolves this controversy. Obviously, the relative occurrence of paraphasic errors in spontaneous language production and repetition will reflect the distribution of damage between the two systems. It may also, as Plaut et al. (1996) point out, reflect the degree to which both routes were developed in the first place in a particular patient. A patient who relies disproportionately on the semantic-acoustic-articulatory route for naming is going to be particularly susceptible to the development of paraphasic errors in spontaneous language and naming given a dominant perisylvian lesion, whether it is visible on imaging studies, as in cortical aphasias, or invisible, as in nonthalamic subcortical aphasias. Several authors have described a form of transcortical motor aphasia that may reflect a complementary deficit (Alexander & Schmitt, 1980; McCarthy & Warrington, 1984; Rubens, 1975), a concept that actually dates back to Lichtheim (1885). These patients are relatively nonfluent in spontaneous language production and, despite the absence of articulatory distortion (as seen in patients with Broca's aphasia), their production of major lexical items is extremely effortful. They do not make phonemic paraphasic errors and their repetition is preserved. No cogent hypothesis has been offered to account for this deficit. However, in the PDP model we have been discussing, this pattern of deficit would occur if the semantic-acoustic-articulatory pathway were completely disrupted and the semantic-articulatory pathway partially disrupted. Alternatively, this pattern of deficit could occur in any patient who had failed to develop the semantic-acoustic-articulatory network, and then incurred damage to the semantic-articulatory network, again, whether it is visible on imaging studies, as in cortical aphasia, or invisible, as in nonthalamic subcortical aphasia.

We have made this long digression to emphasize the plausibility of pervasive dual network mechanisms underlying language function, including the most essential language function of all, the capacity for spontaneous output and naming. The importance of the point is that the product of dual networks is likely to be mutually reinforcing, but when one of the networks is damaged, not only is mutual reinforcement lost but there is a possibility for interference, as we posited in optic aphasia. The relevance for treatment is that in the aphasic patient, it may be important to explicitly recognize the existence of dual networks and conduct two different, network-specific, rehabilitation strategies. For example, in the patient with conduction aphasia (cortical or nonthalamic subcortical) with substantial anomia, rehabilitation of the acoustic-articulatory network could potentially improve anomia by reducing interference from the semantic-acoustic-articulatory network with names more successfully generated via the semantic-articulatory network.

"Gatekeeper" Networks

The prototypic gatekeeper network is that which underlies articulatory motor phonemic representations. In principle, these can be accessed via the acoustic route (repetition), the orthographic route (reading aloud), or the semantic route (naming to confrontation, naming to definition). The interface between these various sources of input with articulatory motor representations may be different. It is not clear which might provide the best route for rebuilding articulatory motor representations. The optimal route may vary from patient to patient and it is possible that a two- or three-pronged

rehabilitation approach (mutually reinforcing) would be preferable. Our understanding of neural structure is not adequate to make predictions and, ultimately, this is an empirical question to be answered in each patient uniquely.

Grammar

Earlier in this chapter we introduced the concept that grammatic function substantially involves procedural memory. If this hypothesis is correct, it has strong implications for rehabilitation of grammatic impairment (whether due to cortical or nonthalamic subcortical aphasia). Procedural memory does not have the instantaneous, single-exposure learning facility provided by the hippocampal system in the realm of declarative memory. Procedural memory is acquired through practice. Thus, if grammatic skills do depend primarily on procedural memory, rehabilitation of grammatic dysfunction would have to entail massed practice conducted over extended periods of time daily. The therapeutic requirements resemble those associated with rehabilitating systems that have but modest intrinsic capacity for generalization, e.g., lexical-semantic, but for entirely different reasons. With grammatic rehabilitation, a modest number of construction types are incrementally developed over very large numbers of trials. With lexical-semantic rehabilitation, a very large number of exemplars are developed all at once, a few at a time.

NONLINGUISTIC BEHAVIORAL DISORDERS RELEVANT TO THE REHABILITATION PROCESS

Over the last 10 years, our estimates of the fundamental plasticity of the adult cerebrum have increased one hundred fold. In principle, it seems that any type of cerebral dysfunction might be susceptible to rehabilitation. However, there are several fundamental cerebral systems whose function appears to be critical to the very conduct of the rehabilitation process. We suggest that, when these systems are substantially impaired, any rehabilitation, but particularly rehabilitation of the level of sophistication and refinement of speech therapy, becomes problematic and prognosis for meaningful advances in therapy becomes relatively poor. These systems include arousal, attention, and frontal systems function. Faced as we are with overwhelming pressures to optimize the utilization of our treatment resources, it is important to identify these types of deficits ahead of time.

Arousal

Impairment in arousal typically reflects dysfunction of the midbrain reticular formation. There are a host of disorders that commonly produce transient dysfunction of the reticular formation (metabolic disorders, drugs, infections, and intracerebral masses). However, patients most often develop *persistent* dysfunction because of embolism to the top of the basilar artery, which occludes small vessels supplying the reticular formation, as well as one or both posterior cerebral arteries (hence abnormalities in vision such as hemianopia or cortical blindness). Infarcts of the midline thalamus, some of which produce aphasia, often extend caudally into the midbrain reticular formation. These patients often experience lethargy which, although most severe initially (to the point of coma), often persists for months or years. There is no treatment that has been shown to be effective in mitigating this lethargy. Because these patients behave as if constantly half asleep, they are unable to engage fruitfully in rehabilitation efforts and their long-term prognosis for an active, interactive life is very poor.

Attention

Arousal is a necessary substrate for attention, so patients with impaired arousal will have impaired attention. Patients with frontal system dysfunction will also often have a disorder of intentional or deliberate attention, even though their level of arousal is normal. Thus, they are limited in their ability to sustain focused attention and they tend to be very distractible. This behavior will substantially undermine any rehabilitation program. This type of impairment is most often seen with degenerative processes implicating the dorsolateral frontal lobes bilaterally but it may also be a feature of patients with midline thalamic lesions.

Patients with nondominant hemisphere dysfunction, most often due to parietal lobe lesions (cortical or nonthalamic subcortical) and occasionally due to thalamic lesions, will often exhibit a hemispatial disorder of attention known as hemispatial neglect, in which they fail to attend or respond to any stimuli presented in the left hemispace. This same disorder is sometimes seen with dominant hemisphere lesions but is characteristically much less severe in these circumstances. Nevertheless, even patients with dominant hemisphere lesions (cortical, subcortical, or thalamic) without apparent right hemispatial neglect may benefit from presentation of stimuli in the left hemispace, for reasons that are still poorly understood and controversial (Coslett et al., 1993; Nadeau et al., 1997; Nadeau & Heilman, 1991).

Frontal Systems Dysfunction

Frontal systems dysfunction may impede therapy in other ways. The precise impact depends on the locus of the predominant pathology. Patients with midline frontal systems dysfunction tend to be akinetic in their general behavior and nonfluent in their language. They are typically poorly motivated, cannot carry out multi-step commands, and may actively resist any type of intervention by caretakers. Patients with orbitofrontal system dysfunction may superficially appear to be normal but they tend to be irresponsible, cannot be relied upon to sustain goal-oriented activity, and tend to be socially inappropriate. Both these types of patients pose major challenges for any type of rehabilitation program.

Patients with dorsolateral frontal system dysfunction may retain strong motivation and exhibit excellent cooperation in rehabilitation programs. The side of the lesion often assumes major importance. Patients with dominant hemisphere lesions, for example, patients with Broca's or global aphasia, are often excellent candidates for speech therapy. However, patients with nondominant hemisphere lesions (seldom seen for aphasia rehabilitation) often exhibit anosognosia (denial of illness) or anosodiaphoria (lack of concern for illness). These patients are poorly motivated to participate in any rehabilitation program because, put simply, they either do not recognize the problem or they do not care about it.

Frontal systems disorders manifested in these ways are rarely a significant problem in patients with nonthalamic subcortical aphasia unless there are bilateral lesions. However, midline thalamic lesions are almost uniformly associated with prominent frontal systems dysfunction. When not lethargic, these patients often appear superficially to be quite normal in their general demeanor. However, they typically exhibit the most profound lack of motivation, to the point of perpetually placing obstacles in the way of any rehabilitation efforts ("I'm too tired"; "I have another appointment in 2 hours"; "I'm too busy"; "I think I've already done enough of that this week"). Thus, they reflect some blend of midline and orbitofrontal systems dysfunction.

Concept Formation

Spoken language depends on the translation of concepts into the articulatory motor sequences that will produce sounds that are intelligible to others. Concepts can be generated in two fundamentally different ways. First, if we look at something, a concept is automatically elicited as the visual input automatically generates a distributed representation in cerebral association cortices corresponding to that concept. Second, we have the power to intentionally generate a distributed representation corresponding to a concept from within—a fragment of a process we refer to as thinking. Some rare patients, usually with bilateral lesions, may exhibit impairment in their ability to automatically generate distributed concept representations in response to specific types of sensory input. They will be unable to name or describe the properties or use of objects they are observing. This disorder, most often seen after lesions of visual pathways, is termed agnosia. Other patients exhibit selective impairment in their ability to generate distributed concept representations from within. These patients will typically appear to be profoundly nonfluent in spontaneous language, tending either not to respond or to respond with single words or short phrases. However, when asked to describe a complex picture (in which case distributed concept representations are automatically generated from without), they typically perform nearly normally. This disorder is termed adynamic aphasia (Gold et al., 1997). It is characteristically seen with frontal lobe lesions, most often affecting the dominant frontal lobe or bilateral in location. It may be seen with nonthalamic subcortical infarcts, and patients with thalamic infarcts associated with aphasia may exhibit some features of adynamic aphasia, although rarely in these cases is the disorder seen in its fullest form. Although effective speech therapy is not absolutely precluded in such patients, spontaneous language is unlikely to become fluent because of the more fundamental underlying deficit (Huntley & Rothi, 1988).

FUTURE TRENDS

The proposed mechanisms of thalamic aphasia discussed in this chapter, although both cogent and supported by lesion studies, have yet to be tested empirically. Whether or not our application of the declarative/procedural dichotomy to language processes in general, and subcortical aphasias in particular, in the hopes of clarifying fundamental mechanisms, will ultimately be vindicated also remains to be seen. PDP models have so far been something of a tour de force as neurally motivated models of higher neural function and in their capacity for generating voluminous output in the testing of specific hypotheses about neural network structure and function. They have provided key insights into the neural processes that might be behind information processing models. They have proven remarkably successful in emulating behavior in normal and brain-impaired individuals. As we have seen, they compare very favorably with information-processing models in their highly specific implications for rehabilitation strategies. Nevertheless, we are at the dawn of the PDP age. Further development of PDP models and elaboration in these models of the declarative/procedural dichotomy will lead to abundant further insights into neural network function. Models will become considerably more accurate in the degree to which they emulate neural network function. PDP learning algorithms will advance from predominantly heuristic algorithms to biologically plausible (e.g., Hebbian) algorithms—a crucial step to understanding the impact of rehabilitation. Finally, the predictions of PDP research for aphasic phenomenology and rehabilitation outcome will be tested empirically—thus providing us feedback on the hypotheses implicitly encoded in PDP network structure.

KEY POINTS

Subcortical aphasia is logically divided into thalamic and nonthalamic types. Aphasia due to thalamic lesions appears to reflect dysfunction of cortical systems involved in language as a result of damage to the thalamic mechanisms for selectively engaging cortical neuronal networks. It is characterized almost exclusively by lexical-semantic dysfunction. Aphasia due to nonthalamic subcortical lesions predominantly reflects damage to the cortex, inapparent on structural imaging studies, that is caused by ischemia in the distal territory of the middle cerebral artery, the proximal occlusion of which is directly responsible for the visible subcortical lesion. Nonthalamic subcortical infarcts may therefore be associated with any type of aphasia and nonthalamic subcortical aphasia is not fundamentally different from cortical aphasia.

In considering therapy for subcortical aphasias, and indeed for aphasia in general, we have considered aphasia from a neural systems perspective incorporating the fundamental concepts underlying PDP models. A PDP conceptualization of brain function, which is almost certainly biologically valid, has many specific implications for language function, dysfunction, and rehabilitation. Principles important for rehabilitation include:

1. The intrinsically limited generalization in therapy involving links between auto-associator and pattern associator networks, e.g., those supporting lexical-semantic function.
2. The intrinsic generalizability of therapy involving pattern associator networks, e.g., those underlying phonologic processing and reading aloud.
3. The importance of maximizing opportunities for Hebbian learning by maximizing the clarity and explicitness of input and desired output and minimizing delay between stimulus presentation and feedback.
4. The need to explicitly recognize the dual network instantiation of many if not most linguistic functions, recognize the capacity for dysfunction in one network to interfere with the output of another network, and take advantage of the potentially mutually reinforcing effect of dual network rehabilitation.
5. The possibility of multiple approaches to the rehabilitation of gatekeeper networks, such as those underlying articulatory motor output.
6. The likelihood that grammatic impairment substantially involves deficits in procedural memories and thus must be treated with extensive practice acquired through a large number of trials.

We have closed with a brief review of the disorders in fundamental underlying brain systems such as arousal, attention, and frontal systems function, that are likely to seriously undermine any rehabilitation effort, and of adynamic aphasia, a disorder of endogenous concept formation, which is likely to substantially limit effectiveness of speech therapy.

References

Alexander, M.P. & Schmitt, M.A. (1980). The aphasia syndrome of stroke in the left anterior cerebral artery territory. *Archives of Neurology, 37,* 97–100.

Coltheart, M., Curtis, B., Atkins, P., & Haller, M. (1993). Models of reading aloud: Dual-route and parallel-distributed-processing approaches. *Psychological Review, 100,* 589–608.

Conway, T., Heilman, P., Gonzalez-Rothi, L.J., Alexander, A.W., Adair, J., & Crosson, B. et al. (1998). Treatment of a case of phonological alexia with agraphia using the auditory discrimination in depth (ADD) program. *JINS, 4,* 608–620.

Coslett, H.B., Schwartz, M.F., Goldberg, G., Haas, D., & Perkins, J. (1993). Multi-modal hemispatial deficits after left hemisphere stroke. *Brain, 116,* 527–554.

Fuster, J.M. (1991). The prefrontal cortex and its relation to behavior. *Progress in Brain Research, 87,* 201–211.

Gold, M., Nadeau, S.E., Jacobs, D.H., Adair, J.C., Gonzalez-Rothi, L.J., & Heilman, K.M. (1997). Adynamic aphasia: A transcortical motor aphasia with defective semantic strategy formation. *Brain and Language, 57,* 374–393.

Goldman-Rakic, P.S. (1990). Cellular and circuit basis of working memory in prefrontal cortex of nonhuman primates. *Progress in Brain Research, 85,* 325–336.

Goldstein, K. (1948). *Language and language disorders.* New York: Grune & Stratton.

Hebb, D.O. (1949). *The organization of behavior.* New York: Wiley.

Huntley, R.A. & Rothi, L.J. (1988). Treatment of verbal akinesia in a case of transcortical motor aphasia. *Aphasiology, 2,* 55–66.

Lichtheim, L. (1885). On aphasia. *Brain, 7,* 433–484.

McCarthy, R. & Warrington, E.K. (1984). A two-route model of speech production: Evidence from aphasia. *Brain, 107,* 463–485.

McGurk, H. & MacDonald, J. (1976). Hearing lips and seeing voices. *Nature, 264,* 746–748.

Moran, J. & Desimone, R. (1985). Selective attention gates visual processing in extrastriate cortex. *Science, 229,* 782–784.

Nadeau, S.E. & Crosson, B. (1997). Subcortical aphasia. *Brain and Language, 58,* 355–402, 436–458.

Nadeau, S.E., Crosson, B., Schwartz, R.L., & Heilman, K.M. (1997). Gaze-related enhancement of hemispheric blood flow in a stroke patient. *Journal of Neurology, Neurosurgery, and Psychiatry, 62,* 538–540.

Nadeau, S.E. & Heilman, K.M. (1991). Gaze-dependent hemianopia without hemispatial neglect. *Neurology, 41,* 1244–1250.

Plaut, D.C. (1996). Relearning after damage in connectionist networks: Toward a theory of rehabilitation. *Brain and Language, 52,* 25–82.

Plaut, D.C., McClelland, J.L., Seidenberg, M.S., & Patterson, K. (1996). Understanding normal and impaired word reading: Computational principles in quasi-regular domains. *Psychological Review, 103,* 56–115.

Ramón y Cajal, S. (1923). *Recuerdos de mi vida.* Madrid: Pueyo.

Roeltgen, D.P. & Heilman, K.M. (1984). Lexical agraphia: Further support for the two-system hypothesis of linguistic agraphia. *Brain, 107,* 811–827.

Rubens, A.B. (1975). Aphasia with infarction in the territory of the anterior cerebral artery. *Cortex, 11,* 239–250.

Rumelhart, D.E., Smolensky, P., McClelland, J.L., & Hinton, G.E. (1986). Schemata and sequential thought processes in PDP models. In J.L. McClelland, D.E. Rumelhart, the PDP Research Group (eds.), *Parallel distributed processing, Vol. 2* (pp. 7–57). Cambridge, MA: MIT Press.

Shuren, J. & Heilman, K.M. (1993). Non-optic aphasia. *Neurology, 43,* 1900–1907.

Squire, L.R. (1987). *Memory and the brain.* New York: Oxford University Press.

Squire, L.R. (1992). Declarative and non-declarative memory: multiple brain systems supporting learning and memory. *Journal of Cognitive Neuroscience, 4,* 232–243.

Tanzi, E. (1893). I fatti e le induzioni nell'odierna istologia del sistema nervoso. *Riv. Sper. Freniatr. Med. Leg. Alienazioni Ment, 19,* 419–472.

Weiller, C., Willmes, K., Reiche, W., Thron, A., Insensee, C., & Buell, U., et al. (1993). The case of aphasia or neglect after striatocapsular infarction. *Brain, 116,* 1509–1525.

Chapter 20

Primary Progressive Aphasia

Malcolm R. McNeil and Joseph R. Duffy

Because aphasia is most commonly caused by stroke, what we understand about its nature, assessment, diagnosis, prognosis, and management is overwhelmingly based on data derived from people in whom it was stroke induced. In spite of this, clinicians recognize that the conditions of closed and penetrating head injuries, tumors, surgical complications, and infection are relatively common causes of aphasia. All of these etiologies are nearly always acute or subacute in their onset characteristics. Assuming adequate medical management of the neurologic cause of aphasia, its natural (i.e., untreated) course is usually thought of as one of sudden or subacute onset, with severity greatest early post-onset, followed by decelerating physiological improvement, ultimately to a point at which the disorder is considered resolved, improving minimally without intervention and thus considered to be in its chronic state.

Until about 18 years ago, most speech-language pathologists and neurologists would have considered aphasia as incompatible with a diagnosis of degenerative central nervous system (CNS) disease. The generally accepted principle was that degenerative neurologic diseases (e.g., Alzheimer's disease, Pick's disease) impair cognitive functions diffusely, and rarely or never in a *focal* or selective way. Thus, any aphasic-like difficulties in individuals with degenerative CNS disease were presumably embedded within a constellation of cognitive difficulties that might include, but always extended beyond, the language domain.

It is now recognized that aphasia can announce the presence of degenerative neurologic disease, and that it may be the only manifestation of CNS disease for a substantial period of time or perpetually. When this happens, the condition is referred to as *primary progressive aphasia* or *PPA*. In this chapter, PPA will be defined, and (a) the criteria for its diagnosis reviewed, (b) its common presenting histories and basic demographics discussed, (c) the characteristics of the aphasia and associated motor speech impairments summarized, (d) common neuroimaging findings and the variety of possible underlying autopsy-based pathologic diagnoses reviewed, and (e) theoretical and philosophical aspects of management

as well as the meager treatment efficacy data will be summarized and discussed.

BASIC DEFINITION AND TERMINOLOGY

We reserve the term aphasia for the deficits of language processing that cross levels or domains of language (semantics, syntax, morphology, phonology) as well as language modalities (listening, reading, writing, talking, and gesturing). These deficits are not attributable to sensory or motor deficits (although they often coexist with such deficits) or to a loss of the representations or rules of the language. They are due to deficits of the cognitive apparatus used to buffer, activate, and inhibit, in precisely timed patterns, the rules and representations of the language. Aphasia, in the absence of other CNS deficits, is caused by relative focal damage to the language dominant hemisphere(s) (usually the left) and is most often (but need not be, and is not in the case in PPA) of sudden onset. However, when language or communication deficits are imbedded within a constellation of other cognitive deficits (e.g., those seen in dementia and in persons with closed brain injury), particularly (but not only) at its onset, it is *not* considered aphasia. The reasons for these inclusion and exclusion criteria are both theoretical and clinical, having implications for epidemiological and other forms of research on prognosis, assessment, and intervention. Although it is beyond the scope of this chapter to discuss aphasia definitions and their inclusionary and exclusionary criteria in detail, such discussions can be found in Darley (1982), McNeil (1988, 1989), and Mesulam (1987). However, in order to use the term *aphasia*, modified by its onset and time-course, evidence is required that other cognitive deficits that cross nonlinguistic specific domains of knowledge, such as procedural memory deficits; altered personality; visual perceptual impairments; altered personal, temporal, or spatial orientation; or psychiatric illness, are not present, or are not accounted for by a single (common) etiology.

Primary progressive aphasia (PPA) can be defined as *aphasia of insidious onset, gradual progression, and prolonged course, without evidence of nonlanguage computational impairments that are shared by a common etiology to the aphasia, and due to a degenerative condition that presumably and predominantly involves*

472

the left (language dominant) perisylvian region of the brain (modified from Duffy, 1987). Because concomitant nonlanguage processing and computational impairments are often (perhaps nearly 50% of the time) revealed in later states of the progressive disorder, the term PPA is used for the aphasic impairments during the time that the concomitant impairments are not manifest. At the point when these impairments are detectable and the criteria for another diagnosis is met (e.g., dementia), the diagnosis changes from one of PPA to one of PPA plus the other disorder (especially if the symptoms are attributable to more than one etiology). In the case of dementia, the diagnosis changes from PPA to dementia, if the language impairment is consistent with its diagnosis. Because aphasia is a behavioral manifestation of neurologic disease, it is important to remember that *PPA is a clinical syndrome and not a reflection of a particular underlying brain pathology.* This principle will be discussed when the underlying histopathology associated with PPA is addressed.

Similar to many clinical disorders, particularly early in the history of their recognition, definition, and study, PPA has had a number of aliases, some of which can be considered synonymous with PPA, others which—under careful scrutiny—probably represent other diagnostic entities. The terms *slowly progressive aphasia* (e.g., Duffy, 1987; Kempler et al., 1990; Kushner, 1990; Poeck & Luzzatti, 1988) and *progressive aphasia without dementia* (e.g., Heath et al., 1983; Mesulam, 1982; Scheltens et al., 1990) probably refer to the same clinical entity as PPA; they seem to have succumbed to PPA as the preferred diagnostic label.[1] In contrast, terms such as *aphasic (or dysphasic) dementia, nonfamilial dysphasic dementia, familial aphasia,* and *hereditary dysphasic dementia* (e.g., Cole et al., 1979; Kobayashi et al., 1990; Mehler, 1988; Morris et al., 1984) may or may not be synonymous with PPA as defined here. At least some of the cases in reports using those labels have had evidence of widespread impairment of cognition early in their course. As discussed above, it should be noted in this context that *PPA does not include patients in whom language impairment or aphasia is just a prominent manifestation of dementia.* It includes only patients in whom aphasia is the only cognitive impairment, or in whom impairment in other cognitive functions is equivocal (or attributable to another etiology) from a formal diagnostic or from a personal or significant other awareness standpoint.[2]

Finally, it is important to recognize that PPA can be considered a subcategory of what are now often referred to as *asymmetric cortical degeneration syndromes* (Caselli, 1995; Caselli & Jack, 1992; Caselli et al., 1992) or *focal cortical atrophy syndromes* (Black, 1996). These labels have emerged with the recognition of a variety of isolated cognitive deficits—such as visual agnosia (e.g., DeRenzi, 1986), prosopagnosia (e.g., Tyrrell et al., 1990), and limb apraxia (e.g., Azouvi et al., 1993; Dick et al., 1989; Piccirilli et al., 1990)—that can be associated with degenerative neurologic disease, of which PPA may be the most common. Caselli (1995) argues for the term *asymmetric*, as opposed to *focal*, because, although these cases may present with a progressing focal neurologic syndrome, more diffuse abnormalities often can eventually be demonstrated clinically and histopathologically.

HISTORIC PERSPECTIVE

Although modern interest in PPA was sparked by a paper by Mesulam in 1982, isolated or relatively isolated progressive language impairment in association with probable or confirmed degenerative neurologic disease seems to have been recognized since the late 1800s. For example, Pick published a paper in 1892 titled "On the relation between aphasia and senile atrophy of the brain." In 1913–14, Mingazzini published a paper titled "On aphasia due to atrophy of the cerebral convolutions." Ironically, Maurice Ravel (1872–1937), whose *Bolero* musically chronicles a slow progression to a climactic conclusion, developed a relatively focal progressive neurological disease at 52 years of age, with prominent aphasia, apraxia, agraphia, alexia, and loss of musical creativity (Henson, 1988). In a review article, Poeck and Luzzatti (1988) identified 19 cases in the literature before 1950 that today might be labeled PPA.

There is no doubt, however, that Mesulam's 1982 summary of six cases with slowly progressive aphasia without other cognitive deficits is the modern seminal work on the topic. It generated interest in PPA in particular, but also in the general concept that a variety of focal cognitive deficits can be associated with degenerative neurologic disease. Since then, many single or multiple case studies have been published, as well as subsequent reviews of their cumulative meaning. For example, Duffy and Petersen (1992) reviewed 54 cases of PPA that were described in 28 papers in the English literature between 1977–90, Mesulam and Weintraub (1992) reviewed 63 cases, Westbury and Bub (1997) summarized 112 cases that have appeared in the English and French literature, and Rogers and Alarcon (1999) reviewed 147 cases from 57 articles. Each of the reviews encompasses those articles and cases included in the earlier reviews, and have included

---

[1] We adhere to the term *primary* modifying the progressive nature of the aphasia with acknowledgment that it is philosophically inconsistent with our criteria for the syndrome's identification. We adhere to this term in order to avoid the advancement of yet another term to describe the emerging literature on this etiologically based category of aphasia. We believe that it is important to recognize that the term does not, in our definition, imply that the aphasic signs and symptoms are simply the most obvious, prevalent, or severe deficit that is accompanied by deficits in other cognitive domains. If other such deficits are validly and reliably identifiable and attributable to a common etiology, then the diagnosis of PPA is probably not appropriate.

[2] We *do* believe it is reasonable to include within the scope of the definition of PPA people in whom neuropsychological examination raises questions about impairment

of cognitive functions beyond the language domain, but in whom there is no such evidence during basic clinical examination, and no complaint of such impairment by the patient or by those with whom the patient is well known.

essentially all published literature since Mesulam's first discussion of the syndrome. Unfortunately, each review interprets admissible and inadmissible cases and aggregates the literature idiosyncratically. Therefore, it is difficult to treat each of these reviews as a systematic accumulation of PPA data. Nonetheless, it is important to examine the cumulative epidemiological evidence to the degree possible. These data are discussed in the Basic Demographics section of this chapter and are summarized in Table 20–2.

There is considerable variability in the degree to which published case studies have met current criteria for the diagnosis of PPA. However, the large number of such cases, and the commonalities among them, are now sufficient to have established that PPA, although representing an uncommon clinical phenomenon, is not an extremely rare one. Today, case presentations that simply support the existence of PPA probably are no longer publishable. Of importance now are studies that improve and refine our understanding of its typical and atypical language manifestations, associated nonlanguage clinical characteristics, clinical course, neuroimaging and other laboratory correlates, histopathology, and responses to behavioral and medical interventions.

DIAGNOSTIC CRITERIA

The criteria for the diagnosis of PPA suggested by Weintraub et al. (1990) seem generally accepted at this time. They include the following: (1) a minimum 2-year history of language decline; (2) prominent language deficits with relative preservation of other mental functions (patients with prominent language deficits in the first 2 years but who also have verifiable memory, attention, or visuospatial deficits would not meet criteria; such patients might meet criteria for a diagnosis of probable Alzheimer's Disease [AD]); (3) independence in activities of daily living; (4) a full neurologic workup has excluded other causes of aphasia (e.g., stroke, tumor, infection, metabolic disturbances); (5) comprehensive speech-language and neuropsychological evaluation have yielded results consistent with the complaint and clinical neurological examination (see footnote #2 in this regard).

While there is some consensus on these criteria for the diagnosis of PPA, some of the assumptions are worthy of discussion. Of particular importance is the 2-year history before a diagnosis of PPA can be made. This criterion has been set in order to reduce the number of false-positive diagnoses of PPA (or the false-negative diagnoses of dementia). The assumption is that an isolated deficit in the domain of language that has endured for a minimum of 2 years will increase the likelihood that the behaviors are not the initial signs of a more general cognitive deficit. In fact, the epidemiological research to support this assumption has not been conducted. In addition, a 2-year hiatus in the diagnosis can delay aphasia management and general life planning. It seems that the diagnosis of PPA can and should be made without regard to the duration of its existence, recognizing that the diagnosis can be altered or discarded at such time that the criteria for PPA are no longer met.

A second assumption imbedded within the diagnostic criteria is that the language deficit is disproportional to any other nonlinguistic deficits (see footnote #1). Again, the degree to which nonlinguistic functions are or are not relatively spared would be the degree to which they meet the criteria for the diagnosis of aphasia. That is, the criteria for the diagnosis of aphasia of any etiology or *type* are the same as those required for the diagnosis of PPA. It is important to remember that the definition of PPA provided here is the definition for these adjectives (i.e., "primary" and "progressive") to aphasia. The definition and criteria for aphasia of any "type" are still required for the valid diagnosis of PPA.

The third assumption of preserved *activities of daily living* (ADL) is included in order to help exclude those persons with cognitive deficits outside of the language domain such as in personality, memory, or attention. Persons with aphasia certainly have deficits of ADL that involve language and communication. In addition, some individuals' reactions to their aphasia can affect ADL outside of the language and communication domains. For example, reactive depression can certainly impair ADL and embarrassment or frustration with failed communicative interactions can dissuade persons with aphasia from participation in a variety of social and familial roles. If reduced ADL is taken at face value as a criterion for rejection of the diagnosis of PPA, it could lead to a decrease in the legitimate diagnosis of PPA and the false-positive diagnosis of dementia. It thus seems appropriate to modify this criterion to permit inclusion of persons with reduced ADL abilities that are a direct or indirect consequence of the aphasia.

A fourth assumption is that the diagnosis of PPA requires a relatively focal or asymmetric degenerative process, one that is progressive and one that is of unknown etiology. It is based on the assumption of an etiology that excludes stroke, tumor, infection, and metabolic disturbances. Stroke is focal, of known etiology, and nonprogressive. Tumor is focal, of known etiology, and progressive. Infection and metabolic disorders may or may not be focally localized, and are of known etiology, and nonprogressive when they are appropriately treated. Table 20–1 summarizes these distinctions.

It has been argued that PPA often is a precursor to generalized dementia or AD, and that it is simply a variant of degenerative diseases that typically present with a broader spectrum of deficits (e.g., Gordon & Selnes, 1984; Poeck & Luzzatti, 1988). The evidence to date suggests that it often is *not* a variant of other degenerative diseases and that it requires a separate diagnosis and management. Regardless of the ultimate outcome in a given case, the early prominence of aphasia and its relative isolation for long periods of time justify its distinction from the typical behavioral characteristics of common dementing illnesses. The people affected by

TABLE 20–1

Aphasia Etiology by Symptom Distribution, Lesion Distribution, Medical Diagnosis, Disease Course, and Medical Treatment

Aphasia Associated With	Symptom Distribution	Lesion Distribution	Neuropathological Diagnosis	Lesion Course	Etiological Treatment
PPA etiologies	Isolated to language only	Focal	Unknown	Progressive	Untreatable
VASCULAR	Typically isolated	Focal	Known	Static (non-progressive)	Some early treatment
INFECTION (BACTERIAL)	Typically general	Focal or diffuse	Known	Progressive until treated	Treatable
INFECTION (VIRAL)	Typically general	Focal or diffuse	Known	Progressive	Untreatable
METABOLIC	Typically general	Focal or diffuse	Known	Progressive until treated	Treatable
TUMOR	Typically isolated	Focal or diffuse	Known	Progressive	Treatable
TRAUMA	Typically general	Focal, Multi-focal, or diffuse	Known	Static	Some early treatment

the disease must cope with a different set of problems than generalized dementia for an extended period of time, the prognosis may be different, the underlying pathology may be different, and management approaches may vary considerably (Duffy & Petersen, 1992).

TYPICAL CLINICAL PRESENTATION

How do people with PPA present clinically? What is their history and how do they behave? Initial diagnosis hinges strongly on answers to these questions, so it is important to recognize typical presenting features.

People with PPA often present clinically many months or a year or more after the onset of language difficulty. Occasionally, they associate the onset with a specific event, giving the onset a superficially acute appearance; in such cases, more often than not, the event was one with significant language demands or psychological stress (e.g., giving a group presentation). Most frequently, however, the *onset is insidious*, and the patient and family are often vague or even disagree about when symptoms first appeared. Unlike people with AD, however, those with PPA often are aware of the problem before their family, friends, or work colleagues are.

Presenting *speech and language complaints can be strikingly similar to those of people with stroke-induced aphasia*. The classic refrain of the person with aphasia that "I know what I want to say but I can't find the words!" is heard commonly as the initial symptom and primary complaint. Westbury and Bub (1997) reported that word-finding difficulty was the most common presenting complaint among the 112 cases of PPA they reviewed.[3]

People with *PPA rarely deny their deficits.* In fact, *they are the ones who usually initiate the search for diagnosis and treatment*, rather than their families. They *do not complain of memory disturbances* outside the verbal domain, and they are *not disoriented*. They and their significant others *do not report significant personality changes*, although *expressions or frank evidence of frustration and reactive depression are common*. If work demands are not language based, *job performance can be unchanged. Daily routine activities* (e.g., grooming, driving, shopping, exercising, and record keeping) *are typically unaffected*. Conversely, if language demands for job performance or daily routine activities (e.g., reading, writing, and calculations for record keeping) are high, especially those involving rapid or large-capacity language processing and extemporaneous production and comprehension, difficulty with job performance or routine daily activities can be the initial situations that reveal early signs or symptoms.

To summarize, the initial clinical presentation of people with PPA can be strikingly different from those with AD or other degenerative diseases that induce diffuse impairments of memory, thinking, organization, self-awareness, personality, and ability to succeed in routine social, self-care, and work activities. Conversely, they can be strikingly similar to stroke-induced and other *static* etiologies for aphasia.

---

[3] This complaint alone may not assist differential diagnosis, however, because it is also a common presenting complaint in patients with probable AD.

CHARACTER OF THE APHASIA

It appears that any *type* of aphasia is possible in PPA. The types reported in the literature include fluent and non-fluent, Broca's, Wernicke's, anomic, and transcortical types (e.g., Karbe et al., 1993; Kertesz et al., 1998; Turner et al., 1996). Even pure word deafness has been reported (Mesulam, 1982; Otsuki et al., 1998; Philbrick et al., 1994). Published case reports before 1990 suggested that the aphasia in PPA was most often fluent, anomic, or Wernicke-like, with only about 20% of patients described as nonfluent or Broca-like (Duffy & Petersen, 1992). However, since 1990, nonfluent aphasia seems to be considered by some to be a prominent hallmark of the syndrome (e.g., Kirshner & Bakar, 1995). It is unlikely that there has been a true shift over time in the distribution of aphasia types associated with PPA. The change more probably reflects stricter adherence to criteria for diagnosis of PPA, or publication bias. For example, it is likely that nonfluent cases are diagnostically more convincing as representing isolated language impairment because language impairment in clinically probable AD, at least in its earlier stages, is typically fluent (Weintraub et al., 1990). Another possibility is that clinicians and editors recently have been more inclined to report nonfluent aphasia as unique simply because the earlier descriptions of PPA were weighted to people with fluent verbal characteristics. Only when large series of patients are reported, using strict diagnostic criteria, will the *true* characterization of the aphasia in PPA be established.

BASIC DEMOGRAPHICS

Gender Ratio and Age of Onset

Table 20–2 summarizes the reviews of Duffy and Petersen (1992), Westbury and Bub (1997), and Rogers and Alarcon (1999). From these reviews it is apparent that more men than women are affected, with an approximate 2:1 male to female ratio (Duffy & Petersen, 1992; Westbury & Bub, 1997). It also appears that the age of onset of PPA is highly variable, covering nearly all adult years, but onset is most often sometime between 40 and 75, with average age of onset across reviews converging on 60.5 years (Duffy & Petersen, 1992; Rogers & Alarcon, 1999; Westbury & Bub, 1997).

Ages of Aphasia Onset and Other Cognitive Deficits

Among the cases reported in the literature, the duration from onset of symptoms of aphasia to the emergence of more widespread impairment of cognitive functions, when they do occur, has varied from 1 to more than 15 years,[4] with an average duration across reviews of 5 years. Duffy and Petersen's (1992) review found that approximately 50% of persons with PPA eventually developed nonaphasic cognitive impairments. Rogers and Alarcon's (1999) review reported that an overall average of 45.7% (46.8% averaged across reviews) progressed to nonaphasic cognitive impairments. There is, however, a growing sentiment that, although many patients have isolated language symptoms for an average of about 5 years after onset, and for as long as 15 years, the great majority will eventually experience symptoms in areas such as memory, personality, or mood (Green et al., 1990). Many of the exceptions, especially when onset is later in life, may be those who succumb to unrelated, acute, or more rapidly progressive conditions (e.g., heart attack, carcinoma, stroke) before the PPA advances to affect other cognitive functions.

Life Expectancy From PPA Onset

Although relatively few cases have been reported, the evidence summarized by Rogers and Alarcon (1999) suggests that the average age of death for persons with PPA is 67.4 years, with a 7.6-year standard deviation and a range from 48 to 84 years. The difference between the number of years of isolated language symptoms preceding the onset of nonlinguistic cognitive deficits and the average time from symptom onset to death is 2.4 years. This duration represents the average time from onset of general cognitive deficits to death. However, this duration spans the considerable range of 1 to 17 years.

Prognostic Factors: The "Fluency" Dimension

The problems with the subclassification of PPA are those that are also present for classification of aphasia with sudden onset (Darley, 1982; McNeil, 1982, 1988; Schwartz, 1984). Specifically, the problem with using fluency or nonfluency as valid adjectives for aphasia is that they (1) are without theoretical motivation as a descriptor of language pathology, (2) are not assigned by a set of uniform criteria across users (e.g., compare the criteria for their assignment on the AAT, the WAB, and the BDAE) and have been found to be unreliably assigned to patients (Trupe, 1984), and (3) as typically applied, are more likely the result of concomitant sensorimotor speech pathologies (dysarthria or apraxia of speech) than the result of a language-specific impairment.

With the above formidable caveats, PPA reported with nonfluent verbal output characteristics (i.e., Broca's aphasia, agrammatism or telegraphic speech, brief and unelaborated

---

[4]Cases of less than 2 years' duration would not meet the Mesulam and Weintraub criteria for a diagnosis of PPA and, if embraced on initial evaluation, might be labeled as having "possible PPA." However, as stated, the diagnosis of PPA is best made on the

coherence of both inclusionary criteria for aphasia of any type, and exclusionary criteria for the disorders with which it is most likely confused (e.g., dementia, conversion disorder).

TABLE 20–2

Demography/Epidemiology of PPA

	Mean	Range	Standard Deviation
Age of Onset (Yrs)	Late 50s[1,2]	40–70[1,2]	
Fluent Aphasia	56.8[3]	40–69[3]	7.1[3]
Nonfluent Aphasia	62[3]	40–81[3]	8.5[3]
"Undetermined" Aphasia	62.6[3]	17–81[3]	13.2[3]
Average	60.5[3]	17–81	9.6[3]
Gender Ratio (M:F)	~2:1[1,2]		
Duration of Isolated Language Signs & Symptoms to Onset of Cognitive Impairment or Death (Yrs)			
Fluent Aphasia	5.6[3]	2–20[3]	3.9[3]
Nonfluent Aphasia	4.8[3]	1.5–14[3]	2.5[3]
"Undetermined" Aphasia	4.8[3]	1.5–11[3]	3.0[3]
Average	5.1[3]	1.5–20[3]	3.1[3]
Duration of Isolated Language Signs & Symptoms to Onset of Cognitive Impairment (Yrs)	5.3[1]	1–15[1]	
Fluent Aphasia	6.6[3]	6–9[3]	
Nonfluent Aphasia	4.3[3]	1.5–14[3]	
"Undetermined" Aphasia	3.7[3]	1.5–11[3]	
Average (across reports)	5.0	1–15	
Percentage Progressing to Nonaphasic Cognitive Impairment	50[1]		
Fluent Aphasia	27[3]		
Nonfluent Aphasia	37[3]		
"Undetermined" Aphasia	73[3]		
Average (across reports)	46.8		
Average Time From Symptom Onset to Death (Yrs)[5]			
Fluent Aphasia	8.8[3]	4–17[3]	
Nonfluent Aphasia	6.8[3]	3–13[3]	
"Undetermined" Aphasia	6.5[3]	3–12[3]	
Average	7.4[3]	3–17[3]	
Average Age at Death			
Fluent Aphasia	65.1[3]	62–67[3]	2.0[3]
Nonfluent Aphasia	68.4[3]	48–84[3]	9.9[3]
"Undetermined" Aphasia	69.0[3]	58–84[3]	11.0[3]
Average	67.4[3]	48–84[3]	7.6[3]

[1] Duffy & Petersen (1992)
[2] Westbury & Bub (1997)
[3] Rogers & Alarcon (1999)
[4] These data were computed from those presented by Rogers & Alarcon (1999). These data include those individuals who remained aphasic only and those that progressed to a diagnosis of dementia. The reader should interpret these and the other data reported here cautiously, as they are based on a retrospective analysis of published reports and on small subject samples.

verbal expression, hesitant and/or aprosodic speech) deserves some special comment because it is generally *unexpected* in the earlier stages of probable AD. In addition, its demographics, localization, and causes may differ from PPA associated without these spoken output characteristics (by default, usually termed *fluent*). For example, Black (1996) suggests that nonfluent PPA tends to progress from the perisylvian region in an anterior direction and is usually associated with "frontotemporal degeneration," a non-AD pathologic condition characterized by spongioform degeneration with gliosis and neuronal loss, sometimes with Pick cells and bodies. Clinically, Duffy and Petersen's (1992) review found that persons described as nonfluent or having Broca's aphasia tended to be younger as a group than those described as fluent. However, as summarized in Table 20–2, Rogers and Alarcon (1999) reported a 62-year average age of onset for persons with *nonfluent* aphasia as compared with 56.8 for *fluent* and 62.6 for unclassified patients. Duffy and Petersen (1992) also reported that the *nonfluent* group tended to have a longer duration of their aphasia before spread to other cognitive functions; however, Rogers and Alarcon's (1999) analysis suggests that the *fluent* group has a 2.3-year longer duration than the *nonfluent* group before the spread to other cognitive functions when a spread does occur. Duffy and Petersen also noted that, at the time, there were fewer autopsied cases of people with *nonfluent* PPA, raising the possibility that survival duration is longer in the *nonfluent* subgroup.[5] Again, the Rogers and Alarcon's (1999) analysis suggests that the *fluent* group had a 2-year longer survival rate than the *nonfluent* group from symptom onset to death.

It seems that distinguishing among persons with and without concurrent speech and language production (e.g., agrammatic or motor speech) impairments and aphasia could be relevant to the demographics of resistance to nonaphasic cognitive impairment, survival, etiology, and perhaps, response to management efforts. It is essential, however, that such distinctions be made on the basis of careful definitions and descriptions of what constitutes *fluent* and *nonfluent* and other types of aphasia, and with the recognition that many, if not most patients probably do not fit neatly into any single category. As will be discussed in following sections, it is also important—perhaps more important—to distinguish among aphasia, apraxia of speech, and dysarthria in studies of PPA.

DEFICITS THAT MAY ACCOMPANY PPA

Other neurologic signs and symptoms can accompany PPA. Dysarthria, dysphagia, right central facial droop or weakness, nonverbal oral apraxia (NVOA), and sometimes, right extremity weakness or clumsiness, may be evident (e.g., Fuh et al., 1994; Kavrie & Duffy, 1994; McNeil, 1998). In addition to apraxia of speech (AOS) and NVOA, limb apraxia may be present, either bilaterally or in the right upper extremity alone. Extrapyramidal (basal ganglia) deficits such as rigidity have also been reported (Duffy & Petersen, 1992). In their review, Rogers and Alarcon (1999) summarize reported

concomitant deficits such as agnosia, depression, hearing loss, and stuttering and diseases such as corticobasal degeneration, corticonigral degeneration, and motor neuron disease.

NEUROIMAGING CORRELATES

The neurologic workup of persons with possible PPA is similar to that for most patients with suspected degenerative CNS diseases such as AD. The results of neuroimaging studies that are conducted as part of such workups are sometimes normal, supporting conclusions that the disorder does not stem from stroke, tumor, or other conditions known to cause focal lesions. In other cases, neuroimaging may identify lateralized, bilateral, or diffuse changes.

In a retrospective study of 13 patients with PPA, Sinnatamby et al. (1996) concluded that MRI and SPECT are the imaging modalities of choice for a neuroradiologic evaluation for patients with suspected PPA. MRI is sensitive to atrophy in the temporal neocortex, and SPECT can reveal functional abnormalities before the appearance of atrophy. This conclusion is supported in the reviews of Duffy and Petersen (1992) and Westbury and Bub (1997). Duffy and Petersen (1992) reported that, in cases for which EEG was conducted, 55% were normal, 18% had bilateral or diffuse abnormalities, 9% had predominant left hemisphere abnormalities, and 18% had left hemisphere abnormalities only. CT scans were normal in 28%, 11% were diffusely abnormal, 21% had left-greater-than-right abnormalities, and 40% had left hemisphere abnormalities only. MRI was normal in 42%, showed left-greater-than-right abnormalities in 17%, and 42% had left hemisphere abnormalities only. Similarly, Westbury and Bub (1997) found that 56% of patients with abnormalities on MRI had left hemisphere abnormalities only, with the remainder having bilateral abnormalities; the left hemisphere abnormalities were most often in the Sylvian fissure or temporal lobe. Of the few patients (12) in the Duffy and Petersen (1992) review who had SPECT or PET, all showed left hemisphere hypoperfusion. Westbury and Bub (1997) reported that 97% of their patients with PPA who underwent PET or SPECT had abnormalities, and that 69% of the abnormalities were in the left hemisphere only; the remaining 31% were bilateral. Most of the left hemisphere abnormalities were in the temporal and/or frontal lobe.

Recently, Abe et al. (1997), in a study of five patients with PPA, reported that clinical signs of nonfluent aphasia were associated with MRI and SPECT evidence of left frontal and perisylvian atrophy, whereas clinical signs of fluent aphasia were associated with left superior, middle, and inferior temporal gyri, hippocampus, and parahippocampal gyrus atrophy. In addition, Anderson et al. (1997) reported that six patients with asymmetric temporal lobe atrophy and progressive Wernicke's aphasia deteriorated over a 6-year

---

[5] For a possible exception, see the report of McNeil et al. (1995) who described the case of a patient with PPA with concomitant spastic dysarthria without other motor impairments, whose survival from onset to death was less than 3 years. This report also highlights the importance of accurate differential diagnosis of the speech production impairments that are often used to classify the "nonfluency."

period, developed frontal lobe dysfunction, and eventually, bilateral temporal lobe atrophy and dementia. When abnormalities were bilateral, they most often involved the frontal lobe.

For patients with a clinical diagnosis of PPA it thus appears that neuroimaging studies, when abnormal, tend to show left hemisphere abnormalities or left-greater-than-right hemisphere abnormalities. The fact that a substantial number of patients have bilateral abnormalities suggests that their underlying disease is not confined to the left hemisphere, even if their clinical syndrome is at the time of assessment. This finding tends to support the contention that PPA and related syndromes may best be thought of as asymmetric rather than focal diseases. As the current best estimates suggest that only about 50% of the reported patients with PPA progress in signs and symptoms to those compatible with the diagnosis of dementia, it will be important in future research to determine whether those with anatomic and physiologic evidence of bilateral disease are those that eventually progress to such a diagnosis and those with left hemisphere disease only are those that remain aphasic only.

HISTOLOGIC PATHOLOGY

There have been only a few case reports with autopsy results for people with PPA. The numbers are sufficient, however, to support a conclusion that PPA can be associated with a variety of pathologic diagnoses. In a sense, this is not surprising because anatomic localization and not histopathology determine the clinical manifestations of neuropathologic processes. Thus, the pathologic heterogeneity associated with PPA suggests that it can be caused by several disease entities whose initial or prominent effects happen to be, for unexplained reasons, located in and shared with those in the areas of the brain that when affected result in language processing deficits consistent in pattern and specificity with aphasia.

PPA has been reported in people with autopsy-confirmed pathologic diagnoses of AD (e.g., Engel & Fleming, 1997; Green et al., 1996; Kempler et al., 1990) and Pick's disease (e.g., Craenhals et al., 1990; Fukui et al., 1996; Graff-Radford et al., 1990; Holland et al., 1985), clinical conditions typically associated with significant cognitive, memory, or personality disturbances. However, these do not represent a majority of the autopsied cases (Westbury & Bub, 1997), and it seems clear that the great majority of patients with PPA will not have a histologic diagnosis of AD (Mesulam et al., 1997).

Of interest, PPA has also been associated with autopsy-confirmed pathologic diagnoses of corticobasal degeneration (CBD), progressive supranuclear palsy (PSP), amyotrophic lateral sclerosis (ALS), corticonigral degeneration, and Creutzfelt-Jakob (CJD) disease (e.g., Arima et al., 1994; Mandell et al., 1989; Sakurai et al., 1996; Shuttelworth

et al., 1985; Yamanuchi et al., 1986),[6] all of whose common clinical characteristics include motor disturbances. The descriptions of the speech and language characteristics of these cases are quite variable, but a number of them were reported to have had *nonfluent* verbal output characteristics and AOS, frequently with an accompanying dysarthria.

Perhaps the most frequent autopsy findings in PPA are of cellular changes that do not correspond to well-known specific clinical or pathologic conditions. Histopathology for a number of PPA cases includes entities such as focal spongioform degeneration (e.g., Kirshner et al., 1987; Scholten et al., 1995; Schwartz et al., 1998), focal neuronal achromasia (e.g., Lippa et al., 1991), nonspecific cortical degeneration (e.g., Scheltens et al., 1994; Scholten et al., 1995), and "dementia lacking specific histology" (e.g., Turner et al., 1996). Turner et al. (1996) concluded from the autopsy findings of three patients with *nonfluent* PPA, plus a review of the literature, that the most common pathology underlying *nonfluent* PPA is dementia lacking specific pathology. This general conclusion was also reached in a *Primary Progressive Aphasia Newsletter* (Informational Topic, 1996) published by the Memory Disorders Research Core at Northwestern University. It reported that approximately 60% of the pathology in patients with PPA shows nonspecific focal degeneration with spongioform changes and gliosis. Approximately 20% of patients were reported to have AD and approximately 20% had Pick's disease. Westbury and Bub's (1997) review indicated that Pick's disease represented about 13% of cases and AD, 19% of cases. Thirty-eight percent of all autopsied cases showed spongioform changes, some also with neuronal loss.

Kertesz and colleagues (Kertesz, 1997; Kertesz et al., 1994; Kertesz & Munoz, 1997) have proposed that the common pathology underlying PPA belongs to disorders captured by the concept of *Pick complex*. This generic concept includes neurodegenerative diseases associated with focal cortical degeneration such as PPA, frontal lobe dementia, and corticonigral and corticobasal degeneration.

Finally, little is known about the possible genetic basis or risk factors for PPA. However, a recent study by Mesulam et al. (1997) reported apolipoprotein E genotyping results for 12 patients with PPA. This was pursued because the E4 allele is a risk factor for AD, so it provided an opportunity to determine if PPA shares a risk factor with AD. The pattern of allele distribution in PPA patients was different than that found for patients with a clinical diagnosis of probable AD, or a histologic diagnosis of AD, and was similar to that of control patients. As a result, the authors concluded that these findings provide neurobiologic support for the clinical distinction between PPA and probable AD, in agreement

---

[6]Because most patients with CJD die within 2 years, they would not meet the Mesulam and Weintraub (1992) criteria for PPA diagnosis. Regardless, it is important to recognize that a progressive aphasia can announce the presence of CJD.

with evidence that most patients with PPA do not have the histopathology of AD.

PRIMARY PROGRESSIVE APRAXIA OF SPEECH (PPAOS)

Because apraxia of speech is often, and perhaps always, a component of the syndrome of Broca's aphasia (McNeil & Kent, 1990), it is reasonable to ask if its presence in PPA is important to factors such as emergence of nonlanguage cognitive impairments, survival, etiology, or management. AOS also is of interest because progressive AOS, in the absence of aphasia and nonaphasic cognitive impairment, has been reported in the literature and encountered by the authors frequently enough to tentatively label such occurrences as *primary progressive AOS*, or *PPAOS*. PPAOS can be defined tentatively as *AOS of insidious onset, gradual progression, and prolonged course, in the absence of nonlanguage cognitive impairments, and sometimes in the absence of aphasia, for a substantial period of time or perpetually, due to a degenerative condition that presumably involves the left hemisphere's apparatus for translating the phonologic aspects of language into the learned kinematic parameters necessary for their expression through speech.*[7]

There are only a small number of published case reports of what does or may represent PPAOS (e.g., Broussolle et al., 1996; Chapman et al., 1997; Cohen et al., 1993; Fukui et al., 1996; Hart et al., 1997; Tyrrell et al., 1991). It is possible, however, that in nearly 20% of the PPA cases that have been reported (i.e., cases described as *nonfluent* or Broca's aphasia), patients have had AOS, and perhaps no aphasia at all, as we define aphasia and AOS.

Chapman et al. (1997) recently presented the case of a person with a 6-year history of progressive motor speech difficulty that included AOS and hypokinetic dysarthria in the absence of aphasia or dementia, and a strong family history of similar difficulties suggestive of an autosomal dominant pattern of inheritance. They argued that the isolated involvement of motor speech processes is distinguishable from both PPA and the dementia of AD, and that the small number of such single cases in the literature may reflect a failure to properly distinguish between the processes of speech and language. Thus, a number of patients labeled as having PPA may actually have had a motor speech problem without true language processing impairment.

Further support for the existence of PPAOS comes from Kavrie and Duffy (1994), who summarized the cases of eight patients seen at the Mayo Clinic over a 7-year period who had a progressive AOS. Six of the eight were also dysarthric; five had no evidence of aphasia, and the remaining three had only equivocal evidence of aphasia. All of their

patients had an obvious nonverbal oral apraxia. Similarly, Broussolle et al. (1996) summarized the cases of eight patients who had what they called a slowly progressive speech production deficit that included "speech apraxia," orofacial apraxia, dysarthria, and dysprosody, but without deficits in language or nonlanguage cognitive abilities. Neuroimaging findings demonstrated left-greater-than-right frontal lobe abnormalities, predominantly in the posterior inferior frontal region. Finally, and anecdotally, one of the authors (JRD) has now seen more than 35 patients whose predominant symptom of degenerative neurologic disease has been AOS. A majority of them also were dysarthric (most often hypokinetic and/or spastic), and the dysarthria was often as severe as the AOS. A majority also were aphasic, but the AOS always was more prominent than the aphasia in this group.

It may be that PPAOS should be considered another variant of the asymmetric cortical degeneration syndromes (Broussolle et al., 1996). Similar to PPA, it may herald more specific neurologic diseases. It is unlikely to represent a single neurologic disease. However, it has been our observation that when it is prominent and is accompanied by significant dysarthria, it tends to progress in a direction that results in clinical diagnoses with prominent motor (e.g., PSP, CBD, ALS) rather than cognitive manifestations. Whether these clinical diagnoses reliably predict ultimate histologic diagnosis remains to be determined.

The distinction between PPAOS and PPA may be relevant to prognosis and possibly management, especially if it is found to have predictive value relative to underlying histopathology. That is, decisions about medical/pharmacological management often depend on relative certainty or predictions about the ultimate clinical or pathologic diagnosis. As a result, existing or future pharmacological treatments for probable AD likely will be different than those for PSP, ALS, and other degenerative sensorimotor disorders.

MANAGEMENT OF PPA

As with all intervention for aphasia, the consideration of treatment for PPA requires both philosophical and scientific inspection. This inspection has taken the form of a number of frequently asked questions. Duffy (1988) asked: 1) Should persons with PPA receive speech-language services at all? 2) If the answer to the first question is affirmative, under what conditions should treatment be given? 3) What should be the nature of the management efforts? 4) What are the criteria for success? To these queries we might ask what there is about PPA that is similar to or different from other forms of aphasia treatment and what there is about it that would require different criteria for intervention initiation, treatment type, and expected or acceptable consequences to the treatment.

---

[7]The reader is referred to McNeil et al. (1997) for a detailed definition and discussion of the nature of AOS.

Once the theoretical/philosophical definition of what aphasia is and is not has been answered, we can begin to address the questions raised above that make the progressive form different from a *static* or nonprogressive form of aphasia. If the fundamental definition of aphasia is the same (as we have argued that it must be, or the diagnosis is incorrect), then it is only the progressive nature of the disorder that demands our differential consideration for treatment implementation. That is, does the progressive nature of the disorder obviate the consideration of treatment? If it does, it would be a rare exception among progressive disorders of speech and language that is not considered for intervention simply because of its degenerative nature. Likewise, the life expectancy of the individual has been raised as an issue in the decision to initiate treatment, especially for degenerative disorders. It seems to us that a decision to initiate or withhold treatment based only on the duration of life expectancy is ethically indefensible. On these bases alone, the question of whether PPA should be exempt from treatment consideration can be dismissed. Therefore, the question becomes one of whether the patient under consideration has the motivation, financial and other (e.g., transportation) resources, level of linguistic and other cognitive mechanisms (e.g., attention and memory), and the potential for language and communication learning and maintenance necessary to support the type of treatment to be initiated. When these determinations have been made, secondary questions can be asked about the potential to benefit from the specific intervention procedure, and the process or treatment milieu for specific and well-defined treatment goals.

To our knowledge, the treatment data (administered under experimental conditions that allow the examination of its efficacy) for only two patients with PPA have been published (McNeil et al., 1995; Schneider et al., 1996). One other uncontrolled case study (Murray, 1998) describes a sequence of treatments administered to one person with PPA, and a book chapter (Rogers et al., In Press) describes the rationale and a detailed plan for the treatment of persons with PPA. The experimental data are of course too limited to provide guidance for the treatment of subsequent patients. However, what has become apparent from these experiments and from the treatment pundits is that the same array of treatment options remains available to persons with PPA as to those persons with nonprogressive aphasia. To the degree that this is true, it also is apparent that these options are in large measure governed by the same clinical and theoretical considerations and biases. That is, whether treatment potential is determined by an assessment of the patient's activity limitations and restrictions in social participatory roles alone, or whether it is based on the evaluation of the presumed underlying mechanisms for the communication disorder (impairment level assessment), represents a major clinical/theoretical bias. Likewise, the type of intervention selected, in great measure, is determined by this bias. Other issues involve the commitment to treat areas of deficit in order to improve them temporarily or to maintain them as long as possible, or alternatively to direct intervention toward the expected decline in abilities with augmentative/alternative communication as the goal and the method. Each of these considerations and biases can be found among the publications reviewed below.

McNeil et al. (1995) published the first experimental attempt to assess the efficacy of treatment for a person with PPA. They evaluated the effects of treatment directed to dysnomia, the primary sign and symptom in a patient with PPA of recent onset. The patient presented with mild spastic dysarthria, nonverbal oral apraxia, aphasia that crossed all modalities and levels of language, and no apraxia of speech. In the context of a single-subject multiple-baseline design, data were derived that demonstrated improved word-finding ability when that was the focus of treatment (Lexical-Semantic Activation Inhibition Treatment; L-SAIT), declines in language abilities that were not treated, and stable nonlanguage cognitive performance. The most effective treatment for the patient was a combination of behavioral treatment plus dextroamphetamine. Although this particular patient's course of degeneration was atypically short, and dominated toward its end by severe spastic dysarthria and dysphagia, the impairment-focused treatment was efficacious and bolstered the patient's interpersonal and intrapersonal communication for some time. While generalization to untreated and progressively deteriorating areas of language performance were evidenced to some degree, secondary benefits of treatment were observed. During the periods in which he was receiving treatment, he had an additional purpose and goal for his life and his otherwise unfilled time. Though of no obvious consequence to his life expectancy, his demonstrated improvements in language and communication gave him a sense of control that was not available to him in other areas of his life. This benefit was acquired with full knowledge that his treatment would not retard the progressive disease underlying his aphasia. Augmentative communication was not an acceptable modality to this patient, and other potential forms of treatment became unreasonable due to the rapid progression of his underlying disease.

Also in the context of a single-subject experimental multiple-baseline design, Schneider et al. (1996) presented data for a person with PPA demonstrating that oral and oral plus gestural training of verb tense were learned and generalized to untreated verbs within tense, but not across tenses. This impairment-level–directed treatment for agrammatism using gestural plus oral responding resulted in higher levels of correct oral sentence production than did verbal responding alone. Although generalization to untreated areas of language and communication was not robust, the gestural responding was generalized and was maintained for a 3-month period following the withdrawal of treatment. This maintenance was achieved in the context of declines in other language functions.

Murray (1998) presented a detailed case study (without experimental control) describing a series of treatments administered to a single subject with *nonfluent* PPA. The patient presented 1 year post-onset of self-described "stuttering," with the complaint of increased "slurring" of speech and word-finding difficulties. Although impaired across all modalities, the patient's progressing deficits during the course of treatment were characterized by agrammatism, anomia, phonemic paraphasia, apraxia of speech, and auditory comprehension deficits. Treatment was first administered over an 11-month period and was directed at her auditory and reading comprehension. It was described as consisting of "traditional stimulus-response activities which were designed to stimulate and facilitate...". The second treatment involved 24 1-hour sessions over a 4-month period and used the "back to the drawing board" program (Morgan & Helm-Estabrooks, 1987), a treatment that involves drawing pictures for communicative purposes and claims to be both an alternative communication method and a deblocker of speaking and writing. The third treatment involved both individual and aphasia support group treatment. Individual treatment in this phase "focused on improving communication interactions between D.D. and her spouse" and involved identifying turn-taking and repair skills. The patient also was trained and appeared to use an augmentative communication device (Dyna Vox), though with poor situational generalization.

Although the lack of experimental control in this case study obviates the attribution of any change to the treatments that were administered, it clearly describes the change of treatment focus and technique as the patient's signs and symptoms changed over the course of her language processing decline. This changing sequence of treatment goals and methods may represent the most common practice in the treatment of aphasia of any etiology. In order for this to represent a generalizable model for best practice in the planning and implementation of intervention for PPA, it will require the same level of evidence as for the treatment of aphasia of any etiology. It does, however, illustrate the apparent frequently used and perhaps necessary adaptations of treatment goals and methods that follow careful observation of patient change that accompanies any efficacious treatment.

Rogers et al. (in press) present a detailed description of *proactive management* for PPA that they believe will minimize activity limitations and participation restrictions as well as maximize communication competence as speech and language decline. This is accomplished by "...early intervention focused on the development and training of augmentative and alternative communication (AAC)." In addition to the early training in AAC, patient and family education and family/partner intervention is advocated, with particular attention being paid to activity and participation limitations in both patient assessment and treatment planning and implementation. It is the inherent

assumption of this approach that AAC is both an efficacious method of treatment for aphasia and the inevitable treatment modality for persons with PPA. In terms of evidence-based practice, neither of these assumptions stands on firm ground. AAC treatment efficacy and effectiveness data for aphasia are essentially nonexistent. Additionally, aphasia patient compliance data, an issue in AAC training for all communication disorders, is in need of verification and perhaps improvement.

It seems clear to us that Rogers et al's (in press) call for assessment of PPA that de-emphasizes the understanding of the nature of the impairment (for treatment planning purposes) and shifts it toward the individual's communication needs, partners, and environments, and that prescribes the early initiation of AAC as the target of treatment, is potentially problematic or at the least premature. One problem is that it may be destined to nonacceptance from a substantial segment of the PPA patient population. A second problem is that this approach neglects the potential to improve and/or maintain specific language processing functions that underlie both the interpersonal and intrapersonal communication deficits (and consequently communicative and other activities and participatory limitations) for a substantive period of time. That is, it neglects the fact that many, if not most patients with PPA decline at a rate and at a level sufficient to support and maintain independent language and communication skills, supporting communicative activity and social participation for many years. It may be that planning for AAC may be on firmer ground when the progressive disorder is motor in nature (PPAOS or dysarthria) or when PPA is accompanied by a progressive motor speech impairment. It seems to us a much more rational and palatable approach, depending on the rate of decline and the impairment level of the patient, to direct treatment at the hypothesized deficits, at compensatory strategies, at psychosocial concomitants of the disorder, at environmental influences (e.g., significant others and caregivers), and when communicatively appropriate, accepted by the patient, and trained before their use is necessary, at augmentative and alternative communication systems. One difference between the management of persons with PPA and those of aphasia with a more static course is the need for clear patient and family education and counseling that emphasizes the progressive nature of this disorder. As with other etiologies, counseling that spans the course of the treatment and the accompanying patient and family changes is essential.

Similar to these treatment recommendations, Thompson (PPA Newsletter, 1997) provided the following useful guidelines for the treatment of PPA: (1) Early speech-language-cognitive evaluation is important, as are frequent follow-ups to establish the pattern of decline. (2) Early treatment may focus on impaired functions but be adjusted as decline occurs. (3) AAC should be introduced early, when they most easily learn them, to be used as the need arises. (4) Family members/significant others must be involved—to enhance awareness of successful strategies and to practice with the patient. (5) Treatment will not reverse progression of the disease, but may enhance communication ability.

In summary, there is no a priori theoretical or philosophical reason to withhold language and communication treatment from persons with PPA if the usual criteria for treatment candidacy are met. It is, however, too early in the accumulation of scientific evidence to determine whether treatment for persons with PPA is predictably efficacious and whether it will follow the same principles of management as aphasia resulting from other etiologies and of other natural courses. It has been demonstrated that persons with PPA can improve on language and communication tasks with impairment-directed treatments that are typical of and efficacious for persons with *static* aphasia. It is reasonable but untested as to whether persons with PPA can learn, will use if learned, and will benefit from augmentative and alternative communication devices. Patient and family counseling and communication training are likely integral parts to any successful aphasia regimen.

KEY POINTS

1. Aphasia of insidious onset, gradual progression, and prolonged course, without evidence of nonlanguage computational impairments, and due to a degenerative condition that presumably and predominantly involves the language dominant perisylvian region of the brain, is known as primary progressive aphasia (PPA). The criteria for the diagnosis of aphasia of any etiology or type are the same as those required for the diagnosis of PPA. The disorder does not include patients in whom language impairment is just a prominent manifestation of dementia. PPA is a clinical syndrome and not a reflection of a particular underlying brain pathology.

2. Currently applied criteria for the diagnosis of PPA include a minimum of a 2-year history of language decline; prominent language deficits with relative preservation of other mental functions; independence in activities of daily living, a full neurologic workup that has excluded other causes of aphasia; comprehensive speech-language and neuropsychological evaluation that has yielded results consistent with the complaint; and clinical neurological examination. It should be noted that the 2-year history criterion is somewhat arbitrary—a working diagnosis of PPA may be justified without regard to duration of the aphasia. In addition, reduced ADL that can be explained by the aphasia should not preclude a diagnosis of PPA.

3. The initial clinical presentation of people with PPA can be very different from that of people with Alzheimer's Disease (AD) or other degenerative diseases that induce diffuse cognitive impairments. It can be strikingly similar to stroke-induced and other static etiologies for aphasia, with the exception of its temporal course.

4. More men than women have PPA. Age of onset is highly variable but averages about 60 years. The duration from onset of aphasia symptoms to the emergence of more widespread impairment of cognitive functions is also highly variable but averages about 5 years. About 45% of patients with reported cases have eventually developed nonaphasic cognitive impairments, but an emerging general consensus is that the great majority eventually experience symptoms in areas such as memory, personality, or mood if they live long enough.

5. Apraxia of speech, nonverbal oral apraxia, dysarthria, dysphagia, right central facial droop or weakness, right extremity weakness or clumsiness, rigidity, agnosia, and depression have been reported in persons with PPA.

6. MRI and SPECT are commonly used for the neuroradiologic evaluation of people with PPA. When abnormal, they tend to show left hemisphere abnormalities or left-greater-than-right hemisphere abnormalities.

7. PPA can be associated with a variety of specific histopathologic diagnoses, including AD, corticobasal degeneration, progressive supranuclear palsy, motor neuron disease, and Creutzfelt-Jakob disease. However, perhaps the most frequent autopsy findings are of cellular changes that do not correspond to well-known specific clinical or pathologic conditions (e.g., nonspecific focal degeneration with spongiform changes and gliosis, nonspecific cortical degeneration). Most patients with PPA will not have a histologic diagnosis of AD.

8. Apraxia of speech (AOS) may be the initial, only, or prominent manifestation of degenerative neurologic disease. Similar to PPA, it may herald more specific neurologic diseases, and is unlikely to represent a single neurologic disease. Distinguishing between a progressive AOS and PPA may be relevant to prognosis, management, and perhaps underlying histopathology.

9. Efficacy and outcome data regarding management of PPA are very limited but there are no a priori theoretical or philosophical reasons to withhold language and communication treatment from persons with PPA if the usual criteria for treatment candidacy are met.

10. It is premature to draw conclusions about whether treatment for persons with PPA is generally effective, but it has been demonstrated that some affected persons can improve on language and communication tasks with impairment-directed treatments that

are typical of and efficacious for persons with static aphasia. It is reasonable but untested as to whether persons with PPA can learn, will use if learned, or will benefit from augmentative and alternative communication devices and strategies.

11. For persons with PPA and their families, there is a need for education and counseling that emphasizes the progressive nature of the disorder and the fact that behavioral treatment to maximize communication ability cannot be expected to retard or reverse progression of the disease.

12. In general, it appears that the most rational approach to management of PPA is to gauge the rate of decline and the level of impairment, and then to direct treatment at the hypothesized deficits, at compensatory strategies, at psychosocial concomitants of the disorder, and at environmental influences (e.g., significant others and caregivers). When communicatively appropriate, accepted by the patient, and trained before their use is necessary, management may also address augmentative and alternative communication systems, particularly if substantive motor speech deficits accompany the PPA.

Information Resources

- *National Aphasia Association* (website contains information about PPA)
  National Aphasia Association
  156 Fifth Avenue, Suite 707
  New York, NY 10010
  Phone: 1-800-922-4622
  http://www.aphasia.org/NAAppa.html
- *Primary Progressive Aphasia Newsletter*: a newsletter about PPA published through:
  The Cognitive Neurology and Alzheimer's Disease Center
  320 East Superior Street
  Searle 11-450
  Chicago, IL 60611-3008
  Phone: 312-908-9339; fax 312-908-8789
  http://www.brain.nwu.edu/core/ppal.htm
- *Rare Dementia Registry*: a registry made up of individuals who have been diagnosed with a rare dementing illness; includes their primary caregiver. PPA is one of several rare dementias listed on the registry. The registry functions as a telephone support group. The database is confidential; names are shared with other registered families only. The service is provided by the:
  Alzheimer's Association, Greater Phoenix Chapter
  1028 East McDowell Road
  Phoenix, AZ 85006-2622
  Phone: 602-528-0550; 1-800-392-0550
  http://aztec.asu.edu/alz.phoenix

References

Abe, K., Ukita, H., & Yanagihara, T. (1997). Imaging in primary progressive aphasia. *Neuroradiology, 39*(8), 556–559.

Andersen, C., Dahl, C., Almkvist, O., et al. (1997). Bilateral temporal lobe volume reduction parallels cognitive impairment in progressive aphasia. *Archives of Neurology, 54*(10), 1294–1299.

Arima, K., Uesugi, H., Fujita, I., Sakurai, Y., Oyanagi, S., Andoh, S., Izumiyami, Y., & Inose, T. (1994). Corticonigral degeneration with neuronal achromasia presenting with primary progressive aphasia; ultrastructural and immunocytochemical studies. *Journal of the Neurological Sciences, 127*(2), 186–197.

Azouvi, P., Bergego, C., Robel, L., Marlier, N., Durand, I., & Held, J.P. et al. (1993). Slowly progressive apraxia: Two case studies. *Journal of Neurology, 240*, 347–350.

Black, S.E. (1996). Focal cortical atrophy syndromes. *Brain & Cognition, 31*(2), 188–229.

Broussolle, E., Bakchine, S., Tommasi, M., Laurent, B., Bazin, B., Cinotti, L., Cohen, L., & Chazot, G. (1996). Slowly progressive anarthria with late anterior opercular syndrome: A variant form of frontal cortical atrophy syndromes. *Journal of Neurological Sciences, 144*(1–2), 44–58.

Caselli, R.J. (1995). Focal and asymmetric cortical degeneration syndromes. *The Neurologist, 1*(1), 1–19.

Caselli, R.J. & Jack, C.R. Jr. (1992). Asymmetric cortical degenerative syndromes: A proposed clinical classification. *Archives of Neurology, 49*, 770–780.

Caselli, R.J., Jack, C.R., Jr., Petersen, R.C., Wahner, H.W., & Yanagihara, T. (1992). Asymmetric cortical degenerative syndromes: Clinical and radiologic correlations. *Neurology, 42*, 1462–1468.

Chapman, S.B., Rosenberg, R.N., Weiner, M.F., & Shobe, A. (1997). Autosomal dominant progressive syndrome of motor-speech loss without dementia. *Neurology, 49*(5), 1298–1306.

Cohen, L., Benoit, N., Van Eekhout, P., Ducarne, B., & Brunet, P. (1993). Pure progressive aphemia. *Journal of Neurology, Neurosurgery, & Psychiatry, 56*(8), 923–924.

Cole, M., Wright, D., & Banker, B.Q. (1979). Familial aphasia due to Pick's disease. *Annals of Neurology, 6*, 158.

Craenhals, A., Raison-Van Ruymbeke, A.M., Rectem, D., Seron, X., & Laterre, E.C. (1990). Is slowly progressive aphasia actually a new clinical entity? *Aphasiology, 4*(5), 485–509.

Darley, F.L. (1982). *Aphasia*. Philadelphia: WB Saunders.

DeRenzi, E. (1986). Slowly progressive visual agnosia or apraxia without dementia. *Cortex, 22*, 171–180.

Dick, J.P., Snowden, J.S., Northen, B., Goulding, P.J., & Neary, D. (1989). Slowly progressive apraxia. *Behavioral Neurology, 2*, 101–114.

Duffy, J.R. (1987). Slowly progressive aphasia. *Clinical Aphasiology, 16*, 349–356.

Duffy, J.R. (1988). Primary progressive aphasia syndrome. Seminar presented to the First National Conference of the National Aphasia Association, Chicago.

Duffy, J.R. & Petersen, R.C. (1992). Primary progressive aphasia. *Aphasiology, 6*(1), 1–15.

Engel, P.A. & Fleming, P.D. (1997). Primary progressive aphasia, left anterior atrophy, and neurofibrillary hippocampal pathology: Observations in an unusual case. *Neuropsychiatry, Neuropsychology, & Behavioral Neurology, 10*(3), 213–218.

Fuh, J.L., Liao, K.K., Wang, S.J., & Lin, K.N. (1994). Swallowing difficulty in primary progressive aphasia: A case report. *Cortex, 30*(4), 701–705.

Fukui, T., Sugita, K., Kawamura, M., Shiota, J., & Nakano, I. (1996). Primary progressive apraxia in Pick's disease: A clinicopathologic study. *Neurology, 47*, 467–473.

Gordon, B., Selnes, O. (1984). Progressive aphasia without dementia: Evidence of more widespread involvement. *Neurology, 34*, 102.

Graff-Radford, N.R., Damasio, A. R., & Hyman, B.T. et al. (1990). Progressive aphasia in a patient with Pick's disease: A neuropsychological, radiologic, and anatomic study. *Neurology, 40*, 620–626.

Green, J., Morris, J.C., Sandson, J., McKeel, D.W., & Miller, J.W. (1990). Progressive aphasia: A precursor of global dementia. *Neurology, 40*, 423–429.

Green, J.D., Patterson, K., Xuereb, J., & Hodges, J.R. (1996). Alzheimer disease and nonfluent progressive aphasia. *Archives of Neurology, 53*(10), 1072–1078.

Hart, R.P., Beach, W.A., & Taylor, J.R. (1997). A case of progressive apraxia of speech and non-fluent aphasia. *Aphasiology, 11*(1), 73–82.

Heath, P.D., Kennedy, P., & Kapur, N. (1983). Slowly progressive aphasia without generalized dementia. *Annals of Neurology, 13*, 687–688.

Henson, R.A. (1988). Maurice Ravel's illness: A tragedy of lost creativity. *British Medical Journal, 296*, 1885.

Holland, A.L., McBurney, D.H., Moossy, J., & Reinmuth, O.M. (1985). The dissolution of language in Pick's disease with neurofibrillary tangles: A case study. *Brain and Language, 24*, 36–58.

Informational topic. (1996, July). *Primary Progressive Aphasia Newsletter, 1*, 1–5.

Karbe, H., Kertesz, A., & Polk, M. (1993). Profiles of language impairment in primary progressive aphasia. *Archives of Neurology, 50*(2), 193–201.

Kavrie, S.H. & Duffy, J.R. (1994, November). Primary progressive apraxia of speech. Paper presented at the annual convention of the American Speech-Langauge-Hearing Association, New Orleans, LA.

Kempler, D., Metter, E.J., Riege, W.H., Jackson, C.A., Benson, D.F., & Hanson, W.R. (1990). Slowly progressive aphasia: Three cases with language, memory, CT and PET data. *Journal of Neurology, Neurosurgery, and Psychiatry, 53*(11), 987–993.

Kertesz, A. (1997). Frontotemporal dementia, Pick disease, and corticobasal degeneration: One entity or 3? *Archives of Neurology, 54*, 1427–1429.

Kertesz, A., Davidson, W., & McCabe, P. (1998). Primary progressive semantic aphasia: A case study. *Journal of the International Neuropsychological Society, 4*(4), 388–398.

Kertesz, A., Hudson, L., MacKenzie, I.R.A., & Munoz, D.G. (1994). The pathology and nosology of primary progressive aphasia. *Neurology, 44*, 2065–2072.

Kertesz, A. & Munoz, D.G. (1997). Primary progressive aphasia. *Clinical Neuroscience, 4*(2), 95–102.

Kirshner, I.I. & Bakar, M. (1995). Syndromes of language dissolution in aging and dementia. *Comprehensive Therapy, 21*(9), 519–523.

Kirschner, H.S., Tanridga, O., Thurman, L., & Whetsell, W.O. (1987). Progressive aphasia without dementia: Two cases with focal spongiform degeneration. *Annals of Neurology, 22*, 527–532.

Kobayashi, K., Kurachi, M., Gyoubu, T., Imao, G., & Nakamura, J. (1990). Progressive dysphasic dementia with localized cerebral atrophy: Report of an autopsy. *Clinical Neuropathology, 9*(5), 254–261.

Kushner, M. (1990). MRI and ^{123}I-iodoamphetamine SPECT imaging of a patient with slowly progressive aphasia. *Functional Neuroimaging, 2*(4), 17–19.

Lippa, C.F., Cohen, R., Smith, T.W., & Drachman, D.A. (1991). Primary progressive aphasia with focal neuronal achromasia. *Neurology, 41*(6), 882–886.

Mandell, A.M., Alexander, M.P., & Carpenter, S. (1989). Creutzfeldt-Jakob disease presenting as isolated aphasia. *Neurology, 39*, 55–58.

McNeil, M.R. (1982). The nature of aphasia in adults. In N.J. Lass, L.V. McReynolds, J. Northern, & D.E. Yoder (eds.), *Speech, language and hearing, Vol. II: Pathologies of speech and language* (pp. 692–740). Philadelphia, WB Saunders.

McNeil, M.R. (1988). Aphasia in the adult. In N.J. Lass, L.V. McReynolds, J. Northern & D.E. Yoder (eds.), *Handbook of speech-language pathology and audiology* (pp. 738–786). Toronto: BC Decker.

McNeil, M.R. (1989). Some theoretical and clinical implications of operating from a formal definition of aphasia. Paper presented to the Annual Meeting of the Academy of Aphasia.

McNeil, M.R. (1998). The case of the lawyer's lugubrious language: Dysarthria plus primary progressive aphasia or dysarthria plus dementia? *Seminars in Speech and Language, 19*(1), 49–57.

McNeil, M.R. & Kent, R.D. (1990). Motoric characteristics of adult apraxic and aphasic speakers. In G.R. Hammond (ed.), *Cerebral control of speech and limb movements* (pp. 349–386). New York: North Holland.

McNeil, M.R., Robin, D.A., & Schmidt, R.A. (1997). Apraxia of speech: Definition, differentiation, and treatment. In M.R. McNeil (ed.), *Clinical management of sensorimotor speech disorders* (pp. 311–344). New York: Thieme.

McNeil, M.R., Small, S.L., Masterson, R.J., & Fossett, T.R.D. (1995). Behavioral and pharmacological treatment of lexical-semantic deficits in a single patient with primary progressive aphasia. *American Journal of Speech-Language Pathology, 4*, 76–87.

Mehler, M.F. (1988). Mixed transcortical aphasia in nonfamilial dysphasic dementia. *Cortex, 24*, 545–554.

Mesulam, M.M. (1982). Slowly progressive aphasia without dementia. *Annals of Neurology, 11*, 592–598.

Mesulam, M.M. (1987). Primary progressive aphasia: Differentiation from Alzheimer's disease. *Annals of Neurology, 22*, 533–534.

Mesulam, M.M., Johnson, N., Grujic, Z., & Weintraub, S. (1997). Apolipoprotein E genotypes in primary progressive aphasia. *Neurology, 49*, 51–55.

Mesulam, M.M. & Weintraub, S. (1992). Spectrum of primary progressive aphasia. In M.N. Rossor (ed.), *Bailliere's clinical neurology, Vol. 1, Unusual dementias* (pp. 583–609). London: Baillière Tindall.

Mingazzini, G. (1914). On aphasia due to atrophy of the cerebral convolutions. *Brain, 36,* 493–524.

Morgan, A. & Helm-Estabrooks, N. (1987). Back to the drawing board: A treatment program for nonverbal aphasic patients. *Clinical Aphasiology, 16,* 34–39.

Morris, J.C., Cole, M., Branker, B., & Wright, D. (1984). Hereditary dysphasic dementia and the Pick-Alzheimer spectrum. *Annals of Neurology, 16,* 455–466.

Murray, L.L. (1998). Longitudinal treatment of primary progressive aphasia: A case study. *Aphasiology, 12*(7/8), 651–672.

Otsuki, M., Soma, Y., Sato, M., Homma, A., & Tsuji, S. (1998). Slowly progressive pure word deafness. *European Neurology, 39*(3), 135–140.

Philbrick, K.L., Rummans, T.A., Duffy, J.R., Kokmen, E., & Jack, C.R. (1994). Primary progressive aphasia: An uncommon masquerader of psychiatric disorders. *Psychosomatics, 35*(2), 138–141.

Piccirilli, M., D'Alessandro, P., & Ferroni, A. (1990). Slowly progressive apraxia without dementia. *Dementia, 1,* 222–224.

Pick, A. (1892). Über die Beziehungen der senilen Hirnatrophie zur Aphasie. *Prager Medizinische Wochenschrift, 17,* 165–167.

Poeck, K. & Luzzatti, C. (1988). Slowly progressive aphasia in three patients. *Brain, 111,* 151–168.

Rogers, M.A. & Alarcon, N.B. (1999). Characteristics and management of primary progressive aphasia. *ASHA Special Interest Division Neurophysiology and Neurogenic Speech and Language Disorders, 9*(4), 12–26.

Rogers, M.A., King, J.M., & Alarcon, N.B. (In Press). Proactive management of primary progressive aphasia. In D.R. Beukelman, K. Yorkston, & J. Reichle (eds.), *Augmentative communication for adults with neurogenic and neuromuscular disabilities.* Baltimore, MD: Brookes.

Sakurai, Y., Hashida, H., Uesugi, H., Murayama, S., Bando, M., Iwata, M., Momose, T., & Sakuta, M. (1996). A clinical profile of corticobasal degeneration presenting as primary progressive aphasia. *European Neurology, 36*(3), 134–137.

Scheltens, P.H., Hazenberg, G.J., Lindeboom, J., Valk, J., & Wolters, E.C. (1990). A case of progressive aphasia without dementia: "Temporal" Pick's disease? *Journal of Neurology, Neurosurgery, and Psychiatry, 53,* 79–80.

Scheltens, P.H., Ravid, R., & Kamphorst, W. (1994). Pathologic findings in a case of primary progressive aphasia. *Neurology, 44*(2), 279–282.

Schneider, S.L., Thompson, C.K., & Luring, B. (1996). Effects of verbal plus gestural matrix training on sentence production in a patient with primary progressive aphasia. *Aphasiology, 10*(3), 297–317.

Scholten, I.M., Kneebone, L.A., Denson, L.A., Fields, C.D., & Blumbergs, P. (1995). Primary progressive aphasia: Serial linguistic, neuropsychological and radiological findings with neuropathological results. *Aphasiology, 9*(5), 495–516.

Schwartz, M.F. (1984). What the classical aphasia categories can't do for us, and why. *Brain and Language, 21,* 3–8.

Schwartz, M.F., DeBlesser, R., Poeck, K., & Weis, J. (1998). A case of primary progressive aphasia: A 14-year follow-up study with neuropathological findings. *Brain, 121,* 115–126.

Shuttleworth, E.C., Yates, A.J., & Paltan-Ortiz, J. (1985). Creutzfeld-Jakob disease presenting as progressive aphasia. *Journal of the National Medical Association, 77,* 649–656.

Sinnatamby, R., Antoun, N.A., Freer, C.E., Miles, K.A., & Hodges, J.R. (1996). Neuroradiological findings in primary progressive aphasia: CT, MRI and cerebral perfusion SPECT. *Neuroradiology, 38*(3), 232–238.

Thompson, C.K. (1997). *Primary Progressive Aphasia Newsletter-Readers Section, 2,* 1–6.

Trupe, E.H. (1984). Reliability of rating spontaneous speech in the Western Aphasia Battery: Implications for classification. *Clinical Aphasiology, 13,* 55–69.

Turner, R.S., Kenyon, L.C., Trojanowski, J.Q., Gonatas, N., & Grossman, M. (1996). Clinical, neuroimaging, and pathologic features of progressive nonfluent aphasia. *Annals of Neurology, 39*(2), 166–173.

Tyrrell, P.J., Kartsounis, L.D., Frackowiak, R.S.J., Findley, L.J., & Rosser, M.N. (1991). Progressive loss of speech output and orofacial dyspraxia associated with frontal lobe hypometabolism. *Journal of Neurology, Neurosurgery, and Psychiatry, 54,* 351–357.

Tyrrell, P.J., Warrington, E.K., Frackowiak, R.S.J., & Rosser, M.N. (1990). Progressive degeneration of the right temporal lobe studied with positron emission tomography. *Journal of Neurology, Neurosurgery, and Psychiatry, 53,* 1046–1050.

Weintraub, S., Rubin, N.P., & Mesulam, M.M. (1990). Primary progressive aphasia: Longitudinal course, neurological profile, and language features. *Archives of Neurology, 47*(12), 1329–1335.

Westbury, C. & Bub, D. (1997). Primary progressive aphasia: A review of 112 cases. *Brain and Language, 60*(3) 381–406.

Yamanouchi, H., Budka, H., & Vass, K. (1986). Unilateral Creutzfeldt-Jakob disease. *Cortex, 24,* 545–554.

Chapter 21

Clinical Intervention for Global Aphasia

Richard K. Peach

Since the publication of the last edition of this text, there have been a number of positive developments reported in the literature regarding rehabilitation for persons with global aphasia. Several papers have appeared that extend the application of nonverbal strategies (e.g., gesture, drawing) to improve the communication abilities of global aphasic individuals (Doyle & DeRuyter, 1995; Rao, 1995; Ward-Lonergan & Nicholas, 1995). In some cases, the global aphasic patient's efficiency in using these alternate communication strategies has been found to rival that of less severe, nonverbal aphasic individuals (e.g., Broca's aphasia) or exceed that of other severe aphasics (e.g., Wernicke's aphasia) who rely upon verbal strategies (Marshall et al., 1997). Gestural-assisted programs such as computerized visual communication (C-ViC) have been shown to be successful in training comprehension of a variety of lexical categories (e.g., verbs, prepositions) although generalization to oral production of these items has been limited (Weinrich et al., 1989, 1993). Lesion site patterns identified by CT scans have been used to predict a priori which global aphasic patients might demonstrate such successful outcomes when using C-ViC (Naeser et al., 1998).

Despite these developments, there continue to be claims in the rehabilitation literature that speech-language treatment does not improve recovery in patients with global aphasia (see, e.g., Nagaratnam et al., 1996). What is more perplexing is that such claims are based upon studies, such as that of Sarno and Levita (1979), that were performed 20 years ago. While the prognosis for recovery of premorbid speech-language abilities is poor indeed following global aphasia, these individuals do make significant improvements in communication skills with treatment during the first year post-onset (Nicholas et al., 1993). Occasionally, those improvements exceed the outcomes observed in other aphasia types (i.e., Broca's & Wernicke's aphasia) that are associated with better prognoses for improvement (Basso & Farabola, 1997, Kertesz & McCabe, 1977).

These different viewpoints arise from the different standards that are used to evaluate treatment-related outcomes in global aphasia. Those who find little evidence for positive outcomes often base their conclusions upon studies that document a failure of these patients to evolve to less severe forms of the disorder in the years following its onset and treatment. A premium in these circles is placed on the reestablishment of oral-verbal skills. Others, however, find positive treatment outcomes in the global aphasic patients' improved use of gesture, writing, and drawing to accompany their reduced vocabularies. The net result of these strategies has been increased functional communication. Reports such as that of a young individual with global aphasia who returned to work using such alternate communication means (Raderstorf et al., 1984) strongly reinforce the substantial improvement that can be associated with speech-language and other treatments following this disorder.

The unmasking of the benefits achieved with speech-language treatment for global aphasia is attributable, in part, to the emphasis over the past decade on case-based studies of treatment outcome. Early large group studies using standardized aphasia batteries to test for treatment effects have given way to the analyses of individual patient profiles using appraisal instruments that are better suited for investigating severe aphasia (see, e.g., Nicholas et al., 1993). Nonetheless, it is clear that not all people with global aphasia show the kinds of dramatic improvement that have been reported in studies such as those cited above.

The central questions regarding outcomes following global aphasia, then, concern discovering the patient characteristics that can be associated with various prognoses and applying these in treatment planning (Peach, 1992). Some recent studies have attempted to do this by examining outcomes with regard to the patterns of lesion sites producing global aphasia (Basso & Farabola, 1997; Kumar et al., 1996; Naeser, 1994; Okuda et al., 1994). Others have investigated the role of an accompanying hemiplegia (Keyserlingk et al., 1997; Nagaratnam et al., 1996). Still others have employed positron emission tomography (PET) to identify predictors that might account for the large amount of variability observed in recovery from aphasia generally, and global aphasia specifically (Heiss et al., 1993; Okuda et al., 1994).

These developments are encouraging especially since the largest percentage of aphasic patients referred for speech-language services is composed of those presenting with global aphasia (Sarno & Levita, 1981). Despite the poor prognosis for recovery of oral language skills following global aphasia, clinicians now have more tools than ever to make informed decisions regarding whether and how to treat global aphasic individuals and the impact that this treatment will have on the patients' communication skills.

OBJECTIVES

Following the completion of this chapter, the reader will be able to identify the features of global aphasia, its etiology, the patterns of evolution and outcome in global aphasia, and some factors that are related to recovery from this syndrome. The reader will also be able to provide a rationale for early intervention with these patients, describe contemporary goals for assessment, and develop treatment plans that exploit the residual language capacity and/or other functional abilities of patients with global aphasia. Finally, the reader will be able to identify current testing measures and treatment programs that emphasize functional communication and are appropriate for assessing and treating global aphasic patients.

FEATURES

Incidence

Global aphasia may be one of the most frequently occurring types of aphasia. Previously, incidence rates between 10 and 40.6% have been reported for global aphasia (Basso et al., 1987; Brust et al., 1976; Collins, 1986; De Renzi et al., 1980; Eslinger & Damasio, 1981; Kertesz, 1979; Kertesz & Sheppard, 1981). Some recent reports, however, suggest that the incidence rate during the acute stage may be even higher. Scarpa et al. (1987) reported an incidence of 55.1% in an acute sample. All of the 108 aphasic patients included in the Scarpa et al. (1987) study were assessed between 15 and 30 days post-onset and were right handed with a single left hemisphere lesion. When these data are combined, they provide evidence indicating that global aphasic patients are prominent among aphasic patients as a whole. As a result, they constitute a significant demand upon the resources of clinical aphasiologists from the acute stages of illness through the time of maximal recovery.

Characteristics

Age and Sex

There appears to be no observable difference in the distribution of global aphasia when patients are compared by either age or sex (Habib et al., 1987; Scarpa et al., 1987; Sorgato et al., 1990). In relation to sex, Davis (1983) suggested that there is a general bias toward males in the data generated among Veterans Affairs Medical Centers due to the nature of the population seen at these hospitals. Further studies including more representative patient distributions may be necessary for reliable data regarding the influence of sex on global aphasia. Regarding age, Sorgato et al. (1990) reported no effect of age on aphasia types, including global aphasia. The older patients in their sample, however, did tend to show atypical aphasias including global aphasia from brain damage that was restricted to either anterior or posterior areas. Nonetheless, age and sex may not be considered to have a differential effect on the incidence of global aphasia.

Site of Lesion

Cerebrovascular lesions producing global aphasia have been described as involving Broca's (posterior frontal) and Wernicke's (superior temporal) areas (Kertesz, 1979) or alternatively, both the prerolandic and postrolandic speech zones (Goodglass & Kaplan, 1983). The global aphasic subjects described by Murdoch et al. (1986) exhibited large lesions extending from the cortical surface inferiorly to subcortical areas including the basal ganglia, internal capsule, and thalamus. Basso and Farabola's (1997) global aphasic subject had damage to the left frontal operculum, Wernicke's area, the premotor area, the supramarginal gyrus, inferior and superior parietal lobules, angular gyrus, and Heschl's gyri. All of these global aphasia-producing lesions involved the cortex and were extensive, dominating the left hemisphere. However, numerous exceptions have been reported in the literature suggesting that such an extensive lesion may not be necessary to produce a global aphasia.

Mazzocchi and Vignolo (1979) found global aphasia in 3 of 11 cases following lesions that were confined to anterior regions. In 4 additional cases, the lesions were deep and confined to the insula, the lenticular nucleus, and the internal capsule. Varying lesion effects also were described by Cappa and Vignolo (1983). Basso et al. (1985) observed global aphasia following discrete lesions confined to anterior (sparing of postrolandic centers) or posterior cortical sites. Lüders et al. (1991) produced global aphasia during electrical stimulation of the basal temporal region. This region has its white matter in contact with the white matter deep to Wernicke's area, thereby favoring close interaction between these two areas. Further, Basso et al. (1985) reported other forms of aphasia following lesions that would have been suggestive of global aphasia.

Global aphasia has also been described in patients with lesions restricted to subcortical regions. Alexander et al. (1987) found global aphasia in association with one lesion or a series of primarily subcortical lesions that collectively damaged the striatum-anterior limb of the internal capsule; the anterior, superior, anterior-superior, and extra-anterior periventricular white matter; and the temporal isthmus. Yang et al. (1989) also identified global aphasia in patients with lesions involving the internal capsule, basal ganglia, thalamus, and anterior-posterior pariventricular white matter. Okuda et al. (1994) described four patients with global aphasia who had lesions in the putamen, posterior internal capsule, temporal isthmus, and periventricular white of the left hemisphere. Kumar et al. (1996) observed global aphasia in their patient following a left thalamic hemorrhage.

Ferro (1992) and Basso and Farabola (1997) investigated the influence of lesion site on recovery from global aphasia. Ferro examined 54 subjects initially during either the first month (34 subjects), third month (7 subjects), or 6 months post-onset (13 subjects). He then followed up each patient at 3, 6, and 12 months and yearly thereafter when possible. The lesions in his group of global aphasic subjects were grouped into five types with differing outcomes. Type 1 included patients with large pre- and postrolandic middle cerebral artery infarcts. These patients had a very poor prognosis. The remaining four groups were classified as follows: type 2, prerolandic; type 3, subcortical; type 4, parietal; and type 5, double frontal and parietal lesion. Patients in these latter groups demonstrated variable outcomes, improving generally to Broca's or transcortical aphasia. Complete recovery was observed in some cases with type 2 and 3 infarcts. In contrast to these findings, Basso and Farabola investigated recovery in 3 cases of aphasia based on the patients' lesion patterns. One patient had global aphasia from a large lesion involving both the anterior and posterior language areas while 2 other patients had Broca's and Wernicke's aphasia from lesions restricted to either the anterior or posterior language areas, respectively. The patient with global aphasia was found to recover better than did his 2 aphasic counterparts while his overall outcome was considered to be outstanding. Based on these observations, Basso and Farrabola concluded that group recovery patterns based on aphasia severity and site of lesion may not be able to account for the improvement that is observed occasionally in individual patients.

Language

The hallmark of global aphasia is a loss of language comprehension with concomitant deficits in expressive abilities (Damasio, 1991; Davis, 1983; Kertesz, 1979). Wallace and Stapleton (1991) suggested that the linguistic deficit in global aphasia has been traditionally interpreted as a loss of language competency, i.e., the knowledge for linguistic rules and operations. According to these authors and others (Rosenbek et al., 1989), the recent clinical evidence demonstrating preserved areas of language functioning in global aphasia suggests that the loss for these patients may be viewed more

appropriately as a variable mix of competence and performance deficits.

Comprehension

Several isolated areas of relatively preserved comprehension following global aphasia have been identified in the literature. These include recognition of specific word categories (McKenna & Warrington, 1978; Wapner & Gardner, 1979), familiar environmental sounds (Spinnler & Vignolo, 1966), and famous personal names (Van Lancker & Klein, 1990; Yasuda & Ono, 1998; but see also Forde & Humphreys, 1995 for a report of relatively impaired access to personal names following global aphasia). In the case of famous personal names, Yasuda and Ono (1998) found a distinct advantage for comprehending these items when reading versus listening. They attributed this finding to the nonsemantic, referential nature of personal names and the probable processing of these stimuli in these patients' intact right hemispheres. Global aphasic subjects also show relatively better comprehension for personally relevant information (Wallace & Canter, 1985; Van Lancker & Nicklay, 1992).

Wallace and Stapleton (1991) analyzed the responses of global aphasic subjects on the auditory comprehension portion of the *Boston Diagnostic Aphasia Examination (BDAE)* (Goodglass & Kaplan, 1983) to identify patterns of preserved and impaired performance. While their results generally supported previous claims that distinct patterns of preserved components are absent in global aphasia, nonetheless, two or three of their subjects did evidence differential performance within and across tasks. Interestingly, the scores for each of these subjects were collected during the acute stage of their recovery. The authors speculate that differential auditory comprehension performance during acute aphasia may be a useful prognostic indicator.

Expression

It has been suggested that global aphasic patients may be most severely impaired in their expressive abilities. This may be due to the greater contributions of the right hemisphere for comprehension than for expressive behaviors (Collins, 1986). The verbal output of many global aphasic patients primarily consists of stereotypic recurring utterances or speech automatisms (Kertesz, 1979). Stereotypes have been described as being either nondictionary verbal forms (unrecognizable) or dictionary forms (word or sentence) (Alajouanine, 1956).

Blanken et al. (1990) examined 26 patients demonstrating the nondictionary forms of speech automatisms. Of these cases, 24 were classified as being global aphasic. The other patients demonstrated signs more closely associated with Broca's and Wernicke's aphasia. Although speech automatisms were frequently associated with comprehension disturbances, the observed variability in language comprehension among these patients suggests that speech automatisms cannot be used to infer the presence of severe comprehension deficits. Blanken et al. (1990) proposed that speech automatisms relate only to speech output and do not necessarily indicate the presence of severe comprehension deficits.

Cognition

The cognitive abilities of brain-damaged patients are often assessed by administration of *Raven's Coloured Progressive Matrices (RCPM)* (Raven, 1965), a nonverbal test of analogical reasoning. Conflicting results have been reported regarding aphasic subjects' performances relative to that of nonaphasic left brain–damaged patients. Some studies have found that aphasic subjects perform at lower levels (Basso et al., 1981; Basso et al., 1973; Colonna & Faglioni, 1966) while others have failed to show any significant difference between these two groups (Arrigoni & De Renzi, 1964; Piercy & Smith, 1962). Collins (1986) has reported significant positive correlations between the language ability of global aphasic subjects and their performance on the RCPM. The subjects in the Collins study were in the early stages of recovery and eventually these subjects achieved RCPM scores similar to those of less severe aphasics.

Using a new version of the RCPM, modified to minimize the potential effect of unilateral spatial neglect, Gainotti et al. (1986) compared acute and chronic subjects with varying types of aphasia with normal controls, right hemisphere–damaged subjects, and nonaphasic left hemisphere–damaged subjects. In the Gainotti et al. (1986) study, the aphasic subjects performed worse than the other groups. Further, the global aphasic and Wernicke aphasic patients scored the poorest in comparison with the other aphasic groups (anomic, Broca, and conduction). These results were similar to those obtained by Kertesz and McCabe (1975). Gainotti et al. (1986) did not obtain differences relative to severity of aphasia, but did link poor performance on the RCPM to the presence of receptive semantic-lexical disturbances. Gainotti et al. (1986) conclude that "a specific relationship exists in aphasia between cognitive nonverbal impairment and breakdown of the semantic-lexical level of integration of language" (p. 48).

Rossor et al. (1995) demonstrated relatively preserved calculation skills in a patient with global aphasia secondary to progressive atrophy of the left temporal lobe. Together with previous reports of selective impairment of calculation in patients with intact language skills, the authors posited that this double dissociation reflects a functional independence between the two domains of behavior, i.e., that calculation skills are not dependent upon the language processing system. Since selective impairment of calculation skills has been associated with left parietal lesions, the authors also suggested that lesions producing language disturbances that spare the parietal lobe may be associated with preserved calculation skills.

Communication

The presence of recurring utterances among individuals with global aphasia was addressed previously. There are those who exhibit only recurring consonant-vowel (CV) syllables (for example, do-do-do or ma-ma-ma). As described by Collins (1986), these global aphasic patients often give the impression of somewhat preserved communicative abilities in that they may make use of the suprasegmental aspects of speech. The use of suprasegmentals in conversational turn-taking may appear to indicate that the aphasic patient is producing utterances with some communicative intent. DeBlesser and Poeck (1984) studied a group of global aphasic patients and found that they did not exhibit prosodic variability to the extent necessary for conveying communicative intent. The utterances used for analysis, however, were limited to those elicited during formal testing and may not have reflected the spontaneous use of inflection to convey intent (Collins, 1986). DeBlesser and Poeck (1985) subsequently analyzed the spontaneous utterances of a group of global aphasic subjects with output limited to CV recurrences. Utterances were sampled during interviews in which the examiner asked a series of open-ended questions. The length of the utterances and their pitch contours were analyzed for variability. The authors concluded that both length and pitch appeared to be stereotypical and that the prosody of these patients did not seem to reflect communicative intent. The appropriateness of these CV-recurring utterances with regard to turn-taking remains questionable. These findings highlight the marked discrepancy that exists between research outcomes and clinical reports. DeBlesser and Poeck (1985) suggest that the contributions to conversation for which these patients are credited may be, in fact, the result of the communicative partner's need for informative communication rather than the patient's use of prosodic elements to convey intent.

In a study by Herrmann et al. (1989), a group of chronic and severe nonfluent aphasic subjects were described in terms of their communication strategies and communicative efficiency. The patients presented with either severe Broca's or global aphasia (50%). The results showed that the efficiency of the patients' communication depended upon the type of question to which they were asked to respond. As might be expected, superior performance was observed for responses to yes/no questions ("Did your illness occur suddenly?") when compared with interrogative pronoun questions ("How long have you had language problems now?") and narrative requests ("Tell me what happened to you after you took ill."). Herrmann et al. (1989) reported that the patients used mostly gesture in their responses to the yes/no questions. The other types of questioning require increased verbal output and thus created the need for more complex communicative responses from the patients.

In examining the communication strategies utilized, Herrmann et al. (1989) found that patients rarely took initiative or expanded on topics. The most frequent strategies reported by these authors were those enabling the patients to secure comprehension (e.g., indicating comprehension problems, requesting support for establishing comprehension). Herrmann et al. (1989) concluded that this population relies most heavily on nonverbal communication.

Marshall et al. (1997) also investigated the efficiency of different communicative strategies utilized by three severely aphasic patients. A Broca aphasic patient communicated primarily through writing and drawing; a Wernicke aphasic patient communicated primarily through speaking; and a global aphasic patient with apraxia of speech communicated primarily through gesturing with a few single words. Marshall et al. assessed each patient's communicative efficiency and the degree of communicative burden assumed by a partner during a declarative message exchange task that was evaluated using a visual analog scale. The investigators also analyzed the effects of context and shared knowledge on efficiency in communicative interactions by varying the extent of the raters' awareness of the message contents (no knowledge, partial, or full knowledge). Their results demonstrated that the efficiency of the global aphasic patient's communication approximated that of the most efficient patient (the Broca patient). Also, the burden imposed by his gestural strategy was nearly as low as the Broca aphasic's writing and drawing. These findings provide support for the effectiveness of the nonverbal strategies used by patients with global aphasia and further reinforce their training as a target of rehabilitation.

Affect

Depression following aphasia has been "underrecognized and undertreated" (Masand & Chaudhary, 1994). Masand and Chaudhary suggest this might be due to a heavy reliance on verbal responses for establishing a diagnosis of depression. Also, patients with global aphasia tend to be excluded from treatment studies because of their severe comprehension deficits. In a case report of a chronic, global aphasic patient hospitalized for deteriorating mental status, these authors describe positive benefits from administration of the psychostimulant methylphenidate for treatment of his major depression. From a pretreatment state characterized by drowsiness and lethargy, sad affect, and an inability to participate in his care, the patient improved within 72 hours of achieving a therapeutic dose (15 mg/day) to become more alert, smiling, attentive, and actively involved in his care. These changes resulted in his improved candidacy for rehabilitation and, upon referral, he reportedly made significant gains in speech-language treatment that included producing single words, following simple commands, and imitating

gestures. Discontinuation of his medications, including the methylphenidate, secondary to two generalized tonic-clonic seizures, resulted in a return to his previous apathetic state within 1 week.

ETIOLOGY

As described, the majority of lesions producing global aphasia are extensive and involve both prerolandic and postrolandic areas. The blood supply for these areas is via the middle cerebral artery. The middle cerebral artery is the largest branch of the internal carotid artery, branching at the point of the Sylvian fissure. Due to the extent of the lesion, global aphasia most commonly results from a cerebrovascular event, the locus of which is in the middle cerebral artery at a level inferior to the point of branching. Further, the event causing global aphasia is more commonly thrombotic than embolic (Collins, 1986).

Not all occurrences of global aphasia are due to a cerebrovascular event in the middle cerebral artery. Interestingly, Wells et al. (1992) reported a temporary case of global aphasia due to simple partial status epilepticus. The aphasia lasted during a period in which there were periodic lateralized epileptiform discharges. Wells et al. (1992) reported that the patient's language returned to near normal during the 24 hours following the seizures. A case of rapidly developing global aphasia and personality change in a young woman secondary to demyelinating disease is also described in the case records of the Massachusetts General Hospital (Anonymous, 1996). MRI scan of the brain with gadolinium showed multiple enhancing white matter lesions predominating in the subcortical and periventricular white matter, the posterior limb of the left internal capsule, and the corona radiata and centrum semiovale bilaterally. Treatment with corticosteroids resulted in minimal improvements; administration of cyclophosphamide, an anti-inflammatory/immunologic agent, produced steady improvement. No other information was provided regarding her speech-language outcome.

RECOVERY

The outlook for recovery from global aphasia tends to be bleak. Kertesz and McCabe (1977) reported that the group of global aphasic subjects in their study generally demonstrated limited language recovery, a pattern similar to that reported by Wapner and Gardner (1979). When assessing the language recovery that does occur, better improvement is demonstrated in comprehension than in expression (Lomas & Kertesz, 1978; Prins et al., 1978). With regard to recovery of nonverbal cognitive abilities, Kertesz and McCabe (1975) found a precipitous and parallel rate of improvement for RCPM and language performance during the first 3 months post-onset. During the next 3 months, RCPM performance continued to increase substantially, surpassing language performance that was only mildly improved from levels attained at the end of the first 3 months. Patients appeared to reach a plateau in both RCPM and language performance during the period between 6 and 12 month post-onset. Overall, RCPM performance in the global aphasic patients did not exceed approximately 50% of the maximum attainable score.

In relation to the recovery observed in other aphasia types, Kertesz and McCabe (1977) described global aphasia as having the lowest recovery rate. With regard to the temporal aspects of recovery in global aphasia, differences have been reported depending upon whether the subjects were receiving speech and language treatment. For global aphasic patients not receiving treatment, improvement appears to be greatest during the first months post-onset (Kertesz & McCabe, 1977; Pashek & Holland, 1988). Siirtola and Siirtola (1984) observed the greatest improvement in their untreated subjects during the first 6 months post-onset.

Global aphasic patients receiving treatment, however, demonstrate substantial improvements during the first 3 to 6 months but also continued improvement during the period between 6 and 12 months or more post-onset (Kertesz & McCabe, 1977; Nicholas et al., 1993; Sarno & Levita, 1979, 1981). In the study of Kertesz & McCabe (1977), significantly greater improvement was noted in treated versus untreated global aphasics during this period, although the authors attributed this gain at least partially to subject heterogeneity. In the studies of Sarno and Levita (1979, 1981), improvement was most accelerated between 6 and 12 months post-stroke. Nicholas et al. (1993) found different patterns of recovery for language and nonlanguage skills following longitudinal administration of the Boston Assessment of Severe Aphasia (BASA) (Helm-Estabrooks et al., 1989), an instrument developed specifically to evaluate communication performance in severe aphasia. Substantial improvements in praxis and oral-gestural expression were noted only in the first 6 months post-onset while similar improvements in auditory and reading comprehension were observed only between 6 and 12 months post-onset. Based upon these findings, the authors stressed the need for analyzing subsets of communication skills rather than overall scores to evaluate recovery from global aphasia.

Evolution

The majority of patients with global aphasia will not recover to less severe forms of the disorder. Some patients, however, will improve to the extent that they evolve into other aphasia syndromes. A number of studies have documented these changes using a variety of assessment instruments and testing schedules.

Six studies used the Western Aphasia Battery (WAB) (Kertesz, 1982) to assess language performance during the acute period of recovery and at regular intervals up to 1 year (or more) post-onset. Kertesz and McCabe (1977) tested 93 aphasic subjects between 0 to 6 weeks post-onset and found that 5 of their 22 global aphasic subjects progressed to other syndromes including Broca's, transcortical motor, conduction, and anomic aphasia after 1 year or more. Siirtola and Siirtola (1984) classified aphasic subjects within the first 2 weeks after hospitalization. At 1 year post-onset, 6 global aphasic subjects from among 14 had evolved to other syndromes including Broca's, conduction, anomic, and Wernicke's aphasia or, in the case of 1 subject, had recovered completely. Holland et al. (1985) followed 15 patients for 1 year who had been classified as global aphasic immediately after stroke. In this study, classifications were based upon results obtained from the WAB as well as from clinical impressions. Several patterns were observed at the end of the first year: 2 patients (in their 30s) returned to normal language functioning, 2 (in their 40s) evolved to Broca's aphasia, 2 (59 and 61 years of age) evolved to anomic aphasia, 2 (in their 70s) evolved to Wernicke's aphasia, and 2 (in their 80s) remained global aphasic. The 5 remaining subjects died during the course of the study. Pashek and Holland (1988) described the evolution of 11 global aphasic subjects from among a larger group of 32 subjects who were followed for at least 6 months. While language performance was assessed by repeated administration of the WAB, these aphasic subjects were classified on the basis of descriptive criteria rather than WAB typology. All subjects were evaluated within the first 5 days after stroke. Four of these patients evolved to less severe syndromes including Broca's, Wernicke's, and anomic aphasia. Two patients evolved to a less severe but unclassifiable aphasic syndrome. One subject recovered normal language and 2 subjects demonstrated symptoms of dementia. Mark et al. (1992) reported the 1 year outcomes of 13 patients initially classified as global aphasic at 7 to 10 days post-onset. One patient was no longer aphasic while 7 patients recovered to a less severe form of aphasia. Among the latter, 2 patients recovered to Wernicke's aphasia, 2 patients recovered to conduction aphasia, and 3 recovered to anomic, Broca's, and transcortical motor aphasias respectively. Finally, 9 of 13 global aphasic patients followed by McDermott et al. (1996) evolved to other forms of aphasia. Seven of these patients evolved to Broca's aphasia and 2 evolved to Wernicke's aphasia.

Nicholas et al. (1993) assessed 17 patients with global aphasia, as well as 7 other patients with severe aphasia, for 2 years after the onset of their aphasia to describe the patterns of recovery. Patients were scheduled for testing with the BASA at 1 to 2 months after the onset of their aphasia and at every 6-month anniversary of their strokes thereafter up to 24 months. Of the patients with global aphasia initially, 4 changed classification during this period while the remaining 13 continued to be classified as having global aphasia. For the patients who did evolve, 1 changed to a mild Wernicke's aphasia and 3 changed to mixed nonfluent aphasia.

Sarno and Levita (1979) investigated recovery from global aphasia using selected subtests of the Neurosensory Center

TABLE 21–1

Proportion of Global Aphasic Subjects Evolving to Less Severe Aphasia Syndromes or Normal Language with Time of Initial Testing After Cerebral Injury

Study	N	Initial Testing	% Evolved[a]
Holland, Swindell, and Forbes (1985)	10	Immediately	80
Pashek and Holland (1988)	11	0–5 days	64
Mark, Thomas, and Berndt (1992)	13	7–10 days	62
Siirtola and Siirtola (1984)	14	0–2 weeks	43
Kertesz and McCabe (1977)	22	0–6 weeks	23
McDermott, Horner, and DeLong (1996)	13	0–6 weeks	69
Sarno and Levita (1979)	11	4 weeks	0
Sarno and Levita (1981)	7	4 weeks	0
Nicholas, Helm-Estabrooks, Ward-Lonergan, and Morgan (1993)	17	1–2 months	24
Reinvang and Engvik (1980)	7	2–5 months	57

[a] Endstage assessments were completed between 6 to 12 months post-injury in all studies except Kertesz and McCabe (1977), Reinvang and Engvik (1980), Nicholas et al. (1993), and McDermott et al. (1996). Only 10 of the global aphasic subjects studied by Kertesz and McCabe (1977) were assessed at 1 year or more post-onset. Specific data for the global aphasic subjects of Reinvang and Engvik (1980) were not reported; the mean time post-onset for the endstage observations of all aphasic subjects in their study was 7.5 months with a minimum time of 3 months post-onset. Fifteen of the 17 global aphasic subjects followed by Nicholas et al. (1993) were assessed at 24 months post-onset. Final testing for the remaining two subjects was completed at 18 months post-onset. Re-evaluation for the 13 global aphasic subjects tested by McDermott et al. (1996) occurred approximately between 1 and 6 months post-onset with a minimum intervening period of at least 30 days.

Comprehensive Examination for Aphasia (NCCEA) (Spreen & Benton, 1977) and the Functional Communication Profile (Sarno, 1969). Classification of aphasia was based upon clinical impressions as well as language test scores. In this study, the earliest language observations were collected at 4 weeks post-onset with a variation of no greater than plus or minus 1 week. Repeated testing was continued until 1 year after the stroke. In contrast to the above studies, none of these 14 global aphasic subjects evolved to another type of aphasia by the end of the year. Similar results were observed in a follow-up study of 7 global aphasic subjects (Sarno & Levita, 1981).

One apparent explanation for the discrepancies among these studies might be the greater instability of language scores and, therefore, aphasia classifications obtained during the first 4 weeks after stroke versus those obtained after the first month post-onset. McDermott et al. (1996) found greater magnitudes of change scores and frequencies of aphasia-type evolution in subjects tested during the first 30 days post-onset versus those tested in the second 30 days post-onset. Aphasia tends to be more severe during the acute stage, giving observers an initial impression of global aphasia. But this symptomatology may be fleeting and result in a seemingly greater potential for patients to evolve to a less severe aphasia syndrome following this early period (see Table 21–1).

However, Holland et al. (1985) and Pashek and Holland (1988) found that global aphasic patients who do progress to

some other form of aphasia demonstrate changes that extend into the first months post-onset. In some cases, the global aphasia may not begin to evolve until after the first month has passed. Additionally, Reinvang and Engvik (1980) assessed their aphasic subjects initially between 2 and 5 months after their injuries (mean = 3 months) and found that four of the seven global aphasic subjects had evolved to a less severe Broca's, conduction, or unclassifiable syndrome at retesting. The retesting was completed no sooner than 1 month after initial testing with a mean time of 7.5 months after injury and a range of 3 to 30 months. Based upon these findings, the discrepancies in recovery from global aphasia reported in these studies do not appear to be simply the result of the time at which the initial language observations were recorded. Apparently, evolution from global aphasia is the result of a complex interaction among a number of heretofore incompletely understood factors.

Prognostic Factors

Age

Following global aphasia, a patient's age appears to have an impact on recovery: the younger the patient, the better the prognosis (Holland et al., 1985; Pashek & Holland, 1988). Age may also relate to the type of aphasia at 1 year post-stroke. For example, in the study reported by Holland et al. (1985), younger global aphasic patients evolved to a nonfluent Broca's aphasia while older patients evolved to increasingly severe fluent aphasias with advancing age. Their oldest patients remained global aphasic (see above).

Whether age can be considered a prognostic indicator has yielded differing conclusions. Advanced age has been found to have a negative influence on recovery (Holland & Bartlett, 1985; Holland et al., 1989; Marshall & Phillips, 1971; Sasanuma, 1988) and to be an insignificant predictor of recovery (Hartman, 1981; Kertesz & McCabe, 1977; Sarno, 1981; Sarno & Levita, 1971). Pashek and Holland (1988) noted specifically that age appeared to predict a poor prognosis for change in global aphasia but they also identified a number of exceptions to this rule. Thus, age can not be considered an absolute predictor. The variability in evolution patterns and age effects identified by these authors is intriguing and suggests the need for further large-scale research studies in this area.

Hemiplegia

Occasionally, global aphasia occurs without an accompanying hemiparesis (Bogousslavsky, 1988; Ferro, 1983; Van Horn & Hawes, 1982). Motor abilities may be preserved following dual discrete lesions occurring in the frontal and temporoparietal regions, a single frontotemporoparietal lesion, or a single temporoparietal lesion. Absence of a hemiparesis in global aphasia may be a positive indicator for recovery (Legatt et al., 1987; Tranel et al., 1987). Tranel et al. (1987) described global aphasic patients with dual discrete lesions (anterior and posterior cerebral) that spared the primary motor area. These patients' global aphasia improved significantly within the first 10 months post-onset. Deleval et al. (1989) reported two cases of global aphasia without hemiparesis following discrete prerolandic lesions. Though both of these patients exhibited mild right arm weakness initially, this motor disturbance cleared within 48 hours of onset. Deleval et al.'s (1989) patients showed rapid recovery yet they continued to exhibit what the authors referred to as a residual motor aphasia. Basso and Farabola's (1997) patient experienced global aphasia and a right hemiparesis that cleared within a few days following a single, left frontotemporal lesion. Though severely aphasic at the initiation of treatment 40 days post-onset, the patient's language outcome 2.5 years later was described as "outstanding." Nagaratnam et al. (1996) examined language recovery at 3 months post-stroke in 12 patients diagnosed with global aphasia without hemiparesis 4 to 8 days after onset. Eight patients with single lesions in either anterior language cortex or posterior language cortex recovered to no more than mild levels of impairment. Four patients with lesions in both anterior and posterior language areas continued to have severe language impairments. Keyserlingk et al. (1997) found that chronic global aphasic patients with no history of hemiparesis secondary to a

single, large lesion of the left perisylvian region did not fare any better with regard to language outcome than did their global aphasic counterparts with hemiparesis from the time of onset. The critical difference between the two groups for motor, but not language function, depended upon the degree to which the patients' lesions extended into the subcortical white matter and nuclei.

Radiologic Findings

CT scans may provide another prognostic tool. In a two-part study, Pieniadz et al. (1983) investigated the relationship between hemispheric asymmetries and recovery from aphasia. The first part of the study involved the analysis of hemispheric asymmetry in a large group of aphasic subjects and in a group of nonaphasic control subjects. The results demonstrated significant similarity and consistency in hemispheric asymmetry for both groups. The most frequent asymmetry involved left-greater-than-right occipital width. Frontal width was greater in the right hemisphere than in the left hemisphere. Length was also greater in the left occipital region. For frontal length, the hemispheres were typically equal.

In the second part of the Pieniadz et al. (1983) study, recovery patterns were examined in a group of global aphasic subjects. These researchers found larger right occipital widths and lengths on CT scans for subjects demonstrating superior recovery of single word comprehension, repetition, and naming. Pieniadz et al. (1983) suggested that these atypical asymmetries may indicate a right hemisphere dominance for language. Evaluation of hemispheric asymmetries may be used, therefore, to predict recovery of single word functions, with atypical patterns suggesting superior long-term gains.

Naeser et al. (1990) used CT scans to compare lesion location and language recovery in a group of global aphasic subjects. The primary foci in the Naeser et al. (1990) study were recovery of comprehension abilities and differentiation between temporal lobe lesions involving Wernicke's area and those restricted to the subcortical temporal isthmus. The subjects in this study had either frontal, parietal, and temporal lobe lesions or lesions involving the frontal and parietal lobes with temporal lobe lesions restricted to the subcortical temporal isthmus. The results of Naeser et al. (1990) showed significantly better recovery of auditory comprehension for the group without damage to Wernicke's area (lesions limited to subcortical temporal isthmus). Over the course of 1 to 2 years, the majority of these subjects reportedly obtained auditory comprehension scores on the BDAE (Goodglass & Kaplan, 1983) that were consistent with only mild to moderate comprehension deficits (Naeser et al., 1990). None of the subjects in this study made significant gains in speech output.

A severe group of global aphasic subjects, with extreme loss of both verbal and nonverbal communication (including comprehension), was studied by De Renzi et al. (1991). De Renzi et al. (1991) found a variety of lesion patterns, only 35% of which involved the entire language area. Attempts to correlate specific types of lesions with some recovery of language abilities were unsuccessful. For the patients who showed some comprehension improvement, there was no common lesion pattern.

Mark et al. (1992) evaluated CT scans obtained from global aphasic patients in a routine acute-care setting to assess their viability for predicting language performance at 1 year post-onset. The scans were measured for lesion volume, total occipital asymmetry, and the cerebral volume occupied by the lateral ventricles and correlated with WAB (Kertesz, 1982) Aphasia Quotients and auditory comprehension scores. No clear relationship was found between acute imaging of the patients' lesions and their aphasia outcomes.

Language Scores

Collins (1986) has used scores obtained from global aphasic patients on the Porch Index of Communicative Ability (PICA) (Porch, 1981) to predict recovery. According to Collins (1986), global aphasic patients will invariably obtain scores below the 25th percentile. However, high intra- and intersubtest variability suggest at least the potential for recovery. Variability in this instance is defined as the difference between the mean score for a PICA subtest and the highest score within that subtest. A total variability score is derived by adding the variability scores for all PICA subtests. Variability scores above 400 suggest excellent potential for recovery while scores below 200 suggest poor potential for recovery.

Using medical and PICA data, Collins (1986) suggests that global aphasic patients demonstrating some variability within subtests and variability scores around 100, but relatively flat scores across all modalities, have a poor prognosis for recovery. Imitation, copying, and matching may be better than other test behaviors. Patients showing additional variability such that their variability scores are well above 100 and have greater divergence among modality scores, have a fair prognosis for recovery. Performance is generally characterized by mostly correct object matching, good copying skills, the ability to name one or two of the objects, and production of some differentiated responses on the verbal subtests. Significant increases in overall variability relative to the previous two categories and occasionally higher scores (7 or above) on auditory comprehension, reading, and naming subtests are consistent with a good prognosis for recovery. One patient described by Collins (1986) achieved a variability score over 400 while still performing at the 9th percentile.

Collins' recommendations should be tempered by recent work. Wertz et al. (1993) tested the influence of PICA intrasubtest variability on prognosis for improvement in aphasia. Negative and nonsignificant correlations were obtained between variability scores at 1 month post-onset and improvement in PICA overall performance at 6 and 12 months post-onset. In addition, no significant differences in improvement were found at 6 and 12 months post-onset between two groups with high variability (over 350) and low variability (under 300) at 1 month post-onset. Wertz et al. (1993) concluded that intrasubtest variability has no influence on prognosis.

For other aphasia measures, it generally appears that a lack of variability between auditory comprehension scores and other language scores may be viewed as a negative indicator. The more performance differs among tasks, the better the outlook. Further, higher test scores, i.e. less severe impairment, are consistent with a better prognosis. Within auditory comprehension scores, global aphasic patients who make yes-no responses to simple questions, regardless of their accuracy, seem to have a better outcome at 1 year post-onset than those who cannot grasp the yes-no format (Marks et al., 1992).

INTERVENTION

Before discussing clinical intervention for global aphasia, a few introductory remarks are provided in support of the management strategies that follow. The issues addressed here include some influences regarding the timing of intervention for global aphasia, the nature of the language assessment, and the behavioral targets for treatment.

Influences Regarding the Timing of Intervention

As described previously, the prognosis for recovery from global aphasia is generally poor (Kertesz & McCabe, 1977). Nonetheless, approximately one-fourth to three-fourths or more of these global aphasic patients will recover to a less severe aphasic or normal condition by the end of the first year after their stroke. Do these findings argue against early intervention for global aphasia? Should practitioners withhold assessment and treatment for these patients until a stable language profile is achieved? Clinicians have opposed withholding early treatment (Collins, 1986) and there are a number of current reasons to continue to do so.

Prognostic Limitations

Primary among the reasons for advocating early intervention is the inability to identify accurately those global aphasic patients who will evolve to less severe syndromes and those who will not. Even if it could be established that withholding early treatment from patients who have a high or low probability for good recovery is an acceptable clinical practice, current methodologies prevent clinicians from accurately identifying the recovery potential for these patients to make such decisions. Global aphasia cannot be reliably discriminated in the early stage (Wallesch et al., 1992) and any general conclusions about recovery in individual patients are "premature" (Basso & Farabola, 1997). Conflicting findings with regard to many of the factors identified above continue to present problems for estimating clinical prognosis.

Information derived from technological applications is assisting with this problem. The potential for recovery of auditory comprehension following global aphasia can be estimated by examining the CT scan lesion site patterns for these patients. As described earlier, better recovery can be expected at 1 to 2 years post-onset in patients whose temporal lesions spare Wernicke's area and involve only the subcortical temporal isthmus. Patients having temporal lesions that include more than half of Wernicke's cortical area, however, will likely continue to demonstrate moderate to severe comprehension deficits at 1 to 2 years after their injuries (Naeser et al., 1990). Recovery of spontaneous speech in severely nonfluent stroke patients with left middle cerebral artery (MCA) infarction can be estimated from the extent of lesion in two subcortical white matter areas: the medial subcallosal fasciculus (initiation of spontaneous speech) and the middle third of the periventricular white matter (motor/sensory aspects of spontaneous speech) (Naeser et al., 1989). For patients with lesions outside the left MCA, Naeser et al. (1989) suggest examining other specific structures as well, e.g., supplementary motor area, cingulate gyrus.

While these findings provide a promising approach to prognosis for global aphasia, their application appears to warrant discretion on several accounts when making decisions regarding early intervention for global aphasia. For example, the findings of Naeser et al. (1989) are limited in the current context because many of the patients in their most severe subject groups were not global aphasic. In addition, exceptions to expected patterns of recovery exist even in patients who meet the suggested neuroanatomical profiles (Naeser et al., 1989). Finally, the lack of clear CT scan patterns that could be associated with recovery from global aphasia in other studies (DeRenzi et al., 1991) suggests that these approaches are in need of further data before they can be applied rigorously.

Besides CT scan analysis, patients' levels of alertness or attention at the outset of global aphasia might also be assessed to predict superior recovery. Patients who are initially more alert or have better attention appear to show greater recovery from their global aphasia (Kertesz & McCabe 1977; Sarno & Levita, 1981). However, since the evidence for these latter findings is primarily anecdotal, their application as a clinical guideline is tenuous until additional information becomes available. These observations, along with differing profiles in the evolution of global aphasia, underscore the fact that global aphasic patients are a heterogeneous group. It is evident that research is needed to identify the particular factors and the way that they interact to account for better recovery. Clinicians might then more accurately identify the subgroups of global aphasic patients who will

demonstrate substantial language recovery and those who will not. This information can then be applied in management decisions regarding treatment (Ferro, 1992; Sarno et al., 1970).

In the absence of accurate techniques for predicting recovery from global aphasia, the most powerful reasons for providing early treatment are (1) the latent recovery observed in those patients who receive acute speech and language treatment and (2) the greater effects that are observed for aphasic patients generally when treated during the acute period of recovery. As described previously, global aphasic patients receiving early treatment, as a group, show continued language improvement during the period between 6 and 12 months post-onset (Kertesz & McCabe, 1977; Nicholas et al., 1993; Sarno & Levita, 1979, 1981) that is not observed in untreated patients (Pashek & Holland, 1988; Siirtola & Siirtola, 1984). Recent meta-analyses of the aphasia treatment literature have provided convincing evidence that outcomes for patients with severe aphasia are much greater when treatment is begun immediately after onset rather than during the postacute period (Robey, 1998). Until more is known about the individual global aphasic patient, these data suggest that clinicians should continue to intervene at the earliest opportunity to assist these patients at a time when such treatments may be most crucial to long-term recovery.

Treatment Objectives

A second reason for early intervention in global aphasia concerns the purpose of treatment. In deliberating this issue, consider a scenario where the clinical limitations described above no longer applied in predicting recovery from global aphasia. With full awareness of whether a patient will experience a good versus a minimal recovery, which outcome would suggest the need for early treatment? For patients who are expected to evolve to a less severe aphasia, would treatment be deferred necessarily to obtain the more stable language profile that might subserve a more effective long-term management plan? Or might treatment be initiated immediately to accelerate the patient's anticipated recovery? For patients who are not expected to demonstrate substantial recovery, would treatment be withheld due to the poor prognosis to allocate clinical and financial resources more effectively? Or would these patients become primary candidates for treatment to develop a functional communication system from the outset of their aphasia that will provide them the primary means through which they will communicate subsequently? When considering the purpose of treatment in either case, the arguments for early intervention with global aphasic patients, no matter their outcome, are more compelling than otherwise. The recovery patterns per se following global aphasia, therefore, do not provide an adequate rationale for postponing aphasia treatment for these patients.

Global aphasia will be greatest during the acute phase of recovery. Often, as alluded to above, treatment during this phase focuses on the remediation of language deficits via stimulation of disrupted cognitive processes. However, depending upon the degree to which the condition renders the patient unable to communicate even the most basic of needs, the first goals of treatment also focus on establishing some means of communication, no matter how simple. Some methods to accomplish this would include establishing reliable yes/no responding or a basic vocabulary of functional items through oral or gestural means such as head nodding, eye blinking, and pointing to pictures or specific icons. Interestingly, the activities associated with establishing these communication systems may, in and of themselves, be considered stimulatory for language. Clinicians also provide information to family, friends, and healthcare staff during this phase regarding the patient's particular language profile, i.e., preserved versus deficient areas, his prognosis, and suitable ways to improve communication with the patient. Early intervention in global aphasia, therefore, has the multiple purposes of language stimulation directed toward cerebral reorganization and recovery, identification of successful communication strategies, and patient, family, and staff counseling. None of these activities can or should be deferred until a stable language profile is achieved.

Goal Revisions

Global aphasic patients do demonstrate varying improvements in linguistic, extralinguistic, and nonverbal communicative functioning (Mohr et al., 1973; Kenin & Swisher, 1972; Prins et al., 1978; Wapner & Gardner, 1979; Sarno & Levita, 1979, 1981). As discussed, these improvements may result in recovery to a less severe form of aphasia in some cases, while in others the changes may be insufficient at as much as 1 year post-onset to suggest reclassification to another form of aphasia (Sarno & Levita, 1979, 1981). For this latter group, improvement can be anticipated in at least one of these categories, especially that of functional communication.

Most, if not all clinical aphasiologists recognize the dynamic nature of aphasia. Early testing, therefore, is viewed only as a measure of the patient's language functioning at a single point in time that will be used to establish a baseline for intervention during the acute period. Because of recovery, frequent probes for improvement in treated and untreated behaviors during this early period as well as re-evaluation using formal instruments is not only encouraged, but expected.

Withholding early treatment while awaiting more stable language profiles to improve treatment planning does not acknowledge that establishing and revising short-term treatment goals are inherent principles of aphasia rehabilitation. Whether treatment is provided before or after the first month post-onset, this process will be repeated regularly throughout the term of the patient's rehabilitation, regardless of the type of aphasia. There is little sense, therefore, in declaring this process to be less valid in global aphasia when treatment is initiated before the first month after injury.

Clinicians have much to offer global aphasic patients and their families during the acute period of recovery. When patients improve, the treatment objectives reflect this change; when they fail to change, concerted rehabilitative efforts continue in the areas of the patients' greatest functional communicative needs.

The Nature of the Assessment

Assessment of aphasic individuals encompasses more than simple diagnosis. Ideally, assessment provides a profile of not only the patients' areas of weakness, but also their strengths. Reasonable treatment plans require both types of data. Formal tests provide one method for gathering such data and, in addition, facilitate discussion of patient findings among colleagues. To that end, Collins (1986, p. 62) provides a summary of the severity ratings for a number of these tests that are suggestive of global aphasia. But formal tests may sometimes be inadequate for treatment planning (Rosenbek et al., 1989), especially in the case of severely impaired patients such as those with global aphasia. Little can be gained about patients' preserved areas of communicative functioning from test scores that are consistently near the floor for a given test. For these patients, information regarding their residual communicative capacities may be more readily available from a variety of informal (i.e., nonstandardized) measures. Such measures consist of patient observation to determine functional communication and the diverse methods for cuing behaviors that, when logically varied, allow a practical test of approaches that result in the most favorable responses. Methods that are successful in eliciting target behaviors are incorporated into treatment and provide an initial approach for developing subsequent behaviors.

Contemporary approaches include both formal and informal measures of assessment to establish a communication profile for the global aphasic patient. From a practical point of view, initial contact with the patient should be preceded by a review of medical records and interviews with knowledgeable others to glean information about the patient's communicative status. To the degree possible, a formal language assessment should be completed using a standardized aphasia battery, sampling behaviors across tasks at least minimally in each language domain (i.e., speaking, listening, reading, writing) and describing the patient's responses to each item. Given this baseline, assessment continues through what might be viewed as diagnostic treatment to identify the conditions which further promote successful language performance. Included here would be an analysis of patient responses during interviews focusing on familiar topics or in selected situations and the evaluation of hierarchical cues within language tasks.

In this "qualitative" approach, as described by Helm-Estabrooks (1986), neither type of language assessment (formal or informal) is seen as simply augmenting the other. For the global aphasic patient, both types are deemed mandatory to adequately describe communication functioning. A host of procedures are available to accomplish these objectives. These will be reviewed in the following sections.

The Behavioral Targets for Treatment

Because the impairment in aphasia is, first and foremost, a linguistic one, the primary target for aphasia treatment traditionally has been that of language performance. As a result, the success of intervention has been most often evaluated by the extent of changes occurring exclusively in the aphasic patient's grammatical and lexical behaviors. In such an approach, the potential for these changes is diminished with increases in the initial severity of the language impairment. Too often, this approach has resulted in an underestimation of what has been accomplished regarding recovery of communication skills.

Nowhere might this problem be more prevalent than in the case of the global aphasic patient. Since Sarno et al. (1970) suggested that severe aphasic stroke patients don't benefit from speech and language treatment, many health care providers have taken a rather pessimistic view with regard to rehabilitation outcomes in this group of patients. However, Sarno et al.'s conclusions, as well as others like them, were based solely upon statistical comparisons of pre- and post-treatment language scores and failed to account for positive changes that may have occurred in other communication behaviors. In a subsequent study involving global aphasic patients, Sarno and Levita (1981) examined the changes occurring not only in language scores, but also in communication performance as assessed by the Functional Communication Profile. These authors observed clinically significant improvements in the patients' language scores that were nonetheless insufficient to warrant reclassification to another aphasia syndrome. Inspection of nonverbal communication abilities revealed recovery of alternate skills (e.g., gesture, pantomime, and other extralinguistic behaviors) that exceeded the reported language changes. According to Sarno and Levita (1981), these improvements resulted in limited but effective communication by the end of the first year after stroke. Nicholas et al. (1993) also found significant improvements in the communication skills of their global aphasic patients during the first year post-stroke even though the majority of them did not change classification.

These findings have given way to a treatment approach that exploits the residual language capacity (Wapner & Gardner, 1979) and/or other functional abilities of these patients to improve communication and the patient's quality of life. Clinicians no longer attend exclusively to improving

propositional speech in global aphasic patients during or after the acute period of recovery. Such an emphasis is apparent in many of the treatment methods that have been developed recently for global aphasic patients.

ASSESSMENT

Assessment of communication functioning in patients with global aphasia is best achieved using both formal and informal measures. These measures are summarized in Table 21–2.

TABLE 21–2

Formal and Informal Measures for Assessment of Global Aphasia

Formal Assessment

General Language
Aphasia Diagnostic Profiles
Aphasia Language Performance Scales
Boston Assessment of Severe Aphasia
Boston Diagnostic Aphasia Examination
Examining for Aphasia—Third Edition
Language Modalities Test for Aphasia
Minnesota Test for Differential Diagnosis of Aphasia
Neurosensory Center Comprehensive Examination for Aphasia
Porch Index of Communicative Ability
Sklar Aphasia Scale—Revised 1983
Western Aphasia Battery

Modality-Specific
Auditory Comprehension Test for Sentences
Boston Naming Test
Functional Auditory Comprehension Test
Nelson Reading Test
Reading Comprehension Battery for Aphasia—Second Edition
Token Test
Revised Token Test

Functional Communication
ASHA Functional Assessment of Communication Skills for Adults
Communication Activities of Daily Living—Second Edition
Functional Communication Profile

Informal Measures

General Language
Auditory Comprehension Assessment (Edelman, 1984)
Behavioral Assessment (Salvatore & Thompson, 1986)

Functional Communication
Assessment of Communicative Effectiveness in Severe Aphasia (Cunningham et al., 1995)
Communicative Effectiveness Index (Lomas et al., 1989)
Functional Rating Scale (Collins, 1986)
Natural Communication (Holland, 1982)

Formal Test Measures

General Language

The language features of global aphasia are described in a previous section. Some standardized aphasia test batteries that specifically address global aphasia in their classification schemes include the *Language Modalities Test for Aphasia* (Wepman & Jones, 1961), the *Minnesota Test for Differential Diagnosis of Aphasia* (irreversible aphasia syndrome) (Schuell, 1974), the *Boston Diagnostic Aphasia Examination* (Goodglass & Kaplan, 1983), the *Sklar Aphasia Scale* (Sklar, 1983), and the *Western Aphasia Battery* (Kertesz, 1982). Additional batteries that comprehensively assess language performance to provide the clinical data for a diagnosis of global aphasia include *Examining for Aphasia—Third Edition* (Eisenson, 1994), the *Porch Index of Communicative Abilities* (Porch, 1981), the *Neurosensory Center Comprehensive Examination for Aphasia* (Spreen & Benton, 1977), and the *Aphasia Language Performance Scales* (Keenan & Brassell, 1975). The performance pattern for global aphasic patients on any of the tests identified above is generally one of severe impairment in all language abilities.

Information derived from a number of modality-specific assessment instruments can also be combined to arrive at a diagnosis of global aphasia. These tests include the following: auditory comprehension—the *Token Test* (De Renzi & Vignolo, 1962), the *Auditory Comprehension Test for Sentences* (Shewan & Canter, 1971; Shewan, 1979), the *Revised Token Test* (McNeil & Prescott, 1978), and the *Functional Auditory Comprehension Task* (LaPointe & Horner, 1978; LaPointe et al., 1985); reading comprehension—the *Reading Comprehension Battery for Aphasia—Second Edition* (LaPointe & Horner, 1998) and the *Nelson Reading Test* (Nelson, 1962; Nicholas et al., 1985); and naming—the *Boston Naming Test* (Goodglass & Kaplan, 1983).

Unlike the foregoing instruments, the *Boston Assessment of Severe Aphasia (BASA)* (Helm-Estabrooks et al., 1989) was developed "for the specific purpose of identifying and quantifying preserved abilities that might form the beginning steps of rehabilitation programs for severely aphasic patients" (p. 1). The BASA assesses performance on 61 items in 15 areas: social greetings and simple conversation; personally relevant yes/no question pairs; orientation to time and place; bucco-facial praxis; sustained phonation and singing; repetition; limb praxis; comprehension of number symbols; object naming; action picture items; comprehension of coin names, famous faces, emotional words, phrases, and symbols; visuospatial items, and signature. Responses are scored for response modality (verbal, gestural, or both), communicative quality (fully communicative, partially communicative, noncommunicative, unintelligible, irrelevant, incorrect, or unreliable, or task refused or rejected), affective quality, and perseveration. Raw scores are summed according to seven clusters of items: auditory comprehension, praxis, oral-gestural expression, reading comprehension, gesture recognition, writing, and visuo-spatial tasks. Norms are provided to convert the total raw score and item cluster raw scores to standard scores and percentile ranks. "Because an important goal of the BASA is to help determine whether a severe case of aphasia may be classified as global," (p. 42) two separate sets of norms are provided, one for cases of severe aphasia and one for global aphasia.

Functional Communication

Three measures for the formal assessment of functional communication include the *Functional Communication Profile (FCP)* (Sarno, 1969), *Communication Activities of Daily Living—Second Edition (CADL-2)* (Holland et al., 1998), and the *Functional Assessment of Communication Skills for Adults (ASHA FACS)* (Frattali et al., 1995). The FCP assesses 45 communication behaviors in a conversational situation that are considered to be common functions of everyday life. Behaviors are rated as normal, good, fair, or poor and transformed to raw scores within five dimensions: movement, speaking, understanding, reading, and other behaviors. The raw scores are converted to a percentage and a weighted score representing the patient's performance relative to normal behavior for that dimension. An overall score is obtained by summing the weighted scores to represent the patient's percentage of normal communication.

The CADL-2 includes 50 items that assess communication skills in structured, simulated daily activities. It includes a series of context-dependent items that evoke a variety of speech acts and verbal interchanges as well as other items that assess functional reading, writing, and math. Responses can be communicated by a variety of verbal and nonverbal means and are scored as correct, adequate, or wrong. The CADL-2 has high inter- and intra-rater reliability and includes standard scores and performance norms.

The ASHA FACS contains 43 items that assess functional communication in four areas: social communication; communication of basic needs; reading, writing, and number concepts; and daily planning. A 7-point quantitative scale rates the frequency of behaviors. A 5-point qualitative scale rates the adequacy, appropriateness, and promptness of an individual's responses as well as the relative sharing of communication burden with the partner. The ASHA FACS has been found to be reliable and valid for use with adult aphasia resulting from left-hemisphere stroke and adult cognitive communication disorders resulting from traumatic brain injury. It is available in both a paper and pencil version and a computerized version.

Informal Measures

General Language

As described previously, informal measures of language assessment are conducted following formal assessment with a standardized battery to identify the conditions that further promote successful language performance. Such measures aim to identify isolated areas of preserved performance such as those found above under features of comprehension. Hierarchical cues are used to evaluate such residual areas within language tasks.

Salvatore and Thompson (1986) provide an example of informal assessment procedures designed to assess verbal and nonverbal communication systems in global aphasic patients. The model used in their approach uses one stimulus to evoke a variety of responses. When stimuli are presented to evoke all levels of responding, stimulus-response relations that are preserved and those that are impaired are identifiable. For example, patients may be asked to provide several responses to a pictured stimulus including matching it to an identical picture and both writing and saying its name. Responses are analyzed in different modes including gesturing, drawing, reading, writing, and verbalizing. A matrix is developed to categorize the various relations that are tested. The results of the assessment provide important information that provides a basis for treatment.

Edelman (1984) provides an outline for the assessment of comprehension in global aphasia that specifically takes into account research findings identifying areas of residual function in global aphasia and factors that facilitate understanding. The suggested framework permits a systematic evaluation of understanding both contextually and acontextually while manipulating variables found to be facilitative. Performance is assessed using commands and questions at simple linguistic levels. Commands are divided into two sections. Those relating to self involve whole body movements, limb movements, and orofacial movements. Those relating to objects in the environment are divided into object recognition and object manipulation. These tasks are assessed respectively in a natural verbal context ("Have you any water?"; "Can you pass the tissues?") and acontextually ("Show me the comb"; "Pick up the comb"). Questions require affirmation or negation only and include those relating to self and those of less personal saliency. Responses are accepted when communicated either verbally or nonverbally. In addition, hierarchical cuing is incorporated, consisting of repetition, utterance expansion, and gestural accompaniment, and scored using a modified PICA system.

Functional Communication

A number of informal procedures that can be used to systematically evaluate the functional communication of global aphasic patients have also appeared in the literature. Holland (1982) developed a procedure to score observations of natural communication in normal family interactions. The categories of behaviors included verbal and nonverbal output, reading, writing, and math, and other communicative behaviors such as talking on the phone and singing. The verbal behaviors were further subcategorized to capture the form, style, conversational dominance, correctional strategies, and metalinguistics of the production. Holland's (1982) procedure is "primarily concerned with the frequency and form of successful and failed verbal and nonverbal communicative acts" (p. 52).

Lomas et al. (1989) constructed the Communicative Effectiveness Index (CETI) using communicative situations provided by aphasic patients and their families that were thought to be important in day-to-day life. The CETI quantitatively assesses aphasic persons' performance over time in 16 situations using judgments provided by spouses or significant others. Performance is rated relative to the aphasic persons premorbid abilities using a visual analog scale. The situations range from getting somebody's attention to describing or discussing something in depth. The index was found to be internally consistent, to have acceptable test-retest and interrater reliability, and to be a valid measure of functional communication when compared with other measures. The authors conclude that the CETI is an instrument that is capable of measuring the functional changes occurring during the aphasic patient's recovery that have been difficult to measure previously.

Cunningham et al. (1995) developed the Assessment of Communicative Effectiveness in Severe Aphasia (ACESA). It consists of two sections: a structured conversation and an assessment of the patient's ability to convey information about objects and pictures. Gesture, facial expression, speech, symbolic noise, and intonation are accepted ways for conveying information. Communicative effectiveness is rated using separate scales of recognizability for verbal and nonverbal responses. In an initial study to test the reliability of the instrument, test–retest reliability and intrarater reliability were found to be good. The authors suggested therefore that the tool can be useful for assessing change in communicative effectiveness when it is scored by the same person. Low interrater reliability, however, suggested that the tool needs further modifications before it can be used confidently for other clinical and/or research purposes.

Finally, a less systematic but often effective assessment of functional communication can be derived from patient interviews or questionnaires completed by individuals who are familiar with the global aphasic patient. Collins (1986) reviews several of these questionnaires and provides one such example, an adaptation of the FCP called the Functional Rating Scale.

TREATMENT

Given the poor outcome in chronic global aphasia (Kertesz & McCabe, 1977; Sarno & Levita, 1981) and the negative results that have been reported for treatment programs aimed specifically at remediating verbal skills (Sarno et al., 1970), treatment for these patients largely emphasizes compensatory rather than stimulatory approaches to

---

TABLE 21–3

Treatment Approaches for Global Aphasia

Stimulation Approaches

Auditory Comprehension
Matching pictures
Eliciting appropriate responses
Playing cards

Verbal Expression
Associating meaning with speech movements
Conversational prompting
Voluntary Control of Involuntary Utterances

Compensatory Approaches

Gestural Programs
Amer-Ind Code
Visual Action Therapy
Pantomime
Limited manual sign systems

Gestural-Assisted Programs
Preparatory training
Communication Boards
Blissymbols
Drawing
Computer-Aided Visual Communication
Lingraphica

---

language rehabilitation (Peach, 1993). Compensatory approaches utilize strategies that exploit the patient's residual linguistic and nonlinguistic cognitive skills to increase successful communication. Stimulatory approaches utilize structured methods that are carefully controlled for levels of difficulty to provide a context that will facilitate successful language responses and shape succeeding language behaviors of increasing complexity. Both approaches, however, may be utilized appropriately in treatment during the course of recovery from global aphasia. Table 21–3 provides a summary of these approaches.

Stimulation Approaches

Auditory Comprehension

Collins (1986, 1997) suggests that a realistic goal for treatment with the global aphasic patient consists of improving auditory comprehension, supplemented with contextual cues, to permit consistent comprehension of one-step commands in well-controlled situations. For the most severe comprehension deficits, picture matching, accompanied by the clinician's production of the name of the items to be matched, may provide the most basic level of auditory stimulation. Even in those cases where the patient has no understanding of the auditory stimulus accompanying the pictures, it is assumed that the response elicited by

the matching task evokes auditory representations of the visual stimuli which may underlie subsequent association of meaning with the name of the pictures (Peach, 1993). Complexity may be increased within this task by (a) increasing the size of the response field, (b) moving from pairing real objects to realistic pictures of objects to line drawings of the objects, (c) matching objects to pictures and pictures to objects, a technique which is incorporated in Visual Action Therapy (Helm-Estabrooks et al., 1982), and (d) using sets of pictures that represent nouns with decreasing frequency of occurrence in language usage. As performance improves, these tasks may be followed by word recognition for objects, pictures, or body parts and responding to simple questions.

Marshall (1986) provides an approach to treating auditory comprehension in global aphasic patients that is presented in four phases: (a) eliciting responses, (b) eliciting differentiated responses, (c) eliciting appropriate responses, and (d) eliciting accurate responses. In the first phase, clinicians focus on attending, pointing, and yes/no responding; at a minimum, the clinician should help the patient to express himself or herself through head nods, smiles, or frowns. Patients who cannot respond to spoken messages may engage in visual matching or orientation tasks. They may also be provided spoken messages accompanied by gestures. Questions and statements about personally relevant topics may comprise one of the best ways to elicit responses during this phase. In the second phase, the materials and techniques to elicit responses are not unlike those used in the first phase. At this time, however, the clinician accepts and reinforces any response that is different from the previous response given for those stimuli, e.g., varied facial expressions, head nods, gestures, and stereotypic utterances. To do this, the clinician records the patient's responses to a standard set of simple questions, looking for a variety of responses between stimuli and from session to session. With progress, the patient will move into the third phase, demonstrating appropriate responses with occasional accurate responses such as pointing to a calendar when asked to show the date, saying "yes" instead of "no," and shrugging the shoulders when asked how he or she is feeling. Other appropriate responses consist of performing one command for another, production of jargon in response to a question or request for information. Marshall suggests that for some patients, appropriate responses may represent their best performance and should therefore be encouraged by clinicians and others in the patient's environment. Finally, in the fourth phase, clinicians seek accurate responses to such tasks as object and picture identification, following commands, and responding to yes/no and wh- questions. Nonverbal responses may be facilitated with accompanying props including pages with words and numbers written on them; a clock with movable hands; a calendar; a road atlas; lists of families, relatives and friends; and a communication notebook.

Collins (1986, 1997) has designed a program to treat auditory comprehension using playing cards. The approach is based on the observation that global aphasic patients can often recognize names that contain two salient features (e.g., "queen of hearts"), differentiate cards by suit, and place cards in a sequence when they are unable to perform similarly with other stimuli. Although not all patients achieve the highest levels of performance, Collins suggests that portions of the program are useful at some stage for most patients.

Verbal Expression

Despite conclusions that traditional treatment focused on verbal communication skills may be ineffective for global aphasia (Sarno & Levita, 1981; Salvatore & Thompson, 1986), short-term attempts to establish or expand verbal expression with global aphasic patients may be a legitimate therapeutic activity during both the acute and chronic phases of recovery (Rosenbek et al., 1989). Rosenbek et al. (1989) do this by first attempting to associate meaning with speech movements. To do this, patients use available methods (e.g., showing fingers, pointing, gesturing, writing, matching, selecting objects) to confirm the meaning of any successfully elicited verbalizations. Included among these may be serial productions, imitated words and phrases, or automatic, meaningful responses to conversations relating to a variety of topics. As described previously, conversational topics that are personally relevant will improve performance (Van Lancker & Klein, 1990; Van Lancker & Nicklay, 1992; Wallace & Canter, 1985). Patients who succeed in these tasks are taught to produce at least a small repertoire of useful spoken or spoken plus gestured responses. They suggest that these items include at least one greeting, the words yes and no, a few proper names, single words that express important needs, and perhaps one or more phrases, especially if they appear in the patient's spontaneous verbal productions. Imitation, either alone or supplemented by gesture and reading, is used to establish these responses (see also Collins, 1986, 1997 for a detailed approach to establishing an unequivocal yes/no response). Imitated responses are then practiced in more functional contexts using questions or practical situations to facilitate response generalization.

Conversational prompting, a method reported by Cochran and Milton (1984), uses modeling, expansion, and feedback to develop the verbal responses of severe aphasic patients in conversational contexts. Props and written cues are provided to facilitate verbal expression. Ten conversational levels are identified ranging from concrete, structured contexts (e.g., manipulating objects, acting out, and describing sequences) to more open contexts (e.g., structured interview, structured discussion). A cuing hierarchy is described to promote language retrieval. With its emphasis on conversational interaction, this technique may be particularly useful in developing contextually appropriate communication for global aphasic patients. It may also provide a suitable means for overcoming some of the problems traditionally associated with the generalization of trained responses to conversational contexts.

As described above, the verbal output of many global aphasic patients consists primarily of stereotypic recurring utterances or speech automatisms. For many of these patients, productive usage of single words or phrases may not be a realistic goal. The treatment program Voluntary Control of Involuntary Utterances (VCIU) (Helm & Barresi, 1980; Helm-Estabrooks & Albert, 1991) can be used with these patients to bring these stereotypies into more productive usage. In this program, words that are involuntarily and inappropriately produced in the contexts of testing and treatment are identified and used as later targets in treatment. The words are trained in a sequence including oral reading, confrontation naming, and finally, conversational usage until a vocabulary of between 200 to 300 words is established.

Compensatory Approaches

Gestural Programs

Amer-Ind Code

Probably the best known of the gestural programs is Amer-Ind Code (Rao, 1986; Skelly, 1979). Amer-Ind Code is adapted from American Indian sign, a gestural system based on the concepts underlying words rather than on the word themselves (Skelly et al., 1975). According to Rao and Horner (1980), Amer-Ind is concrete, pictographic, highly transmissible, easily learned, agrammatic, and generative. The system can be applied in aphasia rehabilitation as an alternative means of communication, as a facilitator of verbalization, and as a deblocker of other language modalities (Rao, 1986). A few reports have demonstrated the usefulness of Amer-Ind Code as an alternative means of communication (Rao et al., 1980, 1995; Tonkovich & Loverso, 1982). The approach might also be combined with other nonverbal means of communication (e.g., drawing) (see below) to increase a severe patient's communicative effectiveness (Rao, 1995). However, the greatest utility of the technique appears to be as a facilitator of verbalization though reports of its effectiveness vary (Hanlon et al., 1990; Hoodin & Thompson, 1983; Kearns et al., 1982; Rao & Horner, 1978; Raymer & Thompson, 1991; Skelly et al., 1974). Rosenbek et al. (1989) describe a treatment program for gestural reorganization that utilizes Amer-Ind Code as the primary system of gestures and has as its end goal verbalization without gestural accompaniment.

Visual Action Therapy (VAT)

VAT (Helm-Estabrooks & Albert, 1991; Helm-Estabrooks et al., 1982; Helm-Estabrooks et al., 1989; Ramsberger & Helm-Estabrooks, 1989) utilizes gestures to reduce apraxia and improve the patient's verbal expression or ability to use symbolic gestures as a means of communication. Three programs constitute the approach including proximal limb, distal limb, and bucco-facial VAT. A hierarchical procedure is used in each program to "move the patient along a performance continuum from the basic task of matching pictures and objects to the communicative task of representing hidden items with self-initiated gestures" (Helm-Estabrooks & Albert, 1991, p. 178). The authors suggest that the method produces improvements not only in the area of pantomime, as indicated by formal assessments, but also in the areas of auditory and reading comprehension, verbal repetition, and graphic copying.

Conlon and McNeil (1991) proposed that the efficacy of VAT has not been established due to experimental limitations in the original work of Helm-Estabrooks et al. (1982). Therefore, they investigated the effects of VAT on the communication abilities of two global aphasic patients. Using a modified program for experimental purposes, positive treatment effects were observed on most steps of the program for their first subject and on about half the steps for their second subject. While these results were generally consistent with those of Helm-Estabrooks et al. (1982), generalization of these effects to untreated items was not observed. This lack of generalization suggested that the learned behaviors did not influence performance on untreated but similar behaviors. Conlon and McNeil determined that VAT is not effective in achieving the program's stated purpose of establishing "symbolic representation" as defined by Helm-Estabrooks et al. (1982). These authors concluded that further research is needed before VAT can be confidently recommended for the treatment of global aphasic patients.

Some other gestural programs include pantomime; limited manual sign systems for hospitals and nursing homes such as manual shorthand, manual self-care signals, or a hand-talking chart; gestures for yes and no; eye-blink encoding; and pointing (Silverman, 1989). Silverman offers a number of suggestions for the selective use of each of these approaches. For example, pantomime may be appropriate for the aphasic patient who cannot use Amer-Ind Code. Limited manual sign systems may be used initially on an interim basis until other communication systems can be developed but may ultimately provide the only means of communication in the most severely impaired patients (for example, see Coelho, 1990, 1991). Pointing is desirable for the patient who is going to use a communication board.

Gestural-Assisted Programs

Silverman also describes gestural communication strategies assisted by nonelectronic or electronic means. Strategies using nonelectronic assistance include transmission of messages by communication boards, manipulation of symbol sequences, and drawing. One of the most prominent gestural-assisted strategies in the rehabilitation of global aphasic patients using electronic means is computer-aided visual communication (C-ViC) (Weinrich et al., 1989).

Preparatory Training

Alexander and Loverso (1993) developed a specific treatment program for global aphasia that supports the capacity to make categorical and associational semantic discriminations while being sufficiently easy to allow an understanding of the nature and purpose of the tasks. They contend that treatment of this sort establishes a necessary precondition for subsequent treatment with gestural-assisted programs utilizing iconic/substitutional language (e.g., communication boards, C-ViC). Twenty-four common everyday objects, realistic pictures of those objects, and realistic pictures of the locations in which those objects would be found, were used as treatment stimuli. The stimuli were described as being representationally similar to those adopted for communication boards or C-ViC. Eight hierarchically arranged treatment levels were identified beginning with object to object matching in a field of 1 and increasing to picture sorting into locatively related groups. Two of five global aphasic patients studied reached the proposed goal of treatment—demonstration of semantic capacity across categorical and associational boundaries. The remaining global aphasic patients were unable to recognize the nature of the response required at more complex levels. The authors concluded that, even if only 40% of the patients respond successfully to the program, these patients constitute the appropriate group for substituted language systems.

Salvatore and Nelson (1995) described a training model for establishing equivalence relationships among visual stimuli that may have potential for use with gestural-assisted programs like those described below. In their study, four severely aphasic subjects learned novel symbolic relationships and generalized these to untrained relationships. The authors suggested that demonstrations of such generalization may be used as an indicator of the patient's ability to benefit from further treatment efforts.

Communication Boards

Communication boards vary in type and complexity. For severely impaired patients, a typical board will contain personally relevant words and pictures, numbers, and the alphabet. Specific treatment is required for effective use of the board. Collins (1986, 1997) suggests a training procedure where target items are identified in isolation, then after an imposed delay, and finally from among increasing numbers of foils until a temporary ceiling is obtained for the number of items contained on one board. Alternative boards containing pictures within only one domain, e.g., family, familiar objects, may be used to increase the number of items available to the patient.

Bellaire et al. (1991) investigated the acquisition, generalization, and maintenance effects of picture communication board training. Although their two subjects were not global aphasic, their findings have potential application to the treatment of this population.

Treatment and acquisition probes were administered in a traditional treatment room while generalization probes and training occurred during a coffee hour in a nursing home care unit. Pictures were divided into three sets for communicating social responses, requests for food and other items, and personal information. Stimulus presentations were followed by a 5-second response interval. If an accurate response was not observed, cues consisting of a verbal cue, a model, and a physical assist were provided. Subjects received response-contingent verbal feedback. Generalization training was conducted using a role-playing procedure in the treatment room using a script employed during the coffee hour probes or within the coffee hour setting. Maintenance data were collected for up to 6 months.

Following treatment, requesting and personal information responses were acquired but not social responses. No response generalization to untrained responses was observed nor was there generalization of board use during the coffee hour. Of the two procedures for training generalization, only training within the actual coffee hour setting resulted in generalized use of all responses except for social responses. Based upon these results, the authors recommended that (a) communication boards include primarily pictures that communicate specific content items and (b) treatment for the use of picture communication boards take place in the natural environments where the board is to be used.

Blissymbols

Johannsen-Horbach et al. (1985) assessed the benefits of treating four global aphasic patients with Blissymbols, a visual symbol system of pictograms and ideograms. All patients had previously received at least 6 months of traditional aphasia therapy without significant improvement in expressive language. For the procedures using Blissymbols, patients received individual treatment twice per week for a period of at least 2 months. The program was designed to (a) provide a basic lexicon of nouns, verbs, adverbs, and function words; (b) teach the production and comprehension of simple sentence in the symbol language; and (c) acquaint relatives with the symbol system to use in communicating with the patients. Symbols were introduced verbally along with simultaneous presentation of pictures or objects or the pantomime of the therapist. Training consisted of associating symbols and pictures for nouns, verbs, and function words in multiple-choice arrays and subsequently incorporating these items into Blissymbol sentences.

All patients acquired a symbol lexicon; three patients produced Blissyntactically correct sentences in response to pictures. Two of the patients successfully used the symbols in their communication with their relatives. In an important related finding, three patients evidenced the ability to articulate the correct words while pointing to the corresponding symbols and one patient articulated grammatical sentences. Variable outcomes with regard to continued use of the symbols with these four patients were reported.

The success of some severe aphasics in communicating with novel visual symbol systems has been interpreted as evidence for their superiority relative to the surface forms of natural language. To test this assumption, Funnell and Allport (1989) investigated the ability of two severely aphasic patients (neither of whom appeared to be globally aphasic) to use Blissymbols to communicate in conversational situations. By performing detailed analyses of the patients' abilities to process isolated words during listening, speaking, reading, and writing, the authors were able to compare the patients' use of Blissymbols with their processing of similar forms in natural language. Funnell and Allport (1989) found that the aphasic patients' performance with Blissymbols was entirely consistent with their processing of spoken and written words and that the use of Blissymbols did not provide a channel for communication that was independent of natural language processes. Further inquiry will be necessary to determine whether these findings can be applied to global aphasic patients who have more severely impaired natural language abilities than those of the subjects participating in Funnell and Allport's study.

Drawing

Drawing has received considerable attention both as a communicative medium and as a means to deblock verbal and written communication. Morgan and Helm-Estabrooks (1987; see also Helm-Estabrooks & Albert, 1991) designed a program entitled Back to the Drawing Board (BDB) to teach patients to communicate messages through sequential drawings. Patients are trained to draw cartoons from memory using verbal instruction, demonstration, and practice through copying. The cartoons range from one panel up to three panels. Criterion performance consists of reproducing a recognizable drawing that contains the critical details relevant to the humorous aspects of the cartoon. Treatment outcome is evaluated by increased accuracy in the patients' drawings of nine "accidents of living." Morgan and Helm-Estabrooks provide an operational definition of accuracy to facilitate comparison and interpretation of the drawings. Their posttreatment results for two patients indicated an improved ability to convey information through the use of drawing alone.

Lyon and Sims (1989) undertook a study to determine the degree to which severely aphasic patients can communicate through drawing and to evaluate the effectiveness of a treatment program emphasizing drawing-aided communication. Eight aphasic patients and eight comparable normal adults participated in the study. The eight aphasic subjects were enrolled in a treatment program focused on refining primary drawing skills (form, visual organization, detail, and perspective) within defined communicative contexts. Verbal and graphic cuing and requests for enlargement of distorted parts were used to improve the recognizability of the drawings. The drawings were then placed in a communicative interaction between the patient and a trained interactant who used specific strategies to optimize communicative effectiveness.

Communicative effectiveness was assessed using a 40-item drawing outcome measure to evaluate pre- and post-treatment performance with and without the use of drawings. A scale of communicative effectiveness was designed to rate performance on the outcome measure. A second scale was also designed to rate the recognition of drawings. Pre- and post-treatment performance on the PICA was also used to measure communicative effectiveness.

Following drawing treatment, substantial gains were observed in the aphasic subjects' communicative effectiveness compared with their pretreatment levels. Performance further improved following treatment to 88% of the communicative effectiveness score attained by the normal adults. The aphasic subjects also improved in the recognizability of their drawings following treatment, achieving 65% of the normal adults' scaled value. Based upon these data, the authors concluded that drawing serves as an important facilitator of communication by providing aphasic patients a fixed representation of a concept that is readily available for subsequent modification.

Kearns and Yedor (1992) have pointed out that specific programming may be needed in some cases to establish spontaneous use of drawing for communicative purposes. Ward-Lonergan and Nicholas (1995) described such a program for their global aphasic patient. The program began with BDB (Morgan & Helm-Estabrooks, 1987), progressed to the less structured conversational framework employed in Promoting Aphasics' Conversational Effectiveness (Davis & Wilcox, 1981) (see below), and concluded with an unstructured, interactive approach which they identified as Functional Drawing Training. The patient made substantial progress during the course of the program and, while spontaneous initiation of communicative drawing was still lacking at the end of the treatment, the patient was able to communicate effectively through drawing when given limited encouragement.

Computer-Aided Visual Communication (C-ViC)

C-ViC (Steele et al., 1987; Steele et al., 1989; Weinrich et al., 1989; Steele et al., 1992) provides another promising approach to establishing alternative communication in severely impaired patients. Using procedures similar to those of visual communication (ViC) (Gardner et al., 1976) but in a microcomputer environment, C-ViC is an iconographic system in which patients construct communications by selecting symbols from six "card decks" and arranging them according to certain syntactic conventions. The card decks contain interjections, animate nouns, verbs, prepositions, modifiers, and common nouns. Using C-ViC, global aphasic patients are able to develop a formal visual syntax in the absence of natural language which may be used successfully in a visual communication system (Weinrich et al., 1989). Formal procedures have been developed that extend training from introductory phases which teach the patient to follow simple commands to later phases designed to transfer C-ViC communication skills to use in a home setting (Baker & Nicholas, 1992).

Naeser et al. (1998) investigated the lesion site patterns for 17 severely aphasic patients who had undergone C-ViC training to determine whether these patterns were predictive of communication outcomes following C-ViC treatment. Although some of their patients were not global aphasic, all of the patients did present with little or no spontaneous speech and impaired auditory comprehension. Prior to treatment, all patients were tested with the BASA (Helm-Estabrooks et al., 1989) and underwent noncontrast CT scanning at 3 months or later post-stroke. C-ViC training was initiated no earlier than 3 months after aphasia onset and was continued twice weekly for 6 months to 1 year. Outcomes were based upon a rating scale that was developed to assess the quality of C-ViC generated sentences.

The findings from this study suggested that the lesion site pattern associated with the best response (initiates communication) using C-ViC spares large portions of either posterior systems that include Wernicke's area and the temporal isthmus or anterior systems that include the supplementary motor area and the cingulate gyrus. Moderate responses (responds to questions but does not initiate interactions) were found following lesions that spared posterior systems but involved anterior systems. Patients who demonstrated no response to the program had bilateral lesions that included variable lesions in either left posterior or posterior and anterior systems. The authors also found, however, that prediction of outcome was optimized when these lesion site patterns were combined with behavioral results obtained from pretreatment testing with the BASA (Naeser et al., 1998).

Similar to that reported with other gestural strategies, verbal facilitation has been noted (personal observation) during C-ViC training that produces successful naming not seen in these same patients in other communicative contexts, e.g., conversation, formal testing. While the ultimate goal of C-ViC is not verbalization without computer assistance (as might be the case with some of the foregoing gestural strategies), these observations suggest that C-ViC is a powerful verbal reorganizer that may enhance the language production of patients using this tool.

Lingraphica

The Lingraphica System is a therapy program delivered to patients in a laptop-computer that is used in the clinic and at home (Aftonomos et al., 1997). The computer provides clinicians and patients 144 interactive clinical exercises in nine different categories. The exercises follow a detailed patient care algorithm that suggests clinical pathways through a series of clinical exercises that are individually tailored to each patient's needs.

Two studies have demonstrated positive effects for chronic patients with a wide range of types and severities of aphasia following treatment using the Lingraphica System. Aftonomos et al. (1997) studied the responses to computer-based treatment of 23 aphasic patients who were 6 months to more than 15 years post-onset and who had been discharged from previous courses of speech-language treatment. All patients received 1-hour treatment sessions with a speech-language pathologist using the Lingraphica System and used the system at home (with the exception of 1 patient) for practice between clinical treatment sessions. Comparison of pre-treatment and post-treatment scores on a variety of formal language instruments demonstrated significantly improved performance in multiple modalities. Aftonomos et al. (1999) extended the previous work by assessing the outcomes of computer-based treatment on functional communication as well as formal language tests. Sixty subjects, consisting of 14 patients less than 6 months post-onset and 46 patients more than 6 months post-onset, were administered the WAB and CETI prior to the initiation of treatment. Treatment consisted of 1-hour sessions using the Lingraphica clinical exercises but with a focus on improving the patients' functional communication outside the clinic. The number of treatment sessions ranged from 10 to 132. Post-treatment group results demonstrated significant improvements for all subtests of the WAB and for the CETI. The acute and chronic aphasic groups each made significant improvements on both of the test measures and all of the patients grouped by aphasia category, with the exception of Wernicke and transcortical motor aphasic patients, made significant improvements. Eleven global aphasic patients included in this group had a mean Aphasia Quotient improvement of 6.2 points.

Promoting Aphasics' Communicative Effectiveness (PACE)

The last approach that will be considered here is Promoting Aphasics' Communicative Effectiveness or PACE treatment (Wilcox & Davis, 1978; Davis, 1980; Davis & Wilcox, 1981, 1985; Davis, 1986). Because PACE procedures allow patients to freely choose the channel(s) through which they will communicate, the technique provides opportunities for patients to use a verbal strategy or any of the gestural or gestural-assisted strategies described above, with or without verbal accompaniment, to convey messages. In this way, the approach emulates natural conversation by allowing participants to exchange information through multiple modalities. In addition to free selection, some of the other characteristics of natural conversation that provide guiding principles for PACE treatment include (a) clinician and patient participate equally as senders and receivers of messages, (b) the interaction incorporates the exchange of new information between clinician and patient, and (c) the clinician's feedback is based on the patient's success in communicating a message (Davis & Wilcox, 1985). PACE treatment utilizes a multidimensional scoring system to better capture the full range of behaviors which may be observed in this interactive approach. Generalization of language gains observed following PACE treatment has been demonstrated on formal language assessment instruments. Given its emphasis on the pragmatic aspects of language, PACE is well suited as a means to incorporate compensatory strategies into communication treatment. An additional strength of the approach, however, lies in its use as a framework for incorporating traditional language stimulation techniques into a communicatively dynamic context.

FUTURE TRENDS

It is clear that future clinical research must better identify the conditions under which treatment for global aphasia is maximally effective. To do so, several issues must receive further exploration. One of these concerns outcome from global aphasia and includes (a) identifying the factors that differentially account for evolution in some global aphasic patients to less severe aphasia syndromes, (b) establishing or refining prognostic indicators or profiles that can reliably predict outcome in global aphasia, and (c) specifying the relationships between site and extent of lesion for outcome in global aphasia. A second issue concerns how this outcome information can be better applied to management decisions for global aphasic patients. Naeser (1994) provides one example of the use of outcome information obtained during the acute phase of recovery for these purposes. This approach must be further developed to improve specificity and accuracy. Third, clinicians must continue to identify specific assessment and treatment approaches that are sensitive to the capabilities of global aphasic patients and produce reasonable outcomes in functional communication relative to the time and effort expended during the rehabilitation process. Finally, greater emphasis will be placed on improving not just communication, but the global aphasic patient's overall quality of life. Rehabilitation programs will incorporate increasingly sensitive measures to evaluate the psychosocial outcomes of treatment. Common practice will extend the continuum of care for these patients to support groups and other community organizations following the completion of formal speech and language treatment.

KEY POINTS

1. Global aphasia may be one of the most frequently occurring types of aphasia; age and sex do not appear to have a differential effect on the incidence of global aphasia.
2. Global aphasia may result from extensive cortical lesions of the dominant hemisphere, lesions confined to either the anterior or posterior cortex, or lesions restricted to subcortical regions. Global aphasic patients with large pre- and postrolandic middle cerebral artery infarcts generally have a poor recovery but some individual patients with this lesion pattern may demonstrate outstanding outcomes.
3. Global aphasic patients have several isolated areas of relatively preserved comprehension including specific word categories, familiar environmental sounds, famous personal names, and personally relevant information. The verbal output of global aphasic patients primarily consists of stereotypic recurring utterances or speech automatisms.
4. Nonverbal cognitive impairment is correlated with the degree of language impairment in global aphasia.
5. Global aphasic patients rely most heavily on nonverbal communication that may be nearly as effective as the communication strategies employed by patients with other types of aphasia.
6. Global aphasia most often results from middle cerebral artery occlusion below the point of branching but cases have occurred from illnesses such as epilepsy and demyelinating disease.
7. Global aphasic patients receiving treatment demonstrate substantial improvements during the first 3 to 6 months post-onset as well as continued improvement during the period between 6 and 12 months or more post-onset. Different patterns of recovery for language and non-language skills may be found during these periods.
8. Evolution from global aphasia is not simply the result of the time at which language is observed initially but is the result of a complex interaction of incompletely understood factors.
9. Younger global aphasic patients and those without accompanying hemiparesis tend to have better prognoses for language recovery.
10. Greater right hemisphere asymmetries are associated with superior recovery of single word language functions. Temporal lobe lesions that are limited to the subcortical temporal isthmus and spare Wernicke's area are associated with significantly better recovery of auditory comprehension following global aphasia.
11. Higher language test scores with greater variability among auditory comprehension and other language scores are consistent with a better prognosis. Global aphasic patients who respond to yes-no questions, regardless of accuracy, may have a better outcome than those who cannot grasp the yes-no question format.
12. In the absence of accurate techniques for predicting recovery from global aphasia, the most powerful reasons for providing early treatment are the latent recovery observed in patients who receive acute speech and language treatment and the greater effects that are observed for aphasic patients generally when treated during the acute period of recovery.
13. Early intervention in global aphasia has the multiple purposes of language stimulation directed toward cerebral reorganization and recovery, identification of successful communication strategies, and patient, family, and staff counseling.
14. Contemporary approaches to assessment include both formal and informal measures to establish a communication profile that documents not only the patients' areas of weakness, but also their strengths.
15. Treatment for global aphasia exploits the residual language capacity and/or other functional abilities of these patients to improve communication and the patient's quality of life.

References

Aftonomos, L.B., Steele, R.D., & Wertz, R.T. (1997). Promoting recovery in chronic aphsaia with an interactive technology. *Archives of Physical Medicine & Rehabilitation, 78*, 841–846.

Aftonomos, L.B., Appelbaum, J.S., & Steele, R.D. (1999). Improving outcomes for persons with aphasia in advanced community-based treatment programs. *Stroke, 30*, 1370–1379.

Alajouanine, M.S. (1956). Verbal realization in aphasia. *Brain, 79*, 1–28.

Alexander, M.P., Naeser, M.A., & Palumbo, C.L. (1987). Correlations of subcortical CT lesion sites and aphasia profiles. *Brain, 110*, 961–991.

Alexander, M.P. & Loverso, F.L. (1993). A specific treatment for global aphasia. *Clinical Aphasiology, 21*, 277–289.

Anonymous (1996). Weekly clinicopathological exercises: Case 8-1996: A 28 year old woman with the rapid development of a major personality change and global aphasia [Case records of the Massachusetts General Hospital]. *New England Journal of Medicine, 334*, 715–720.

Arrigoni, G. & De Renzi, E. (1964). Constructional apraxia and hemispheric locus of lesion. *Cortex, 1*, 170–197.

Baker, E. & Nicholas, M. (1992). *C-ViC training manual.* Unpublished manuscript.

Basso, A. & Farabola, M. (1997). Comparison of improvement of aphasia in three patients with lesions in anterior, posterior, and antero-posterior language areas. *Neuropsychological Rehabilitation, 7,* 215–230.

Basso, A., Capitani, E., Luzzati, C., & Spinnler, H. (1981). Intelligence and left hemisphere disease: The role of aphasia, apraxia and size of lesion. *Brain, 104,* 721–734.

Basso, A., De Renzi, E., Faglioni, P., Scotti, G., & Spinnler, H. (1973). Neuropsychological evidence for the existence of cerebral areas critical to the performance of intelligence tasks. *Brain, 96,* 715–728.

Basso, A., Della Sala, S., & Farabola, M. (1987). Aphasia arising from purely deep lesions. *Cortex, 23,* 29–44.

Basso, A., Lecours, A.R., Moraschini, S., & Vanier, M. (1985). Anatomoclinical correlations of the aphasias as defined through computerized tomography: Exceptions. *Brain and Language, 26,* 201–229.

Bellaire, K.J., Georges, J.B., & Thompson, C.K. (1991). Establishing functional communication board use for nonverbal aphasic subjects. *Clinical Aphasiology, 19,* 219–227.

Blanken, G., Wallesch, C.W., & Papagno, C. (1990). Dissociations of language functions in aphasics with speech automatisms (recurring utterances). *Cortex, 26,* 41–63.

Bogousslavsky, J. (1988). Global aphasia without other lateralizing signs. *Archives of Neurology, 45,* 143.

Brust, J.C., Shafer, S.Q., Richter, R.W., & Bruun, B. (1976). Aphasia in acute stroke. *Stroke, 7,* 167–174.

Cappa, S.F. & Vignolo, L.A. (1983). CT scan studies of aphasia. *Human Neurobiology, 2,* 129–134.

Cochran, R.M. & Milton, S.B. (1984). Conversational prompting: A sentence building technique for severe aphasia. *Journal of Neurological Communication Disorders, 1,* 4–23.

Coelho, C.A. (1990). Acquisition and generalization of simple manual sign grammars by aphasic subjects. *Journal of Communication Disorders, 23,* 383–400.

Coelho, C.A. (1991). Manual sign acquisition and use in two aphasic subjects. *Clinical Aphasiology, 19,* 209–218.

Collins, M. (1986). *Diagnosis and treatment of global aphasia.* San Diego, CA: College-Hill.

Collins, M.J. (1997). Global aphasia. In L.L. LaPointe (ed.), *Aphasia and related neurogenic language disorders* (2nd ed.) (pp. 133–150). New York: Thieme.

Colonna, A. & Faglioni, P. (1966). The performance of hemisphere-damaged patients on spatial intelligence tests. *Cortex, 2,* 293–307.

Conlon, C.P. & McNeil, M.R. (1991). The efficacy of treatment for two globally aphasic adults using Visual Action Therapy. *Clinical Aphasiology, 19,* 185–195.

Cunningham, R., Farrow, V., Davies, C., & Lincoln, N. (1995). Reliability of the assessment of communicative effectiveness in severe aphasia. *European Journal of Disorders of Communication, 30,* 1–16.

Damasio, A. (1991). Signs of aphasia. In M.T. Sarno (ed.), *Acquired aphasia* (2nd ed.) (pp. 27–43). San Diego: Academic Press.

Davis, G.A. (1980). A critical look at PACE therapy. *Clinical Aphasiology, 10,* 248–257.

Davis, G.A. (1983). *A survey of adult aphasia.* Englewood Cliffs, NJ: Prentice-Hall.

Davis, G.A. (1986). Pragmatics and treatment. In R. Chapey (ed.), *Language intervention strategies in adult aphasia* (2nd ed.) (pp. 251–265). Baltimore: Williams & Wilkins.

Davis, G.A. & Wilcox, J. (1981). Incorporating parameters of natural conversation in aphasia. In R. Chapey (ed.), *Language intervention strategies in adult aphasia* (pp. 169–194). Baltimore: Williams & Wilkins.

Davis, G.A. & Wilcox, M.J. (1985). *Adult aphasia rehabilitation: Applied pragmatics.* San Diego: College-Hill.

De Renzi, E. & Vignolo, L.A. (1962). The token test: A sensitive test to detect receptive disturbances in aphasics. *Brain, 85,* 665–678.

De Renzi, E., Colombo, A., & Scarpa, M. (1991). The aphasic isolate: A clinical-CT scan study of a particularly severe subgroup of global aphasics. *Brain, 114,* 1719–1730.

De Renzi, E., Faglioni, P., & Ferrari, P. (1980). The influence of sex and age on the incidence and type of aphasia. *Cortex, 16,* 627–630.

deBlesser, R. & Poeck, K. (1984). Aphasia with exclusively consonant-vowel recurring utterances: Tan-Tan revisited. In F.C. Rose (ed.), *Advances in neurology: Vol. 42. Progress in aphasiology* (pp. 51–57). New York: Raven Press.

deBlesser, R. & Poeck, K. (1985). Analysis of prosody in the spontaneous speech of patients with CV-recurring utterances. *Cortex, 21,* 405–416.

Deleval, J., Leonard, A., Mavroudakis, N., & Rodesch, G. (1989). Global aphasia without hemiparesis following prerolandic infarction. *Neurology, 39,* 1532–1535.

Doyle, M. & DeRuyter, F. (1995). Augmentative and alternative communication intervention for persons with severe aphasia. *Topics in Stroke Rehabilitation, 2*(1), 29–39.

Edelman, G.M. (1984). Assessment of understanding in global aphasia. In F.C. Rose (ed.), *Advances in neurology: Vol. 42. Progress in aphasiology* (pp. 277–289). New York: Raven.

Eisenson, J. (1994). *Examining for aphasia* (3rd ed.). Austin, TX: Pro-Ed.

Eslinger, P.J. & Damasio, A.R. (1981). Age and type of aphasia in patients with stroke. *Journal of Neurology, Neurosurgery and Psychiatry, 44,* 377–381.

Ferro, J.M. (1983). Global aphasia without hemiparesis. *Neurology, 33,* 1106.

Ferro, J.M. (1992). The influence of infarct location on recovery from global aphasia. *Aphasiology, 6,* 415–430.

Forde, E. & Humphreys, G.W. (1995). Refractory semantics in global aphasia: On semantic organisation and the access-storage distinction in neuropsychology. *Memory, 3*(3/4), 265–307.

Frattali, C., Holland, A.L., & Thompson, C.K. (1995). *Functional assessment of communication skills for adults.* Rockville, MD: American Speech-Language-Hearing Association.

Funnell, E. & Allport, A. (1989). Symbolically speaking: Communicating with Blissymbols in aphasia. *Aphasiology, 3,* 279–300.

Gainotti, G., D'Erme, P., Villa, G., & Caltagirone, C. (1986). Focal brain lesions and intelligence: A study with a new version of Raven's colored matrices. *Journal of Clinical and Experimental Neuropsychology, 8,* 37–50.

Gardner, H., Zurif, E.B., Berry, T., & Baker, E. (1976). Visual communication in aphasia. *Neuropsychologia, 14,* 275–292.

Goodglass, H. & Kaplan, E. (1983). *The assessment of aphasia and related disorders* (2nd ed.). Philadelphia: Lea & Febiger.

Habib, M., Ali-Cherif, A., Poncet, M., & Salamon, G. (1987). Age-related changes in aphasia type and stroke localization. *Brain and Language, 31*, 245–251.

Hanlon, R.E., Brown, J.W., & Gerstman, L.J. (1990). Enhancement of naming in nonfluent aphasia through gesture. *Brain and Language, 38*, 298–314.

Hartman, J. (1981). Measurement of early spontaneous recovery from aphasia with stroke. *Annals of Neurology, 9*, 89–91.

Heiss, W.D., Kessler, J., Karbe, H., Fink, G.R., & Pawlik, G. (1992). Cerebral glucose metabolism as a predictor of recovery from aphasia in ischemic stroke. *Archives of Neurology, 50*, 958–964.

Helm, N.A. & Barresi, B. (1980). Voluntary control of involuntary utterances: A treatment approach for severe aphasia. *Clinical Aphasiology, 10*, 308–315.

Helm-Estabrooks, N. (1992). *Aphasia diagnostic profiles.* Chicago: Riverside Publishing.

Helm-Estabrooks, N. (1986). Severe aphasia. In J.M. Costello & A.L. Holland (eds.), *Handbook of speech and language disorders* (pp. 917–934). San Diego, CA: College-Hill.

Helm-Estabrooks, N. & Albert, M.L. (1991). *Manual of aphasia therapy.* Austin, TX: Pro-Ed.

Helm-Estabrooks, N., Fitzpatrick, P.M., & Barresi, B. (1982). Visual action therapy for global aphasia. *Journal of Speech and Hearing Disorders, 47*, 385–389.

Helm-Estabrooks, N., Ramsberger, G., Brownell, H., & Albert, M. (1989). Distal versus proximal movement in limb apraxia. *Journal of Clinical and Experimental Neuropsychology, 7*, 608.

Helm-Estabrooks, N., Ramsberger, G., Morgan, A.R., & Nicholas, M. (1989). *Boston Assessment of Severe Aphasia.* Chicago: Riverside Press.

Herrmann, M., Koch, U., Johannsen-Horbach, H., & Wallesch, C.W. (1989). Communicative skills in chronic and severe nonfluent aphasia. *Brain and Language, 37*, 339–352.

Holland, A.L., Fratalli, C.M., & Fromm, D. (1998). *Communication Activities of Daily Living* (2nd ed.). Austin, TX: Pro-Ed.

Holland, A.L. (1982). Observing functional communication of aphasic adults. *Journal of Speech and Hearing Disorders, 47*, 50–56.

Holland, A.L. & Bartlett, C.L. (1985). Some differential effects of age on stroke-produced aphasia. In H.K. Ulatowska (ed.), *The aging brain: Communication in the elderly* (pp. 141–155). San Diego, CA: College-Hill.

Holland, A.L., Greenhouse, J.B., Fromm, D., & Swindell, C.S. (1989). Predictors of language restitution following stroke: A multivariate analysis. *Journal of Speech and Hearing Research, 32*, 232–238.

Holland, A.L., Swindell, C.S., & Forbes, M.M. (1985). The evolution of initial global aphasia: Implications for prognosis. *Clinical Aphasiology, 15*, 169–175.

Hoodin, R.B. & Thompson, C.K. (1983). Facilitation of verbal labeling in adult aphasia by gestural, verbal or verbal plus gestural training. *Clinical Aphasiology, 13*, 62–64.

Johannsen-Horbach, H., Cegla, B., Mager, U., Schempp, B., & Wallesch, C.W. (1985). Treatment of global aphasia with a nonverbal communication system. *Brain and Language, 24*, 74–82.

Kearns, K., Simmons, N.N., & Sisterhen, C. (1982). Gestural sign (Amer-Ind) as a facilitator of verbalization in patients with aphasia. *Clinical Aphasiology, 12*, 183–191.

Kearns, K.P. & Yedor, K. (1992, June). Artistic activation therapy: Drawing conclusions. Paper presented at the Clinical Aphasiology Conference, Durango, CO.

Keenan, J.S. & Brassell, E.G. (1975). *Aphasia language performance scales.* Murphreesboro, TN: Pinnacle Press.

Kenin, M. & Swisher, L.P. (1972). A study of patterns of recovery in aphasia. *Cortex, 8*, 56–68.

Kertesz, A. (1979). *Aphasia and associated disorders: Taxonomy, localization, and recovery.* Orlando, FL: Grune & Stratton.

Kertesz, A. (1982). *Western Aphasia Battery.* New York: Grune & Stratton.

Kertesz, A. & McCabe, P. (1975). Intelligence and aphasia: Performance of aphasics on Raven's Coloured Progressive Matrices (RCPM). *Brain and Language, 2*, 387–395.

Kertesz, A. & McCabe, P. (1977). Recovery patterns and prognosis in aphasia. *Brain, 100*, 1–18.

Kertesz, A. & Sheppard, A. (1981). The epidemiology of aphasia and cognitive impairment in stroke. *Brain, 104*, 117–128.

Keyserlingk, A.G., Naujokat, C., Niemann, K., Huber, W., & Thron, A. (1997). Global aphasia—with and without hemiparesis. *European Neurology, 38*, 259–267.

Kumar, R., Masih, A.K., & Pardo, J. (1996). Global aphasia due to thalamic hemorrhage: A case report and review of the literature. *Archives of Physiology, Medicine, and Rehabilitation, 77*, 1312–1315.

LaPointe, L.L. & Horner, J. (1978, Spring). The functional auditory comprehension task (FACT): Protocol and test format. *FLASHA Journal*, pp. 27–33.

LaPointe, L.L. & Horner, J. (1998). *Reading comprehension battery for aphasia* (2nd ed.). Austin, TX: Pro-Ed.

LaPointe, L.L., Holtzapple, P., & Graham, L.F. (1985). The relationships among two measures of auditory comprehension and daily living communicative skills. *Clinical Aphasiology, 15*, 38–46.

Legatt, A.D., Rubin, M.J., Kaplan, L.R., Healton, E.B., & Brust, J.C.M. (1987). Global aphasia without hemiparesis: Multiple etiologies. *Neurology, 37*, 201–205.

Lomas, J. & Kertesz, A. (1978). Patterns of spontaneous recovery in aphasic groups: A study of adult stroke patients. *Brain and Language, 6*, 388–401.

Lomas, J., Pickard, L., Bester, S., Elbard, H., Finlayson, A., & Zoghaib, C. (1989). The communicative effectiveness index: Development and psychometric evaluation of a functional communication measure for adult aphasia. *Journal of Speech and Hearing Disorders, 54*, 113–124.

Lüders, H., Lesser, R.P., Hahn, J., Dinner, D.S., Morris, H.H., Wyllie, E., & Godoy, J. (1991). Basal temporal language area. *Brain, 114*, 743–754.

Lyon, J.G. & Sims, E. (1989). Drawing: Its use as a communicative aid with aphasic and normal adults. *Clinical Aphasiology, 18*, 339–355.

Mark, V.W., Thomas, B.E., & Berndt, R.S. (1992). Factors associated with improvement in global aphasia. *Aphasiology, 6*, 121–134.

Marshall, R.C. (1986). Treatment of auditory comprehensive deficits. In R. Chapey (ed.), *Language intervention strategies in adult aphasia* (2nd ed.) (pp. 370–393). Baltimore: Williams & Wilkins.

Marshall, R.C., Freed, D.B., & Phillips, D.S. (1997). Communicative efficiency in severe aphasia. *Aphasiology, 11*(4/5), 373–385.

Marshall, R.C. & Phillips, D.S. (1971). Prognosis for improved verbal communication in aphasic stroke patients. *Archives of Physical Medicine and Rehabilitation, 64*, 597–600.

Masand, P. & Chaudhary, P. (1994). Methylphenidate treatment of postroke depression in a patient with global aphasia. *Annals of Clinical Psychiatry, 6*(4), 271–274.

Mazzocchi, F. & Vignolo, L.A. (1979). Localization of lesions in aphasia: Clinical CT scan correlations in stroke patients. *Cortex, 15*, 627–654.

McDermott, F.B., Horner, J., & DeLong, E.R. (1996). Evolution of acute aphasia as measured by the Western Aphasia Battery. *Clinical Aphasiology, 24*, 159–172.

McKenna, P. & Warrington, E.K. (1978). Category-specific naming preservation: A single case study. *Journal of Neurology, Neurosurgery, and Psychiatry, 41*, 571–574.

McNeil, M.R. & Prescott, T.E. (1978). *Revised Token Test*. Baltimore: University Park Press.

Mohr, J.P., Sidman, M., Stoddard, L.T., Leicester, J., & Rosenberger, P.B. (1973). Evolution of the deficit in total aphasia. *Neurology, 23*, 1302–1312.

Morgan, A.L.R. & Helm-Estabrooks, N. (1987). Back to the Drawing Board: A treatment program for nonverbal aphasic patients. *Clinical Aphasiology, 17*, 64–72.

Murdoch, B.E., Afford, R.J., Ling, A.R., & Ganguley, B. (1986). Acute computerized tomographic scans: Their value in the localization of lesions and as prognostic indicators in aphasia. *Journal of Communication Disorders, 19*, 311–345.

Naeser, M.A. (1994). Neuroimaging and recovery of auditory comprehension and spontaneous speech in aphasia with some implications for treatment in severe aphasia. In A. Kertesz (ed.), *Localization and neuroimaging in neuropsychology* (pp. 245–295). San Diego, CA: Academic Press.

Naeser, M.A., Baker, E.H., Palumbo, C.L., Nicholas, M., Alexander, M.P., Samaraweera, R., Prete, M.N., Hodge, S.M., & Weissman, T. (1998). Lesion site patterns in severe, nonverbal aphasia to predict outcome with a computer-assisted treatment program. *Archives of Neurology, 55*, 1438–1448.

Naeser, M.A., Gaddie, A., Palumbo, C.L., & Stiassny-Eder, D. (1990). Late recovery of auditory comprehension in global aphasia: Improved recovery observed with subcortical temporal isthmus lesion vs Wernicke's cortical area lesion. *Archives of Neurology, 47*, 425–432.

Naeser, M.A., Palumbo, C.L., Helm-Estabrooks, N., Stiassny-Eder, D., & Albert, M.L. (1989). Severe non-fluency in aphasia: Role of the medial subcallosal fasciculus plus other white matter pathways in recovery of spontaneous speech. *Brain, 112*, 1–38.

Nagaratnam, N., Barnes, R., & Nagaratnam, S. (1996). Speech recovery following global aphasia without hemiparesis. *Journal of Neurologic Rehabilitation, 10*, 115–119.

Nelson, M.J. (1962). *The Nelson Reading Test*. Boston: Houghton-Mifflin.

Nicholas, L.E., MacLennan, D.L., & Brookshire, R.H. (1985). Validity of multi-sentence reading comprehension subtests in aphasia tests. *Clinical Aphasiology, 15*, 29–37.

Nicholas, M.L., Helm-Estabrooks, N., Ward-Lonergan, J., & Morgan, A.R. (1993). Evolution of severe aphasia in the first two years post onset. *Archives of Physical Medicine and Rehabilitation, 74*, 830–836.

Okuda, B., Tanaka, H., Tachibana, H., Kawabata, K., & Sugita, M. (1994). Cerebral blood flow in subcortical global aphasia: Perisylvian cortical hypoperfusion as a crucial role. *Stroke, 25*(7), 1495–1499.

Papanicolaou, A.C., Moore, B.D., Deutsch, G., Levin, H.S., & Eisenberg, H.M. (1988). Evidence for right-hemisphere involvement in recovery from aphasia. *Archives of Neurology, 45*, 1025–1029.

Pashek, G.V. & Holland, A.L. (1988). Evolution of aphasia in the first year post-onset. *Cortex, 24*, 411–423.

Peach, R.K. (1992). Efficacy of aphasia treatment: What are the real issues? *Clinics in Communication Disorders, 1*, 7–10.

Peach, R.K. (1993). Clinical intervention for aphasia in the United States of America. In A. Holland & M. Forbes (eds.), *Aphasia therapy: World perspectives* (pp. 335–369). San Diego, CA: Singular Publishing Group.

Pieniadz, J.M., Naeser, M.A., Koff, E., & Levine, H.L. (1983). CT scan cerebral hemispheric asymmetry measurements in stroke cases with global aphasia: Atypical asymmetries associated with improved recovery. *Cortex, 19*, 371–391.

Piercy, M. & Smith, V.O.G. (1962). Right hemisphere dominance for certain non-verbal intellectual skills. *Brain, 85*, 775–790.

Porch, B.E. (1981). *Porch Index of Communicative Ability* (3rd ed.). Palo Alto, CA: Consulting Psychologists Press.

Prins, R.S., Snow, E., & Wagenaar, E. (1978). Recovery from aphasia: Spontaneous speech versus language comprehension. *Brain and Language, 6*, 192–211.

Raderstorf, M., Hein, D.M., & Jensen, C.S. (1984). A young stroke patient with severe aphasia returns to work: A team approach. *Journal of Rehabilitation, 50*(1), 23–26.

Ramsberger, G. & Helm-Estabrooks, N. (1989). Visual Action Therapy for bucco-facial apraxia. *Clinical Aphasiology, 18*, 395–406.

Rao, P.R. (1986). The use of Amer-Ind code with aphasic adults. In R. Chapey (ed.), *Language intervention strategies in adult aphasia* (2nd ed.) (pp. 360–367). Baltimore: Williams & Wilkins.

Rao, P.R. (1995). Drawing and gesture as communication options in a person with severe aphasia. *Topics in Stroke Rehabilitation, 2*, 49–56.

Rao, P.R. & Horner, J. (1978). Gesture as a deblocking modality in a severe aphasic patient. *Clinical Aphasiology, 8*, 180–187.

Rao, P.R. & Horner, J. (1980). Nonverbal strategies for functional communication in aphasic persons. In M.S. Burns & J.R. Andrews (eds.), *Neuropathologies of speech and language: Diagnosis and treatment* (pp. 108–133). Evanston, IL: Institute for Continuing Professional Education.

Rao, P.R., Basili, A.G., Koller, J., Fullerton, B., Diener, S., & Burton, P. (1980). The use of Amer-Ind code by severe aphasic adults. In M.S. Burns & J.R. Andrews (eds.), *Neuropathologies of speech and language: Diagnosis and treatment* (pp. 18–35). Evanston, IL: Institute for Continuing Professional Education.

Raven, J.C. (1965). *Guide to using the Coloured Progressive Matrices*. London: H.K. Lewis.

Raymer, A.M. & Thompson, C.K. (1991). Effects of verbal plus gestural treatment in a patient with aphasia and severe apraxia of speech. *Clinical Aphasiology, 20*, 285–295.

Reinvang, I. & Engvik, H. (1980). Language recovery in aphasia from 3 to 6 months after stroke. In M.T. Sarno & O. Hook (eds.), *Aphasia: Assessment and treatment* (pp. 79–88). New York: Masson.

Robinson, R.G. & Benson, D.F. (1981). Depression in aphasic patients: Frequency, severity, and clinical-pathological correlations. *Brain and Language, 14,* 282–291.

Robey, R.R. (1998). A meta-analysis of clinical outcomes in the treatment of aphasia. *Journal of Speech, Language, and Hearing Research, 41,* 172–187.

Rosenbek, J.C., LaPointe, L.L., & Wertz, R.T. (1989). *Aphasia: A clinical approach.* Austin, TX: Pro-Ed.

Rosser, M.N., Warrington, E.K., & Cipolotti, L. (1995). The isolation of calculation skills. *Journal of Neurology, 242,* 78–81.

Salvatore, A.P. & Nelson, T.R. (1995). Training novel language systems in severely aphasic individuals: How novel is it? *Clinical Aphasiology, 23,* 267–278.

Salvatore, A.P. & Thompson, C.K. (1986). Intervention for global aphasia. In R. Chapey (ed.), *Language intervention strategies in adult aphasia* (2nd ed.) (pp. 403–418). Baltimore: Williams & Wilkins.

Sarno, M.R. & Levita, E. (1971). Natural course of recovery in severe aphasia. *Archives of Physical Medicine and Rehabilitation, 52,* 175–178.

Sarno, M.R. & Levita, E. (1979). Recovery in treated aphasia during the first year post-stroke. *Stroke, 10,* 663–670.

Sarno, M.T. (1969). *The functional communication profile: Manual of directions* (Rehabilitation Monograph 42). New York: New York University Medical Center, Institute of Rehabilitation Medicine.

Sarno, M.T. (1981). Recovery and rehabilitation in aphasia. In M.R. Sarno (ed.), *Acquired aphasia* (pp. 485–529). New York: Academic Press.

Sarno, M.T. & Levita, E. (1981). Some observations on the nature of recovery in global aphasia after stroke. *Brain and Language, 13,* 1–12.

Sarno, M.T., Silverman, M.G., & Sands, E.S. (1970). Speech therapy and language recovery in severe aphasia. *Journal of Speech and Hearing Research, 13,* 607–623.

Sasanuma, S. (1988). Studies in dementia: In search of the linguistic/cognitive interaction underlying communication. *Aphasiology, 2,* 191–193.

Scarpa, M., Colombo, A., Sorgato, P., & De Renzi, E. (1987). The incidence of aphasia and global aphasia in left brain-damaged patients. *Cortex, 23,* 331–336.

Schuell, H.M. (1974). *The Minnesota test for differential diagnosis of aphasia* (rev. ed.). Minneapolis, MN: University of Minnesota Press.

Shewan, C.M. (1979). *Auditory comprehension test for sentences.* Chicago: Biolinguistics Clinical Institutes.

Shewan, C.M. & Canter, G.J. (1971). Effects of vocabulary, syntax, and sentence length on auditory comprehension in aphasic patients. *Cortex, 7,* 209–226.

Signer, S., Cummings, J.L., & Benson, D.F. (1989). Delusion and mood disorders in patients with chronic aphasia. *Journal of Neuropsychiatry, 1,* 40–45.

Siirtola, T. & Siirtola, M. (1984). Evolution of aphasia. *Acta Neurologica Scandinavica, 69*(Suppl. 98), 403–404.

Silverman, F.H. (1989). *Communication for the speechless* (2nd ed.). Englewood Cliffs, NJ: Prentice Hall.

Skelly, M. (1979). *Amer-Ind gestural code based on universal American Indian hand talk.* New York: Elsevier.

Skelly, M., Schinsky, L., Smith, R., Donaldson, R., & Griffin, P. (1974). American Indian Sign (Amerind) as a facilitator of verbalization for the oral-verbal apraxic. *Journal of Speech and Hearing Disorders, 39,* 445–456.

Skelly, M., Schinsky, L., Smith, R., Donaldson, R., & Griffin, P. (1975). American Indian sign: Gestural communication for the speechless. *Archives of Physical Medicine and Rehabilitation, 56,* 156–160.

Sklar, M. (1983). *Sklar aphasia scale* (revised). Los Angeles, CA: Western Psychological Services.

Sorgato, P., Colombo, A., Scarpa, M., & Faglioni, P. (1990). Age, sex, and lesion site in aphasic stroke patients with single focal damage. *Neuropsychology, 4,* 165–173.

Spinnler, H. & Vignolo, L. (1966). Impaired recognition of meaningful sounds in aphasia. *Cortex, 2,* 337–348.

Spreen, O. & Benton, A.L. (1977). *Neurosensory center comprehensive examination for aphasia* (rev. ed.). Victoria, BC: University of Victoria.

Steele, R.D., Kleczewska, M.K., Carlson, G.S., & Weinrich, M. (1992). Computers in the rehabilitation of chronic, severe aphasia: C-ViC 2.0 cross-modal studies. *Aphasiology, 6,* 185–194.

Steele, R.D., Weinrich, M., Kleczewska, M.K., Carlson, G.S., & Wertz, R.T. (1987). Evaluating performance of severely aphasic patients on a computer-aided visual communication system. *Clinical Aphasiology, 17,* 46–54.

Steele, R.D., Weinrich, M., Wertz, R.T., Kleczewska, M.K., & Carlson, G.S. (1989). Computer-based visual communication in aphasia. *Neuropsychologia, 27,* 409–426.

Tonkovich, J.D. & Loverso, F.L. (1982). A training matrix approach for gestural acquisition by the agrammatic patient. *Clinical Aphasiology, 12,* 283–288.

Tranel, D., Biller, J., Damasio, H., Adams, H.P., & Cornell, S.H. (1987). Global aphasia without hemiparesis. *Archives of Neurology, 44,* 304–308.

Van Horn, G. & Hawes, A. (1982). Global aphasia without hemiparesis: A sign of embolic encephalopathy. *Neurology, 32,* 403–406.

Van Lancker, D. & Klein, K. (1990). Preserved recognition of familiar personal names in global aphasia. *Brain and Language, 39,* 511–529.

Van Lancker, D. & Nicklay, C.K.H. (1992). Comprehension of personally relevant (PERL) versus novel language in two globally aphasic patients. *Aphasiology, 6,* 37–61.

Wallace, G.L. & Canter, G.J. (1985). Effects of personally relevant language materials on the performance of severely aphasic individuals. *Journal of Speech and Hearing Disorders, 50,* 385–390.

Wallace, G.L. & Stapleton, J.H. (1991). Analysis of auditory comprehension performance in individuals with severe aphasia. *Archives of Physical Medicine and Rehabilitation, 72,* 674–678.

Wallesch, C.W., Bak, T., & Schulte-Monting, J. (1992). Acute aphasia—patterns and prognosis. *Aphasiology, 6,* 373–385.

Wapner, W. & Gardner, H. (1979). A note on patterns of comprehension and recovery in global aphasia. *Journal of Speech and Hearing Research, 29,* 765–772.

Ward-Lonergan, J. & Nicholas, M. (1995). Drawing to communicate: A case report of an adult with global aphasia. *European Journal of Disorders of Communication, 30,* 475–491.

Weinrich, M., Steele, R., Carlson, G.S., Kleczewska, M., Wertz, R.T., & Baker, E.H. (1989). Processing of visual syntax in a globally aphasic patient. *Brain and Language, 36,* 391–405.

Weinrich, M., Steele, R., Kleczewska, M., Carlson, G.S., Baker, E.H., & Wertz, R.T. (1989). Representation of "verbs" in a computerized visual communication system. *Aphasiology, 3,* 501–512.

Wells, C.R., Labar, D.R., & Solomon, G.E. (1992). Aphasia as the sole manifestation of simple partial status epilepticus. *Epilepsia, 33,* 84–87.

Wepman, J.M. & Jones, L.V. (1961). *The language modalities test for aphasia.* Chicago: Education-Industry Service.

Wertz, R.T., Dronkers, N.F., & Hume, J.L. (1993). PICA intrasubtest variability and prognosis for improvement in aphasia. *Clinical Aphasiology, 21,* 207–211.

Wilcox, M.J. & Davis, G.A. (1978, November). Procedures for promoting communicative effectiveness in an aphasic adult. Symposium conducted at the annual meeting of the American Speech and Hearing Association, San Francisco, CA.

Yang, B.J., Yang, T.C., Pan, H.C., Lai, S.J., & Yang, F. (1989). Three variant forms of subcortical aphasia in Chinese stroke patients. *Brain and Language, 37,* 145–162.

Yasuda, K. & Ono, Y. (1998). Comprehension of famous personal and geographical names in global aphasic subjects. *Brain and Language, 61,* 274–287.

Chapter 22

Cognitive Neuropsychological Approaches to Rehabilitation of Language Disorders: Introduction

Argye E. Hillis

OBJECTIVES

The purpose of this chapter is to (1) describe the normal cognitive mechanisms (mental representations and processes) necessary to accomplish a given language task, such as naming or reading, which together comprise cognitive neuropsychological models of those language tasks; (2) describe an approach to assessment and treatment of aphasic individuals that begins with identifying, in each patient, the cognitive mechanisms that are impaired and those that are intact, within a cognitive neuropsychological model of the affected language task; (3) provide examples of this general approach that have resulted in functional gains in communication abilities; (4) delineate the uses and limitations of this approach to clinical management of aphasic persons; and (5) speculate on the future trends in the areas of cognitive science and language rehabilitation.

DEFINITION

This section provides illustrations of a general approach to assessment and treatment of specific language tasks that makes use of cognitive analyses and models developed within the discipline of cognitive neuropsychology—a branch of psychology that seeks to understand normal human cognitive mechanisms through evidence from how cognitive mechanisms are modified by brain damage. This approach begins, for each individual patient, with identifying which cognitive processes and representations underlying the language task are impaired and which processes and representations are intact. Treatment then focuses either on remediation of the impaired cognitive processes or compensation via the intact cognitive processes or both. This framework involves consideration of the patient's performance of the task in light of a model of the cognitive processes and representations that underlie normal performance of the task. It should be emphasized that the treatment procedures themselves are not based on models from cognitive neuropsychology, but are based on principles of learning, clinical experience with the sorts of input that successfully elicit better performance, and other skills, talents, and knowledge of the clinician—just like other therapy strategies in speech-language pathology. In fact, the selection of the chapter contributors reflects the fact that this approach has its foundations in the integration and cooperation across the professions of cognitive neuropsychology, speech-language pathology, behavioral neurology, and other professions within the discipline of cognitive science. Related areas include cognitive psychology (a branch of psychology devoted to the study of normal cognitive processing), psycholinguistics (a branch of psychology devoted to the study of rules and representations that underlie normal language comprehension and production), and linguistics (a profession devoted to investigation of the structure and computation of language). No one profession can lay claim to the sort of rehabilitation described in this section, although clinicians in each profession can engage in it equally. Consider the background of the authors. Leslie Gonzalez-Rothi and Anastasia Raymer are speech-language pathologists who have worked with Kenneth Heilman and numerous other behavioral neurologists and neuropsychologists at the Gainesville VA Medical Center. Anastasia Raymer (along with Rita Berndt & Charlotte Mitchum) also worked in the Cognitive Neuropsychology Laboratory at Johns Hopkins. Rita Berndt, a cognitive neuropsychologist, and Charlotte Mitchum, a speech-language pathologist, have had a long and enormously productive collaboration in the Neurology Department at University of Maryland Hospital. Pelagie Beeson is a speech-language pathologist who has worked with behavioral neurologists, neuropsychologists, and other aphasiologists at the National Center for Neurogenic Communication Disorders in Tuscon, Arizona. Finally, I am a behavioral neurologist, who was previously both a speech-language pathologist and a researcher in the cognitive neuropsychology laboratory at Johns Hopkins University. Therefore, together, we represent the three major professions that have contributed to this approach, and we have each enjoyed productive cross-disciplinary interactions.

PRINCIPLES AND PROCEDURES OF THE "COGNITIVE NEUROPSYCHOLOGICAL" APPROACH

The goal of cognitive neuropsychological research is to develop models of normal language processes, in the form of "information-processing models" of specific language tasks. A model of this type specifies the mechanisms for solving the necessary computational problems of a particular task, such as naming, as a sequenced set of representations (i.e., stored visual, orthographic, semantic, or phonological information) and the processes required to compute each representation from the preceding one. So, for example, we might propose that picture naming involves, at the very least, the following: discrimination of the lines, edges, and shadings of the picture to develop a representation of the visual image; matching the computed visual representation to a stored representation of the physical structure of the object (i.e., accessing "the structural/visual description"); accessing stored information about the set of instances with a particular name (i.e., accessing a "semantic representation"); accessing the stored pronunciation (the "phonological representation") of the word to which it corresponds; and activating representations of the motor programs involved in articulating the word.

One such information-processing model of the lexical system is schematically depicted in Figure 22–1. This figure depicts some of the principal cognitive processes underlying reading, spelling, and naming, understood as a series of transformations of mental representations. It is important to note that although each component is dedicated to a particular aspect of lexical processing, some of the components are involved in more than one lexical task. For example, both

reading and naming involve computing the phonological representation of a word for output from a semantic representation. Hence, if computation of the phonological representation were to be disrupted by brain damage, it should be manifest as impairment in both reading and naming, although the consequences for output may be somewhat different in the two tasks. In the case of reading, additional information about the pronunciation of the name is available from the printed word. Therefore, if the patient is unable to compute "chair" from the semantic representation of CHAIR, he or she will be unable to name the pictured chair but may yet be able to correctly read chair on the basis of letter-to-sound correspondence mechanisms (i.e., by "sounding out" the word).

Motivation for proposing specific representations and processes comes from considering the computational requirements of the cognitive task, and the proposals are supported by empirical evidence from studies of normal subjects and from single case studies of brain-damaged subjects. To illustrate, evidence for proposing separate mechanisms for computing phonological and graphemic representations of words from a semantic representation comes from patients who show good comprehension of printed and spoken words (indicating adequate access to the semantic representation) and are able to write the corresponding written word (in dictation or picture-naming tasks), but are not able to access the pronunciation of the same word. Such a pattern of performance (reported in Caramazza & Hillis, 1990; Ellis et al., 1983; Hier & Mohr, 1977) is inconsistent with an alternative proposal that computation of the graphemic representation first requires computation of the phonological representation. Thus, such models are constrained by patterns of performance of brain-damaged patients that cannot be otherwise explained by proposing specific loci of damage to the existing model. The subsequent chapters will cite cases that provide evidence for proposing those components of lexical processing that are involved in naming (Raymer & Gonzalez-Rothi, Chapter 23, this volume; see also Hillis, 1994), reading and writing (Beeson & Hillis, Chapter 25, this volume; see also Ellis, 1982; Goodman & Caramazza, 1986; Coltheart et al., 1980; Hillis & Caramazza, 1992; Patterson et al., 1985) et al., and sentence processing (Mitchum & Berndt, Chapter 24, this volume; see also Garrett, 1980).

In turn, the models guide our understanding of patterns of performance by aphasic individuals. That is, language disorders resulting from brain damage (which disrupts previously normal language) can be characterized by proposing deformations of one or more of the constituent mental representations or processes underlying language tasks. For example, imagine a patient who understands spoken and written words and writes the names of pictures adequately but is unable to say the correct names, despite unimpaired motor skills for articulating the correct name. We might propose in this case that the patient is unable to retrieve the accurate

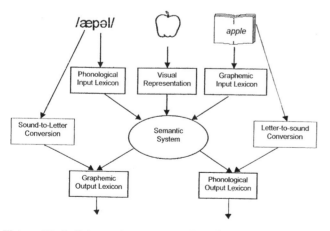

Figure 22–1. Schematic representation of the components of lexical processing.

pronunciation of the word from among the stored pronunciations of all words he or she knows ("the phonological output lexicon"). Therefore, a pattern of performance that indicates a proposed locus of disruption in the lexical system at the level of the phonological output lexicon would include (1) demonstrated access to the semantic system from printed and spoken words (i.e., intact reading and auditory comprehension) and from pictures, and (2) access to printed words from semantics (i.e., intact written expression of names and of self-generated ideas), but (3) failure to access the phonological representation from pictures or objects (impaired oral naming) or from written words (impaired oral reading). This example illustrates that the data crucial to proposing a specific locus of damage include the patient's profile of performance across lexical tasks in all modalities. To understand a patient's writing, for example, we need to know about his or her reading, comprehension, and speech, as well as performance on various spelling tasks. In addition, an analysis of the types of errors made in the affected task(s) and the stimulus parameters that influence performance (e.g., word frequency, part of speech, word length, and so on) may be required, as illustrated in several cases in the following chapters.

Basic Assumptions

There are a few basic assumptions of cognitive neuropsychological research, which if proved to be incorrect would undermine the usefulness of this approach for understanding normal language processing. First, the universality assumption states that everyone has essentially "the same" cognitive processes. Certainly, there may be different modes of learning and thinking that reflect variable reliance on one type of processing relative to another, but we all start out with the same types of mental representations and processes. Secondly, the "transparency assumption" states that brain-damaged patients also have basically the same cognitive processes, except for a focal modification at some level(s) of representation or processing, "transparently" revealed by the pattern of performance in various tasks. In other words, brain damage does not result in new types of mental representations or operations, although it may change *which* of our normal components we rely on to accomplish a task. For example, referring to Figure 22–1, normal oral reading of a word like *yacht* is accomplished by accessing a representation in the "phonological output lexicon" (the repository of stored "pronunciations" of familiar words). However, when there is damage to the phonological output lexicon a patient may now read aloud via letter-to-sound conversion mechanisms. This local modification in the system is transparently revealed by pronunciation of the word yacht as "yached" (/jæ+S/t/☐). Normally, oral reading of English is likely to be accomplished by an interaction of the two mechanisms (access to the phonological output lexicon from semantics

and letter-to-sound conversion mechanisms; see Hillis & Caramazza, 1991, & 1995), although some readers may rely more on one or the other, at least in learning to read.

Different Types of Cognitive Models

The classical cognitive neuropsychological model is the so-called "serial" or "box and arrow" schematic representation of the cognitive representations and their interactions that underlie a given task, such as reading, spelling, naming, or sentence production. These representations and processes do not necessarily correspond to locations in the brain. Rather, they represent distinct functional components of a cognitive operation. Several models of this type are illustrated in the following chapters, and a "serial" model of the lexical system is shown in Figure 22–1. The basis for proposing each level of representation comes from patients whose performance of the task, and pattern of performance across tasks, can be understood by proposing selective damage to that cognitive component and dependence on the other "spared" components. Such schema are described as serial because it was initially assumed that processing at each level of representation was completed before processing at the next level of representation was started. In serial models, feedback from one level to a prior level of representation, and integration of the various components were not considered. However, several cognitive mechanisms may interact to select or "access" a specific lexical representation at a subsequent level (Hillis & Caramazza, 1991, 1995; Patterson, et al., 1994) and that information may "cascade" from one level to the next, such that several representations are simultaneously active and contributing to the final output (Humphreys et al., 1988).

The concepts of integration and feedback are best seen in more recent, "computational models" of specific language tasks. This type of model is a computer simulation of the cognitive representations and procedures that underlie the task, utilizing several levels of "nodes" with feedback and feedforward connections between each level. In some of these models, the strength of the connections between nodes is not "programmed in," but is learned through many repeated simulations. Evidence for postulating specific characteristics of each model comes from patients whose pattern of performance can be simulated by "damaging" the simulation in some way (e.g., by reducing the connection strength between two levels of nodes). It is likely that each of these types of serial and computational models is likely to capture some of the characteristics of normal language processing.

Application of Models to Treatment

Focusing Treatment

The clinician's primary goal in understanding the patient's deficit is to focus treatment on just those levels of processing that are impaired or to identify methods that will allow the patient to process language successfully by "getting around" the deficit. Thus, the predominant usefulness of cognitive models is in identifying the level(s) of processing that are impaired in each patient, so that therapy can be directed toward remediation of that component and/or strategies to compensate for the loss of that component. Among the first illustrations of this application was a study by Byng and Coltheart (1986) showing that selective damage to particular components of the reading system in their patient could be treated successfully by focusing treatment on the impaired component (see Beeson & Hillis, Chapter 25, this volume). Additional notable examples of studies in which cognitive analyses have been used to focus intervention are described in the subsequent chapters in this section. In each case, a model of the normal processes underlying the treated task served to pinpoint the patient's deficit and thereby to focus intervention. For example, patient JJ (reported in Hillis & Caramazza, 1991), whose pattern of performance across lexical tasks indicated a disruption at the level of the semantic system, showed more improvement in naming performance when treatment tasks explicitly required semantic processing (printed word/picture matching) than when treatment tasks did not overtly require semantic processing (oral reading with phonological cues). In contrast, patient HW, whose naming impairment could be localized to the phonological output lexicon, showed greater improvement in naming performance as a consequence of the facilitated oral reading treatment than as a consequence of treatment using printed word/picture matching to enhance semantic processing (see Hillis & Caramazza, 1994, for details and discussion). Raymer and co-workers (Raymer et al., 1993; see also Thompson et al., 1991; McNeil et al., 1999) also reported that phonological strategies to facilitate naming (e.g., using rhyming word cues) improved naming performance of patients whose impairment was localized to the phonological output lexicon. Additional reports of treatment focused on specific components of the naming process are reported by Raymer and Gonzalez-Rothi in Chapter 23 (this volume). However, many types of naming treatment described in the literature, including those that directly facilitate production of the name in response to the picture, might improve naming at either the level of the semantic system or the level of the phonological output lexicon or both (e.g., Hillis, 1989; Howard et al., 1985; Linebaugh, 1983; Thompson & Kearns, 1981).

Another use of cognitive neuropsychological models has been in the prediction of patterns of generalization across tasks and across items. For example, in Chapter 25 of this volume, we (Beeson & Hillis) describe a patient, HG, whose performance across lexical tasks could be explained by assuming that she had partial damage to semantic representations of words and profound damage to the phonological forms of

words (Hillis, 1994, 1990). In various tasks, such as written and spoken naming, repetition, written word/picture matching, and spoken word/picture matching, HG made semantic errors, such as "tulip" named or understood as "rose." However, her errors were inconsistent. Tulip might be named on one occasion as "rose" and on another occasion as "daisy." Furthermore, when shown a picture of a tulip she would accept the name "rose," "daisy," "tulip" or any other flower as the name of the picture. This pattern can be explained by assuming that HG accessed underspecified semantic representations, or meanings, of words. In this case, she might have had a semantic representation of "tulip" that consisted of a partial set of features that define tulip. While the normal semantic representation of "tulip" might include all of the features that jointly define a tulip and allow it to be distinguished from all other flowers, such as <flower> <bulb>, <upright petals>, <slender, upright leaves>, <spring blooming>, <dutch>; HG's semantic representation might include only <flower> and <spring blooming>. Therefore, she would accept any word that corresponded to these features in word/picture verification. Furthermore, her underspecified semantic representation would access all spoken and written word forms (phonological representations and orthographic representations) that correspond to these features, so that a picture of tulip might be named as any one of many spring flowers. In addition, HG mispronounced nearly every word in all tasks with spoken output (repetition, oral reading, spoken naming). This aspect of HG's performance was attributed to an additional deficit in accessing phonological representations for output. Initially, treatment focused on her semantic impairment (see Chapter 25, this volume), by teaching her the features that distinguish semantically related words, for certain categories of words, such as foods and clothing. Based on the model in Figure 25–1, it was predicted that treatment (teaching/improving specific semantic representations) should improve her performance of all tasks that involve the semantic component—e.g., spoken and written naming, and spoken and written word comprehension. And, indeed, although treatment engaged the task of written naming, her reduction in semantic errors generalized to tasks of spoken naming and spoken and written word comprehension. However, the treatment was expected to be specific to the trained categories of words. That is, teaching her features that distinguish various types of clothing should not reduce her semantic errors in naming or understanding of furniture. And, consistent with this prediction, her gains generalized to untrained items within the trained categories, but not to untrained categories. Furthermore, the treatment of semantic representations utilizing the task of written naming was not expected to improve her pronunciation of words in spoken output, and it did not. Subsequent therapy directed toward teaching her accurate pronunciations by re-establishing phonological representations (or access to them) in the task of oral reading did result in more accurate pronunciations in not only oral reading, but also in oral naming and repetition. In this case, treatment was item specific, as expected, since re-teaching a phonological representation of "tulip" would only improve pronunciation of tulip. Behrmann and Lieberthal (1989) reported comparable generalization results—improvement in categorization of *untreated items* within *treated categories*—of a therapy strategy that also focused on teaching semantic distinctions among related items. Their patient, like HG, showed a pattern of performance consistent with damage to the semantic system, as indicated in particular by his category-specific impairment in comprehension (but unlike HG he showed some improvement of items in one of the untrained categories). Additional reports in the literature of item-specific treatment include treating reading of functors using association with visually/phonologically similar content words (Hatfield, 1983) and improving printed word recognition by reinforcing correct word/nonword, semantic, and phonological decisions about the "treated" set of words (Hillis, 1993). These reports are consistent with the hypothesis that if treatment influences specific representations (or access to them), performance involving the target representations (treated stimuli) should improve across tasks, but performance would not be expected to improve for other representations (of untreated words).

A different type of generalization concerns changes in performance across treated and untreated stimuli. Here, we would expect that if treatment influences a general processing mechanism (say, holding representations in a short-term memory system), processing should improve across all stimuli that are subject to that mechanism. Many examples of therapy that influenced both treated and untreated stimuli have been reported, such as improving reading speed by reinforcing rapid semantic decisions about printed words ("gestalt processing") (Gonzalez-Rothi & Moss, 1989), improving comprehension of sentences (Byng & Coltheart, 1986), improving use of a self-correction strategy in spelling (Hillis & Caramazza, 1987), and improving use of sublexical letter-to-sound conversion mechanisms or "phonological assembly" to improve oral reading (Berndt & Mitchum, 1994; de Partz, 1986; Hillis, 1993) or sound-to-letter conversion mechanisms to improve spelling (Carlomagno et al., 1994; Hillis Trupe, 1986). The problem in making predictions as to whether or not to expect improvement across stimuli is that we have no way of knowing, a priori, how treatment affects processing. Indeed, we might instead use treatment results to propose whether a general mechanism or specific representations were affected by our treatment (see Goodman-Schulman et al., 1990, for discussion and illustration).

Finally, we always work toward ensuring that treatment effects generalize to other tasks and settings outside the therapy session. For example, patient HG (above) showed dramatically improved use of trained words not only during therapy, but also in the job setting (documented by her job coach), at home (documented by her mother), and in restaurants (observed by her therapist). Hinckley and colleagues (1999) also reported that treatment that focused on specific cognitive skills—"the cognitive neuropsychological approach"—resulted in better generalization of improvements to untrained tasks, such as the *Communicative Abilities in Daily Living* (CADL; Holland, 1980) than treatment that focused on a particular functional activity.

Limitations

Several authors have argued that cognitive neuropsychological models are simply models of cognitive tasks, not models of rehabilitation. That is, current models of cognitive processing provide no direct motivation for specific treatment strategies. For example, knowing the patient's level of disruption in the naming process does not guide the clinician as to how to treat the problem (see Caramazza, 1989; Caramazza & Hillis, 1991; Wilson & Patterson, 1990, for discussion). In fact, such knowledge does not even guide the clinician as to what to treat. Should we treat the damaged component of processing, or should we try to exploit the preserved components in the hopes for more functional, but not normal, language processing? The models alone do not help us in this regard, because they do not specify which components are subject to remediation, nor how the system might be reorganized following damage to circumscribed parts. Hence, choices of treatment must rely (as usual) on the clinician's intuitions about what might help, the goals of the person seeking therapy, and ongoing evaluation of treatment effects. Empirical reports of improvement in functioning associated with specific treatment approaches in well-described cases of damage to selective components of language processing might give the clinician hope that a particular component is treatable, but valid predictions about improvement in a different case of damage to the same component would also require evidence as to the patient characteristics that influence outcome and nature of damage to the impaired component (see Hillis, 1993; Hillis & Caramazza, 1994, for detailed discussion). In fact, even patients who have the "same" deficit with respect to the level of representation in some cognitive task do not consistently respond to the same treatment. It is not clear, from considering the model, whether the differential response to treatment is due to different forms of damage to the same component or due to different overall learning abilities, motivation, or other patient characteristics.

Another limitation in applying these sorts of models to treatment is that the analyses required to determine the patient's level of damage are often extremely time consuming and may not be cost effective (Schwartz, 1998). That is, with the recent limitations on the number of reimbursable therapy visits, and requirements to document improvement in each visit, it is often impractical to spend hours of time testing a patient to precisely pinpoint which components of each task are impaired. However, in other cases, such extensive evaluation may be justifiable. For instance, in the case of HG, whose deficits were quite complicated, it was difficult to know where to even begin treatment until damage to specific components of lexical processing were identified. She had undergone years of unfocused therapy for "cortical deafness" and other inaccurate psychiatric and language diagnoses, with virtually no improvement in language or communication, prior to careful analysis of her impairments. She made useful, albeit slow, gains after delineating her deficits.

It has also been argued that treatment based on cognitive neuropsychological models fails to generalize across tasks and across items (for evidence for and against this claim, see Schwartz, 1998). Recall HG, a patient described earlier in this chapter as having a semantic impairment, demonstrated by identical rates and types of semantic errors in a lexical tasks (oral naming, written naming, auditory word/picture matching, written word/picture matching, and writing to dictation). HG's improvements in oral production were item specific, and her improvements in semantic processing were limited to trained categories of words (see also Hillis, 1998). Although this failure of generalization to untrained items or categories is far from ideal, item-specific gains are better than no gains. Furthermore, as mentioned above, HG's gains served a significant function. She gradually regained a functional vocabulary for daily activities (such as dining out and riding public transportation) and a vocabulary specific to the job for which she was training (as a stock clerk in a fabric store). Her item-specific gains, which generalized well across settings, thus permitted HG to obtain and maintain a job and independence in activities of daily living.

Similarly, the "phonological" therapy with a patient HW (see above and Chapter 25, this volume) that involved cued oral reading treatment seemed to result in improved access to specific phonological representations in the output lexicon, irrespective of the setting. Like patient HG, patient HW produced mostly fluent speech with few content words before this item-specific therapy was initiated more than 5 years post-stroke. Her impairment was localized to the "phonemic output lexicon" (Fig. 22–1), because (1) she showed flawless performance in auditory word/picture and written word/picture matching tasks and was able to define both words and pictures she could not name, indicating that her processing of words and pictures was unimpaired through the level of the semantic system; (2) she produced accurate or recognizable written names of 100% of pictures, even though she could not produce the spoken name, indicating that semantics and access to the graphemic output lexicon were intact; and (3) she had perfect fluency, articulation, and repetition of words she could not name, ruling out a motor speech deficit as the basis for her impaired spoken naming. HW's improvements in producing a trained set of words using the "phonological" therapy were sufficiently rapid that she was

able to receive treatment for many sets of words she selected. She was also observed to use trained words in conversation at home, in restaurants, and over the telephone in follow-up calls. In describing the "Cookie Theft" picture from the *Boston Diagnostic Aphasia Examination*, HW improved in the number of accurate content units produced, from 5 before the phonological treatment to 12 after treatment (cf. Yorkston & Beukelman, 1980, for description of content units). Furthermore, not only were her gains maintained more than a year after treatment, but additional gains were achieved: She produced 15 content units. The further progress was probably achieved in part through HW's oral reading practice with her husband providing cues.

In contrast to item-specific gains that generalize across settings resulting from therapy for naming and other oral production tasks, gains that generalize across tasks but often not to other settings have been reported for sentence production/comprehension therapies (see Mitchum & Berndt, Chapter 24, this volume). Several authors have reported not only generalization of improvements from comprehension to production (or vice versa), but also generalization across trained and untrained sentence types.

Perhaps a more important limitation of conclusions reached about the results of a given treatment for an individual patient is that it is not possible to determine, a priori, which other patients will respond to the same treatment in the same way. Ideally, we would like to be able to conclude that treatment of a specific component of cognitive processing would help all patients with damage to that component. Unfortunately, such conclusions are not possible in light of our current levels of theory. As noted previously, we have no way of knowing how any specific mechanisms are actually modified by our interventions (see Caramazza & Hillis, 1991, for discussion). Thus, the observation that a "semantic" approach was associated with improved naming in a patient with a semantic deficit does not directly imply that all patients with semantic deficits will show improved naming with that treatment. Earlier studies have shown that sometimes patients with putatively "the same" locus of impairment do not respond to the same treatment approach, but different approaches have been beneficial for individuals, and sometimes patients with different loci of damage in the lexical system respond to the same treatment (Hillis, 1993; Hillis & Caramazza, 1994). This finding is not unexpected, since the characteristics of the patient and the form of impairment at any given level of processing that may influence treatment outcomes have yet to be precisely defined. Although studies have identified recovery as a function of a variety of individual factors, these studies have not been integrated with (a) the specific cognitive mechanisms that are impaired in the patient, and (b) the cognitive mechanisms that might be influenced by the treatment.

This inability to predict whether a particular patient will benefit from a given treatment strategy is certainly not specific to the approach described in this chapter, which relies on a cognitive analysis of patient performance but applies equally to other "schools" of treatment.

In summary, information-processing models of specific language tasks are useful for understanding the nature of impairment consequent to brain damage in individual patients but do not constitute a theory of language rehabilitation. The latter would require motivated hypotheses about how mental representations or transformations are modified, how particular interventions bring about these modifications, and how particular patient characteristics influence response to treatment. Moreover, a theory of rehabilitation would need to specify the interactions among these variables, in order to make predictions about results of a given treatment approach.

INTRODUCTION TO THE CHAPTERS IN THIS SECTION

Scope of the Section

There has been no attempt to cover every domain of cognition in this section, nor even every domain of language. Instead, I have chosen to include chapters on those domains that have received the most attention in the cognitive neuropsychological literature. Therefore, there are chapters on spoken word comprehension and naming, written word comprehension and production (reading and writing), and sentence comprehension and production. Perhaps as a consequence of the number of studies in these areas, the models in these domains are the most clearly articulated and most well (although not universally) accepted. Although each chapter will discuss models of tasks limited to that domain (e.g., a model of the cognitive processes underlying reading), it is important to understand that there is a great deal of overlap in the cognitive representations and processes that underlie reading, writing, naming, word comprehension, and sentence comprehension and production. For example, as discussed in the case of HG, we believe that a single set of phonological representations (a phonological output lexicon) is accessed in the course of all tasks that have spoken word output: oral reading, oral naming, repetition, oral sentence production, and spoken conversation. Similarly, a single semantic system is engaged in a variety of tasks that involve comprehension and/or production of words. Therefore, identifying the patient's problem in oral naming may require assessment of oral reading, comprehension, and written naming, and so on. It is probably never possible to be sure of the level of damage by assessing performance on only one task.

It is also crucial to note that other cognitive abilities, such as attention and memory, are engaged in every language task. Impairments of sustained attention, selective attention, spatial attention, and/or short- or long-term memory can affect performance on any given language task. Although there

are models and theories of each of these areas, we have not addressed them, since the focus of this book is on language intervention. Other important domains that have received much attention in the psychological literature are procedural and episodic memory, and the so-called "executive functions" such as planning, judgment, organization (sequencing, switching and maintaining tasks, etc.). Investigations in these domains have not yielded the types of models of specific component cognitive representations of the type we are considering in these chapters. Nevertheless, awareness of deficits in these areas is often helpful in understanding patients' responses or failure of response to particular treatment strategies.

Content of the Chapters

In Chapter 23, Anastasia Raymer and Leslie Gonzalez-Rothi describe clinical diagnosis and treatment of spoken word comprehension and production. They identify impairments at different levels of cognitive processing that result in poor auditory word comprehension and/or poor oral naming. The authors further report rehabilitation strategies that rely on this type of diagnosis, made in view of a cognitive neuropsychological model of word comprehension and naming. In the next chapter (24), Charlotte Mitchum and Rita Berndt discuss evaluation and rehabilitation of sentence comprehension and production based on cognitive neuropsychological models of sentence processing. They focus on issues of the relationship between theory and therapy and issues of generalization. Finally, in Chapter 25, Pelagie Beeson and I describe how to identify an individual patient's underlying deficit in comprehension or production of written words. We focus on assessment and treatment of reading and spelling at the single word level, and show how treatment can generalize to improved reading and spelling in untrained tasks.

FUTURE TRENDS

As noted, this section illustrates the integration of speech-language pathology with cognitive neuropsychology and behavioral neurology. The authors have been involved in integrative research centers in Gainesville, Tucson, and Baltimore. Other excellent interdisciplinary centers for aphasia research and rehabilitation exist in Philadelphia, Ann Arbor, and Pittsburgh in the United States, and in Belgium (the Brussels Neuropsychological Rehabilitation Unit), the United Kingdom, Italy, the Netherlands, France, Germany, and Australia (see Appendix for contact person and names of several such centers). Many centers are also collaborating with other disciplines in the field of cognitive science, such as artificial intelligence, linguistics, and neuroscience. For example, interdisciplinary collaboration at Moss Rehabilitation and Temple University, at Carnegie Mellon, and elsewhere have led to the development of computational models of naming that have been useful in understanding various forms of naming impairment. It is expected that such collaborations are only a hint of what may come. Several authors have predicted that computational models of language may become important in directing rehabilitation as well (Plaut, 1996). Certainly, computational models are helping us to understand learning and recovery, two crucial aspects of rehabilitation. Functional imaging techniques (such as functional magnetic resonance imaging [fMRI], positron emission tomography [PET], magnetic resonance perfusion, and spectroscopy) have been used in many studies to shed light on physiologic aspects of learning and recovery. Perhaps more importantly, anticipated advances in cognitive neuroscience in understanding how the brain recovers through reorganization of neural representation (Jenkins & Merzenich, 1987; Jenkins et al., 1990), and how the brain changes with learning, through changes in neural synaptic strength and genetic expression (Kandel et al., 1995), will surely contribute to developing an interdisciplinary theory of aphasia rehabilitation.

▶ *Acknowledgments*–This work was supported in part by NIH grant DC00174-01 and a National Stroke Association Fellowship Award. The author is grateful to Pelagie Beeson, Charlotte Mitchum, Roberta Chapey, Anastasia Raymer, and Leslie Gonzalez Rothi for helpful comments on an earlier draft.

KEY POINTS

Chapters 23 to 25 will illustrate how a particular aphasic patient's therapy can be guided by pinpointing his or her impairment to one more components of a model of the cognitive processes underlying the specific language task to be treated. This approach to intervention has its foundations in the fields of cognitive neuropsychology, speech-language pathology, and behavioral neurology.

1. The strategies utilized are not truly model-based interventions, since the strategies themselves rely more on clinical intuitions and experience than on the model of the language task to be treated.
2. Reference to a model of the task being treated often allows the therapist to understand when, how, and why a particular therapy procedure is likely to have an effect on performance.
3. Models can also sometimes help us to understand why therapy "works" for some aphasic individuals and not for others.
4. Future developments through cooperative efforts in these fields, as well as in other areas of cognitive neuroscience, may further guide our models and our therapies.

GLOSSARY

Behavioral neurology—branch of neurology devoted to understanding the neural mechanisms of behavior and cognition.

Cognitive neuropsychology—branch of psychology devoted to understanding normal cognitive processes through the study of people who have sustained brain damage.

Computational model—computer simulation of a particular task.

Lexical processing—mental representations and processes involved in comprehension and production of single words in various modalities.

Graphemic representation—stored spelling of a word.

Phonological representation—stored "sound" of a word.

Semantic representation—stored meaning of a word.

References

Behrmann, M. & Lieberthal, T. (1989). Category-specific treatment of a lexical-semantic deficit: A single case study of global aphasia. *British Journal of Communication Disorders, 24,* 281–299.

Berndt, R. & Mitchum, C. (1994). Approaches to the rehabilitation of "phonological assembly": Elaborating the model of nonlexical reading. In G.W. Humphreys & M.J. Riddoch (eds.), *Cognitive Neuropsychology and Cognitive Rehabilitation* (pp. 503–526).

Byng, S. & Coltheart, M. (l986). Aphasia therapy research: Methodological requirements and illustrative results. In E. Hjelmquist & L.-G. Nilsson (eds.), *Communication handicap: Aspects of psychological compensation and technical aids.* North-Holland: Elsevier Science Publishers B.V.

Caramazza, A. & Hillis, A.E. (1990). Where do semantic errors come from? *Cortex, 26,* 95–122.

Caramazza, A. & Hillis, A.E. (1991). For a theory of remediation of cognitive deficits. *Neuropsychological Rehabilitation, 3,* 217–234.

Caramazza, A. (1989). Cognitive neuropsychology and rehabilitation: An unfulfilled promise? In T. Seron & G. DeLoche (eds.), *Cognitive approaches in rehabilitation* (pp. 383–398). Hillsdale, NJ: LEA.

Carlomagno, S., Iavarone, A., & Colombo, A. (1994). Cognitive approaches to writing rehabilitation. In M.J. Riddoch & G. Humphreys (eds.), *Cognitive neuropsychology and cognitive rehabilitation* (pp. 485–502). London: Lawrence Erlbaum Associates.

Coltheart, M., Patterson, K., & Marshall, J.C. (1980). *Deep dyslexia.* London: Routeledge and Kegan Paul.

de Partz, M.P. (1986). Re-education of a deep dyslexic patient: Rationale of the method and results. *Cognitive Neuropsychology, 3,* 149–177.

Ellis, A.W., Miller, D., & Sin G. (1983). Wernicke's aphasia and normal language processing: A case study in cognitive neuropsychology. *Cognition, 15,* 111–114.

Ellis, A.W. (1982). Spelling and writing (and reading and speaking). In A.W. Ellis (ed.), *Normality and pathology in cognitive functions.* London: Academic Press.

Garrett, M.F. (1980). Levels of processing in sentence production. In B. Butterworth (ed.), *Language production Vol. 1.* New York: Academic Press.

Goodglass, H. & Kaplan, E. (1972). *The Boston Diagnostic Aphasia Examination.* Philadelphia, PA: Lea & Febiger.

Gonzalez-Rothi, L. & Moss, S. (October, 1989). Alexia without agraphia: A model-driven therapy. Paper presented at Academy of Aphasia, Santa Fe, NM.

Goodman, R.A. & Caramazza, A. (1986). Phonologically plausible errors: Implications for a model of the phoneme-grapheme conversion mechanism in the spelling process. In G. Augst (ed.), *Proceedings of the International Colloquium on Graphemics and Orthography* (pp. 300–325).

Goodman-Schulman, R.A., Sokol, S., Aliminosa, D., & McCloskey, M. (October, 1990). Remediation of acquired dysgraphia as a technique for evaluating models of spelling. Paper presented at the Academy of Aphasia, Baltimore, MD.

Hatfield, M.F. (1983). Aspects of acquired dysgraphia and implications for re-education. In C. Code & D.J. Muller (eds.), *Aphasia therapy* (pp. 157–169). London: Edward Arnold.

Hier, D.B. & Mohr, J.P. (1977). Incongruous oral and written naming. *Brain and Language, 4,* 115–126.

Hillis, A.E. (1998). Treatment of naming disorders: New issues regarding old therapies. *Journal of the International Neuropsychological Society, 4,* 648–660.

Hillis Trupe, A.E. (1986). Effectiveness of retraining phoneme to grapheme conversion. In R.H. Brookshire (ed.), *Clinical aphasiology, 1986* (pp. 163–171). Minneapolis, MN: BRK.

Hillis, A.E. (1989). Efficacy and generalization of treatment for aphasic naming errors. *Archives of Physical Medicine and Rehabilitation, 70,* 632–636.

Hillis, A.E. (1990). Effects of a separate treatments for distinct impairments within the naming process. In T. Prescott (ed.), *Clinical aphasiology, Vol. 19* (pp. 255–265). Austin, TX: Pro-Ed.

Hillis, A.E. (1993). The role of models of language processing in rehabilitation of language impairments. *Aphasiology, 7,* 5–26.

Hillis, A.E. (1994). Contributions from cognitive analyses. In R. Chapey (ed.), *Language intervention strategies in adult aphasia (3rd ed.)* (pp. 207–219). Baltimore: Williams and Wilkins.

Hillis, A.E. & Caramazza, A. (1987). Model-driven treatment of dysgraphia. In R.H. Brookshire (ed.), *Clinical aphasiology, 1987* (pp. 84–105). Minneapolis, MN: BRK.

Hillis, A. & Caramazza, A. (1992). The reading process and its disorders. In D.I. Margolin (ed.), *Cognitive neuropsychology in clinical practice* (pp. 229–261). Oxford: University Press.

Hillis, A.E. & Caramazza, A. (1991). Mechanisms for accessing lexical representations for output: Evidence from a category-specific semantic deficit. *Brain and Language, 40,* 106–144.

Hillis, A.E. & Caramazza, A. (1994). Theories of lexical processing and theories of rehabilitation. In M.J. Riddoch & G. Humphreys (eds.), *Cognitive neuropsychology and cognitive Rehabilitation* (pp. 449–484). Hove: LEA.

Hillis, A.E. & Caramazza, A. (1995). Converging evidence for the interaction of semantic and phonological information in accessing lexical information for spoken output. *Cognitive Neuropsychology, 12,* 187–227.

Hinckley, J.J., Patterson, J., & Carr, T.H. (June, 1999). Differential effects of context- and skill-based treatment approaches: Preliminary findings. Paper presented at Clinical Aphasiology Conference, Key West, FL.

Holland, A. (1980). *Communicative Abilities in Daily Living (CADL).* Baltimore, MD: University Park Press.

Howard, D., Patterson, K., Franklin, S., Orchard-Lisle, V., & Morton, J. (1985). The facilitation of picture naming in aphasia. *Cognitive Neuropsychology, 2,* 42–80.

Humphreys, G.W., Riddoch, M.J., & Quinlan, P.T. (1988). Cascade processes in picture identification. *Cognitive Neuropsychology, 5,* 67–104.

Jenkins, W.M., Merzenich, M.M., & Recanzone, G. (1990). Neocortical representational dynamics in adult primates: Implications for neuropsychology. *Neuropsychologia, 28,* 573–584.

Jenkins, W.M. & Merzenich, M.M. (1987). Reorganization of neocortical representations after brain injury: A neurophysiological model of the bases of recovery from stroke. In F.J. Seil & B.M. Carlson (eds.), *Progress in brain research, 71* (pp. 249–266).

Kandel, E.R., Schwartz, J.H., & Jessell, T.M. (1995). *Essentials of neural science and behavior.* Stamford, CT: Appleton and Lange.

Linebaugh, C. (1983). Treatment of anomic aphasia. In C. Perkins (ed.), *Current therapies for communication disorders: Language handicaps in adults.* New York: Thieme-Stratton.

McNeil, M.R., Matunis, M., Just, M., Carpenter, P., Haarman, H., Rosenblatt, H., & Langer, E. (June, 1999). Paper presented at Clinical Aphasiology Conference, Key West, FL.

Patterson, K., Graham, M., & Hodges, J. (1994). The impact of semantic memory loss on phonological representations. *Journal of Cognitive Neuroscience, 6,* 57–69.

Patterson, K.E., Coltheart, M., & Marshall, J.C. (1985). *Surface dyslexia.* London: LEA.

Plaut, D. (1996). Relearning after damage in connectionist networks: Toward a theory of rehabilitation. *Brain and Language, 52,* 25–82.

Raymer, A.M., Thompson, C.K., Jacobs, B., & LeGrand, H.R. (1993). Phonological treatment of naming deficits in aphasia: Model-based generalization analysis. *Aphasiology, 7,* 27–53.

Schwartz, M. (October, 1998). Psycholinguistic theory and aphasia rehabilitation: When worlds collide. Paper presented at Academy of Aphasia, Santa Fe, NM.

Thompson, C. & Kearns, K. (1981). Experimental analysis of acquisititon and generalization of naming behaviors in a patient with anomia. In R.H. Brookshire (ed.), *Clinical aphasiology conference, Vol. 10* (pp. 35–45).

Thompson, C.K., Raymer, A., & leGrand, H. (1991). Effects of phonologically based treatment on aphasic naming deficits: A model-driven approach. In T. Prescott (ed.), *Clinical aphasiology, Vol. 20* (pp. 239–259). Austin, TX: Pro-Ed.

Wilson, B.A. & Patterson, K. E. (1990). Rehabilitation and cognitive neuropsychology. *Applied Cognitive Psychology, 4,* 247–260.

Yorkston, K. & Beukelman, D. (1980). An analysis of connected speech samples of aphasic and normal speakers. *Journal of Speech and Hearing Disorders, 45,* 27–36.

APPENDIX 22-1
Selected Interdisciplinary Centers for Aphasia Research and Rehabilitation

Name and Location	Contact Person, telephone, e-mail
Aphasia Research Center Boston VA Medical Center Boston University Medical School 150 South Huntington Ave. Boston, MA 02130 USA	Martin L. Albert, MD (617) 232-9500 e-mail: malbert@bu.edu
The Aphasia Research Center Moss Rehabilitation Hospital 1200 W. Tabor Road Philadelphia, PA 19141 USA	Myrna Schwartz, Ph.D. Ruth Fink, Ph.D. (215) 456-9605 e-mail: mschwar@vm.temple.edu
Birkbeck College Department of Psychology University of London Malet Street London WC1E 7HX	Wendy Best, Ph.D. w.best@psych.bbk.ac.uk
Clinical Communication Studies City University Northampton Square London, England EC1V 0HB UK	Sally Byng, Ph.D. 0171-477-8000 e-mail: s.c.byng@city.ac.uk
Georgetown Institute for Cognitive and Computational Sciences Georgetown University Medical Center 3970 Reservoir Rd. NW Washington, DC 20007 USA	Rhoda Friedman, Ph.D. (202) 784-4134 rfried01@medlib.georgetown.edu
Instituto di Scienze Neurologiche Universita Degli Studi di Napoli I Facolta Di Medicina E Chirurgia 80131 Napoli Via Pansini 5 ITALY	Sergio Carlomagno, Ph.D.
National Center for Neurogenic Communication Disorders University of Arizona Tuscon, AZ 85721-0071 USA	Audrey Holland, Ph.D. Pelagie Beeson, Ph.D. (520) 621-9878 Pelagie@u.arizona.edu

Name and Location	Contact Person, telephone, e-mail
School of Behavioural Sciences	Max Coltheart, Ph.D.
Macquaire University	Lyndsey Nickels, Ph.D.
Sydney, New South Wales 2109	612-9850-8448
AUSTRALIA	lyndsey@frogmouth.bhs.mq.edu.au
VA RR&D Brain Rehabilitation Research Center-151A	Leslie Gonzalez Rothi, Ph.D.
Gainesville VA Medical Center	(904) 376-1611
Gainesville, FL 32608	gonazlj@medicine.ufl.edu
USA	

Chapter 23

Cognitive Approaches to Impairments of Word Comprehension and Production

Anastasia M. Raymer
and Leslie J. Gonzalez Rothi

OBJECTIVES

Our objectives are to describe a model of lexical processing that represents the mechanisms involved in word comprehension and production; delineate impairments in lexical comprehension and production with respect to breakdown at specific stages in lexical processing; illustrate the application of this lexical model in clinical interactions for assessment, recovery analysis, and treatment of lexical impairments; and consider the limitations and future trends in the use of lexical models in the clinical setting.

DEFINITION

Impairments of word comprehension and, in particular, word retrieval, are pervasive symptoms among patients with acquired aphasia (Goodglass & Kaplan, 1983). However, the cognitive and neural bases for lexical impairments vary among patients. Traditional methods of aphasia syndrome classification may not be effective in disentangling the distinct mechanisms of lexical failure across patients (Byng et al., 1990; Raymer et al., 1995a). Rather, in recent years, researchers have applied a cognitive neuropsychological approach to describe the diverse lexical impairments that patients may incur (Ellis & Young, 1988; Rothi et al., 1991).

The initial goal of research in cognitive neuropsychology was to use studies of brain-impaired subjects to provide a converging body of evidence to support work in cognitive psychology attempting to explain the complex system of processes/structures involved in performing cognitive tasks (Ellis et al., 1983; Ellis & Young, 1988). However, researchers such as Coltheart (1984) recognized the value that a cognitive approach may play in the rehabilitation process as well.

Many other clinical researchers have echoed his sentiments that a cognitive neuropsychological approach may provide a strategic theoretical foundation motivating clinical practice with patients with acquired cognitive disorders (Byng et al., 1990; Hillis, 1993; Howard & Patterson, 1989; Mitchum, 1992; Raymer et al., 1995a). Although researchers have completed cognitive neuropsychological studies across a variety of cognitive and linguistic domains, this chapter will focus specifically on a model of lexical processing and its implications for assessment and management of impairments related to comprehension and production of spoken words.

In the cognitive neuropsychological (CN) approach, clinicians use a systematic assessment to characterize lexical impairments with respect to a model of lexical processing. In turn, researchers use this framework to develop rational treatments that either target impaired lexical mechanisms, or take advantage of spared mechanisms to circumvent lexical impairments (Rothi, 1998). Thus, the CN approach is largely an impairment-oriented approach (Lux, 1999). Some clinicians, however, have expressed skepticism that impairment-oriented treatments have any influence on the use of verbal communication in functional settings (Lyon, 1996; Wilson, 1997, 1999). We propose that the CN approach, when applied with methodological rigor, has implications for practice in aphasia assessment and treatment, including management of impairments related to lexical comprehension and production.

MODEL OF LEXICAL PROCESSING

Figure 23–1 depicts a model of lexical processing, developed on the basis of studies of normal and brain-impaired individuals, that forms the basis for this discussion of lexical impairments for spoken words. Although the details vary to some extent across versions of such models, the general features are the same. The model includes a complex system of distributed and interconnected modules that allow for processing of different types of lexical information in cascade fashion (Rapp & Caramazza, 1998; Humphreys et al.,

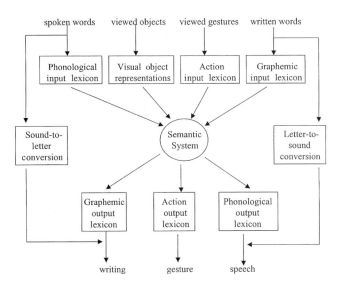

spoken words viewed objects viewed gestures written words

| Phonological input lexicon | Visual object representations | Action input lexicon | Graphemic input lexicon |

Sound-to-letter conversion

Semantic System

Letter-to-sound conversion

Graphemic output lexicon | Action output lexicon | Phonological output lexicon

writing gesture speech

Figure 23–1. Model of lexical processing.

1988). Following the activation of peripheral sensory structures with some form of sensory input such as spoken and written words or viewed objects and gestures, cognitive mechanisms in the central nervous system are triggered for processing and reacting to that input. Subsequently, peripheral motor processes allow for planning and executing a response to the stimulus in the form of speech, writing, or gesture. The focus of this chapter is on the mechanisms involved in processing spoken words, so the description will center on the more central mechanisms critical for phonological lexical processing. However, because lexical tasks often incorporate visual object stimuli, we will also consider the mechanism responsible for object recognition.

To acquire skill in any behavior implies that the person is more efficient in the production of that behavior than in the production of less skilled behaviors. The central nervous system can increase efficiency by storing information that the individual has previously experienced such that subsequent processing experiences with that information can be expedited (Rothi et al., 1991). Therefore, rather than reconstructing a new representation with each experience (assembled knowledge), previously assembled representations in the lexical system can be activated from memory and re-utilized (addressed knowledge). Thus, there must be some stored memory that is formed by experience with a stimulus. The model of lexical processing in Figure 23–1 indicates that lexical abilities are dependent upon the integrity of a number of different types of stored representations. We will review the mechanisms proposed to make up this complex system and the types of impairments we might observe associated with dysfunction of these mechanisms. In the course of the discussion, we will address issues of controversy for the proposed model. Finally, we will mention the neurological site of lesion often associated with dysfunction of the lexical

mechanisms to suggest neural regions critically associated with the stages of lexical processing.

Recognition Level

Mechanisms

Following early sensory processing, stimulus recognition processes allow for activation of representations that closely correspond to the input stimulus. Recognition is the point in information processing when a stimulus becomes uniquely distinguishable and familiar compared to all other physically similar stimuli (Tyler, 1987). Stimulus recognition is not the point at which a stimulus is understood or comprehended. Instead, recognition is better thought of as the point at which a stimulus is identified as previously experienced and familiar. It allows the individual to say "yes" when asked whether a stimulus is a real object or a real word. It does not yet allow the individual to state what that object or word means. Recognition level processes provide a processing advantage to allow us to react quickly to whatever form the stimulus exemplar may take. For example, if the word is spoken with an accent or written in an unusual font, or if an object or gesture is viewed from an unusual orientation, stimulus recognition mechanisms allow for the quick realization that the stimulus is familiar in spite of input perturbations.

A number of lines of empirical and theoretic evidence to be reviewed below support the notion that recognition level processes are modality specific (Caramazza & Miceli, 1990; Ellis & Young, 1988); that is, separate modules represent knowledge for different types of familiar sensory stimuli, as shown in Figure 23–1. The phonological and graphemic input lexicons are stores of familiar spoken and written words, respectively. The visual object representations are stored memories of familiar objects. The action input lexicon is the store of familiar viewed actions (Rothi et al., 1991, 1997a). Other mechanisms for processing in other sensory modalities such as taction or olfaction also may exist.

Impairments

Agnosia is the term used for failure as a result of brain damage to recognize a sensory stimulus that is not attributable to dysfunction of peripheral sensory mechanisms. Agnosia can affect sensory modalities separately or in combinations (Farah, 1990; Feinberg et al., 1986). The fractionation of these systems can occur within modalities by type of stimulus as well. For example, within vision, researchers have described isolated recognition failures specific to orthography (Déjerine, 1891), objects (Bauer, 1993), colors (Benton & Tranel, 1993), and pantomimes (Rothi et al., 1986). Therefore, the fractionation of these forms of agnosia underscores the notion that recognition systems are sensory and material specific as well as neuroanatomically distinct and distributed. Deficits related to two of these sensory/material specific recognition systems depicted in Figure 23–1 are relevant to this chapter.

Visual Object Representation Impairments

Impairments related to the mechanism of visual object representations will affect performance in any lexical task that requires the patient to process viewed objects. For example, on clinical examination, patients will be impaired in picture naming, and they may have difficulty in word-to-picture matching tasks to test comprehension. In contrast, the same patient may be able to name in response to other sensory inputs such as to spoken definitions, or to demonstrate comprehension with printed word-to-word matching tasks.

Impairments of object processing may take different forms depending upon which stage of object processing is affected (see Farah, 1990, for a complete review). Dysfunction of early visual processes involved in developing a percept for the viewed object (Marr, 1982) prior to activation of visual object representations may lead to apperceptive or integrative forms of visual agnosia (Lissauer, 1890/1988; Riddoch & Humphreys, 1987a; Shelton et al., 1994; Warrington & Taylor, 1978). These patients, who have adequate visual acuity, may be unable to copy a line drawing or even to match simple drawings. They achieve little meaning from viewed pictures. However, their stored knowledge of what objects should look like appears to be intact as they may be able to answer questions about the visual characteristics of named objects in visual imagery tasks. In contrast, patients with impairment of the visual object representations themselves, including some individuals identified with visual associative agnosia (Lissauer, 1890/1988), demonstrate adequate performance in visual tasks dependent upon early visual processes such as matching line drawings or copying a figure. Errors in naming may include visual misperceptions (e.g., 'pen' for dart), or failures to respond ('I don't know') (Farah, 1990). Patients may be impaired in tasks requiring knowledge of the structure of a visual stimulus, such as distinguishing familiar from nonsense objects (visual object decision), or drawing from memory.

A phenomenon that is often discussed in the realm of the visual object agnosias is optic aphasia, a syndrome first described by Freund (1889). Some patients experience naming failure restricted to the visual modality (modality-specific), as in visual agnosia. However, they may be able to describe the function of viewed objects, sort objects into categories, or gesture the appropriate use for the object they are unable to name, arguing against a visual agnosia in which meaning is not appreciated for viewed objects. Some researchers consider optic aphasia a mild form of associative agnosia (Bauer, 1993; Chanoine et al., 1998; Iorio et al., 1992). Others have

attributed optic aphasia to a visual-to-semantic access impairment (Hillis & Caramazza, 1995a, 1995b; Riddoch & Humphreys, 1987b). They suggest that the modality-specific object naming impairment arises because, although visual object processing mechanisms are intact, the visual object representations are unable to activate the full semantic representations for viewed objects. Thereby, some semantic information is available regarding a picture for the patient to sort by category or to provide an appropriate gesture, but the full semantic representation must be activated for accurate picture naming to occur.

An alternative account of optic aphasia has consequences for the model depicted in Figure 23–1. Some researchers have proposed that optic aphasia arises due to an impairment of a direct, nonsemantic means to activate the phonological output lexicon from the object input mechanism, leaving the inherently unstable visual-to-semantic route of processing intact (Davidoff & De Bleser, 1993; Ratcliff & Newcombe, 1982). Other researchers have also argued for a nonsemantic route for object naming on the basis of studies in patients with Alzheimer's disease. Specifically, some patients show better object naming than expected in spite of documented impairments in word comprehension or name to definition tasks (Hodges & Patterson, 1995; Kremin et al., 1994; Raymer et al., 1995b; Shuren et al., 1993). While these types of data suggest that a nonsemantic visual-phonological process may exist, this proposal remains highly controversial.

The critical point for this discussion is that modality-specific object naming failures may involve different stages of impairment in the mechanism storing visual object representations. The clinician must assess the full range of abilities in visual and verbal tasks to determine what aspect of visual object processing has been affected in a given patient, as those differences may have important consequences for management of the impairment (Greenwald et al., 1995).

Two recent papers have analyzed lesion locations reported for patients with visual agnosia and optic aphasia (Iorio et al., 1992; Schnider et al., 1994). Those studies suggest critical brain regions responsible for the neural representation of object knowledge. Although bilateral posterior cerebral artery lesions were commonly reported, researchers have also described visual associative agnosia in a number of patients with unilateral left posterior mesial cortex infarctions. Schnider and colleagues proposed that the distinction between optic aphasia and associative agnosia relates to the integrity of the splenium of the corpus callosum. Patients with visual agnosia tend to have less splenial damage than do those with optic aphasia, and apparently access and employ the impaired left posterior hemisphere, which apparently is a critical region for object recognition. Patients with optic aphasia, in contrast, have more extensive splenial lesions preventing access to the damaged left hemisphere, and rely on the right hemisphere's contribution to visual and semantic processing in order to perform an array of semantic tasks (Coslett & Saffran, 1989, 1992; Raymer et al., 1997b).

Phonological Input Lexicon Impairments

Selective damage affecting the phonological input lexicon (Figure 23–1) will lead to impairments in all tasks requiring patients to process a spoken word such as auditory word-to-picture matching tasks, naming to spoken definitions, or gesturing to verbal command. The same patients may demonstrate preserved comprehension for written words (Ellis et al., 1983). In contrast to the visual system, fewer reports have been published about patients with retained hearing acuity but impairments related to phonological input processing stages. On the basis of the literature describing patients with pure word deafness, some general parallels may be seen between the impairments of object processing and impairments of phonological processing (Franklin, 1989; Polster & Rose, 1998; Vignolo, 1982). Some patients seem to have a pre-lexical apperceptive impairment that affects processing of phonemic and other types of acoustic stimuli (Buchman et al., 1986; Buchtel & Stewart, 1989), whereas other patients may retain the ability to recognize nonlinguistic acoustic stimuli (Takahashi et al., 1992).

Some patients identified with Wernicke's aphasia also may have impairments related to the phonological input lexicon. Patients with Wernicke's aphasia described by Ellis and colleagues (1983) and by Semenza and colleagues (1992) had modality-specific auditory comprehension impairment. Because the patients had retained comprehension for written material, semantic processing appeared to be intact and the auditory comprehension impairment presumably related to presemantic, phonological lexical stages of processing. Some early theories had proposed that the processing of the orthographic form of a word occurred subsequent to phonological activation (Caplan, 1993). However, if this dependency of orthographic processing upon phonological processing exists, patients with phonological input lexicon dysfunction should necessarily have corollary reading comprehension impairments. Thereby, patients with selective impairment for phonological input provide further evidence for separate, parallel input mechanisms for graphemic and phonological lexical processing.

The phonological correlate of optic aphasia may be represented in some patients with word meaning deafness (Kohn & Friedman, 1986). For example, Franklin and colleagues (1996) described a patient who could process the phonological components of words as indicated by preserved ability to discriminate and repeat words, and to perform auditory lexical decision which presumably depends upon the integrity of the phonological input representations. Although the patient demonstrated intact reading comprehension, he had difficulty in auditory comprehension tasks, particularly for abstract, low-frequency words. Franklin and colleagues attributed the failure to an impairment in activating the full semantic specification for spoken words, an argument similar to that proposed by Hillis and Caramazza (1995a) for optic aphasia.

Some studies have described the neural correlates of phonological input lexicon impairments. Individuals with pure word deafness typically have lesions affecting bilateral temporal or subcortical left hemisphere lesions affecting input to Wernicke's area (Polster & Rose, 1998), suggesting that these regions are important for prelexical stages of phonological processing. Some cases of Wernicke's aphasia associated with left posterior perisylvian lesions including Wernicke's area lesions (Kertesz et al., 1993; Weiller et al., 1995) may be characterized by an impairment of the phonological input lexicon. Therefore, it appears that the posterior portion of the left superior temporal cortex is a critical neural region subserving phonological lexical input knowledge.

Semantic Processing

Mechanism

Once a recognition-level representation achieves sufficient activation, it initiates activity in the semantic system (Figure 23–1). Semantic representations contain stored world knowledge shared by speakers of a language including meanings for words, objects, or actions. The semantic system can be accessed from any input modality and can access any output mode that is appropriate. Semantic representations presumably involve a network of information about words, objects, and ideas that includes superordinate, coordinate, associated, and subordinate relationships.

Discussion in cognitive neuropsychology continues regarding the structure of the semantic system. Some proposals view semantic representations as modality independent in that a single unitary semantic system provides meaning for a stimulus, regardless of input modality or output mode (Caramazza et al., 1990; Caramazza & Shelton, 1998; Hillis et al., 1990; Rapp et al., 1993; Riddoch et al., 1988). A contrasting view holds that the semantic system is structured into subsystems for different sensory modalities or output modes (Allport, 1985; Paivio, 1971, 1986; Saffran, 1997; Shallice, 1988). A discussion of impairments related to semantic processing may shed light on the preferred interpretation.

Impairments

A patient with a semantic impairment will have difficulty performing any tasks that require semantic mediation including comprehension of spoken and written words, interpreting the meanings of objects and gestures, and spoken and written picture naming (Ellis et al., 1992). Performance in oral word reading and writing to dictation may also be affected if alternative sublexical letter-sound conversion mechanisms are unavailable for decoding or encoding written words. If the unitary semantics system proposal is correct, the performance of individuals with brain damage leading to semantic system impairment should demonstrate quantitatively and qualitatively similar impairments across lexical tasks. Researchers have described this association of impairments in some patients with vascular lesions (Hillis et al., 1990; Howard & Orchard-Lisle, 1984) and progressive neurological impairments (Chertkow et al., 1989; Hodges & Patterson, 1996; Lambon Ralph et al., 1995; Raymer & Berndt, 1996). For example, Hillis and colleagues (1990) described the performance of their patient, KE, who produced the same proportion of semantic errors across all lexical tasks, and proposed that the impairment represented a dysfunction of a unitary semantic mechanism.

Other patients demonstrate lexical impairments that appear to represent dysfunction related to the semantic system, but dysfunction seems associated with disruption in stages of input to or output from the semantic system. Hart and Gordon (1990) described three patients who had difficulties with word comprehension in the context of preserved oral naming. They attributed this pattern to impairment of the input stage of semantic processing. In contrast, Raymer and colleagues (Raymer et al., 1997a; Raymer et al., 1997c) described patients who had no difficulty with word comprehension, but significant parallel patterns of word retrieval impairment across verbal and written output modes for both modalities of input tested (pictures, spoken definitions). They attributed this pattern of impairments to dysfunction at a common late stage in semantic processing prior to activating subsequent mode-specific output lexicons.

Researchers have also described individuals with aphasia whose naming and comprehension impairments fractionate, demonstrating selective preservation or selective impairment, for specific semantic categories. Patients have impairments for categories such as living and nonliving things (Bunn et al., 1998; Montanes et al., 1995; Silveri et al., 1997; Warrington & McCarthy, 1983), fruits and vegetables (Hart et al., 1985; Farah & Wallace, 1992), tools (Ochipa et al., 1989), animals (Caramazza & Shelton, 1998; Ferreira et al., 1997; Hart & Gordon, 1992; Hillis & Caramazza, 1991), and medical terminology (Crosson et al., 1997). At first look, one might use these unusual dissociations to infer that the semantic system is structured in a fashion that represents these specific categories of knowledge. However, Warrington and her colleagues (Warrington & McCarthy, 1983, 1987, 1994; Warrington & Shallice, 1984) have entertained a more principled account of these interesting dissociations. They attributed semantic category dissociations to the type of semantic information that is a defining characteristic for that category. They propose that category-specific deficits arise because the semantic system is structured along lines of sensory modalities and output

modes in a complex network of subsystems (Allport, 1985; Saffran, 1997). Disruption of selective subsystems leads to impairments affecting semantic categories for which that subsystem contributes critical semantic information. So, for example, because visual semantic information may be critical for distinguishing exemplars within the category of animals, impairment of the visual semantic subsystem results in category-specific impairment for animals (Warrington & Shallice, 1984).

In contrast, Caramazza and colleagues (Caramazza et al., 1994; Caramazza & Shelton, 1998) have argued that the semantic subsystems view does not entirely account for observations in patients with category-specific impairments. They question how impairment to a selective subsystem of semantic processing, for example, visual semantics, could lead to impairment for individual semantic categories such as fruits and vegetables, without also affecting other categories for which visual knowledge is a critical characteristic (Caramazza et al., 1994). Rather, Caramazza and Shelton (1998) proposed that category-specific impairments arise because of texturing in the interconnections of properties comprising semantic representations for members of a category of objects. If critical shared properties happen to be localized in a neural region that is damaged by neurologic disease, any concepts that include those properties in their semantic representations will be affected. In particular, items within certain natural categories such as plants or animals may have a number of highly interconnected properties, making all exemplars of the category vulnerable upon neurological injury.

Investigations of patients with category-specific semantic impairments have led some researchers to support the view that the semantic system is structured along modality/mode-specific lines. The semantic subsystems theory has more difficulty accounting for patients like those of Hillis and colleagues (1990) who had a more generalized impairment of semantic processing that affects all categories of objects across all lexical tasks. Because of these more generalized semantic impairments, it would seem prudent at this time to proceed with the assumption that the semantic system is a unitary system that processes information for all input modalities and output modes. There is some texture to the structure of semantic representations so that strategically placed neural lesions may result in impairments for selective categories of information (Caramazza & Shelton, 1998).

Regarding neural correlates of semantic system impairments, lesion analyses in patients with semantic dysfunction provide clues as to the neural instantiation of semantic knowledge. In particular, left hemisphere posterolateral cortical regions appear to play a critical role as these regions are implicated in individuals with degenerative dementias leading to semantic dysfunction (Graham et al., 1998; Hodges et al., 1992; Kertesz et al., 1998). Left posterior regions also are implicated in patients with acute vascular lesions. Hart and

Gordon (1990) reported that the left posterior temporal/inferior parietal cortex was affected in their patients with impairments affecting input to semantic processing (comprehension impairment with preserved word retrieval). In contrast, patients with an impairment affecting the semantic output stage (cross-modal word retrieval impairment with preserved comprehension) had discrete lesions confined to the left inferior temporal/occipital cortex junction or Brodmann's area 37 (Foundas et al., 1998; Raymer et al., 1997a). Therefore, although individuals with significant semantic impairments often have large left hemisphere lesions, left posterior perisylvian regions appear to play a critical role in semantic processing.

In addition, the left thalamus also seems to be implicated in the complex semantic network. Transcortical sensory aphasia, a syndrome associated with semantic dysfunction, is observed in many individuals with vascular lesions affecting the left thalamic nuclei (Crosson, 1992). Raymer et al. (1997c) reported that their two patients with left thalamic infarcts had a cross-modal word retrieval impairment implicating dysfunction in the process of semantic activation of lexical output representations.

Neural regions associated with category-specific impairments also suggest critical regions representing specific aspects of semantic knowledge. Viral encephalitis, which has a predilection for damage in the anterior and mesial temporal cortex, has been associated with impairments for the category of living items (Warrington & Shallice, 1984). Damasio and colleagues (1996) investigated lesion locations associated with impairments for three different semantic categories: (1) persons: left temporal pole lesions; (2) animals: left inferotemporal lesions; (3) tools: left temporal-parietal-occipital lesions. Finally, Crosson and colleagues (1997) reported a category-specific naming impairment for medical terminology associated with a left thalamic hemorrhage. Findings from these lesion studies provide further support that left posterior temporal-parietal-occipital and thalamic regions play a critical role in the neural representation of semantic mechanisms.

Output Lexicons

Mechanism

Once recognition has occurred and meaning has been activated for a word, object, or gesture, a response is initiated with activation of the output lexicons (Figure 1). As in recognition level structures, the output lexicons are modality specific as there are separate stores for familiar spoken and written words as well as for gestures (Rothi et al., 1991a, 1997a). In this discussion, we will focus on the store of spoken words, the phonological output lexicon. The nature and organization of the stored phonological

information is not completely understood. However, there is some indication that words are stored in phonologically similar groupings and that root morphemes are separated from affixes (e.g., walk+ -ed, -ing, -s) (Badecker & Caramazza, 1991; De Bleser & Cholewa, 1998; Miceli & Caramazza, 1988). Word class distinctions (e.g., nouns and verbs) also appear to be represented at the level of the output lexicon (Caramazza & Hillis, 1991; Caramazza & Miozzo, 1997).

Impairments

In the case of dysfunction related to the phonological output lexicon, the patient will be impaired in all verbal tasks dependent upon the integrity of the stored phonological representations. Patients will have difficulty in all oral naming tasks (e.g., picture naming, name to definitions). They may even have difficulty in oral reading, particularly for exception words (e.g., choir, yacht), as sublexical processes are insufficient to derive accurate pronunciations for those words. Production errors may take a variety of forms including semantic errors (Caramazza & Hillis, 1991), phonemic paraphasias (Kay & Ellis, 1987), and neologisms (Kohn et al., 1996). The variation in the forms of verbal errors represents the differential impairments that may occur at one stage of processing, in this case the phonological output lexicon. Some individuals may have greater difficulty activating the output lexicon (Caramazza & Hillis, 1991; Le Dorze & Nespoulous, 1989; Miceli et al., 1991) leading to semantic or no response errors. Others may have a disturbance affecting the internal structure resulting in neologistic responses (Kohn et al., 1996) or post-lexical phonemic processes leading to phonemic paraphasias (Ellis et al., 1992).

Researchers have inferred key features of the structure of the lexical system from observed lexical dissociations across patients with brain damage. For example, some patients demonstrate retained auditory comprehension for words they are unable to pronounce (Kay & Ellis, 1987; Maher et al., 1994; Nickels & Howard, 1995). Such a dissociation has been interpreted as evidence for the input/output distinction for the phonological lexicons. Similarly, some patients have selective impairments for phonological output in the context of retained performance in written word production (Bub & Kertesz, 1982; Caramazza & Hillis, 1990). A dissociation of this sort provides support for the distinction between phonological and graphemic output lexicons, the latter remaining intact in some patients with phonological output impairments. However, neurological injury usually affects multiple lexical mechanisms so patients may be impaired in a variety of lexical tasks (e.g., impairments of both verbal and written output, e.g., Caramazza et al., 1983; Miceli et al., 1991; impairments of both phonological input and output, e.g., Ellis et al., 1983, Kohn et al., 1996).

Whereas many studies of lexical retrieval impairments have focused largely on noun retrieval (Gainotti et al., 1986; Goodglass et al., 1969; Kay & Ellis, 1987; Kohn & Goodglass, 1985; Kohn et al., 1996; Le Dorze & Nespoulous, 1989), other studies have also identified disturbances for verb retrieval in some patients (Damasio & Tranel, 1993; Ellsworth & Raymer, 1998; Miceli et al., 1984; Zingeser & Berndt, 1990). Caramazza and Hillis (1991) described two patients with contrasting word retrieval impairments for specific grammatical categories that provide evidence for the nature of lexical knowledge in the output lexicons. Specifically, one patient was more impaired in writing verbs than nouns, but had intact performance for both nouns and verbs in speaking tasks. The second patient was more impaired in oral production of verbs than nouns, with intact writing for both verbs and nouns. Hillis and Caramazza (1995c) reported about a third patient who was more impaired in oral production of nouns than verbs, indicating that verbs are not simply more difficult than nouns in some unknown variable. Caramazza and Hillis proposed that this pattern of dissociation provides evidence that the grammatical class distinction observed only within a specific mode of output is represented at the level of the output lexicon.

Distinct neural regions appear to be associated with impairments affecting the phonological output lexicon. In particular, researchers typically have described noun retrieval impairments in patients with fluent aphasia and left posterior perisylvian cortex lesions often including temporal regions (Damasio & Tranel, 1993; Miozzo et al., 1994). In contrast, verb retrieval impairments have been associated with nonfluent aphasia and left frontal lesions (Caramazza & Hillis, 1991; Damasio & Tranel, 1993; Kohn et al., 1996; Miceli et al., 1984; Zingeser & Berndt, 1990).

In summary, studies examining impairments of lexical processing in a variety of patients with aphasia have provided evidence for a complex, distributed system of lexical processing as depicted in Figure 23–1. The lexical system is fractionated so that there are separate phonological and graphemic mechanisms as well as distinct mechanisms subserving lexical input and lexical output. All of these mechanisms store our repository of representations for familiar words within that modality/mode of processing. These lexical mechanisms interact by way of a semantic system whereby meaning is applied for lexical input and output. In addition, distinct brain regions are involved in the neural representation of lexical knowledge. Overall, it is the left hemisphere that plays the key role in representing lexical knowledge, although the right hemisphere may contribute to certain aspects of lexical-semantic processing (Joanette & Goulet, 1998). Although controversies persist regarding details of processing and representation in the lexical system, this general model provides a rational theoretical basis for guiding clinical management in patients with lexical impairments.

CLINICAL APPLICATIONS OF THE LEXICAL MODEL

The model of lexical processing provides a framework to explore the implications of the cognitive neuropsychological (CN) approach for the clinical process. The CN framework has definite implications for the form of the lexical assessment. In addition, researchers have applied this approach to analyses of lexical recovery and treatment. The CN approach also has direct implications for predictions regarding generalization of treatment effects.

Assessment

The goal of assessment within cognitive neuropsychology is to characterize a patient's language impairments with respect to a cognitive model. The model of lexical processing in Figure 23–1 provides a basis for discussion of impairments specifically related to spoken word comprehension and production. On the basis of their assessment, clinicians will describe impairments with respect to the lexical mechanism implicated in the pattern of spared and impaired performance. Arguably, cognitive models have had their greatest contribution to clinical practice in the realm of assessment (Schwartz & Whyte, 1992). For example, Raymer et al. (1995a) depicted how a CN analysis played a significant role in distinguishing the lexical impairments of two patients whose standardized aphasia assessments acutely indicated anomic aphasia. However, when clinicians evaluated the profound word retrieval impairments in greater detail, it became clear that the two patients had distinctive differences in the cognitive mechanisms for their word retrieval impairments. One patient had an impairment affecting semantic activation of the output lexicons (Raymer et al., 1997a). The other had impairments affecting at least two stages of lexical processing: visual object activation of the semantic system, and semantic activation of the output lexicons (Raymer et al., 1997b). Assessment results then had consequences for treatment for the word retrieval impairment in the second patient (Greenwald et al., 1995). The challenge to clinicians is to tailor assessments to assess the integrity of the lexical mechanisms.

General Considerations

Mode/Modality Comparisons

A key concept in an assessment geared to identify impairments in the lexical system is mode/modality comparison. The lexical assessment should include a variety of single word processing tasks in which the clinician systematically varies input modalities and output modes, and analyzes patterns of performance for tasks sharing modalities/modes of processing. Typical input modalities of interest will include auditory, verbal, written, viewed objects, and possibly, viewed gestures.

TABLE 23–1

Lexical Tasks to Include in Assessment

Output Tasks	Input Tasks
*Oral picture naming	*Auditory word-to-picture matching
*Written picture naming	*Written word-to-picture matching
*Oral naming to spoken definitions	Auditory word-picture verification
Written naming to spoken definitions	Written word-picture verification
*Oral word reading	*Semantic associates matching
*Writing to dictation	Auditory lexical decision
Name to tactile object presentation	Written lexical decision
Name to environmental sounds	Category sorting
Gesture to command	
Gesture to viewed objects	

*Indicates key tasks in the general lexical assessment.

TABLE 23–2

Linguistic Factors That May Affect Performance for Items Within Lexical Tasks with Selected Normative References

Word frequency (Francis & Kucera, 1982)
Grammatical category (noun, verb, functor)
Semantic category (living items, fruits, animals)
Lexicality (word, nonword)
Regularity (Berndt et al., 1987; regular spelling—mat, exceptional spelling—yacht)
Age of acquisition (Gilhooly & Logie, 1980)
Imageability (Gilhooly & Logie, 1980; Coltheart, 1981)
Operativity (Coltheart, 1981; tools and objects tools act upon)
Length (syllable length, phoneme length)
Familiarity (Snodgrass & Vanderwart, 1980)

Modes of output will include speech, writing, and gesture. Table 23–1 lists a number of lexical tasks that result when combining modalities and modes. Using this principle, we created the Florida Semantics Battery (Raymer et al., 1990) to use in assessments for patients with lexical impairments. Other researchers have developed similar experimental batteries (e.g., Hillis et al., 1990). Published psycholinguistic tests now are available that allow systematic assessment of lexical processing (e.g., Psycholinguistic Assessment of Language Processing Abilities, Kay et al., 1992; Psycholinguistic Assessment of Language, Caplan, 1993). The lexical assessment typically will include key tasks such as oral picture naming, written picture naming, naming to spoken definition, oral word reading, writing to dictation, auditory word comprehension, and written word comprehension, among others.

Lexical Stimuli

A second critical consideration in lexical assessment is the selection of appropriate stimulus material. As tasks contrast modalities/modes of processing, it is important, to the extent possible, to employ the same set of stimuli across tasks. For example, the Florida Semantics Battery incorporates the same set of 120 nouns across tasks. (See Appendix 23-1 for the full set of 120 nouns.) Patients complete blocks of stimuli systematically across experimental tasks to control for effects of repeated exposure to the same stimuli. In this way, the clinician can attribute differences observed across tasks to the modality of processing and not to differences in stimulus

variables. On the other hand, there will be times when the clinician wants to evaluate performance for contrasting sets of materials, for example, contrasting performance for nouns versus verbs (e.g., Zingeser & Berndt, 1990). In this case, care must be taken in selecting stimuli matched on independent linguistic factors that experimental studies have demonstrated may affect lexical performance, as shown in Table 23–2. Clinicians should be sensitive to differences across semantic categories (e.g., animals, tools, etc.) and grammatical class (nouns, verbs, functors). In early studies examining factors influencing word retrieval, investigators often discussed the effect of word frequency, as higher frequency words are named better than lower frequency words (e.g., Howes, 1964; Goodglass et al., 1969; norms from Francis & Kucera, 1982). Experimental studies often have reported word frequency effects on lexical performance (e.g., Howard et al., 1984; Kay & Ellis, 1987; Raymer et al., 1997a; Raymer et al., 1997c; Zingeser & Berndt, 1988). However, recent carefully controlled studies have demonstrated that word frequency has a less potent effect on lexical processing than do factors such as imageability, length, familiarity, and especially, age of acquisition (Feyereisen et al., 1988; Hirsh & Ellis, 1994; Lambon Ralph et al., 1998; Nickels & Howard, 1994, 1995). Words learned early in life are particularly resilient under conditions of brain damage. Therefore, the clinician should evaluate the effect such variables have on their patient's performance as certain factors may have implications for materials chosen for use in treatment.

Comprehension Tasks

In tasks assessing comprehension of single words, at times it can be difficult to detect an impairment. For example, in word-to-picture matching tasks, individuals may respond correctly to an item on the basis of only basic semantic information if a target picture (e.g., "apple") and the distractor pictures are unrelated (e.g., apple, chair, hammer, dress) (Raymer & Berndt, 1996). For this reason it is important to evaluate comprehension performance in the context of semantically related distractors as well (e.g., apple, orange, banana, grapes), which will require subjects to activate more specified semantic information to derive the correct answer.

A more sensitive task to assess comprehension can be picture-word verification in which the patient sees a picture and must decide (yes-no) whether a given word is the correct label. Hillis and colleagues (1990), using this task, systematically varied the distractor word across conditions. For example, for a picture of an apple, on different trials the patient hears the correct word (apple), a semantically related word (orange), or an unrelated word (table). If the patient has a suspected impairment affecting phonological input, a phonologically related word (opal) might also be a useful distractor. An item is scored as correct only if the patient responds correctly in all conditions. A simple modification in distractor conditions may allow the examiner to identify subtle lexical impairments that otherwise may be overlooked in assessment.

Error Patterns Across Lexical Tasks

Another key concept to consider in the lexical assessment is the pattern of errors produced across tasks. Mitchum and colleagues (1990) described a response analysis system for coding the types of lexical errors clinicians may observe in their patients with aphasia. Table 23-3 provides a list of some typical errors observed for verbal responses in lexical tasks. The types of errors may provide important clues as to the mechanism underlying a patient's lexical impairment. However, whereas within-task error analyses allow some insight into the mechanism of a lexical failure, it is the comparison of error patterns across tasks that allows one to hypothesize about the locus of deficit. The same quantitative and qualitative pattern of errors should be observed in all tasks that necessarily require processing by the impaired mechanism. For example, a deficit of semantic processing will affect performance in all comprehension and naming tasks (e.g., Hillis et al., 1990). A phonological output lexicon dysfunction will result in parallel patterns of impairment in all verbal production tasks (e.g., oral naming of pictures and oral reading of single words if sublexical processes also are impaired) (Caramazza & Hillis, 1990).

Examination of the type of error itself within one lexical task is not sufficient to distinguish the level of lexical impairment responsible for the error. Semantic errors in picture naming are a case in point (Hillis & Caramazza, 1995b). For example, for the target picture of a carrot, semantic naming errors may include responses such as "vegetable" (superordinate), "celery" (coordinate), or "rabbit" (associated). On the surface, one might assume that these errors

---

TABLE 23-3

Types of Production Errors Commonly Observed in Lexical Tasks

Error Type	Description
Visual	In object naming, names of objects sharing visual characteristics, e.g., "pencil" for screwdriver; in oral reading, words which share orthography, e.g., "chain" for choir
Semantic	
Superordinate	Semantic category name for the viewed object/word
Coordinate	Name of alternative item within the semantic category, e.g., "apple" for pear
Associate	Words bearing some relationship (e.g., function, location, attribute) to the target picture/word, e.g., "pound" for hammer
Circumlocution	Description of the semantic attributes of the object/word
Phonemic	Response sharing phonemic attributes of target; at times is a real word, e.g., "trick" for truck, or nonword, e.g., "trut" for truck
Unrelated	Responses bearing no relationship to target, e.g., "cow" for lamp
No Response	Refusal or inability to retrieve response, e.g., "I don't know"

---

represent semantic system dysfunction (Figure 23-1). Indeed, in some patients, semantic errors may represent semantic system impairment (Hillis et al., 1990; Raymer, 1997a; Howard & Orchard-Lisle, 1984). However, Caramazza and Hillis (1990) described a patient who produced semantic errors only for oral picture naming and oral word reading, but none in written picture naming and writing to dictation. They interpreted this mode-specific impairment as a disturbance at the level of the phonological output lexicon. In contrast, patients with optic aphasia often produce large numbers of semantic errors in picture naming tasks (oral and written), but no semantic errors in naming to definition (Hillis & Caramazza, 1995a; Raymer et al., 1997b). Such a pattern may represent an impairment of visual object activation of the semantic system. These observations underscore the need to analyze error patterns across lexical tasks to develop an accurate hypothesis regarding the source of the lexical error (Raymer & Rothi, in press).

Stage-Specific Analyses

Many lexical tasks involve processing at multiple stages in the lexical system. It is necessary to contrast performances across tasks sharing processing at one stage to develop a precise hypothesis about the nature of the impairment affecting performance at that stage. In this section we will review tasks that the clinician may administer to assess performance at each lexical stage. (See Rothi et al., 1997b, for a description of assessment techniques for the action system.) The review will include tasks that involve multiple stages of processing, as well as tasks that more specifically target processing at a particular stage.

Visual Object Representation Tasks

Tasks that require processing of familiar pictures will depend upon the integrity of visual object representations. Therefore, general tasks such as object naming and word-to-picture matching provide an initial screening for this mechanism. Object recognition impairment is suspected if performance improves for contrasting tasks when no picture or object processing is necessary (e.g., name to definitions, word-to-word matching), or when patient responses in picture naming represent visually similar objects (e.g., "pencil" for screwdriver). Tasks that target processing by visual object representations more directly require subjects to determine familiarity of objects or to use knowledge of the visual form of objects. Object-nonsense object decision, which requires a subject to decide whether a viewed stimulus is a familiar object, presumably depends on an intact visual object representation. Similarly, drawing from memory also may tap this object recognition process. As described above, impairments of object recognition may take a number of forms; therefore, a full range of object processing tasks, such as copying and matching line drawings, may be necessary to distinguish early object processing impairments from impairments affecting visual object representations themselves. The key feature, however, is that impairment will be specific to the visual modality. When other verbal mechanisms are assessed, performance may be intact.

Phonological Input Lexicon Tasks

Any tasks requiring lexical processing through the auditory verbal channel will require activation of the phonological input lexicon. Testing will include tasks that are part of the general lexical assessment such as auditory word-to-picture matching (especially in the presence of phonological or semantic distractors), naming to spoken definitions, and gesture to verbal command. As in visual object representations, stage-specific phonological tasks require patients to process auditory aspects of familiar phonological stimuli. Auditory lexical decision in which patients decide whether a given stimulus is a real or nonsense word is such a task. Additional phonological tasks such as phoneme discrimination, repetition, or identification of familiar environmental sounds may be useful to determine whether the impairment for phonological lexical information relates to pre-lexical auditory

impairments. A modality-specific dysfunction is suspected if performance improves when stimuli are presented through other nonphonological modalities such as written or viewed object input and when responses to phonological stimuli suggest misperception or confusion with phonologically related words.

Semantic System Tasks

All lexical comprehension and production tasks presumably depend upon adequate processing by the semantic system, regardless of input modality and output mode. Therefore, semantic impairment will affect performance across tasks. However, performance for oral reading and writing to dictation of regularly spelled words may be spared even in the face of semantic impairments if sublexical print-sound conversion processes remain intact. In practice, it may be possible for a neurological lesion to cause extensive damage to lexical input and output stages simultaneously, leading to mode/modality-consistent impairments that mimic semantic dysfunction. Therefore, it can be useful to administer additional semantic tasks that require more specific processing of semantic attributes of stimuli or that avoid the use of lexical stimuli. Sorting objects by category and systematically manipulating the distance between categories may help detect semantic impairment. Asking patients to provide definitions for words also taxes semantic processing. The Florida Semantics Battery (Raymer et al., 1990) includes a semantic associates subtest patterned after the Pyramids and Palm Trees Test (Howard & Patterson, 1992) to assess semantic processing. The semantic associates task requires subjects to match a target item (e.g., carrot) to a semantically related item from three choices (e.g., associate—rabbit; distractors—squirrel, cake). The clinician can contrast object and verbal modalities of presentation, requiring matching of viewed objects to viewed objects, spoken object names to spoken object names, viewed objects to spoken object names, and spoken object names to viewed objects. This test can be sensitive to more subtle impairments in semantic activation (e.g., Raymer et al., 1997b).

Because semantic impairments can fractionate along the lines of specific semantic categories, it is useful to include tasks that are structured according to this dimension. The Florida Semantics Battery incorporates semantic category distinctions as it tests items from 12 different semantic categories (see Appendix 23-1). Within standard aphasia tests currently available, an astute examiner may notice either impairment or spared performance related to selective categories by noting errors and exploring category distinctions with additional testing with relevant materials. It is also helpful to ask patients whether they notice problems for specific categories. During an extended hospitalization, one patient complained he was experiencing great difficulty with medical words. Careful examination substantiated his complaint of a selective impairment for medical terminology (Crosson et al., 1997).

Clinicians may find it useful to develop informal sets of stimuli that include items from a variety of semantic categories that stress different types of semantic content. For example, visual information is purportedly an important characteristic of living categories such as animals, fruits, and vegetables; action output/operativity is relevant to categories of garage tools, kitchen implements, and office implements. Results of testing that identifies selective categories of difficulty for a patient may allow the clinician to streamline efforts in rehabilitation.

Phonological Output Lexicon Tasks

On the general lexical assessment, tasks requiring verbal production of familiar words will require activation of the phonological output lexicon. Impairment in oral naming, oral word reading, or repetition tasks in the context of good performance in auditory and reading comprehension, written naming, and writing to dictation leads one to suspect impairment of the phonological output lexicon (Caramazza & Hillis, 1990). However, this dissociation may arise with subsequent post-lexical dysfunction (e.g., apraxia of speech). To further evaluate the integrity of the phonological output lexicon, it may be necessary to administer tasks that require phonological lexical processing in particular. One such task is rhyme verification for picture pairs. The patient views two pictures and must determine whether their names rhyme (e.g., whale-nail). The rhyming task will prove difficult for individuals who fail to activate a full lexical representation for the pictures. Word-nonword repetition is a task that may also help decipher whether an impairment stems from the phonological output lexicon or beyond. Patients with post-lexical impairments often have greater difficulty for nonword stimuli (Kahn et al., 1998), whereas patients with lexical impairments may have greater difficulty with word stimuli than nonword stimuli (Hillis et al., 1999).

Summary of Assessment

Overall, the CN approach to assessment of lexical function is distinguished by its systematic examination of patterns of performance across modalities of input and modes of output. Rather than employing a specific assessment protocol, assessment will be individualized on the basis of demonstrated deficits in preliminary testing. Additional testing will proceed as the clinician develops hypotheses regarding suspected levels of impairment.

The CN assessment approach has a number of advantages (Raymer et al., 1995b). Many patients with extensive neurological lesions have dysfunction affecting multiple levels in the lexical system. An in-depth assessment will frequently suggest not only what mechanisms are impaired, but

also what mechanisms are spared in lexical processing. In addition, the clinician may identify specific linguistic factors that affect performance across tasks. These types of information may be especially beneficial as the clinician turns toward devising treatments for each patient.

Some clinicians may argue that in these days of limited resources, it is unrealistic to promote such a lengthy assessment. However, the clinician may adapt these methods using a more circumscribed set of available materials. For example, it might be possible to select 10 stimuli representing a variety of semantic categories and to vary mode/modality of processing for key lexical processing tasks listed in Table 23–1. A systematic assessment may indeed be more cost effective as clinicians understand their patients' impairments and direct treatments in the most expeditious manner.

Recovery of Lexical Impairments

Researchers have described diverse lexical impairments in individuals with a variety of neurologic disorders. In general, etiology of the brain disorder and size and extent of brain lesion will have greatest influence on the prognosis for recovery of lexical impairment among these individuals (Rothi, 1997). For example, lexical-semantic impairments described in patients with degenerative dementias, whether from Alzheimer's disease or more selective cortical atrophy leading to semantic dementia, are unlikely to improve and are apt to worsen over time. In contrast, recovery from lexical impairments related to acute neurologic etiologies such as stroke is more favorable. The extent of lexical recovery may relate to size and site of neurological lesion. Larger cortical lesions are associated with more limited recovery of lexical skills (Knopman et al., 1984; Naeser et al., 1987). In contrast, lexical impairments related to subcortical thalamic lesions typically resolve more quickly (Crosson, 1992).

Recently, investigators have described more detailed analysis of language recovery to identify lexical factors predictive of recovery from aphasia. Recovery analyses described by Kohn and colleagues (1996) and Laiacona and colleagues (1997) provide information to help clinicians predict which patients are likely to recover from lexical impairment. Kohn and colleagues examined recovery of neologistic verbal output in four subjects with lexical impairment related to the phonological output lexicon, only two of whom demonstrated substantial improvement after 6 months. The distinguishing characteristic in the nonrecovering subjects was a perseverative phonemic pattern in their neologisms at onset. The authors proposed that the patients who recovered had an impairment that affected retrieval of representations from the phonological output lexicon whereas the two with no recovery had substantial loss of phonological representations.

Laiacona and colleagues (1997) described recovery of lexical abilities in two patients with category-specific lexical impairments for living items as compared to nonliving items. One patient was initially less impaired than the other and had normal performance for nonliving items across tasks. One year later, that patient had improved to normal levels of performance for living items as well. In contrast, a second patient was initially severely impaired across categories, with an advantage for items in the nonliving category. After 2 years, performance had improved significantly only for the category of nonliving items and living items remained severely impaired. The authors proposed that distinct mechanisms of word retrieval failure led to differential resolution of the category-specific impairments in the two patients. Similar to the argument of Kohn and colleagues (1996), an impairment characterized by loss of semantic representations was associated with more limited recovery than an impairment that affected semantic system access to intact lexical output representations.

Recovery analyses may serve to distinguish hypotheses generated to account for lexical impairments in individuals with similar patterns of lexical impairments. Miceli and colleagues (1991) described a patient with impaired word retrieval in oral and written naming tasks and intact performance in comprehension tasks. They attributed the impairment to co-occurring deficits of the phonological and graphemic output lexicons. Raymer et al. (1997a) described a patient with a similar pattern of lexical performance. However, they opted for a more parsimonious proposal that the impairment arose at a late stage in semantic processing as semantic representations activate subsequent lexical output mechanisms. When Raymer and Rothi (2000) assessed the pattern of recovery for their patient, parallel patterns of improvement, qualitatively and quantitatively, were evident for both oral and written naming, as might be predicted if the impairment arose at a common stage in lexical processing. These parallel recovery patterns across output modes further substantiate the original proposal that the lexical impairment for speech and writing related to a common stage in processing.

Although fewer studies have assessed recovery from a CN perspective, those to date have demonstrated the implications of such analyses. Recovery analyses may allow researchers to confirm and contrast interpretations made regarding lexical impairments observed early after a neurological lesion. Over time, clinicians may use knowledge derived from recovery analyses to direct clinical efforts toward lexical processes that are predicted to recover. And finally, recovery analyses may ultimately provide additional evidence to validate proposed models of lexical processing (Martin, 1996).

Treatment

A number of clinical researchers have voiced optimism that CN models may provide a sound theoretical foundation from which to develop rational treatments for patients with aphasia

(Coltheart, 1984; Mitchum, 1992; Raymer et al., 1995b; Riddoch & Humphreys, 1994; Seron & Deloche, 1989). Of course, cognitive models are not the sole determinant of decisions made in the treatment for patients with aphasia (Caramazza & Hillis, 1993; Hillis, 1993). Clinicians also weigh a number of other medical, neurological, and social factors as they develop a plan of management for a given patient. Intervention may be indicated in patients with neurological etiologies for which some amount of recovery is expected (Raymer & Rothi, 2000), while it may be less beneficial in individuals with diseases that are expected to worsen (degenerative dementias) (e.g., McNeil et al., 1995). Moreover, the type of intervention strategy chosen should relate to the chronicity of the lexical impairment. Rothi (1995) proposed that restitutive strategies, which encourage restoration of functioning in a manner compatible with normal language processing, are appropriate in early stages of recovery from a neurological injury when neurophysiologic processes of recovery are operational. Substitutive strategies that attempt to circumvent the dysfunction using intact cognitive mechanisms will be beneficial during either acute or chronic stages of impairment.

Cognitive models of lexical processing lend themselves well toward the restitutive/substitutive distinction. Restitutive treatments would target lexical processes which clinicians have identified as impaired following the systematic lexical assessment. Substitutive treatments would incorporate processes that assessment has indicated remain intact in lexical processing. Clinical researchers have applied the CN approach in a number of lexical studies, some of which used a restorative approach, and others of which used a substitutive approach as deemed appropriate on the basis of patterns of preserved performance across lexical tasks.

Treatments for Comprehension Impairments

The process of word comprehension in which meaning is applied to a lexical referent involves activation of both the phonological input lexicon and the semantic system. Restitutive treatments for auditory comprehension might target those mechanisms, whereas substitutive treatments would use alternative processes to accomplish comprehension. A small number of studies have applied a CN approach in the treatment of auditory comprehension impairments.

Restitutive Comprehension Treatments

Morris and colleagues (1996) described a phonological treatment for a patient with impairments of auditory comprehension arising at a prelexical phonological stage of processing. In their treatment, the patient participated in a series of tasks in which he was to process different types of phonemic information including phoneme-grapheme matching, phoneme discrimination, auditory-word to picture and auditory-word to written-word matching and verification, and nonsense CV syllable discrimination. As needed, the clinician provided additional lip-reading cues and hand signals (substitutive strategies) to embellish the phonemic input. Following 6 weeks of twice weekly treatment, the patient demonstrated significant improvements in a variety of phonological tasks, but no improvement in written word comprehension and picture naming tasks that did not involve phonological input processing. Although it is not clear at which stage in phonological processing the treatment had its effect, it is evident that the effect was modality specific and not due to spontaneous recovery.

Grayson and colleagues (1997) implemented a semantic treatment for a patient with severe deficits of lexical comprehension related to dysfunction at both phonological and semantic stages of processing. They chose first to target the semantic impairment by having the patient execute a number of lexical tasks that require semantic processing: auditory word and written word to picture-matching, in which they systematically increased the number and relatedness of distractors; category-sorting for pictures and written words of increasing semantic relatedness; and associated-matching of written words. Following 4 weeks of treatment, the patient improved in other word-picture matching tasks, but not in a phoneme discrimination task. Subsequently, the clinicians added a phonological component to their semantic treatment as they asked the patient to perform a word-picture matching task using all rhyming word foils. Following 4 additional weeks of treatment, improvement was seen in auditory word-picture matching tasks as well as a nonword phoneme discrimination task, suggesting that repeated exposure to the treatment tasks affected both phonological and semantic processing.

Behrmann & Lieberthal (1989) applied a similar semantic treatment in a patient with category-specific comprehension impairments that were particularly severe for the categories of body parts, furniture, and transportation. Clinicians trained the patient on superordinate and specific semantic details about the three targeted categories and then had the patient perform visual and verbal matching tasks applying the semantic information. Following treatment, their patient demonstrated improved categorization of items in the trained categories as well as one untrained category. Little improvement was noted in other semantic processing tasks.

In summary, requiring patients to complete tasks that require some form of phonological or semantic decisions appears to affect future processing abilities for spoken input. Although we cannot be certain, it appears that these improvements relate to changes in phonological input and semantic stages of lexical processing.

Substitutive Comprehension Treatments

Substitutive treatments for auditory comprehension impairments may take a number of forms, depending upon the modality of input selected. Some researchers have advocated the use of a lip-reading strategy to provide additional visual information during the course of phonological processing (Ellis et al, 1983; Morris et al., 1996). Shindo and colleagues (1991) assessed the effect of lip-reading in four patients with impairments of phonological input processing. All four patients demonstrated an advantage in processing spoken words with lip-reading cues as opposed to that without lip-reading cues. It appears that lip-reading can be an especially useful strategy in patients with intact semantic processing in the presence of phonological processing impairments.

The graphemic input system is another modality for use in patients with phonological processing impairments. For example, Hough (1993) used reading to treat the severe lexical impairment in a patient with Wernicke's aphasia. Although the patient improved in oral naming, no changes were evident in auditory comprehension. Alternative modalities of input may be used to circumvent the impaired phonological input system. However, there is little clear evidence to suggest that the use of alternative input modalities will ultimately improve functioning in the affected phonological input system.

Treatment for Naming Impairments

Researchers have reported many more studies using the CN approach in the treatment of word retrieval impairments. Word retrieval requires both semantic and phonological output stages of lexical processing. Thereby, a number of studies have examined the usefulness of restitutive treatments incorporating various semantic and phonological tasks, either independently or in combination, as shown in Table 23–4. Substitutive treatments, in contrast, have incorporated alternative modes of output to either circumvent

---

TABLE 23–4

Semantic and Phonological Treatments Used to Improve Word Retrieval

Semantic Treatments

Semantic comprehension tasks (e.g., auditory word/picture matching; written word/picture matching; yes/no verification)

Semantic features descriptions (e.g., distinguishing features between similar objects)

Semantic matrix training (e.g., category, function, attribute, associates)

Phonological Treatments

Phonological questions tasks (e.g., rhyming comprehension, syllable number verfication, initial phoneme verification)

Oral word reading

Word repetition

Phonological cuing hierarchy (e.g., rhyming word, initial phoneme, repetition)

an impairment or to vicariatively encourage word retrieval through alternative means.

Restitutive Word Retrieval Treatments

Semantic Treatments. Recognizing the common role the semantic system plays in both word comprehension and word retrieval, a number of researchers have applied comprehension treatments in an attempt to facilitate word retrieval. Byng and colleagues (1990) described a treatment for a patient with a severe aphasia that crossed input and output modalities and implicated a semantic impairment. The patient participated in semantic processing tasks requiring picture categorization with increasingly related categories, and word-picture matching with increasingly difficult semantic distractors (closer semantic relationship to the target). Following this type of semantic comprehension treatment, the patient demonstrated improvement in word retrieval for trained words.

A series of similar studies has evaluated improvements in oral picture naming when subjects complete semantic comprehension tasks (auditory word-picture matching, written word-picture matching, or answering yes-no questions about semantic details of a picture) over multiple treatment sessions. In these studies, the patients also said the word during the performance of the comprehension tasks, adding a phonological component to the treatment (Davis & Pring, 1991; Marshall et al., 1990; Nickels & Best, 1996b; Pring et al., 1990). Following semantic comprehension treatment, a variety of subjects with word retrieval impairments related to either semantic or phonologic dysfunction demonstrated significant improvement in word retrieval abilities.

Noting that the earlier studies incorporated phonological output in the performance of semantic comprehension tasks, two subsequent studies contrasted treatments in which semantic comprehension tasks were performed with and without phonologic production of target words to determine the role that the phonologic output component played in the treatment (Drew & Thompson, 1999; Le Dorze et al., 1994). The findings of both studies indicated that subjects benefited maximally during training in which the comprehension tasks were combined with the phonologic output component of training. Hence, a semantic plus phonological output treatment protocol that parallels the normal process of word retrieval was most effective.

Some patients with semantic dysfunction seem to lack specific details of semantic representations, and thereby produce many semantic errors. Following a lexical assessment that indicated a word retrieval impairment related to underspecified semantic representations, Hillis (1991, 1998) devised a semantic treatment for her patient. She provided her patient with semantic information about target pictures she was unable to name, and contrasted those features with the semantic features of a closely related object. Ochipa and

colleagues (1998) used a similar semantic treatment with their patient with word retrieval impairment stemming from semantic system dysfunction. Patients in both studies demonstrated significant improvements in naming trained pictures as well as generalization to untrained pictures and untrained lexical tasks incorporating semantic processing (written word production). Hillis (1998) also reported that this semantic features treatment was more effective than a traditional cuing hierarchy treatment in her patient.

In another type of semantic treatment, developed on the basis of cognitive theories of how semantic representations are structured, clinicians attempt to improve word retrieval in picture naming using a semantic feature matrix (Haarbauer-Krupa et al., 1985). Clinicians teach subjects to use a viewed matrix of printed cue words (e.g., function, properties, category, etc.) to assist in retrieving semantic information about a target picture along with its name. Following training with a semantic feature matrix, subjects demonstrated improved naming of trained pictures as well as generalization of the strategy to some untrained pictures (Boyle, 1997; Boyle & Coelho, 1995; Lowell et al., 1995; McHugh et al., 1997).

Phonological Treatments. Other studies have used treatment protocols incorporating phonological information to target phonological output stages of word retrieval. A shared phonological output representation may be activated in oral reading, word repetition, and oral picture naming. Capitalizing on this relationship, Miceli and colleagues (1996) had their patient repeatedly read aloud or repeat target words. Both procedures resulted in improved picture naming for trained words in one subject with phonologically based word retrieval failure. Mitchum and Berndt (1994) used a similar phonological rehearsal treatment (incorporating repetition practice) in their patient with a selective verb retrieval impairment. Following training, their subject demonstrated improvements in verb retrieval, but little improvement in the formulation of complete sentences using the trained verbs.

Other studies have incorporated treatments using a hierarchy of phonological cues to assist in retrieving the phonological form of target words. Subjects who were repeatedly exposed to a hierarchy of initial phoneme, rhyme, and word repetition cues demonstrated improvements in word retrieval for trained words (Greenwald et al., 1995; Hillis, 1993, 1998; Raymer et al., 1993). Among these studies, treatment was effective for subjects with either semantic or phonological word retrieval dysfunction, although improvements were more limited in patients with co-occurring semantic impairment (Raymer et al., 1993). Because of concerns that the phonemic hierarchy was effective simply because of a final rehearsal phase in the treatment, Greenwald and colleagues (1995) also administered a simple rehearsal (repetition) phase of treatment, independent of the phonemic hierarchy.

Only mild improvement was evident with simple rehearsal compared to the more noticeable effects of the phonemic cuing hierarchy treatment in both patients.

Robson and colleagues (1998) used a different type of phonological training scheme that paralleled the procedures applied in semantic comprehension treatment. To encourage activation of phonological output representations, they required patients to complete tasks in which they made judgments about phonological information for words, such as the number of syllables and the initial phoneme of words. Their subject demonstrated improvement in retrieving words when trained with this strategy and showed some generalization of the process in naming untrained pictures.

Semantic Plus Phonological Treatments. Finally, some studies have incorporated both semantic and phonological aspects of lexical processing in their treatments to encourage the normal multistage process of word retrieval. As noted above, semantic comprehension treatment was more effective when combined with phonological production of the corresponding target words (Drew & Thompson, 1999; Le Dorze et al., 1994). Marshall and colleagues (1998) used a combination of semantic comprehension tasks and phonological lexical processing tasks to train verb retrieval for their subject with selective verb retrieval impairment. Following treatment, their subject not only improved verb retrieval for trained verbs, but also increased the use of grammatical sentences incorporating those verbs.

Object Recognition Treatment. Finally, for some patients, picture naming failure stems from impairments in visual-semantic stages of processing (Hillis & Caramazza, 1995a; Raymer et al., 1997b). Greenwald and colleagues (1995) applied a treatment for object-semantic processing in two patients with inordinate word retrieval impairment in the visual modality (both patients also had an additional lexical impairment affecting semantic to lexical output stages). In their visual treatment, the patients first named the category of the viewed object, then verbalized distinctive visual features for that object. Once the clinician summarized the visual-semantic information, the patients completed a rehearsal phase for the target word. Although both patients improved using this technique, one showed marked improvements in object naming following this visual-semantic treatment, but little generalization to untrained words.

Contrasting Restitutive Treatments. Fewer investigations have directly contrasted the effects of different restitutive treatments within individuals to determine the most effective strategy. Howard and colleagues (1985) sequentially evaluated separate treatments requiring subjects to answer questions about either semantic or phonological information for target pictures. Their group results indicated that both treatments led to improved naming for trained words, with an advantage of semantic over phonological

treatment. Because they reported results for the group as a whole, however, it is not clear how each subject responded individually to the two treatments and whether some subjects actually found the phonological treatment more effective or whether some subjects did not benefit from treatment.

Ennis and colleagues (1999) recently completed a study contrasting the effects of a semantic question hierarchy versus a phonological question hierarchy in four individuals with aphasia. In the semantic question hierarchy, subjects answered three yes/no questions about the category, a coordinate object, and an associated word for each training word. In the phonological question hierarchy, the subjects answered three yes/no questions about the number of syllables, the initial phoneme, and a rhyming word for each training word. Both treatments ended with a common rehearsal phase. Effects of semantic treatment surpassed phonological treatment in improving noun retrieval for two subjects with primarily phonological word retrieval impairments. In contrast, effects of phonological treatment were greater than semantic treatment in a third patient with semantic + phonological impairment. A fourth subject showed no effect for either treatment.

Ellsworth and Raymer (1998) used a similar paradigm in which they contrasted phonological and semantic question training hierarchies for one subject with selective verb retrieval impairment. Their hierarchy included only two yes/no questions as it is difficult to identify a semantic category for verbs, and the number of syllables varies depending on the morphological form of the verb (run, running). Both treatments led to improvements in verb retrieval for trained verbs and increases in the use of grammatical sentences incorporating those trained verbs. Training hierarchy effects surpassed the effects observed when the subject was administered a simple repetition treatment, in keeping with the findings of Greenwald et al. (1995) in training noun retrieval. Maintenance of treatment effects over time was greatest for verbs trained with the phonological treatment.

In summary, the findings of a number of studies indicate that different types of restitutive semantic and phonological treatments are effective in improving word retrieval for trained words. However, one observation is that there is little direct correlation between type of word retrieval impairment (semantic or phonological) and most effective type of treatment (Hillis, 1993). Either semantic or phonological treatment seems to improve word retrieval in individuals with either semantic or phonological impairments. These findings are compatible with the interactive nature of semantic and phonological processing in the course of word retrieval (Humphreys et al., 1988). In fact, the best restitutive treatments are those that combine semantic and phonological information during the course of training to encourage the overall process of word retrieval (Drew & Thompson, 1999; Le Dorze et al., 1994).

Substitutive Word Retrieval Treatments

An alternative approach to rehabilitation of word retrieval impairments is to devise treatments that either circumvent the impaired lexical mechanism or develop an alternative means to vicariatively mediate word retrieval using other cognitive mechanisms. For example, the use of semantic circumlocution to describe a concept when a word retrieval failure occurs would be a substitutive semantic strategy to circumvent failure at the subsequent stage of phonological lexical retrieval. Some treatment studies have evaluated the effects of methods to vicariatively activate word retrieval.

Graphemic Mechanisms. Some patients with word retrieval impairments stemming from failure to access the phonological output lexicon nevertheless may be able to access some knowledge about the word's spelling. In turn, using print-to-sound conversion processes, it may be possible to generate the appropriate spoken form of the word. Bruce and Howard (1987) reported a treatment study in which they applied this strategy with their patient who had some retained graphemic knowledge for words he was unable to produce. The patient typed the letters into a computer and the computer in turn generated the initial phoneme of the word. Over time the patient improved word retrieval for practiced words even in the absence of the computer-generated phonemic cues.

Hillis (1989) trained subjects to use alternative sublexical print-to-sound conversion processes to support impaired word retrieval processes as well. The two subjects in her studies demonstrated selective verb retrieval impairments, one for spoken verb retrieval and the other for written verb retrieval. One subject learned to use a sound-to-print cuing hierarchy to improve her written verb retrieval. The second subject was not able to apply the reverse print-to-sound process to improve spoken verb retrieval, however. In contrast, Nickels (1992) reported that her patient improved word retrieval skills using a similar graphemic training technique, in spite of impaired print-to-sound conversion abilities. Translation of the initial phoneme was sufficient to self-cue the correct phonological output.

Hillis (1998) described a remarkable patient who spontaneously used retained print-to-sound conversion abilities to support her impaired word retrieval. This patient often mispronounced words using regularized pronunciations (e.g., /brid/ for bread) when a word retrieval failure occurred. Listeners who were familiar with her maladaptive technique could often perform a reverse translation and figure out the word the patient was attempting to say. To circumvent this awkward strategy, Hillis taught her patient to pronounce regularized spellings of common words with exceptional spellings (e.g., kwire for choir). Improvements in oral reading also were evident in oral naming of the same words.

Gesture. An alternative method that researchers have applied to mediate word retrieval is the use of the action output lexicon through pantomime. Luria (1970) originally referred to such a process as "intersystemic gestural re-organization," using intact gesture abilities to activate the impaired language system. Cognitive models of lexical and praxis processing recognize the interactive nature of the two systems (Rothi et al., 1991a, 1997a), suggesting that gesture may be useful to mediate activation of lexical retrieval. A desirable consequence of gestural facilitation with pantomimes is that should verbal processes not improve with training, the patient has benefited from practice with an alternative functional communication mode. A number of studies developed using traditional therapy procedures have demonstrated positive effects of verbal + gestural training in individuals with aphasia (e.g., Hoodin & Thompson, 1983; Kearns et al., 1982; Raymer & Thompson, 1991). Recent studies have examined factors that may optimize gestural training effects.

Pashek (1997) investigated the effect of hand (left versus right) in verbal + gestural training, reasoning that the handedness of gestures may facilitate improvements in an asymmetrical manner. However, her subject demonstrated improvements in retrieval of words trained with both left and right hand gestures. At 6-month follow-up, the subject maintained word retrieval improvements, but tended to use the dominant right hand for all gestures. Early gesture studies primarily used nouns as training stimuli. Pashek (1998), recognizing the differences between nouns and verbs in neural-cognitive representation, compared the effectiveness of verbal + gestural training for nouns versus verbs. Her findings in one subject with mild limb apraxia suggested that whereas gestural training led to improvements in both classes of words, improvement was greater for verbs than for nouns.

One problem with earlier gesture studies is that the integrity of the action mechanisms (limb apraxia) was often not well documented in the subjects with aphasia. Patients with severe limb apraxia may not be able to use pantomime as a viable communication mode, as their gestures are often unrecognizable. Raymer (1999) completed a recent pilot study of verbal + gestural training, examining differences between verbs and nouns in a patient with severe word retrieval impairment and severe limb apraxia. Whereas the treatment had no effect on verbal output, the patient's limb apraxia improved noticeably so that trained gestures were now recognizable for communication. The gesture improvements were greater when attempting to produce verbs as opposed to nouns.

In summary, alternative intact mechanisms of the lexical system may be used to support communication attempts in individuals with word retrieval impairments. Some substitutive treatments may over time act vicariatively to improve spoken word retrieval. At other times, the substitutive strategy remains the primary means of communication as word retrieval improvement is not forthcoming. It is critical that a systematic lexical assessment takes place to identify potential substitutive modes of communication in the event of a lexical impairment.

Summary of Treatment Research

Studies have demonstrated that restitutive treatments are effective for improving performance in individuals with impairments of either lexical comprehension or production. Other studies have shown that substitutive treatments also can benefit word comprehension and retrieval in some patients. Whereas most patients benefit from the treatments described in research studies, occasionally researchers report findings for subjects who did not benefit from the chosen treatment regime (Boyle & Coelho, 1995; Hillis, 1993; Hillis & Caramazza, 1994; Raymer et al., 1993). For example, Ennis and colleagues (1999) found that her patient who showed no response to either semantic or phonological treatment hierarchies had an unusual cortical representation of language as suggested by her fluent neologistic aphasia subsequent to a left frontal lesion. Boyle and Coelho (1995) proposed that additional cognitive impairments may have undermined the potential for one of their patients to respond to semantic matrix training. Therefore, other cognitive and neurological factors can influence the potential for response to lexical treatments.

The other remarkable finding of this series of treatment studies is that, whereas patients may present with impairments that implicate either semantic or phonological stages of processing, there is no direct relationship to the type of treatment that will be most effective for treating those stage-specific impairments (Hillis, 1993). Some patients with semantic impairments benefit from treatment that focuses on phonological output and vice versa. Although simple rehearsal of spoken words can help a person improve word retrieval, the most effective treatments were those which engaged either semantic, phonological, and in particular, semantic plus phonological processing within one treatment protocol. That is, treatments that attempted to facilitate the multistage process of word retrieval were often most effective.

Generalization

The CN approach has specific implications for analyzing the generalization of treatment effects for lexical impairments (Hillis, 1993; Raymer et al., 1995b). First, if treatment facilitates processing in a particular lexical mechanism, improvements should be evident in all tasks that require processing by that mechanism. Hereafter, this type of generalization will be referred to as "generalization across tasks." Second, as treatment strengthens targeted lexical representations, semantically or phonologically related lexical representations may benefit from the treatment as well. This type of generalization will be referred to as "generalization to untrained stimuli." A number of treatment studies have examined these two types of generalization.

Generalization Across Tasks

A number of word retrieval studies have examined effects of treatment in other untrained lexical tasks that may benefit from concurrent treatment. Hillis (1991, 1998) examined generalization across untreated lexical tasks following her semantic features treatment for word retrieval. Benefits of semantic treatments should be evident in all tasks involving semantic activation including oral and written naming, comprehension, and possibly oral reading and writing to dictation. Although semantic treatment focused solely on written naming, improvements were also evident in all other lexical tasks as predicted. Likewise, Ochipa and colleagues (1998) reported improvement in written naming following semantic features treatment targeting oral naming. Similarly, benefits of phonological treatments should be evident in oral naming and oral reading, and less likely in written naming and comprehension. So, for example, when Hillis (1991, 1998) trained her patient to pronounce regularized spellings of words with exceptional spellings, her patient improved pronunciation of the same words in picture naming and word repetition as well, but not in written naming.

However, there are times when treatment effects observed in additional lexical tasks are contrary to predictions. For example, Raymer and colleagues (1993) used a phonological cuing hierarchy to train oral picture naming, and observed generalized improvements in oral word reading as well as written picture naming in one patient. In contrast, Greenwald and colleagues (1995) reported improvements in oral picture naming following visual-semantic training, but no improvement in a visual picture associate matching task that they predicted would also improve following training. These patterns of generalization that are contrary to the predicted generalization patterns suggest that the complexity of the mechanisms and the types of processing that occur between mechanisms also influence treatment in important, but as yet unspecified, ways.

Finally, the results of the CN assessment may assist the clinical researcher in selection of tasks to demonstrate that the effects of treatment indeed result from treatment and not from spontaneous recovery (Raymer et al., 1995b). The clinician can identify other independent areas of cognitive/linguistic impairment that should not be affected by treatment and probe performance over time. The clinician demonstrates control when treatment improves performance in the targeted task, but not in the untreated task.

Generalization to Untrained Stimuli

Generalization to untrained stimuli may be generated in two ways. Some treatments affect a lexical process, teaching patients to use this process or strategy to improve performance for a set of trained stimuli. If the patient learns this strategy or improves this process, performance should be affected when applying that process for all stimuli, trained or untrained.

This type of generalization has been explored more often in treatment studies for reading and writing (Berndt, 1992; DePartz, 1986; Hillis, 1993; Rothi & Moss, 1989). An example of such a process that affects word retrieval abilities may be semantic feature matrix training in which clinicians train patients to use a matrix of cue words to encourage the recall of semantic information for a target word and ultimately word retrieval. Boyle and Coelho (1995; Boyle, 1997) and Lowell and colleagues (1995) reported that their subjects who responded to semantic feature matrix training also demonstrated improvements in naming untrained pictures as well. It may be that the patients learned to self-generate semantic information whenever a word retrieval failure occurred, thereby leading to accurate activation of the lexical response for untrained stimuli.

A second way in which generalization might occur to untrained stimuli is at the level of the lexical representations. Consider the account that Caramazza and Shelton (1998) gave for category-specific semantic impairments. They proposed that category-specific deficits arise when features of semantic representations, shared by a number of items within a semantic category, are rendered dysfunctional by a strategically placed neurological lesion. All items within one semantic category that incorporate the shared feature as part of their semantic representations will be affected. Moving to the treatment domain, if training somehow restores features or representations to a more optimal state, then all items sharing those features should be affected. Therefore, generalization may be evident in predictable ways to items that share semantic or phonological features. It may be this type of effect that can account for generalization to semantically related items found after semantic feature training (Hillis, 1991, 1998; Ochipa et al., 1998). Ennis and colleagues (1999) noted that following semantic question hierarchy treatment, two of her patients demonstrated generalization to a small number of untrained items that shared either semantic or phonemic characteristics with trained words. Behrmann and Lieberthal (1989) evaluated generalization of category-specific semantic comprehension treatment to naming of untrained items within trained and untrained categories. They observed generalization to untrained items within one trained category, as might be predicted. But they also noted improved naming in one untrained category, which cannot be completely explained on the basis of this hypothesis.

More often than not, improvements in trained lexical tasks seem to be item specific and little generalization of improvement is evident for untrained stimuli. For example, Raymer and colleagues (1993) systematically assessed generalization of the effects of a phonological cuing hierarchy to items that were either semantically or phonologically related to trained pictures. However, they observed no clear patterns of response generalization among the patients. It is interesting that studies showing more positive generalization to untrained items typically incorporated

semantic treatments. However, not all semantic treatments led to response generalization (Pring et al., 1993). Because there is no indisputable reason to predict generalization to untrained items, it would be sensible to select treatment words that respect the functional needs of each individual patient. For example, Hillis (1998) used a cuing hierarchy to train her patient to retrieve the names of different types of fabrics after the patient took a job at a fabric store.

Functional Outcomes of Impairment-Oriented Treatments

The primary dependent variable in treatment studies for lexical impairments in aphasia has been percent improvement in the trained lexical task or in other lexical tasks sharing the same lexical mechanism. However, a final means of generalization of critical importance is generalization of treatment effects to functional language and communication situations outside the treatment setting, the ecological validity of treatments. Treatment studies for verb retrieval often report improvements in the formulation of complete sentences as a consequence of the verb retrieval treatment (Ellsworth & Raymer, 1998; Marshall et al., 1998), although some patients have additional syntactic impairments that impede sentence production (Mitchum & Berndt, 1994; also see Chapter 18). However, those effects are typically assessed within the structured clinical setting.

Fewer studies have investigated the generalization of lexical improvements to functional communication settings. Hillis (1998) reported anecdotal evidence that her patient's impairment-oriented treatments led to improved functional communication as observed in dinner and phone conversations and shopping trips. Her patient also identified specific functional vocabulary for use in treatment. Selected other treatment studies have reported quantitative evidence with implications for functional communication. Boyle and Coelho (1995) reported no changes in conversational speech measures of words per minute and information units conveyed per minute following successful semantic matrix training for noun retrieval. However, a family member judged that the patient improved on a rating scale of communicative effectiveness (Lomas et al., 1989), which may indicate the functional gains of lexical treatment. Ellsworth and Raymer (1998) examined conversational output following verb retrieval treatment in their patient with aphasia. Using quantitative production analysis of lexical and grammatical use (Saffran et al., 1989), they noted changes toward more normal proportions of nouns/verbs and nouns/pronouns following treatment. They documented few other noticeable changes in grammatical and lexical use in the patient's conversation, although she claimed that she communicated better in her home environment (e.g., using the telephone).

Overall, the functional consequences of treatments using the CN approach have not been well studied. Some studies have provided quantitative measures that suggest that treatments directed at specific lexical impairments have positive consequences for the patient's daily communication needs. However, further documentation of the functional outcomes of CN studies certainly are warranted.

Limitations of Cognitive Approach

While this discussion has focused largely on the positive ramifications of the CN approach for the clinical rehabilitation process, the CN approach has some recognized shortcomings. Surely, the systematic, in-depth assessment of lexical abilities advocated in this approach proves tremendously difficult to accomplish in many clinical settings. However, clinicians may find it possible to use this approach in a more condensed format to accumulate the information necessary to make informed treatment decisions. Clinicians may be able to complete a series of lexical tasks with a more circumscribed set of materials in the course of diagnostic treatment in an attempt to characterize lexical abilities more specifically. It may prove advantageous for clinicians to accurately characterize impairments, but in addition, to identify retained lexical abilities, as the clinician may capitalize upon those retained abilities to devise appropriate substitutive treatments for lexical impairments. Furthermore, observations of overall patterns of impairments may eventually allow clinicians to develop better prognoses for their patients with impairments. For example, disturbed oral naming in the presence of preserved oral word reading skills seemed to be predictive of best response to word retrieval treatments (Raymer et al., 1993; Pring et al., 1990).

Although one of the initial goals of the CN approach was to identify more rational treatments which target identified impairments in the lexical system (e.g., semantic treatments for semantic impairments, and so forth), the findings to date do not support this notion. But the considerable body of research certainly has suggested a more favorable course to follow when attempting restorative treatments with patients with aphasia. Treatments that encourage activation of multiple stages in the lexical process (Figure 23–1) in the course of one treatment protocol appear to be most effective. Although the lexical mechanisms are distinct and distributed, they are highly interactive in the course of lexical processing. Results of various studies suggest that treatments that encourage the interactions of the stages of lexical processing seem to be most worthwhile.

Some clinicians have argued that the CN approach, which emphasizes impairment-oriented treatments, has few consequences for overcoming the disabling and handicapping conditions posed by aphasia (Wilson, 1999). Because earlier treatment studies often neglected to report the functional aftermath of lexical treatments, this argument may have some merit. Substitutive treatments that researchers have generated on the basis of lexical theories definitely encourage

progress in functional communication in a variety of patients. Recent studies have attempted to improve methods to document the substantial impact that impairment-oriented treatments have for patients and their families.

Hillis (1993) noted that although an assessment may help the clinician to characterize the nature of the patient's impairment, it does not help determine what specific strategy will be most effective; that is, how to treat the impairment. As noted above, a number of additional neurological, cognitive, and social factors also must play a role in this type of treatment decision. As researchers accrue a greater body of knowledge about treatment effects across patients, clinicians may be better at making predictions about who, what, and how to treat.

FUTURE TRENDS

A review of the limitations of the CN approach to lexical treatment suggests a number of areas for future research. Continued research is necessary contrasting treatments in the same patients in crossover designs. Much of the treatment literature has reported the effects of one type of treatment, so clinicians are unable to judge whether that treatment was as effective as other possible treatment options. Some recent studies have implemented these types of designs to add to the body of knowledge of what clinicians know are the most beneficial treatments across patients.

Also, the impairment-oriented approach to aphasia treatment has received much criticism and skepticism. Therefore, future studies must incorporate methods to evaluate the functional consequences of treatments for daily communication situations. Finally, recent studies using neuroimaging techniques have evaluated patterns of brain activation before and after treatment for aphasia and dyslexia (Adair et al., 1998; Belin et al., 1996; Small et al., 1998). Imaging studies are beginning to document the neural changes associated with successful behavioral treatments. Continued research in each of these areas will advance the effectiveness and the efficiency of clinical practice for our patients with aphasia.

KEY POINTS

1. The lexical system is a complex, distributed system of modules that store information in sensory modality-specific and output mode-specific mechanisms that interact by way of a semantic system.
2. Lexical impairments take many forms depending on which component of the lexical system is affected.
3. Assessment focuses on mode/modality comparisons across lexical tasks. Patterns of performance, quantitatively and qualitatively, help the clinician develop an informed hypothesis about the nature of lexical impairments.

4. Recovery analyses may assist clinicians in predicting which patients will recover and in which direction, and may serve to confirm hypotheses generated on initial assessment.

5. Restitutive treatments target impaired lexical mechanisms. Treatments that are putatively semantic in nature and others that focus on phonological aspects of lexical information have induced changes in auditory comprehension and word retrieval in a variety of patients. However, contrary to early predictions of the cognitive neuropsychological approach, there is not a direct correspondence between types of impairments and most effective treatments. Treatments that incorporate multiple stages of the lexical process seem most beneficial.

6. Substitutive treatments capitalize on retained aspects of lexical processing to either circumvent an impairment at some stage in lexical processing or to vicariatively mediate activation of the impaired mechanism.

7. Generalization of treatment effects is observed across all tasks for which the mechanism facilitated by treatment plays a necessary role in accurate performance. Generalization of treatment effects to untrained stimuli has been more limited, although there are indications that semantic treatments incite greater generalization to untrained semantically related words.

8. Less research has been focused on the functional outcomes of these impairment-oriented treatments.

GLOSSARY

Category-specific semantic impairments: disturbance in comprehension or production for selective semantic categories, with preserved performance for other categories.

Lexical system: complex, distributed set of mechanisms storing representations for familiar words, objects, and actions, as well as processes for decoding and encoding unfamiliar stimuli.

Lexical decision: task in which patient decides whether a given stimulus is a familiar real word/object, or a nonsense word or object.

Optic aphasia: visual modality-specific impairment in naming viewed objects in presence of basic semantic processing indicated through circumlocutions or gestures associated with unnamed object.

Phonological input lexicon: mechanism-storing representations for familiar spoken words that have been previously heard.

Phonological output lexicon: mechanism-storing representations for familiar spoken words that have been previously produced.

Pure word deafness: auditory modality-specific impairment in processing spoken input.

Recognition: point in stimulus processing at which stimulus is distinguished, familiar, and previously experienced.

Restitutive treatments: strategies that encourage restoration of functioning in a manner compatible with normal language processing.

Semantic system: lexical mechanism responsible for storing meaning representations for familiar words, objects, and gestures.

Substitutive treatments: strategies that attempt to circumvent a dysfunctional language mechanism using other intact language and cognitive processes.

Visual agnosia: failure as a result of brain damage to recognize a viewed stimulus that is not due to peripheral sensory visual disorder.

Visual object representations: mechanism-storing memories for familiar objects that have been previously seen.

Word meaning deafness: impairment in ability to apply meaning to heard words despite intact phonological processing.

REVIEW QUESTIONS

1. What is modality specificity as it relates to the model of lexical processing?
2. What is the difference between the phonological input lexicon, the semantic system, and the phonological output lexicon?
3. A dysfunction of the phonological input lexicon will result in a pattern of impairment in which lexical tasks and preserved performance for what other lexical tasks?
4. What is the pattern of lexical performance seen in patients with optic aphasia?
5. What is a category-specific impairment? For what semantic categories might we observe category-specific impairments?
6. What is the purpose of mode/modality comparisons in the cognitive neuropsychological assessment?
7. The presence of semantic errors in naming may represent dysfunction at which three stages of lexical processing?
8. Describe one stage-specific assessment task to target processing in each of the following: visual/structural descriptions, phonological input lexicon, semantic system, and phonological output lexicon.
9. How are analyses of lexical recovery useful in clinical practice?

10. Describe restitutive and substitutive treatments that may be useful to improve functioning in an individual with phonological input lexicon impairment.

11. Why are semantic comprehension tasks useful as a restitutive treatment for word retrieval impairments?

12. What are three different tasks a patient may practice to encourage restoration of functioning in the phonological output stage of word retrieval?

13. How can the graphemic system be used in a substitutive strategy for word retrieval impairments?

14. How do models of lexical processing assist in predicting generalization effects to untrained tasks?

15. What are some functional consequences that have been described for impairment-oriented cognitive neuropsychological treatments?

References

Adair, J.C., Nadeau, S.E., Conway, T.W., Rothi, L.J.G., Heilman, P., Green, I.A., & Heilman, K.M. (1998). Change in functional neuroanatomy after successful treatment of phonologic alexia. *Journal of the International Neuropsychological Society, 4*, 50 (abstract).

Allport, D.A. (1985). Distributed memory, modular subsystems and dysphasia. In S. Newman & R. Epstein (eds.), *Current perspectives in dysphasia* (pp. 32–60). Edinburgh: Churchill Livingstone.

Badecker, W. & Caramazza, A. (1991). Morphological composition in the lexical output system. *Cognitive Neuropsychology, 8*, 335–367.

Bauer, R.M. (1993). Agnosia. In K.M. Heilman & E. Valenstein (eds.), *Clinical neuropsychology* (3rd ed.) (pp. 215–278). New York: Oxford University Press.

Belin, P., Van Eeckhout, Ph., Zilbovicius, M., Remy, Ph., Francoois, C., Guillaume, S., Chain, F., Rancurel, G., & Samson, Y. (1996). Recovery from nonfluent aphasia after melodic intonation therapy: A PET study. *Neurology, 47*, 1504–1510.

Benton, A. & Tranel, D. (1993). Visuoperceptual, visuospatial, and visuoconstructive disorders. In K.M. Heilman & E. Valenstein (eds.), *Clinical neuropsychology* (3rd ed.) (pp. 165–213). New York: Oxford University Press.

Behrmann, M. & Lieberthal, T. (1989). Category-specific treatment of a lexical-semantic deficit: A single case study of global aphasia. *British Journal of Disorders of Communication, 24*, 281–299.

Berndt, R.S., Reggia, J.A., & Mitchum, C.C. (1987). Empirically derived probabilities for grapheme-to-phoneme correspondences in English. *Behavior Research Methods, Instruments, and Computers, 19*, 1–9.

Berndt, R.S. (1992). Using data from treatment studies to elaborate cognitive models: Non-lexical reading, an example. In NIH Publication no. 93-3424: *Aphasia treatment: Current approaches and research opportunities* (pp. 47–64).

Boyle, M. (1997, November). Semantic feature analysis treatment for dysnomia in two aphasia syndromes. Poster presented at the annual meeting of the American Speech-Language-Hearing Association, Boston, MA.

Boyle, M. & Coelho, C.A. (1995). Application of semantic feature analysis as a treatment for aphasic dysnomia. *American Journal of Speech-Language Pathology, 4*, 94–98.

Bruce, C. & Howard, D. (1987). Computer-generated phonemic cues: An effective aid for naming in aphasia. *British Journal of Disorders of Communication, 22*, 191–201.

Bub, D. & Kertesz, A. (1982). Evidence for lexicographic processing in a patient with preserved written over oral single word naming. *Brain, 105*, 697–717.

Buchman, A.S., Garron, D.C., Trost-Cardmone, J.E., Wichter, M.D., & Schwartz, M. (1986). Word deafness: One hundred years later. *Journal of Neurology, Neurosurgery, Psychiatry, 49*, 489–499.

Buchtel, H.A. & Stewart, J.D. (1989). Auditory agnosia: Apperceptive or associative disorder? *Brain and Language, 37*, 12–25.

Bunn, E.M., Tyler, L.K., & Moss, H.E. (1998). Category-specific semantic deficits: The role of familiarity and property type reexamined. *Neuropsychology, 12*, 367–379.

Byng, S., Kay, J., Edmundson, A., & Scott, C. (1990). Aphasia tests reconsidered. *Aphasiology, 4*, 67–91.

Caplan, D. (1993). *Language: Structure, processing and disorders.* Cambridge, MA: MIT Press.

Caramazza, A., Berndt, R.S., & Basili, A.G. (1983). The selective impairment of phonological processing: A case study. *Brain and Language, 18*, 128–174.

Caramazza, A. & Hillis, A. (1993). For a theory of remediation of cognitive deficits. *Neuropsychological Rehabilitation, 3*, 217–234.

Caramazza, A. & Hillis, A.E. (1991). Lexical organization of nouns and verbs in the brain. *Nature, 349*, 788–790.

Caramazza, A. & Hillis, A.E. (1990). Where do semantic errors come from? *Cortex, 26*, 5–122.

Caramazza, A., Hillis, A.E., Leek, E.C., & Miozzo, M. (1994). The organization of lexical knowledge in the brain: Evidence from category- and modality-specific deficits. In L. Hirschfeld & S. Gelman (eds.), *Mapping the mind: Domain specificity in cognition and culture* (pp. 68–84). New York: Cambridge University Press.

Caramazza, A., Hillis, A.E., Rapp, B.C., & Romani, C. (1990). The multiple semantics hypothesis: Multiple confusions? *Cognitive Neuropsychology, 7*, 161–189.

Caramazza, A. & Miceli, G. (1990). Structure of the lexicon: Functional architecture and lexical representation. In J.L. Nespoulous & P. Villiard (eds.), *Morphology, phonology, and aphasia* (pp. 1–19). New York: Springer-Verlag.

Caramazza, A. & Miozzo, M. (1997). The relation between syntactic and phonological knowledge in lexical access: Evidence from the 'tip-of-the-tongue' phenomenon. *Cognition, 64*, 309–343.

Caramazza, A. & Shelton, J.R. (1998). Domain-specific knowledge systems in the brain: The animate-inanimate distinction. *Journal of Cognitive Neuroscience, 10*, 1–34.

Chanoine, V., Ferreira, C.T., Demonet, J.F., Nespoulous, J.L., & Poncet, M. (1998). Optic aphasia with pure alexia: A mild form of visual associative agnosia? A case study. *Cortex, 34*, 437–448.

Chertkow, H., Bub, D., & Seidenberg, M. (1989). Priming and semantic memory loss in Alzheimer's disease. *Brain and Language, 36*, 420–446.

Coltheart, M. (1984). Editorial. *Cognitive Neuropsychology, 1*, 1–8.

Coltheart, M. (1981). The MRC psycholinguistic database. *Quarterly Journal of Experimental Psychology, 33A*, 497–505.

Coslett, H.B. & Saffran, E.M. (1992). Optic aphasia and the right hemisphere: A replication and extension. *Brain and Language 43*, 148–161.

Coslett, H.B. & Saffran, E.M. (1989). Preserved object recognition and reading comprehension in optic aphasia. *Brain, 112*, 1091–1110.

Crosson, B. (1992). *Subcortical functions in language and memory*. New York: Oxford University Press.

Crosson, B., Moberg, P.J., Boone, J.R., Rothi, L.J.G., & Raymer, A.M. (1997). Category-specific naming deficit for medical terms after dominant thalamic/capsular hemorrhage. *Brain and Language, 60*, 407–440.

Damasio, A.R. & Tranel, D. (1993). Nouns and verbs are retrieved with differently distributed neural systems. *Proceedings of the National Academy of Sciences, USA, 90*, 4957–4960.

Damasio, H., Grabowski, T.J., Tranel, D., Hichwa, R.D., & Damasio, A.R. (1996). A neural basis for lexical retrieval. *Nature, 380*, 499–505.

Davidoff, J. & De Bleser, R. (1993). Optic aphasia: A review of past studies and reappraisal. *Aphasiology, 7*, 135–154.

Davis, A. & Pring, T. (1991). Therapy for word-finding deficits: More on the effects of semantic and phonological approaches to treatment with dysphasic patients. *Neuropsychological Rehabilitation, 1*, 135–145.

De Bleser, R. & Cholewa, J. (1998). Dissociations between inflection, derivation, and compounding: Neurolinguistic evidence for morphological fractionations within the lexical system. In E.G. Visch-Brink & R. Bastiaanse (eds.), *Linguistic levels in aphasiology* (pp. 231–243). San Diego, CA: Singular Publishing Group.

Déjerine, J. (1891). Sur un cas de cécité verbale avec agraphie, suivi d'autopsie. *Comptes Rendus Hebdomadaires des Séances et Memoires de la Societé de Biologie, 3*, 197–201.

DePartz, M.P. (1986). Re-education of a deep dyslexic patient: Rationale of the method and results. *Cognitive Neuropsychology, 3*, 149–177.

Drew, R.L. & Thompson, C.K. (1999). Model-based semantic treatment for naming deficits in aphasia. *Journal of Speech, Language, & Hearing Research, 42*, 972–989.

Ellis, A.W., Kay, J., & Franklin, S. (1992). Anomia: Differentiating between semantic and phonological deficits. In D.I. Margolin (ed.), *Cognitive neuropsychology in clinical practice* (pp. 207–227). New York: Oxford University Press.

Ellis, A.W., Miller, D., & Sin, G. (1983). Wernicke's aphasia and normal language processing: A case study in cognitive neuropsychology. *Cognition, 15*, 111–144.

Ellis, A.W. & Young, A.W. (1988). *Human cognitive neuropsychology*. East Sussex, UK: Lawrence Erlbaum.

Ellsworth, T.A. & Raymer, A.M. (1998). Contrasting treatments for verb retrieval impairment in aphasia: A case study. *ASHA Leader, 3*(16), 84 (abstract).

Ennis, M.R. (1999). Semantic versus phonological aphasia treatments for anomia: A within-Subject Experimental Design. Unpublished doctoral dissertation. University of Florida: Gainesville.

Farah, M.J. (1990). *Visual agnosia*. Cambridge, MA: MIT Press.

Farah, M.J. & Wallace (1992). Semantically-bounded anomia: Implications for the neural implementation of naming. *Neuropsychologia, 30*, 609–621.

Feinberg, T.E., Rothi, L.J.G., & Heilman, K.M. (1986). Multimodal agnosia after unilateral left hemisphere lesion. *Neurology, 36*, 864–867.

Ferreira, C.T., Giusiano, B., & Poncet, M. (1997). Category-specific anomia: Implication of different neural networks in naming. *Neuroreport, 6*, 1595–1602.

Feyereisen, P., Van Der Borght, F., & Seron, X. (1988). The operativity effect in naming: A re-analysis. *Neuropsychologia, 26*, 401–415.

Foundas, A.L., Daniels, S.K., & Vasterling, J.J. (1998). Anomia: Case studies with lesion localization. *Neurocase, 4*, 35–43.

Francis, W.N. & Kucera, H. (1982). *Frequency analysis of English usage: Lexicon and grammar*. Boston: Houghton Mifflin.

Franklin, S. (1989). Dissociations in auditory word comprehension; Evidence from nine fluent aphasic patients. *Aphasiology, 3*, 189–207.

Franklin, S., Turner, J., Ralph, M., Morris, J., & Bailey, P. (1996). A distinctive case of word meaning deafness. *Cognitive Neuropsychology, 13*, 1139–1162.

Freund, C.S. (1889). Ueber optische aphasie und seelendblindheit. *Archiv fur Psychiatrie Nervenkrankheiten, 20*, 276–297, 371–416.

Gainotti, G., Silveri, M.C., Villa, G., & Miceli, G. (1986). Anomia with and without lexical comprehension disorders. *Brain and Language, 29*, 18–33.

Gilhooly, K.J. & Logie, R.H. (1980). Age-of-acquisition, imagery, concreteness, familiarity and ambiguity measures of 1944 words. *Behavioral Research Methods and Instrumentation, 12*, 395–427.

Goodglass, H., Hyde, M.R., & Blumstein, S. (1969). Frequency, pictureability and availability of nouns in aphasia. *Cortex, 5*, 104–119.

Goodglass, H. & Kaplan, E. (1983). *Boston Diagnostic Aphasia Examination* (2nd ed.). Philadelphia: Lea & Febiger.

Graham, K., Patterson, K., & Hodges, J.R. (1998). Semantic dementia and pure anomia: Two varieties of progressive fluent aphasia. In E.G. Visch-Brink & R. Bastiaanse (eds.), *Linguistic levels in aphasiology* (pp. 49–68). San Diego, CA: Singular Publishing Group.

Grayson, E., Hilton, R., & Franklin, S. (1997). Early intervention in a case of jargon aphasia: Efficacy of language comprehension therapy. *European Journal of Disorders of Communication, 32*, 257–276.

Greenwald, M.L., Raymer, A.M., Richardson, M.E., & Rothi, L.J.G. (1995). Contrasting treatments for severe impairments of picture naming. *Neuropsychological Rehabilitation, 5*, 17–49.

Haarbauer-Krupa, J., Moser, L., Smith, G., Sullivan, D.M., & Szekeres, S.F. (1985). Cognitive rehabilitation therapy: Middle stages of recovery. In M. Ylvisaker (ed.), *Head injury rehabilitation: Children and adolescents* (pp. 287–310). San Diego, CA: College Hill Press.

Hart, J., Berndt, R.S., & Caramazza, A. (1985). Category specific naming deficit following cerebral infarction. *Nature, 316*, 439–440.

Hart, J. & Gordon, B. (1990). Delineation of single-word semantic comprehension deficits in aphasia, with anatomical correlation. *Annals of Neurology, 27*, 226–231.

Hart, J. & Gordon, B. (1992). Neural subsystems for object knowledge. *Nature, 359*, 60–64.

Hillis, A.E. (1991). Effects of separate treatments for distinct impairments within the naming process. In T. Prescott (ed.), *Clinical Aphasiology, Vol. 19* (pp. 255–265). San Diego, CA: College Hill Press.

Hillis, A.E. (1989). Efficacy and generalization of treatment for aphasic naming errors. *Archives of Physical Medicine & Rehabilitation, 70*, 632–636.

Hillis, A.E. (1993). The role of models of language processing in rehabilitation of language impairments. *Aphasiology, 7*, 5–26.

Hillis, A.E. (1998). Treatment of naming disorders: New issues regarding old therapies. *Journal of the International Neuropsychological Society, 4*, 648–660.

Hillis, A.E., Boatman, D., Hart, J., & Gordon, B. (1999). Making sense out of jargon: A neurolinguistic and computational account of jargon aphasia. *Neurology, 53*, 1813–1824.

Hillis, A.E. & Caramazza, A. (1991). Category-specific naming and comprehension impairment: A double dissociation. *Brain, 114*, 2081–2094.

Hillis, A.E. & Caramazza, A. (1995a). Cognitive and neural mechanisms underlying visual and semantic processing: Implications from "optic aphasia." *Journal of Cognitive Neuroscience, 7*, 457–478.

Hillis, A.E. & Caramazza, A. (1995b). The compositionality of lexical semantic representations: Clues from semantic errors in object naming. *Memory, 3*, 333–358.

Hillis, A.E. & Caramazza, A. (1995c). Representation of grammatical categories of words in the brain. *Journal of Cognitive Neuroscience, 7*, 396–407.

Hillis, A.E. & Caramazza, A. (1994). Theories of lexical processing and theories of rehabilitation. In G. Humphreys & M.J. Riddoch (eds.), *Cognitive neuropsychology and cognitive rehabilitation* (pp. 449–484). London: Lawrence Erlbaum.

Hillis, A.E., Rapp, B., Romani, C., & Caramazza, A. (1990). Selective impairment of semantics in lexical processing. *Cognitive Neuropsychology, 7*, 191–243.

Hirsh, K.W. & Ellis, A.W. (1994). Age of acquisition and lexical processing in aphasia: A case study. *Cognitive Neuropsychology, 11*, 435–458.

Hodges, J.R. & Patterson, K. (1995). Is semantic memory consistently impaired early in the course of Alzheimer's disease? Neuroanatomical and diagnostic implications. *Neuropsychologia, 33*, 441–459.

Hodges, J.R. & Patterson, K. (1996). Nonfluent progressive aphasia and semantic dementia: A comparative neuropsychological study. *Journal of the International Neuropsychological Society, 2*, 511–524.

Hodges, J.R., Patterson, K., Oxbury, S., & Funnell, E. (1992). Semantic dementia: Progressive fluent aphasia with temporal lobe atrophy. *Brain, 115*, 1783–1806.

Hodges, J.R., Patterson, K., & Tyler, L.K. (1994). Loss of semantic memory: Implications for the modularity of mind. *Cognitive Neuropsychology, 11*, 505–542.

Hoodin, R.B. & Thompson, C.K. (1983). Facilitation of verbal labeling in adult aphasia by gestural, verbal or verbal plus gestural training. In R.H. Brookshire (ed.), *Clinical aphasiology conference proceedings* (pp. 62–64). Minneapolis, MN: BRK.

Hough, M. (1993). Treatment of Wernicke's aphasia with jargon: A case study. *Journal of Communication Disorders, 26*, 101–111.

Howard, D. & Orchard-Lisle, V. (1984). On the origin of semantic errors in naming: Evidence from the case of a global aphasic. *Cognitive Neuropsychology, 1*, 163–190.

Howard, D. & Patterson, K. (1992). *Pyramids and palm trees.* Bury St. Edmunds, UK: Thames Valley Publishing.

Howard, D., Patterson, K. (1989). Models for therapy. In X. Seron & G. Deloche (eds.), *Cognitive approaches in neuropsychological rehabilitation* (pp. 39–64). Hillsdale, NJ: Lawrence Erlbaum.

Howard, D., Patterson, K., Franklin, S., Morton, J., & Orchard-Lisle, V. (1984). Variability and consistency in picture naming in aphasic patients. In F.C. Rose (ed.), *Advances in neurology, Vol. 42: Progress in aphasiology* (pp. 163–276). New York: Raven Press.

Howard, D., Patterson, K., Franklin, S., Orchard-Lisle, V., & Morton, J. (1985). Treatment of word retrieval deficits in aphasia. *Brain, 108*, 817–829.

Howes, D. (1964). Application of the word-frequency concept to aphasia. In A.V.S. DeReuck & M. O'Connor (eds.), *Disorders of language* (pp. 47–75). Boston: Little, Brown.

Humphreys, G.W., Riddoch, M.J., & Quinlan, P.T. (1988). Cascade processes in picture identification. *Cognitive Neuropsychology, 5*, 67–103.

Iorio, L., Falanga, A., Fragassi, N.A., & Grossi, D. (1992). Visual associative agnosia and optic aphasia: A single case study and a review of the syndromes. *Cortex, 28*, 23–37.

Joanette, Y. & Goulet, P. (1998). Right hemisphere and the semantic processing of words: Is the contribution specific or not? In E.G. Visch-Brink & R. Bastiaanse (eds.), *Linguistic levels in aphasiology* (pp. 19–34). San Diego, CA: Singular Publishing Group.

Kahn, H.J., Stannard, T., & Skinner, J. (1998). The use of words versus nonwords in the treatment of apraxia of speech: A case study. ASHA Special Interest Division 2: *Neurophysiology and Neurogenic Speech and Language Disorders, 8*(3), 5–10.

Kay, J. & Ellis, A. (1987). A cognitive neuropsychological case study of anomia: Implications for psychological models of word retrieval. *Brain, 110*, 613–629.

Kay, J., Lesser, R. & Coltheart, M. (1992). *PALPA: Psycholinguistic Assessments of Language Processing in Aphasia.* East Sussex, England: Lawrence Erlbaum.

Kearns, K.P., Simmons, N.N., & Sisterhen, C. (1982). Gestural sign (Amer-Ind) as a facilitator of verbalization in patients with aphasia. In R. Brookshire (ed.), *Clinical aphasiology conference proceedings* (pp. 183–191). Minneapolis, MN: BRK.

Kertesz, A., Davidson, W., & McCabe, P. (1998). Primary progressive semantic aphasia: A case study. *Journal of the International Neuropsychological Society, 4*, 388–398.

Kertesz, A., Lau, W.K., & Polk, M. (1993). The structural determinants of recovery in Wernicke's aphasia. *Brain and Language, 44*, 153–164.

Knopman, D.S., Selnes, O.A., Niccum, N., & Rubens, A.B. (1984). Recovery of naming in aphasia: Relationship to fluency, comprehension, and CT findings. *Neurology, 34*, 1461–1470.

Kohn, S.E. & Friedman, R. (1986). Word meaning deafness: A phonological-semantic dissociation. *Cognitive Neuropsychology, 3*, 291–308.

Kohn, S.E. & Goodglass, H. (1985). Picture-naming in aphasia. *Brain and Language, 24*, 266–283.

Kohn, S.E., Smith, K.L., & Alexander, M.P. (1996). Differential recovery from impairment to the phonological lexicon. *Brain and Language, 52*, 129–149.

Kremin, H., Beauchamp, D., & Perrier, D. (1994). Naming without picture comprehension? Apropos the oral naming and semantic comprehension of pictures by patients with Alzheimer's disease. *Aphasiology, 8*, 291–294.

Laiacona, M., Capitani, E., & Barbarotto, R. (1997). Semantic category dissociations: A longitudinal study of two cases. *Cortex, 33,* 441–461.

Lambon Ralph, M.A., Ellis, A.W., & Franklin, S. (1995). Semantic loss without surface dyslexia. *Neurocase, 1,* 363–369.

Lambon Ralph, M.A., Graham, K.S., Ellis, A.W., & Hodges, J.R. (1998). Naming in semantic dementia—what matters? *Neuropsychologia, 36,* 775–784.

Le Dorze, G., Boulay, N., Gaudreau, J., & Brassard, C. (1994). The contrasting effects of a semantic versus a formal-semantic technique for the facilitation of naming in a case of anomia. *Aphasiology, 8,* 127–141.

Le Dorze, G., & Nespoulous, J.-L. (1989). Anomia in moderate aphasia: Problems in accessing the lexical representation. *Brain and Language, 37,* 381–400.

Lissauer, H. (1890/1988). A case of visual agnosia with a contribution to theory. *Cognitive Neuropsychology, 5,* 153–192.

Lomas, J., Pickard, L., Bester, S., Elbard, H., Finlayson, A., & Zoghaib, C. (1989). The communicative effectiveness index: Development and psychometric evaluation of a functional communication measure for adult aphasia. *Journal of Speech and Hearing Disorders, 54,* 113–124.

Lowell, S., Beeson, P.M., & Holland, A.L. (1995). The efficacy of a semantic cueing procedure on naming performance of adults with aphasia. *American Journal of Speech-Language Pathology, 4,* 109–114.

Luria, A.R. (1970). *Traumatic aphasia.* The Hague: Mouton.

Lux, J.B. (1999). Towards a common language for functioning and disablement: ICIDH-2 (The international classification of impairments, activities, and participation). *ASHA Special Interest 2: Neurophysiology and Neurogenic Speech and Language Disorders, 9*(1), 8–10.

Lyon, J. (1996). Optimizing communication and participation in life for aphasic adults and their prime caregivers in natural settings: A use model for treatment. In G.L. Wallace (ed.), *Adult aphasia rehabilitation* (pp. 137–160). Boston, MA: Butterworth-Heinemann.

Maher, L.M., Rothi, L.J.G., & Heilman, K.M. (1994). Lack of error awareness in an aphasic patient with relatively preserved auditory comprehension. *Brain and Language, 46,* 402–418.

Marr, D. (1982). *Vision.* New York: W.J. Freeman.

Marshall, J., Pound, C., White-Thomson, M., & Pring, T. (1990). The use of picture/word matching tasks to assist word retrieval in aphasic patients. *Aphasiology, 4,* 167–184.

Marshall, J., Pring, T., & Chiat, S. (1998). Verb retrieval and sentence production in aphasia. *Brain and Language, 63,* 159–183.

Martin, N. (1996). Cognitive approaches to recovery and rehabilitation in aphasia. *Brain and Language, 52,* 3–6.

McHugh, R.E., Coelho, C.A., & Boyle, M. (1997, November). Semantic feature analysis as a treatment for dysnomia: A replication. Poster presented at the annual convention of the American Speech-Language-Hearing Association, Boston, MA.

McNeil, M.R., Small, S.L., Masterson, R.J., & Fossett, T.R.D. (1995). Behavioral and pharmacological treatment of lexical-semantic deficits in a single patient with primary progressive aphasia. *American Journal of Speech-Language Pathology, 4,* 76–87.

Miceli, G., Amitrano, A., Capasso, R., & Caramazza, A. (1996). The treatment of anomia resulting from output lexical damage: Analysis of two cases. *Brain and Language, 52,* 150–174.

Miceli, G. & Caramazza, A. (1988). Dissociations of inflectional and derivational morphology. *Brain and Language, 35,* 24–65.

Miceli, G., Giustollisi, L., & Caramazza, A. (1991). The interaction of lexical and non-lexical processing mechanisms: Evidence from anomia. *Cortex, 27,* 57–80.

Miceli, G., Silveri, M.C., Villa, G., & Caramazza, A. (1984). On the basis for the agrammatic's difficulty in producing main verbs. *Cortex, 20,* 207–220.

Miozzo, A., Soardi, M., & Cappa, S.F. (1994). Pure anomia with spared action naming due to a left temporal lesion. *Neuropsychologia, 32,* 1101–1109.

Mitchum, C.C. (1992). Treatment generalization and the application of cognitive neuropsychological models in aphasia therapy. In NIH Publication No. 93-3424: *Aphasia treatment: Current approaches and research opportunities* (pp. 99–116).

Mitchum, C. & Berndt, R.S. (1994). Verb retrieval and sentence construction: Effects of targeted intervention. In M.J. Riddoch & G. Humphreys (eds.), *Cognitive neuropsychology and cognitive rehabilitation* (pp. 317–348). Hove: Erlbaum.

Mitchum, C.C., Ritgert, B.A., Sandson, J., & Berndt, R.S. (1990). The use of response analysis in confrontation naming. *Aphasiology, 4,* 261–280.

Montanes, P., Goldblum, M.C., & Boller, F. (1995). The naming impairment of living and nonliving items in Alzheimer's disease. *Journal of the International Neuropsychological Society, 1,* 39–48.

Morris, J., Franklin, S., Ellis, A.W., Turner, J.E., & Bailey, P.J. (1996). Remediating a speech perception deficit in an aphasic patient. *Aphasiology, 10,* 137–158.

Naeser, M.A., Helm-Estabrooks, N., Haas, G., Auerbach, S., & Srinivasan, M. (1987). Relationship between lesion extent in Wernicke's area on computed tomographic scan and predicting recovery of comprehension in Wernicke's aphasia. *Archives of Neurology, 44,* 73–82.

Nickels, L. (1992). The autocue? Self-generated phonemic cues in the treatment of a disorder of reading and naming. *Cognitive Neuropsychology, 9,* 155–182.

Nickels, L. & Best, W. (1996a). Therapy for naming disorders (Part I): Principles, puzzles, and progress. *Aphasiology, 10,* 21–47.

Nickels, L. & Best, W. (1996b). Therapy for naming disorders (Part II): Specifics, surprises, and suggestions. *Aphasiology, 10,* 109–136.

Nickels, L. & Howard, D. (1995). Aphasic naming: What matters? *Neuropsychologia, 33,* 1281–1303.

Nickels, L. & Howard, D. (1994). A frequent occurrence: Factors affecting the production of semantic errors in aphasic naming. *Cognitive Neuropsychology, 11,* 289–320.

Ochipa, C., Maher, L.M., & Raymer, A.M. (1998). One approach to the treatment of anomia. *ASHA Special Interest Division 2: Neurophysiology and Neurogenic Speech and Language Disorders, 15*(3), 18–23.

Ochipa, C., Rothi, L.J.G., & Heilman, K.M. (1989). Ideational apraxia: A deficit in tool selection and use. *Annals of Neurology, 25,* 190–193.

Paivio, A. (1971). *Imagery and verbal processes.* New York: Holt, Rinehart, & Winston.

Paivio, A. (1986). Mental comparisons involving abstract attributes. *Memory & Cognition, 2,* 199–208.

Pashek, G.V. (1997). A case study of gesturally cued naming in aphasia: dominant versus nondominant hand training. *Journal of Communication Disorders, 30,* 349–366.

Pashek, G.V. (1998). Gestural facilitation of noun and verb retrieval in aphasia: A case study. *Brain and Language, 65,* 177–180.

Polster, M.R. & Rose, S.B. (1998). Disorders of auditory processing: Evidence for modularity in audition. *Cortex, 34,* 47–65.

Pring, T., Hamilton, A., Harwood, A., & Macbride, L. (1993). Generalization of naming after picture/word matching tasks: Only items appearing in therapy benefit. *Aphasiology, 7,* 383–394.

Pring, T., White-Thomson, M., Pound, C., Marshall, J., & Davis, A. (1990). Picture/word matching tasks and word retrieval: Some follow-up data and second thoughts. *Aphasiology, 4,* 479–483.

Rapp, B.C. & Caramazza, A. (1998). Lexical deficits. In M.T. Sarno (ed.), *Acquired aphasia* (3rd ed.) (pp. 187–227). San Diego, CA: Academic Press.

Rapp, B.C., Hillis, A.E., & Caramazza, A. (1993). The role of representations in cognitive theory: More on multiple semantics and the agnosias. *Cognitive Neuropsychology, 10,* 235–249.

Ratcliff, G. & Newcombe, F. (1982). Object recognition: Some deductions from clinical evidence. In A.W. Ellis (ed.), *Normality and pathology in cognitive functions* (pp. 147–171). London: Academic Press.

Raymer, A.M. (1999, November). Verbal+gestural treatment: Effects for severe limb apraxia. Paper presented at the annual meeting of the American Speech-Language-Hearing Association, San Francisco.

Raymer, A.M. & Berndt, R.S. (1996). Reading lexically without semantics: Evidence from patients with probable Alzheimer's disease. *Journal of the International Neuropsychological Society, 2,* 340–349.

Raymer, A.M., Foundas, A.L., Maher, L.M., Greenwald, M.L., Morris, M., Rothi, L.J.G., & Heilman, K.M. (1997a). Cognitive neuropsychological analysis and neuroanatomic correlates in a case of acute anomia. *Brain and Language, 58,* 137–156.

Raymer, A.M., Greenwald, M.L., Richardson, M.E., Rothi, L.J.G., & Heilman, K.M. (1997b). Optic aphasia and optic apraxia: Case analysis and theoretical implications. *Neurocase, 3,* 173–183.

Raymer, A.M., Maher, L.M., Foundas, A.L., Rothi, L.J.G., & Heilman, K.M. (2000). Analysis of lexical recovery in an individual with acute anomia. *Aphasiology, 14,* 901–910.

Raymer, A.M., Maher, L.M., Greenwald, M.L., Morris, M., Rothi, L.J.G., & Heilman, K.M. (1990). The Florida Semantics Battery. Unpublished test.

Raymer, A.M., Moberg, P., Crosson, B., Nadeau, S.E., & Rothi, L.J.G. (1997c). Lexical-semantic deficits in two patients with dominant thalamic infarction. *Neuropsychologia, 35,* 211–219.

Raymer, A.M. & Rothi, L.J.G. (2000). Semantic system. In L.J.G. Rothi, B. Crosson, & S. Nadeau (eds.), *Aphasia and language: Theory to practice.* New York: Guilford Press.

Raymer, A.M., Rothi, L.J.G., & Greenwald, M.L. (1995a). The role of cognitive models in language rehabilitation. *NeuroRehabilitation, 5,* 183–193.

Raymer, A.M., Rothi, L.J.G., & Heilman, K.M. (1995b). Nonsemantic activation of lexical and praxis output systems in Alzheimer's subjects. *Journal of the International Neuropsychological Society, 1,* 147 (abstract).

Raymer, A.M. & Thompson, C.K. (1991). Effects of verbal plus gestural treatment in a patient with aphasia and severe apraxia

of speech. In T.E. Prescott (ed.), *Clinical aphasiology, Vol. 12* (pp. 285–297). Austin, TX: Pro-Ed.

Raymer, A.M., Thompson, C.K., Jacobs, B., & LeGrand, H.R. (1993). Phonologic treatment of naming deficits in aphasia: Model-based generalization analysis. *Aphasiology, 7,* 27–53.

Riddoch, M.J. & Humphreys, G.W. (1987a). A case of integrative visual agnosia. *Brain, 110,* 1431–1462.

Riddoch, M.J. & Humphreys, G.W. (1994). Cognitive neuropsychology and cognitive rehabilitation: A marriage of equal partners? In M.J. Riddoch & G.W. Humphreys (eds.), *Cognitive neuropsychology and cognitive rehabilitation* (pp. 1–15). London: Erlbaum.

Riddoch, M.J. & Humphreys, G.W. (1987b). Visual object processing in optic aphasia: A case of semantic access agnosia. *Cognitive Neuropsychology, 4,* 131–185.

Riddoch, M.J., Humphreys, G.W., Coltheart, M., & Funnell, E. (1988). Semantic systems or system? Neuropsychological evidence re-examined. *Cognitive Neuropsychology, 5,* 3–25.

Robson, J., Marshall, J., Pring, T., & Chiat, S. (1998). Phonologic naming therapy in jargon aphasia: Positive but paradoxical effects. *Journal of the International Neuropsychological Society, 4,* 675–686.

Rothi, L.J.G. (1995). Behavioral compensation in the case of treatment of acquired language disorders resulting from brain damage. In R.A. Dixon & L. Backman (eds.), *Compensating for psychological deficits and declines: Managing losses and promoting gains* (pp. 219–230). Mahwah, NJ: Lawrence Erlbaum.

Rothi, L.J.G. (1998). Cognitive disorders: Searching for the circumstances of effective treatment: introduction by the symposium organizer. *Journal of the International Neuropsychological Society, 4,* 593–594.

Rothi, L.J.G. (1997). Transcortical motor, sensory, and mixed aphasia. In L.L. LaPointe (ed.), *Aphasia and related neurogenic language disorders* (2nd ed.) (pp. 91–111). New York: Thieme Medical Publishers.

Rothi, L.J.G. & Moss, S. (1989). Alexia without agraphia: A model driven treatment. Paper presented at the annual meeting of the Academy of Aphasia, Santa Fe, NM.

Rothi, L.J.G., Mack, L., & Heilman, K.M. (1986). Pantomime agnosia. *Journal of Neurology, Neurosurgery and Psychiatry, 49,* 451–454.

Rothi, L.J.G., Ochipa, C., & Heilman, K.M. (1991a). A cognitive neuropsychological model of limb praxis. *Cognitive Neuropsychology, 8,* 443–458.

Rothi, L.J.G., Ochipa, C., & Heilman, K.M. (1997a). A cognitive neuropsychological model of limb praxis and apraxia. In L.J.G. Rothi & K.M. Heilman (eds.), *Apraxia: the neuropsychology of action* (pp. 29–49). East Sussex, UK: Psychology Press.

Rothi, L.J.G., Raymer, A.M., & Heilman, K.M. (1997b). Limb praxis assessment. In L.J.G. Rothi & K.M. Heilman (eds.) *Apraxia: the neuropsychology of action* (pp. 61–73). East Sussex, UK: Psychology Press.

Rothi, L.J.G., Raymer, A.M., Maher, L.M., Greenwald, M., & Morris, M. (1991b). Assessment of naming failures in neurological communication disorders. *Clinics in Communication Disorders, 1,* 7–20.

Saffran, E.M. (1997). Aphasia: Cognitive neuropsychological aspects. In T.E. Feinberg & M.J. Farah (eds.), *Behavioral neurology and neuropsychology* (pp. 151–165). New York: McGraw-Hill.

Saffran, E.M., Berndt, R.S., & Schwartz, M.F. (1989). The quantitative analysis of agrammatic production: Procedure and data. *Brain and Language, 37,* 440–479.

Schnider, A., Benson, D.F., & Scharre, D.W. (1994). Visual agnosia and optic aphasia: Are they anatomically distinct? *Cortex, 30,* 445–457.

Schwartz, M.F. & Whyte, J. (1992). Methodologial issues in aphasia treatment research: The big picture. In NIH Publication No. 93-3424: *Aphasia treatment: Current approaches and research opportunities* (pp. 17–23).

Semenza, C., Cipolotti, L., & Denes, G. (1992). Reading aloud in jargonaphasia: An unusual dissociation in speech output. *Journal of Neurology, Neurosurgery, & Psychiatry, 55,* 205–208.

Seron, X. & Deloche, G. (eds.) (1989). *Cognitive approaches in neuropsychological rehabilitation.* Hillsdale, NJ: Erlbaum.

Shallice, T. (1988). *From neuropsychology to mental structure.* Cambridge, MA: Cambridge University Press.

Shelton, P.A., Bowers, D., Duara, R., & Heilman, K.M. (1994). Apperceptive visual agnosia: A case study. *Brain and Cognition, 25,* 1–23.

Shindo, M., Kaga, K., & Tanaka, Y. (1991). Speech discrimination and lip reading in patients with word deafness or auditory agnosia. *Brain and Language, 40,* 153–161.

Shuren, J., Geldmacher, D., & Heilman, K.M. (1993). Nonoptic aphasia: Aphasia with preserved confrontation naming in Alzheimer's disease. *Neurology, 43,* 1900–1907.

Silveri, M.C., Gainotti, G., Perani, D., Cappelletti, J.Y., Carbone, G., & Faxio, F. (1997). Naming deficits for non-living items: Neuropsychological and PET study. *Neuropsychologia, 35,* 359–367.

Small, S.L., Flores, D.K., & Noll, D.C. (1998). Different neural circuits subserve reading before and after therapy for acquired dyslexia. *Brain and Language, 62,* 298–308.

Snodgrass, J.G. & Vanderwart, M. (1980). A standardised set of 260 pictures: Norms for name agreement, image agreement, familiarity and visual complexity. *Journal of Experimental Psychology: Human Perception and Performance, 6,* 174–215.

Takahashi, N., Kawamura, M., Shinotou, H., Hirayama, K., Kaga, K., & Shindo, M. (1992). Pure word deafness due to left hemisphere damage. *Cortex, 28,* 295–303.

Tyler, L.K. (1987). Spoken language comprehension in aphasia: A real-time processing perspective. In M. Coltheart, G. Sartori, & R. Job (eds.), *The cognitive neuropsychology of language* (pp. 145–162). London: Lawrence Erlbaum.

Vignolo, L.A. (1982). Auditory agnosia. *Philosophical Transactions of the Royal Society (London), 298,* 49–57.

Warrington, E.K. & McCarthy, R.A. (1987). Categories of knowledge: Further fractionation and an attempted integration. *Brain, 110,* 1273–1296.

Warrington, E.K. & McCarthy, R.A. (1983). Category-specific access dysphasia. *Brain, 100,* 1273–1296.

Warrington, E.K. & McCarthy, R.A. (1994). Multiple meaning systems in the brain: A case for visual semantics. *Neuropsychologia, 32,* 1465–1473.

Warrington, E. & Shallice, T. (1984). Category specific semantic impairments. *Brain, 107,* 829–854.

Warrington, E. & Taylor, (1978). Two categorical stages of object recognition. *Perception, 7,* 695–705.

Weiller, C., Isensee, C., Rijntjes, M., Huber, W., Muller, S., Bier, D., Dutschka, K., Woods, R.P., Noth, J., & Diner, H.C. (1995). Recovery from Wernicke's aphasia: A positron emission tomographic study. *Annals of Neurology, 37,* 723–732.

Wilson, B.A. (1997). Cognitive rehabilitation: How it is and how it might be. *Journal of the International Neuropsychological Society, 3,* 487–496.

Wilson, B.A. (1999). *Case studies in neuropsychological rehabilitation.* New York: Oxford University Press.

Zingeser, L.B. & Berndt, R.S. (1988). Grammatical class and context effects in a case of pure anomia: Implications for models of language production. *Cognitive Neuropsychology, 5,* 473–516.

Zingeser, L.B. & Berndt, R.S. (1990). Retrieval of nouns and verbs in agrammatism and anomia. *Brain and Language, 39,* 14–32.

APPENDIX 23-1
Stimuli from the Florida Semantics Battery (Raymer et al., 1990)

Body Parts	Frequency	Transportation	Frequency	Vegetables	Frequency	Fruits	Frequency
ankle	15 MF	airplane	21 MF	broccoli	1 LF	apple	15 MF
elbow	17 MF	jeep	16 MF	celery	4 LF	cherry	6 LF
wrist	16 MF	van	22 MF	lettuce	1 LF	lemon	4 LF
ear	67 HF	bus	42 HF	peas	24 MF	peach	4 LF
nose	65 HF	truck	80 HF	potato	30 HF	pineapple	9 MF
chin	25 MF	canoe	8 LF	carrot	5 LF	banana	4 LF
thumb	14 MF	sailboat	4 LF	corn	38 HF	grapes	10 MF
arm	217 HF	boat	123 HF	onion	19 MF	orange	15 MF
leg	126 HF	train	86 HF	pepper	13 MF	pear	8 LF
teeth	102 HF	wagon	72 HF	pumpkin	2 LF	raisin	1 LF

Kitchen Utensils	Frequency	Clothing	Frequency	Animals	Frequency	Personal Items	Frequency
fork	20 MF	mitten	2 LF	deer	13 MF	brush	36 HF
pan	16 MF	robe	10 MF	mouse	20 MF	mirror	27 MF
spoon	6 LF	sweater	18 MF	turtle	9 MF	razor	15 MF
cup	58 HF	dress	63 HF	cow	46 HF	toothbrush	6 LF
knife	86 HF	shoe	58 HF	fish	281 HF	towel	17 MF
jar	19 MF	pants	9 MF	frog	2 LF	comb	6 LF
skillet	2 LF	scarf	4 LF	pig	14 MF	perfume	11 MF
bottle	90 LF	coat	52 HF	cat	42 HF	soap	25 MF
glass	128 HF	hat	71 HF	dog	147 HF	toothpaste	2 LF
plate	44 HF	suit	64 HF	horse	203 HF	tissue	54 HF

Furniture	Frequency	Office Items	Frequency	Tools	Frequency	Musical Instruments	Frequency
crib	8 LF	book	100 HF	axe	19 MF	accordian	1 LF
shelf	20 MF	newspaper	43 HF	hammer	6 LF	drum	20 MF
stool	8 LF	phone	46 HF	pliers	1 LF	guitar	10 MF
bench	42 HF	scissors	1 LF	saw	8 LF	harp	1 LF
desk	69 HF	tape	39 HF	shovel	8 LF	trumpet	5 LF
hammock	5 LF	clip	6 LF	clamp	2 LF	bell	17 MF
sofa	9 MF	pen	13 MF	hoe	1 LF	flute	3 LF
bed	139 HF	ruler	13 MF	rake	8 LF	harmonica	0 LF
chair	89 HF	stamp	8 LF	screwdriver	1 LF	piano	32 HF
table	242 HF	pencil	38 HF	wrench	1 LF	violin	9 MF

Includes 120 nouns from 12 different semantic categories. Frequencies based on Francis & Kucera, 1982.

HF–40 highest frequency words; range 32–242.

MF–40 middle frequency words; range 9–25.

LF–40 lowest frequency words; range 0–8.

Chapter 24

Cognitive Neuropsychological Approaches to Diagnosing and Treating Language Disorders: Production and Comprehension of Sentences

Charlotte C. Mitchum
and Rita Sloan Berndt

Models of normal language can be very useful in the diagnosis and treatment of aphasia, especially in cases where the goal of therapy is to restore normal language function. At the very least, a conception of how the language system operates normally provides a basis for interpreting how brain damage has altered normal processing. For planning therapy, a concept of the components involved in normal language can guide the selection of therapy materials and can influence the design of therapy tasks. Unfortunately, the application of a theoretical model of normal language to diagnosis and treatment of impaired (aphasic) language is limited by two factors. First is the lack of a complete model of normal language function to serve as a standard reference. Second is the lack of a complete understanding of how aphasic language deviates from normal language. Given these limitations, it might be reasonable to end our discussion of model-driven therapy at this point. We could say that we simply do not know enough about either normal or aphasic language to compare the two (Caramazza, 1989; Wilson & Patterson, 1990). However, a number of recent studies have demonstrated that therapy can be guided even by a partial model of sentence processing. Moreover, the interpretation of treatment response in the context of a model of normal sentence processing has enlightened our understanding of how therapy affects language function.

OBJECTIVES

In conjunction with the other chapters of this section, we describe a cognitive neuropsychological approach to aphasia, with particular emphasis on sentence processing impairments. The objectives of this chapter are (1) to describe a theoretical model of normal sentence production and comprehension; (2) to illustrate how aphasic sentence processing is interpreted in the context of the normal theory; and (3) to demonstrate how such an interpretation can be used to guide language therapy. A final discussion draws some conclusions regarding the current state and future direction of this approach.

NORMAL SENTENCE PROCESSING

Normal speakers produce and comprehend sentences with little apparent conscious effort. Nevertheless, the cognitive operations that support sentence processing must be remarkably complex. To utter even a single sentence requires, at the very least, the integration of the products of lexical retrieval, syntactic formulation, phonological encoding, and articulation. Comprehension similarly is achieved by the interaction of a number of separate operations. Exactly how the interaction of these components yields a coherent message is not entirely understood. There are various theories of normal sentence processing that attempt to describe the inner structure of language in a manner that demonstrates the temporal unfolding of cognitive events. Such theories, though controversial, can be very useful for the speech-language clinician interested in understanding how aphasic language deviates from language that is unimpaired (Byng, 1988; Davis, 1993; Dell et al., 1997; Humphreys & Riddoch, 1994; Mitchum & Berndt, 1995; Seron & Deloche, 1989; Schwartz, 1987). For a full perspective on this issue, see also Caramazza (1989); Hillis (1993); and Wilson & Patterson (1990).

Sentence Production

The range of operations governing sentence production stretch from the creation of an intended message to its ultimate articulation. Even in the absence of a formal theory, it would seem likely that sentences are produced by means of a series of fairly independent stages. Thoughts form a rough, preverbal idea of what one wants to say. Although all thoughts may be candidates for verbal expression, they do not seem to be lexically specified or grammatically well formed. It is especially clear that many thoughts never become phonologically encoded. For selected thoughts, however, we seem to readily convert the unspecified message into an ordered utterance that contains both lexical content—comprised of open-class words (e.g., nouns, verbs, adjectives, adverbs) and grammatical structure—comprised of closed-class words (e.g., functors, articles, prepositions). The utterance is made known using an articulatory code common to both speaker and listener. However, this informal description tells us little about how these events are coordinated. That is, how do we construct a verbal sentence from thought? Importantly, for the speech-language pathologist, what has gone wrong in aphasic sentence production?

Speech Error Data

Models of normal sentence production are based in part on the premise that errors produced by normal speakers are not random, but rather show patterns indicative of how words are retrieved and how sentences normally are formed. Speech error analysis is complex and sometimes controversial, and will not be exhaustively reviewed here (for more detail see Fromkin, 1971; Garrett 1975, 1980; Levelt, 1989; Stemberger, 1985). We will, however, consider how normal speech errors can constrain theoretical accounts of lexical retrieval and grammatical construction.

For many years, retrieval of a word from the mental lexicon was viewed as an all-or-none event. That is, it was assumed that a single lexical entry stored all aspects of a word, including its meaning and phonology. This assumption was undermined by evidence that normal speakers experiencing a "tip-of-the-tongue" state could express knowledge of word meaning, and segmental information (e.g., first sound[s], number of syllables), despite being unable to say the word (Brown & McNeil, 1966). Evidence such as this indicates that partial word retrieval sometimes occurs. Contemporary theories of lexical retrieval in sentence production provide for separate access to word meaning and phonological form (Bock & Levelt, 1994; Dell, 1986; Garrett, 1988; Levelt, 1989).

Although words are produced serially in sentences, speech errors indicate that they are not planned serially. In some utterances, the grammatical elements of the sentence are produced in their proper places despite the misplacement of lexical content. Errors of this type may involve the exchange of content words within the same grammatical category (e.g., "why did the *horn* blow its *train*?"), or reflect an exchange across grammatical form class (e.g.,

"I went to get a *cash checked*.") (examples from Garrett, 1980, 1982). Grammatical stranding errors occur with both free-standing (e.g., articles) and bound (e.g., inflections) grammatical morphemes. Production of these sorts of errors is taken as evidence that such grammatical elements comprise a "sentential frame" which is constructed at least partially independently of the lexical content of the sentence.

A Theoretical Model

The model of normal sentence production most widely applied to the interpretation of aphasic sentence production has been developed by Garrett (1975, 1982, 1988). Based in psycholinguistic theory, the model is derived from an interpretation of normal speech errors; it attempts to account for the specific mental operations that govern sentence production. Garrett (1984) describes five distinct levels of mental representation that are required to construct a well-formed and meaningful sentence. These include (1) the Message level; (2) the Functional level; (3) the Positional level; (4) the Phonetic level; and (5) the Articulatory level. A basic schematic of the theoretical model is shown in **Figure 24–1**. The levels of information representation achieved during sentence production are designated from top to bottom, in serial order. The arrows indicate the general direction of processing; the boxes encompass processing demands required to achieve each level of representation.

The focus of attention in Garrett's model is on the middle processing levels, where grammatical information is translated from Message-to-Functional-to-Positional Levels. This is not to diminish the importance of the more peripheral levels involving input to the Message, or Phonetic and Articulatory encoding. It is strictly a matter of avoiding overinterpretation of the normal speech error data that supports the basic theory. We have sketched an elaborated version of the expanded model of normal sentence production offered in Garrett (1988), with examples included to illustrate how the model accounts for the ability to produce a sentence to convey the message that a girl is kicking a boy (Figure 24–2).

Message Level Representation

A raw, preverbal concept of some information the speaker wishes to convey forms the Message Level representation. Garrett (1982) describes the Message Level representation as conceptual and nonlinguistic. Other theories of normal production view the preverbal message as containing relevant information linked to the speaker's perception of an event. For example, Levelt (1989) and Bock & Levelt (1994) identify Message Level "event roles" which govern the thematic relations among entities in the message by identifying "who" is doing "what" to "whom."

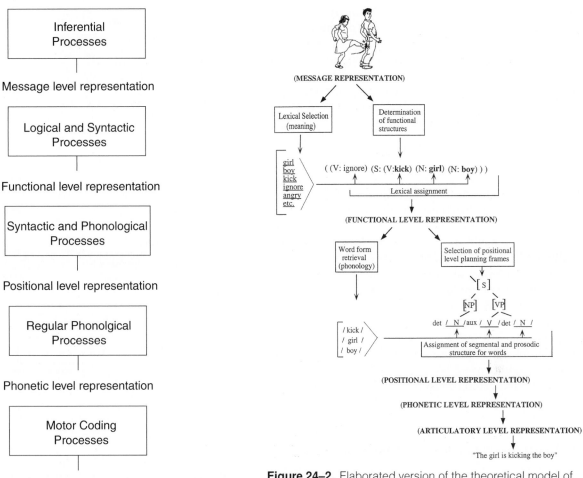

Figure 24–1. Basic theoretical model of normal sentence production. (Redrawn with permission from Garrett, M.F. [1984]. The organization of processing structure for language production: Applications to aphasic speech. In D. Caplan, A.R. Lecours, & A. Smith (eds.), *Biological perspectives on language* [p. 174]. Cambridge, MA: MIT Press.

Figure 24–2. Elaborated version of the theoretical model of normal sentence production (Reprinted with permission from Garrett, M.F. (1988). Processes in language production. In F.J. Newmeyer (ed.), *Linguistics: The Cambridge Survey: III. Language: Psychological and biological aspects* (pp. 69–96). Cambridge, UK: Cambridge University Press.) The model has been modified here with an exemplary utterance.

Functional Level Representation

Representations at the Functional Level encode the conceptual content of the message. Abstract lexical entries (specifying word meanings but not pronunciation) are selected to correspond to various elements of the message. Functional structures designate the grammatical class of the content words. For example, if a person intends to convey that a little boy is kicking a little girl, the Functional Level representation provides the information that the sentence must encode a verb, two nouns representing young people of a particular gender, and a name for the object that is central to the action (Figure 24–2). Multiple possibilities may be generated, including more than one option for the central action (verb). This is an important feature of the model since it allows for multiple forms of a similar message. For example, a person attempting to describe the picture shown in Figure 24–2

could easily encode one of (at least) two possible messages: (a) "The girl is *kicking* the boy" or (b) "The boy is *ignoring* the girl." Either sentence (a) or (b) is an accurate and reasonable description of the depicted scene. The choice of verb may result from the desire to highlight either "the girl" or "the boy" as the topic of the message. Importantly, the choice of verb clearly dictates which noun will serve as thematic agent (i.e., the noun "doing" the action), thus placing some constraint on the eventual structure of the sentence.

Positional Level Representation

A hierarchy of syntactic constituents (NP, VP, PP) impose order on the sentence elements at the Positional Level. The chosen lexical content is phonologically specified and inserted into a sentence frame formed by bound and free grammatical elements (e.g., determiner, auxiliary verb). Segmental and prosodic contours are imposed on the sentence. The details of how the lexical content is inserted, and of how the grammatical morphemes are composed into a phrasal frame, are largely unspecified in Garrett's (1980) model. The critical point, supported by the occurrence of "stranding" errors (see previously), is that the lexical content is obtained independently of the grammatical frame.

Sentence Comprehension

The goal of sentence production is to articulate an internally driven message by converting the abstract conceptual information into a linguistically structured utterance. For sentence comprehension, the goal is to deconstruct an externally received utterance into an abstract conceptual message. Viewed this way, comprehension can be conceived of as the serial inverse of production (Byng, 1986; Berndt, 1998; Saffran et al., 1980b). This characterization of sentence comprehension assumes that sentence production and comprehension may engage at least some of the same cognitive representations. The precise relationship between production and comprehension of language is a critical issue for speech-language pathologists, but is not clearly delineated by the model.

The Model Applied to Sentence Comprehension

Since the model of sentence production proposed by Garrett (1988) was not designed to account for sentence comprehension, we have taken some liberty in renaming the components of the model. The terminology is intended to reflect the events involved in translating from an ordered array of lexical and syntactic information to an unordered cognitive code that carries a specific message. For comprehension, as in production, grammatical processing mediates between sentence structure (at the Positional Level) and sentence meaning (at the Message Level). In Figure 24–3, we have sketched levels of representation that correspond to the production model described above. For sentence comprehension, the model begins at the bottom, with the conversion of an acoustic signal to a phonologic code.

Positional Level Representation

The segmental and prosodic contours of the signal are decomposed at the Positional Level. Phrasal frames are identified by parsing the sentence into syntactic constituents that organize the lexical and grammatical content of the sentence. This process involves conversion of the incoming string of words into a representation of the constituent structure of a sentence (see Mitchell, 1994, for review). Specific phonological word forms of the lexical content are identified at this level.

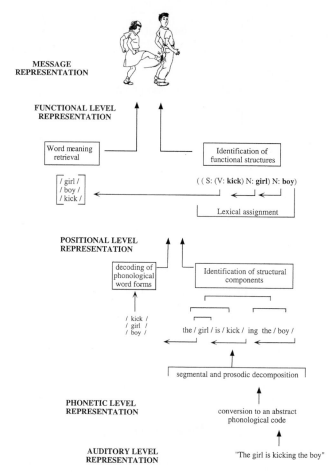

Figure 24–3. Theoretical model of normal sentence comprehension adapted from a model of normal sentence production (Reprinted with permission from Garrett, M.F. (1988). Processes in language production. In F.J. Newmeyer (ed.), *Linguistics: The Cambridge Survey: III. Language: Psychological and biological aspects* (pp. 69–96). Cambridge, UK: Cambridge University Press.)

Functional Level Representation

At the Functional Level, the lexical information is identified semantically, and interpreted thematically. This translation between the Positional and Functional Levels allows the listener to understand the central action and the logical roles of those elements involved in the action. In Figure 24–3, this yields the information that a young female is taking her foot and moving it swiftly toward the leg of a young male. If all goes well, the results of this decoding process serve to establish in the listener the message intended by the speaker.

USING THE MODEL TO INTERPRET APHASIC SENTENCE PROCESSING

Reference to a theoretical framework has provided a valuable mechanism for sorting out the array of aphasic production problems, ranging from impaired word retrieval in anomic aphasia, to the telegraphic utterances of Broca's aphasia and fluent aberrations associated with Wernicke's & jargon aphasia (Garrett, 1982; Goodglass, 1993; Schwartz, 1987). The model has even been used to elucidate the nature of residual linguistic function in global aphasia (Shelton et al., 1996). At the same time, it is increasingly clear that there is no theoretical model of production that can fully account for all the problems observed in aphasic language (Berndt, 2000). Even the most detailed models tend to remain underspecified. For example, Garrett (1980, 1988) has little to say regarding how the representational levels of his model are actually created. A more explicit description of processing mechanisms is offered by Levelt (1989) and Bock & Levelt (1994), but even these theories fall short of the detail needed to account for all aphasic language symptoms.

The underspecification of the processes that yield a representational level makes it difficult to locate the source of aphasic symptoms unambiguously within the theoretical model (Caramazza & Hillis, 1989). Berndt (2000) suggests that mapping aphasic production onto the normal production model is further complicated by the nature of the breakdown in aphasia. That is, aphasic speech patterns often reflect the interaction of multiple language impairments, which are compounded by additional cognitive limitations, and the masking of deficits through the use of compensatory strategies. Despite these challenges, numerous studies have uncovered patterns of production that are interpretable (more or less) within the theoretical framework of a normal production model (Byng, 1986; Caramazza & Hillis, 1989; Garrett, 1982; Goodglass, 1993; Mitchum & Berndt, 1994; Schwartz, 1987). Such model-driven interpretations of aphasic language production have been directed primarily at the type of disorder associated with agrammatic sentence production.

Agrammatic Production

The basic symptoms associated with agrammatic production include (1) reduced phrase length; (2) simplified syntactic complexity; (3) poor production of main verbs; and (4) omission and/or substitution of free and bound grammatical morphemes (Berndt & Caramazza, 1980; Saffran et al., 1989; Saffran et al., 1980a). The focus on grammatical encoding of sentences has interested language theoreticians who assume that the grammatical processing required for normal sentence formulation breaks down in aphasia in a highly systematic manner. A considerable amount of literature has emerged over the past 20 years regarding the study of "agrammatic" production.

Interpreting the Production Impairment

It was once thought that the deficit underlying agrammatism could be attributed to a singular impairment affecting a "phonologic" (Kean, 1982) or "syntactic" (Berndt &

Caramazza, 1980) processor. Such views have given way to the general consensus that agrammatic production varies among aphasic speakers (Saffran et al., 1989); that the co-occurrence of core symptoms of agrammatic production is more "probable" than "fixed" (Kolk & Heeschen, 1985); and that aspects of agrammatic production can appear in fluent speech (Caramazza & Miceli, 1991; Kolk & VanGrunsven, 1985; Mitchum & Berndt, 1994). Current research no longer attempts to explain a "prototypical" pattern of agrammatic production, but tries to account instead for the wide range of patterns associated with grammatical processing deficits. In the context of Garrett's normal production model (1980, 1988), the symptoms of agrammatism can be viewed in terms of the ability to achieve the series of representational levels necessary to drive sentence formulation.

The Message Level

The identification of a Message Level impairment depends on what is attributed to this level of representation. In Garrett's scheme the Message representation is largely unspecified. This characterization might be taken to imply that assignment of thematic roles to verb arguments is normally accomplished as part of the Functional Level representation, where lexical content is assigned to a functional structure (e.g., Schwartz, 1987). However, it cannot be assumed from this interpretation that thematic role assignment originates at the Functional Level (Byng, 1986). As noted above, some theories of normal sentence production describe the preverbal message as containing a conceptualized set of "event roles," which are the rough equivalent of thematic roles (Bock & Levelt, 1994). In this characterization, the Message Level representation is the primary source of information regarding "who" does "what" to "whom."

Some investigators studying aphasia therapy have developed experimental tests specifically designed to assess the aphasic speaker's ability to perceive event roles in action pictures (Byng, 1986, 1988; Marshall et al., 1993; Nickels et al., 1991). Such tests measure the ability to extract predicate (e.g., verb) information from pictures (e.g., sorting action vs. nonaction pictures), and to recognize fine distinctions in verb meaning (e.g., distinguishing the equivalence of two depictions of "pouring" compared to a distracter picture showing "dripping"). Other tasks assess the ability to recognize the relationship between the action and actors (or objects) depicted (e.g., "point to the person who is pouring something"). These types of tests attempt to isolate pre–Functional Level operations that contribute to sentence production, and have been used to identify impaired event role perception.

It might be presumed that a severe deficit of message formation would result in a person's having little or nothing to say. The lack of production, however, does not always indicate that Message Level information is unavailable. Weinrich and colleagues have shown that even severely impaired aphasic speakers (classified as "global") can demonstrate intact Message Level representations. Using a computerized iconic communication device (C-ViC), patients select lexical items from a limited iconic vocabulary and place them into a "sentence" formed with a serial-array of retrieved icons (Weinrich et al., 1995). Additional studies have shown remarkable appreciation of the thematic roles of noun icons in the "sentences" formed by these severely aphasic speakers (Weinrich et al., 1995). These studies show that the removal of the phonological and morphological constraints on language (accomplished by using the computerized system) can allow for demonstration of relatively intact representation of the Message and Functional Level information needed for sentence production.

The Functional Level

A major feature of the Functional Level representation is the retrieval of word meaning. Word finding impairments in aphasia can be sensitive to grammatical class. For example, several studies have demonstrated differential patterns of retrieval for object names (nouns) and action names (verbs) (Goodglass et al., 1966; Miceli et al., 1984; Zingeser & Berndt, 1990). Poor production of lexical verbs, in particular, has been implicated in the sentence production impairment observed in aphasia (Saffran et al., 1980b; Saffran et al., 1989; Berndt et al., 1997). Consider, for example, the following excerpt from an aphasic speaker (L.R.) in a task where she is asked to describe a scene at a beach where a boy is pouring sand on a girl:

> L.R.: "the girl is in the sand…the boy is motionless."
> Ex: "tell me about how they are interacting" (points to boy and girl)
> L.R.: "the girl in the sand…the man…the girl is in the sand…(L.R. points in the picture to where the sand is being poured)…the girl is in the sand…pouring the woman…man…two separate…equal but…the girl is in the sand."

Although poor verb retrieval is highly correlated with impaired sentence production, there is little evidence to indicate that it actually *causes* the grammatical disturbance in sentence production. In some cases, impaired verb retrieval does not co-occur with grammatical production errors, thus providing evidence against a causal interpretation (Berndt et al., 1997; Caramazza & Hillis, 1989; Kremin & Basso, 1993).

Berndt and coworkers (1997) concluded that one of the problems in explicating a causal relationship is that poor verb retrieval can exercise its influence in a variety of ways, and may implicate deficits at multiple locations within the normal production process. For example, it would be predicted (from Garrett's model) that sentence production impaired by poor verb retrieval would benefit from having the verb provided. Berndt et al. (1997) found that some, but not all verb-impaired speakers showed improved sentence production when given a verb to use in a sentence. For those who

showed improvement, the problem in sentence production was resolved by making the phonological form of the verb available (i.e., upon hearing it spoken aloud by the examiner). For those who did not show improved sentence production, it was apparent that additional problems undermined sentence construction.

Another contribution of the Functional Level representation involves the selection of functional structures. The association of lexical items from specific grammatical categories (noun, verb) with specific syntactic roles (subject, object) prepares the representation for conversion into an ordered grammatical form at the Positional Level. The erroneous productions of some aphasic speakers suggests an inability to integrate lexical content with the grammatical elements of a sentence frame—a problem that could arise from an inability to assign nouns to the grammatical roles of subject/object. For example, picture description tasks (where the target is known to the listener) sometimes elicit sentences with incorrect noun order. Shown a picture of a *girl* kicking a *boy*, the response "the boy is kicking the girl" is a clear violation of the target meaning; the response assigns the role of agent to the boy. Role reversal errors are infrequent in spontaneous aphasic speech (Menn & Obler, 1990). Carefully constructed tests are needed to elicit these error types (see Schwartz et al., 1995). Tasks designed to constrain the response to a noncanonical sentence structure also increase the frequency of word order errors (Caramazza & Berndt, 1985). For example, when shown a picture of a girl kicking a boy, the aphasic speaker can be asked to produce a sentence starting with the nonagentive noun, in this case "the boy." A tendency to maintain canonical word order yields the response "the boy is kicking the girl." Even when the error is recognized, the aphasic speaker may find it impossible to integrate noncanonical word order with a compatible surface structure (such as the passive sentence "The girl is kicked by the boy."). The following example from aphasic speaker S.T. indicates that the problem of expressing thematic role relations is not necessarily due to a lack of structural options, or to poor interpretation of the picture stimulus:

> picture: *A girl leading a sheep by a leash.*
> instruction: "Describe this picture by telling me a sentence that starts with 'the girl'."
> response: "the little girl is being pulled along by the sheep…that's not good." [says the same sentence twice more, then studies the picture.]
> instruction: "Try again."
> response: "the little girl is being pulled forward by the sheep…but that's wrong because the sheep is actually behind….the little girl is following the sheep on a leash….the little girl is taking the sheep on a walk."

In some cases, word order errors are produced even in nonreversible sentences, thus yielding a clearly anomalous response, such as "the apple is eating the boy" or "the wall is painting the girl."

The Positional Level

Realization of a Positional Level representation is the final critical step of grammatical encoding. Although this aspect of sentence production appears especially vulnerable in aphasia, it is not easy to predict how a deficit specific to this level of processing would manifest itself. One problem is the difficulty in distinguishing between a deficit located at this level and one that emerges from failure to elaborate the information that feeds into this level (i.e., from the Message and Functional Levels). Caramazza & Hillis (1989) argued that an impairment arising from the Positional Level would be evident when the symptoms of agrammatic production co-occur with intact single word retrieval and normal sentence comprehension. This profile suggests that Functional Level operations (word meaning retrieval and thematic role mapping) are fully operational for comprehension, thus localizing the symptom to a point where the grammatical elements of the sentence are realized for production. (Such a case is reported in Mitchum et al., 2000).

Exactly how the grammatical elements are derived at the Positional Level is left largely unspecified in Garrett's (1982, 1988) model of normal sentence production. Some patterns of agrammatic production clearly indicate that the speaker has the ability to retrieve grammatical function words, but does not seem to know where to place them to form a structural sentence frame (Berndt et al., 1997). For example, when asked to use the word "soap" in a sentence, aphasic speaker M.L. attempted several constructions before settling on a final response:

> M.L.: "the boy in the soap and...no, the boy and his wash the soap...the boy is washing the soap."

Further support that a variety of grammatical structures are available, but underutilized, comes from recent investigation of structural sentence "priming." Several studies have shown that some aphasic speakers can produce a specific structure immediately after hearing a sentence that serves as a model or "prime" (Saffran & Martin, 1997). Hartsuiker & Kolk (1998) obtained experimental evidence that this syntactic priming effect may be diminished when the participants are told explicitly to model the previous sentence. When the same task is given without overt instruction to use the "model," the effect of priming is very robust for both active and passive sentence types. This finding implies that the construction of a Positional Level representation may be undermined by conscious effort in aphasic production. Interestingly, the inverse was observed for control subjects: priming was facilitated when they were explicitly asked to match the structure of the model sentence structure.

Asyntactic Comprehension

There are several classes of sentence comprehension impairments observed in aphasia that arise from various different underlying disorders (see Saffran, in press). Those associated with syntactic processing impairment have been well studied within the constraints of cognitive neuropsychology. The main focus has been on a comprehension disorder described as "asyntactic," which is observed in the context of intact comprehension of word meanings. Identification of this deficit requires testing with carefully designed materials that force syntactic processing of sentences.

Patterns of Asyntactic Comprehension

One of the most commonly used testing procedures used to uncover asyntactic sentence comprehension requires matching a spoken sentence to a picture. To force syntactic processing, the lexical content is the same for both the target and foil (distracter). An example of such a task using a two-picture–one-sentence format is illustrated in Figure 24–4. It is also possible to design essentially the same test using one picture and one sentence with a required "yes" vs. "no" response.

Consider the two series of stimuli (L) and (S) with respect to the target sentence "the girl is kicking the boy." The tasks are superficially similar: A target picture is paired with a foil (nontarget picture) and presented for viewing. A sentence is spoken (e.g., "The girl is kicking the boy") and the patient is instructed to point to the picture that best depicts the spoken sentence. In the *lexical* contrast condition (series "L"; left side top and bottom are presented together), it is possible to identify the top picture as the target on the basis of recognizing that the word "boy," and not "ball" was used in the target sentence. In series "S," a *syntactic* foil is presented with the target picture. In this condition, all the content words are the same; importantly, either noun could carry out the

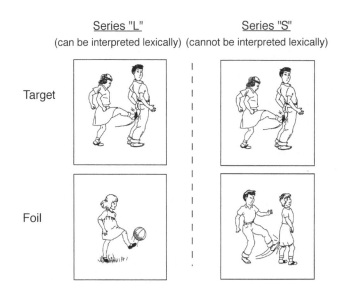

Series "L"   Series "S"
(can be interpreted lexically) (cannot be interpreted lexically)

Target

Foil

Figure 24–4. Examples of stimuli used to assess comprehension of sentences based on lexical ("L") or structural ("S") cues to meaning.

stated action (i.e., the sentence is "semantically reversible"). Upon hearing the target sentence "The girl is kicking the boy," the listener who is dependent upon lexical/semantic interpretation of sentences will find it very difficult to identify the matching picture. Because this arrangement forces the listener to attend to the syntactic sentence structure (word order, verb inflection), poor performance in the "S" condition is taken as evidence of an "asyntactic" approach to sentence comprehension.

Studies of sentence comprehension are complicated by the application of strategic responses to the assessment tasks that mask the symptoms of asyntactic comprehension. Aphasic listeners rarely refuse to respond in the sentence-picture matching test. All things being equal, performance predicted by chance in a forced choice task with two pictures is 50% across all (active and passive) trials. However, performance often reflects some partial comprehension that employs a heuristic (or strategy) for "interpreting" the sentence. In the absence of rule-based syntactic constraints on sentence comprehension, response patterns in the picture-sentence matching task have been attributed to preferential assignment of agent to animate nouns (in mixed animacy conditions) (Saffran et al., 1980b), or assignment of the first-mentioned noun to the role of thematic agent (Ansell & Flowers, 1982). Some response patterns have indicated reliance on the spatial arrangement of noun referents in the picture (Chatterjee et al., 1995). The inconsistent application of these sorts of strategies makes interpretation of test performance especially difficult. For example, the first-noun-as-agent strategy predicts perfect performance on active sentences (e.g., the girl is kicking the boy), but results in consistently incorrect responses to noncanonical sentences (e.g., passives, such as "the boy is kicked by the girl") where the first noun is not the thematic agent.

Interpreting the Comprehension Impairment

Current investigations of asyntactic sentence comprehension propose a variety of possible explanations of the impairment. Some accounts point to a diminished general resource that undermines the ability to sustain complex cognitive manipulations, such as those required for syntactic processing (Miyake et al., 1994), or to limitations of language-relevant memory systems (Caplan & Waters, 1995; Martin, 1995). Others identify asynchrony in the delicate timing operations that coordinate syntactic and lexical processing (Frazier & Freiderici, 1991; Haarmann & Kolk, 1991; Kolk & VanGrunsven, 1985). Linguistic theories predict specific performance patterns on the basis of the surface structure of certain sentence types (Grodzinsky, 1984). However, as in production, close examination of the data challenges any explanation of comprehension impairment that attempts to identify a single source of dysfunction for all patterns of asyntactic comprehension.

The model of normal comprehension (described previously) offers a rough framework for interpreting individual patterns of aphasic performance (Berndt, 1998; Byng, 1986, 1988; Saffran & Schwartz, 1988; Schwartz et al., 1995).

The Positional Level

At the Positional Level, comprehension involves parsing of the auditory sentence into its syntactic constituents. Through the 1980s, a variety of accounts of asyntactic comprehension were directed at some form of a parsing impairment arising from poor processing of grammatical morphemes (Bradley et al., 1980) or an inability to decompose the phrasal structure of the positional (grammatical) frame (Caplan & Futter, 1986). However, these accounts were undermined by a series of studies initiated by Linebarger et al. (1983) showing that many aphasic listeners, including those with serious impairments of sentence comprehension, correctly judged whether or not a sentence was grammatical. This was an important demonstration that the ability to dissect the syntactic structure into phrasal constituents such as NP, VP, PP could be operationally normal despite the inability to comprehend similar sentences (see also Schwartz et al., 1987).

The ability to judge whether or not a sentence is grammatical even when sentence meaning cannot be understood provides a strong demonstration that asyntactic sentence comprehension does not arise from a general inability to perceive, or to parse the basic structure of the incoming sentence. Instead, the problem in such cases appears to arise from linking the grammatically parsed sentence to its underlying meaning. The ability to judge sentence grammaticality is one of several clinical features that distinguishes asyntactic comprehension from other forms of aphasic sentence comprehension (such as Wernicke's aphasia) in which performance is generally poor (Saffran, in press).

The Functional Level

If the ability to parse a sentence into its syntactic constituents is indicative of successful processing at the Positional Level, it becomes crucial to determine how comprehension is made vulnerable at the Functional Level. According to our specification of the Functional Level representation (see Figure 24–3), a deficit could arise from at least two sources: (1) a failure in interpreting word meaning, or (2) an inability to decipher the lexical-thematic role relations.

The use of lexical contrasts in sentence comprehension tests (e.g., series "L" described previously) is one method used to rule out a failure of word meaning interpretation. Failure to distinguish among lexical contrasts may warrant further investigation of single-word comprehension as the source of poor sentence interpretation. The opposite pattern (good performance in lexical distracter conditions and poor performance in reversible sentence conditions) points to a specific inability to appreciate thematic role relations expressed in the sentence. In semantically reversible sentences, such information is dictated by the sentence (surface) structure.

The Mapping Deficit Hypothesis

A series of studies investigated the problem of word order in agrammatic production and in asyntactic comprehension. Saffran et al. (1980a,b) concluded that a fundamental problem undermining production was an inability to produce surface structure orders (NP V NP) to reflect the underlying thematic roles (agent/patient) that link structure to meaning. Schwartz et al. (1980) similarly concluded that asyntactic comprehension stemmed from an inability to recover the relational structure of sentences from the surface sentence structure. Further studies have demonstrated that the deficit does not arise from failure to obtain representations associated with sentence meaning or structure (Linebarger et al., 1983; Schwartz et al., 1987). The deficit is identified as one of *mapping* between the intact Functional and Positional Level representations.

There are two variants of thematic mapping implicated by the mapping deficit hypothesis (Saffran et al., 1980a; Saffran & Schwartz, 1988; Schwartz et al., 1987). "Lexical" mapping refers to the exploitation of verb-specific mapping information, and fulfills the requirements needed to assign thematic agent to grammatical subject. A "procedural" mapping operation governs thematic role assignment for sentences that require the interpretation of structural cues (word order, verb morphology) in order to relate the surface structure NPs to underlying sentence meaning. Saffran & Schwartz (1988) suggest that impaired "lexical" mapping explains aphasic sensitivity to the argument structure of verbs, even in canonical sentences where the deep and surface structure roles are aligned. "Procedural" mapping impairment is the source of difficulties inherent in sentences in that require a shift of verb arguments from their (deep) grammatical representations to their surface structure realization, i.e., noncanonical sentences.

APPLYING THE MODEL TO TREATMENT OF APHASIA

Therapy studies designed using the cognitive neuropsychological approach have consistently demonstrated that it is possible to change the sentence-processing abilities of aphasic patients (Mitchum et al., in press). Participants in cognitive neuropsychological treatment studies tend to be chronically aphasic, showing stable, residual cognitive-linguistic impairments that (in many cases) are not responsive to traditional speech-language therapy. Nevertheless, in these experimental treatments, it has been common to observe a significant change in language function within the first few sessions of treatment. Although there have been some attempts to describe the clinical potential of these treatment studies, the endeavor remains largely oriented to research.

Components of a Cognitive Neuropsychological Treatment Study

As yet, there is no set protocol for cognitive neuropsychological assessment or intervention (but see Schwartz et al., 1995). There is, however, some general uniformity in the fundamental design across various studies.

Baseline

A pre-therapy series of tests is selected or designed using the theoretical model as a guide. An attempt is made to isolate and test the function of each subcomponent that contributes to a processing domain. For example, sentence production (in a picture description task) minimally requires perception of the picture stimulus, formation of Message, Functional and Positional Level representations, and articulation of the response. Impaired processing could arise from a disturbance at one (or more) of these subcomponents. As tests are completed, the investigator attempts to identify "where" and/or "how" normal processing has failed, thus forming a "hypothesis" of the possible underlying cause of impaired processing (Byng & Coltheart, 1986; Seron & Deloche, 1989).

The types of tasks that reveal these highly specific problems are not typically found in standardized measures. Instead, they are mostly created by researchers who are trained to select stimuli, and to design tasks that either support or disconfirm a working hypothesis of the nature of the deficit as it relates to a model of normal language function (Mitchum, 1994; Mitchum & Berndt, 1992). Some tests are published (Bishop, 1982; Kay et al., 1992; Howard & Patterson, 1992), while others are unique to the assessment at hand (e.g., Byng, 1988; Jones, 1986; Mitchum et al., 1995; Mitchum, 1991).

Therapy

It is generally agreed that even the most explicit model-based analysis of language dysfunction does not reveal what to do in therapy (Byng, 1988; Hillis, 1993; Mitchum & Berndt, 1992; Wilson & Patterson, 1990). Nevertheless, reference to a theory of normal language processing provides a basis for predicting how various stimuli will influence processing, and how stimulus complexity can be systematically manipulated over the course of intervention (Mitchum, 1991; Mitchum et al., 1995). For example, the selection of verbs that function equally as transitive and intransitive can be used to build sentence production skills systematically from S+V, to V+S, and finally S+V+O sentences without changing the lexical (verb) content of the practice materials (Crystal, 1984). Rather than serving simply as a stimulus-response mechanism, therapy tasks motivated by normal processing models are designed to convey information to the patient about how the stimuli can be processed.

Outcome

A post-therapy assessment is obtained to measure changes in performance that are attributable to the intervention. The success of therapy is measured by the ability to accomplish the therapy task, as well as by the generalization of learned skills to untreated materials and conditions of processing (Mitchum, 1991; Mitchum et al., 1995). The model assists in predicting which language and cognitive functions may be functionally related to the operation(s) targeted in therapy. It can be expected that functionally related operations will show some change in processing as an indirect consequence of treatment. Some studies also assess a theoretically unrelated cognitive function before and after therapy as a means of demonstrating that post-therapy changes were, in fact, specific to the therapy, and not the result of a coincidental general improvement in cognitive function (see Byng & Coltheart, 1986).

Interpretation

Treatment studies guided by and interpreted from a normal language model serve to highlight the strength and weakness of the normal theory. Some results can support, and even inform the developing model (e.g., Berndt & Mitchum, 1993; Mitchum et al., 1995). In any case, a retrospective analysis of the original hypothesis provides a means of interpreting the effects of therapy (Byng et al., 1994). This aspect of the intervention study provides valuable insight regarding the predictive power of assessment materials, and furthers our understanding of how cognitive functions respond to intervention. For example, patterns of generalization can reflect widespread changes in cognitive function (Mitchum et al., 1995), or may reveal the application of strategies that simply allow for successful response to the therapy task (e.g., Haendiges et al., 1996).

Sentence Processing Therapy

Several examples of the model-driven approach to sentence processing therapy are described below. Although the details of treatment differ widely, each of these studies is structured around the premise of the Mapping Deficit Hypothesis (see previously). Treatment is designed to improve mapping between sentence structure and sentence meaning. In the context of Garrett's model, the general goal of therapy is to establish a link between the Functional and Positional Level representations of the sentence. The review below focuses only on the basic outcome of mapping therapy studies in order to draw some general conclusions of the effect of this treatment approach. Further details, particularly regarding assessment tests and therapy procedures, are available in the published studies.

Sentence Production Therapy: Functional to Positional Level Mapping

Verb Retrieval and Sentence Production

Even the most severely impaired aphasic speakers respond well to therapy to improve verb retrieval (Fink et al., 1997; Weigle-Crump & Koenigsnecht, 1973; Weinrich et al., 1997). However, research has shown that despite the strong correlation between poor verb retrieval and poor sentence construction, the sentence production abilities of agrammatic speakers are not necessarily improved by the availability of lexical verbs. This has been shown both in cases in which verb retrieval is unimpaired (Caramazza & Hillis, 1989; Maher et al., 1995; Marshall et al., 1998), and when agrammatic speakers are given a verb to use in a sentence (Berndt et al., 1997; Caplan & Hanna, 1998). This suggests that therapy to improve retrieval of single words may have no impact on the ability to produce the same words in sentences, at least for verbs.

Mitchum and Berndt (1994) and Mitchum et al. (1993) studied the relationship between verb retrieval therapy and sentence production in two chronic aphasic speakers. In terms of superficial symptoms of aphasia, M.L. (7 years post-onset) and E.A. (8 years post-onset) were clinically different. M.L. was fluent, yet showed all the features associated with agrammatic production: reduced phrase structure, use of simple sentence structures, poor verb retrieval in sentence production and impaired use of verb-related grammatical morphemes. Comprehension was asyntactic (Mitchum & Berndt, 1994). E.A. was severely nonfluent. Although he could not produce sentences verbally, his attempts at written sentence production revealed the same pattern of response elicited verbally from M.L. (see Mitchum et al., 1993).

For both M.L. and E.A., it was hypothesized that facile availability of verbs would improve sentence production if, in fact, poor verb retrieval was a source of the sentence production impairment. The same technique to improve verb retrieval was used to elicit a verbal (M.L.) or written (E.A.) response: repeated naming of action pictures using several exemplars of a small set of action verbs. As criterion performance was reached for each verb (correct response initiated within 3 seconds), a new verb was added systematically until eight verbs were easily named in a rapid, random presentation. The treatment successfully established facile retrieval of eight verbs, and criterion level naming was sustained for at least 1 month following therapy. Nevertheless, the effect on sentence production was limited to a slight increase in attempts to include a verb in sentences, with no improvement in sentence structure.

For example:

Picture: *a man cutting a rope.*
M.L. before therapy: "Tom was takin' a rope and takin' a scissors."
after therapy: "Tom is a hope and then the bends".

Even in the few responses that included a relevant verb, both patients demonstrated difficulty incorporating the verb into a sentence:

Picture: *a woman kissing a baby.*
M.L. before therapy: "My wife was very pretty because these a baby".
after therapy: "The mother and her baby are...the mother is very...the kiss".
Picture: *a girl riding a bike.*
E.A. before therapy: "THE GIRL IS THE BIKE" (written response)
after therapy: "THE GIRL WAS RIDE BY HIS BIKE" (written response)

The finding that improved verb retrieval does not generalize spontaneously to improved sentence production has been replicated (Reichmann-Novak & Rochon, 1997; Weinrich et al., 1997a). Even in cases where improved verb retrieval is accompanied by changes in the number of verb arguments produced with the verb, there is no effect on the grammatical structure of attempted sentences (Byng et al., 1994; Marshall et al., 1993).

In a recent study of verb retrieval therapy, Marshall et al. (1998) reported an immediate effect of improved verb retrieval on sentence production. Treatment targeted the nonfluent, agrammatic production of a chronic aphasic speaker (E.M.). However, the results of therapy may be attributable to the relative nature of her language impairment. Although her production was similar to that of other patients studied (poor verb retrieval along with impaired use of grammatical morphemes), her intact ability to comprehend semantically reversible sentences indicated that she could process thematic role relations, at least for comprehension. It is possible that the availability of Functional Level information enhanced the outcome of E.M.'s production therapy compared to the other patients described above.

It is also significant that the therapy described in Marshall et al. (1998) was qualitatively different from the simple picture naming therapy used in the other studies. For E.M., therapy focused on semantic tasks to establish verb meaning. Tasks paired nouns and verbs based on functional relational similarities (i.e., E.M. was asked to "access verbs from provided nouns," or "to generate verbs in response to a spoken scenario," Marshall et al., 1998, p. 174). Although sentence production was not overtly practiced, the pairing of nouns and verbs in therapy may have engaged (or stimulated) the processing of predicate-argument relations

at the Functional Level representation of normal sentence production.

The different effects of single-word retrieval therapy on sentence production demonstrate how various therapies can "exercise" the components of the production process. The therapies that practice simple stimulation of action words with pictures may address only a part of the verb's lexical representation. If the therapy task stimulates only production of the phonological word form (devoid of semantic and thematic requirements), it may address problems of retrieval at the Positional Level, while leaving the earlier (Functional Level) representations of the sentence production process "untouched" by intervention. If there is an indication of additional impairment involving the Functional Level representation (e.g., if sentence comprehension is poor), the treatment predictably would not affect sentence production. These findings stress the value of directing sentence processing therapy at the earliest level(s) of processing that may be impaired.

Grammatical Frame Construction

The findings from verb retrieval therapy studies clearly have indicated that verb availability does not automatically drive the construction of a Positional Level planning frame. This result prompted Mitchum et al. (1993; see also Mitchum et al., 1994) to reconsider their interpretation of the essential problem underlying the impaired sentence production of M.L. and E.A. A second therapy tested the hypothesis that the verb was of no use to an aphasic speaker if there was no grammatical frame available for verb insertion. This hypothesis led to a therapy designed to improve production of the (Positional Level) planning frame.

Although a task of sentence repetition might "practice" production of Positional Level planning frames, it was considered crucial to link grammatical frame construction to earlier levels of processing. The goal was to provide a therapy task that would initiate construction of a planning frame in a natural manner. A treatment to force grammatical frame construction targeted sentences in which verb morphology contrasted future, present, and past tense action. Sentences were matched to sequential action pictures (e.g., the horse /will jump/, /is jumping/, /has jumped/ the fence). A pretest verified that both M.L. and E.A. appreciated the logical order of three sequential depictions of a simple action. Therapy focused on a series of tasks to assist them in producing a sentence to describe each event in the sequence. The goal was to establish general availability of three different grammatical frames.

As shown in Figure 24–5, M.L. and E.A. learned to produce the trained grammatical "frames" for both trained and untrained stimuli, and applied the skill in other tasks of production. Moreover, both M.L. and E.A included a wide range of (untreated) verbs in the post-therapy sentences they

example series of sequential action pictures

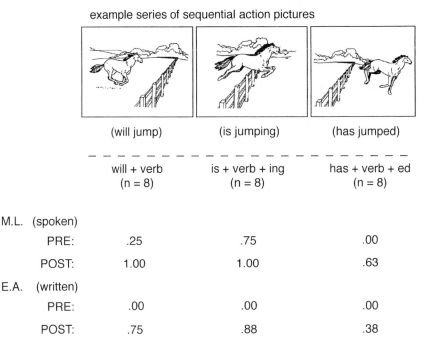

	will + verb (n = 8)	is + verb + ing (n = 8)	has + verb + ed (n = 8)
M.L. (spoken)			
PRE:	.25	.75	.00
POST:	1.00	1.00	.63
E.A. (written)			
PRE:	.00	.00	.00
POST:	.75	.88	.38

Figure 24–5. Example of training materials used in a treatment to improve production of grammatical sentence frames (Mitchum et al., 1993; Mitchum & Berndt, 1994). Proportion of sentences produced with the targeted verb form from two patients, before and after therapy, are shown.

produced. All responses used trained sentence structures, or some close alternative. No generalization to noncanonical structures, such as passive, was obtained.

Direct Training of Passive Sentence Production

Two recent studies have used Garrett's production model to interpret the results of direct training in passive sentence production. Riechman-Novak and Rochon (1997) provided therapy to an agrammatic speaker (D.L.) who demonstrated very poor lexical verb retrieval, limited production of grammatical morphemes, and impaired production and comprehension of semantically reversible sentences. The treatment used the picture naming task described by Mitchum and Berndt (1994) and Mitchum et al. (1993) to improve lexical verb retrieval, and yielded a similar outcome: action verb naming improved with therapy but had no effect on sentence production. This result was followed by a treatment that focused on construction of grammatical frames using a combination of the sequential pictures therapy described in Mitchum and Berndt (1994) and the sentence-query paradigm of Schwartz et al. (1994; described below). The results yielded an increase in the production of passive sentence structures, but at the expense of (previously intact) active sentence production. This result demonstrates that changes obtained in response to therapy do not always reflect substantive improvement of sentence processing.

Another direct passive production therapy targeted an unusual pattern of production observed in a chronic aphasic speaker (Mitchum et al., in press). A.L., who was 1 year post-onset, demonstrated intact sentence comprehension. His production of active sentences was flawless. The preservation of these abilities made his *in*ability to produce passive sentences all the more striking. In picture description tasks, A.L. could easily produce an S+V+O sentence when allowed to start his response with the agentive noun (e.g., "the girl is kicking the boy"). Nevertheless, he found it impossible to produce a sentence when constrained to start with the nonagentive noun. Whenever possible, he made use of verbs and or sentence structures that avoided passive sentence production (Table 24–1). When he was unable to use this avoidance strategy, his responses showed a striking deficit of verb retrieval. This yielded a pattern of intact verb retrieval for active sentences, but not for passive sentences, to describe the same pictures. Since thematic mapping was intact for comprehension, this production pattern indicated that production-specific thematic mapping rules were available for the expression of active sentence structures, yet remained unavailable for production of passive sentences. This profile is highly consistent with many of the post-therapy production patterns that have been reported (e.g., Byng et al., 1994; Marshall et al., 1998; Schwartz et al., 1994). The occurrence of this profile in A.L. before treatment provides an important demonstration that the pattern is not exclusively a result of the limited effects of intervention.

TABLE 24-1

Sample of A.L.'s Responses in a Picture Description Task.

Stimulus	Active	Passive
girl kicking a boy	"The girl is kicking the boy."	"The boy is perturbed because the girl is kicking the boy."
man drinking tea	"The man is drinking from the cup."	"The tea is hot."
man cutting a rope	"The man is cutting the rope."	"The rope is...piecemeal."
boy eating an apple	"The boy is eating the apple."	"The apple...is paramount."
girl riding bike	"The girl is riding the bike."	"The bike is...not very pretty."
boy pushing a box	"The boy is fixing the boxes."	"The box......."
horse jumping a fence	"The horse is jumping."	"The fence......"

Responses are Constrained by the Requirement That the Sentences Start with the Agent Noun (for Active Targets) or Nonagent Noun (for Passive Targets). The Same Picture is Used in Separate Test Sessions to Elicit Each Type of Sentence.

Therapy to improve A.L.'s production of passive sentences focused on two levels (Mitchum et al., in press). It was hypothesized that intact mapping for sentence comprehension might place A.L. among the rare good candidates for direct production therapy without the need to attend to Functional Level representations (which presumably were intact to support mapping for sentence comprehension). A therapy exploited his intact sentence repetition by practicing repetition of active and passive sentences. Despite the achievement of fluent and errorless repetition of passive sentences, this approach yielded no change in his ability to form passive sentences in tasks of picture description. A second treatment focused on the generation of sentence structures to express a particular meaning, i.e., the treatment targeted the mapping from Functional to Positional Level representations. A treatment task using word anagrams capitalized on A.L.'s intact reading and comprehension of active sentences. The goal of treatment was to demonstrate to A.L. that actives and passive sentences can express essentially the same meaning, but require different grammatical frames. Initially, passive sentences were "produced" by arranging anagram words into a passive sentence to express the same meaning as the active (model) sentences. As therapy progressed, the tasks grew increasingly difficult by forcing random anagram "production" of actives and passives, and eventually culminated (over 12 1-hour therapy sessions) in his ability to produce verbal counterparts (active or passive) to spoken model sentences. Post-therapy assessments showed a significant improvement in A.L.'s production of passive sentences in picture descriptions tasks, with no concurrent decline in active sentence production.

The successful outcome of A.L.'s production therapy was attributed to the focus on linking sentence meaning (which he obtained via intact comprehension of active sentences) and sentence structure (which he gained in exercises involving anagram manipulations). This was contrasted with the poor results obtained from repetition therapy in which no attempt was made to link production of the passive sentence structures to any form of sentence meaning. We view this finding as further evidence in favor of the general view that therapy must attempt to link early levels of linguistic processing to later production in order to establish changes in production that are not stimulus dependent, but rather are driven by the speaker's desire to express a message.

Sentence Comprehension Therapy: Positional to Functional Level Mapping

Sentence-Query Therapy

One of the first treatment studies to target a hypothesized mapping deficit was designed for a man who was 6 years post-onset of aphasia. Jones (1986) outlined a series of diagnostic tests that led her to attribute B.B.'s impaired sentence processing to an inability to exploit lexical mapping rules. Comprehension of semantically reversible sentences was poor. His speech was nonfluent and agrammatic. Although he readily produced verbs in tasks of picture naming, he was unable to use verbs in sentences. Occasionally, with a great deal of help, he was able to produce a simple SVO sentence.

Therapy was carried out in a series of steps over the course of about 9 months. Using B.B.'s intact ability to parse written sentences into NP, VP phrases, Jones describes a therapy that forced B.B. to parse the sentence, identify the lexical verb, then systematically determine the argument relations of the verb by answering questions regarding specific thematic roles. A focus on "input" was maintained by having B.B. use color-coded markings on the written sentence to identify (first) the lexical verb, and systematically respond to queries regarding "who is doing the action" and "to whom the action is done." Stimuli were selected to be progressively more challenging. Initial exercises used nonreversible sentences, then reversible sentences. Adjectives and prepositional phrases gradually were added and, finally, passive sentences were introduced.

TABLE 24-2

Examples of Responses from B.B. in a Task of Spoken Picture Description Before and After Therapy Designed to Improve Reversible Sentence *Comprehension*

Target Sentence	Response Before Therapy	Response After Therapy
The boy is kicking the ball	eh...um...push...pu...no...ball...no	eh..kick the ball...boy is kicking the ball
The boy is riding the bike	girl..no boy...bike...well...um...boy	The girl....is riding...a bike
The girl is writing a letter	writing../r/../r/..read...girl	Letter! the girl....is writing...a letter..to eh..friend.
The boy is painting a picture	eh..boy..no girl..um don't know.	The boy is...painting...eh..a picture... a house. Good!
The boy is digging the garden	/g/../g/..don't know (cue) garden...boy..is no	The boy...is digging...his garden.
The boy is eating an apple	boy..no (pointing to apple) drink...no	Eating an apple..eh..the girl...no boy... is eating an apple.

(Reprinted with permission from Jones, 1986).

Following therapy, B.B.'s ability to interpret active and passive semantically reversible sentences was significantly improved from baseline. Although Jones describes therapy as strictly targeting sentence comprehension, changes in sentence production were noted. Post-therapy sentences produced by B.B. revealed an increased number of sentences that included a lexical main verb with at least two (noun) arguments (Table 24–2).

An Expansion of Sentence-Query Therapy

To address the goal of developing a generally applicable approach to sentence processing therapy, Schwartz et al. (1994) greatly expanded the treatment used by Jones (1986). The therapy included three distinct phases that systematically varied verb type and sentence structure. This was planned as a means of assessing how intervention using a particular verb type and/or sentence structure would generalize to comprehension of untrained verbs and sentences (Table 24–3). To test the general applicability of the therapy, they selected a group of treatment candidates who showed various symptoms of impaired thematic mapping in production and/or comprehension.

Schwartz and colleagues completed the therapy program with five aphasic speakers and one person with asyntactic comprehension, but intact grammatical production. The outcome was variable among the group, despite the fact that the same therapy was given to patients showing the same essential symptom (i.e., impaired comprehension and/or production of reversible sentences). Although the treatment primarily targeted reversible sentence comprehension, significant improvement in comprehension was noted for only two of the six who were treated. However, as observed for B.B. (Jones, 1986), the comprehension-based therapy yielded significant gains in sentence production. Increased use of main verbs and verb arguments was observed in all but the most severely impaired of the group.

The findings of Schwartz et al. (1994) clearly indicate improved thematic mapping between the grammatical subject and the thematic agent for production and comprehension of reversible active sentences. Nevertheless, the treatment had little effect on the production and comprehension of passive sentences. Schwartz et al. (1994) hypothesized that the demands of the training task may have overtaxed patients, thus limiting the effectiveness of training for some patients in some conditions. In a follow-up to the original sentence-query therapy study, Fink et al. (1998) provided therapy to an additional 9 aphasic speakers selected for evidence of agrammatic production and some degree of asyntactic sentence comprehension. This treatment used only transitive verbs and, importantly, introduced a variety of modifications to facilitate comprehension of all semantically reversible sentence types, including passive structures. The initial phase of the study first trained canonical (active), then noncanonical (passive and object cleft) sentences. Seven of the nine study participants responded to training, but only 1 person showed a pattern of change indicative of improved sentence comprehension. Fink and colleagues interpreted the patterns of change in sentence processing for 5 of the group as reflecting a weak task heuristically related to overgeneralization of the response being trained. That is, training with active sentences led to an interpretation of all sentences (including noncanonical) as thematically mapping subject noun to the role of agent; training with passives led to all sentences (including canonical) mapping object noun to the role of agent. A second group of 6 agrammatic speakers (nonparticipants in the first study) showed a similar task-specific response to the query condition. Schwartz et al. (1994) concluded that their attempt to accommodate more therapy candidates by reducing the demands of the noncanonical phase of sentence-query therapy was successful with only a very small percentage of the 15 candidates selected for treatment.

TABLE 24–3

Design of Stimulus Materials Used in a Therapy to Improve Comprehension of Reversible Sentences. Phases A and B Contrasted Different Verb Types (Action vs. Emotion) in Canonical Sentences. Phases A and C Contrasted Different Action Verbs in Canonical vs. Noncanonical Sentences.

Phase A: Action Verbs in Canonical Sentences

Target Structures:	*Examples:*
1) Subj and Obj NPs	Susan drinks the soda.
2) Adj in Sub position	The old man is fixing it.
3) Adj in Obj position	Ann washed the playful child.
4) Complex Subj NP	Tommy's grandfather built the wall.
5) Complex Obj NP	Jan called the person in charge.
6) Complex Subj and Obj NPs	The girl from the office was helping Mary's daughter.

Phase B: Emotion Verbs in Canonical Sentences

Target structures (same as above)
Target verbs used in sentences (see, know, love, want, hear, need, believe, like, forget, hate)

Phase C: Action Verbs in Noncanonical Sentences

Target Structures:	*Examples:*
1) Passive	Ann was pushed by the neighbor.
2) Cleft object	It was the window that John cleaned this morning.
3) Cleft subject	It was Sam that cut Joe.
4) Object relative (embedded in obj NP)	They saw the play that Tom wrote.
5) Object relative (embedded in subj NP)	The bus that the girl rode was yellow.
6) Subject relative (embedded in subj NP)	The girl that kissed the picture was sad.

(Reprinted with permission from Schwartz et al., 1994).

To date, the findings of the several approaches to mapping therapy have demonstrated that therapy designed to improve sentence *comprehension* often yields substantially improved *production* of semantically reversible, canonical sentences (Byng et al., 1994; Nickels et al., 1991; Schwartz et al., 1994). For the most part, production changes have been attributed to improved verb retrieval with a correlated increase in the number of noun arguments included in a sentence. The general finding is limited to the mapping of thematic agent to grammatical subject, even when an attempt is made to train other mapping possibilities (Schwartz et al., 1994). The few participants who also learned to map thematic agent to grammatical object (e.g., for passive sentences) were relatively mildly impaired in associated language functions.

Implicit Feedback Therapy

A different series of studies targeted the asyntactic comprehension of three aphasic speakers (Berndt & Mitchum, 1997; Haendiges et al., 1996; Mitchum et al., 1995). The treatment candidates were selected on the basis of showing poor comprehension of semantically reversible (active/passive) sentences. Though they differed broadly in speech fluency, naming, and other skills, all demonstrated poor sentence production, with characteristics of impaired thematic mapping in attempted sentence productions. Preliminary attempts to use a sentence-query approach were met with difficulty interpreting the *wh*-probe questions (Mitchum et al., 1995). A treatment paradigm was designed with the goal to instill an implicit realization that active and passive sentences could express the same meaning using different structural forms.

A treatment similar to the standard picture-matching procedure used to identify asyntactic comprehension was devised. An active or passive sentence was spoken and a picture verification response was required. In one version of the task, a spoken sentence was matched (by pointing) to one of two pictures (the target vs. its semantic-reversal as a foil). Another version of the task paired one picture with a spoken sentence. Active and passive sentences were interspersed in a random series of "yes" and "no" (i.e., matching, nonmatching) trials. The element of therapy added to the basic matching task was a systematic feedback procedure (Figure 24–6). If a spoken sentence was correctly matched to a picture, the correct response was acknowledged and reinforced as the therapist pointed (simultaneously) to each pictured element while saying the correct sentence as "feedback." Incorrect responses were immediately identified as incorrect, and followed up with the correct sentence spoken as the relevant action and actor were pointed out. The treatment stimuli included 10 transitive verbs controlled for a variety of factors to prevent the use of nonlinguistic strategies (e.g., spatial order of the nouns, number of active vs. passive sentence trials, etc.).

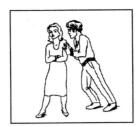

FEEDBACK: (For correct responses)

Spoken Sentence	Target response	Actual response	Feedback
(active)			
"The man is pushing the woman"	yes	"yes"	"That's right. The man is pushing the woman."
"The woman is pushing the man"	no	"no"	"That's right, it's the other way. The man is pushing the woman."
(passive)			
"The woman is pushed by the man"	yes	"yes"	"That's right. The woman is pushed by the man."
"The man is pushed by the woman"	no	"no"	"That's right, it's the other way. The woman is pushed by the man."

FEEDBACK: (For incorrect responses)

Spoken Sentence	Target response	Actual response	Feedback
(active)			
"The man is pushing the woman"	yes	"no"	"It's yes. The man is pushing the woman."
"The woman is pushing the man"	no	"yes"	"No. It was wrong. The man is pushing the woman."
(passive)			
"The woman is pushed by the man"	yes	"no"	"It's yes. The woman is pushed by the man."
"The man is pushed by the woman"	no	"yes"	"No. It was wrong. The woman is pushed by the man."

Figure 24–6. Example of the implicit feedback training procedure for improving active and passive reversible sentence comprehension. The patient looks at the picture as the sentence is spoken. Feedback is contingent upon each response.

Two of the three participants in the sentence comprehension therapy reached criterion performance with the treatment materials, and the third participant improved to within a very close range. A unique learning pattern was exhibited by each of the participants. Considerable gains were observed in the post-therapy comprehension of active and passive reversible sentences.

Various patterns of post-therapy generalization were demonstrated among the group. M.L. showed the strongest evidence of generalized improvement, with excellent performance in a variety of (untrained) comprehension tests (Mitchum et al., 1995). His only failure in the generalization measures were with very long sentences that arguably were beyond his auditory retention span. E.A. showed similar strong gains in treatment (Haendiges et al., 1996). However, his ability to comprehend passive sentences appeared to rely on the full expression of the "by" phrase. This outcome was interpreted as successful, but only for helping E.A. to establish a superficial strategy for detecting the structural cues of the noncanonical sentence form. F.M., who routinely performed just below criterion level in therapy,

showed limited generalization (Berndt & Mitchum, 1997). An analysis of the sentences he learned to comprehend (active and passive) showed an effect of sensitivity to specific verbs. That is, the sentences that F.M. easily learned contained verbs that required active agents and relatively stationary patients (or themes) (e.g., wash, splash, find, hold, hit). The verbs to which he responded poorly in training and assessment depicted relatively equal activity levels for both agent and patient (theme) (e.g., tow, pay, follow, chase). It is noteworthy that similar findings of sensitivity to specific verbs in response to sentence production therapy have been reported (Byng et al., 1994; Marshall et al., 1997). These results suggest that treatment outcome for both production and comprehension may be influenced by the semantic and/or thematic properties of the verbs used in treatment.

Contributions from Mapping Therapy Studies

Our understanding of the effects of thematic mapping therapy is far from complete. Nonetheless, collected attempts to structure therapy from a specific model of normal language function has enlightened our understanding of sentence processing impairments in aphasia.

The Nature of the Mapping Impairment

The details of how thematic role relations are linked to sentence structures are not well understood. In Schwartz's (1987) interpretation of Garrett's model, the assignment of grammatical roles is complete when a Functional Level representation has been created. However, as Byng (1986) has emphasized, it is unclear how, and at what point, thematic roles are available. The implication is that thematic mapping information is available from earlier, Message Level representations (Bock & Levelt, 1994). Mapping therapy data appear to support an early (Message Level) locus of thematic mapping. Several studies have shown that patients selected for mapping therapy on the basis of "asyntactic comprehension" differ widely in their response to mapping therapy (Byng et al., 1994; Schwartz et al., 1994; Mitchum et al., in press). Although a variety of factors can undermine outcome, it is clear in some cases that the comprehension deficit is associated with a fundamental inability to derive a conceptual-linguistic understanding of the pictured event (Byng et al., 1994; Marshall et al., 1993).

Saffran and Schwartz (1988) suggested that the mapping function may be different for different sentence types. Verb-centered mapping therapies (e.g., sentence-query therapies), which arguably stress verb-stated mapping rules, frequently report improved processing of active sentences accompanied rarely by any change in passive sentence processing (Byng et al., 1994; Schwartz et al., 1994). Passive sentence processing, however, has responded to therapy focused on the surface structure cues to sentence meaning (word order and structural morphology), with no special attention to the verb (Mitchum et al., 1995; Haendiges et al., 1996; Berndt & Mitchum, 1997; Mitchum et al., in press). This finding suggests that different approaches to mapping therapy exercise different mapping functions. Verb-centered mapping treatment affects lexical mapping functions, perhaps linking Functional Level grammatical role relations to conceptual (Message Level) meaning. The attention to surface structure may better accommodate the mapping requirements needed to mediate between the Positional Level representation and sentence meaning.

The Relationship between Production and Comprehension

The findings from thematic mapping therapy have some bearing on the issue of the sentence production/comprehension relationship. Treatments stressing verb-centered mapping have consistently reported spontaneous generalization from comprehension to production. The main finding—predicted from enhanced use of lexical mapping rules—is an increased number of verb arguments produced in sentences (Byng, 1986; Schwartz et al., 1994). Significant production changes have not emerged from comprehension therapy targeting the structural interpretation of sentence meaning (e.g., the implicit-feedback approach). The results thus far suggest that lexically stated mapping rules are relevant to both production and comprehension, whereas procedural operations exercise over modality-specific domains.

The Therapy Process

Mapping therapy studies demonstrate how intervention can be guided by a model of normal sentence processing. This approach assists in interpreting the underlying problems that give rise to surface symptoms, thus allowing treatment to target relevant subcomponents of sentence processing. The most successful treatments were those that attempted to link together the full range of processing subcomponents, rather than attempting to isolate therapy within a single component.

FUTURE TRENDS

We suggested that the cognitive neuropsychological studies of sentence processing disorders have been conducted largely as a research endeavor. Nevertheless, there is some expectation that aspects of these intervention studies should be clinically relevant. What they have shown, collectively, is that (1) remarkable changes in complex cognitive functions (such as sentence processing) can be obtained even in cases of chronic aphasia; (2) the changes obtained are arguably related to a course of intervention, and not to a generalized improvement of cognitive function; and (3) specific subcomponents of processing appear to respond selectively to different approaches to therapy.

The challenge ahead for this research endeavor is to broaden the base of fundamental research studies that explore the cognitive response to language intervention. The most immediate issues in sentence processing therapy studies include improving the predictive power of pre-therapy assessments tests, and refining our ability to interpret the diverse range of intervention outcomes. Another application of this methodology, as yet unexplored, is its ability to predict and interpret traditional approaches to the treatment of sentence processing impairments. In some cases, the unexplained and variable results commonly obtained in therapy would benefit from the level of scrutiny applied to cognitive neuropsychological interventions.

▶ *Acknowledgment*–The preparation of this paper was supported by grant R01-DC00262 from the National Institute on Deafness and Other Communication Disorders to the University of Maryland School of Medicine.

KEY POINTS

1. Although theoretical models of normal sentence processing are incomplete, they can provide some understanding of the mental operations involved in the production and comprehension of sentences. We described a model of sentence production that has been used to interpret aphasic sentence processing and, more recently, has served as a guide to treatment of sentence processing disorders.

2. Impaired production and comprehension of sentences observed in aphasia can be interpreted in the context of normal sentence processing models. Abnormal patterns of language processing can be attributed to failure to obtain necessary mental representations, or to an inability to make use of available information. In general, patterns of aphasic production and comprehension do not appear to reflect selective impairment to components of the normal sentence processing models. Even so, the model provides a context for interpreting how the complex symptoms of language impairment may be functionally related. For example, we discussed various ways in which the inability to retrieve verbs can interfere with sentence production.

3. An interpretation of aphasic language in the context of normal language does not dictate what to do to improve language processing. Nevertheless, we describe several sentence processing treatment studies that demonstrate how a model of normal sentence processing can sharpen the focus of treatment, assist in task design, and guide the selection of therapy materials.

4. Treatment studies based on a cognitive neuropsychological interpretation of sentence processing impairments in aphasia are largely conducted as a research endeavor. Although the treatment approaches described here may have some clinical application, the goal of these studies is not to demonstrate the efficacy of a particular therapy. Rather, the motivation for cognitive neuropsychological treatment research is to develop a basis for interpreting how cognitive functions respond to intervention. For example, many of the studies of therapy designed to improve thematic mapping had little impact on the functional communication abilities of the treated patients. Nevertheless, studying the response to therapy enhanced the interpretation of the deficit, and led to a refined understanding of the cognitive functions that support sentence processing. While the immediate application of individual cognitive neuropsychological treatment studies may be limited, it is important to recognize the possible contribution of this research to a better understanding of cognitive intervention in general.

References

Ansell, B.J. & Flowers, C.R. (1982). Aphasic adults' use of heuristic and structural linguistic cues for sentence analysis. *Brain and Language, 96*, 64–72.

Berndt, R.S. (2000). Sentence Production. In B. Rapp (ed.), *Handbook of cognitive neuropsychology*, Philadelphia: Psychology Press.

Berndt, R.S. (1991). Sentence processing in aphasia. In M.T. Sarno (ed.), *Acquired aphasia* (2nd ed.). New York: Academic Press.

Berndt, R.S. (1998). Sentence processing in aphasia. In M.T. Sarno (ed.), *Acquired aphasia* (3rd ed.) (pp. 229–267). San Diego, CA: Academic Press.

Berndt, R.S. & Caramazza, A. (1980). A redefinition of the syndrome of Broca's aphasia: Implications for a neuropsychological model of language. *Applied Psycholinguistics, 1*, 225–278.

Berndt, R.S., Haendiges, A.N., Mitchum, C.M., & Sandson, J. (1997). Verb retrieval in aphasia. 2. Relationship to sentence processing. *Brain and Language, 56*, 107–137.

Berndt, R.S., Haendiges, A.N., & Wozniak, M.A. (1997). Verb retrieval and sentence processing: Dissociation of an established symptom association. *Cortex, 33*, 99–114.

Berndt, R.S. & Mitchum, C.C. (1993). Approaches to the rehabilitation of phonological assembly: Elaborating the model of nonlexical reading. In G. Humphreys & J. Riddoch (eds.), *Cognitive neuropsychology and cognitive rehabilitation*. London: Erlbaum.

Berndt, R.S. & Mitchum, C.C. (1997). An experimental treatment of sentence comprehension. In N. Helm-Estabrooks & A. Holland (eds.), *Approaches to the treatment of aphasia*. San Diego, CA: Singular Publication Group.

Berndt, R.S., Mitchum, C.C., & Haendiges, A.N. (1996). Comprehension of reversible sentences in "agrammatism": A meta-analysis. *Cognition, 58*, 289–308.

Berndt, R.S., Mitchum, C.C., & Wayland, S. (1997). Patterns of sentence comprehension in aphasia: A consideration of three hypotheses. *Brain and Language, 60*, 197–221.

Bishop, D.V.M. (1982). *Test for the Reception of Grammar (TROG)*. London: Medical Research Council.

Bock, K. & Levelt, W. (1994). Language production. Grammatical encoding. In M.A. Gernsbacher (ed.), *Handbook of psycholinguistics*. San Diego, CA: Academic Press.

Bradley, D.C., Garrett, M.F., & Zurif, E.B. (1980). Syntactic deficits in Broca's aphasia. In D. Caplan (ed.), *Biological studies of mental processes*. Cambridge, MA: MIT Press.

Brown, R. & McNeil, D. (1966). The "tip-of-the-tongue" phenomenon. *Journal of Verbal Learning and Verbal Behavior, 5*, 325–337.

Byng, S. (1986). Sentence processing deficits in aphasia: Investigation and remediation. Unpublished doctoral dissertation, University of London.

Byng, S. (1988). Sentence processing deficits: Theory and therapy. *Cognitive Neuropsychology, 5*, 629–676.

Byng, S. & Coltheart, M. (1986). Aphasia therapy and research: Methodological requirements and illustrative results. In E. Hjelmquist & L.-G. Nilsson (eds.), *Communication handicap: Aspects of psychological compensation and technical aids*. North Holland: Elsevier Science Publishers, B.V.

Byng, S., Nickels, L., & Black, M. (1994). Replicating therapy for mapping deficits in agrammatism: Remapping the deficit? *Aphasiology, 8*, (4), 315–342.

Caplan, D. & Futter, C. (1986). Assignment of thematic roles to nouns in sentence comprehension by an agrammatic patient. *Brain and Language, 27*, 117–134.

Caplan, D. & Hanna, J.E. (1998). Sentence production by aphasic patients in a constrained task. *Brain and Language, 63*, 184–218.

Caplan, D. & Waters, G.S. (1995). Aphasic disorders of syntactic comprehension and working memory capacity. *Cognitive Neuropsychology, 12*, 637–649.

Caramazza, A. (1989). Cognitive neuropsychology and rehabilitation: An unfulfilled promise? In X. Seron & G. Deloche (eds.), *Cognitive approaches in neuropsychological rehabilitation.* Hillsdale, NJ: Lawrence Erlbaum.

Caramazza, A. & Berndt, R.S. (1985). A multicomponent deficit view of agrammatic Broca's aphasia. In M.L. Kean (ed.), *Agrammatism.* New York: Academic Press.

Caramazza, A. & Hillis, A.E. (1989). The disruption of sentence production: Some dissociations. *Brain and Language, 36*, 625–650.

Caramazza, A. & Hillis, A.E. (1993). For a theory of remediation of cognitive deficits. *Neuropsychological Rehabilitation, 3*, 217–234.

Caramazza, A. & Miceli, G. (1991). Selective impairment of thematic role assignment in sentence processing. *Brain and Language, 41*, 402–436.

Chatterjee, A., Maher, L.M., Gonzalez-Rothi, L.J., & Heilman, K.M. (1995). Asyntactic thematic role assignment: The use of a temporal-spatial strategy. *Brain and Language, 49*, 125–139.

Crystal, D. (1984). *Linguistic encounters with language handicap.* New York: Basil Blackwell.

Davis, G.A. (1993). *A survey of adult aphasia and related language disorders* (2nd ed.). Upper Saddle River, NJ: Prentice Hall.

Dell, G.S. (1986). A spreading activation theory of retrieval in sentence production. *Psychological Review, 93*, 283–321.

Dell, G.S., Schwartz, M.F., Martin, N., Saffran, E.M., & Gagnon D.A. (1997). Lexical access in aphasic and nonaphasic speakers. *Psychological Review, 104*, 801–838.

Fink, R.B., Schwartz, M.F., & Myers, J.L. (1998). Investigations of the sentence query approach to mapping therapy. Abstracts of the Academy of Aphasia. *Brain and Language, 65*, 203–207.

Fink, R.B., Schwartz, M.F., Sobel, P.R., & Myers, J.L. (1997). Effects of multilevel training on verb retrieval: Is more always better? *Brain and Language, 60*, 41–44.

Frazier, L. & Friederici, A.D. (1991). On deriving the properties of agrammatic comprehension. *Brain and Language, 40*, 51–66.

Fromkin, V.A. (1971). The non-anomalous nature of anomalous utterances. *Language, 47*, 27–52.

Garrett, M.F. (1975). The analysis of sentence production. In G.H. Bower (ed.), *The Psychology of learning and motivation* (pp. 133–177). London: Academic Press.

Garrett, M.F. (1980). Levels of processing in sentence production. In B. Butterworth (ed.), *Language production, Vol. 1* (pp. 170–220). London: Academic Press.

Garrett, M.F. (1982). Production of speech: Observations from normal and pathological language use. In A. Ellis (ed.), *Normality and pathology in cognitive functions* (pp. 19–76). London: Academic Press.

Garrett, M.F. (1984). The organization of processing structure for language production: Applications to aphasic speech. In D. Caplan, A.R. Lecours, & A. Smith (eds.), *Biological perspectives on language* (p. 174). Cambridge, MA: MIT Press.

Garrett, M.F. (1988). Processes in language production. In F.J. Newmeyer (ed.), *Linguistics: The Cambridge Survey: III. Language: Psychological and biological aspects* (pp. 69–96). Cambridge, UK: Cambridge University Press.

Goodglass, H. (1993). *Understanding aphasia.* San Diego, CA: Academic Press.

Goodglass, H., Klein, B., Carey, P., & Jones, K. (1966). Specific semantic word categories in aphasia. *Cortex, 2*, 74–89.

Grodzinsky, Y. (1984). The syntactic characterization of agrammatism. *Cognition, 42*, 143–180.

Haarmann, H.J. & Kolk, H.H.J. (1991). A computer model of the temporal course of agrammatic sentence understanding: The effects of variation in severity and sentence complexity. *Cognitive Science, 15*, 49–87.

Haendiges, A.N., Berndt , R.S., & Mitchum, C.C. (1996). Assessing the elements contributing to a "mapping" deficit: A targeted treatment study. *Brain and Language, 52*, 276–302.

Hartsuiker, R.J. & Kolk, H.H.J. (1998). Syntactic facilitation in agrammatic sentence production. *Brain and Language, 62*, 221–254.

Heeschen, C. & Kolk, H. (1988). Agrammatism and paragrammatism. *Aphasiology, 2*, 299–302.

Hillis, A.E. (1993). The role of models of language processing in rehabilitation of language impairments. *Aphasiology, 7*, 5–26.

Howard, D. & Patterson, K. (1992). The Palm Trees and Pyramid Test: A test of semantic access from words and pictures. Bury St. Edmonds, UK: Thames Valley Test Company.

Humphreys, G.W. & Riddoch, M.J. (1994). *Cognitive neuropsychology and cognitive rehabilitation.* Hove, UK: Lawrence Erlbaum.

Jones, E.V. (1986). Building the foundations for sentence production in a non-fluent aphasic. *British Journal of Disorders of Communication, 21*, 63–82.

Kay, J., Lesser, R., & Coltheart, M. (1992). *Psycholinguistic assessment of language processing in aphasia.* Hove, UK: Lawrence Erlbaum.

Kean, M.L. (1982). Grammatical representations and the description of language processing. In D. Caplan (ed.), *Biological studies of mental processes* (pp. 239–268). New York: Academic Press.

Kolk, H.H.J. & Heeschen, C. (1985). Agrammatism versus paragrammatism: A shift of behavioral control. Presented at a meeting of the Academy of Aphasia, October 1985, Pittsburgh, PA.

Kolk, H.H.J. & van Grunsven, M.M.F. (1985). Agrammatism as a variable phenomenon. *Cognitive Neuropsychology, 2*, 347–384.

Kremin, H. & Basso, A. (1993). Apropos the mental lexicon: The naming of nouns and verbs. In F.J. Stachowiak, R. deBleser, G. Deloche, R. Kaschel, H. Kremin, P. North, L. Pizzamiglio, L. Robertson, & B. Wilson (eds.), *Developments in the assessment and rehabilitation of brain damaged patients—Perspectives from a European concerted action.* Tubingen: Narr Verlag.

Levelt, W.J.M. (1989). *Speaking: From intention to articulation.* Cambridge, MA: MIT Press.

Linebarger, M.C., Schwartz, M.F., & Saffran, E.M. (1983). Sensitivity to grammatical structure in so-called agrammatic aphasics. *Cognition, 13,* 361–392.

Maher, L.M., Chatterjee, A., Rothi, L.J., & Heilman, K.M. (1995). Agrammatic sentence production: The use of a temporal-spatial strategy. *Brain and Language, 49,* 105–124.

Marshall, J., Chiat, S., & Pring, T. (1997). An impairment in processing verbs' thematic roles: A therapy study. *Aphasiology, 11,* 855–876.

Marshall, J., Pring, T., & Chiat, S. (1993). Sentence processing therapy: Working at the level of the event. *Aphasiology, 7,* 177–199.

Marshall, J., Pring, T., & Chiat, S. (1998). Verb retrieval and sentence production in aphasia. *Brain and Language, 63,* 159–183.

Martin, R. (1995). Working memory doesn't work: A critique of Miyake et al.'s capacity theory of aphasic comprehension deficits. *Cognitive Neuropsychology, 12,* 623–636.

Menn, L. & Obler, L.K. (1990). Cross-language data and theories of agrammatism. In L. Menn & L.K. Obler (eds.), *Agrammatic aphasia, Vol. 2.* Amsterdam: John Benjamins.

Miceli, G., Silveri, M.C., Villa, G., & Caramazza, A. (1984). On the basis for the agrammatics' difficulty in producing main verbs. *Cortex, 20,* 207–220.

Mitchell, D.C. (1994). Sentence parsing. In M.A. Gernsbacher (ed.), *Handbook of psycholinguistics* (pp. 375–409). San Diego, CA: Academic Press.

Mitchum, C.C. (1991). Treatment generalization and the application of cognitive neuropsychological models in aphasia therapy. *NIH monographs: Aphasia treatment: Current approaches and research opportunities* (pp. 99–116).

Mitchum, C.C. (1994). Traditional and contemporary views of aphasia: Implications for clinical management. *Topics in Stroke Rehabilitation, 1,* 14–36.

Mitchum, C.C. & Berndt, R.S. (1992). Clinical linguistics, cognitive neuropsychology and aphasia therapy. *Clinical Linguistics and Phonetics, 6,* 3–10.

Mitchum, C.C. & Berndt, R.S. (1994). Verb retrieval and sentence construction: Effects of targeted intervention. In G. Humphreys & J. Riddoch (eds.), *Cognitive neuropsychology and cognitive rehabilitation.* London: Lawrence Erlbaum.

Mitchum, C.C. & Berndt, R.S. (1995). The cognitive neuropsychological approach to treatment of language disorders. *Neuropsychological Rehabilitation, 5,* 1–16.

Mitchum, C.C., Greenwald, M.L., & Berndt, R.S. (2000). Cognitive treatments of sentence processing disorders: What have we learned? *Neuropsychological Rehabilitation,* 311–336.

Mitchum, C.C., Haendiges, A.N., & Berndt, R.S. (1993). Model-guided treatment to improve written sentence production: A case study. *Aphasiology, 7,* 71–109.

Mitchum, C.C., Haendiges, A.N., & Berndt, R.S. (1995). Treatment of thematic mapping in sentence comprehension: Implications for normal processing. *Cognitive Neuropsychology, 12,* 503–547.

Miyake, A., Carpenter, P.A., & Just, M.A. (1994). A capacity approach to syntactic comprehension disorders: Making normal adults perform like aphasic patients. *Cognitive Neuropsychology, 11,* 671–717.

Nickels, L., Byng, S., & Black, M. (1991). Sentence processing deficits: A replication of treatment. *British Journal of Disorders of Communication, 26,* 175–199.

Reichman-Novak, S. & Rochon, E. (1997). Treatment to improve sentence production: A case study. *Brain and Language, 60,* 102–105.

Saffran, E.M. (1982). Neuropsychological approaches to the study of language. *British Journal of Psychology, 73,* 317–337.

Saffran, E.M. (in press). Effects of language impairment on sentence comprehension. In R.S. Berndt (ed.), *Handbook of neuropsychology, Vol. 2. Language and aphasia.* The Netherlands: Elsevier.

Saffran, E.M., Berndt, R.S., & Schwartz, M.F. (1989). The quantitative analysis of agrammatic production: Procedure and data. *Brain and Language, 37,* 440–479.

Saffran, M. & Martin, N. (1997). Effects of structural priming on sentence production in aphasics. *Language and Cognitive Processes, 12,* 877–882.

Saffran, E.M. & Schwartz, M.F. (1988). 'Agrammatic' comprehension it's not: Alternatives and implications. *Aphasiology, 2,* 389–394.

Saffran, E.M., Schwartz, M.F., & Marin, O. (1980a). The word order problem in agrammatism: Production. *Brain and Language, 10,* 263–280.

Saffran, E.M., Schwartz, M.F., & Marin, O.S.M. (1980b). Evidence from aphasia: Isolating the components of a production model. In B. Butterworth (ed.), *Language production, Vol. 1* (pp. 221–241). New York: Academic Press.

Schwartz, M.F. (1987). Patterns of speech production deficit within and across aphasia syndromes: Application of a psycholinguistic model. In M. Coltheart, G. Sartori, & R. Job (eds.), *The Cognitive neuropsychology of language.* Hillsdale, NJ: Lawrence Erlbaum.

Schwartz, M.F., Saffran, E.M., & Marin, O.S.M. (1980). The word order problem in agrammatism: Comprehension. *Brain and Language, 10,* 249–262.

Schwartz, M.F., Fink, R.B., & Saffran, E.M. (1995). The modular treatment of agrammatism. *Neuropsychological Rehabilitation, 5,* 93–127.

Schwartz, M.F., Linebarger, M.C., Saffran, E.M., & Pate, D.S. (1987). Syntactic transparency and sentence interpretation in aphasia. *Language and Cognitive Processes, 2,* 85–113.

Schwartz, M.F., Saffran, E.M., Fink, R.B., Myers, J.L., & Martin, N. (1994). Mapping therapy: A treatment programme for agrammatism. *Aphasiology, 8,* 9–54.

Seron, X. & Deloche, G. (1989). *Cognitive approaches in neuropsychological rehabilitation.* Hillsdale, NJ: Lawrence Erlbaum.

Shelton, J.R., Weinrich, M., McCall, D., & Cox, D.M. (1996). Differentiating global aphasic patients: Data from in-depth language assessments and production training using C-VIC. *Aphasiology, 10,* 319–342.

Stemberger, J.P. (1985). An interactive activation model of language production. In A. Ellis (ed.), *Progress in the psychology of language, Vol. 1* (pp. 143–186). London: Lawrence Erlbaum.

Weigle-Crump, C. & Koenigsknecht, R.A. (1973). Tapping the lexical store of the adult aphasic: Analysis of the improvement made in word retrieval skills. *Cortex, 9,* 410–418.

Weinrich, M., McCall, D., & Weber, C. (1995). Thematic role assignment in two severely aphasic patients: Associations and dissociations. *Brain and Language, 48,* 221–227.

Weinrich, M., McCall, D., Weber, C., Thomas, K., & Thornberg, L. (1995). Training on an iconic communication system for severe aphasia can improve natural language production. *Aphasiology, 9,* 343–364.

Weinrich, M., Shelton, J.R., Cox, D.M., & McCall, D. (1997a). Remediating production of tense morphology improves verb retrieval in chronic aphasia. *Brain and Language, 58,* 23–45.

Weinrich, M., Shelton, J.R., McCall, D., & Cox, D.M. (1997b). Generalization from single sentence to multisentence production in severely aphasic patients. *Brain and Language, 58,* 327–352.

Wilson, B. & Patterson, K.E. (1990). Rehabilitation and cognitive neuropsychology: Does cognitive psychology apply? *Applied Cognitive Psychology, 4,* 247–260.

Zingeser, L. & Berndt, R.S. (1990). Retrieval of nouns and verbs by agrammatic and anomic aphasics. *Brain and Language, 39,* 14–32.

Chapter 25

Comprehension and Production of Written Words

Pelagie M. Beeson and Argye E. Hillis

OBJECTIVES

The purpose of this chapter is to delineate the processes necessary for reading and spelling familiar and unfamiliar words; describe assessment procedures for the comprehension and production of written words, with particular emphasis on single-word processing; describe the nature of acquired impairments of reading and writing; and provide a description of treatment procedures (and illustrative case reports) for specific impairments to the component processes for reading and writing words.

INTRODUCTION

Despite the fact that most individuals with aphasia have impaired comprehension and production of written words, treatment directed toward the improvement of reading and writing abilities is often quite limited. This may reflect the prominence of spoken communication in our daily lives, thus placing a lower priority on rehabilitation of written communication. In today's society, however, face-to-face communication is increasingly replaced by written communication in forms such as electronic mail, automated banking machines, and on-line and mail-order catalogues. Thus, the functional consequences of reading and writing impairments can be quite significant.

The limited attention given to reading and writing rehabilitation may also reflect, in part, restricted knowledge of treatment approaches to acquired alexia and agraphia in comparison to the treatment of language in the spoken modality. Thus, the purpose of this chapter is to provide numerous approaches that have been shown to be effective for treating reading and writing impairments. Our approach to treatment begins with an effort to understand the nature of a patient's impairment by determining what processes and representations necessary for reading and writing are impaired, and

what skills are spared. Therefore, we begin with a review of the component processes that support reading and writing, and then describe how impairments to specified representations and processes result in reading and writing disturbances. Specific patients will be presented to demonstrate how hypotheses were formulated regarding the nature of the impairment and the logic by which the treatment approach was selected or devised. These impairment-based approaches constitute a central component of treatment plans that have as their ultimate goal the facilitation of meaningful, functional changes in patients' lives.

READING

Reading of familiar words is typically accomplished with relative ease as we recognize a string of letters as a word and comprehend its meaning. Despite the myriad of possible writing styles, we are able to recognize the letter identities that comprise a written word. The word "apple," for example, is activated by any of the following font styles: apple = `apple` = *apple* = apple = apple. In each case, the letter combination is recognized as the spelling for a word that we know. Our vocabulary of written words is variously referred to as the *visual input lexicon, orthographic input lexicon,* or *graphemic input lexicon* (the term that we will use here, as shown in **Figure 25–1**). Graphemes are letters or letter clusters that correspond to a single phoneme, for example, *f* and *ph* are both graphemes for the sound /f/. The graphemic input lexicon is the mental store of letter strings that we recognize as familiar words.

Under normal circumstances, representations in the graphemic input lexicon activate the appropriate word meaning in the semantic system so that we comprehend the words that we read. As we read aloud (and often when reading silently), we access the stored representations for word pronunciations in the *phonological output lexicon.* In turn, this activated representation accesses the component phonemes of the word, and they are held in a short-term storage mechanism referred to as the *phonological buffer.* The sequence of phonemes is held in the phonological buffer as we plan the appropriate articulatory movements. This cascade of events is referred to as reading via the *lexical-semantic route* because we derive semantic meaning by activation of words in the

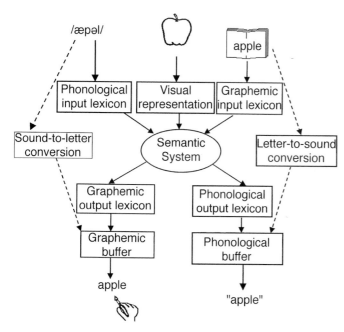

Figure 25–1. Schematic representation of the component representations and processes for single-word reading and writing. The solid lines depict lexical-semantic routes and the dashed lines indicate sublexical routes.

lexicon. In terms of Figure 25–1, this route is as follows: written word (*apple*) → graphemic input lexicon → semantic system → phonological output lexicon → phonological buffer → spoken word ("apple").

It also appears possible to read without meaning (see Greenwald & Berndt, 1998, for the strongest evidence to date). We can all recall those occasions when we are reading aloud without apprehending the meaning of the words. In that case, the graphemic input lexicon directly addresses the phonological output lexicon, and meaning is bypassed. This is a lexical route because whole words are processed, but it is a nonsemantic route because word meanings are not activated. If we persist with a nonsemantic approach to reading, we will fail to grasp the meaning of the text, as is the case with some brain-damaged individuals, particularly those with dementia (Schwartz et al., 1987; but also see Hillis & Caramazza, 1991a, 1995a).

When we attempt to read unfamiliar words, there is no corresponding representation to access in our graphemic input lexicon, so we may take advantage of our knowledge of relatively predictable relations between letters and sounds. In this way, we convert letters (or clusters of letters) to the appropriate sounds and assemble them to produce plausible attempts at their pronunciation. This approach is depicted in Figure 25–1 (with dashed lines) as the *letter-to-sound conversion* route; it is also referred to as *grapheme-to-phoneme conversion* or *orthography-to-phonology conversion*. This reading process is considered a *sublexical*, or *nonlexical*, reading route because it does not depend on activation of words in

our lexicon. Although we typically use this sublexical route to read unfamiliar words, it can be used if we are asked to read pronounceable nonwords or pseudowords, like "flig" or "merber," for example. When brain damage causes reading failure via the lexical-semantic route, patients may rely on this sublexical approach for reading words and nonwords alike. An obvious feature of the sublexical route is that it only works well if the letter-to-sound correspondences are predictable. Because there is a large number of irregularly spelled words in English, the sublexical route is susceptible to error. For example, the word "lamb" might be mispronounced because of failure to appreciate the silent 'b.' Proper names, like the first names of the authors of this chapter, also present a challenge because the sound-to-letter correspondences may be difficult to predict: Pelagie = /pe₁la₁ʒɪ'/; Argye = /ar'dʒɪ/.

Impairments of Reading

Neurological damage can disturb the processes necessary for reading in a variety of ways. In order to isolate the source of the reading impairment, it is helpful to examine performance on tasks that are dependent upon specified representations and processes. Considerable information can be gained from the examination of performance on tasks that require processing of single words presented variously in spoken, written, and pictured forms with spoken, written, or nonverbal (pointing) responses. As discussed in Chapter 22, some processing components are specific to reading (e.g., visual analysis of letter strings, graphemic input lexicon, and letter-to-sound conversion), whereas other components are shared with other lexical processing tasks. For example, semantic processing is necessary for auditory comprehension tasks, writing, and oral naming, as well as reading. Similarly, the phonological output lexicon is accessed for both oral naming and oral reading tasks. By contrasting performance for single-word comprehension and production in written and spoken modalities, the hypothesized locus (or loci) of impairment may be isolated.

In addition to examining performance across language modalities, it is also informative to determine the influence of various lexical features on reading accuracy (and reading speed, in some cases). Clues regarding the location of damage can be obtained by examining what types of words pose the greatest problem for reading. Carefully constructed word lists that control for lexical features such as word length, part of speech, frequency of use, and concreteness (or imagery) are useful to discern the nature of the impairment, as shown in Table 25–1. Controlled word lists are available in the *Psycholinguistic Assessments of Language Processing in Aphasia* (PALPA; Kay et al., 1992), the Battery of Adult Reading Function (Rothi et al., 1986), and the Johns Hopkins University (JHU) Dyslexia Battery (Goodman & Caramazza, 1986). The latter two lists were previously unpublished and difficult to obtain, so the JHU Dyslexia Battery

TABLE 25–1

Primary Features of Various Acquired Dyslexia Profiles

Locus of Damage	Example Syndrome	Effect					
		Word Length Short > Long	Spelling Regularity Reg > Irreg	Frequency HF > LF	Imageability/ Concreteness HI > LI	Word Class N > F	Inability to Read Nonwords
Access to Graphemic Input Lexicon	Letter-by-Letter Reading	X					
Graphemic Input Lexicon	Surface Dyslexia		X	X			
Semantics & Letter-to-Sound Conversion	Deep Dyslexia			X	X	X	X
Access to Phonological Output Lexicon	Surface Dyslexia		X	X			
Access to Phonological Output Lexicon & Letter-to-Sound Conversion	Deep Dyslexia			X			X

X = significant effect; Reg = regular spelling; Irreg = irregular/exceptional spelling; HF = high frequency; LF = low frequency; HI = high imagery; LI = low imagery; N = nouns; F = functors.

is included in Appendix 25–1. The word lists provide contrasts of lexical features that allow examination of various processes for reading single words. The information gained from performance on these controlled word lists will be discussed further in the context of specific reading impairments.

When appropriate, reading should also be assessed at sentence and paragraph levels. Sentence and paragraph reading can be screened using subtests from standardized aphasia tests including the *Western Aphasia Battery* (Kertesz, 1982) and the *Boston Diagnostic Aphasia Examination* (Goodglass & Kaplan, 1983). The PALPA (Kay et al., 1992) also provides some sentence comprehension subtests, and the *Reading Comprehension Battery for Aphasia-2* (RCBA-2; LaPointe & Horner, 1998) samples reading for single words, sentences, and paragraphs. In the absence of a comprehensive assessment tool for reading at the paragraph level, some of the tests designed for the examination of developmental reading disorders are useful for examining acquired alexia. For example, the *Gray Oral Reading Test-3* (GORT-3: Wiederholt & Bryant, 1992) provides short essays of graded difficulty that can be used to assess reading rate and accuracy, as well as comprehension. The GORT-3 is particularly useful in that alternate forms (A and B) are available. Another resource for testing text level reading is the *Nelson Reading Skills Test* (Hanna et al., 1977), which provides paragraph-level text.

The pattern of impaired and preserved reading processes will differ among individuals, but there are discernible patterns of impairment that have been recognized as various acquired alexia syndromes (Ellis, 1993; Hillis & Caramazza,

1992; Margolin & Goodman Schulman, 1992). Several patterns of acquired reading impairment will be reviewed here, and clinically proven treatment approaches are reported for each of the various patterns. We will show how the hypothesized nature of the impairment can help to guide the treatment approach. Reading impairments will be reviewed in an order that starts at the processing of visual input and ends with impairments in the spoken production of written language.

Impaired Access to the Graphemic Input Lexicon

In some cases of neurologic damage, patients fail to recognize strings of letters as familiar words, even though the individual letters are perceived. In its pure form, this disorder is specific to reading, while writing remains completely intact, so it is referred to as *pure alexia* or *alexia without agraphia*. Many individuals with pure alexia are able to perceive and name the letters of words that they fail to recognize, and if they spell the word letter-by-letter it often helps them identify the word (see papers in Coltheart, 1998)[a]. For example, a patient may fail to recognize the word *apple* but after spelling it aloud (or subvocally) quickly acknowledges, "oh, apple."

A schematic depiction of the impaired access to the graphemic input lexicon is shown in Figure 25–2 with

---

[a]The neuroanatomical account of letter-by-letter reading is based on the finding that patients with this clinical syndrome often have damage affecting both the left occipital lobe, causing right homonymous hemianopia, and a lesion in the splenium of the corpus collosum, which prevents visual information from the right occipital lobe from efficiently crossing to left hemisphere language areas.

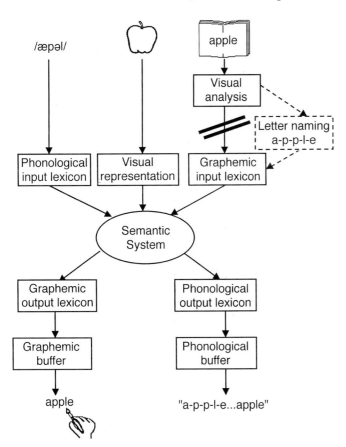

Figure 25–2. Schematic representation of impaired access to the graphemic input lexicon with strategic compensation in the form of letter-by-letter reading. Bold black hash marks indicate disrupted process.

letter-by-letter reading shown as a compensatory strategy. As indicated, the graphemic input lexicon is not impaired, and letter naming may provide an alternative means of activating the graphemic representations. The deficit is specific to the visual modality, so in most cases, individuals with pure alexia are able to quickly recognize words that are spelled aloud to them. Once a word is properly identified, its meaning is easily accessed because there is no impairment of the semantic system. There is also no difficulty in saying the word aloud once it has been recognized.

In pure alexia, access to the graphemic input lexicon is disrupted for all types of words, so that reading accuracy typically is not strongly affected by features such as word frequency, concreteness (or imageability), grammatical class, or regularity of spelling, as is shown in Table 25–1. When words are decoded letter-by-letter, however, there is a marked word length effect so that long words take more time to read and are more prone to errors than short words. In fact, there is often a linear increase in reading time as a function of the number of letters. In some cases, there is also difficulty with letter identification, which limits the effectiveness of letter-by-letter reading even further.

Treatment for Impaired Access to the Graphemic Input Lexicon

Several treatment approaches have been shown to be effective for improving access to the graphemic input lexicon or compensating for the impairment. The approaches discussed here differ with respect to the manner in which preserved abilities are used to compensate for the impairment. The first approach, multiple oral rereading, is thought to strengthen access to the graphemic input lexicon either in a direct manner or via the compensatory letter-naming route. A different treatment approach is appropriate for patients who show impaired letter identification in addition to impaired access to the graphemic input lexicon. Finally, a treatment using brief exposures of single words is described that has been useful for some individuals with pure alexia.

Multiple Oral Rereading. Multiple oral rereading (MOR) entails the use of repeated reading aloud of a given text as a means of facilitating whole-word, rather than letter-by-letter reading. Several researchers have shown this procedure to be effective as a means to increase reading rate in letter-by-letter readers (Beeson, 1998; Moyer, 1979; Tuomainen & Laine, 1991). It was hypothesized that repeated reading of the same text facilitates a shift from letter-by-letter reading to whole-word reading because of clues provided by sentence context and familiarity with the text. This approach is thought to improve or re-establish access to the graphemic input lexicon so that letter-by-letter reading can decrease. Procedures for implementing MOR are described in Table 25–2.

The MOR approach was used with Patient H.L. (reported by Beeson, 1998), who had an acquired reading impairment following a stroke in the left posterior occipitotemporal region. It was evident that H.L.'s impairment was relatively specific to reading in that his processing of information presented via the auditory modality was without error, and his spoken and written output were preserved. By 3 months post-stroke, H.L. was able to correctly name written letters with fair accuracy, and he could recognize most written words by reading them slowly in a letter-by-letter fashion. In contrast, his recognition of words that were orally spelled to him was rapid and accurate. Thus, it appeared that H.L.'s stroke had resulted in impaired access to the word forms in the graphemic input lexicon, so that they were no longer directly activated by the visual representation. H.L.'s letter-by-letter reading strategy provided a means for him to read, but at an incredibly slow rate of about 10 words per minute. He was anxious to improve his reading rate with good accuracy in order to return to work and to be able to read for pleasure.

Passages from the Reading Laboratory by Scientific Research Associates (SRA; Parker, 1976; Parker & Scannell, 1998) were used as stimuli because they include essays and stories of controlled length and complexity. H.L. initially read a given passage orally within the weekly therapy session so that rate and accuracy were documented. H.L. used a

TABLE 25–2

Steps for Implementing Multiple Oral Rereading (MOR) Treatment Approach

A. Initial treatment session(s)

Step 1. Determine reading rate and accuracy for text-level material.

    a. Select a passage of appropriate difficulty, e.g., 100-word segment to be used as practice text.

    b. Ask patient to read the text aloud allowing for letter-by-letter decoding as needed.

    c. Calculate reading rate in words per minute and score reading errors in terms of number of deviations from print (self-corrected errors may be tallied separately).

Step 2. Establish multiple oral rereading procedures.

    a. Have patient reread the practice text, providing assistance as needed to achieve correction of reading errors. Multiple repetitions during therapy session provide opportunity to increase familiarity with text, and should result in increased accuracy.

    b. Establish homework activity.

        1) Provide a copy of the written text for homework.

        2) Agree upon daily homework schedule, e.g., 30 minutes of repeated oral reading of practice text once or twice daily.

        3) Establish a log for recording completion of homework. Patients may time themselves and record the time taken to read the passage, or simply note completion of homework on daily basis.

B. Subsequent therapy sessions

Step 1. Review patient's log to confirm consistency in completing MOR homework.

Step 2. Determine rate and accuracy of reading for practiced text.

    a. Have patient read practiced text aloud.

    b. Keep a graphic plot of reading rate and accuracy.

Step 3. Determine target rate for practiced text, e.g., to achieve 50 wpm or 100 wpm. When target rate is attained (with acceptable accuracy) for practiced text, provide a new passage for MOR homework.

Step 4. Determine reading rate and accuracy for new (previously unread) text.

    a. Provide a new passage (about 100 words) for oral reading to determine if reading rate or accuracy for new material improves.

    b. Calculate and record reading rate and accuracy during each session to determine effectiveness of MOR treatment.

(After Beeson, 1998) Rationale: Multiple oral rereading is thought to improve access to the graphemic input lexicon, so that reliance on letter-by-letter reading decreases and whole-word recognition improves.

letter-by-letter reading approach as needed to identify words. After reading the passage several times within the therapy session, H.L. was given the passage to read repeatedly as homework for a minimum of 30 minutes daily. With repeated readings, and thus familiarity with the text, H.L. increased his reading rate for practiced passages from initial rates of about 12 wpm to the criterion rate of 100 wpm. In the context of practiced text, H.L. was able to rapidly recognize whole words. As the criterion rate was achieved for a given passage, new passages were introduced for repeated oral reading as homework.

To test whether MOR resulted in a general improvement in reading (or whether it specifically improved reading of the words in the trained paragraphs), reading rates and accuracy for previously unread passages were sampled during weekly therapy sessions. As desired, H.L. showed steady improvement in reading rate for new text while maintaining a high level of accuracy. H.L.'s improvement in reading rate to about 40 wpm allowed him to return to reading novels for pleasure, but he was unable to return to work due to other health factors. Follow-up testing 2 years after this treatment showed that H.L. had continued to read for pleasure and had become

self-employed in part-time work. By that time, his reading rate had improved to over 100 wpm.

The MOR protocol can be implemented with relatively infrequent treatment sessions because it is heavily dependent upon the patient's accomplishment of reading homework. Weekly or even biweekly sessions may be adequate. Variations in the protocol might include adjustment of the criterion reading rate for practiced text from 100 wpm, to a slower rate, such as 50 words per minute. The repeated reading of text appeared to be an essential component for the treatment of pure alexia; however, the work of Cherney and colleagues (1986) suggests that oral reading treatment *without* multiple rereading may be beneficial for some individuals with aphasia and acquired alexia. They found that oral reading, with clinician support for reading accuracy, was an effective treatment for a heterogeneous group of individuals with aphasia (Cherney et al., 1986). Although the specific locus of the treatment effect was not discernible, these results suggest that the clinical value of oral reading should be further examined.

Beeson and Insalaco (1998) showed that the MOR approach can also benefit individuals who do not fit the classic pure alexia profile, but who have some impairment of access to the graphemic input lexicon. The MOR approach was implemented with two individuals with anomic aphasia who reported slow reading rate as their primary complaint. Both showed a word length effect as well as slower reading rate for functors in comparison to nouns. Their reading rates before treatment ranged from 40 to 60 wpm, which is slow compared to normal adult oral reading rates, which range from 150 to 200 wpm (Rayner & Pollatsek, 1989). Using the MOR approach, both patients were able to improve their reading rate for new text to about 100 words per minute, an increase that was adequate to support pleasure reading. An examination of their reading rate and accuracy for single words before and after treatment showed that the greatest improvement was noted in reading rate for functors, suggesting that MOR may be particularly beneficial for improving recognition of function words for some individuals. This may be due to the syntactic constraints offered by sentence contexts which help to predict functors more than content words.

Cross-Modality Cuing. Letter-by-letter reading cannot be accomplished effectively if a significant number of letter identification errors are made. In some patients, letter identification is facilitated when information regarding the letter shape is provided via another modality. For example, some patients perceive the letters when they are traced on their palm, or when they trace the letter themselves (Seki et al., 1995). Tracing the component letters of a word with one's finger, or copying the written word, are compensatory strategies that can be used by the patient without assistance. It is assumed that the kinesthetic information about spelling provides access to the graphemic input lexicon, which substitutes for activation of the lexicon via the visual input. Thus, the procedure has been referred to as cross-modality cuing.

A positive response to cross-modality cuing was reported by Maher et al. (1998) for patient V.T. who had pure alexia. V.T. had difficulty naming letters, so that letter-by-letter decoding of words was not possible, but V.T. was able to name letters in a word after she traced each letter with her finger. Maher et al. (1998) took advantage of this residual skill, so that V.T. traced letters of words to provide kinesthetic input that resulted in word recognition. Treatment using this motor cross-cuing strategy resulted in improved word recognition and increased reading rate from 20 to 45 wpm in 4 weeks. With practice, V.T. showed improved letter recognition so that every letter did not need to be traced, but simply tracing the first letter or two was adequate to cue word identification.

Brief Exposure. A different approach to treatment for impaired access to the graphemic input lexicon involves the presentation of written words for brief exposures so that letter-by-letter reading is not possible. The motivation for this treatment came from the observation that some individuals with pure alexia retain an ability to derive some meaning from words that they cannot explicitly name (Coslett & Saffran, 1989, 1994).

Rothi and Moss (1992) proposed that their pure alexic patient might be stimulated to use this implicit knowledge gained from brief whole-word "reading" to facilitate reading comprehension and possibly to regain access to the graphemic input lexicon. Single words were presented on a computer screen for brief exposures (e.g., 500 msec), and the patient was asked to make a decision about the word, for example, "Is it an animal?" Although the patient often indicated that he had not actually read the word, he was encouraged to guess. Response accuracy was above chance, indicating some ability to apprehend the whole word at an implicit level. This brief exposure procedure resulted in improved reading rate (following 20 treatment sessions) in Rothi and Moss's patient, suggesting that it facilitated recovery of whole-word reading. However, Rothi and colleagues reported failure of this treatment approach with two other patients (Maher et al., 1998; Rothi et al., 1998), suggesting that it may be useful for a subset of people with pure alexia.

An adaptation of the brief exposure procedure could be implemented using written words presented on cards and shown for brief duration rather than computer presentation. Another variation includes contrasting real words with plausible nonwords, so that the task is to answer the question, "Is this a word?" These variations share the common goal of promoting whole-word apprehension rather than letter-by-letter reading.

Impaired Representations in the Graphemic Input Lexicon

Some reading impairments occur because of an impairment of the representations in the graphemic input lexicon (or impaired access to graphemic representations). It appears as though the individual's vocabulary of written words has eroded, so that visually perceived words that were once familiar now appear unfamiliar and their meaning cannot be derived. If the ability to sound out words is retained, reading may be accomplished by means of the letter-to-sound conversion procedure (i.e., via the sublexical route), as shown in Figure 25–3. This procedure works well for words that have good letter-to-sound correspondences (referred to as regular words), but words that have uncommon letter-to-sound correspondences (i.e., irregular words, such as *yacht*) pose a problem and are often misread. For example, the word "know" might be pronounced /kənoʊ/. Thus, when reading is accomplished via a sublexical rather than lexical route, performance is characterized by greater difficulty reading irregularly spelled words when compared to regularly spelled words, as indicated in Table 25–1. This reading profile has been referred to as *surface alexia* because reading is

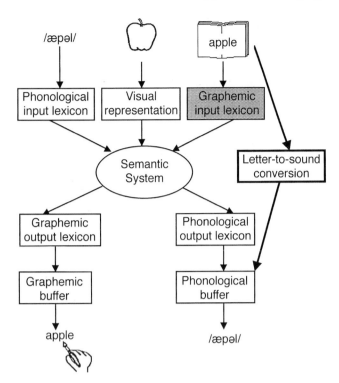

Figure 25–3. Schematic representation of impairment of the graphemic input lexicon (shaded) and reliance on letter-to-sound conversion to decode written words (heavy black lines).

accomplished via phonology rather than meaning, so that it might be thought of as reading "on the surface" (see papers in Patterson et al., 1985)[b]. Because reading is accomplished by sounding-out, nonwords are read with at least fair accuracy. There are no strong effects of lexical-semantic features such as imageability or word class because reading "bypasses" the semantic system. However, the impairment at the level of the graphemic input lexicon should be more notable on low frequency words as opposed to high frequency words, because high frequency words are thought to be more resistant to damage. Word length may have a negative effect on reading accuracy, because longer words provide more opportunities for errors in letter-to-sound conversion, and it may also take longer to sound out a long word rather than a short word; however, a word length effect is not an essential feature associated with impaired representations in the graphemic input lexicon.

Treatment for Impaired Representations in the Graphemic Input Lexicon

Although individuals with an impairment of representations in the graphemic input lexicon (or access to them) have the

---

[b]It should be noted, however, that the surface dyslexia profile may arise when there is damage to other components of the lexical-semantic route, including the semantic system or the phonological output lexicon.

potential to use letter-to-sound correspondences to sound out words, in some cases, they do not use this strategy. In other cases, patients show some ability to use the sublexical route, but need training to more consistently apply the conversion rules. Therefore, treatment may be devoted to training the "sounding out" strategy to strengthen letter-to-sound correspondences. A consequence of over-reliance on the sublexical route is misunderstanding words that sound the same but are spelled differently (i.e., homophones, such as "dear" and "deer"), because access to semantics is gained from the oral reading response. Additionally, words that are spelled the same, but are pronounced differently (i.e., homographs) may be mispronounced for a given context; for example, "lead" might be incorrectly pronounced the same in the phrases, "the lead pipe" and "I will lead the way." Such problem words may need to be specifically trained. Another treatment approach is the use of brief exposures and corrected oral reading trials in order to strengthen representations (or access to them), in an item-specific manner. Patient P.S. (reported by Hillis, 1993) received all three of these treatment approaches, which will be described below.

Strengthening Letter-to-Sound Conversion. Patient P.S. had an acquired reading impairment as the result of damage to the left temporoparietal area due to traumatic injury (for details, see Hillis, 1993). The injury resulted in damage to multiple components of language processing, so that several treatment protocols were implemented over the course of P.S.'s rehabilitation. P.S. had an impairment of oral and written naming and comprehension that was restricted to the categories of animals and vegetables (Hillis & Caramazza, 1992). For all other categories of words, his naming and comprehension were quite good. His spelling and reading, however, were markedly impaired, interfering with his ability to carry out his work as the president of a small contracting company.

On the Johns Hopkins University Dyslexia Battery, P.S. was significantly more accurate in reading high frequency words as opposed to low frequency words, regular words relative to irregular words, and nonwords as opposed to real words. He could read nonwords because any plausible pronunciation of a nonword is considered correct. His reading of real words were nearly all phonologically plausible errors, such as *threat* read as "threet" [Θrit] and *stood* read as "stewed." He could not reliably distinguish real words from nonwords, indicating an impairment in accessing representations in the graphemic input lexicon.

Although P.S. showed some ability to use the sublexical reading route, he was inconsistent in the application of letter-to-sound conversion. Therefore, he was retrained to produce the appropriate phoneme in response to letters as well as digraphs (e.g., ee, ea, oa) that are common in English. To establish proficiency using the sublexical reading procedures, P.S. was trained to read nonword syllables composed of target letters plus one or two other sounds that he produced correctly. For example, to train the pronunciation of *oa* he was trained to read the nonwords *toa* and *poa*. In order to help P.S. cue himself as he attempted to read nonwords, a corpus of key words was identified that P.S. could consistently read correctly. During treatment, each nonword was presented on a card for P.S. to read; if he failed, he was shown his key word on the back of the card and was guided to derive the nonword pronunciation via the key word pronunciation. To illustrate, to teach pronunciation of *oa* in *poa*, he was cued with the key word, *boat*. For letters (and digraphs) having several common manners of pronunciation, the alternative pronunciations were trained as well.

A multiple baseline design showed that P.S. was able to master sets of letter-to-sound correspondences after (but not before) they were entered into treatment. This resulted in item-specific improvement on the targeted words, as well as improvement on untrained regularly and irregularly spelled words. The improvement on irregularly spelled words reflected a benefit from attempting to "sound out" irregular words, thus providing partial phonological information that was adequate to cue word recognition.

There are many possible variations for training letter-to-sound conversions (see Nickels, 1992). The specific procedures used with P.S. might be modified to suit a particular patient. The training of letter-to-sound correspondences has the potential to be an effective strategy for reading many words (rather than a specific set of words), so it is worthwhile to determine if a given patient can relearn the associations. The first step is to establish a set of key words that the patient can read successfully, and at least one key word should be linked to each grapheme. A list of phoneme-grapheme pairs is included in Appendix 25–2, ordered by frequency of occurrence in English words that can be used to guide the choice of targets (see Berndt et al., 1987, for details). Because the predictability of letter-to-sound correspondences is stronger for consonants than vowels, it may be most effective to establish key words for consonants first. For some patients, it may be too much of an effort to train the vowels at all. Although the time required to re-establish the letter-to-sound associations may be considerable, much of the work can be accomplished by self-drill outside of the therapy session. An approach to establishing key words is described in Table 25–3.

TABLE 25–3

Establishing Key Words That Are Associated With Specific Graphemes

A. Initial treatment sessions
  Step 1. Determine what grapheme-phoneme pairs will be targeted for training.
    a. Select consonants first because they have more consistent letter-to-sound correspondences than vowels.
    b. Select frequently occurring consonants (see Appendix 25–2); proceed to less frequent consonants and vowels as appropriate for a given patient. For example, train consonants in sets of 5 at a time:

Set 1. r, t, n, s, l

Set 2. k, d, m, p, b

Set 3. f, sh, v, g, z

  Step 2. For each target grapheme, assist the patient in identifying a key word that begins with the grapheme.
    a. If possible, find key words that the patient can consistently say correctly, example, "Ron" for r.
    b. If the patient does not have a key word available for a given grapheme, a word should be agreed upon and trained for consistency of production.
    c. Construct stimulus cards that have a grapheme on one side (e.g., R-r) and the associated key word on the other side (e.g., Ron).

B. Establish homework procedures
    a. Using stimulus cards, the patient should look at the grapheme and say the name of the key word (Look at key word on back of the card only as necessary for cuing).
    b. Establish frequency of homework (e.g., daily practice).

C. Subsequent therapy sessions
    a. Review ability to retrieve key word for each targeted grapheme.
    b. Target additional graphemes as appropriate.

D. Subsequent treatment
    Select (or develop) subsequent protocol to take advantage of key words for deriving phonology from written words (for reading) or deriving graphemes from phonology (for writing).

Rationale: to develop a corpus of key words that can be used to assist the patient in retrieving phonology from written words.

Brief Exposures. A procedure adapted from the brief exposure approach used by Rothi and Moss (1992) was also implemented with patient P.S. In this case, the rationale for the use of brief exposure of written words was to facilitate processing at the level of the graphemic input lexicon, as opposed to relying on the sublexical reading route. P.S. was presented a corpus of target words (contrasted with nonwords) for 200-msec durations. P.S. was asked to read the words (but not the nonwords), and corrective feedback was provided. He improved from 22 to 92% in correct oral reading of the word lists, and from 0 to 80% in correct oral reading of the same words when they were presented in paragraphs. His accuracy in recognizing the trained words and rapidly distinguishing them from the nonwords improved to 100%. Therefore, the procedure resulted in item-specific mastery of 50 target words, which were drawn from a vocabulary necessary for P.S.'s vocation. Thus, it appeared that brief presentations coupled with corrected oral reading served to strengthen specific graphemic representations (or access to them). It is also possible that treatment served to build new graphemic representations, rather than strengthen degraded representations, but that distinction is difficult to determine.

Training Homophones and Homographs. Finally, P.S. received treatment to help him disambiguate *homographs*, words that are spelled the same but have different pronunciations and meanings, for example /ter/ (as in 'to tear a page') and /tir/ (as in 'tear drop'). P.S. had difficulty with such words because the differences in pronunciation could not be derived via the sublexical reading route. Word pairs that could not be correctly read aloud on the basis of letter-to-sound correspondence rules were selected for treatment. He was also trained to disambiguate *homophones*, word pairs that are pronounced the same but have different spellings and meanings, such as *stake* and *steak*. One word from each homographic or homophonic pair was targeted for treatment. The target word was presented in print with its written definition that was read aloud by the clinician. P.S. was asked to write the target word in a sentence. During each session, prior to treatment, oral reading, spelling, and comprehension (as assessed by use of the word in sentence contexts) were probed. P.S. improved on all tasks for the trained words, and also improved his oral reading for the untrained members of the word pairs. Therefore, the pairing of the graphemic representations with semantics served to strengthen P.S.'s ability to read via the lexical-semantic route, allowing him to disambiguate homographs and homophones. This procedure, like the use of brief exposures, resulted in item-specific learning; therefore, it was important to select words of functional value for the patient.

Impairment of Semantics and Letter-to-Sound Conversion

Many individuals with left hemisphere damage experience disruption of several processes critical for reading.

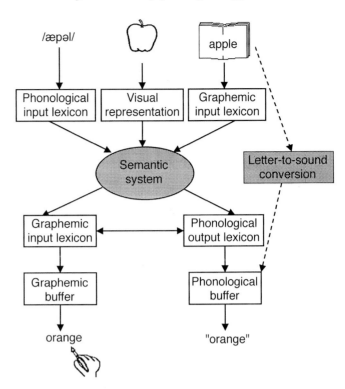

Figure 25–4. Schematic representation of impairments to the semantic system and letter-to-sound conversion resulting in a semantic error (*orange* for *apple*). Note the semantic error was also made in writing due to the impairment of the central semantic system.

Concomitant impairment of semantics and letter-to-sound conversion (as shown in Figure 25–4) is not uncommon in individuals with aphasia. When lexical and sublexical processes are disrupted, patients have difficulty recognizing written words and activating their meaning, and are also unable to sound out words using letter-to-sound correspondence rules. Reading is accomplished via a damaged lexical-semantic route because sublexical processes are unavailable. In most cases, the weakened lexical-semantic route results in the following profile: high frequency words are read better than low frequency words; concrete (high imagery) words are read better than abstract (low imagery) words; and nouns are read better than adjectives and verbs, which are read better than functors. This profile may reflect the fact that concrete, high frequency nouns have the strongest semantic representations and therefore are most resistant to damage. Abstract, low frequency words or functors have the weakest semantic representations, or semantic representations that have a great deal of overlap with other words (and are thus easily confused). For example, the meaning of "belief" is difficult to define and overlaps considerably with the meaning of many other words: confidence, conviction, credence, creed, notion, thought, concept, faith, religion, hope, idea, presumption, principle, trust, and so on. In contrast, the meanings of concrete nouns like *fork* do not overlap so much with other meanings. In addition to the word class effect, unfamiliar words and nonwords cannot be read because of the inability to use the sublexical processes to derive the appropriate sound for a given letter. The reading impairment is characterized by a variety of error types including semantic errors (apple → orange), visual errors (soul → soup), inflectional errors (walked → walking), and functor word substitutions (until → between). This reading profile has been referred to as deep dyslexia (Coltheart et al., 1987). It has been suggested that deep dyslexia may reflect reading from the right hemisphere, which appears to be a plausible hypothesis particularly for patients with extensive left hemisphere lesions (Coltheart et al., 1987; Patterson et al., 1989).[c]

Treatment for Impaired Semantics and Letter-to-Sound Conversion

Individuals with impaired semantics and concomitant impairment of the letter-to-sound conversion mechanism may benefit from treatment directed at either, or both, the lexical-semantic and sublexical routes. We will first review an approach to strengthening the link between written words and their associated meaning; then we will revisit an approach to teaching letter-to-sound correspondences.

Improving Semantics. Patient J.J., who was described by Hillis and Caramazza (1991a,b, 1994), showed an impairment of semantics that affected his reading (as well as writing and spoken naming). J.J. was a right-handed man who had a stroke involving the left temporal lobe and basal ganglia. At 9 months post-stroke, he made frequent semantic errors on oral and written naming in response to pictured or written stimuli (although he showed spared knowledge for animals). J.J. showed impairment of letter-to-sound conversion, but he was able to use the sublexical route to some extent so that oral reading was better than oral naming.

A set of 40 words from two semantic categories was selected for treatment. The semantic treatment entailed presentation of one printed word from the set, along with pictures of items depicting all 40 of the words. J.J. was asked to point to the picture corresponding to the written word. Incorrect responses were corrected, and the items in error were presented again after intervening items, until J.J.'s response to that word was correct. Although pronunciation was not specifically trained, J.J.'s oral reading of the trained words improved rapidly, concurrent with his improved comprehension of the trained words. The effect on oral reading achieved with this semantic treatment was significantly stronger than the effect of cued oral reading practice of the trained words (see Hillis & Caramazza, 1994). In contrast to J.J., a different patient with damage to the phonological output lexicon,

H.W., showed significantly greater effects with cued oral reading treatment (described below) than with this semantic treatment, demonstrating the utility of aiming treatment at the impaired component of the process.

Teaching Letter-to-Sound Conversion. Individuals who rely on an impaired lexical-semantic route for reading are additionally disadvantaged if they cannot derive phonological information from the written word. If they can sound out even the initial phoneme, it may serve to cue correct production or block the production of semantic errors in reading. An approach to retraining letter-to-sound conversion was discussed earlier in this chapter in the context of patient P.S. who had an impairment of the graphemic input lexicon. A different approach proved successful for patient S.P. (reported by dePartz, 1986), who showed impairment of semantics and letter-to-sound conversion.

Patient S.P. had a significant Wernicke's aphasia as the result of a parietotemporal intracerebral hemorrhage. S.P. was totally alexic and agraphic with relatively preserved auditory comprehension for word/picture matching. DePartz documented that S.P. was unable to use the letter-to-sound conversion mechanism in that he showed no difference in error rates for regularly and irregularly spelled words, and he could not read nonwords. S.P.'s single-word reading was significantly better for high frequency, concrete words as opposed to low frequency, abstract words, and nouns were read with greater accuracy than words from other grammatical classes. There was no evidence of an impairment at the level of the graphemic input lexicon in that S.P. could distinguish real words from nonwords on a lexical decision task; nor did word length have an effect on his reading accuracy. S.P.'s reading included semantic errors (e.g., *round* for *circle*), visual errors, derivational errors, and substitutions of one function word for another. S.P.'s overall profile was consistent with that of deep dyslexia due to the impairment of both the semantic system and the nonlexical reading route, as well as the presence of semantic errors (Coltheart et al., 1987; Newcombe & Marshall, 1984).

S.P. received treatment that was directed toward retraining letter-to-sound conversion abilities so that he could sound out words. The first phase of treatment was devoted to establishing single letter-to-sound correspondences. The treatment procedure took advantage of S.P.'s ability to read some words via the lexical route. Using a procedure similar to that described in Table 25–3, S.P. developed a corpus of key words (or "code words") to help him retrieve the phonology for a given letter (e.g., his wife's name, Carole, was the key word for C). With assistance, S.P. selected a key word for each letter of the alphabet, and was ultimately able to say the appropriate key word in response to each letter. The next step was to train S.P. to speak only the first sound of the key word in response to its associated letter. This training required S.P. to say the code word with the first sound prolonged, and then say only the first phoneme (for example, "Carole". . ./k/).

---

[c]It is important to note that the deep dyslexia profile can be seen in patients with damage anywhere in the lexical-semantic route who have concomitant impairment to letter-to-sound conversion. For example, reading performance of patients with damage to the phonological output lexicon and letter-sound conversion can fit the deep dyslexia profile (Caramazza & Hillis, 1990; Hillis & Caramazza, 1995b)

After S.P. was able to derive single phonemes from each key word, he was trained to read three- or four-letter, one-syllable words and nonwords by deriving the component sounds and blending them to produce a word (or nonword). Mastery of these skills allowed S.P. to read regularly spelled words; additional treatment procedures were implemented to address difficulties created by different pronunciations of letters and irregularly spelled words (see dePartz, 1986). In some patients, mastery of regular letter-to-sound associations provides the necessary additional information to support the impaired lexical-semantic reading route, so that treatment addressing the nuances of irregular spellings is not necessary.

Impaired Access to Phonological Output Lexicon

Oral reading may be disrupted by an impairment that is specific to accessing the phonological output lexicon. Impaired access to the phonological output lexicon affects naming of objects in a similar manner because the phonological output lexicon is common to the two tasks. In both modalities, high frequency words are more likely to be retrieved than low frequency words. The written word may be helpful to cue speech production if phonology can be derived from the letters (as shown in Figure 25–5), but dependence on the sublexical reading route can result in regularization errors for irregularly spelled words, resulting in another variant of surface alexia (see Table 25–1). Some patients have concomitant impairment of letter-to-sound conversion mechanisms,

so that they cannot make use of sublexical information for reading; in such cases, the impaired access to the phonological output lexicon is characterized only by a frequency effect.

Treatment for Impaired Access to the Phonological Output Lexicon

Initial attempts to improve access to the phonological output lexicon might be directed toward taking advantage of letter-to-sound correspondences. Unfortunately, some patients fail to improve when treatment is directed toward the sublexical route. In such cases, alternative treatment to stimulate access to the phonological representations for specific written words may be successful.

Strengthening Letter-to-Sound Conversion. Phonological information obtained via letter-to-sound conversion may be adequate to reduce or block phonological errors in oral reading. Treatment procedures for strengthening the sublexical reading route (that were reviewed in the context of damaged graphemic input lexicon and the damaged semantic system) may also be employed to compensate for impairments of the phonological output lexicon.

Cued Oral Reading. Patient H.W. (reported by Hillis, 1993; Hillis & Caramazza, 1994), a right-handed, 64-year-old woman, sustained left parietal and occipital strokes resulting in fluent aphasia and a persistent reading impairment. When tested at 2.5 years post-stroke on the JHU Dyslexia Battery, her oral reading was significantly affected by word frequency and grammatical class. She correctly read 38% of nouns compared with 18% of verbs. The majority of her reading errors were semantic errors or omissions. The semantic errors were not accounted for by a semantic deficit, because H.W.'s comprehension of words was intact and her written naming was relatively preserved, even for words that elicited semantic errors in oral naming and oral reading. It was hypothesized that H.W.'s semantic errors arose as a result of failed activation of the appropriate entry in the phonologic output lexicon. Additional testing revealed that H.W.'s pattern of significantly poorer naming of verbs compared to nouns was evident on all tasks that required oral output, but verb comprehension was good. Thus, it was apparent that she had damage at the level of the phonological output lexicon, affecting verb production more than nouns. H.W. was unable to read nonwords, suggesting damage to the letter-to-sound conversion mechanism as well. She did not respond well to initial treatment efforts to improve her letter-to-sound conversion abilities, so an alternate approach was implemented that served to improve access to oral reading in an item-specific manner.

During treatment, H.W. was presented written words (transitive verbs) for oral reading. Phonemic cuing and repetition were provided as needed to elicit correct production of the written words. A multiple baseline design provided

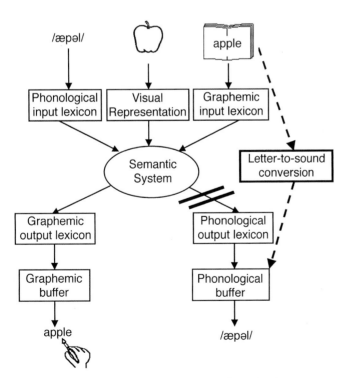

Figure 25–5. Schematic representation of impaired access to the phonological output lexicon. Bold black hash marks indicate disrupted process.

evidence that H.W. improved her ability to orally read (and orally name) the set of treated words. There was no generalization to an untrained set of words until they were entered into treatment, suggesting that the treatment influenced only access to those phonological representations that were activated in treatment. The fact that oral naming improved in response to treatment of oral reading confirmed the hypothesized locus of damage to the phonological output lexicon that is common to both tasks.

The success of this procedure is best explained as a lowering of the activation threshold in the phonological output lexicon as a consequence of the increased frequency of production in the training context. This stimulation effect is a familiar result of effective hierarchical cuing and mass practice effects. Despite the lack of generalization to other words, H.W. benefited from the item-specific improvement of single-word reading and naming. In this case, improvement was observed in both reading and oral naming. For several years thereafter, H.W. practiced oral reading each day with her husband providing cues, allowing her continued steady improvement in oral reading and oral naming for over a decade. She is still improving, 10 years later, and now has only mild anomia.

Summary of Treatments for Acquired Reading Impairments

Reading disturbances may reflect impairments to the component processes necessary for comprehension and production of written words. Degraded representations (or impaired access to representations) may occur at the level of the graphemic input lexicon, semantics, or the phonological output lexicon. Similarly, the sublexical reading route that allows for sounding out of words may be impaired. These impairments may occur in isolation or in various combinations. Numerous treatment approaches have been shown to be effective in strengthening lexical-semantic representations and processes, improving letter-to-sound conversion abilities, as well as developing alternative strategies to support reading. Even when reading processes are not fully restored, item-specific improvements and the retrieval of partial information can serve to improve functional reading skills. It is also worth noting that several treatment approaches might be implemented in sequence, so that improved skills are incorporated in successive treatment stages. For example, initial treatment efforts may focus on lexical-semantic processes, while a later stage of treatment may include strengthening the sublexical route. In this way, progressive approximation of normal reading processes is maximized, and appropriate strategic compensations are established.

SPELLING

The act of expressing our ideas in writing involves clarifying our thoughts, formulating sentences, and sequentially translating each word to its written form according to the spelling conventions for the language. Writing calls upon a multitude of cognitive, linguistic, and perceptual-motor processes. We will focus here primarily on the processes that are specific to single-word spelling. The motivation to write a word most often reflects self-activation of a semantic concept; but in clinical situations, we may ask a patient to write a word that we dictate (i.e., in response to auditory input), write the name of a pictured item, or even copy a printed word.

Under normal circumstances, our semantic representation activates a written word in our mental dictionary. This collection of spellings that we know is referred to as the *graphemic output lexicon* (Figure 25–1), or it may also be referred to as the *orthographic output lexicon* or the *visual output lexicon* (Ellis, 1993). As we prepare to write a word and as a word is written, it is held in short-term storage in the *graphemic output buffer*, which may be called, simply, the *graphemic buffer*. The information is held in the graphemic buffer as a series of graphemes, which are generic, abstract, letter representations (as opposed to specific upper or lower case exemplars in particular writing styles). The representation in the graphemic buffer allows implementation of spelling in several forms—handwriting, typing, or oral spelling. Written spelling requires implementation of peripheral processes whereby the specific letter forms (referred to as *allographs*) are selected and motor movements are planned and executed. The selection of a particular letter form is referred to as the *allographic conversion* process. Finally, graphic motor programs are implemented in order to write the component letters of a word.

As is the case with reading, spelling may be accomplished using an alternate route that relies on our knowledge of sound-to-letter correspondences, as shown in Figure 25–1. When a word is unfamiliar (or a nonword), spelling can be derived by sounding out the word and converting from sounds to letters, a process that is also referred to as *phoneme-to-grapheme conversion*. This sound-to-letter conversion is considered a nonlexical, or sublexical process, because spellings are assembled rather than retrieved as whole words. Assembled spellings are likely to reflect regular spelling rules, so that irregularly spelled words might be regularized, for example, "cough" might be spelled as *coff*. This sublexical route can provide an important compensatory spelling strategy when the lexical-semantic spelling route is impaired.

Impairments of Spelling

The processes necessary to spell words can be disrupted by damage to central linguistic processes as well as more peripheral components of the writing process (Ellis, 1993; Rapcsak & Beeson, 2000). A comprehensive assessment of writing includes examination of spontaneous writing, written naming, writing to dictation, and copying. A sample of spontaneous writing may be obtained by asking a patient to compose a short narrative; however, it may be preferable to request a

TABLE 25–4

Primary Features of Various Acquired Agraphias

Locus of Damage	Example Syndrome	Effect					
		Word Length Short > Long	Spelling Regularity Reg > Irreg	Frequency HF > LF	Imageability/ Concreteness HI > LI	Word Class N > F	Inability to Read Nonwords
Semantics & Sound-to-Letter Conversion	Deep Agraphia			X	X	X	X
Graphemic Output Lexicon	Surface (or Lexical) Agraphia		X	X			
Graphemic Output Lexicon & Sound-to-Letter Conversion	Global Agraphia			X			X
Graphemic Buffer	Graphemic Buffer Agraphia	X					

X = significant effect; Reg = regular spelling; Irreg = irregular/exceptional spelling; HF = high frequency; LF = low frequency; HI = high imagery; LI = low imagery; N = nouns; F = functors.

written description of a standard picture, such as the picnic scene from the WAB (Kertesz, 1982) or the cookie theft picture from the BDAE (Goodglass & Kaplan, 1983). The use of a standard stimulus allows for comparison over time, and also provides referent information that may be helpful to discern the intended content and spellings. Written narratives allow for examination of semantic organization, syntactic structure, word choice, as well as single-word spelling.

There are several sources of standardized stimuli that can be used to assess single-word writing. Standardized aphasia tests, such as the WAB and BDAE, offer a small set of items for initial screening of writing. A comprehensive assessment of single-word writing requires the use of controlled word lists, such as those included in the PALPA (Kay et al., 1992) or the Johns Hopkins University Dysgraphia Battery (Goodman & Caramazza, 1986; Appendix 25–1). These lists allow for independent evaluation of various lexical features including word frequency, imagery, grammatical class, spelling regularity, word length, morphological complexity, and nonword spelling. Assessment of oral spelling, typing, spelling with anagram letters, and copying may be indicated to discern whether central or peripheral spelling processes are impaired. Given that clinical evaluations are typically constrained by time and finances, it is important to select writing subtests that serve to test hypotheses regarding the locus of damage to the spelling system, so that an appropriate treatment approach is selected.

Characteristic patterns of acquired agraphia may result when certain processes are disturbed, as shown in Table 25–4, in a manner similar to that described relative to acquired alexia. Several patterns of acquired spelling impairments will be described, with greatest attention given to the central (or

linguistically based) writing impairments that often accompany aphasia. Treatment approaches directed toward particular components of the writing process are described in the context of specific patients.

Impaired Semantics and Sound-to-Letter Conversion

Spontaneous writing provides the expression of a concept or semantic representation. It has been hypothesized that our semantic representations are made up of sets of features that define the concept, as discussed in Chapter 10. For example, our semantic representation of *apple* might include <fruit>, <round>, <red>, <juicy>, <sweet>. If this representation is damaged, or in some way underspecified, it may result in the retrieval of the incorrect graphemic representation. For example, if the semantic representation included <fruit>, <round>, <juicy>, <sweet>, but failed to include <red>, then it might activate *orange* (as shown in Figure 25–6). Such semantic errors may be observed in writing, but also may be evident in other output modalities, such as spoken production.

The combined profile of written semantic errors and poor *phoneme-to-grapheme conversion* ability has been called *deep dysgraphia*, or *deep agraphia*, which is the analog of deep dyslexia.[d] As shown in Table 25–4, these impairments result in spelling that is influenced by lexical features including

---

[d]Selective impairment of the phoneme-to-grapheme conversion mechanism has been termed *phonological agraphia*, in reference to the inability to use phonology to assist in nonlexical spelling. A truly selective impairment of that nature would have relatively little consequence in the presence of a well-functioning lexical-semantic spelling route. Therefore, the impairment of grapheme-to-phoneme conversion ability will be discussed only in the context of concomitant spelling impairments.

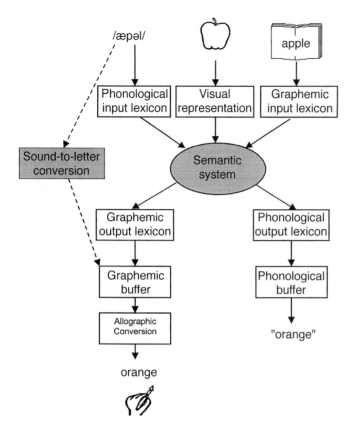

Figure 25–6. Schematic representation of impairments of the semantic system and the sound-to-letter conversion mechanism, as might result in a written semantic error (*orange* for *apple*). Note that a semantic error also was made in the spoken production due to the central semantic impairment.

concreteness/imageability (concrete words are spelled with greater accuracy than abstract words), word class (nouns are spelled with greater accuracy than functors), and frequency (high frequency words are spelled with greater accuracy than low frequency words) (Rapcsak et al., 1991). There is not an influence of spelling regularity because of minimal ability to perform sound-to-letter conversion; this also makes the spelling of nonwords impossible. In addition to semantic errors, patients typically produce morphological errors (e.g., *walking* for *walked*), functor substitutions (e.g., *since* for *about*), and visually similar misspellings (*storm* for *store*). Written semantic errors might be blocked or corrected if phonological information is available to guide retrieval of the graphemic representation. For example, if the initial letter "a" is activated, it may be adequate to block the semantic error "orange" in favor of "apple" (Bub & Kertesz, 1982).

Treatment for Impaired Semantics and
Sound-to-Letter Conversion

Individuals with impairment to both semantics and sound-to-letter conversion may benefit from treatment directed

toward either the lexical-semantic or sublexical spelling routes. Effective remediation of semantic impairments may result in improved responses on oral naming and repetition tasks, as well as writing. Strengthening of the sound-to-letter conversion mechanism would ideally provide a means of writing via phonology, and even partial writing of the word form may serve to block semantic errors or support activation of the graphemic output lexicon.

Treatment to Improve Semantics. Hillis (1991) described an approach to improve lexical semantics in patient H.G., a 22-year-old woman who had experienced massive left fronto-parietal damage resulting in severe language impairment. At 7 years post-onset she had persistent impairment of her semantic system so that semantic errors were prominent in writing, as well as in oral naming, spelling to dictation, repetition, spoken word-to-picture matching, and written word-to-picture matching. The presence of H.G.'s semantic errors (such as *pants* for *shirt*) on all tasks suggested an underspecification of the features necessary to distinguish among items in the same semantic category. Treatment was directed toward clarifying the semantic distinctions among written words as they were matched to corresponding pictures. When errors were made, corrective feedback was offered that highlighted distinctive features of the target in contrast to other members of the semantic category. For example, if *shirt* was written incorrectly as *pants*, then gestures, pointing, and simple verbal explanation highlighted the distinction of *shirt* as clothing for the upper body and *pants* as clothing for the legs.

A multiple baseline design showed that as H.G. improved her written naming of pictured items, she also improved her performance on other tasks for the trained items (such as oral naming). This generalization to other tasks, including comprehension, provided evidence that improvement occurred at the level of the semantic system. H.G. also showed generalized improvement to untrained items in the same semantic category as trained items, indicating that treatment resulted in richer semantic representations, allowing for more accurate distinctions among items in the treated categories. As expected, improved performance did not generalize to items in untrained semantic categories. H.G.'s response to treatment demonstrated the value of training specific items to a level of mastery. It is unlikely that comparable results would have been achieved if semantic treatment had shifted from one category to another without achieving mastery in any category.

Teaching Sound-to-Letter Conversions. Semantic errors in writing might be avoided or self-corrected if a patient at least has some ability to translate the initial sounds of a word into the corresponding graphemes. For example, if the intended target word is *movie*, but the patient incorrectly writes *TV*, the error might be self-corrected if the initial phoneme /m/ is converted to the grapheme *m*. If a patient has impairment of both the semantic system and sound-to-letter conversion abilities, but has some ability to say words, it may be worthwhile to provide treatment to improve sound-to-letter conversion abilities.

One illustrative case is that of patient J.S., a 36-year-old woman with severe aphasia following a motor vehicle accident and subsequent stroke affecting the left posterior frontal, anterior parietal, and superior temporal lobes (Hillis Trupe, 1986). J.S. had limited verbal output and used single written words to communicate. She showed relatively good comprehension of spoken and written words, but semantic errors were common in her writing. She showed little ability to associate phonemes to graphemes. In order to improve J.S.'s ability to generate spellings for single words and to reduce her written semantic errors, a treatment hierarchy similar to that depicted in Table 25–5 was implemented to re-establish the association between 30 sound-to-letter correspondences. The initial step in developing the treatment plan was to identify key words that J.S. could reliably spell. As discussed in the context of reading treatment, the key words served as a means to develop sound-to-letter correspondences. As J.S. mastered the phoneme-to-grapheme correspondences, she was able to self-cue spellings and block semantic errors. As a result of treatment, J.S. was able to use partial information from the sublexical route in combination with a partially damaged lexical-semantic system to more reliably derive the correct single words for written communication.

Impairment of the Graphemic Output Lexicon

In many cases of acquired agraphia, patients appear to have lost the graphemic representations for words, or have degraded representations, so that they show partial knowledge of word forms that they once knew. Low frequency

---

TABLE 25–5

Cuing Hierarchy for Teaching Phoneme-to-Grapheme Conversion

A. Initial treatment sessions
   a. Select target graphemes to be trained, for example, four sets of five graphemes (See Appendix 25.2).
   b. Establish one key word that patient can write for each grapheme (See procedures in Table 25–3).

B. Implement cuing hierarchy to train targeted graphemes.
   Note that step 1 is the most difficult task. If patient cannot respond correctly, proceed to step 2, then subsequent steps as needed. Follow the instructions to ascend the hierarchy when correct responses are achieved.
   1. "Write the letter that makes the sound /phoneme/."
      a. If correct, move on to the next target phoneme.
      b. If in error, proceed to step 2.
   2. Provide an array of letters (5 or more) including the correct target and say, "Point to the letter that makes the sound /phoneme/."
      a. If correct, remove array of letters and go to step 1.
      b. If incorrect, proceed to step 3.
   3. "Think of a word that starts with /phoneme/." or "Think of your key word for /phoneme/."
      "Now point to the first letter of your key word" (from array of letters).
      a. If correct, say, "Yes, a word that starts with /phoneme/ is [key word]. [Key word] starts with the letter [target letter]." For example, "Yes, a word that starts with /b/ is baby. Baby starts with the letter B." Rearrange the letters in the array and go back to step 2.
      b. If incorrect, go to step 4.
   4. "A word that starts with /phoneme/ is [key word]. Point to the letter that makes the first sound of [key word]."
      a. If correct, rearrange the array of letters and go back to step 2.
      b. If incorrect, go to step 5.
   5. "Write your key word for /b/. Write [key word]."
      "Now point to the letter that makes the first sound of [key word]."
      a. If correct, rearrange letters in the array and go back to step 2.
      b. If incorrect, go to step 6.
   6. Clinician writes the key word for the target sound /phoneme/, and says, for example, "The letter B makes the first sound of *baby*. /b/ is the first sound of *baby*. B makes the sound /b/. Point to the letter B. Now copy the letter B." Return to step 2.

C. Repeat the probe and cuing hierarchy for all targeted letters. Record responses only to initial trials of step 1 to determine progress. Probe each letter at least 3 to 5 times per session.

D. Once single letters are reliably written in response to their associated phoneme, provide spoken words and ask the patient to write the first letter of the word.
   For example, "Write the first letter for the word 'basketball.'"

E. Determine next appropriate protocol to develop and take advantage of phoneme-to-grapheme conversion abilities.

(After Hillis Trupe, 1986). Rationale: to train the ability to derive graphemes from their associated phonemes.

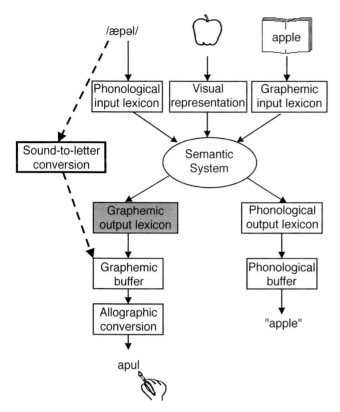

Figure 25–7. Schematic representation of impairment to the graphemic output lexicon showing reliance on the sound-to-letter conversion mechanism resulting in a phonologically plausible spelling error.

words are typically more vulnerable to impairment than high frequency words. If sound-to-letter conversion abilities are spared, as shown in Figure 25–7, spelling may be accomplished using the knowledge of sound-to-letter correspondences. This provides a useful strategic compensation, but over-reliance on the sublexical spelling route results in errors in the spelling of words that have irregular spellings, so that *knight* and *yacht* might be spelled as *nite* and *yot*. This spelling pattern is referred to as *surface agraphia* in reference to the pattern of "writing how it sounds" (i.e., "on the surface"); it is also referred to as *lexical agraphia* in reference to the damaged lexicon for writing (see Table 25–4). Surface agraphia is also characterized by the relatively spared ability to spell nonwords, thus confirming the ability to use the sublexical spelling route.

For many individuals with aphasia, impairments to lexical spelling processes are accompanied by impairment to sublexical spelling processes as well. In such cases, there is little ability to take advantage of sound-to-letter correspondences to resolve spelling difficulties, so that spelling is not characterized by the regularity effect that is the hallmark of surface agraphia, and nonword spelling is not possible. Impairment to the graphemic output lexicon with concomitant impairment to the sublexical spelling system is not characterized as a particular agraphia syndrome, but

when the damage is extensive, the resulting profile might be considered a variant of *global agraphia.*[e] As indicated in Table 25–4, such an impairment profile might be characterized by a limited number of correctly spelled words of relatively high frequency, and a complete inability to spell nonwords. Despite the complexity and severity of such global agraphia profiles, several case reports have documented successful treatments designed to strengthen specific graphemic representations (or access to the representations) in severely aphasic individuals.

Taking Advantage of Sound-to-Letter Correspondences

Teaching Sound-to-Letter Correspondences. When the graphemic output lexicon is impaired, spelling treatment may be designed to maximize the use of the sublexical spelling route to resolve spelling difficulty. This is a particularly useful approach when patients have access to phonological representations for words that they are unable to write, but they are not generating plausible spellings of words via sound-to-letter correspondences. Hillis and Caramazza (1994, 1995c) described patient S.J.D. who had an impairment of the graphemic output lexicon with preserved oral naming ability. Despite the fact that S.J.D. could say the words that she wanted to write, her ability to make sound-to-letter conversions was limited, so that she could not derive information from phonology to guide her spelling. Her written spellings also contained semantic errors. In order to increase her use of the sublexical spelling route, S.J.D. was trained 30 sound-to-letter correspondences in a manner similar to that given to patient J.S. (discussed above) using key words. After treatment, S.J.D. was able to derive the first letter or two of problem words, which served to cue her retrieval of the words and to block semantic errors in writing.

Training a Problem-Solving Approach to Spelling. When there is an over-reliance on the sublexical spelling route, errors are likely to occur on irregularly spelled words and homophones. In some cases, plausible misspellings derived by sound-to-letter conversion may provide written cues that help patients resolve their own spelling errors. Two patients (S.V. and S.W.) with mild anomic aphasia and persistent spelling problems were recently reported who responded to treatment that focused on a problem-solving approach to spelling errors (Beeson et al., 2000). When they encountered spelling difficulty, both individuals were often capable of generating plausible or partial spellings. They learned to inspect and self-correct spelling errors by evaluating their written attempts relative to their lexical knowledge. Both patients also made use of an electronic speller that was accepting of plausible misspellings as a last resort to resolve

---

[e]There is not a generally accepted criterion for the term *global agraphia*. Impairment to the graphemic output lexicon and the nonlexical spelling processes might also accompany impairment to the semantic system, as well as additional impairments to the graphemic output buffer and allographic conversion processes.

their spelling difficulties. The problem-solving strategies proved useful for self-correction of spelling errors, but in addition, Beeson et al. (2000) documented that, following the implementation of homework-based writing treatment employing the problem-solving approach, both individuals showed improved spelling abilities.

Strengthening the Graphemic Output Lexicon

Item-specific training to strengthen representations in the graphemic output lexicon may be used to teach correct spellings for irregularly spelled words (Hillis & Caramazza, 1987) and homonyms (Behrman, 1987). Hillis and Caramazza (1987) showed that repeated, corrected practice served to improve spelling of targeted words. Behrman (1987) used a task that involved matching pictures and written words followed by written naming of the picture. She also employed homework that required selection of the appropriate homonym to complete printed sentences. The treatment was successful in improving spelling of homophones and some untreated irregularly spelled words, but did not generalize to untreated homophones.

Anagram and Copy Treatments. Several effective treatment protocols have been reported that include the task of arranging anagram letters to spell target words (Beeson, 1999; Hillis, 1989). An approach called Anagram & Copy Treatment (ACT) was used to develop a corpus of functional single words to supplement spoken and gestural communication in patient S.T., a man with severe Wernicke's aphasia (Beeson, 1999). As depicted in Figure 25–8, the treatment procedure consists of a task hierarchy to elicit correct spelling of the target words by the arrangement of anagram letters followed by repeated copying of the word with the goal of strengthening the mental representation of the written word. After correct anagram arrangement and copy of the word, recall trials require repeated recall of the correct spelling of each target word. The ACT approach relies heavily on the completion of daily homework (at least 30 minutes per day) that involves repeated copy of target words presented with line drawings of the target word. Typically, five new words are learned at one time.

This protocol was initiated with patient S.T. when he was 4 years post-onset of aphasia due to a large left temporo-parietal stroke. A multiple baseline design documented that sets of words were learned only when they were entered into treatment. During the first 10 weeks, S.T. learned 17 words that he was able to use in conversational interaction.

Copy and Recall Treatment. A variation of the ACT protocol was subsequently implemented with S.T. that relied only on homework-based, repeated copy of target words. Personally relevant words were selected by S.T. and his wife (e.g., movie, iced tea), and were written by S.T. in a notebook. S.T. was also able to select target words using a picture

dictionary. On a daily basis, S.T. repeatedly copied the target words, and then self-tested his recall of the spelling for those words by covering up the written example and attempting to recall the spelling, a procedure referred to as Copy and Recall Treatment (CART). In this way, S.T. was able to master additional sets of words, so that his corpus of written words approached 100. He was then able to carry on telegraphic, written "conversation" using the words he had relearned. Periodic testing showed that S.T. appeared to acquire only those words that he targeted to learn, confirming that the improved spelling was item specific. Despite this limitation, the CART approach proved to be highly functional because S.T. continued to expand his written vocabulary to include many proper names of family, friends, favorite restaurants, and the like, allowing for specific, meaningful exchange of information.

Impairment of the Graphemic Buffer

The graphemic representation that is derived either from the graphemic output lexicon or via the sublexical sound-to-letter conversion process is held in short-term storage while letter forms are selected and the implementation of writing is initiated. It has been documented that some patients have an impairment of this graphemic buffer, so that information decays at an abnormally rapid rate (Miceli et al., 1985; Hillis & Caramazza, 1995d). As shown in Figure 25–9, the graphemic buffer receives the output from the lexical-semantic and sublexical routes, so that an impairment of the graphemic buffer will affect all writing tasks including spontaneous writing, written naming, writing to dictation, and delayed copying. Damage to the graphemic buffer affects spelling of all word types, so that there are no effects of frequency, imagery, grammatical class, or regularity of spelling (Table 25–4). In contrast, word length has a significant effect on performance in that short words tend to be more accurately spelled than long words due to the increased demand on the storage capacity for longer words. Damage to the graphemic buffer tends to result in loss of information about the identity and serial ordering of letters so that spelling errors consist of letter omissions (e.g., sweater → *sweatr*), substitutions (e.g., peanut → *peanul*), transpositions (e.g., painter → *painetr*), and additions (e.g., flower → *flowaer*). In the case of left hemisphere brain damage, the initial letters of the word are most likely to be correct, with errors occurring toward the end or in the middle of words (Katz, 1991; Caramazza et al., 1987; Hillis & Caramazza, 1989, 1995d).

Treatment for Impairment of the Graphemic Buffer

In cases of selective impairment of the graphemic output buffer, the spared cognitive processes for spelling may provide a means to compensate (or self-correct) for spelling errors. Hillis & Caramazza (1987) reported such a case—patient D.H., who had a mild anomic aphasia with persistent spelling impairment affecting about 50% of all written words.

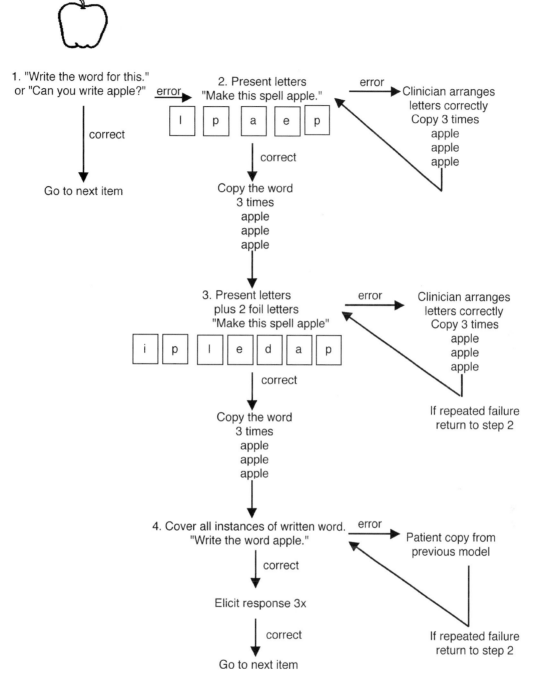

Figure 25–8. Schematic depiction of Anagram and Copy Treatment (ACT).

D.H. made predominantly single-letter spelling errors on the ends of words on all spelling tasks (written naming, writing to dictation, and oral spelling). Given that D.H. had preserved ability to use the sound-to-letter conversion mechanism, and also had a relatively intact graphemic output lexicon, a treatment protocol was devised to take advantage of those skills. D.H. was trained to examine spellings in order to self-correct them. A search strategy to detect errors included examining spellings to evaluate the accuracy (i.e., comparing to representations in his graphemic lexicon), focusing on the ends of words (where most of his errors occurred), and also sounding out each word as it was written (to call attention to phonologically implausible misspellings). D.H. was responsive to this treatment so that he improved his self-correction of spelling in written narratives. Although D.H. still made many spelling errors, his ability to self-correct his errors allowed him to return to previous employment.

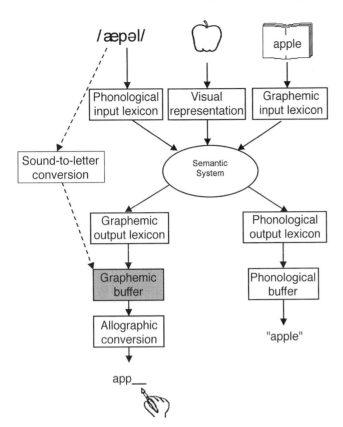

Figure 25–9. Schematic representation of impairment to the graphemic output buffer resulting in loss of information for the rightmost part of the word.

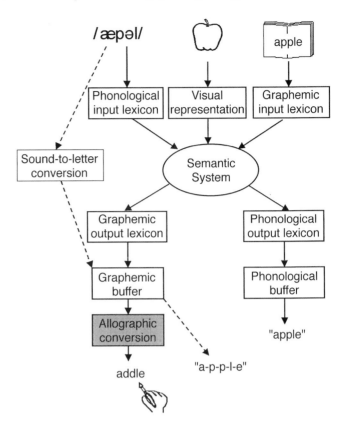

Figure 25–10. Schematic representation of impairment to the allographic conversion mechanism resulting in errors of letter selection in writing. Preserved ability to perform oral naming is indicated.

Impairment of Allographic Conversion

Writing requires the conversion of each grapheme (i.e., abstract letter identity) into a particular letter shape, or allograph, in order to form the string of letters for a word. There are many ways to write a given grapheme, including upper or lowercase, print or cursive, and individual variations in writing style. Therefore, each time a word is written, the appropriate letter shape must be selected for that instance. This stage of writing, the allographic conversion process, is specific to written spelling, and is not required for oral spelling (Figure 25–10). Some patients show a selective impairment of the allographic conversion process so that they can spell aloud, but are impaired in the selection and generation of the correct letter shapes in handwriting (Margolin, 1984; Ramage et al., 1998). Oddly enough, this impairment may be specific to letter case (upper or lowercase; DeBastiani & Barry, 1986; Kartsounis, 1992) or style (print vs. cursive; Hanley & Peters, 1996). The characteristic features include incorrect letter selection resulting in well-formed, but incorrect letters, and may also result in disturbed letter formation. In either case, the writing errors are accompanied by preserved oral spelling.

When examining allographic conversion processes, it is useful to ask patients to transcode printed words from lower

to uppercase and vice versa (see Appendix 25–1). Performance on this task may be compared to direct copy of single words. If graphomotor skills appear preserved for copy, but performance on the transcoding task is impaired, it is suggestive of an impairment at the level of allographic conversion.

Treatment for Allographic Conversion Impairment

It makes sense that treatment for individuals with impaired allographic conversion processes should attempt to take advantage of superior oral spelling abilities. Pound (1996) presented such a patient, J.A., who had impaired letter selection, with better (but not perfect) oral spelling. J.A. was somewhat unusual in that she also showed a notable word length effect suggestive of a graphemic buffer impairment as well. During treatment, patient J.A. was instructed to orally spell each target word before attempting to write it. She was then instructed to self-dictate each letter as she wrote one letter at a time. This procedure was successful because J.A. was capable of writing single letters with fair accuracy; letter selection errors occurred only as she attempted to write the entire word. J.A. was instructed to examine her written words one letter at a time as she orally spelled the word again. She was to self-correct any noted errors, and was prompted to use an alphabet card if a model was needed. Finally, J.A. was to inspect the entire word to check it against her graphemic representation for the word. This procedure proved effective in improving J.A.'s written spelling. Although her spelling was not flawless, it more closely approximated her oral spelling, which tended to show regularity effects suggestive of use of sound-to-letter correspondences. A similar self-dictation procedure was reported by Ramage et al. (1998) that also resulted in improved written spelling in an individual with anomic aphasia and persistent impairment of writing.

Summary of Treatment for Spelling Impairments

Spelling impairments can result from damage to one or more of the critical components of the cognitive processes that support written spelling. Individual case reports demonstrate that treatments directed toward lexical-semantic and sublexical spelling processes can improve spelling abilities of individuals with acquired writing impairments. In some cases, treatments serve to strengthen damaged or degraded representations, including conceptual semantic representations or the graphemic representations (i.e., spellings), and the access to those representations. In other cases, the sublexical sound-to-letter conversion processes are strengthened to support the damaged lexical spelling route. Finally, other treatments improve the operation of the graphemic buffer or allographic conversion processes that ultimately initiate the graphic motor plans for writing. The more peripheral sensorimotor impairments of writing (such as those resulting from cerebellar damage, subcortical lesions, and disorders of praxis) were not discussed here because they are less likely to accompany aphasia, but these disorders are reviewed elsewhere (Rapcsak & Beeson, 2000).

CLOSING COMMENTS

In this chapter, we have sought to provide a framework for assessing reading and spelling, and using the assessment findings to select or design rational treatments. The treatment approaches focused on those components of the reading or spelling process that are impaired or can be used more efficiently to compensate for damaged components. The illustrative evaluation and therapy methods we have described surely do not exhaust the possibilities for improving processing at each level. However, the general approach to identifying, in each patient, what processes are impaired and what processes are spared in the tasks of reading or spelling should provide a springboard for designing other focused treatments. As illustrated by some cases, sequential treatment approaches may be warranted to develop and take full advantage of improved skills and compensatory strategies. It is worth emphasizing that it is essential to carefully monitor a patient's progress so that only effective interventions are pursued. Additionally, it is assumed that specific treatment approaches are tailored to appropriately meet the functional needs of the patient.

FUTURE TRENDS

In the next few decades, our understanding of the cognitive processes that support reading and writing will advance in ways that influence our treatment approaches for acquired alexia and agraphia. We expect that knowledge gained from behavioral research will be complemented by that gained from endeavors such as functional neuroimaging, computer modeling of normal and disordered language processes, and pharmacological interventions. For example, functional neuroimaging studies of regional brain activation during language tasks provide a window to examine normal language processes as well as recovery from brain damage (Karbe et al., 1998; Mimura et al., 1998; Weiller et al., 1995). In fact, researchers have begun to explore the use of functional magnetic resonance imaging to study changes in regional brain activation following behavioral treatments. For example, Small and colleagues (1998) provided evidence of a shift in the region of brain activation during reading following successful treatment in a patient with acquired alexia. Such research should serve to inform our understanding of recovery mechanisms and enhance our ability to design treatment approaches that better match specific patients.

Currently, attempts are being made to use computer modeling to simulate the effects of brain damage and test different treatment approaches (see, for example, Plaut, 1996). Although it may seem far-fetched at the moment, it may be reasonable to expect that such computer modeling ultimately would allow us to "test" treatment approaches for a given patient to determine that which is likely to be most successful. Such a procedure (if it proved valid) would clearly serve to maximize efficiency and effectiveness of behavioral treatments.

Regarding pharmacologic intervention, recent successes in the treatment of acute stroke have served to reduce the extent of brain damage resulting from stroke. Research is in progress to determine if behavioral treatments might be potentiated by specific drugs administered concurrent with behavioral treatment. Although supportive evidence is sparse to date, it is reasonable to consider that future behavioral treatments may be delivered in the context of pharmacological treatment that maximizes the effects of behavioral intervention.

The foregoing comments reflect our optimistic view of the advancement of treatment approaches for reading and writing. However, our enthusiastic view of future possibilities does not blind us to the trend toward limited provision of rehabilitation services for individuals with persistent language impairments. We recognize that speech-language pathologists may find little time available to adequately address reading and writing impairments. We emphasize, however, that many of the approaches that we have reviewed here are heavily reliant on structured homework tasks that can be implemented and monitored within relatively constrained therapy time. Therefore, we suggest that service delivery models extend beyond the treatment session and take full advantage of structured tasks that can be accomplished by the patient between treatment sessions. We also recognize that some patients are best able to respond to reading and writing treatments at relatively long post-onset times, when they typically are no longer receiving treatment. Therefore, we suggest that speech-language pathologists educate and advocate for patients to obtain such services when they are deemed appropriate, regardless of the time post-onset of the impairment. Our experience shows that improved reading and writing abilities can result in significant gains in functional communication and improved quality of life.

KEY POINTS

1. Neurological damage can disturb the processes necessary for reading and writing in a variety of ways. Careful examination of the component processes for reading and writing can serve to isolate the locus (or loci) of impairment and thus guide the treatment procedures.
2. Treatment for acquired reading and writing impairments include approaches that strengthen weakened processes and representations, and those that encourage the development and use of strategies to compensate for impaired processes.
3. Reading impairments can result from impairment to any or all of the following processes or representations: visual processing of written words, the graphemic input lexicon (the store of known written words), the semantic system, the phonological processes necessary for speech production (for oral reading), and the processes necessary to convert letters to the corresponding sounds.
4. Treatment for acquired reading impairments may be directed toward the lexical-semantic processes, so that the links between written words and their meanings are strengthened. Conversely, treatment may be directed toward strengthening the sublexical route for reading whereby letters are converted to their associated sounds, and word pronunciations are assembled.
5. Writing impairments can result from impairment to any or all of the following processes or representations: the semantic system, the graphemic output lexicon (the store of spellings), the graphemic buffer that temporarily holds graphemic information for writing, the conversion processes necessary to select and form specific letters, and the graphic motor processes necessary for the implementation of writing.
6. Similar to reading, treatment for writing impairments may be directed toward lexical-semantic processes, toward sublexical spelling processes, or both.
7. Some treatment approaches result in item-specific improvements, whereas other approaches result in the development of strategies that are of general benefit. Both approaches are valid.

GLOSSARY

alexia without agraphia—an acquired reading impairment that is not accompanied by an impairment of writing; also called pure alexia. It is often characterized by a letter-by-letter reading approach.

allographic conversion—the process whereby an abstract graphemic representation is converted to a specific physical manifestation of a given grapheme.

allographs—the different forms that a grapheme can take, that is, the various ways one can write a given letter by varying, for example, font, case, script, and handwriting styles.

deep agraphia (deep dysgraphia)—an acquired writing impairment that is characterized by the presence of written semantic errors, as well as effects of word frequency (high better than low), imagery (high better than low), and grammatical class (nouns better than functors).

deep alexia (deep dyslexia)—an acquired reading impairment that is characterized by the presence of semantic errors in reading, as well as reading performance that is better for high frequency, concrete nouns in comparison to low frequency, abstract words.

global agraphia—an acquired impairment of writing that disrupts lexical and sublexical spelling processes to such an extent that few words are spelled correctly and it is difficult to detect lexical influences on spelling accuracy.

grapheme—the abstract representation of a letter's identity, e.g., *F* and *f* are letters that both represent the grapheme *f*. A grapheme is a letter or letter cluster that corresponds to a single phoneme.

grapheme-to-phoneme conversion mechanism—a mental process whereby a written word is sounded out by associating each letter identity with its corresponding sound.

graphemic input lexicon—the corpus of written words that one recognizes.

graphemic output buffer—the short-term storage mechanism for holding graphemes as one selects the specific allographs (letter form and style) and implements graphic motor programs.

graphemic output lexicon—the corpus of words that one knows how to spell.

homographs—words that are spelled the same but pronounced differently, for example, the adjective *lead* as in "a lead pipe" and the verb *lead* as in "lead the group"

letter-to-sound conversion—the process of reading aloud by converting a letter (or letter cluster) to the corresponding sound.

letter-by-letter reading—an approach to reading whereby letters are identified in serial order; typically observed as a compensatory reading approach in individuals with pure alexia.

lexical agraphia (surface agraphia)—an acquired writing impairment that is characterized by an over-reliance on sound-to-letter conversion processes; typical errors include regularization of irregularly spelled words (e.g., *yot* for *yacht*).

lexical-semantic route—a means of processing information whereby lexical entries for words are activated along with their corresponding meanings.

nonlexical route—a means of information processing that does not rely on activation of lexical representations, for example, nonlexical reading can be accomplished by converting letters to their corresponding sounds and nonlexical writing can be accomplished by converting sounds to their corresponding letters.

orthographic input lexicon—the collection of mental representations for written words that one recognizes; also called the visual input lexicon or the graphemic input lexicon.

orthographic output lexicon—the collection of mental representations for spellings that one knows; also called the graphemic output lexicon.

orthography-to-phonology conversion—the process of reading aloud by converting a letter (or letter cluster) to the corresponding sound; also referred to as letter-to-sound conversion.

phoneme-to-grapheme conversion—the process of writing by means of deriving spelling based on knowledge of sound-to-letter correspondences.

phonological agraphia—an acquired impairment of spelling that is characterized by the inability to write nonwords due to impairment of the sublexical sound-to-letter conversion processes.

phonological alexia—an acquired impairment of reading that is characterized by an inability to read nonwords due to impairment to the sublexical letter-to-sound conversion processes.

phonological buffer—the short-term storage mechanism whereby phonemes are held while articulatory planning for speech production is accomplished.

phonological output lexicon—the collection of phonological representations for words that one can produce.

pure alexia—an acquired reading impairment that is not accompanied by an impairment of writing. It results from a disruption of visual input from accessing the appropriate abstract word form representation, so that words are visually perceived, but not recognized.

semantic paralexias—reading errors that are semantic in nature, for example, reading *bus* as "car."

sublexical route—a means of information processing that does not rely on activation of lexical representations, for example, reading that is accomplished by converting letters to their corresponding sounds or writing that is accomplished by converting sounds to their corresponding letters.

surface agraphia (lexical agraphia)—an acquired writing impairment that is characterized by an over-reliance on sound-to-letter conversion processes; typical errors include regularization of irregularly spelled words (e.g., *yot* for *yacht*).

surface alexia (surface dyslexia)—an acquired reading impairment characterized by reading according to letter-to-sound correspondence rules so that irregularly spelled words (such as yacht) tend to be mispronounced.

visual input lexicon—the collection of mental representations for written words that one recognizes; also called orthographic input lexicon or graphemic input lexicon.

visual output lexicon—the collection of mental representations for spellings that one knows, also called orthographic output lexicon or graphemic output lexicon.

▶ *Acknowledgment*–The work of the first author (PMB) was supported, in part, by Multipurpose Research and Training Grant DC-01409 from the National Institute on Deafness and Other Communication Disorders (NIDCD), and the work of the second author (AEH) was supported by a fellowship award from the National Stroke Association, a K23 award DC00174-01 from the NIDCD to Johns Hopkins University School of Medicine, and R01-NS22201 from the National Institute on Neurologic Disorders and Stroke to Harvard University. The authors wish to thank Roberta Goodman-Schulman and Alfonso Caramazza for generously sharing the Johns Hopkins Dyslexia and Dysgraphia Batteries.

References

Beeson, P.M. (1998). Treatment for letter-by-letter reading: A case study. In N. Helm-Estabrooks & A.L. Holland (eds.), *Approaches to the treatment of aphasia* (pp. 153–177). San Diego, CA: Singular.

Beeson, P.M. (1999). Treating acquired writing impairment. *Aphasiology, 13*, 367–386.

Beeson, P.M. & Insalaco, D. (1998). Acquired alexia: Lessons from successful treatment. *Journal of the International Neuropsychological Society, 4*, 621–635.

Beeson, P.M., Rewega, M., Vail, S., & Rapcsak (2000). Problem-solving approach to agraphia treatment: Interactive use of lexical and sublexical spelling routes. *Aphasiology, 14,* 551–565.

Behrmann, M. (1987). The rites of righting writing: Homophone remediation in acquired dysgraphia. *Cognitive Neuropsychology, 4,* 365–384.

Berndt, R.S., Reggia, J.A., & Mitchum, C.C. (1987). Empirically derived probabilities for grapheme-to-phoneme correspondences in English. *Behavior Research Methods, Instruments, & Computers, 19,* 1–9.

Bub, D. & Kertesz, A. (1982). Deep agraphia. *Brain and Language, 17,* 146–165.

Caramazza, A. & Hillis, A.E. (1990). Where do semantic errors come from? *Cortex, 26,* 95–122.

Caramazza, A., Miceli, G., Villa, G., & Romani, C. (1987). The role of the graphemic buffer in spelling: Evidence from a case of acquired dysgraphia. *Cognition, 26,* 59–85.

Cherney, L.R., Merbitz, C.T., & Grip, J.C. (1986). Efficacy of oral reading in aphasia treatment outcome. *Rehabilitation Literature, 47,* 112–117.

Coltheart, M., Patterson, K., & Marshall, J.C. (eds.) (1987). *Deep dyslexia* (2nd ed.). London: Routledge & Kegan Paul.

Coltheart, M. (ed.). (1998). Pure alexia: Letter-by-letter reading. Hove, East Sussex, UK: Psychology Press.

Coslett, H.B. & Saffran, E.M. (1989). Evidence for preserved reading in pure alexia. *Brain, 112,* 327–259.

Coslett, H.B. & Saffran, E.M. (1994). Mechanisms of implicit reading in alexia. In M.J. Farrah & G. Ratcliff (eds.), *The Neuropsychology of high-level vision* (pp. 299–330). Hillsdale, NJ: Lawrence Erlbaum.

De Bastiani, P. & Barry, C. (1986). After the graphemic buffer: Disorders of peripheral aspects of writing in Italian patients. *Cognitive Neuropsychology, 6,* 1–23.

de Partz, M.P. (1986). Re-education of a deep dyslexic patient: Rationale of the method and results. *Cognitive Neuropsychology, 3,* 147–177.

Ellis, A.W. (1993). *Reading, writing and dyslexia: A cognitive analysis.* Hillsdale, NJ: Lawrence Erlbaum.

Goodglass, H. & Kaplan, E. (1976, rev. 1983). *The assessment of aphasia and other disorders.* Philadelphia: Lea & Febiger.

Goodman, R.A. & Caramazza, A. (1986, unpublished). *The Johns Hopkins University Dyslexia and Dysgraphia Batteries.*

Greenwald, M.L. & Berndt, R. (1998). Letter-by-letter access without semantics or specialized letter name phonology (abstract). *Brain and Language, 65,* 149–152.

Hanley, J.R. & Peters, S. (1996). A dissociation between the ability to print and write cursively in lower-case letters. *Cortex, 32,* 737–745.

Hanna, P.R., Hanna, J.S., Hodges, R.E., & Rudorf, E.H. (1966). *Phoneme-grapheme correspondences as cues to spelling improvement.* Washington, DC: US Department of Health, Education, and Welfare.

Hanna, G., Schell, L.M., & Schreiner, R. (1977). *The Nelson Reading Skills Test.* Chicago, IL: Riverside.

Hillis Trupe, A.E. (1986). Effectiveness of retraining phoneme to grapheme conversion. In R.H. Brookshire (ed.), *Clinical aphasiology* (pp. 163–171). Minneapolis, MN: BRK.

Hillis, A.E. (1989). Efficacy and generalization of treatment for aphasic naming errors. *Archives of Physical Medicine and Rehabilitation, 70,* 632–636.

Hillis, A.E. (1991). Effects of a separate treatments for distinct impairments within the naming process. In T. Prescott (ed.), *Clinical aphasiology, Vol. 19* (pp. 255–265). Austin, TX: Pro-Ed.

Hillis, A.E. (1993). The role of models of language processing in rehabilitation of language impairments. *Aphasiology, 7,* 5–26.

Hillis, A.E. & Caramazza, A. (1987). Model-driven treatment of dysgraphia. In R.H. Brookshire (ed.), *Clinical aphasiology* (pp. 84–105). Minneapolis, MN: BRK.

Hillis, A.E. & Caramazza, A. (1989). The graphemic buffer and attentional mechanisms. *Brain and Language, 36,* 208–235.

Hillis, A.E. & Caramazza, A. (1991a). Mechanisms for accessing lexical representations for output: Evidence from a category-specific semantic deficit. *Brain and Language, 40,* 106–144.

Hillis, A.E. & Caramazza, A. (1991b). Category-specific naming and comprehension impairment: Theoretical and clinical implication. In T. Prescott (ed.), *Clinical aphasiology, Vol. 20* (pp. 191–200). Austin, TX: Pro-Ed.

Hillis, A.E. & Caramazza, A. (1992). The reading process and its disorders. In D.I. Margolin (ed.), *Cognitive neuropsychology in clinical practice.* New York: Oxford University Press.

Hillis, A.E. & Caramazza A. (1994). Theories of lexical processing and rehabilitation of lexical deficits. In M.J. Riddoch & G.W. Humphreys (eds.), *Cognitive neuropsychology and cognitive rehabilitation.* Hillsdale, NJ: Lawrence Erlbaum.

Hillis, A.E. & Caramazza, A. (1995a). Converging evidence for the interaction of semantic and phonological information in accessing lexical information for spoken output. *Cognitive Neuropsychology, 12,* 187–227.

Hillis, A.E. & Caramazza, A. (1995b). The compositionality of lexical-semantic representations: Clues from semantic errors in object naming. *Memory, 3,* 333–358.

Hillis, A.E. & Caramazza, A. (1995c). "I know it but I can't write it": Selective deficits in long and short-term memory. In R. Campbell (ed.), *Broken memories: Neuropsychological case studies* (pp. 344–365). London: Blackwell.

Hillis, A.E. & Caramazza, A. (1995d). Spatially-specific deficits in processing graphemic representations in reading and writing. *Brain and Language, 48,* 263–308.

Karbe, H., Thiel, A., Weber-Luxenburger, G., Herholz, K., Kessler, J., & Heiss, W.-D. (1998). Brain plasticity in poststroke aphasia: What is the contribution of the right hemisphere? *Brain and Language, 64,* 215–230.

Kartsounis, L.D. (1992). Selective lower-case letter ideational dygraphia. *Cortex, 28,* 145–150.

Katz, R.B. (1991). Limited retention of information in the graphemic buffer. *Cortex, 27,* 111–119.

Kay, J., Lesser, R., & Coltheart, M. (1992). *Psycholinguistic Assessments of Language Processing in Aphasia* (PALPA). East Sussex, England: Lawrence Erlbaum.

Kertesz, A. (1982). *Western Aphasia Battery.* New York: Grune & Stratton.

LaPointe, L.L. & Horner, J. (1998). *Reading Comprehension Battery for Aphasia* (2nd ed.). Austin, TX: Pro-Ed.

Maher, L.M., Clayton, M.C., Barrett, A.M., Schober-Peterson, D., & Rothi, L.J.G. (1998). Rehabilitation of a case of pure alexia:

Exploiting residual abilities. *Journal of the International Neuropsychological Society, 4,* 636–647.

Margolin, D.I. (1984). The neuropsychology of writing and spelling: Semantic, phonological, motor and perceptual processes. *Quarterly Journal of Experimental Psychology, 36A,* 459–489.

Margolin, D.I. & Goodman-Schulman, R. (1992). Oral and written spelling impairments. In D.I. Margolin (ed.), *Cognitive neuropsychology in clinical practice.* New York: Oxford University Press.

Miceli, G., Silveri, M.C., & Caramazza, A. (1985). Cognitive analysis of a case of pure dysgraphia. *Brain and Language, 25,* 187–212.

Mimura, M., Kato, M., Kato, M., Sano, U., Kojima, T., Naeser, M., & Kashima, H. (1998). Prospective and retrospective studies of recovery in aphasia: Changes in cerebral blood flow and language functions. *Brain, 121,* 2083–2094.

Moyer, S.B. (1979). Rehabilitation of alexia: A case study. *Cortex, 15,* 139–144.

Newcombe, F. & Marshall, J.C. (1984). Task and modality-specific aphasias. In F.C. Rose (ed.), *Advances in neurology, Vol. 42: Progress in aphasiology.* New York: Raven Press.

Nickels, L. (1992). The autocue? Self-generated phonemic cues in the treatment of a disorder of reading and naming. *Cognitive Neuropsychology, 9,* 155–182.

Patterson, K. (1992). Reading, writing, and rehabilitation: A reckoning. In M.J. Riddoch & G.W. Humphries (eds.), *Cognitive neuropsychology and cognitive rehabilitation* (pp. 425–448). Hillsdale, NJ: Lawrence Erlbaum.

Patterson, K.E., Marshall, J.C., & Coltheart, M. (1985). *Surface dyslexia.* London: Lawrence Erlbaum.

Patterson, K., Vargha-Khadem, F., & Polkey, C.E. (1989). Reading with one hemisphere. *Brain, 112,* 510–530.

Plaut, D.C. (1996). Relearning after damage in connectionist networks: Toward a theory of rehabilitation. *Brain and Language, 52,* 25–82.

Pound, C. (1996). Writing remediation using preserved oral spelling: A case for separate output buffers. *Aphasiology, 10,* 283–296.

Ramage, A., Beeson, P.M., & Rapcsak, S.Z. (June, 1998). Dissociation between oral and written spelling: Clinical characteristics and possible mechanisms. *Clinical Aphasiology Conference.*

Rapcsak, S.Z. & Beeson, P.M. (2000). Agraphia. In L.J.G. Rothi, B. Crosson, & S. Nadeau (eds.), *Aphasia and language: Theory and practice.* New York: Guilford.

Rapcsak, S.Z., Beeson, P.M., & Rubens, A.B. (1991). Writing with the right hemisphere. *Brain and Language, 41,* 510–530.

Rayner, K. & Pollatsek, A. (1989). *The Psychology of reading.* Hillsdale, NJ: Lawrence Erlbaum.

Rothi, L.J.G., Coslett, H.B., & Heilman, K.M. (1986, unpublished test). *Battery of Adult Reading Function, Experimental Edition.*

Rothi, L.J.G. & Moss, S. (1992). Alexia without agraphia: Potential for model assisted therapy. *Clinical Communication Disorders, 2,* 11–18.

Rothi, L.J.G., Greenwald, M., Maher, L.M., & Ochipa, C. (1998). Alexia without agraphia: Lessons from a treatment failure. In N. Helm-Estabrooks & A.L. Holland (eds.), *Approaches to the treatment of aphasia* (pp. 179–202). San Diego, CA: Singular Publishing Group.

Schwartz, M.F., Saffran, E.M., & Marin, O.S.M. (1987). Fractionating the reading process in dementia: Evidence for word-specific print-to-sound associations. M. Coltheart, K. Patterson, & J.C. Marshall (eds.), *Deep dyslexia* (2nd ed.) (pp. 259–269). New York: Routledge & Kegan Paul.

Seki, K., Yajima, M., & Sugishita, M. (1995). The efficacy of kinesthetic reading treatment for pure alexia. *Neuropsychologia, 33,* 595–609.

Small, S.L., Flores, D.K., & Noll, D.C. (1998). Different neural circuits subserve reading before and after therapy for acquired dyslexia. *Brain and Language, 62,* 298–308.

Parker, D.H. & Scannell, G. (1998). *Scientific Research Associates Reading Laboratory 1C.* Columbus, OH: McGraw-Hill.

Parker, D.H. (1976). *Scientific Research Associates Reading Laboratory, Mark II series.* Scientific Research Associates, Inc.

Tuomainen, J. & Lain, M. (1991). Multiple oral rereading technique on rehabilitation of pure alexia. *Aphasiology, 5,* 401–409.

Wiederholt, J.L. & Bryant, B.R. (1992). *Gray Oral Reading Tests* (3rd ed.) (GORT-3). Austin, TX: Pro-Ed.

Weiller, C., Isensee, C., Rijntjes, M., Huber, W., Muller, S., Bier, D., Dutschka, K., Woods, R.P., Noth, J., & Diener, H.C. (1995). Recovery from Wernicke's aphasia: A positron emission tomography study. *Annals of Neurology, 37,* 723–732.

APPENDIX 25–1
Stimuli from Johns Hopkins University Dyslexia and Dysgraphia Batteries (Goodman & Caramazza, 1986)

The following word lists are controlled for lexical features including grammatical word class, frequency of occurrence in written English, concreteness, regularity of spelling based on sound-to-letter correspondences, and word length. Nonwords are also provided that are pseudohomophones (i.e., nonword spellings that are homophones with real words) and nonhomophones (i.e., pronouncible nonwords derived by altering real words by one grapheme). The words are grouped on the basis of their relevant features, so that the contrasts are apparent; however, items within a given list should be presented in random order during test administration. In many cases, the same word lists can be used to assess reading and writing, but as indicated below, some lists are specific to the Dyslexia or Dysgraphia Batteries.

The Dyslexia Battery consists of oral reading of words and nonwords. The Dysgraphia Battery includes writing to dictation, written naming of pictures, and transcoding by letter case (e.g., upper to lowercase), and copying of single words. Writing to dictation is accomplished by presenting a word or nonword auditorily and the patient is asked to first repeat the stimulus aloud and then write it.

1. Grammatical Word Class
   List composition: 104 words (28 nouns, 28 adjectives, 28 verbs, 20 functors)
   a. Dyslexia Battery
     Task: oral reading
   b. Dysgraphia Battery
     Task: writing to dictation

Word	Class	Frequency	# Letters	Word	Class	Frequency	# Letters
body	noun	HF	4	jury	noun	LF	4
child	noun	HF	5	bugle	noun	LF	5
music	noun	HF	5	digit	noun	LF	5
noise	noun	HF	5	faith	noun	LF	5
ocean	noun	HF	5	glove	noun	LF	5
space	noun	HF	5	grief	noun	LF	5
bottom	noun	HF	6	motel	noun	LF	5
church	noun	HF	6	career	noun	LF	6
column	noun	HF	6	pillow	noun	LF	6
friend	noun	HF	6	priest	noun	LF	6
length	noun	HF	6	sleeve	noun	LF	6
member	noun	HF	6	stripe	noun	LF	6
nature	noun	HF	6	threat	noun	LF	6
street	noun	HF	6	lobster	noun	LF	7
loud	adj	HF	4	brisk	adj	LF	5
tiny	adj	HF	4	cheap	adj	LF	5
angry	adj	HF	5	crisp	adj	LF	5
broad	adj	HF	5	loyal	adj	LF	5
fresh	adj	HF	5	rigid	adj	LF	5
happy	adj	HF	5	sleek	adj	LF	5
short	adj	HF	5	vivid	adj	LF	5
afraid	adj	HF	6	absent	adj	LF	6
bright	adj	HF	6	decent	adj	LF	6
common	adj	HF	6	fierce	adj	LF	6
hungry	adj	HF	6	quaint	adj	LF	6
strong	adj	HF	6	severe	adj	LF	6

Word	Class	Frequency	# Letters	Word	Class	Frequency	# Letters
certain	adj	HF	7	strict	adj	LF	6
strange	adj	HF	8	vulgar	adj	LF	6
begin	verb	HF	5	deny	verb	LF	4
bring	verb	HF	5	adopt	verb	LF	5
carry	verb	HF	5	annoy	verb	LF	5
hurry	verb	HF	5	greet	verb	LF	5
learn	verb	HF	5	argue	verb	LF	5
solve	verb	HF	5	merge	verb	LF	5
speak	verb	HF	5	spoil	verb	LF	5
spend	verb	HF	5	borrow	verb	LF	6
become	verb	HF	6	pierce	verb	LF	6
bought	verb	HF	6	preach	verb	LF	6
caught	verb	HF	6	reveal	verb	LF	6
decide	verb	HF	6	sought	verb	LF	6
happen	verb	HF	6	starve	verb	LF	6
listen	verb	HF	6	conquer	verb	LF	7
both	functor	HF	4	since	functor	HF	5
into	functor	HF	4	these	functor	HF	5
only	functor	HF	4	those	functor	HF	5
what	functor	HF	4	under	functor	HF	5
about	functor	HF	5	while	functor	HF	5
above	functor	HF	5	before	functor	HF	6
after	functor	HF	5	enough	functor	HF	6
could	functor	HF	5	rather	functor	HF	6
often	functor	HF	5	should	functor	HF	6
shall	functor	HF	5	though	functor	HF	6

2. Word Concreteness List

List composition: 42 nouns (21 concrete, 21 abstract)
a. Dyslexia Battery
Task: oral reading
b. Dysgraphia Battery
Task: writing to dictation

Word	Feature	Frequency	# Letters	Word	Feature	Frequency	# Letters
cabin	concrete	HF	5	beauty	abstract	HF	6
cattle	concrete	HF	6	danger	abstract	HF	6
engine	concrete	HF	6	method	abstract	HF	6
valley	concrete	HF	6	moment	abstract	HF	6
window	concrete	HF	6	sister	abstract	HF	6
kitchen	concrete	HF	7	system	abstract	HF	6
village	concrete	HF	7	science	abstract	HF	7
college	concrete	MF	6	mercy	abstract	LF	5
dollar	concrete	MF	6	basis	abstract	MF	5
insect	concrete	MF	6	advice	abstract	MF	6
palace	concrete	MF	6	degree	abstract	MF	6
planet	concrete	MF	6	effort	abstract	MF	6
spider	concrete	MF	6	theory	abstract	MF	6
turkey	concrete	MF	6	courage	abstract	MF	7
salad	concrete	LF	5	success	abstract	MF	7
bullet	concrete	LF	6	belief	abstract	LF	6
fabric	concrete	LF	6	horror	abstract	LF	6
oyster	concrete	LF	6	status	abstract	LF	6
parent	concrete	LF	6	talent	abstract	LF	6
journal	concrete	LF	7	offense	abstract	LF	7
sparrow	concrete	LF	7	pursuit	abstract	LF	7

3. Word Frequency
    List composition: Use responses from any or all of the following lists
        Grammatical Class List (nouns, adjectives, verbs only) = 42 HF and 42 LF
        Word Concreteness List (concrete and abstract) = 14 HF, 14 MF, and 14 LF
        Word Length List = 35 HF and 35 LF
    a. Dyslexia Battery
      Task: oral reading
    b. Dysgraphia Battery
      Task: writing to dictation

4. Nonwords
    a. Dyslexia Battery
      Task: oral reading
      List composition: 34 pseudohomophones and 34 nonhomophones
    b. Dysgraphia Battery
      Task: writing to dictation
      List composition: 34 nonhomophones (* indicates 20 nonwords to be used for oral spelling task with real words in list 7)

Reading Only			Reading and Writing		
Nonword	Type	# Letters	Nonword	Type	# Letters
berd	pseudohomophone	4	berk	nonhomophone	4
bole	pseudohomophone	4	boke*	nonhomophone	4
groe	pseudohomophone	4	troe	nonhomophone	4
hert	pseudohomophone	4	herm*	nonhomophone	4
lern	pseudohomophone	4	lorn*	nonhomophone	4
meen	pseudohomophone	4	feen*	nonhomophone	4
noys	pseudohomophone	4	foys	nonhomophone	4
rewt	pseudohomophone	4	dewt*	nonhomophone	4
snoe	pseudohomophone	4	snoy	nonhomophone	4
sune	pseudohomophone	4	sume	nonhomophone	4
breth	pseudohomophone	5	bruth	nonhomophone	5
ghurl	pseudohomophone	5	ghurb	nonhomophone	5
kroud	pseudohomophone	5	kroid	nonhomophone	5
kwene	pseudohomophone	5	kwine*	nonhomophone	5
lytes	pseudohomophone	5	pytes	nonhomophone	5
phait	pseudohomophone	5	phoit*	nonhomophone	5
reech	pseudohomophone	5	reesh*	nonhomophone	5
skurt	pseudohomophone	5	skart*	nonhomophone	5
cherch	pseudohomophone	6	chench*	nonhomophone	6
hunnee	pseudohomophone	6	hannee*	nonhomophone	6
kattul	pseudohomophone	6	kittul	nonhomophone	6
lemmun	pseudohomophone	6	remmun*	nonhomophone	6
merder	pseudohomophone	6	merber*	nonhomophone	6
mursee	pseudohomophone	6	murnee*	nonhomophone	6
phlore	pseudohomophone	6	phloke	nonhomophone	6
sircle	pseudohomophone	6	sarcle*	nonhomophone	6
windoe	pseudohomophone	6	wundoe	nonhomophone	6
wissel	pseudohomophone	6	wessel	nonhomophone	6
consept	pseudohomophone	7	donsept*	nonhomophone	7
haytrid	pseudohomophone	7	haygrid*	nonhomophone	7
kuntre	pseudohomophone	7	kantree*	nonhomophone	7
sertain	pseudohomophone	7	sortain	nonhomophone	7
teybull	pseudohomophone	7	teabull*	nonhomophone	7
mushrume	pseudohomophone	8	mushrame*	nonhomophone	8

5. Regularity of Spelling
    a. Dyslexia Battery—Letter-to-Sound Regularity
      List composition: 60 words with regular spelling and 30 words with irregular (exception) spelling
      Task: oral reading

Reading Only

Word	Regularity	Frequency	# Letters
but	regular	HF	3
base	regular	HF	4
bone	regular	HF	4
cook	regular	HF	4
cool	regular	HF	4
cord	regular	HF	4
corn	regular	HF	4
days	regular	HF	4
face	regular	HF	4
feed	regular	HF	4
feel	regular	HF	4
five	regular	HF	4
grow	regular	HF	4
home	regular	HF	4
life	regular	HF	4
lift	regular	HF	4
list	regular	HF	4
main	regular	HF	4
meat	regular	HF	4
nine	regular	HF	4
paid	regular	HF	4
race	regular	HF	4
sand	regular	HF	4
save	regular	HF	4
seen	regular	HF	4
thin	regular	HF	4
wake	regular	HF	4
shell	regular	HF	5
still	regular	HF	5
these	regular	HF	5
gut	regular	LF	3
boot	regular	LF	4
dare	regular	LF	4
dean	regular	LF	4
dock	regular	LF	4
dome	regular	LF	4
fern	regular	LF	4
fowl	regular	LF	4
gull	regular	LF	4
hike	regular	LF	4
jays	regular	LF	4
math	regular	LF	4
mode	regular	LF	4
mush	regular	LF	4
peat	regular	LF	4
pest	regular	LF	4
pill	regular	LF	4
pose	regular	LF	4
rave	regular	LF	4
rust	regular	LF	4
sock	regular	LF	4
teak	regular	LF	4
tile	regular	LF	4
wail	regular	LF	4
weld	regular	LF	4
greed	regular	LF	5

Reading Only

Word	Regularity	Frequency	# Letters
eye	exception	HF	3
two	exception	HF	3
once	exception	HF	4
sign	exception	HF	4
view	exception	HF	4
earth	exception	HF	5
front	exception	HF	5
ghost	exception	HF	5
knife	exception	HF	5
laugh	exception	HF	5
piece	exception	HF	5
sword	exception	HF	5
friend	exception	HF	6
school	exception	HF	6
tongue	exception	HF	6
axe	exception	LF	3
heir	exception	LF	4
limb	exception	LF	4
quay	exception	LF	4
tsar	exception	LF	4
aisle	exception	LF	5
choir	exception	LF	5
chute	exception	LF	5
corps	exception	LF	5
fraud	exception	LF	5
gauge	exception	LF	5
seize	exception	LF	5
sieve	exception	LF	5
weird	exception	LF	5
brooch	exception	LF	6

Reading Only

Word	Regularity	Frequency	# Letters
moose	regular	LF	5
pouch	regular	LF	5
stink	regular	LF	5
stint	regular	LF	5

b. Dysgraphia Battery—Sound-to-Letter Probability
   List composition: 30 words with high-probability spelling and 80 words with low-probability spelling
   (Probability based on likely phoneme-grapheme conversion)
   Task: writing to dictation

Writing Only

Word	Probability	Frequency	# Letters
best	HIGH	HF	4
dust	HIGH	HF	4
fact	HIGH	HF	4
flat	HIGH	HF	4
hard	HIGH	HF	4
land	HIGH	HF	4
soft	HIGH	HF	4
spot	HIGH	HF	4
stop	HIGH	HF	4
cloud	HIGH	HF	5
count	HIGH	HF	5
drive	HIGH	HF	5
point	HIGH	HF	5
round	HIGH	HF	5
trade	HIGH	HF	5
grab	HIGH	LF	4
mend	HIGH	LF	4
plot	HIGH	LF	4
rent	HIGH	LF	4
twin	HIGH	LF	4
wept	HIGH	LF	4
blame	HIGH	LF	5
bribe	HIGH	LF	5
broom	HIGH	LF	5
chant	HIGH	LF	5
crime	HIGH	LF	5
grave	HIGH	LF	5
hound	HIGH	LF	5
trout	HIGH	LF	5

Writing Only

Word	Probability	Frequency	# Letters
book	LOW	HF	4
dead	LOW	HF	4
free	LOW	HF	4
give	LOW	HF	4
gone	LOW	HF	4
grew	LOW	HF	4
head	LOW	HF	4
keep	LOW	HF	4
love	LOW	HF	4
move	LOW	HF	4
snow	LOW	HF	4
stay	LOW	HF	4
talk	LOW	HF	4
true	LOW	HF	4
type	LOW	HF	4
shoe	LOW	HF	4
skin	LOW	HF	4
tree	LOW	HF	4
want	LOW	HF	4
blood	LOW	HF	5
check	LOW	HF	5
chief	LOW	HF	5
cross	LOW	HF	5
dance	LOW	HF	5
fence	LOW	HF	5
field	LOW	HF	5
fight	LOW	HF	5
floor	LOW	HF	5
fruit	LOW	HF	5
group	LOW	HF	5
knife	LOW	HF	5
learn	LOW	HF	5
leave	LOW	HF	5
noise	LOW	HF	5
share	LOW	HF	5
sheep	LOW	HF	5
speak	LOW	HF	5
voice	LOW	HF	5
breath	LOW	HF	6
bright	LOW	HF	6
beak	LOW	LF	4
crow	LOW	LF	4
debt	LOW	LF	4

	Writing Only		
Word	Probability	Frequency	# Letters
dumb	LOW	LF	4
germ	LOW	LF	4
jeep	LOW	LF	4
jerk	LOW	LF	4
junk	LOW	LF	4
kiss	LOW	LF	4
lamb	LOW	LF	4
loaf	LOW	LF	4
myth	LOW	LF	4
skip	LOW	LF	4
toss	LOW	LF	4
urge	LOW	LF	4
worm	LOW	LF	4
yawn	LOW	LF	4
budge	LOW	LF	5
cheer	LOW	LF	5
cloak	LOW	LF	5
crawl	LOW	LF	5
glove	LOW	LF	5
gross	LOW	LF	5
knock	LOW	LF	5
ledge	LOW	LF	5
lodge	LOW	LF	5
moose	LOW	LF	5
phase	LOW	LF	5
pulse	LOW	LF	5
rinse	LOW	LF	5
sauce	LOW	LF	5
shack	LOW	LF	5
shove	LOW	LF	5
skull	LOW	LF	5
thief	LOW	LF	5
tread	LOW	LF	5
vague	LOW	LF	5
weave	LOW	LF	5
sketch	LOW	LF	6
sneeze	LOW	LF	6

6. Word Length

a. Dyslexia Battery

List composition: 70 words (14 each of 4-letter, 5-letter, 6-letter, 7-letter, 8-letter words balanced for frequency)

Task: oral reading

b. Dysgraphia Battery

List composition: 70 words (14 each of 4-letter, 5-letter, 6-letter, 7-letter, 8-letter words balanced for frequency)

Task: writing to dictation

Word	# Letters	Frequency	Word	# Letters	Frequency
baby	4	HF	edit	4	LF
copy	4	HF	evil	4	LF
iron	4	HF	jury	4	LF
lady	4	HF	odor	4	LF
open	4	HF	pity	4	LF
poem	4	HF	riot	4	LF
unit	4	HF	ruin	4	LF
color	5	HF	avert	5	LF

Word	# Letters	Frequency	Word	# Letters	Frequency
party	5	HF	cable	5	LF
power	5	HF	drama	5	LF
ready	5	HF	elbow	5	LF
seven	5	HF	fluid	5	LF
solid	5	HF	igloo	5	LF
value	5	HF	urban	5	LF
center	6	HF	excess	6	LF
future	6	HF	fumble	6	LF
letter	6	HF	pigeon	6	LF
pretty	6	HF	pirate	6	LF
reason	6	HF	shower	6	LF
region	6	HF	tragic	6	LF
travel	6	HF	vision	6	LF
brother	7	HF	absence	7	LF
machine	7	HF	curtain	7	LF
million	7	HF	cushion	7	LF
problem	7	HF	leopard	7	LF
provide	7	HF	rooster	7	LF
special	7	HF	sincere	7	LF
trouble	7	HF	suspend	7	LF
complete	8	HF	chipmunk	8	LF
language	8	HF	frequent	8	LF
mountain	8	HF	instinct	8	LF
pressure	8	HF	nuisance	8	LF
question	8	HF	province	8	LF
surprise	8	HF	schedule	8	LF
thousand	8	HF	scramble	8	LF

7. Oral Spelling and Copy Tasks—Dysgraphia Battery Only

List composition: 42 words (21 HF and 21 LF including nouns, adjectives, verbs, functors)

a. Oral spelling—ask the patient to spell the word aloud

b. Copy

1) Cross-case transcoding—present written words in uppercase and ask patient to copy in lowercase

2) Direct copy—present written words in lowercase and ask patient to copy in lowercase

Word	Class	Frequency	# Letters	Word	Class	Frequency	# Letters
poem	noun	HF	4	faith	noun	LF	5
length	noun	HF	6	glove	noun	LF	5
moment	noun	HF	6	grief	noun	LF	5
street	noun	HF	6	fabric	noun	LF	6
window	noun	HF	6	talent	noun	LF	6
fresh	adj	HF	5	pursuit	noun	LF	7
happy	adj	HF	5	brisk	adj	LF	5
afraid	adj	HF	6	crisp	adj	LF	5
bright	adj	HF	6	rigid	adj	LF	5
hungry	adj	HF	6	absent	adj	LF	6
bring	verb	HF	5	quaint	adj	LF	6
carry	verb	HF	5	severe	adj	LF	6
since	verb	HF	5	strict	adj	LF	6
speak	verb	HF	5	argue	verb	LF	5
listen	verb	HF	6	bring	verb	LF	5
provide	verb	HF	7	greet	verb	LF	5
what	functor	HF	4	spoil	verb	LF	5
under	functor	HF	5	borrow	verb	LF	6
enough	functor	HF	6	pierce	verb	LF	6
rather	functor	HF	6	starve	verb	LF	6
though	functor	HF	6	suspend	verb	LF	7

8. Written Naming—Dysgraphia Battery Only
Line drawings of the following 52 items are presented for written naming

Word	Frequency	# Letters	Word	Frequency	# Letters	Word	Frequency	# Letters
car	HF	3	tie	MF	3	cane	LF	4
bear	HF	4	flag	MF	4	comb	LF	4
bell	HF	4	pipe	MF	4	drum	LF	4
fish	HF	4	shoe	MF	4	lamb	LF	4
foot	HF	4	lamp	MF	4	broom	LF	5
iron	HF	4	tent	MF	4	glass	LF	5
rope	HF	4	brush	MF	5	glove	LF	5
glass	HF	5	canoe	MF	5	nurse	LF	5
money	HF	5	pilot	MF	5	razor	LF	5
plant	HF	5	shirt	MF	5	onion	LF	5
table	HF	5	thumb	MF	5	skirt	LF	5
train	HF	5	basket	MF	6	snail	LF	5
watch	HF	5	castle	MF	6	spoon	LF	5
bottle	HF	6	cheese	MF	6	tiger	LF	5
church	HF	6	orange	MF	6	witch	LF	5
doctor	HF	6	rocket	MF	6	anchor	LF	6
island	HF	6	thread	MF	6	carrot	LF	6
						guitar	LF	6

9. Nonwords—Additional list for Dyslexia Battery

Nonword	Type	# Letters	Nonword	Type	# Letters
ded	pseudohomophone	3	ner	nonhomophone	3
dert	pseudohomophone	4	buke	nonhomophone	4
gard	pseudohomophone	4	cest	nonhomophone	4
gerl	pseudohomophone	4	dree	nonhomophone	4
groe	pseudohomophone	4	feve	nonhomophone	4
hert	pseudohomophone	4	fute	nonhomophone	4
lern	pseudohomophone	4	gand	nonhomophone	4
meen	pseudohomophone	4	gree	nonhomophone	4
rufe	pseudohomophone	4	leng	nonhomophone	4
snoe	pseudohomophone	4	nuck	nonhomophone	4
sune	pseudohomophone	4	pesh	nonhomophone	4
turm	pseudohomophone	4	plen	nonhomophone	4
werd	pseudohomophone	4	tink	nonhomophone	4
werk	pseudohomophone	4	trin	nonhomophone	4
wite	pseudohomophone	4	vece	nonhomophone	4
breth	pseudohomophone	5	plent	nonhomophone	5
munny	pseudohomophone	5	sheem	nonhomophone	5
reech	pseudohomophone	5	taght	nonhomophone	5
shure	pseudohomophone	5	thalk	nonhomophone	5
whall	pseudohomophone	5	thell	nonhomophone	5
whife	pseudohomophone	5	tuddy	nonhomophone	5
merder	pseudohomophone	6	jenior	nonhomophone	6
sircle	pseudohomophone	6	sloser	nonhomophone	6
consept	pseudohomophone	7	resords	nonhomophone	7
sertain	pseudohomophone	7	sountry	nonhomophone	7

APPENDIX 25–2
Rank Order of Phoneme Occurrences in Word Corpus and the Common Associated Graphemic Representations

Rank of Occurrence[a]	International Phonetic Alphabet	Keyboard-Compatible Representation	Probable Grapheme[b]	Example
1	/r/	r	r	rat
2	/t/	t	t	tea
3	/n/	n	n	no
4	/s/	s	s	sun
5	/ɪ/	ih	i	pill
6	/ə/	uh	o, a	button, about
7	/l/	l	l	lake
8	/k/	k	k, c	key, cat
9	/i/	ee	ee, ea	bee, eat
10	/æ/	ae	a	apple
11	/ɛ/	eh	e	egg
12	/d/	d	d	dog
13	/m/	m	m	man
14	/p/	p	p	pen
15	/ɚ/	er	er	mother
16	/o/	o	oa, o	boat, open
17	/b/	b	b	book
18	/e/	ay	a-e	ape
19	/a/	ah	a	father
20	/f/	f	f	fan
21	/ʃ/	sh	sh	shoe
22	/v/	v	v	van
23	/ai/	ai	i, i-e	find, ice
24	/ʌ/	uh+	u	up
25	/g/	g	g	goat
26	/z/	z	z	zebra
27	/dʒ/	dj	j	joke
28	/ɔ/	aw	aw, o	saw, soft
29	/h/	h	h	hat
30	/w/	w	w	window
31	/ŋ/	ng	ng	ring
32	/tʃ/	tch	ch	chin
33	/u/	oo	oo	food
34	/ð/	th–	th	then
35	/aʊ/	au	ou, ow	house, owl
36	/ʊ/	u	oo	book
37	/ɔɪ/	oy	oy	boy
38	/θ/	th+	th	thin
39	/j/	y	y	yellow
40	/ʒ/	zh	g	rouge

[a] Rank of occurrence was calculated from a corpus of 17,310 English words by Hanna et al. (1967) with modifications made by Berndt et al. (1987).
[b] Phoneme-to-grapheme correspondences were taken from Berndt et al. (1987) who used the Hanna et al. (1967) data to calculate probability estimates for pronunciation of particular graphemes. The graphemes presented here reflect only the most probable spellings (see Berndt et al. for a complete listing of graphemes for each phoneme).

Chapter 26

Treatment of Underlying Forms: A Linguistic Specific Approach for Sentence Production Deficits in Agrammatic Aphasia

Cynthia K. Thompson

This chapter will discuss a recently developed and researched treatment for sentence production deficits seen in individuals with agrammatic aphasia. The approach is based on linguistic theory and uses the underlying canonical form of complex sentences to improved sentence production.

OBJECTIVES

The objectives of this chapter are to summarize the literature regarding the type of language difficulties shown by patients with agrammatic aphasia; provide a brief discussion of theories of agrammatism; detail the theoretical basis of and rationale for treatment of underlying forms; describe methods for clinical assessment of agrammatism; detail methods used to train sentence production and comprehension; discuss the acquisition and generalization effects of treatment of underlying forms; highlight changes in narrative discourse that result from treatment; and present functional imaging (fMRI) data showing local change in blood oxygenation in activated cerebral tissue prior to and following treatment.

Agrammatism has been characterized as a symptom complex seen in the context of nonfluent Broca's aphasia. It is typically associated with a frontal opercular lesion, occupying Brodmann's areas 44 and 45, the adjacent premotor and motor regions, underlying white matter, the basal ganglia, and the insula (Damasio, 1991; Damasio & Damasio, 1989.[a]

The disorder refers to a pattern of sentence production that reflects an absence of grammatical structure. Individuals with agrammatism speak effortfully and make grammatical errors, but often convey adequate messages by using structurally impoverished strings of content words. Detailed descriptions of agrammatic language production have shown that individuals with agrammatism evince difficulty producing closed-class words, i.e., free-standing grammatical morphemes such as prepositions, articles, pronouns, and auxiliary verbs (Caramazza & Hillis, 1989; Goodglass, 1976; Menn & Obler, 1989; Miceli et al., 1989; Saffran et al., 1989). As well, morphological markers of inflectional and derivational processes are simplified or left out of the agrammatic patients' discourse. In addition to problems with closed-class words, individuals presenting with agrammatic patterns also have difficulty with some open-class words. They tend to over-rely on nouns, resulting in an impoverishment in verb production (Kohn et al., 1989; Miceli et al., 1983; Saffran et al., 1989; Thompson et al., 1997; Thompson et al., 1994; Kim & Thompson, 2000; Zingeser & Berndt, 1990). Further, a preference for production of simple verbs (e.g., intransitive verbs such as *sleep*) versus more complex verbs is prevalent (e.g., dative verbs such as *send*) (Thompson et al., 1997). This problem with verb production is important to understanding and treating agrammatic aphasic individuals' sentence production deficits.

Agrammatic aphasic individuals also present with difficulty producing grammatical sentences. They produce primarily short, simple, subject-verb (SV) and subject-verb-object (SVO) structures that are often grammatically ill formed. Sentence constituents (e.g., noun phrases [NPs]) also are often misordered around the verb (Caplan & Hanna, 1999; Goodglass et al., 1993; Saffran et al., 1989). In addition, verbs and verb arguments often are missing. Notably,

---

[a]The lesion site associated with agrammatism can vary greatly. Vanier and Caplan (1990) reported lesions based on CT scans from 20 cross-linguistic cases of agrammatism, ranging from small lesions located in the frontal lobe or outside of the frontal lobe, sparing the entirety of the perisylvian lateral cortex, to middle-sized lesions affecting both cortical and subcortial structures, to large lesions affecting the entire perisylvian area and other structures in the distribution of the middle cerebral artery.

agrammatic aphasic individuals have great difficulty producing complex sentences in which noun phrases (NPs) have been moved out of their canonical order (i.e., SVO in English) (Saffran et al., 1989; Thompson et al., 1995).

Consider the following language sample produced by a patient diagnosed with nonfluent Broca's aphasia with agrammatism, illustrating many of the characteristics noted in the literature. The patient is telling the story of Cinderella.

Patient 1: Male, 41 years old

Cinderella uh ... scrubing and uh ... hard worker and wants to go a ball. Step fa ... mother uh I want to go. Can't do it. Not ... no well why not? I don't know. Because uh I uh uh ... scrubing uh uh whatchacallit uh uh working ... object and so clean out bad.

Cinderella uh seems like animals love her. Because uh dress ... Horse help her. And stepmother uh uh ... ruin dress. I don't know why. Probably because cute. Mad because uh uh ... stepmother really ugly. Dress broken and now can't do it because what dress? Mother Teresa ... not exactly ... uh uh magic godmother! That's it. Godmother dress don't worry I can fix it. And ... beautiful.

Now carriage where? I don't know how do you go here? Because castle big. Probably uh mountain castle. How do you get uh here? Oh don't worry. I can uh ... pumpkin and uh ... servants and horse and beautiful carriage and so magic. But, better midnight be here because uh uh pumpkin carriage gone. Midnight be here.

Prince see prince oh my god! I think loves uh uh uh uh uh prince ... Cinderella dance. I think probably uh prince uh uh ... loves her. Midnight uh clock uh Cinderella hear clock oh my god! Goodbye. Prince where you going? I'm sorry. can't well stay. Slipper fall. Prince got it uh ... slipper. And duke uh order prince uh ... find out can fit all the kingdom. A woman see can do it.

Now duke uh uh home where uh ... stepmother. Prince can't uh uh stepmother fitting no slipper? No! stepmother slipper uh ... not can't be do it. Now stepmother. I don't know why. Should know not uh probably not uh ball because uh where's dress? But stepmother decided not want to uh ... duke not want to see. That's it. oh no! Actually Cinderella where? Well locked. I wonder why. Sure enough obviously fits because Cinderella uh ... magic uh ... girl. And duke finally found it. And probably uh prince and Cinderella married and happy. What's it? You know happy I don't know. That's it.

Agrammatic aphasic individuals also present with deficits in comprehension, although general descriptions of the disorder suggest that comprehension remains relatively spared (Goodglass, 1976; also see deBlesser, 1987 for historical review). They show particular difficulty comprehending complex, noncanonical sentences such as passive sentences and object relative clauses (e.g., *The artist was chased by the thief; The man saw the thief who the policeman chased*), but less difficulty is noted in comprehending active sentences or those with subject relative clauses (e.g., *The thief chased the artist; The man saw the policeman who chased the thief*) (Berndt et al., 1996; Berndt, 1987; Caplan et al., 1985; Caplan & Hildebrandt, 1988; Grodzinsky, 1986; Nespoulous et al., 1988; Saffran & Schwartz, 1988; Schwartz et al., 1985; Schwartz et al., 1987). This pattern of comprehension impairment is referred to as asyntactic comprehension. It is important to note that these patients often show particular difficulty with semantically reversible sentences (i.e., those in which two nouns are equally probable candidates for the thematic role of *agent* of the action; e.g., the *thief* in *The thief chased the artist*). Agrammatic aphasic individuals also have difficulty understanding sentences with complex verbs, or those with more than one verb (Caplan et al., 1985; Caplan & Hildebrandt, 1988; Caramazza & Zurif, 1976; Nespoulous et al., 1988; Schwartz et al., 1980).

In addition to sentence comprehension deficits, individuals showing agrammatic patterns of language breakdown also have difficulty judging the grammar of some sentence types, especially those with movement of phrasal constituents such as wh-questions and subject-raising structures (Grodzinsky & Finkel, 1998).[b] Other studies of grammaticality judgment, however, have shown largely preserved ability in agrammatic aphasia (Linebarger et al., 1983).

Notably, there is heterogeneity among the characteristics considered to be part of the symptom complex of agrammatic aphasia and dissociations among the primary characteristics of agrammatism have been reported. Three types of grammatical disturbances were described some years ago by Tissot et al. (1973), including (a) fragmented, halting, and limited speech output without major structural errors, (b) a primarily morphological impairment in which bound and free-standing grammatical morphemes are missing but word order is intact, and (c) a primarily constructional impairment in which complete sentences are rarely produced, but grammatical morphemes are not impaired. More recent literature has further detailed patterns of impairment in agrammatic patients. For example, patients have shown differential deficits in bound, but not free-standing morphemes (Miceli & Mazzuchi, 1990; Saffran et al., 1989) and within these classes some elements and not others have been affected (Friedmann & Grodzinsky, 1997; Nespoulous et al., 1988; Miceli et al., 1989; Thompson et al., in press). Some patients show problems affecting only grammatical morphemes, but not sentence structure per se and vice versa (Berndt, 1987; Schwartz et al., 1980). Finally, some (but not all) agrammatic patients present patterns of asyntactic comprehension.

---

[b]Notably, Grodzinsky and Finkel (1998) reported similar grammaticality judgment errors in patients with Wernicke's aphasia, and, in both Broca's and Wernicke's subject groups, variability in performance was noted across subjects.

Because of the heterogeneity that exists among patients diagnosed with agrammatism, the diagnostic category of agrammatism has been challenged (Badecker & Caramazza, 1985; Miceli et al., 1989). Indeed, it cannot be questioned that patients presenting with language behaviors indicative of agrammatism vary in terms of the specific impairments that they present. Of importance here, however, is not whether or not the disorder exists, because in fact we believe that it does. Instead, given the variability of language disruption patterns seen in agrammatism, it is important both in research and in clinical practice to carefully delineate the specific language behaviors that are disrupted in individual cases because patients presenting with differing agrammatic error patterns may require different treatment approaches. As described below, the agrammatic patients appropriate for the type of treatment described here show asyntactic comprehension patterns and sentence structural deficits in production involving the retrieval and proper concatenation of sentence constituents.

THEORIES OF AGRAMMATISM

Many theoretical accounts have been offered to accommodate the performance patterns seen in agrammatism, including linguistic explanations that place the impairment within specific aspects of the syntactic representation that patients can generate (Grodzinsky, 1986, 1995, 2000; Mauner et al., 1993). Other explanations locate the impairment in operations that "map" syntactic roles of nouns to thematic (semantic) roles such as *agent of the action* (Schwartz et al., 1987). Still other theories have suggested that error patterns seen in agrammatism reflect an adaptation to short-term memory limitations, changes in the thresholds of word activation, or an increase in noise in the system (Kolk et al., 1985).

Recent theories also have used linguistic tree structures to locate production deficits seen in agrammatism (Friedmann & Grodzinsky, 1997; Hagiwara, 1995). Hagiwara (1995), for example, observed that aphasic subjects who demonstrate impairments at lower levels of the tree show impairments affecting all structures higher in the tree. Hagiwara, therefore, suggested that projections of higher levels in the tree are dependent on successful projection of lower levels.

Models of normal sentence production also have been used to determine where in the process of sentence planning breakdowns occur in agrammatic aphasia (Bock, 1987; Garrett, 1980, 1984). Garrett's model, for example, includes several stages of sentence planning, from an early conceptual, or inferential, stage where the ideas to be expressed in a sentence are generated to an articulatory stage where the motor codes for production of the sentence are accessed. Using this model, agrammatism has been cast as a disorder resulting from disruption of one of two possible stages of sentence planning: (1) the "functional" level of processing, where open-class words including verbs and their arguments are accessed and thematic roles are assigned (Thompson et al., 1993), and (2) the "positional" level, a stage where bound and free-standing morphemes are placed in sentence frames together with content words and the phonology of these elements is specified (Caramazza & Hillis, 1989). The exact locus of the deficit, however, remains under debate. Clearly, given the different patterns of impairment seen in individuals with agrammatism, it is likely that different aspects of sentence planning may be involved in different patients.

TREATMENT OF AGRAMMATISM

A Philosophy of Intervention

Treatment for aphasia is not an exact science. Until recently, research investigating the effects of certain treatments for certain aphasic deficits was rare. Early attempts to document the effects of treatment were undertaken with groups of aphasic patients (often with no control group) who presented with a wide variety of language impairments. Nonspecific treatment, for example, "traditional, individual stimulus-response type treatment of speech and language deficits in all communicative modalities" (Wertz et al., 1981, p. 583) was provided for the patients, and language changes noted on standardized tests following treatment were documented. The limitations of this approach to documentation of treatment effects are apparent given the above discussion regarding the different language deficit patterns seen in agrammatism. Aphasic patients are not all the same, even those diagnosed as having a particular aphasic syndrome. Therefore, it follows that all aphasic patients will not respond optimally to the same treatment. Further, standardized tests do not capture specific changes within the language-processing system. Indeed, improvements in language have been documented in patients who have not demonstrated improvement on standardized tests (Thompson, 1989).

The importance of studying language breakdown in individual patients with aphasia has recently gained popularity, precisely because of the heterogeneity evident among aphasic individuals. For example, in the cognitive neuropsychological literature, the case study approach has been widely used to delineate deficit patterns within and across language domains in aphasic patients (Caramazza, 1986). While this approach has been subject to criticism (Bates et al., 1991), it has heightened awareness of individual patterns of language disruption that may occur in aphasic individuals, and it has provided information for formulating models of language processing that will later need to be experimentally examined and verified.

In the treatment domain, individual aphasic patients also have come into focus. Recent examinations of treatment effects have used single-subject experimental paradigms in which experimental control is demonstrated by comparing performance patterns across phases of a study (e.g., between baseline and treatment phases) in individual subjects, rather than comparing performance patterns between groups of subjects as in group experimental designs. Importantly, however, these designs require replication of treatment effects across subjects presenting with similar language disruption patterns (Kearns, 1986; Kearns & Thompson, 1991; McReynolds & Thompson, 1986; Thompson & Kearns, 1991). Single-subject experimental research, therefore, does not mean research with an *n* of one. Because this approach requires close examination of individual subjects' performance, it has brought us closer to understanding the effects of certain treatments for certain language deficits.

The treatment approach presented here (i.e., treatment of underlying forms for sentence production and comprehension) has been extensively researched using single-subject experimental research design. In this work certain language behaviors (i.e., sentences) are selected for analysis based on their linguistic characteristics. Production (and comprehension) of the sentences is then tested prior to treatment in a baseline phase. Treatment then is applied to one structure, while the others are tested for generalization. In this way we have been able to chart patterns of generalization across sentence types and have, thus, learned how certain structures are related to one another. We also have examined generalization to spontaneous discourse and have found that treatment influences the grammar and content of spoken language.

Generalization is an important and often overlooked aspect of aphasia treatment. Although aphasiologists have historically assumed that generalization is a natural and expected outcome of treatment (e.g., Schuell et al., 1964), this has turned out to be an erroneous assumption. Indeed, well-controlled treatment research has indicated that generalization sometimes does not occur. Clearly, if generalization to untrained responses does not occur as a result of treatment, then "in theory we must endeavor to train all responses that the aphasic patient will ever use . . . . and if generalization across contexts does not occur . . . our treatment may be deemed unsatisfactory, because it is this carryover of responding from the clinic to natural contexts that is the ultimate goal of treatment" (Thompson, 1989, p. 83). Therefore, in the design of treatment for agrammatism (as well as for all other aphasias) target structures need to be selected and measured in a variety of language contexts in the baseline or pretreatment phase. Treatment is then applied to only one or to a few of these structures in one or more contexts. Periodically, throughout the treatment phase generalization is measured (a) to untrained structures and (b) in the untrained language contexts. If generalization does not occur as a natural outcome of treatment, then steps must be taken to facilitate generalization (see Thompson, 1989, for review of these methods).

TABLE 26–1	

Helm-Elicited Language Program for Syntax Stimulation Sentence Types

Sentence Type	Sample Sentence
1. imperative intransitive	Sit down.
2. imperative transitive	Drink your milk.
3. wh-interrogative	Where are my shoes?
4. declarative transitive	He teaches school.
5. declarative intransitive	He swims.
6. comparative	He's taller.
7. passive	The car was towed.
8. yes-no questions	Did you watch the news?
9. direct and indirect object	He brings his mother flowers.
10. embedded sentences	She wanted him to be rich.
11. future	He will sleep.

Approaches to Treatment

Treatment for agrammatic aphasia has received little attention in the literature and few treatment approaches have been advanced. For example, treatment research concerned with establishing methods for improving access to grammatical morphemes—either bound or free standing—is limited to a handful of studies (see for example, Cannito & Vogel, 1987; Kearns & Salmon, 1984) and the effects of such training on sentence production have not been addressed.

Treatment concerned directly with improving production of sentences—e.g., training production of certain sentence types—has received a bit more attention, although research in this area is limited as well. For example, syntax stimulation (Helm-Estabrooks et al., 1981; Helm-Estabrooks & Ramsberger, 1986) and direct production treatment approaches (Thompson & McReynolds, 1986; Wambaugh & Thompson, 1989) focus on instruction and practice in producing certain sentence types. The *Helm-Estabrooks Language Program for Syntax Stimulation* (HELPPS; Helm-Estabrooks, 1981), for example, is focused on training a set of sentences shown by Goodglass et al. (1972) to be difficult for agrammatic aphasic individuals to produce (see Table 26–1). One sentence type is trained at a time, beginning with that considered to be the easiest (e.g., imperative intransitives such as *Sit down*). Research concerned with establishing the efficacy of this approach has indicated that patients improve in their ability to produce trained sentences. However, less impressive findings have been reported with regard to generalization across sentence types. That is, training individual sentence types does not always influence production of others (Doyle et al., 1987; Fink et al., 1995; Salvatore et al., 1983).

Direct production treatment has resulted in similar performance patterns. For example, we (Thompson &

TABLE 26–2

Example of Sentence Types Targeted by Schwartz et al. (1994) for Treatment Using Mapping Therapy

Sentence Type	Sample Sentence
1. Simple Subject and Object NPs	Susan drinks the soda.
2. Adjective in Subject NP	The old man is fixing it.
3. Adjective in Object NP	Ann washed the playful child.
4. Complex Subject NP	Tommy's grandfather built the wall.
5. Complex Object NP	Jan called the person in charge.
6. Complex Subject and Object NPs	The girl from the office was helping Mary's daughter.

McReynolds, 1986) trained four agrammatic aphasic individuals to produce *what*-questions and, although all subjects improved in their ability to produce these questions, training had no effect on production of *who*, *where*, or *when* questions.

The noted lack of generalization across sentence types that often results in using syntax stimulation and/or direct production approaches led researchers to take a different—more theoretical—direction in developing treatment methods for sentence production deficits. Instead of focusing directly on the surface representation of sentences, these treatments focus on aspects of production (or processing) that are thought to be awry in agrammatic aphasia. For example, Loverso and colleagues (Loverso et al., 1986) developed a method known as *verb as core* treatment. It is based on the premises that (a) access to verbs is often disrupted in agrammatic aphasia and (b) verbs are central to sentence production. In this approach, patients are trained to produce verbs together with specific sentence constituents (usually NPs) that are assigned various thematic roles by the verb (e.g., *agent*, *theme*) in simple, active sentences. Results of research investigating the effects of this treatment have indicated improved verbal scores using the *Porch Index of Communicative Abilities* (PICA [Porch, 1973]). However, the extent to which this treatment influences (a) production of various sentence types, including complex sentences, (b) the grammaticality of sentences, or (c) aspects of sentence production in spontaneous discourse has not been investigated.

Another treatment for sentence level deficits designed to improve both comprehension and production of sentences in individuals with agrammatic aphasia is *mapping therapy* (Byng, 1988; Jones, 1986; Schwartz et al., 1994). Like *verb as core* training, this approach is theoretically motivated. It is based on the notion that difficulty comprehending semantically reversible sentences such as *The boy is chased by the girl* represents a deficit in mapping semantics onto syntax, as discussed previously (see Theories of Agrammatism). Mapping therapy is thereby designed to alleviate this mapping deficit. It focuses on the thematic roles of sentence NPs in both simple, active canonical sentences and in more complex, noncanonical sentences (see Table 26–2). Presented with sentences in written form, patients are asked to underline the *agent*, *theme*, etc. in response to questions concerning the logical subject and the logical object (e.g., "Which one is doing the V-ing"? and "What is she/he V-ing"?). Results of treatment research using this method have shown improved comprehension of both canonical and noncanonical sentence forms. However, like syntax stimulation and direct production approaches, improvement has been constrained largely to the types of sentences entered into treatment. For example, Schwartz et al. (1994) used mapping therapy to train canonical (SVO) sentences with action verbs and various padding (i.e., additions of modifying words and phrases to the subject and/or object NP) and found improved canonical sentence comprehension (and production), yet little improvement on noncanonical sentences (i.e., passives, object relatives).

The lack of noteworthy generalization across sentence types found in the aforementioned studies may be related to the nature of the sentences entered into treatment and to the treatment strategy itself. Treatment of underlying forms is a linguistic approach which was developed in consideration of both the lexical and syntactic properties of sentences trained and those selected for analysis of generalization. In addition, the linguistic properties of sentences were considered in development of the treatment. As discussed later on (see Theoretical Framework section), subjects with agrammatic Broca's aphasia appear to have normal access to verbs and thematic information; however, they do not always assign thematic roles normally, nor do they use them fully in their sentence productions. Further, these patients do not appear to normally process sentences with moved constituents (i.e., they do not establish trace-antecedent relations)—and it is likely that such binding relations are also not established in production. Therefore, like mapping therapy, treatment of underlying forms begins with tasks concerned with establishing and improving knowledge and access to the thematic role information around verbs using the canonical (S-V-O) form of target sentences.[c] Next, operations involved in establishing trace-antecedent relations in complex sentences are exploited. Finally, to test the effects of treatment, generalization is evaluated to sentences that are similar to those trained in terms of their semantic and syntactic properties. It turns out that when the linguistic underpinnings of complex sentences are considered successful generalization across sentences that are different in their surface form, but that are similar in their underlying linguistic properties, results.

In addition, the complexity of structures trained appears to be relevant to generalization. That is, training more complex structures first results in generalization to less complex structures that are in a subset relation to trained structures (see later section, The Role of Syntactic Complexity: Optimal Order for Promoting Generalization). From this point of view it is not surprising that treatments that progress from simple sentences to more difficult ones (e.g., syntax stimulation, mapping therapy) have shown little generalization across sentence types.

Theoretical Framework

As noted above, the treatment of underlying forms approach is based on aspects of formal linguistic theory (e.g., Chomsky 1986, 1991, 1993, 1995)[d] as well as the results of psycholinguistic and neurolinguistic research (Caplan et al., 1985; Caplan & Futter, 1986; Caplan & Hildebrandt, 1988; Frazier & Clifton, 1989; Shapiro et al., 1991; Shapiro et al., 1993; Shapiro & Levine, 1990; Swinney & Zurif, 1995; Zurif, 1993). The theoretical basis of this approach has been detailed previously (see, for example, Shapiro, 1997 for review; Shapiro & Thompson, 1994; Thompson & Shapiro, 1994; Thompson et al., 1997). Therefore, only crucial background information is summarized here.

Verbs and Their Influence on Sentences

Argument Structure

Most sentences can be considered representations of relations between a verb and its arguments. Verbs are central

to the sentence as much of the core information contained within sentences is determined by the verb. That is, verbs are acquired together with knowledge that they can (and sometimes must) occur with particular structures. For example, when the verb *hit* is learned, it also is learned that someone or something must be hit. Additionally, it is learned that someone must do the hitting. The number of participants that go into the 'action' described by the verb are called *arguments* of the verb. Arguments are typically NPs (though they can also be sentential clauses, prepositional phrases, or adjectival phrases) that fill *argument positions* (typically, subject, object, and indirect object positions). Each argument of a verb is assigned a *thematic role* (e.g., *agent, theme, goal*). The verb *hit* assigns a two-place argument structure as in (1); therefore, it is a two-place verb. *Zack* is assigned the thematic role of *agent* and *the ball* is assigned the role of *theme*.

1. [Zack] AGENT [VP hit [the ball THEME]]

Indeed, there are several different types of verbs—determined (a) by the number of participants (i.e., arguments) that go into the action described by the verb, and (b) by the number of different argument structure arrangements that are possible given a certain verb. Table 26–3 highlights several types of verbs and their argument structure. In contrast to the transitive verb *hit*, which requires two participants and so selects a two-place argument structure, the verb *put* requires three participants and thus entails a three-place argument structure.

2. [Zack] [VP put [the shirt] [in the closet]]

Note that in (1) one of the arguments (*the ball*) appears within the domain of the verb phrase (VP), and in (2) two of the arguments (*the shirt*, and *in the closet*) fall within the VP. These are internal arguments; the subject (i.e., *Zack*) is the external argument in both sentences. The verb *know* also takes a two-place argument structure, though the second argument can have a different syntactic realization. Consider:

3. [Zack] [VP knew [NP the answer]]

4. [Zack] [VP knew [CP that the painter was excellent]]

In (3) the internal argument is an NP (i.e., *the answer*); in (4) it is a sentential complement (i.e., *that the painter was excellent*).

Another important point about verb arguments is that they must be present in sentences in order for the sentences to be grammatical. This principle, known as the Projection Principle (Chomsky, 1986), requires that the lexical information associated with the verb be represented in sentences. Sentences like *Zack hit* and *Zack put the car* are, therefore, ungrammatical because all of the arguments of the verb are not represented.

Importantly, recent psycholinguistic and neurolinguistic research has shown that a verb's argument structure and its thematic representations influence sentence processing. Both normal and Broca's aphasic subjects appear to access

---

[c] We note that both *verb as core* (Loverso et al., 1986) and *mapping therapy* (Jones, 1986; Byng, 1988; Schwartz et al., 1994) focus on the thematic roles of sentence NPs. Our approach, however, departs from theirs in that we require production and comprehension (vs. strictly comprehension in *mapping therapy*) of the verb and its arguments as well as adjuncts contained in target sentences. Additionally, we also exploit the movement operations involved in creating grammatically correct noncanonical sentences and emphasize how thematic roles are retained in the s-structure of complex sentences in which NPs have been moved out of their canonical positions.

[d] The theoretical constructs that we exploit are integral to Government-Binding Theory, the Principles and Parameters (P & P) frameworks, and the Minimalist Program (Chomsky, 1986, 1993, 1995; Marantz, 1995), but they also have their counterparts in other linguistic theories. For example, X-bar theory, subcategorization, and argument structure are part of Generalized Phrase Structure Grammar (GPSG) (Gazdar et al., 1985) and Lexical Functional Grammar (LFG) (Bresnan, 1992). Noncontinuous dependencies of the sort that we target in our treatment studies are also considered in GPSG (e.g., the category SLASH, which effectively connects one part of the tree to another) and LFG (i.e., functional control).

TABLE 26-3

Types of Verbs and Their Argument Structure

Verb Type	Sample Verb	Argument Structure	Sample Sentence
Simple Verbs			
Obligatory One-Place	*sleep*	Agent	[Zack] slept.
Obligatory Two-Place	*hit*	Agent, Theme	[Zack] hit [the fence].
Obligatory Three-Place	*put*	Agent, Theme, Goal	[Zack] put [the shirt] [in the closet].
Complex Verbs			
Alternating Three-Place	*give*	Agent, Theme, Goal	[Zack] gave [the book] [to Matt].
		Agent, Goal, Theme	[Zack] gave [Matt] [the book].
Optional Three-Place	*send*	Agent, Theme	[Zack] sent [the letter].
		Agent, Theme, Goal	[Zack] sent [the letter] [to Frederick].
Complement	*know*	Agent, Theme	[Zack] knew [the painter].
		Agent, Sentential	[Zack] knew [that the painter was good].

not only the verb, but also its thematic representations when listening to sentences (e.g., Shapiro et al., 1987; Shapiro et al., 1991; Shapiro & Levine, 1990; Shapiro et al., 1993; Tanenhaus et al., 1989). That is, reaction times (RTs) are longer when more complex verbs (i.e., those taking more possible argument structure arrangements; e.g., alternating three-place verbs like *give* and complement verbs) are encountered in the sentence than when simple verbs (e.g., obligatory one- and two-place verbs) are heard. Such findings suggest that when the verb is encountered and accessed during the temporal unfolding of a sentence, so too are its thematic properties. The fact that Broca's aphasic individuals retain this ability after brain damage is crucial to our treatment approach.

Arguments and Adjuncts

The distinction between arguments and *adjuncts* also is important. As discussed above, phrases which are assigned a thematic role by the verb are called its arguments. Arguments, unlike adjuncts, form part of the verb's lexical entry. Although both arguments and adjuncts can be represented as similar forms (i.e., prepositional phrases), adjuncts are not selected by the verb. Consider (5) and (6) below. In (5) the prepositional phrase is an argument of the verb *put*. Without it, the sentence is not grammatical. In (6) the prepositional phrase is an adjunct. It adds to the meaning, but is not part of the verb's lexical representation.

5. Zack put the book *on the table*
6. Tim kissed the girl *in the park*

In (5) the verb *put* assigns three thematic roles to its arguments—*agent* to the NP *Zack*, *theme* to the NP *the book*, and *goal* to the prepositional phrase (PP) *on the table*. Without the PP the sentence is ungrammatical. The two-place transitive verb *kiss* in (6) assigns only two thematic roles—*agent* to the NP *Tim*, and *theme* to *the girl*. The

PP *in the park* is a locative adjunct; its "meaning" is not inherent in the verb's representation. Even without the adjunct, the sentence is grammatical.

Phrasal geometry also distinguishes between arguments and adjuncts in that adjunct PPs frequently show attachment ambiguities, which sometimes renders them semantically ambiguous. For example, (6) can mean something like "It was *the girl in the park* (not some other girl) that Tim kissed" in which case the adjunct PP, *in the park*, is attached to (i.e., modifies) the noun phrase *the girl*. But it can also mean something like "It was *in the park* (not somewhere else) where Tim *kissed the girl*." In this case the PP attaches to the VP. Unlike the adjunct PP in (6), the argument PP in (5) is unambiguous; it carries one and only one possible interpretation: the location of the 'action' described by the verb.

Again, it turns out that the presence of adjuncts in sentences influences how sentences are processed. When normal subjects encounter an adjunct prepositional phrase like *in the park* (as in [6]) while listening to a sentence, reaction times (i.e., processing load) are increased relative to when an argument prepositional phrase (e.g., *on the table*, as in [5]) is encountered (Shapiro et al., 1993).

Formation of Noncanonical Sentences

In the English language sentences take the form of SVO. When sentences appear in this simple form they are considered to be *canonical*. But, many sentences in English are noncanonical. Consider the following:

7. Zack kissed Joelle. (active)
8. Who did Zack kiss? (wh-question)
9. Joelle was kissed by Zack. (passive)
10. It was Joelle who Zack kissed. (object cleft)

Despite appearing in different positions in the sentence, *Zack* is the *agent* and *Joelle* (or *Who*) is the *theme* (or *patient*) in all sentences. As discussed previously, the Projection Principle and the lexical entry for *kiss* require it to have a direct object argument to which the *patient* role is assigned. Accordingly, it appears that only (7) is grammatical in that it has a direct object; (8) through (10) appear ungrammatical as there is no overt direct object following the verb.

Importantly, however, sentences (8) though (10) are derived from their simple canonical form. Skipping the details, formation of noncanonical sentences requires movement of sentence constituents from d-structure (an underlying form)—where they receive their thematic role assignments—to s-structure.[e] This transformation is referred to as *move-alpha*. Once moved, the moved constituent is linked (co-indexed) with the position from which it was derived and the thematic role, originally assigned in the d-structure, is inherited by the moved constituent. According to syntactic theory there is a dependency relationship between the empty direct object position (gap) and the antecedent of the trace (i.e., the moved sentence constituent).

There are two types of movement subsumed under the general rule *move-alpha*: wh-movement and NP-movement. Wh-movement is involved in wh-questions (8) and object clefts (10); NP-movement is involved in passives (9) and other types of sentences. Both types of movement relate the d-structure of a sentence, a pure representation of lexical information, with the s-structure representation. NP-movement moves an NP from an argument position to another argument position, leaving behind an NP-trace, whereas wh-movement involves displacement of wh-phrases from argument or adjunct positions to nonargument positions. (See later section, *Training and Generalization of Wh-Movement vs. NP-Movement Structures* for details about the two types of movement.)

For example, an approximation of the underlying structure (d-structure) for a wh-question (e.g., 8) is shown in (11):

11. [Zack AGENT] kissed [who THEME]

Who is in the direct object argument position and is assigned the thematic role of theme by *kiss*. To derive the noncanonical surface form, *who* is moved to the sentence initial position, leaving behind a *trace* (*t*) in the direct object argument position, as illustrated in (12):

12. [Who i THEME] did [Zack AGENT] Kiss [*t* i THEME]

When non-brain-damaged individuals process sentences, it appears that they "reaccess" the moved NP in the vicinity of the trace—well after the moved constituent has occurred in the sentence (e.g., Swinney & Osterhaut, 1990). That is, they "hold on to" the moved NP such that it can be assigned its proper thematic role once the verb in the sentence is heard; thus, normal subjects are able to assign the proper thematic

roles to sentence NPs even when they are encountered in noncanonical order. Importantly, agrammatic Broca's aphasic patients do not show normal co-referencing between elements in sentences with moved sentence constituents. That is, they have difficulty properly assigning thematic roles to arguments that have been moved out of their canonical positions (Caplan & Futter, 1986; Grodzinsky, 1990; Schwartz 1987; Swinney & Zurif, 1995; Zurif et al., 1993).

Argument and Adjunct Movement

The example above (12) illustrates movement of an argument, the direct object NP. Wh-movement also can apply to adjuncts, as in (13).

13. Matt fixed the car [in the garage] → Where i did Matt fix the car *t* i ?

In this example, the moved wh-expression, *where*, corresponds to a locative adjunct. Thus, a co-referential relation is established between the trace in the adjunct position and *where*.

Assessment of Agrammatism

The first step in assessment of agrammatism is to administer a standardized aphasia test battery such as the *Western Aphasia Battery* (WAB; Kertesz, 1982) or the *Boston Diagnostic Aphasia Examination* (BDAE; Goodglass & Kaplan, 1983). Aphasic individuals appropriate for treatment of underlying forms show profiles on these tests consistent with a diagnosis of Broca's aphasia. Most individuals evince mild to moderately severe aphasia; aphasia quotients (AQs) on the WAB range from around 65 to 85. In a recent study by Ballard and Thompson (1999), we studied individuals with agrammatism with somewhat lower AQs, i.e., as low as 54. Results showed that subjects with less severe impairment (i.e., AQs of at least 65) respond most favorably to treatment.

Assessment of grammatical aspects of agrammatic aphasia presents a challenge. Because various aspects of sentence production may be involved in these patients, an in-depth assessment of the impairment is imperative, including testing of both comprehension and production of verbs and verb arguments as well as various sentence types. Unfortunately, at present, published assessment tools are not available for accomplishing this and information provided by administering the WAB or BDAE is not adequate for this purpose.

Testing Sentence Comprehension

Available tests for comprehension such as the *Revised Token Test* (McNeil & Prescott, 1978) and the *Auditory Comprehension Test for Sentences* (Shewan, 1981) do not address all types of sentence-level problems that need to be tested with this patient population. Saffran and colleagues developed a test for sentence comprehension, the *Philadelphia Comprehension Battery for Aphasia* ([PCBA] Saffran et al.,

---

[e] The terms *deep structure* and *surface structure* have been replaced by d- and s-structure, respectively in Chomsky's more recent writings.

unpublished). To date, the test has been used primarily for research, but it may be available for clinical use in the future. This test addresses important aspects of sentence comprehension, providing sections for contrasting lexical (single-word) comprehension with comprehension of sentences of several types, including reversible actives, passives, object-relative clause structures, and subject-relative clause structures.

We (Thompson and colleagues) also developed a test for examining sentence comprehension, The *Northwestern Sentence Comprehension Test* (NSCT). Like the PCBA, this test examines active sentences, passives, object relatives, and subject relatives. Comprehension of each sentence is tested using a picture-pointing task; two pictures for each item are presented—the target and its semantically reversed counterpart; the patient selects the one corresponding to the sentence. The NSCT differs from the PCBA in that more exemplars of each sentence type (n = 20) are tested. The PCBA tests only five exemplars of each. Sample sentences tested with the NSCT are presented in Appendix 26–1.

Results of testing show a characteristic pattern of asyntactic comprehension in our agrammatic patients. Lexical comprehension is superior to overall sentence comprehension. Comprehension of canonical sentences (i.e., actives and subject relatives) is superior to comprehension of more complex sentences in which NPs are moved out of their canonical position (i.e., passives and object relatives). For example, most subjects show a sharp contrast between comprehension of active sentences (usually 90% correct or better) and passive sentences (usually at chance or below). Finally, semantically reversible sentences are more difficult than nonreversible sentences.

Testing Verbs and Verb Arguments

Another important aspect of testing for agrammatic aphasia is examination of verbs and verb argument structures. Again, no published test is presently available for doing this, although several research laboratories around the world have developed protocols for this purpose (Bastiaanse & Jonkers, 2000; Kim & Thompson, 2000; Masterson & Druks, 1998; Thompson et al., 1997). For example, we (Kim & Thompson, 2000; Thompson et al., 1997) developed a test to examine comprehension and production of verbs of several types, including one-place verbs (i.e., intransitive verbs), two-place verbs (i.e., transitive verbs), and three-place verbs. The verb battery has three subtests: verb comprehension, verb naming, and sentence production. Action pictures are used in all subtests. To test comprehension, subjects are asked to point to the verb named (out of four pictures), and to assess verb naming, they are asked to name the action depicted. To test verbs in sentence contexts, arrows are added to the pictures to denote objects or people that represent arguments of the verb. Sample picture stimuli used to elicit production of single verbs and verbs in sentences are shown in Figure 26–1.

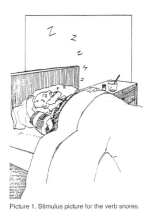
Picture 1. Stimulus picture for the verb snores.

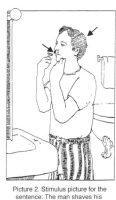
Picture 2. Stimulus picture for the sentence: The man shaves his moustache.

Figure 26–1. Sample picture stimuli for eliciting verbs as singletons (picture 1) and in sentence contexts (picture 2) using the Northwestern University Verb Production Battery. Arrows in picture 2 refer to arguments of the verb.

A list of verbs tested in our verb battery is listed in Appendix 26–2. Agrammatic aphasic subjects show good ability to comprehend verbs of all types; however, they show difficulty producing them both as singletons and in sentence contexts. Interestingly, there often is a hierarchy of difficulty of verb production in agrammatic aphasic patients, based on verb type. That is, one-place verbs are easiest to produce and three-place verbs are the most difficult. For example, subjects produce verbs like *sleep* correctly more often than verbs like *put*. Similarly, sentences with one- or two-place verbs are produced correctly more often than those with three-place verbs. On average, our agrammatic patients produce about 85% of *agents*, 65% of *themes/patients*, and only 20% of *goals/locations* in sentences.

Testing Sentence Production

There are few methods for testing sentence production available to clinicians. One measure that has been used clinically is the story completion test (Gleason et al., 1975; Goodglass et al., 1972). The story completion test examines production of 14 different English sentence structures found to be difficult for agrammatic patients. In our early work with treatment of agrammatism, we often used this method. However, because not all sentence types that are relevant to our approach are included on the test, we no longer recommend using it as the primary test of sentence production.

In order to test sentence production we developed a sentence production priming task. The task entails presentation of a pair of pictures, one depicting the target sentence and the other depicting its semantically reversed counterpart (Figure 26–2). The examiner elicits sentences by modeling the target sentence type using the semantically reversed picture and then asking the patient to produce a similar sentence using the target picture. Using this method several types of sentences are tested for production ability, including

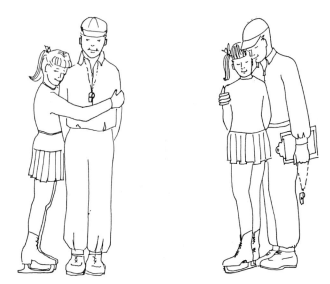

Figure 26–2. Picture pair used to elicit production of target sentence structures. The examiner presents the pictures, shows the patient that in both pictures there is a *skater* and a *coach*, and says: "For this picture (pointing to the picture on the left) you could say *The coach was hugged by the skater*; for this picture (pointing to the picture on the right) you could say . . ." (expected response: *The skater was hugged by the coach*).

actives, passives, object clefts, subject clefts, object relative clause structures, subject relative clause structures, and wh-questions.

Examining Spontaneous Discourse

Analysis of spontaneous discourse is one of the key components of evaluating the patient. Saffran et al. (1989) recommend using a story retelling task, e.g., retelling of *Cinderella*, to collect the language sample. They then code the samples for utterance type, word class, verb inflections, etc. As well, sentence constituents (e.g., noun phrases, verb phrases) are coded. From these data, both lexical and sentence structural analyses are undertaken to derive information such as noun:verb ratio, open class:closed class ratio, noun:pronoun ratio, number of words produced in sentences, mean length of sentences, and the proportion of utterances with complete sentences.

Thompson and colleagues (Thompson et al., 1995) developed a similar method. Patients are asked to tell the story of *Cinderella* or *Red Riding Hood*. We also have asked individuals to watch a silent Charlie Chaplin film and then tell about it. Notably, regardless of elicitation condition, agrammatic aphasic individuals show very similar patterns of language production. Once the sample is collected, it is transcribed and segmented into utterances based on syntactic, prosodic, and semantic criteria. Each utterance then is coded. First, it is determined whether or not an utterance is a sentence (utterances without verbs are not sentences).

Sentences then are coded as simple versus complex based on whether or not phrasal movement and/or embedded clauses are used. The verb(s) in each sentence are then coded with regard to verb type (e.g., one-place, two-place) and morphological complexity, and the presence or absence of verb arguments is noted. Each word in an utterance is then coded for grammatical class (e.g., noun, verb). Results of the analysis yield data such as mean length of utterance (MLU), the proportion of grammatical sentences, the proportion of simple versus complex sentences, the proportion of verbs produced with correct arguments, noun:verb ratio, and open class:closed class ratio, all of which are important for diagnosing agrammatism. Although this coding system is quite complex, it is worthwhile for clinicians to become familiar with analyses of this type not only to diagnose the patient, but also because changes in these language variables are important to document as one of the outcomes of treatment.

In narratives our subjects show decreased mean length of utterance (MLU = 3.0 to 5.5 words). Sentences are ungrammatical and primarily of the simple, active form. Open class:closed class ratios indicate an underuse of closed-class words. In addition, subjects show difficulty with verb production. Noun:verb ratios indicate that they often produce more nouns than verbs and they show a reduction in the proportion of verbs produced with correct argument structure. Further, analysis of verb and verb arguments indicates a preference for producing primarily simple verbs that require accessing simple argument structure arrangements (i.e., one- and two-place verbs).

Treatment of Underlying Forms: Data and Method

The aforementioned psycholinguistic and neurolinguistic facts argue for a principled account of grammatical representations when designing treatment programs. For example, lexical entries at least for verbs seem to be available at d-structure for some, if not all, Broca's aphasic subjects, but they have difficulty properly assigning thematic roles onto arguments that have been moved out of their canonical positions. The problem for these patients lies either in the derivation of s-structure representations (e.g., traces— see Grodzinsky, 1990, 2000) or in the sentence processing routines computing these representations (see, for example, Prather et al., 1991; Zurif et al., 1993). On the production side, it appears that verbs are compromised relative to nouns, and even when used, the lexical entries for verbs are not fully accessible. Further, patients with agrammatic aphasia use primarily simple sentence structures, avoiding complex sentences in which binding relations are essential. Thus, their simple sentence productions could be explained not only by limitations in access to verbs and verb-argument structure, but also by limited access to knowledge concerned with the ways that verb arguments refer to each other when placed in sentence frames. Treatment of underlying forms exploits these strengths and weaknesses and considers the representational similarities and differences underlying the surface realizations of sentences that are the focus of treatment.

The treatment approach utilizes the active, declarative form of noncanonical sentences. Subjects are taught to recognize the verb, its arguments, and the arguments' thematic roles. Then instructions concerning the movement of various sentence constituents are provided and subjects are taken through the proper movement to derive the surface form of target sentences. Additional morphemes required in the surface form of various sentences are provided and inserted into sentence frames. Once the noncanonical form is derived, subjects are required to produce them. Specific procedures for training various sentences types are included in Appendix 26–3.

Training and Generalization of Wh-Movement Structures

Training and Generalization of Wh-Questions

Our treatment approach evolved from early work concerned with wh-question training (e.g., Thompson & McReynolds, 1986; Wambaugh & Thompson, 1989). Wh-questions were selected for treatment because of their noted difficulty for aphasic individuals (Gleason et al., 1975) and because of their importance for requesting information and for participating in conversations. In addition, wh-questions are linguistically interesting, relying on wh-movement, as discussed previously.

It is important here to discuss one of our early studies, as the results derived from it directly influenced the direction of our approach. Briefly, Wambaugh and Thompson (1989) examined the effects of training wh-question production (*what* and *where* questions) in four agrammatic aphasic subjects using direct production treatment. Results indicated that, although generalization within structures occurred (i.e., from *what* constructions to untrained *what* constructions), generalization across structures (i.e., from *what* to *where* constructions) was not forthcoming, even though the two forms are essentially identical in surface form. In keeping with our theoretical framework, we surmised that this lack of generalization across wh-questions could have resulted because of differences in the lexical properties of verbs utilized in the two question types as well as differences in movement operations required. Consider, for example, the following sentence trained by Wambaugh and Thompson (1989):

14. What is he *cooking*?
15. Where is he *sleeping*?

Importantly, the verbs *cook* and *sleep* have different lexical properties. *Cook* is a two-place transitive verb allowing a direct object NP and the thematic roles of *agent*, *theme*, whereas *sleep* is a pure intransitive verb—not taking a direct object NP. To appreciate the structural distinction between these two verb types, consider the following:

16. He is cooking the dinner.
17. He is sleeping in the bed.

As discussed above, the direct object in (16)—*the dinner*—is an argument of the verb. However, in (17), the locative phrase—*in the bed*—is an adjunct. Thus, *what* questions as in (14) are derived from argument movement; *where* questions as in (15) are derived from adjunct movement.

We theorized that the lack of generalization from *what* to *where* questions was related to the distinction between argument and adjunct movement. We further conjectured that, if this were correct, wh-questions that are alike not only in s-structure, but also in their underlying linguistic representation would be better candidates for generalization. For example, we predicted generalization from *what* to *who* questions that are identical in both phrase structure and in argument structure—both constructions require verbs that take a direct object NP. Both questions also rely on argument movement.

Training and Generalization of Argument Movement

In a follow-up study, we (Thompson et al., 1993) investigated generalization across wh-questions requiring argument movement, training two agrammatic aphasic subjects to produce *what* and *who* questions. Consider the following:

18. Zack is helping a friend.
19. Zack is fixing the toy.

Note that in (18) and (19) both the verbs *help* and *fix* take a direct object NP assigned the thematic role of *theme* in d-structure. In addition, to derive a wh-question, both require argument movement as in (20) and (21):

20. Who $_i$ is Zack helping $_{t\,i}$?
21. What $_i$ is Zack fixing $_{t\,i}$?

In treatment, we focused on the underlying lexical and syntactic properties of these wh-questions, rather than focusing treatment simply on their surface representation. Sentences like those in (18) and (19) were used to train the *who* and *what* questions.^{f} In addition, we used sentences with three-place verbs like *give* embedded in NP-V-NP-PP sentences (as in [22]) to train *who*- and *what*-questions (as in [23]).

22. The man is giving money to the boy.
23. What is the man giving to the boy?

Results of treatment indicated, as predicted, that training of selected exemplars of *who* questions resulted not only in improved production of both trained and untrained *who* questions, but also of untrained *what* questions. We attributed this successful generalization to our controlling the lexical properties of verbs as well as the movement operations required for *what* and *who* questions. Interestingly,

---

^{f} We do not claim that declarative sentences like (18) and (19) are, in fact, the d-structure or underlying form for the derived wh-questions in (20) and (21); they simply contain the same thematic properties and thus can be used to help train such notions.

TABLE 26–4

Target Wh-Questions and Active Forms Used to Train Them

Underlying Canonical Form	Wh-Question Trained
Argument Movement Structures	
The soldier is pushing *the woman* into the street.	*Who* is the soldier pushing (*t*) into the street?
The boy is kicking *the cow* in the barn.	*What* is the boy kicking (*t*) in the barn?
Adjunct Movement Structures	
The student is helping the doctor *in the evening*.	*When* is the student helping the doctor (*t*)?
The guard is protecting the clerk *at the store*.	*Where* is the guard protecting the clerk (*t*)?

both subjects showed generalization from more to less "complex" structures. That is, when questions like (23) were trained, generalized production of questions like those in (21) was noted without direct treatment.

Training and Generalization of Argument vs. Adjunct Movement

To further establish the distinction between training wh-questions that utilize argument movement versus those that utilize adjunct movement we (Thompson et al. 1996) trained an additional seven agrammatic aphasic individuals to produce *who*, *what*, *where*, and *when* questions. As previously noted, *who* and *what* questions require similar movement of the argument NP (direct object), whereas *when* and *where* questions require adjunct movement. As in our other treatment work, the primary outcome of interest was generalization across wh-question types.

Using a set of 20 two-place verbs, 80 active sentence stimuli (NP-V-NP-PP) were developed to depict the underlying form of the four question constructions shown in Table 26–4.

Prior to treatment, wh-question production was tested using active sentences and a wh-question elicitation procedure was used to test production of all question types. The active sentence was presented, in written form, on cards.

The patient was asked to read (or repeat) the active sentence and then instructed: "You want to know *the person* the soldier is pushing, so you ask?." The word 'person' was emphasized; rising inflection was used. To elicit *what* questions using the sample stimulus sentence above, the examiner instructed: "You want to know *the thing* the soldier is pushing, so you ask?." On these trials, the word 'thing' was emphasized. To elicit *when* and *where* questions, the same procedure was used except that subjects were instructed to ask about *the time* or *the place*, respectively.

Following baseline testing, patients were trained to produce one wh-question type at a time and the rest were tested

for generalization. In training, the active, canonical form of the target wh-question was again presented. This time each sentence constituent was presented on a separate card as detailed in Appendix 26–3. The examiner then sequentially pointed out the verb and all sentence constituents and the patient was asked to produce them. Next, patients were shown how the sentence constituents move to different sentence positions to form wh-questions, while retaining their thematic roles. Once wh-questions were formed, patients practiced producing them. Finally, the cards were rearranged in their original (canonical) position, and the patient practiced moving them to form a wh-question.

Results of treatment again showed that generalization occurs across structures that are linguistically similar. As predicted, when treatment was applied to wh-questions requiring argument movement (e.g., *what* questions), generalized production of untrained wh-questions was restricted to *who* questions that also rely on argument movement. Notably, neither *who* or *what* question treatment affected production of *where* and *when* questions. Similarly, when treatment was applied to wh-questions requiring adjunct movement (e.g., *where* questions), generalization occurred to untrained wh-questions relying on adjunct movement (e.g., *when* questions), but no effect on *who* or *what* questions was noted.

Some of our subjects had particular difficulty producing the wh-words themselves. For these individuals, we provided wh-morpheme discrimination/production treatment in addition to wh-movement treatment.

Summary of Wh-Question Training Data

We find that the treatment of underlying forms approach to training wh-questions results in improved sentence production in agrammatic aphasics. Also, we see successful generalization to untrained sentences with this approach. Our studies also show that (a) the argument/adjunct distinction seen in both theoretical linguistic and psycholinguistic literature extends to the cross-generalization patterns exhibited by aphasic patients, and that (b) there may be separate processes underlying the production (and perhaps comprehension) of wh-movement constructions. That is, wh-question production requires control of syntactic features of wh-question formation (i.e., movement of the NP itself) and control of lexical features of wh-questions (i.e., wh-morpheme selection).

Training and Generalization of Wh-Movement vs. NP-Movement Structures

As noted above, there is a distinction among certain sentence types, depending on whether they involve the syntactic operations of wh- or NP-movement. Wh-questions and object clefts are wh-movement structures, whereas passive sentences and those with subject raising are NP-movement structures. In our sentence production work, we investigated the effects of training sentences that involve wh-movement on those that involve NP-movement and vice versa (Thompson & Shapiro, 1994; Thompson et al., 1997). Because these two types of movement are quite different, we predicted that treatment applied to sentences relying on one type of movement would not influence sentences relying on the other type. For example, training wh-questions should have no effect on passive sentences. However, because of the linguistic similarities between wh-movement sentences, for example, we thought training one wh-movement structure might affect others, even when the surface structure is different. For example, training object cleft structures might influence wh-questions. Consider, for example, the following sentences:

24. Who has the biker lifted? (wh-question)
25. It was the student who the biker lifted. (object cleft)

Indeed, on the face of it, these two sentences appear to be quite different. The two sentence types, however, are fundamentally similar in that they both rely on wh-movement. As discussed previously in the Theoretical Framework section of this chapter, wh-questions as in (24) are noncanonical sentences derived from an underlying or d-structure as approximated in (26). The symbol ϕ is used here to indicate a movement site that is vacant at d-structure.

26. ϕ the biker lifted [who]

To form a wh-question, *who* (which occupies a direct object argument position), is moved to the front of the sentence. Before movement occurs thematic roles are assigned by the verb to all argument positions. The verb *lift*, for example, assigns a thematic role to *who*. Once movement occurs, a trace (*t*) of the movement is left behind and a chain is formed between the trace and the antecedent (i.e., the moved sentence constituent) of the trace. In this manner, the antecedent to the trace (in this case *who*) and the trace site (i.e., the direct object argument position) are co-indexed as in (27).

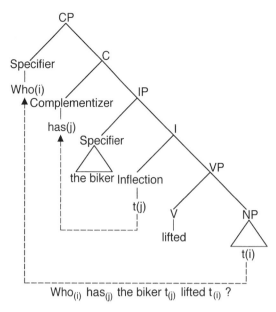

Figure 26–3. Tree diagram illustrating wh-movement in wh-questions. Movement is from the post-verbal NP (direct object) position to the sentence initial position. Subject-auxiliary verb inversion (i.e., verb movement) also is depicted. Shown in the diagram are the basic elements of the tree which include local trees headed by CP (complementizer phrase, formerly known as S'), IP (inflection phrase, formerly S), and VP (verb phrase). Going from the top down, the *specifier* position of the COMP-headed local tree [SPEC CP] is the landing site for the wh-word. The head of CP (the *complementizer* position) is filled with the auxiliary verb when subject-auxiliary verb inversion occurs. The next level down is the local tree headed by IP. Its *specifier* position [SPEC, IP] is the subject position. The local head *Inflection* contains verb tense and agreement information.

27. [$_{CP}$ who$_i$ [$_{C'}$ has [$_{IP}$ the biker lifted $_{t\ i}$]]]

The movment involved in wh-questions is most easily seen by referring to a tree diagram. Figure 26–3 depicts movement of *who* from its postverbal position to the sentence initial position. The place in the tree where *who* lands is called the specifier position of the complementizer phrase (SPEC, CP). The additional operation of subject-auxiliary verb inversion is also required to form a wh-question; this too is illustrated in Figure 26–3.

Now consider the object cleft sentence in (25). As in wh-questions, movement occurs from direct object position to SPEC, CP as shown in (28) and in Figure 26–4.

28. It was the student [ϕ the biker lifted who]

However, unlike wh-questions, object clefts involve movement within an embedded relative clause.

We (Thompson & Shapiro, 1994) trained aphasic subjects to produce *who* questions and tested generalization to object-cleft and passive sentences. At the same time, we

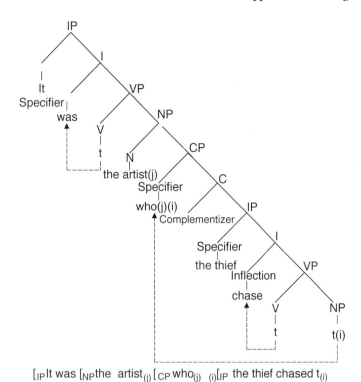

[IP It was [NP the artist(j) [CP who(j) (i)[IP the thief chased t(i)

Figure 26–4. Tree diagram illustrating wh-movement in object clefts. Movement is from the post-verbal NP (direct object) position to the specifier position of COMP [SPEC CP], as in wh-questions. Importantly, movement occurs in an embedded clause. Note that there is a co-referential relation between SPEC CP and the head of the NP (*the artist*).

trained other subjects to produce object-cleft sentences and tested generalization to wh-questions and passives. The active underlying form of sentences, which is identical for all three sentence types (see [29] below), was used for treatment.

29. The student lifted the biker. (active)

The treatment used for wh-questions was like that discussed above; a similar approach was used to train object-cleft sentences (see Appendix 26–3). Following testing of all sentence types using the sentence production priming procedure (see previous section, Assessment of Agrammatism), treatment was begun. Subjects were taught to recognize the verb, its arguments, and their thematic role assignments, and to move sentence constituents to derive the surface form of targeted sentences. Throughout the training period, production of both trained and untrained sentence types was tested using the sentence priming task, and emergent production patterns were recorded.

Results of treatment indicated that all but one patient with agrammatism readily learned to produce both *who* questions and object clefts, and generalization between these two structures was noted. For example, training object clefts resulted in improved production of both object cleft sentences and *who* questions. However, neither object cleft or *who* question training affected production of NP-movement–derived passive sentences.

Ballard and Thompson (1999) and Jacobs and Thompson (2000) found a similar dissociation between wh- and NP-movement–derived sentences. Using our linguistically based approach, treatment of underlying forms, Ballard and Thompson (1999) trained five patients to produce wh-movement structures (i.e., object clefts and/or wh-questions) and tested passive sentences. All subjects improved in production of wh-movement structures, but no change in passive structures was seen. Jacobs and Thompson (2000) trained both object clefts and passive sentences in four patients. Again, all improved on the structures trained, but none showed generalization from object clefts to passives, or from passives to object clefts.

In a complete study examining the relation between wh- and NP-movement, Thomspon et al. (1997) found the same pattern. The wh-movement structures selected for treatment included wh-questions like that in (30) and object-cleft sentences like that in (31).

30. Who did the cop stop? (wh-question)
31. It was the driver who the cop stopped. (object cleft)

In addition, NP-movement structures were selected for treatment and generalization testing. These included passives and subject-raising sentences like those in (32) and (33), respectively.

32. The driver was stopped by the cop. (passive)
33. The cop seems to have stopped the driver. (subject raising)

These NP-movement structures are clearly quite different on the surface. However, like the wh-movement structures discussed above, they are linguistically similar. Unlike wh-movement, which involves movement from an argument position to a non-argument position (i.e., the specifier position of CP), NP-movement involves movement from an argument position to another argument position, the specifier position of IP ([SPEC, IP]). To illustrate the NP-movement involved in passive sentences, once again consider the d-structure approximated in (34).

34. φ was lifted *the student* by the biker.

To derive the passive, the direct object NP (i.e., *the student*) is moved and a trace of this movement is left behind (as in wh-movement). However, the landing site of the moved NP is the empty subject position ([SPEC, IP]) as in (35). Therefore, the trace is co-indexed with the moved sentence constituent that is now in the specifier position of IP rather than with the specifier position of CP as in wh-movement (**Figure 26–5**).

35. [IP The student$_i$ was lifted t$_i$ [by the biker]]

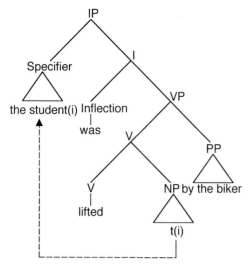

The student(i) was lifted t(i) by the biker.

Figure 26–5. Tree diagram illustrating NP-movement in passives. Note that here the landing site for movement is SPEC IP, the subject position.

NP-movement also is involved in the derivation of what are called subject-raising constructions. In this type of sentence, movement is from the subject position of a sentential complement to subject position of the matrix sentence, as below in (36).

36. φ seems the biker to have lifted the student.
[IP The biker_i seems [t_i to have lifted the student]]

In our study of wh- and NP-movement treatment, agrammatic Broca's aphasic individuals were trained to produce one sentence type at a time using the protocols in Appendix 26–3C for training *who* questions, object-clefts, passives, and subject-raising structures. Results of treatment, again, showed that training wh-movement structures resulted in generalization to other wh-movement structures—that is, we found generalization from object-clefts to wh-questions; however, wh-movement treatment had little influence on production of NP-movement structures. Similarly, when NP-movement structures were trained, generalization occurred to other NP-movement structures (e.g., generalization occurred from passives to subject-raising sentences, and vice versa), but no change in production of object clefts or *who* questions was seen.

Summary of Wh- and NP-Movement Training

Our work concerned with examining wh- and NP-movement structures shows that these are functionally separate processes that influence sentence production. That is, generalization is not seen from sentences relying on one type of movement to sentences relying on the other. Importantly,

however, we find successful generalization across sentences that rely on the same type of movement, even though these sentences are very different in their surface representation. These data show again that the linguistic underpinnings of sentences are important to consider in treatment of sentence production deficits.

The Role of Syntactic Complexity: Optimal Order for Promoting Generalization

Another variable that is related to successful generalization is the complexity of structures trained. Results of our research (Ballard & Thompson, 1999; Thompson et al., 1993; Thompson et al., 1998; Thompson et al., in preparation) show that generalization may be enhanced if the direction of treatment is from more complex to less complex structures, when treated structures encompass processes relevant to untreated ones. While training complex structures prior to training simpler ones may seem counterintuitive, recent studies have suggested that optimal generalization may result from this approach (Eckman et al., 1988; Gierut, 1990; Plaut, 1996).

Close examination of our data reported in earlier studies (i.e., Thompson & Shapiro, 1994; Thompson et al., 1997) showed that for subjects who received wh-movement training, better generalization was noted from object clefts to *who* questions than from *who* questions to object clefts. In consideration of the complexity of these structures, object clefts are the most complex. The two structures are similar in that they both require wh-movement; however, as pointed out above, the movement in object clefts is within an embedded clause. The movement in *who* questions (of the type trained in our studies) occurs in the matrix clause; no embedding is required.

We therefore undertook additional studies to examine the complexity issue. Results showed that, indeed, generalization occurs more readily from object clefts to *who* questions than vice versa. As can be seen in Table 26–5 a total of 17 subjects have been trained to produce one structure or the other across studies. Of the 10 individuals trained to produce object clefts, 8 have shown generalization to wh-questions. In contrast, of the 7 subjects trained to produce who-questions, only 1 showed generalization to object clefts.

The three subjects who did not fit the pattern of generalization expected require some comments. A.H., who showed generalization to object clefts when *who* questions were trained, was unlike the other subjects in that her aphasia did not result from stroke. Instead, she presented with primary progressive aphasia of unknown etiology. In addition, at the time of the study she demonstrated a very mild aphasia (WAB AQ = 93.6). On the other hand, the two subjects who did not show generalization from object clefts to *who* questions were more severely impaired than the other subjects (AQs in the

TABLE 26–5

Generalization Patterns Seen Between Object Cleft Structures, Matrix *Who* Questions, and Passive Sentences.

Subject	Trained Wh-Movement Structure	Untrained Wh-Movement Structure	Untrained NP-Movement Structure
DL+	Object clefts ⟶	*Who* questions ⟶⫽▶	Passives
MD*	Object clefts ⟶	*Who* questions ⟶⫽▶	Passives
Person 1 ∝	Object clefts ⟶	*Who* questions ⟶⫽▶	Pasives
Person 2 ∝	Object clefts ⟶	*Who* questions ⟶⫽▶	Passives
Person 3 ∝	Object clefts ⟶	*Who* questions ⟶⫽▶	Passives
MR Ω	Object clefts ⟶	*Who* questions ⟶⫽▶	Passives
LD Ω	Object clefts ⟶	*Who* questions ⟶⫽▶	Passives
HH**	Object clefts ⟶	*Who* questions ⟶⫽▶	Passives
Person 4 ∝	Object clefts ⟶⫽▶	*Who* questions ⟶⫽▶	Passives
Person 5 ∝	Object cleft ⟶⫽▶	*Who* questions ⟶⫽▶	Passives
AH**	*Who* questions ⟶	Object cleft ⟶⫽▶	Passives
JH Ω	*Who* questions ⟶⫽▶	Object clefts ⟶⫽▶	Passives
GK Ω	*Who* questions ⟶⫽▶	Object clefts ⟶⫽▶	Passives
FP+	*Who* questions ⟶⫽▶	Object cleft ⟶⫽▶	Passives
KD**	*Who* questions ⟶⫽▶	Object cleft ⟶⫽▶	Passives
CH+	*Who* questions ⟶⫽▶	Object cleft ⟶⫽▶	Passives
PR*	*Who* questions ⟶⫽▶	Object cleft ⟶⫽▶	Passives

Note: ⟶ = Successful generalization; ⟶⫽▶ = No generalization.
*Subjects from Thompson et al., 1997.
**Subjects from Thompson and Shapiro, 1994.
+Subjects from Thompson et al., 1998.
∝Subjects from Ballard and Thompson, 1999.
ΩSubjects from Thompson et al., in preparation.

50s). These results suggest that severity of language impairment may have affected treatment outcome.

Effects of Treatment on Discourse Patterns. Changes in discourse characteristics have been noted in several of the aforementioned treatment studies examining treatment of underlying forms. The most important changes noted across subjects include (a) decreases in the proportion of simple sentence productions and a concomitant increase in complex sentence productions, (b) increases in MLU, and (c) increases in the proportion of verbs produced with correct argument structure. Following treatment, subjects also produce proportionately more verbs across discourse samples and, while retaining a preference for producing primarily simple verbs (i.e., one- and two-place verbs), they more often produce these verbs, as well as other more complex verbs, with correct verb argument structure. Notably, Ballard and Thompson (1999) and Jacobs (1996) also have found changes from pre-treatment to post-treatment narrative samples in informativeness and efficiency of production using an analysis method advanced by Nicholas and Brookhire (1993). This finding shows that improved sentence production leads to production of more information

with increased efficiency. Ballard and Thompson (1999) also examined the social validity of treatment by asking naive listeners to rate pre-treatment and post-treatment narrative samples on a number of variables, including content, coherence, sentence length and complexity, and grammaticality. Results showed that listeners perceived positive changes in narrative language production in three of their five subjects.

Neurological Correlates of Improved Sentence Production and Comprehension

We also recently undertook an fMRI study of one of our patients who received treatment focused on wh-movement structures, including object–relative clause constructions, object clefts, and object-extracted wh-questions. The subject was a well-educated, 52-year-old, right-handed gentleman (H.R.) who was 10 years post-onset of a left MCA stroke resulting in aphasia. Extensive language testing at the time of the study showed language behaviors consistent with a diagnosis of agrammatic aphasia. Sentence length and grammaticality was compromised, he produced more open-class than closed-class words, and more nouns than verbs. Language comprehension was largely intact, although he showed the

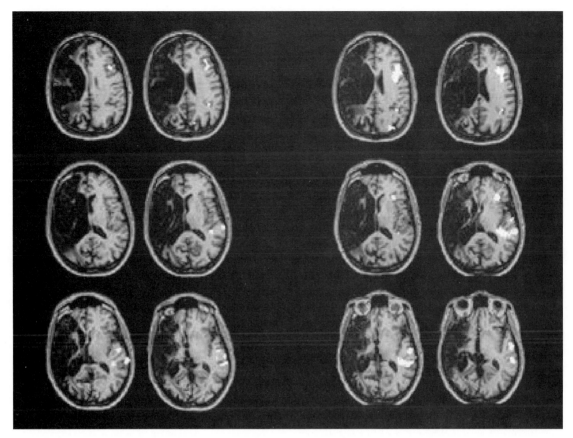

Figure 26–6. Areas of significant activation for sentences versus words prior to and following treatment of complex sentence structures in a patient with agrammatic aphasia.

characteristic pattern of asyntactic comprehension, whereby only comprehension of complex noncanonical sentences was compromised.

Prior to treatment, we undertook an fMRI study of H.R. The task required that he listen to complex object cleft sentences such as *It was the student who the biker lifted* and simpler subject cleft sentences such as *It was the biker who lifted the student* and view pictures. When a sentence matched a picture presented, he pressed a button. Thirty-two contiguous 4-mm axial slices were obtained relative to the AC-PC line using whole-brain echo-planar imaging. Prior to treatment, sentence processing as compared to a single-word control condition resulted in significant activation in the right hemisphere in BA 22 (right homologue of Wernicke's area) and BA 46 (dorsolateral prefrontal cortex).

Following a course of treatment (treatment of underlying forms) which improved H.R.'s production and comprehension of all three sentence types, H.R. once again underwent fMRI. Post-treatment scans showed increased activation in homologous right hemisphere areas in and around Wernicke's area (activation now encompassed BA 22, 21, and 37) and in Broca's area (BA 44 and 45) (Figure 26–6). These changes were associated with marked improvement

in scanner task performance and behavioral testing. These findings are indeed exciting and indicate that improvements in language-processing ability, induced by treatment, can be mapped onto the brain.

CONCLUSIONS

The findings from our work in developing and in testing the effects of treatment of underlying forms indicate that treatment for sentence production deficits in patients with agrammatic aphasia is efficacious when the linguistic underpinnings of (a) the language deficit exhibited by the aphasic individual, (b) the sentences selected for treatment, and (c) the treatment strategy utilized are considered. When lexical and syntactic properties of sentences are not considered, generalization effects are considerably diminished—or are absent, resulting in little or no discernible improvement in sentence production beyond the kind of constructions trained. In addition to the linguistic properties of sentences, we also find that the complexity of structures trained is a factor that needs to be considered in facilitating generalization.

The results of our work have important clinical implications. Because of restrictions in health care presently imposed for aphasic individuals, it is essential that clinicians provide treatment that will result in optimal generalization. Our data suggest that optimal generalization results from treatment when structures that are linguistically similar are selected as treatment targets and when treatment is applied to the most complex of these structures first. While additional data are needed to further substantiate the latter, we conclude that linguistically based treatment, i.e., treatment of underlying forms, may be used successfully for training sentence production in aphasic individuals who present with deficits like those seen in our subjects.

In conclusion, treatment of sentence production deficits as seen in agrammatic aphasia requires careful analysis of *how* and in *what ways* the sentence processing/production system has been affected with brain damage. Application of treatment explicitly designed to address these deficits is recommended. Indeed, the more we learn about the linguistic and psycholinguistic underpinnings of sentence production and comprehension, and the more we learn about aphasic language deficits, the more detailed we can be about the design of treatment.

▶ *Acknowledgment*–The work reported here was supported by the National Institutes on Deafness and Other Communication Disorders (NIDCD) grant RO1-DC01948.

KEY POINTS

The key points of this chapter are as follows:
1. The literature indicates that individuals with agrammatic aphasia show particular deficit patterns that must be carefully tested prior to application of treatment.
2. Consideration of the lexical and syntactic properties of sentences selected for treatment and for generalization analysis is important for obtaining optimal generalization.
3. Generalization from one structure to another occurs when sentences are linguistically related to one another. When sentences are not linguistically related, generalization is limited.
4. Generalization may be enhanced by training more complex structures first. Generalization from more complex structures to simpler ones occurs when simple sentences encompass structures and processes in common with the more complex ones.
5. Treatment improves the grammar, content, and efficiency of spontaneous discourse.
6. Neural correlates of treatment-induced behavioral changes can be mapped onto the brain.

References

Badecker, W. & Caramazza, A. (1985). On consideration of method and theory governing the use of clinical categories in neurolinguistics and cognitive neuropsychology: The case against agrammatism. *Cognition, 20*, 97–126.

Ballard, K.J. & Thompson, C.K. (1999). Treatment and generalization of complex sentence production in agrammatism. *Journal of Speech, Language, and Hearing Research, 42*, 690–707.

Bastiaanse, R. & Jonkers, R. (1998). Verb retrieval in action naming and spontaneous speech in agrammatism and anomic aphasia. *Aphasiology, 11*, 951–969.

Bates, E., Appelbaum, M., & Allard, L. (1991). Statistical contraints on the usage of single cases in neuropsychological research. *Brain and Language, 40*, 295–329.

Berndt, R.S. (1987). Symptom co-occurrence and dissociation in the interpretation of agrammatism. In M. Coltheart, G. Sartori, & R. Job (eds.), *The cognitive neuropsychology of language*. Hillsdale, NJ: Lawrence Erlbaum.

Berndt, R.S., Mitchum, C.C., & Haendiges, A.N. (1996). Comprehension of reversible sentences in "agrammatism": A meta-analysis. *Cognition, 58*, 289–308.

Bock, K. (1987). Coordinating words and syntax in speech plans. In A. Ellis (ed.), *Progress in the psychology of language* (pp. 337–390).

Bresnan, J. (ed.) (1992). *The mental representation of grammatical relations*. Cambridge, MA: MIT Press.

Byng, S. (1988). Sentence processing deficits: Theory and therapy. *Cognitive neuropsychology, 5*, 629–676.

Cannito, M.P. & Vogel, D. (1987). Treatment can facilitate reacquisition of a morphological rule. In R.H. Brookshire (ed.), *Clinical aphasiology conference proceedings* (pp. 23–28). Minneapolis, MN: BRK.

Caplan, D., Baker, C., & Dehaut, F. (1985). Syntactic determinants of sentence comprehension in aphasia. *Cognition, 21*, 117–175.

Caplan, D. & Futter, C. (1986). Assignment of thematic roles to nouns in sentence comprehension by an agrammatic patient. *Brain and Language, 27*, 117–134.

Caplan, D. & Hanna (1998). Sentence production by aphasic patients in a constrained task. *Brain and Language, 63*, 184–218.

Caplan, D. & Hildebrandt, N. (1988). Specific deficits in syntactic comprehension. *Aphasiology, 2*, 255–258.

Caramazza, A. (1986). On drawing inferences about the structure of normal cognitive systems from the analysis of patterns of impaired performance: The case for single patient studies. *Brain and Cognition, 5*, 41–66.

Caramazza, A. & Hillis, A.E. (1989). The disruption of sentence production: Some dissociations. *Brain and Language, 36*, 625–650.

Caramazza, A. & Zurif, E. (1976). Dissociation of algorithmic and heuristic processes in language comprehension: Evidence from aphasia. *Brain and Language, 3*, 572–582.

Chomsky, N. (1986). *Knowledge of language: Its nature, origin, and use*. New York: Praeger.

Chomsky, N. (1991). Some notes on the economy of derivation and representation. In R. Friedin (ed.), *Principles and parameters in comparative grammar*. Cambridge, MA: MIT Press.

Chomsky, N. (1993). A minimalist program for linguistic theory. K.

Hale & S.J. Keyser (eds.), *The view from building 20*. Cambridge, MA: MIT Press.

Chomsky, N. (1995). Bare phrase structure. In G. Webelhuth (ed.), *Government and binding theory and the minimalist program*. London: Basil Blackwell Publishers.

Damasio, H. (1991). Neuroanatomical correlates of the aphasias. In M.T. Sarno (ed.), *Acquired aphasia* (2nd ed.). New York: Academic Press.

Damasio, H. & Damasio, A.R. (1989). *Lesion analysis in neuropsychology*. New York: Oxford University Press.

deBlesser, R. (1987). From agrammatism to paragrammatism: German aphasiological traditions and grammatical disturbances. *Cognitive Neuropsychology, 4*, 187–256.

Doyle, P.J., Goldstein, H., & Bourgeois, M. (1987). Experimental analysis of syntax training in Broca's aphasia: A generalization and social validation study. *Journal of Speech and Hearing Disorders, 52*, 143–155.

Eckman, R.F., Bell, L., & Nelson, D. (1988). On the generalization of relative clause instruction in the acquisition of English as a second language. *Applied Linguistics, 9*, 1–20.

Fink, R., Schwartz, M.F., Rochon, E., Myers, J.L., Socolof, G.S., & Bluestone, R. (1995). Syntax stimulation revisited: An analysis of generalization of treatment effects. Paper presented at the Clinical Aphasiology Conference, OR.

Frazier, L. & Clifton, C. (1989). Successive cyclicity in the grammar and the parser. *Language and Cognitive Processes, 4*, 93–126.

Friedmann, N. & Grodzinsky, Y. (1997). Tense and agreement in agrammatic production: Pruning the syntactic tree. *Brain and Language, 56*, 397–425.

Gazdar, G., Kein, E., Pullum, J., & Sag, I. (1985). *Generalized phrase structure grammar*. Cambridge, MA: Harvard University Press.

Garrett, M.F. (1980). Levels of processing in sentence production. In B. Butterworth (ed.), *Language production, Vol. 1*. New York: Academic Press.

Garrett, M.F. (1984). The organization of processing structure for language production: Applications to aphasic speech. In D. Caplan, A.R. Lecours, & A. Smith (eds.), *Biological perspectives on language* (pp. 172–195). Cambridge, MA: MIT Press.

Gierut, J. (1990). Differential learning of phonological oppositions. *Journal of Speech and Hearing Research, 33*, 540–549.

Gleason, J.B., Goodglass, H., Green, E., Ackerman, N., & Hyde, M.K. (1975). The retrieval of syntax in Broca's aphasia. *Brain and Language, 24*, 451–471.

Goodglass, H. (1976). Agrammatism. In H. Whitaker & H.A. Whitaker (eds.), *Studies in neurolinguistics, Vol. 1* (pp. 237–260). New York: Academic Press.

Goodglass, H., Christiansen, J.A., & Gallagher, R. (1993). Comparison of morphology and syntax in free narrative and structured tests: Fluent vs. nonfluent aphasics. *Cortex, 29*, 377–407.

Goodglass, H., Gleason, J.B., Bernholtz, N.D., & Hyde, M.K. (1972). Some linguistic structures in the speech of a Broca's aphasic. *Cortex, 8*, 191–212.

Goodglass, H. & Kaplan, E. (1983). *The assessment of aphasia and related disorders* (2nd ed.). Philadelphia, PA: Lea & Febiger.

Grodzinsky, Y. (1990). *Theoretical Perspectives on Language Deficits*. Cambridge, MA: MIT Press.

Grodzinsky, Y. (1986). Language deficits and syntactic theory. *Brain and Language, 27*, 135–159.

Grodzinsky, Y. (1995). A restrictive theory of agrammatic comprehension. *Brain and Language, 50*, 27–51.

Grodzinsky, Y. (2000). The neurology of syntax: Language use without Broca's area. *Behavioral and Brain Sciences, 23*.

Grodzinsky, Y. & Finkel, L. (1998). The neurology of empty categories: Aphasics' failure to detect ungrammaticality. *Journal of Cognitive Neuroscience, 10*, 281–191.

Hagiwara, H. (1995). The breakdown of functional categories and the economy of derivation. *Brain and Language, 50*, 92–116.

Helm-Estabrooks, N. (1981). *Helm Elicited Language Program for Syntax Stimulation*. Austin, TX: Exceptional Resources.

Helm-Estabrooks, N., Fitzpatrick, P., & Barresi, B. (1981). Response of an agrammatic patient to a syntax stimulation program for aphasia. *Journal of Speech and Hearing Disorders, 46*, 422–427.

Helm-Estabrooks, N. & Ramsberger, G. (1986). Treatment of agrammatism in long-term Broca's aphasia. *British Journal of Disorders of Communication, 21*, 39–45.

Jacobs, B.J. (1996). Summary of changes in linguistic structure and function aspects of aphasic discourse. Paper presented at the American Speech-Language-Hearing Association Convention, Seattle, WA.

Jacobs, B.J. & Thompson, C.K. (in press). Cross-modal generalization effects of training noncanonical sentence comprehension and production in agrammatic aphasia. *Journal of Speech, Language, and Hearing Research, 43*, 5–20.

Jones, E.V. (1986). Building the foundations for sentence production in a non-fluent aphasic. *British Journal of Disorders of Communication, 21*, 63–82.

Kim, M. & Thompson, C.K. (2000). Patterns of comprehension and production of nouns and verbs in agrammatism: Implications for lexical organization. *Brain and Langauge, 74*, 1–25.

Kearns, K.P. (1986). Flexibility of single-subject experimental designs: Part II. Design selection and arrangement of experimental phases. *Journal of Speech and Hearing Disorders, 51*, 204–214.

Kearns, K.P. & Salmon, S. (1984). An experimental analysis of auxiliary and copula verb generalization in aphasia. *Journal of Speech and Hearing Disorders, 49*, 152–163.

Kearns, K.P. & Thompson, C.K. (1991). Technical drift and conceptual myopia: The Merlin effect. In T.E. Prescott (ed.), *Clinical aphasiology, Vol. 19*. Austin, TX: Pro-Ed.

Kertesz, A. (1982). *The Western Aphasia Battery*. New York: Grune & Stratton.

Kohn, S.E., Lorch, M.P., & Pearson, D.M. (1989). Verb finding in aphasia. *Cortex, 25*, 57–69.

Kolk, H.H. & Van Grunsven, M. (1985). Agrammatism as a variable phenomenon. *Cognitive Neuropsychology, 2*, 347–384.

Kolk, H.H., Van Grunsven, M., & Keyser, A. (1985). On parallelism between production and comprehension in agrammatism. In M.L. Kean (ed.), *Agrammatism* (pp. 165–206). Orlando, FL: Academic Press.

Linebarger, M.C., Schwartz, M.F., & Saffran, E.M. (1983). Sensitivity to grammatical structure in so-called agrammatic aphasics. *Cognition, 13*, 361–394.

Loverso, F.L., Prescott, T.E., & Selinger, M. (1986). Cueing verbs: A treatment strategy for aphasic adults. *Journal of Rehabilitation Research, 25*, 47–60.

Marantz, A. (1995). The minimalist program. In G. Webelhuth (ed.), *Government and binding theory and the minimalist program*. London: Basil Blackwell Publishers.

Masterson, J. & Druks, J. (1998). Description of a set of 164 nouns and 102 verbs matched for printed word frequency, familiarity and age-of-acquisition. *Journal of Neurolinguistics, 11,* 331–354.

Mauner, G., Fromkin, V., & Cornell, T. (1993). Comprehension and acceptability judgments in agrammatism: Disruption in the syntax of referential dependency. *Brain and Language, 45,* 340–370.

Menn, L. & Obler, L. (1989). *Agrammatic aphasia: Cross-language narrative sourcebook.* Baltimore, MD: John Benjamins.

McNeil, M.R. & Prescott, T.E. (1978). *Revised Token Test.* Baltimore, MD: University Park Press.

McReynolds, L.V. & Thompson, C.K. (1986). Flexibility of single-subject experimental designs: Part I. Review of the basics of single-subject design. *Journal of Speech and Hearing Disorders, 51,* 194–203.

Miceli, G. & Mazzucchi, A. (1990). The nature of speech production deficits in so-called agrammatic aphasia: Evidence from two Italian patients. In L. Menn & L.K. Obler (eds.), *Agrammatic aphasia: Cross-language narrative sourcebook.* Baltimore, MD: John Benjamins.

Miceli, G., Mazzucchi, A., Menn, L., & Goodglass, H. (1983). Contrasting cases of Italian agrammatic aphasia without comprehension disorder. *Brain and Language, 19,* 65–97.

Miceli, G., Silveri, M.C., Romani, C., & Caramazza, A. (1989). Variation in the pattern of omissions and substitutions of grammatical morphemes in the spontaneous speech of so-called agrammatic patients. *Brain and Language, 36,* 447–492.

Nespoulous, J.L., Dordain, M., Perron, C., Ska, B., Bub, D., Caplan, D., Mehler, J., & Lecours, A.R. (1988). Agrammatism in sentence production without comprehension deficits: Reduced availability of syntactic structures and/or grammatical morphemes? A case study. *Brain and Language, 33,* 273–295.

Nicholas, L.E. & Brookshire, R.H. (1993). A system for quantifying the informativeness and efficiency of the connected speech of adults with aphasia. *Journal of Speech and Hearing Research, 36,* 338–350.

Plaut, D.C. (1996). Relearning after damage in connectionist networks: Toward a theory of rehabilitation. *Brain and Language, 52,* 25–82.

Porch, B.E. (1973). *The Porch Index of Communicative Abilities: Administration, scoring, and interpretation.* Palo Alto, CA: Consulting Psychologists Press.

Prather, P., Shapiro, L.P., Zurif, E.B., & Swinney, D. (1991). Real time examination of lexical processing in aphasia. *Journal of Psycholinguistic Research, 23,* 271–281.

Saffran, E.M., Berndt, R.S., & Schwartz, M.F. (1989). The quantitative analysis of agrammatic production: Procedure and data. *Brain and Language, 37,* 440–479.

Saffran, E.M. & Schwartz, M.F. (1988). Agrammatic comprehension it's not: Alternatives and implications. *Aphasiology, 2,* 389–394.

Saffran, E.M., Schwartz, M.F., Linebarger, M., Martin, N., & Bochetto, P. (unpublished). *The Philadelphia Comprehension Battery for Aphasia.*

Salvatore, T., Trunzo, M., Holtzapple, P., & Graham, L. (1983). Investigation of the sentence hierarchy of the Helm Elicited Language Program for Syntax Stimulation. In R.H. Brookshire (ed.), *Clinical apahasiology conference proceedings* (pp. 73–84). Minneapolis, MN: BRK.

Schuell, H., Jenkins, J.J., & Jimenez-Pabon, E. (1964). *Aphasia in adults: Diagnosis, prognosis and treatment.* New York: Harper & Row.

Schwartz, M.F., Saffran, E.M., Fink, R.B., Myers, J.L., & Martin, N. (1994). Mapping therapy: A treatment programme for agrammatism. *Aphasiology, 8,* 19–54.

Schwartz, M.F. (1987). Patterns of speech production deficit within and across aphasia syndromes: Application of a psycholinguistic mode. In M. Coltheart, G. Sartori, & R. Job (eds.), *The cognitive neuropsychology of language.* Hillsdale, NJ: Lawrence Erlbaum.

Schwartz, M.F., Linebarger, M.C., & Saffran, E.M. (1985). The status of the syntactic deficit theory of agrammatism. In M.L. Kean (ed.), *Agrammatism* (pp. 83–104). New York: Academic Press.

Schwartz, M.F., Linebarger, M.C., Saffran, E.M., & Pate, D.S. (1987). Syntactic transparency and sentence interpretation in aphasia. *Language and Cognitive Processes, 2,* 85–113.

Schwartz, M.F., Saffran, E.M., & Marin, O. (1980). The word order problem in agrammatism: 1. Comprehension. *Brain and Language, 10,* 249–262.

Shapiro, L.P. (1997). Tutorial: An introduction to syntax. *Journal of Speech, Language, and Hearing Research, 40,* 254–272.

Shapiro, L.P. & Levine, B.A. (1990). Verb processing during sentence comprehension in aphasia. *Brain and Language, 38,* 21–47.

Shapiro, L.P., McNamara, P., Zurif, E., Lanzoni, S., & Cermak, L. (1991). Processing complexity and sentence memory: Evidence from amnesia. *Brain and Language, 42,* 431–453.

Shapiro, L.P., Nagel, H.N., & Levine, B.A. (1993). Preferences for a verb's complements and their use in sentence processing. *Journal of Memory and Language, 32,* 96–114.

Shapiro, L.P. & Thompson, C.K. (1994). The use of linguistic theory as a framework for treatment studies in aphasia. In P. Lemme (ed.), *Clinical aphasiology, Vol. 21.*

Shapiro, L.P., Zurif, E., & Grimshaw, J. (1987). Sentence processing and the mental representation of verbs. *Cognition, 27,* 219–246.

Shewan, C.M. (1981). *Auditory comprehension test for sentences.* Chicago, IL: Biolinguistics Clinical Institutes.

Swinney, D. & Osterhaut, L. (1990). Inference generation during auditory language comprehension. In A. Graesser & G. Bower (eds.), *Inferences and text comprehension.* San Diego, CA: Academic Press.

Swinney, D. & Zurif, E. (1995). Syntactic processing in aphasia. *Brain and Language, 50,* 225–239.

Tannenhaus, M.K., Carlson, G., & Trueswell, J.C. (1989). The role of thematic structure in interpretation and parsing. *Language and Cognitive Processes, 4,* SI211–SI234.

Thompson, C.K. (1989). Generalization in the treatment of aphasia. In L.V. McReynolds & J.E. Spradlin (eds.), *Generalization strategies in the treatment of communication disorders.* Philadelphia, PA: BC Decker.

Thompson, C.K., Ballard, K.J., & Shapiro, L.P. (1998). The role of syntactic complexity in training wh-movement structures in agrammatic aphasia: Optimal order for promoting generalization. *Journal of the International Neuropsychological Society,* 661–674.

Thompson, C.K., Fix, S.C., & Gitelman, D.R. (in press). Selective impairment of morphosyntactic production in a neurological patient. *Brain and Language.*

Thompson, C.K. & Kearns, K.P. (1991). Analytical and technical directions in applied aphasia analysis: The Midas touch. In T. Prescott (ed.), *Clinical aphasiology, Vol. 19* (pp. 31–40). Austin, TX: Pro-Ed.

Thompson, C.K., Lange, K.L., Schneider, S.L., & Shapiro, L.P. (1997). Agrammatic and non-brain damaged subjects' verb and verb argument structure production. *Aphasiology, 11*, 473–490.

Thompson, C.K. & McReynolds, L.V. (1986). Wh-interrogative production in agrammatic aphasia: An experimental analysis of auditory-visual stimulation and direct-production treatment. *Journal of Speech and Hearing Research, 29*, 193–206.

Thompson, C.K. & Shapiro, L.P. (1994). A linguistic-specific approach to treatment of sentence production deficits in aphasia. In P. Lemme (ed.), *Clinical aphasiology, Vol. 21.*

Thompson, C.K., Shapiro, L.P., & Roberts, M.M. (1993). Treatment of sentence production deficits in aphasia: A linguistic-specific approach to wh-interrogative training and generalization. *Aphasiology, 7*, 111–133.

Thompson, C.K., Shapiro, L.P., Tait, M.E., Jacobs, B.J., Schneider, S.L., & Ballard, K.J. (1995). A system for the linguistic analysis of agrammatic language production. *Brain and Language, 124–129.*

Thompson, C.K., Shapiro, L.P., Tait, M.E., Jacobs, B., & Schneider, S.S. (1996). Training Wh-question production in agrammatic aphasia: Analysis of argument and adjunct movement. *Brain and Language, 52*, 175–228.

Thompson, C.K., Shapiro, L.P., Ballard, K.J., Jacobs, B.J., Schneider, S.L., & Tait, M. E. (1997). Training and generalized production of *wh-* and NP-movement structures in agrammatic aphasia. *Journal of Speech and Hearing Research, 40*, 228–244.

Thompson, C.K., Shapiro, L.P., & Kiran, S. (manuscript in preparation). Syntactic complexity as a factor for promoting generalization of sentence production.

Tissot, R.J. & Maunin, (1990). CT-scan correlates of agrammatism. In L. Menn & L. K. Obler (eds.), *Agrammatic aphasia: A cross-language narrative sourcebook.* Philadelphia: John Benjamins.

Vanier, M. & Caplan, D. (1990). CT-scan correlates of agrammatism. In L. Menn & L. Obler (eds.), *Agrammatic aphasia: A cross-language narrative sourcebook* (pp. 37–114). Amsterdam/Philadelphia: John Benjamins.

Wambaugh, J.L. & Thompson, C.K. (1989). Training and generalization of agrammatic aphasic adults: Wh-interrogative productions. *Journal of Speech and Hearing Disorders, 54*, 509–525.

Wertz, R.T., Collins, M.J., Weiss, D., Kurtzke, J.F., Friden, T., Brookshire, R.H., Pierce, J., Holtzapple, P., Hubbard, D.J., Porch, B.E., West, J.A., Davis, L., Matovitch, V., Morley, G. K., & Ressureccion, E. (1981). Veterans Administration cooperative study on aphasia: A comparison of individual and group treatment. *Journal of Speech and Hearing Research, 24*, 580–594.

Zingeser, L. & Berndt, R.S. (1990). Retrieval of nouns and verbs in agrammatism and anomia. *Brain and Language, 39*, 14–32.

Zurif, E., Swinney, D., Prather, P., Solomon, J., & Bushell, C. (1993). On-line analysis of syntactic processing in Broca's and Wernicke's aphasia. *Brain and Language, 45*, 448–464.

APPENDIX 26–1
Northwestern University Sentence Comprehension Test (NSCT)

Sentence Types Tested	Sample Stimulus Sentence	Semantically Reversed Counterpart
Active	The girl tickled the boy.	The boy tickled the girl.
Passive	The boy was tickled by the girl.	The girl was tickled by the boy.
Object Relative	I see the boy who the girl tickled.	I see the girl who the boy tickled.
Subject Relative	I see the girl who tickled the boy.	I see the boy who tickled the girl.

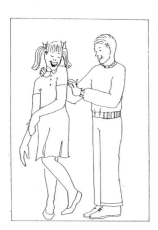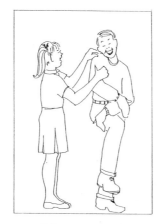

Sample stimulus picture pair used to test all four constructions.

APPENDIX 26-2
Northwestern University Verb Production Battery
Verb Types Tested by Type and Argument Structure

Obligatory One-Place
Argument structure: x[g]
  SKATE
  SNEEZE
  JUMP
  SIT
  PRAY
  SWIM
  RUN
  LISTEN
  LAUGH
  SNORE

Obligatory Two-Place
Argument structure: x, y
  PULL
  CATCH
  WIPE
  PUSH
  WRAP
  SPILL
  ERASE
  CARRY
  STIR
  WEIGH

Obligatory Three-Place
Argument structure: x, y, z
  GIVE
  PUT
  STICK

Optional Two-Place
Argument structure: x; x, y
  DIG
  CLEAN
  EAT
  SWEEP
  SING
  WATCH
  SHAVE
  RIDE
  JUGGLE
  CLIMB

Optional Three-Place
Argument structure: x, y; x, y, z
  SERVE
  BAKE
  THROW
  BUY
  SHOW
  TEACH
  READ
  WRITE
  POUR
  FRY

APPENDIX 26-3
Treatment of Underlying Forms: Treatment Protocols
Training Object-Extracted Wh-Questions (Wh-Movement)

Step 1. Wh-question elicitation. A randomly selected semantically reversible stimulus pair (pictured) is presented—e.g., (a) girl kissing a boy and (b) boy kissing a girl. Wh-question production is elicited using the sentence production priming task (see section, *Assessment of Agrammatism*). If a grammatically correct wh-question is produced, a new stimulus set is presented for elicitation of a new object cleft sentence. When a grammatically correct wh-question is not produced, training steps 2–7 are followed.

Step 2. Sentence constituents comprising the active training sentence are presented on individual cards, together with WHO, WHAT, and ? cards (e.g., THE SOLDIER, IS, PUSHING, THE WOMAN, INTO THE STREET, WHO, WHAT, ?). The verb and verb arguments (thematic roles), and adjunct prepositional phrase are identified by the examiner in the following manner: Pointing to the verb, the examiner explains: "This is *PUSHING*;

---

[g]Variables x, y, z denote the arguments *agent, theme, goal*, respectively.

it is the action of the sentence"; pointing to the agent (subject NP), the examiner explains: "This is *THE SOLDIER*; he is the person doing the pushing"; pointing to the theme (object NP), the examiner explains: "This is *THE WOMAN*; she is the person/thing being pushed"; and finally, pointing to the PP, the examiner explains: "This is *INTO THE STREET*; this is the place/time the pushing occurred."

Step 3. The examiner replaces the theme with either WHO or WHAT, explaining that the person/thing is WHO/WHAT is being pushed. The question mark card then is placed at the end of the card string which forms an echo question (e.g., *THE SOLDIER IS PUSHING* WHO *INTO THE STREET* ?). Subjects then are required to read/repeat the echo question.

Step 4. Subject/auxiliary verb inversion is demonstrated (e.g., *IS THE SOLDIER PUSHING* WHO *INTO THE STREET* ?).

Step 5. The examiner demonstrates movement of the wh-morpheme to the sentence initial position (e.g., WHO *IS THE SOLDIER PUSHING INTO THE STREET* ?) and the subject is instructed to read/repeat the resultant question.

Step 6. Sentence constituents are re-arranged in declarative sentence form together with WHO, WHAT, and ? cards (as in step 2). Steps 3, 4, and 5 are repeated with the subject replacing/selecting/moving the cards to form the correct s-structure representation of the target wh-question. Assistance is provided if needed.

Step 7. Repeat Step 1.

Object Cleft Training (Wh-Movement)

Step 1. A randomly selected semantically reversible stimulus pair (pictured) is presented—e.g., (a) girl kissing a boy and (b) boy kissing a girl. Object cleft sentence production is elicited using the sentence production priming task (see *Assessment of Agrammatism* section). If a grammatically correct object cleft sentence is produced, a new stimulus set is presented for elicitation of a new object cleft sentence. When a grammatically correct object cleft is not produced, training steps 2–7 are followed.

Step 2. Sentence constituents comprising the declarative form of the target sentence (e.g., *The woman kissed the man*) are presented on individual cards (e.g., THE WOMAN, KISSED, THE MAN). Additional sentence element cards needed to form the object cleft (e.g., IT, WAS, WHO) are placed above. The client is instructed to read aloud/repeat the declarative sentence. The verb and verb arguments (thematic roles) are identified in the following manner: Pointing to the verb, the examiner explains: "This is *KISSED*; it is the action of the sentence"; pointing to the agent, the examiner explains: "This is *THE WOMAN*; she is the person doing the kissing"; pointing to the theme, the examiner explains: "This is *THE MAN*; he is the person who is being kissed." The client is asked to verbally identify the verb/action, the agent, and the theme.

Step 3. The WHO card is placed next to the theme card (THE MAN). The clinician explains that to make a new sentence, WHO is added next to THE MAN because THE MAN is the person who was kissed. The client is instructed to read/repeat the sentence in the word order that it now appears on the cards (e.g., THE WOMAN, KISSED, THE MAN, WHO).

Step 4. The theme (THE MAN) and the WHO cards are moved to the sentence initial position; then the IT WAS card is added to the beginning of the sentence. The examiner explains: "To make the correct sentence, these words are moved to the beginning of the

sentence. IT WAS is added to the sentence because it was the man who the woman kissed." The subject is instructed to read/repeat the target sentence (e.g., IT WAS THE MAN WHO THE WOMAN KISSED).

Step 5. Sentence constituents are re-arranged in declarative sentence form together with IT, WAS, WHO cards (as in step 2). Steps 3 and 4 are repeated with the subject replacing/selecting/moving the cards to form the correct s-structure representation of the target object cleft sentence. Assistance is provided as needed.

Step 6. Repeat Step 1.

Training Passive Sentences (NP-Movement)

Step 1. A randomly selected semantically reversible stimulus pair (pictured) is presented—e.g., (a) a girl tickling a boy and (b) a boy tickling a girl. Passive sentence production is elicited using the sentence production priming task (see *Assessment of Agrammatism* section). If a grammatically correct passive sentence is produced, a new stimulus set is presented for elicitation of a new passive sentence. When a grammatically correct passive is not produced, training steps 2–7 are completed.

Step 2. Pictures are removed and sentence constituents comprising the declarative form of the target sentence (e.g., *The girl tickled the boy*) are presented on individual cards (e.g., THE GIRL, TICKLED, THE BOY). Additional sentence element cards needed to form the passive (e.g., WAS, BY) are placed above. The client is instructed to read aloud/repeat the declarative sentence. The verb and verb arguments (thematic roles) are identified in the following manner: Pointing to the verb, the examiner explains: "This is *TICKLED*; it is the action of the sentence"; pointing to the agent, the examiner explains: "This is *THE GIRL*; she is the person doing the tickling"; pointing to the theme, the examiner explains: "This is *THE BOY*; he is the person who is being tickled." The client is asked to verbally identify the verb/action, the agent, and the theme.

Step 3. The verb card (TICKLED) is placed at the end of the card string and the WAS card is placed next to it, resulting in a card string like: THE GIRL, THE BOY, WAS, TICKLED. The examiner explains that a new sentence can be formed about the boy and the girl by moving 'tickled' to the end and adding 'was'—because the boy was tickled. The client is instructed to read/repeat the sentence.

Step 4. The examiner adds the BY card next to the Agent (THE GIRL) and moves both cards to the sentence initial position (e.g., THE BOY, WAS, TICKLED, BY, THE GIRL). The examiner explains that to make the sentence correctly, 'by' is added next to 'the girl' and that both are moved to the end of the sentence because the boy was tickled *by the girl*. The client is instructed to read/repeat the correct sentence.

Step 5. Sentence constituents are re-arranged in declarative sentence form together with WAS, BY cards (as in step 2). Steps 3 and 4 are repeated with the subject replacing/selecting/moving the cards to form the correct s-structure of the target passive sentence. Assistance is provided if needed.

Step 6. Repeat Step 1.

Training Subject-Raising Structures (NP-Movement)

Step 1. A randomly selected semantically reversible stimulus pair (pictured) is presented—e.g., (a) a girl tickling a boy and (b) a boy tickling a girl. Subject-raising sentence production is elicited using a delayed modeling procedure. The subject-raising construction is modeled by the clinician using picture (a) and the client is instructed to produce a similar sentence using picture (b). A 5-sec response interval is provided. If a grammatically correct subject-raising sentence is produced, a new stimulus set is presented for elicitation of a new subject-raising sentence. When a grammatically correct subject-raising sentence is not produced, training steps 2–7 are completed.

Step 2. Pictures are removed and sentence constituents comprising the declarative form of the target sentence (e.g., *The girl tickled the boy*) are presented on individual cards (e.g., THE GIRL, TICK-LED, THE BOY). Additional sentence element cards needed to form the subject-raising structure (e.g., IT, SEEMS, TO HAVE) are placed above. The client is instructed to read aloud/repeat the declarative sentence. The verb and verb arguments (thematic roles) are identified in the following manner: Pointing to the verb, the examiner explains: "This is *TICKLED*; it is the action of the sentence"; pointing to the agent, the examiner explains: "This is *THE GIRL*; she is the person doing the tickling"; pointing to the theme,

the examiner explains: "This is *THE BOY*; he is the person who is being tickled." The client is asked to verbally identify the verb/action, the agent, and the theme.

Step 3. The examiner places the IT and SEEMS cards in sentence initial position while explaining: "A new sentence can be made about the boy and the girl by adding IT SEEMS to the beginning of the sentence." The client is instructed to read/repeat the sentence (e.g., IT, SEEMS, THE GIRL, TICKLED, THE BOY).

Step 4. The examiner replaces the IT card with THE GIRL card and adds TO HAVE in front of the verb while explaining: "In the new sentence, THE GIRL is replaced by IT; TO HAVE is added to the verb to make the correct sentence." The client is instructed to read/repeat the correct sentence (e.g., THE GIRL SEEMS TO HAVE TICKLED THE BOY).

Step 5. Sentence constituents are re-arranged in declarative sentence form together with IT, SEEMS, TO HAVE cards (as in step 2). Steps 3 and 4 are repeated with the subject replacing/selecting/moving the cards to form the correct s-structure of the target passive sentence. Assistance is provided if needed.

Step 6. Repeat Step 1.

Chapter 27

Language-Oriented Treatment: A Psycholinguistic Approach to Aphasia

Donna L. Bandur
and Cynthia M. Shewan

OBJECTIVES

The purpose of this chapter is to define Language-Oriented Treatment (LOT); outline the implementation of LOT; describe the benefits of an LOT approach; highlight the "functional" aspects of LOT; and demonstrate the efficacy of LOT.

Language-Oriented Treatment (LOT) is a psycholinguistic approach to the treatment of aphasia. As such, it strives to enable a person with aphasia to utilize a language processing system, at its maximum functional level. This language-oriented approach is based on the application of psycholinguistic research evidence to treatment, reflecting how language is normally processed and how it is altered in the presence of aphasia. Because of its neurolinguistic underpinnings with respect to theory, application, and evolution, Helm-Estabrooks (1988) has categorized LOT as a neurolinguistic approach to treatment. LOT was developed in the 1970s over a 2-year period by Shewan (1977) with the aim of creating an approach consisting of a structured methodology, coupled with content based on research data from normal and disordered language. In order to acquaint the reader with the climate in which LOT was conceived, a brief history of aphasia treatment will be reviewed.

HISTORY OF APHASIA TREATMENT

Little in the way of what we now know as orthodox treatment for aphasia appeared before the beginning of the 20th century. In the early 1900s, the literature reported a few studies describing treatment (Franz, 1906, 1924; Frazier & Ingham, 1920; Mills, 1904; Weisenburg & McBride, 1935) and even as far back as this, questions were raised, although not answered, relative to the efficacy of treatment.

After World War II, there was a surge of interest in aphasia treatment because of the number of war veterans with aphasia as a result of trauma. The focus of these rehabilitation efforts was on re-education, the approach developed for treatment. Because of the effects of trauma on the personality of these individuals, many psychotherapy groups became a part of rehabilitation efforts (Backus, 1952; Blackman, 1950). Reportedly, these groups provided support and positively influenced both communication and personality adjustment (Aronson et al., 1956; Blackman & Tureen, 1948). Questions of treatment efficacy were raised, but few answers were given. Data, however, with the exceptions of Eisenson (1949) and Wepman (1951), were primarily anecdotal and not statistically supported. In addition, the data available focused on trauma rather than stroke.

In the 1950s, aphasia treatment shifted to dealing with individuals who developed aphasia as a result of stroke. Schuell's work in this era and in the 1960s predominated (Schuell et al., 1964). The data published about treatment were controversial, and whether aphasia treatment was efficacious remained an issue. On the one hand, Vignolo's study (1964) reported the significantly positive effects of treatment, while the study by Sarno et al. (1970) failed to show the positive effects of language treatment.

The 1970s and early 1980s witnessed the publication of several studies, some with and some without control groups, that supported the efficacy of language treatment in aphasia (Basso et al., 1979; Basso et al., 1975; Broida, 1977; Dabul & Hanson, 1975; Deal & Deal, 1978; Hagen, 1973; Prins et al., 1978; Sefer, 1973; Shewan & Kertesz, 1984; Smith et al., 1972; Wertz et al., 1978; Wertz et al., 1981). The ideal study, using a randomized no-treatment control group, was not done, and some believed that only this study would lay to rest their doubts about the efficacy of aphasia treatment. Despite some studies that disputed the efficaciousness of language treatment (David et al., 1982; Meikle et al., 1979), enough evidence had been gathered by 1982 for Darley (1982) to conclude that "the foregoing collage of

629

studies...collectively provides a series of answers and together lays our doubt about efficacy to rest" (p. 175).

However, Darley's proclamation did not convince everyone, and efficacy studies continued throughout the 1980s and into this decade, with the majority favoring the significant and positive effects of treatment (Brindley et al., 1989; Holland & Wertz, 1988; Poeck et al., 1989; Schonle, 1988; Springer et al., 1991; Wertz et al., 1986; Whitney & Goldstein, 1989). In summarizing the results of most large group studies, Holland et al. (1996) described them as demonstrating the value of aphasia treatment, particularly when therapy is frequent and conducted over a lengthy interval. The authors also highlighted the contributions made in recent years by small-group, single-subject experimental studies and individual case studies. These investigations have provided more detailed descriptions of the efficacy of specific approaches when applied to particular language problems. Because the individuals studied in these reports have generally been in the chronic stages of their recovery, language gains realized are not likely to be attributed to spontaneous recovery. Treatment studies examining the application of highly specified procedures for carefully delineated disorders hold much promise in advancing our therapeutic approaches to the myriad of problems manifested in aphasia and in discovering "what works best for whom."

EVOLUTION OF LANGUAGE-ORIENTED TREATMENT

From the foregoing summary, one can see how the landscape of aphasia treatment has in many ways changed. With pressures not only to prove that what we do works and/or results in functional improvements, greater emphasis has also been placed on being able to describe what it is that we do in therapy to effect these changes. When LOT was first conceptualized, the aphasia literature contained few descriptions of treatment that were sufficiently detailed to assure clinicians that they were indeed actually replicating them. While the predominant type of treatment was stimulation therapy, clinicians were finding that some patients did not seem to be improving with this approach. As such, they were seeking alternative methods that were perhaps more clearly defined and incorporated the accumulating research data on how patients with aphasia process language. Because few treatments then had been proven efficacious, efficacy questions were still prevalent, pressuring clinicians to reexamine their treatment approaches and accompanying rationales.

LOT was subsequently designed, outlining a structured methodology in which an individual progressed through steps of increasing difficulty with the content of therapy based on psycholinguistic research data. LOT was pilot tested (Shewan, 1977) on a small group of patients. The resulting promising data led to a full-scale clinical trial described later in this chapter. A decade passed from ideational conception to publication of a book fully describing LOT, complete with treatment guidelines, treatment materials and efficacy data (Shewan & Bandur, 1986). Ongoing research has necessitated modifications particularly to the content of LOT. As further advancements have been made in our understanding of normal language processing, aphasic deficits and the impact of specific treatment procedures, LOT has been refined and in some respects, broadened in scope.

Philosophy and Rationale

Aphasia treatments, with LOT being no exception, are typically based on a theoretical construct of aphasia. Defined here, aphasia represents an impairment in the language system and potentially in the access to the language system. Processes for understanding and producing language are thereby impaired. This theoretical view of aphasia is derived from the work of Zurif and his colleagues (Zurif & Caramazza, 1976; Zurif et al., 1972; Zurif et al., 1976). It is proposed that the linguistic or conceptual knowledge base is not lost in aphasia but can no longer be accessed automatically, at an unconscious level. Language, or at least certain aspects of language, must be mediated by more conscious and explicit mechanisms (Byng, 1995).

In the LOT method, the content of language treatment is important. LOT does not represent indiscriminant stimulation of the language system, with the hope that something takes and improvement occurs. The goal is to provide the patient with a language-processing system that operates at its maximum functional level by applying neurolinguistic findings to treatment.

The content of LOT is based on language materials that are arranged in hierarchies of difficulty that, in turn, reflect research information about how adults with normal language and those with aphasia process language. Because the content and activities are based on and sequenced according to an analysis of the language deficits, opportunities for success are maximized and errors are less random and better understood by both the clinician and the patient. This experience is in contrast to that of providing a "workbook" activity to match a symptom, with consequent frustration when responding appears inconsistent or when the difficulty level fails to match the problem.

LOT is designed to provide a highly individualized and tailored approach to treatment based on the language profile and the interests and goals of the patient. Guidelines, not prescriptions, are detailed in order to assist with organizing and implementing therapy. An effort has been made to maintain a high degree of flexibility with the approach while providing enough structure to allow effective replication.

Content

Implementation of LOT requires the analysis and understanding of the pattern of deficits presented, specific to the

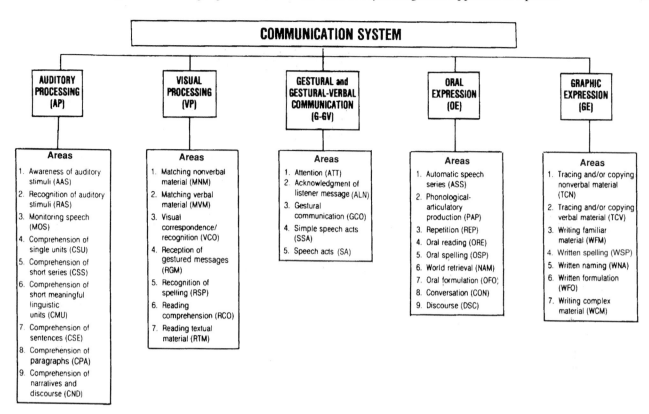

Figure 27–1. Schematic model of the language modalities and areas within these modalities that make up the communication system.

individual presenting them. A hypothesis regarding the underlying nature of the problems is based on available information from normal language processing and that in aphasia. A psycholinguistic approach emphasizes the need for clinicians to ensure that their interpretation of symptoms is guided by theoretical hypotheses rather than relying on intuition and that treatment is individualized with respect to the symptoms displayed by the specific person being treated (Byng, 1992; Albert, 1998). To provide a system whereby the content of language can be described comprehensively and to facilitate data collection, LOT divides the communication system into five modalities, which are non-overlapping and mutually exclusive (Figure 27–1). The five modalities are auditory processing, visual processing, gestural and combined gestural-verbal communication, oral expression, and graphic expression.

Each modality is further subdivided into mutually exclusive areas that collectively encompass the entire modality. With each modality segmented into component parts, a clinician can specify clearly the content of treatment being provided. Rather than advocating a particular breakdown of the communication system, the division was intended to facilitate specifying the content of treatment and to permit its replication.

Within each area of a modality (for example, comprehension of sentences, within auditory processing) treatment materials are organized according to difficulty level, based on the research literature describing how persons with aphasia process language. The goal of language treatment, then, is to improve a patient's language deficits by presenting material that increases in difficulty level, at a pace that the individual can accommodate.

Although the modalities have been delineated to assist in outlining LOT content and areas for potential treatment, it is acknowledged that treatment within one modality or area may be targeted to facilitate performance in another. For example, within the oral expression modality, oral reading would rarely be chosen as a goal, in and of itself. An oral reading task may be selected to achieve a variety of objectives such as self-monitoring, auditory processing, reading comprehension, and so forth. When selecting an activity within an area, it is imperative that it corresponds to the goal that has been established and to consider how responses within an activity, area, or modality might reflect other language processes.

The reader is also cautioned that the content areas within each modality serve only as guidelines for consideration and are not necessarily arranged in a hierarchical order; nor are all of them intended for use with every patient. These content areas are considered as the base in treatment. As our understanding of aphasia evolves, along with knowledge about the effectiveness of specific treatment techniques, these advancements can be incorporated into the content of LOT.

Finally, more than one modality can and typically is treated simultaneously, that is, either within the same session or perhaps within the same activity. Again, LOT was designed to be flexible and promote the use of procedures that facilitate optimal responding by the patient. To this end, the clinician must be cognizant of the many variables that impact performance and design tasks that can meet the goals selected and organize them in ways that allow changes to be measured and documented. By more clearly specifying the elements of treatment, plans and activities can be more easily evaluated and described, thereby enabling replication with other patients.

Methodology

LOT methodology has adopted a paradigm in which the major components are stimulus, response, and reinforcement. In contrast to operant conditioning, however, the goal is not to learn specific stimulus-response connections such as certain words in a word retrieval task or specific sentences in a sentence formulation task. Rather, the paradigm of presenting stimuli, followed by responses with accompanying descriptive feedback enables patients to process or use language at levels appropriate, yet challenging, given their current capabilities. In order to facilitate correct responding, modifications may be made to the stimuli or task requirements as difficulties are encountered. Facilitated problem solving has been used to describe treatment that is characterized by the relationship between a narrow focus in the materials used, what the patient is required to do with them, and the interaction with the clinician (Byng & Black, 1995). This process of adjusting the task in response to the patient at a given point in time has been proposed to be one of the critical elements of therapy.

Approaching treatment from a stimulus-response-reinforcement paradigm allows the clinician to collect data about performance and provides objective feedback to the clinician and patient about progress over time on a particular task. Improvements in treatment may not be quickly translated into changes on standardized test measures. Being able to demonstrate steady gains across a hierarchy of tasks can serve as an invaluable source of reinforcement for the patient and significant others, as well as those who may be questioning the value of financially supporting ongoing treatment. Alternatively, this method provides objective information as to when a procedure may need to be modified or perhaps even abandoned.

Difficulty Levels

In LOT, activities are presented in order of increasing difficulty to optimize opportunities for success and minimize feelings of frustration and failure on the part of the patient. Several variables can affect the difficulty level of a task, such as type of materials incorporated, mode of presentation, complexity of response required, and amount of clinician support provided. Difficulty levels may be based on an analysis of results from standardized testing and systematic probing, in concert with information available from research literature regarding normal and/or disordered language functioning.

The stimuli and their responses in treatment are presented in blocks of 10 items each. To advance the difficulty level of a task, a patient must achieve 70% or more correct on two consecutive blocks of items at the same difficulty level. When this criterion is achieved, the difficulty level of the task is increased to the next level in the hierarchy. If the 70% correct criterion is not achieved, the block of 10 stimulus items is repeated. If 70% correct is still not achieved, the level of difficulty of the task is decreased. If, even with a decrease in the task difficulty, the 70% correct criterion is not obtained, the task is discontinued.

A criterion of 70% correct was chosen to allow flexibility in response performance and to accommodate for some error without unduly delaying progress in treatment. If a particular patient demonstrates the need for a higher criterion, one can be used. The efficacy data reported later in this chapter, however, used the 70% criterion.

Cuing

If a patient cannot generate an independent response, the clinician may accept a cued response as correct. The goal in using a cuing system is to determine which cues are effective, to develop the patient's awareness of those that are helpful, to transfer the responsibility for initiating and providing cues from the clinician to the patient, and to increase the patient's production of independent responses, using self-cuing as necessary.

Criterion Response and Branching

Defining the elements of a correct response is required to advance the difficulty level. The clinician decides what constitutes a correct response, as described earlier. Because the clinician has flexibility in establishing this decision, the definition of a correct response differs for each task. In most tasks, many different levels of response are possible, and what is accepted as correct may change with time and as improvement occurs. For example, early in treatment a clinician may decide that in a naming task, a recognizable production meets criterion. Later, a phonetically correct response may be required to score it as meeting criterion.

When the difference between two adjacent levels of difficulty proves to be too great for a patient to master, the clinician can create levels of intermediate difficulty (branching). Branching constructs a link between the initial tasks and helps the patient to reach the next level. Another situation requiring branching may arise when a clinician wants to divide a large group of equally difficult material into two subgroups in order to provide language processing opportunities with each subgroup and to avoid omitting some materials.

Feedback

Feedback is a crucial aspect to the implementation of LOT. Information regarding the correctness and quality of a response promotes a better understanding of the language impairment and renders it less mysterious. By engaging in mutual problem-solving exchanges and encouraging self-evaluation, the patient becomes an active participant in treatment. The patient can also be a rich source of information and insight for the clinician by providing a different perspective on the nature of the problem by describing, when possible, how a particular response has occurred or was facilitated.

Sequence of Treatment Activities

Activities are sequenced within a given treatment session. With an awareness of proactive and retroactive facilitation and inhibition, a clinician can sequence activities to take as much advantage of facilitation as possible. It is desirable to begin a treatment session with an activity on which the patient performs well. The initial success can lead to increased motivation and reduce the possible effects of fatigue. Generally, the difficulty of activities is increased as the session progresses. If perseveration is noted and persists, the best strategy may be to change the task. Another important consideration is to select an activity that is enjoyable and successful, aiming to conclude the session on a positive note.

Recording Data

Recording data is important in LOT because it is the patient's performance that dictates when tasks should be increased or decreased in difficulty. Two forms (Appendices 27–1 and 27–2) can be helpful in this respect. A LOT Goals Form, if used for each area in each modality, can chart the course of treatment. The difficulty level, the stimuli, the presentation method, cuing, criterion for a correct response, and response method are all recorded. Additional responses are also noted. Using this form, a clinician can show how treatment is changing over time. A LOT Data Record Form specifies the amount of time spent in each session for each area and modality, the difficulty level of the task, the number of items presented, the data collected, and any comments a clinician may wish to record. Glancing at this form indicates what transpired in each session and suggests when the task level should be increased. Again, it may be easiest to record data for each area and each modality using a separate form.

Patient-Clinician Relationship

Although LOT is structured in content and methodology, it is carried out within a caring and positive interpersonal environment. Albert (1998) describes the loss of ability to communicate as tantamount to the loss of personhood and there is evidence to suggest that the self-esteem of individuals who have suffered strokes can contribute to their functional abilities, at least in the early phases of recovery (Chang & MacKenzie, 1998). Le Dorze and Brassard (1995) have reported on the impact of aphasia on both patients and their significant others. Negative communication consequences include increased effort, irritation, frustration, and fatigue in communication, with language disabilities having a marked impact on interpersonal relationships.

Sarno (1997) has described how intensive, long-term rehabilitation which addresses language, communication strategies, functional communication, and psychosocial issues for the first year positively impacts on the quality of life of persons with aphasia. In this context, the importance of the patient-clinician relationship cannot be overstated. Understanding and respecting premorbid personality and lifestyle characteristics of patients are the first steps in developing collaborative, supportive relationships with them and their significant others. Creating a climate for open and honest exchange of ideas and feelings is needed to facilitate mutual goal-setting and a sense of partnership. Skillful clinicians are mindful of how central the therapeutic relationship is to the treatment of aphasia. Helping patients and their support systems understand the loss accompanying aphasia is a necessary component of treatment. This in turn creates the foundation for working through the many challenges and sometimes disappointments that are encountered throughout the rehabilitation process.

Although LOT employs a structured methodology of stimulus-response-reinforcement, in concert with clearly defined hierarchies and scoring systems, this approach does not preclude the establishment of a patient-centered milieu in treatment. The patient and significant others play integral roles in determining goals and activities based on their needs, interests, and abilities. In order to facilitate the transfer of skills to more functional aspects of the patient's life, the clinician must develop an understanding of the impact of aphasia on the whole person and the world in which he or she participates.

IMPLEMENTATION OF LOT

Guiding Principles

In the following sections, a description of each of the modalities will be provided. It is not possible to discuss all of the areas within the confines of this chapter, so only some of them will be highlighted, particularly as they reflect current practice or changes since the inception of LOT. The reader is referred to *Treatment of Aphasia: A Language-Oriented Approach* (Shewan & Bandur, 1986). A complete listing of the areas incorporated in each of the modalities is also found in

Figure 27–1. It is worth noting that this chart reflects the content of LOT at the time of its original development. Since then, approaches to treatment have been refined in some areas and these new or expanded treatment applications will be discussed in the descriptions of the modalities that follow.

The decision as to which modalities and areas to introduce initially in treatment is based on individual patient patterns of performance, a hypothesis regarding the underlying nature of the symptoms, and an application of research information in selecting the most viable approach at that point in time. Particularly with patients with more severe impairments, one might look for *pockets of strength* and capitalize on them early to achieve success and maintain motivation.

At the conclusion of the treatment section, some case illustrations will be provided to demonstrate the practical applications of LOT with patients exhibiting a range of aphasic deficits. These descriptions provide evidence that systematically addressing the underlying problems results in functional improvements.

Generally, aphasia therapy takes place in a face-to-face setting between a clinician and patient. Most often in this interaction, the clinician presents activities and related feedback and modifies tasks according to the patient's responses. The advent of computers has provided another vehicle for providing treatment. At least in some activities, the clinician's role as an activity or feedback provider can be assumed by a computer. Using the LOT paradigm, however, activities must be carefully designed and sequenced according to the psycholinguistic principles described to avoid failure and consequent frustration on the part of the patient.

Computer-Assisted Treatment

The literature reflects varied degrees of improvement in language functioning related to implementation of computerized programs. When evaluating the results of an unsupervised home-based computer program, Petheram (1996) failed to find a relationship between progression through a hierarchy of tasks and improvements on formalized language measures. Amount of time spent on the computer varied widely and appeared to be associated with less frequent opportunities for hobbies or other forms of social interaction. In coupling home- and clinic-based computer instruction, significant improvements have been reported in certain language measures, such as naming in a group of patients with chronic aphasia (Aftonomos et al., 1997). Icons associated with natural lexical items representing various categories were manipulated in a range of activities. The amount of daily home practice (mean, 2.04 hours) was considered to be a significant contributor to the gains realized.

Treatment of reading through the computer medium has been explored (Katz & Wertz, 1997), employing a hierarchy of activities from simple letter matching to sentence comprehension tasks. At the conclusion of treatment, those who had received reading comprehension training demonstrated significantly more improved scores on overall language measures than those who were provided with only computer stimulation tasks.

With many individuals now having computers in their homes, development of carefully structured treatment activities using a hierarchy of difficulty levels could be incorporated into the LOT approach, providing additional avenues for practice. The visual processing and graphic expression modalities are those that would likely best lend themselves to being supplemented with computer practice.

Auditory Processing

General Considerations

Various types of auditory processing problems occur in aphasia, including auditory imperception, pure-word deafness, and auditory agnosia. The most prominent difficulties, however, are generally associated with auditory comprehension, and have consequently received the most attention in designing treatment strategies. In LOT, auditory processing has been divided into two major categories: auditory perceptual processing deficits and auditory comprehension deficits. Generally, auditory perceptual activities are introduced only if success cannot be attained with auditory comprehension tasks. By developing auditory perceptual skills, the patient may learn to tune into the auditory modality and prepare this mechanism for comprehension activities.

The roles of attention and memory in aphasia are intertwined with the impaired language system, making it challenging to separate out their potential effects. Evidence suggests that individuals with aphasia may experience problems with tasks that involve orienting, sustaining, focusing, or dividing their attention, and these difficulties may occur with both visual and auditory input (Murray, 1999). Especially with patients who have more severe impairments and are unresponsive to auditory and/or visual input, directly addressing attentional skills may be the first avenue of treatment. A specific cognitive approach to treatment has been reported with success by Helm-Estabrooks (1998). Attention and concentration activities included cancellation tasks, repeating and alternating graphomotor patterns, and trail making. Other cognitive tasks were incorporated that addressed visual memory, visuoperception, judgment, and semantic knowledge. Post-treatment testing revealed significant gains with auditory comprehension.

Burgio and Basso (1997) have described long-term problems with verbal memory associated with even mild aphasia. Although memory problems were found across all subjects in the acute phase, some individuals showed improved performance over time, with story-retelling as compared to word-list (paired associate) learning. These findings suggest that tasks dependent on verbal memory may not all be equal and may reflect differing processes at work. When activities are introduced at the sentence, paragraph, and discourse levels, their degrees of complexity should be evaluated, keeping in mind the influence of memory variables.

Auditory Perception

Auditory perceptual deficits are addressed in three areas: awareness of nonspeech and speech stimuli, recognition of nonspeech and speech stimuli, and monitoring speech. In establishing awareness of nonspeech and speech stimuli, the patient is required only to respond differentially, but not necessarily to demonstrate recognition of the stimuli. Environmental sounds, music, familiar and unfamiliar speakers, and foreign languages may be used. In recognition of nonspeech and speech stimuli, however, the patient must attach meaning to the stimuli presented, such as matching a telephone ring to its corresponding referent.

In the final area, monitoring speech, activities are incorporated to develop the patient's ability to monitor the accuracy and/or meaningfulness of speech stimuli, whether they are his or her own productions or those of others. There has been a suggestion that auditory comprehension may not be directly tied to monitoring skills, or at least may not totally account for the monitoring problems encountered by patients (Marshall et al., 1998). In this account, ability to detect neologisms was purported to be affected by impaired access to the phonological output lexicon from semantics. Following a course of treatment designed to improve semantic associations between written words and related pictures, significantly improved judgments regarding the accuracy of verbal responses were noted. This approach might be used with those patients who are able to identify clinician errors and those in their own productions off-line, but who persist with erroneous on-line judgments.

Auditory Comprehension

Treatment for auditory comprehension has been divided into six areas. Comprehension of single units deals with stimuli at the single-word level. In designing activities, some important factors related to vocabulary selection are frequency of occurrence, grammatical class, and semantic category. Depending on the type of aphasia, various hierarchies may be established through systematic alteration of both stimuli and response variables. A hierarchy for semantic word categories for three types of aphasia is illustrated in Figure 27–2 (Goodglass et al., 1966; Goodglass & Wingfield, 1993). It has been proposed that auditory comprehension of visually presented stimuli may be negatively impacted if the items depicted represent functionally conceived, man-made objects, e.g., furniture, rather than those that are visually conceived or based on physical properties, e.g., animals (Goodglass, 1993). Finally, evidence from lexical decision tasks indicates that both normal controls and subjects with aphasia experience

	Broca's	Wernicke's	Anomic
Easy	Body parts	Body parts	Body parts
	Actions	Actions	Objects
	Objects	Objects	Actions
	Numbers	Numbers	Numbers
	Colors	Letters	Colors
	Letters	Colors	Letters
Difficult	Geometric forms	Forms	Forms

Figure 27–2. Hierarchies in difficulty levels showing differences according to semantic categories.

greater priming for concrete versus abstract word pairs, suggesting that abstract words may be less rich in semantic representations, thereby making them more difficult to access (Tyler et al., 1995).

In addition to carefully selecting and ordering stimuli, manipulating response variables such as picture relatedness and number of response choices can increase task difficulty (Pierce et al., 1990).

Comprehension of short series might be introduced when memory variables need to be stressed, as the word series themselves do not form a syntactic unit. For example, when presenting a group of numbers, the patient must attend to each item in order to identify the series correctly. Syntactic units are incorporated in the area of comprehension of short meaningful linguistic units, where variables such as word frequency and topic familiarity are important to consider.

Particularly with sentences, stress as a suprasegmental cue has been found to influence performance (Goodglass, 1975, 1976; Kellar, 1978; Pashek & Brookshire, 1980). Patients with severe comprehension problems may obtain information from intonational contour to differentiate among questions, statements, and commands (Boller & Green, 1972; Green & Boller, 1974). Word frequency has been shown to affect comprehension in sentences, with common, frequently occurring vocabulary items facilitating processing.

Sentences that are longer and reflect more complex syntax tend to be more difficult (Shewan, 1979). Altering the canonicity of thematic roles (agent-theme-goal) or incorporating a second verb or proposition in a sentence has been shown to negatively impact comprehension in aphasia (Caplan et al., 1997). Patients also may benefit from the use of context in sentence comprehension activities (Pierce, 1988). Cannito et al. (1996) found that patients in the post-acute phase (5 weeks to 6 months) of their recovery experienced a facilitative effect in processing reversible passive sentences when they followed a paragraph of a predictive nature. Patients in the chronic stages of recovery (greater than 6 months) benefited equally from both predictive and nonpredictive paragraphs preceding sentence presentation. Repetition of key lexical items in the paragraph was believed to reduce the semantic processing load for the target sentences so that more resources could be assigned to understanding the relationships between the nouns. Decreased verbal memory span was also associated with those who were able to make the best use of context. With these findings in mind, sentence comprehension activities might incorporate a hierarchy of sentence types in concert with presentation of predictive and nonpredictive paragraphs, teaching the patient to recognize salient or redundant cues in the narratives and use them to assist with sentence processing.

Individuals with aphasia have demonstrated superior performance on language tasks, including comprehension of yes/no questions (Wallace & Canter, 1985) when personally relevant material is used. Other issues to be considered include situational context, speech rate, emotional content, and topic familiarity.

Although sentence comprehension is influenced by word frequency and syntactic complexity, these variables have less impact on discourse processing (Nicholas & Brookshire, 1995b). Also, a weak link between comprehension of individual sentences and comprehension of discourse has been offered. In analyzing discourse, comprehension has been shown to be superior for main ideas as opposed to details and directly stated information is recalled with greater accuracy than implied, with both normal subjects and those with aphasia.

Pierce and Grogan (1992) describe a number of factors that are normally involved in narrative comprehension. Briefly, they identify the microstructure (words and their relationship to the text) and macrostructure (gist) as the two major text components. A schema is formed by bringing one's own formulation of goals, expectations, and previous experience to the interpretation of the narrative. Schemas will vary among individuals and the macrostructure that is formed is influenced by situational variables, e.g., listening to a news broadcast versus a classroom lecture. Finally, the authors point out that while a text base (meaning of the narrative) is being developed, the listener brings his/her own knowledge and opinions to the topic, which assists with inferencing. In aphasia, it is suggested that with greater coherence or a strong relationship between propositions, comprehension and retention are facilitated. Knowledge about the topic increases inferencing, coherence, and ultimately comprehension. Less cohesive narratives may be better understood by providing a topic theme. Alternatively, recall of details can be facilitated by using narratives with several topic changes.

Some patients may experience difficulty in comprehending referents from contextual information (Chapman & Ulatowska, 1989) and may benefit from specific instruction with processing them. More errors in recalling details of high-ratio dialogues (i.e., ones in which the amount of speaking between the participants is significantly disproportionate) has also been noted. Finally, mode of presentation may affect performance such that audiotape, videotape, and live presentations can have varying impacts, depending on the individual.

When addressing comprehension of paragraphs and comprehension of narratives and discourse, many of the above variables can be manipulated to form individualized hierarchies depending on the nature and degree of the impairment. Identification of the gist, main ideas, and details in narratives of increasing length and decreasing personal relevancy could be considered. Other tasks might include those directed to improving inferencing skills by capitalizing on the patient's knowledge of scripts and developing awareness of and use of contextual cues. Altering the amount of cohesion and/or redundancy within narratives and discourse could be additional factors to control, while varying the response requirements.

Case Study

S.K. is a 24-year-old university student. Following excision of a left temporal occipital arteriovenous malformation, he demonstrated a fluent aphasia, characterized by moderate anomia, auditory and visual processing problems, and a mild agraphia. Formalized testing included administration of the Boston Diagnostic Aphasia Evaluation, the Auditory Comprehension Test for Sentences, the Revised Token Test, and the Boston Naming Test.

Auditory comprehension problems were initially found in S.K.'s comprehension of material at the paragraph level and in his processing of linguistically complex, lengthy instructions. The first treatment area selected was comprehension of paragraphs. Further probing revealed that S.K. experienced increased difficulty when required to make inferences and when the number of facts included within a paragraph was substantially increased.

For the first level of difficulty, the clinician aurally provided short paragraphs consisting of a high degree of redundancy, with S.K. required to answer inferential questions. When a 70% success rate was achieved at this level, difficulty was increased by including more facts in the paragraphs. As treatment progressed, difficulty levels were further adjusted by altering topic familiarity. More complex responses on the part of the patient were gradually introduced, so that prior to questioning by the clinician, S.K. was asked to recall as many details as possible from the paragraph. Further information was then extracted through use of either factual or inferential questions.

Comprehension of narratives and discourse was next developed. Short radio broadcasts were presented, followed by videotaped news segments and lengthier documentaries. Task difficulty was again increased by increasing the complexity of the response and varying the degree of topic familiarity.

S.K. was an active participant in developing treatment goals and hierarchies. He provided detailed feedback on the variables that he found affected his performance and reported on specific situational problems. Following treatment for word retrieval, auditory processing, and written spelling, S.K. returned to university to complete his masters degree.

Sample Activities

Level 1

Stimuli: Paragraphs 60 to 80 syllables in length; high degree of redundancy; high degree of topic familiarity.

Procedure: The paragraph is read aloud by the clinician, followed by inferential questions, requiring a yes/no response.

Level 2

Stimuli: Paragraphs 60 to 80 syllables in length; low degree of redundancy; high degree of topic familiarity.

Procedure: The paragraph is read aloud by the clinician, followed by inferential questions, requiring a yes/no response.

Level 3

Stimuli: Paragraphs 60 to 80 syllables in length; low degree of redundancy; low degree of topic familiarity.

Procedure: The paragraph is read aloud by the clinician, followed by inferential questions, requiring a yes/no response.

Visual Processing

General Considerations

Visual processing refers to the processing of information presented in pictorial, gestural, and/or written forms. As with the auditory modality, this area can be subdivided into visual perception and reading comprehension problems. Patients with aphasia demonstrate reading problems to varying degrees. Those with the most severe language impairments can experience limitations with visual recognition, such that even matching objects, drawings, forms, colors, letters, and words may be compromised. Visual acuity and field deficits can also affect performance, resulting in problems with visual attention, scanning, and tracking.

Inability to comprehend written material due to brain damage is referred to as alexia. When applied to those with aphasia, this term is used only when particular patterns are observed. Alexia without agraphia or pure alexia consists of reading problems with preserved writing. Patients may have difficulty recognizing words, although identification of high-frequency vocabulary and letters may be better. Reading is usually accomplished by using a letter-by-letter approach, making longer words more difficult to decode because of memory load (Goodglass, 1993). Comprehension of oral spelling is typically intact and words traced in the palm of the hand or palpated can often be recognized. Although there is no accompanying agraphia, the patient is unable to read his or her own writing. Both color naming and color name recognition can be impaired.

Alexia with agraphia is characterized by a severe reading impairment, often along with problems in reading musical notes and numbers, and a calculation deficit. Those affected are unable to recognize orally spelled words and are unable to spell words aloud. Tracing or palpating letters is not facilitative (Lecours, 1999). Marked writing problems are usually found in conjunction with a right homonymous hemianopsia.

The term *aphasic alexia* can be used to cover the spectrum of reading disorders that are secondary to the disruption of oral language in aphasia (Goodglass, 1993). Problems with lexical processing and sentence comprehension are often noted.

Although the area of oral reading was initially included under the oral expression modality, it will be addressed here for ease of description and application. Three disorders of oral reading have been described because of their unique pattern of errors (Webb & Love, 1994; Goodglass, 1993). The most salient features of deep dyslexia are substitution of semantically related words bearing no structural or phonological similarity to the targets, with functor words typically being substituted or omitted. From easiest to most difficult to read are nouns, verbs, and adjectives. Failure to read pseudowords is also encountered. Some consider deep dyslexia to be a variant of phonological alexia (Friedman, 1995).

Phonological alexia is characterized by problems with applying grapheme-to-phoneme correspondence rules to enable the reading of pseudowords. Errors involving visually similar words may be encountered.

Various patterns of symptoms have been associated with surface dyslexia. Commonalities reflect difficulties in effectively accessing semantics and whole-word phonology, along with an overuse, but faulty application of phoneme-to-grapheme conversion rules.

Another reported syndrome, although rare, is visual agnosia. Patients experience difficulty recognizing material presented visually (Benson & Geschwind, 1969; Eisenson, 1984) but presentation of stimuli through another modality, e.g., touch and hearing, can meet with success. Breakdown occurs for both verbal and nonverbal material. Writing is generally well preserved.

Many factors such as the individual's educational level, occupation, and avocational interests are considered in determining the extent to which the visual modality is addressed in treatment. In addition, with patients demonstrating severe impairments, this modality may be better preserved than others (Helm & Barresi, 1980; Helm-Estabrooks, 1983) and can serve as an appropriate starting point in treatment.

Visual Perception

Treatment for visual processing is divided into six areas, with the first one dealing specifically with visual perceptual deficits. Area 1, matching nonverbal material, requires the patient to match objects, pictures, and geometric forms. In developing a hierarchy of difficulty, picture complexity and degree of stylization can be adjusted, in addition to altering the stimulus category. The task may then be made more difficult by requiring category recognition.

Area 2 incorporates matching of verbal material such as numbers, letters, and words. Individual hierarchies are established considering variables of length, visual similarity, and size of the stimuli. To tax attention and memory, a series of these items may be introduced.

Area 3, visual correspondence/recognition, demands that the patient recognize different visual forms of the same stimulus. For example, the task may require matching a printed word to a corresponding object or matching trademarks to referents. Other activities in this area might address semantic categories through having the patient make decisions about subordinate-superordinate relationships. Individuals with aphasia may experience even more difficulty in performing categorization tasks that involve functional relationships (e.g., "things that write") as opposed to those consisting of superordinate relations (McCleary & Hirst, 1986).

Visual Comprehension

Area 4 focuses on reception of gestured messages. Although gesture recognition may be a less impaired modality (Porch, 1967), patients with aphasia, as a group, tend to perform more poorly in interpreting pantomimes than do those with normal language abilities. A strong relationship has been found between gesture recognition and the person with aphasia's ability to imitate nonmeaningful movements (Wang & Goodglass, 1992). Pantomime recognition and production are correlated with each other and auditory comprehension, but not with a global measure of aphasia.

One hierarchy that has been suggested for developing comprehension of gestures, in increasing order of difficulty, is associating object, action picture, object pictures, and line drawing to corresponding gestures (Daniloff et al., 1982; Netsu & Marguardt, 1984). Typically, this area would be developed in the context of preparing a patient for a gestural production system. Additional detail will therefore follow in the gestural and gestural-verbal communication modality.

Recognition of spelling is addressed in Area 5. Tasks may involve proofreading activities that include presentation of the patient's written production or those of others, for correction. This activity might be considered a form of monitoring

for those who rely heavily on written communication. Also, individuals with surface dyslexia may benefit from sentence judgment tasks requiring homophone recognition (e.g., "We took our/hour car") (Scott & Byng, 1989).

Reading Comprehension

Reading comprehension activities are initiated in Area 6, where stimuli may consist of single words, phrases, sentences, or paragraphs.

Kay et al. (1996) provide one model of reading which can serve as a point of reference for interpreting the many symptoms associated with alexia. First, abstract letter identification is required before access to the orthographic input lexicon is achieved. Once a word's entry in the orthographic input lexicon is found, the semantic system can be entered to search for the word's representation there. The spoken forms of words are stored in the phonological output lexicon. There is a buffer system consisting of a temporary storage for information while it is being worked on at a given moment in time, such as during sound assembly. When reading aloud, a dual-route model is proposed with one route leading from the orthographic input lexicon to the phonological output lexicon, by way of the semantic system. The nonlexical route, however, uses grapheme-to-phoneme rules allowing readers to read nonwords. Because it is possible to read aloud without comprehension, a third pathway leading directly from the orthographic input lexicon to the phonological output lexicon, without involving semantics is hypothesized.

Investigators tend to agree that the deficits found in pure alexia are associated with prelexical problems and typically intact lexical-orthographic and phonological knowledge (Coslett et al., 1993; Arguin & Bub, 1994). It is hypothesized that the encoding of printed words is forced to be accomplished by the right hemisphere, which is unable to encode individual letters and has limited ability to process low imageability words, morphemes, and functors (Burbaum & Coslett, 1996). This, in turn, forces the patient to analyze individual letters rather than using a more holistic approach in reading words. Additionally, more difficulty in reading lower case as compared to upper case letters may be encountered. Some case studies have demonstrated success in improving reading in pure alexia. One approach (Arguin et al., 1994) addressed what the authors posited as being the underlying problem or the failure of the patient to encode abstract "letter types." Upper and lower case letters of varying fonts were used in matching tasks, followed by speed reading of pronounceable four-letter strings using upper case letters and a font resembling script. Improvements were found with matching tasks in addition to increased speed and accuracy of reading letter strings.

Another method in treating pure alexia has been to capitalize on the tactile-kinesthetic feedback that the patient may be able to utilize (Lott et al., 1994). A treatment hierarchy was established starting with copying sets of individual letters in a uniform way, first, in the palm of the hand, followed by naming of the target and then presentation of cards with printed words for copying and oral production. Reading of both trained and untrained word lists improved with this therapy.

Specific treatment techniques have also been applied to the problems associated with surface and deep dyslexia (Nickels, 1995). In surface dyslexia where the difficulties are thought to occur at the lexical level, pairing words with mnemonic aids such as pictures improved oral reading of irregularly spelled words, using a whole-word approach and generalized to untrained items. Another patient was provided with sentence completion tasks involving homophone selection to establish the route from the visual input lexicon to the semantic system. Improvements were particularly evident with treated homophones and to a lesser extent with those that were untreated. Teaching grapheme-to-phoneme correspondence rules was used successfully with some patients with deep dyslexia. Patients were taught to link letters of the alphabet with specific words that they had selected and then to sound out letters of simple words and nonwords using these learned associations.

Individuals with deep dyslexia are impaired in using grapheme-to-phoneme correspondence rules and in using the whole-word reading route (orthographic input to phonological output lexicons) and must access the semantic route for reading. Closed-class words and pseudowords are read more poorly than open-class words but semantic value does not appear to be the sole contributing factor (Silverberg et al., 1998). Greater accuracy in oral reading was found when comparing list to text forms of presentation particularly for closed-class words. Bound-class morphemes were read more accurately than free-class morphemes especially in the list format, although both again benefited from text presentation. The authors suggest that treatment emphasizing reading in context might be more advantageous than single-word reading or the training of phoneme-to-grapheme correspondence rules.

From the foregoing descriptions of treatment approaches for some of the more clearly defined and studied forms of alexia, efforts have been made to associate the symptomatology with a breakdown in one or more aspects of a model for processing written words. Treatment hierarchies can then be established by altering vocabulary and contextual variables that are known to play specific roles in each of these disorders.

In aphasic alexia, patients may experience problems in distinguishing words that belong to the same category and share a strong connotative quality (e.g., distinguishing among tame domesticated animals) (Goodglass, 1993). Those with impaired lexical semantic processing may find it less difficult to contrast items from different connotative categories. The reading of emotionally laden vocabulary is more successful than that of concrete nouns or abstract nonemotional words when matched for frequency. Task difficulty may be altered by varying the response choices to include auditory, semantic, or visual confusions (Gardner & Zurif, 1976; Van Demark et al., 1982).

When phrases and sentences are introduced, other factors such as syntax and number of content words relevant to length may be considered. Similar to performance in listening, patients benefit from the presentation of predictive and nonpredictive preceding paragraphs to facilitate comprehension of at least certain complex sentence forms (Germani & Pierce, 1992). Altering the degree of redundancy and amount of context can be used in developing a hierarchy for treating various sentence types.

At the paragraph level, overall length can be systematically adjusted while varying individual sentence length, complexity, vocabulary difficulty, and thematic content. In developing or selecting paragraphs, one strives for high passage dependency, which reflects the degree to which accurate responses to questions about the paragraph are dependent on having read the paragraph and not on prior knowledge (Thomas & Jackson, 1997). Other issues affecting passage dependency are the relatedness of the test questions to each other and the plausibility of the answers, given a multiple choice sentence format. Questions involving little-known facts and those requiring more detailed answers would be harder to answer without having read the paragraph on which they are based. It is suggested that if the patient is able to answer less than half of the questions without having read the paragraph, higher passage dependency is indicated.

Area 7 completes this modality with reading textual material. As empirical data are limited, individual hierarchies must be developed considering variables such as overall length, vocabulary, redundancy, grammatical complexity, amount of cohesion, use of anaphoric reference, and familiarity (Shewan & Bandur, 1986). As well, many of the factors outlined in auditory comprehension of narratives and discourse could be incorporated in this section.

Case Study

N.H. is a 69-year-old homemaker who suffered from multiple strokes resulting in left frontal and right parietal occipital lobe infarcts. Administration of the Western Aphasia Battery, the Auditory Comprehension Test for Sentences, and the Boston Naming Test revealed a mild auditory processing problem, a mild verbal dyspraxia, anomia, and moderate visual processing and graphic expression difficulties. Because the patient reported being an avid reader up until the time of her most recent stroke, visual processing activities were introduced simultaneously with activities from other modalities.

Language testing suggested good single-word reading comprehension and ability to read short, simple paragraphs. Additional probing demonstrated reading comprehension to be compromised above a Grade 3 readability level. Degree of abstractness also significantly affected performance. The first difficulty level involved presentation of short paragraphs with a readability level of Grade 3 to Grade 4. The patient was required to read the paragraphs and to reformulate them orally using printed "who, what, when, where, why/how" prompts. Once N.H. was successful in recounting the significant points from the paragraphs at this level, the same length of paragraph was used but the grade level was increased to Grade 5. Over time, paragraph length, abstractness, and grade level were all systematically increased. Newspaper articles and short stories were gradually introduced, with the patient eventually reporting success in reading romance novels for enjoyment.

Sample Activities

Level 1

Stimuli: Paragraphs 75 to 100 syllables in length; Grade 3 to Grade 4 readability; printed "who, what, when, where, why/how" cards.

Procedure: The patient reads the paragraph and orally responds to the "who, what, when, where, why/how" prompts.

Level 2

Stimuli: Paragraphs 75 to 100 syllables in length; Grade 5 readability; printed "who, what, when, where, why/how" prompts.

Procedure: The patient reads the paragraph and orally responds to the "who, what, when, where, why/how" cards.

Level 3

Stimuli: Paragraphs 75 to 100 syllables in length; Grade 5 readability; no printed cues.

Procedure: The patient reads the paragraph and orally provides the relevant information.

Gestural and Gestural-Verbal Communication

General Considerations

Gestural production may prove to be an alternative mode of communication for some patients with severe aphasic impairments or may be used to augment verbal expression attempts. For others, this modality may serve as a starting point in treatment with gradual transition to oral expression activities.

As noted in the previous section, the gestural modality tends to be less affected than others in aphasia (Porch, 1967), although individuals with more severe impairments use fewer complex gestural forms spontaneously in their communication attempts, with gestures becoming nonspecific and unclear (Glosser et al., 1986). As a group, patients with severe aphasia communicate more often and for longer periods of time through nonverbal means than their communication partners (Herrmann et al., 1988). Although pantomime production is reportedly infrequent, at least in untrained users, a greater use of codified gestures has been observed, suggesting perhaps that they require less creativity and praxis skills. Wang and Goodglass (1992) found a strong correlation between auditory comprehension skills and measures of pantomime recognition and expression. Pantomime performance was also strongly linked to the ability to produce meaningless gestures on imitation. Duffy et al. (1994) have proposed that both language and neurophysiological motor and visual processing disorders are tied to pantomime deficits.

Individuals with significant language limitations may be able to acquire some single signs and patients with less involvement may perhaps be capable of acquiring and generalizing simple grammars (Coelho, 1990). Ability to generalize signs has been inversely related to severity of aphasia (Coelho & Duffy, 1987). Aphasia severity may, in fact, be the most significant determinant of successful sign use (Coelho & Duffy, 1986).

Some positive effects on the reception and production of gestures through pantomime training have been described (Schlanger & Freemann, 1979). The Amer-Ind Sign System (Skelly, 1979) has been used with varying reports of success. Rao (1994) has suggested that possible prognostic indicators for success with Amer-Ind code include good pantomime recognition and that limb apraxia is not severe and predominantly ideomotor, rather than ideational in nature.

Finally, use of gestures can facilitate oral speech production for some patients, by serving as a cue for word retrieval or by adding greater descriptive value to verbal output. Individuals may not automatically use this strategy so that specific instruction and coaching may be required for it to be successfully incorporated into communication exchanges.

Social Signals

Area 1, attention, is an elementary step in gestural communication. The patient learns to obtain the attention of a communication partner through eye contact, touch, vocalization, gesture, or a combination of these.

With Area 2, acknowledgment of the message received, some form of gesture, such as a head nod, is developed to indicate that a message has been received, although not necessarily understood.

Gestures

Single gestures and combinations of gestures are used in Area 3, gestural communication. Some investigators have found propositional gestures to be more difficult to acquire than nonpropositional ones (Buck & Duffy, 1980). A possible hierarchy might consist of appropriate facial expressions, conventional gestures, and propositional gestures.

Successful outcomes have been described with Visual Action Therapy (VAT) in improving both apraxia and gestural communication abilities (Helm-Estabrooks et al., 1982). In this nonvocal, visual/gestural program, a hierarchy of activities is used, ranging from tasks such as requiring the patient to match objects and pictures to gesturing the use of items hidden from view. Modifications to VAT were based on the finding that patients experience less difficulty using gestures representing objects involving proximal movements than those involving distal movements (Helm-Estabrooks et al., 1989b). With patients demonstrating severe language problems, VAT may serve as the initial phase in treatment, advancing to implementation of Amer-Ind Code training.

Communicative importance or personal relevancy is one factor that may affect the ease of sign acquisition (Coelho & Duffy, 1986). There is also a tendency for patients to experience less difficulty in learning signs that have a high degree of iconicity, that is, those whose meanings are evident, based on their physical or structural characteristics (Coelho & Duffy, 1986). Other important variables to consider are the stimuli selected to teach the gestures. Objects and action pictures have been found to evoke superior gestural performance to line drawings (Netsu & Marguardt, 1984).

A treatment hierarchy has been described by Rao (1994) for training patients with aphasia in the use of Amer-Ind Code. It consists of a continuum of tasks: demonstration, recognition, imitation, replication, consolidation, retrieval, and initiation. Additional strategies to ensure generalization include involving significant others in the program and encouraging some risk taking on the part of the patient.

Speech Acts

Area 5, simple speech acts, incorporates both message content (proposition) and intent of the speaker (elocutionary force). Elocutionary force is communicated with gestures and/or vocalization to signal a command, statement, or question. Simple pointing gestures may be used to communicate content, such as indicating the action, agent, or object. Area 5, speech acts, includes a combination of verbal and nonverbal communication. Gestures continue, however, to carry the burden of communication, although some verbalization may be produced.

Case Study

A.G. is a 62-year-old retired political consultant who suffered a stroke, with a large left middle cerebral artery infarct, resulting in global aphasia and a right hemiplegia. Initially, the Boston Assessment of Severe Aphasia was administered. Relative strengths were found in the areas of oral-gestural expression, gesture recognition, and visuospatial tasks. A variety of treatment strategies was used to develop oral expression skills, including VAT and Melodic Intonation Therapy (MIT), as well as LOT naming and sentence formulation activities. Functional oral communication skills, however, remained severely limited.

The Amer-Ind Sign System (Skelly, 1979) was next introduced. Because this treatment approach focuses on new learning as opposed to stimulation of previously learned material, a strict LOT paradigm could not apply. Ten common agents and actions were chosen for training. Initially, the clinician provided a gesture, along with an array of four action pictures from which the patient was to select the one associated with the gesture. Once recognition was established, A.G. was required to produce the gesture in response to an action picture. In the next treatment phase, situations were simulated in which A.G. provided the gesture in the absence of the action picture.

The subsequent difficulty level involved encouraging the use of trained gestures in conversational attempts. A.G. consistently progressed through his treatment program, successfully producing gestures that had not even been trained. Continuous encouragement and counseling were needed, however, as A.G. was reluctant to use gestural communication as a substitute for oral speech, even several months post-stroke.

Sample Activities

Level 1

Stimuli: Ten pictured actions, along with 20 foils.
Procedure: The clinician presents an array of four pictures to the patient and produces a gesture corresponding to one of the actions depicted. The patient points to the appropriate picture.

Level 2

Stimuli: The 10 action pictures used in Level 1 for identification.
Procedure: The pictures are presented one at a time and the patient is required to produce the associated gesture.

Level 3

Stimuli: The 10 action pictures used in Levels 1 and 2.
Procedure: A sentence or brief story is aurally presented and the patient is required to complete the sentence with the appropriate gesture (e.g., "When you are hungry, you --------.").

Oral Expression

General Considerations

Oral expression problems vary with respect to both nature and severity in aphasia. Although various oral expression patterns are observed in different types of aphasia, many patients share common areas of difficulty. Problems may be encountered with highly overlearned or automatic speech, with phonological articulatory skills, repetition, oral reading, naming, sentence formulation, and discourse planning/production. Because these areas are not mutually exclusive, limitations involving one area may directly affect another. Treatment may, therefore, simultaneously incorporate two or more areas. In developing a therapeutic plan, the areas of deficit, along with their nature and severity, are carefully examined.

Automatic Speech

Area 1 addresses development of automatic speech series. Activities are designed to facilitate oral speech in those with very limited verbal output. Stimuli such as greetings, number sequences, poems, days of the week, months of the year, and letters of the alphabet may be incorporated.

Voluntary Control of Involuntary Utterances (VCIU) is a treatment approach designed for patients with nonfluent aphasia that attempts to use their stereotypic expressions as a step to develop meaningful propositional speech (Helm & Barresi, 1980). VCIU incorporates a progression through oral reading, confrontation naming, and conversation involving production of the stereotypic words and phrases.

Phonological-Articulatory Production

Misarticulations that occur with aphasia may be the result of phonological problems, articulatory problems, or a combination of both. Phonological-articulatory impairment resulting from an anterior left-hemisphere lesion, in and surrounding Broca's area, is most often termed *verbal dyspraxia*. Posterior left-hemisphere lesions may also result in sound production errors, generally in the form of literal or phonemic paraphasias.

LOT activities in Area 2, phonological-articulatory production are based on Shewan's Content Network (1980) for treating verbal dyspraxia. Separate hierarchies for presentation method, stimulus characteristics, type of response, and facilitation of response variables have been constructed according to difficulty levels. These hierarchies are based on data provided by a variety of researchers. A step-by-step progression towards the goal of achieving spontaneous production of propositional speech is used, as the patient can accommodate. Support provided by the clinician is gradually reduced to ensure that the patient develops more independence in oral speech.

In selecting treatment stimuli, several variables may be critical. At the phoneme level, vowels are easier to produce than consonants, and high-frequency consonants are less difficult than those of low frequency. Distinctive feature characteristics also play a role in ease of production, with nasality and voicing features being less problematic than manner and place. In phoneme selection, the clinician can, therefore, establish a hierarchy incorporating all of these parameters.

When introducing single words, concrete, functional words tend to influence performance positively. Additional variables that may be important to control are word frequency and length. Beyond single words, phrase/sentence length, stress pattern, and linguistic complexity may be systematically varied to increase the difficulty levels in treatment.

Differing presentation methods can also be incorporated into a hierarchy. Combined auditory-visual presentation may facilitate correct speech production more easily than either auditory or visual presentation in isolation.

The clinician may alter the type of response required, such as production following a model, unison production, or production requiring a number of consecutive responses. Facilitating response variables can be manipulated to elicit more accurate productions. For example, associated movements such as finger tapping may accompany speech. Inserting a schwa (//) between consonants in a cluster may enhance performance. Facilitating responses may be used temporarily by some and be required as long-term strategies by others.

As the patient advances within the treatment hierarchy, additional response complexity can be required, while maintaining constant the presentation method, stimuli, and facilitating response variables. More spontaneous productions are incorporated, with the clinician gradually withdrawing assistance.

Repetition

Although the ability to repeat is not an end goal in treatment, this skill is described in Area 3 to facilitate performance of other related speech-language behaviors. For example, repetition tasks may be used in treating verbal dyspraxia and are an important component of Melodic Intonation Therapy (MIT). MIT consists of a hierarchy of three levels in which multisyllabic words and short, high-probability phrases are musically intoned, followed by longer, phonologically complex sentences (Sparks et al., cited in Helm-Estabrooks & Albert, 1991).

When preparing stimuli for repetition activities, many factors can influence performance. Single-word repetition is affected by phonological complexity, frequency of occurrence, semantic class, and if the stimulus is a foreign or pseudoword (Ramsberger, 1996). When abstractness and frequency are controlled, repetition of emotional words is superior to that of nonemotional vocabulary. High-probability (Goodglass &

Kaplan, 1972, 1983) and personally relevant material (Wallace & Canter, 1985) are easier to repeat, as are shorter items (Gardner & Winner, 1978). When sentence-level material is introduced, a hierarchy that varies sentence forms (Goodglass, 1968, 1976) can be used, as patients demonstrate repetition difficulty with increasing syntactic complexity.

Response variables can affect accuracy and/or ease of production. For some individuals, use of a delay prior to initiation of a response can facilitate performance, although for others this strategy may have a negative impact (Gardner & Winner, 1978). It is therefore important for the clinician to determine the direction of this effect prior to its implementation in the treatment program.

Oral Reading and Spelling

As in the previous area, oral reading, Area 4, is most often used as a vehicle for improving other aspects of speech-language skills. Improvements in language functioning, such as reading comprehension, oral expression, auditory comprehension, and written expression, have been described (Cherney et al., 1986; Tuomainen & Laine, 1991). Oral reading of sentences and paragraphs, in unison and independently, have resulted in improved language skills in those with both fluent and nonfluent aphasia. Presentation of scrambled written sentences for oral reading can be used with patients who may demonstrate impulsive responding and poor self-monitoring skills. They can be required to point to each word in the sentence while reading aloud, with sentences being systematically adjusted for length and syntactic complexity.

Some forms of dyslexia have been characterized by differences in oral reading performance. These were described in detail in the visual processing modality, within the area of reading comprehension. Area 5, oral spelling, may be used as an activity to enhance written spelling skills and be practiced as a strategy for word retrieval with some patients.

Word Retrieval

Word-finding problems are associated with all types of aphasia and may also occur in nonaphasic disorders. Benson (1979) has outlined five varieties of anomia associated with aphasia and four nonaphasic types. In developing activities in Area 6, the goal is to facilitate the actual word-retrieval process rather than to teach specific vocabulary items. The clinician first attempts to determine the nature of the word-retrieval problem or where in the process the breakdown appears to occur, establishes the vocabulary level and type with which the patient experiences errors, and determines whether patterns of performance vary across picture description, confrontation naming, and conversational activities.

Word retrieval and how it relates to phonological and semantic activation in connected speech are not well understood. In picture naming tasks, however, various theoretical models for lexical retrieval have been proposed and

integrated (Weinrich et al., 1997b; Goodglass, 1998). Goodglass (1998) attributes word-retrieval problems in aphasia to problems accessing the phonological lexicon, in which phonological strings are stored, because of either a loss or degradation of information at the level of the lemma, which contains semantic and thematic information, or in the output lexicon itself. He suggests that if there is competition at the conceptual stage, related lemmas may be activated, resulting in semantic substitutions. Additionally, words of a higher frequency, or having personal significance for the speaker (Freudian slip) or those associated with a recently used word may be activated. With the activation of two semantically related lemmas, production of another real or nonword reflecting their combined phonological composition may ensue. Semantically and phonologically related errors may be the result of spreading activation in which several semantic options are activated that have a number of competing phonological forms. Reinforcement or inhibition is received depending on the semantic match. Having an appreciation of a model of lexical processing and developing hypotheses regarding the cause of word-retrieval symptoms in a patient can lead to the design of individualized treatment procedures. Responses can be more effectively analyzed, not only enabling the clinician to successively respond on-line but, with explanation, can lead to the patient's developing a greater understanding of how and when errors may occur.

Constructing a hierarchy of stimuli is an important prerequisite in developing word-finding skills. A number of characteristics impacting retrieval have been cited in the literature. Differences in the ability to recall living (animals, food, flowers, body parts) as opposed to nonliving object labels have been described (De Renzi & Lucchelli, 1994). One explanation is that members of living categories are discriminated among each other based on visual features, rendering them more difficult to name, whereas identification of tools is based on functional characteristics. Others have found that when confounding effects are controlled, animacy and operativity do not play significant roles in word retrieval (Howard et al., 1995). There does, however, appear to be a trend for objects experienced through multiple senses to be better named. Many patients also demonstrate greater success in naming objects that are not embedded in a physical context or are separate from their environment.

Semantic and grammatical categories may be differentially affected, depending on the type of aphasia (Goodglass et al., 1966; Berndt et al., 1997). Noun impairments have been specifically associated with severe anomia, although verb retrieval deficits can occur with both Broca's and Wernicke's aphasia. Within the grammatical category of verbs, other factors may be implicated. "Light" verbs (e.g., have, do, come), although frequently used, may generate a number of meanings when activated, which, in turn, render them more difficult to retrieve than "heavy" or more complex verbs (e.g., run, hit, stop) (Breedin et al., 1998).

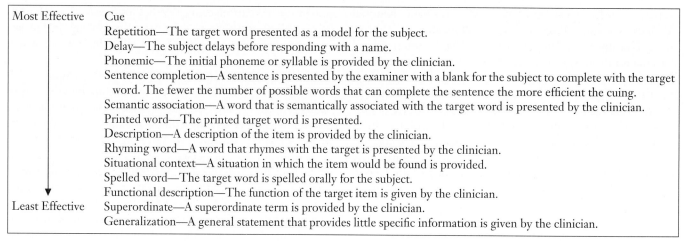

Most Effective	Cue
↓	Repetition—The target word presented as a model for the subject.
	Delay—The subject delays before responding with a name.
	Phonemic—The initial phoneme or syllable is provided by the clinician.
	Sentence completion—A sentence is presented by the examiner with a blank for the subject to complete with the target word. The fewer the number of possible words that can complete the sentence the more efficient the cuing.
	Semantic association—A word that is semantically associated with the target word is presented by the clinician.
	Printed word—The printed target word is presented.
	Description—A description of the item is provided by the clinician.
	Rhyming word—A word that rhymes with the target is presented by the clinician.
	Situational context—A situation in which the item would be found is provided.
	Spelled word—The target word is spelled orally for the subject.
	Functional description—The function of the target item is given by the clinician.
Least Effective	Superordinate—A superordinate term is provided by the clinician.
	Generalization—A general statement that provides little specific information is given by the clinician.

Figure 27–3. Hierarchy of cues according to effectiveness level.

Some additional stimulus variables to consider are word length, frequency, and concreteness. An item may be easier to name if its label is of low uncertainty. Uncertainty indicates the consistency with which an item is called a particular name. Some individuals may be sensitive to prototypicality, or the degree to which an item is characteristic of its class.

Once stimuli have been selected, effective cuing strategies are determined for each patient. Overall, phonemic cues prove to be the most facilitative for the various aphasia types (Li & Williams, 1989). It has been suggested that anomia for common nouns in conduction and Broca's aphasia can occur late in lexical retrieval once semantic activation has occurred and some indication of word form has been established or, in some instances, may reflect unsuccessful lemma retrieval (Beeson et al., 1997). Reporting on the frequently observed tip-of-the-tongue phenomenon, the authors found that these two groups were more successful than chance in identifying the initial letters of target words (names of famous faces). Alternatively, more limited evidence exists to suggest that word form knowledge is intact for patients with Wernicke's and anomic aphasia. Patients with anomia seem to demonstrate a preference for semantic cues as well (Li & Williams, 1990) when verbs are presented. Some findings (Stimley & Noll, 1991) indicate that presentation of semantic cues increases the number of semantic paraphasias, with a decrease in unrelated word errors. Phonemic cue presentation, on the other hand, may increase the number of phonemic paraphasias. Another factor to consider in cue presentation is the use of simultaneous cues (e.g., initial syllable combined with sentence completion format). Particularly with those who demonstrate more severe impairments, combined presentation may be most effective (Huntley et al., 1986). The hierarchy shown in Figure 27–3 is an attempt to integrate the findings of various researchers.

A number of activities and contexts may be employed to assist the patient in developing an understanding of the effectiveness and use of cues. Less difficulty may be encountered in naming pictured stimuli than in providing responses to definition or sentence completion tasks (Berndt et al., 1997), particularly in the presence of auditory comprehension problems. Patients with anomia, on the other hand, may benefit from the presentation of a sentence frame containing a word semantically related to the target (McCall et al., 1997). Both the syntactic context and/or syntactic constraints imposed, supplemented by semantic information, appear to be facilitative.

Differing findings regarding use of real objects, colored photos, or line drawings have been cited, so the clinician may need to alter this presentation variable on an individual basis (Benton et al., 1972; Bisiach, 1966).

As patients advance along a hierarchy, using increasingly difficult levels of vocabulary and cue presentation, responsibility for cuing is shifted from the clinician to the patient. Ultimately, tasks should be implemented that allow practice to occur in meaningful, naturalistic situations. For example, application of PACE (Promoting Aphasics' Communicative Effectiveness) (Davis & Wilcox, 1981), which encourages patients to use multiple channels to communicate, has met with some success in developing effective cuing strategies (Li et al., 1988).

Sentence Formulation

Area 7 focuses on the generation of meaningful units at phrase and sentence levels. A hierarchy of sentence types may be established, such as that found in the Helm Elicited Language Program for Syntax Stimulation (HELPSS) (Helm-Estabrooks, 1981). This approach was developed for use with patients with nonfluent aphasia to improve their use of syntax by training 11 sentence types with a story completion format. Sentence types range from the imperative intransitive to use of the future verb tense.

A hierarchy of sentence types for training might also be created based on order of reappearance in language samples (Ludlow, 1973) elicited from those with aphasia. Difficulty levels can be developed by varying the uses of morphological markers (Goodglass & Berko, 1960) and by varying phrase/sentence length. The stress pattern of a sentence may influence performance of some individuals. Patients with Broca's aphasia, for example, tend to initiate utterances with stressed words. Use of stress in these cases would be an important variable to include in the treatment hierarchy.

Another approach used with treating agrammatism has been mapping therapy (Byng et al., 1994; Marshall, 1995; Schwartz et al., 1994; Thompson & Shapiro, 1995). The mapping deficit hypothesis suggests that some patients are unable to relate sentence form to meaning (Marshall, 1995). The problem can arise from a lexical deficit in which the verb fails to provide information about its thematic structure (goal, agent) or a procedural deficit in which the rules assigning thematic roles to moved argument structures are lost. These limitations occur in both comprehension and production, although patients are generally able to carry out grammaticality judgments, perhaps related to residual syntactic skills. No one particular application of mapping therapy has proven to have qualitatively or quantitatively similar outcomes for all patients, requiring highly individualized implementation. Typically, treatment involves both comprehension and production tasks to encourage explicit analysis of verb-noun relational structures in canonical (example: subject-verb-object) and noncanonical sentence types (Schwartz et al., 1994). Colored lines may be drawn on cards to represent syntactic class (noun phrase and verb), with the patient required to select the appropriate color-coded written phrases to match the cards and corresponding pictured representation (Byng et al., 1994). Eventually, the patient is required to produce the sentence, with prompts from the clinician to enable the development and utilization of self-monitoring and problem-solving skills. Byng et al. described increased verb retrieval with their patients using this method. Other improvements were noted but varied with individuals, perhaps reflecting differing patterns of deficits and/or a need for more customized approaches. Although no specific training in production was provided to their group with chronic, nonfluent aphasia, Schwartz et al. (1994) found that the majority of patients improved on one or more of their production measures following a course of mapping therapy.

Thompson and Shapiro (1995) have treated sentence production deficits in agrammatism by strictly controlling the lexical and syntactic properties of the stimuli and by focusing explicitly on the processes underlying sentence production. Among some of the most notable findings, at the completion of treatment was the presence of more complex sentences in discourse, along with an increase in the number of verbs produced.

Contextual variables such as use of pictured stimuli or conversation may affect the nature of the responses. Some patients produce a greater number of major utterances (subject-predicate) in response to pictures than in conversation (Easterbrook et al., 1982); others may produce more words, depending on the gender bias of the picture (Correia et al., 1990).

The use of C-VIC, a computerized visual communication system, has been widely investigated particularly with respect to its use with patients exhibiting nonfluent aphasia. In this system (Weinrich et al., 1995), patients were introduced to a lexicon consisting of animate nouns, common nouns, verbs, prepositions, and modifiers. Icons with printed words were available to be inserted into slots provided for the patient and clinician/interactant to form simple syntactic constructions. Employing comprehension and formulation tasks, while encouraging subsequent verbalization, subject-verb-object constructions improved both when using C-VIC and in spontaneous speech. Improvements were also noted in the use of locative prepositional phrases (in, on, by). Some patients have demonstrated a positive response through C-VIC training targeting tense inflection (Weinrich et al., 1997a). Gains in retrieving verbs were also a by-product of this approach. Attempts to facilitate the generalization of single-sentence production in C-VIC to narrative production have not been successfully reported to date (Weinrich et al., 1997b).

C-VIC training might be employed as a branch step in LOT to facilitate oral sentence forms with those who are unable to make gains in these abilities using the methods earlier described. For some with severe aphasic limitations, C-VIC might serve as a more permanent avenue of communication. Naeser et al. (1998) studied a group of patients with severe aphasia to isolate factors that might play a role in determining successful candidacy for C-VIC. These authors concluded that the best outcome (ability to initiate communication with C-VIC) was associated with a lesion sparing large portions of either the posterior systems or anterior systems involved in language recovery. Inability to use C-VIC was associated with bilateral lesions. Overall test scores on the Boston Assessment of Severe Aphasia were also good indicators of response to C-VIC, when considered with lesion data.

Conversation and Discourse

Current practice delineates four categories of discourse: conversational, expository, procedural, and narrative. Although conversation is formally addressed in Area 8, many of the parameters affecting performance also apply to other forms of discourse (Area 9) and will be outlined in that section. Unique to conversation, however, are the roles of turn-taking and repair (Ferguson, 1998). Turn-taking was found to be unimpaired in a sample of speakers with fluent aphasia when conversing with both familiar and unfamiliar communication partners. Perkins (1995) suggests that conversational partners respond based on the amount of shared knowledge, degree of linguistic impairment, and individual discourse styles. For example, the presence of significant oral expression difficulties in the context of shared knowledge of a particular topic may result in the glossing over of problematic aspects in conversation rather than working to modify them through collaborative repair. Variability of tolerance for pauses can also be found among communication partners, which can impact turn-taking and repair.

Involvement of significant others in treating conversation has been reported with success by authors incorporating different approaches. Conversational coaching (Holland, 1991) uses prepared scripts, requiring the patient with initial support from the clinician to communicate the story to a significant other. The clinician assists the communication partner in identifying opportunities for and practicing implementation of effective strategies to facilitate the exchange. Using a modified approach in a case report, Boles (1998) selected three aspects of a spouse's conversational style for intervention. With the spouse reducing her rate of speech, percentage of taking turns, and topic shifts, the patient participated more effectively and to a greater extent in conversation.

Drawing on the work of the previously mentioned authors, one might develop a hierarchy of activities in enhancing conversational exchanges between patients and significant others. Communication partners might benefit from specific instruction in dealing appropriately with pauses in conversation, altering their rate of speech, effectively introducing new topics, and modifying their turn-taking. Various forms of conversation could also be introduced, in which the amount of shared knowledge or new information is controlled. Although pragmatic deficits in conversation have been less frequently documented in those with aphasia, some may require instruction and practice in turn-taking, topic maintenance, seeking clarification, and initiating repairs. Treatment in the area of conversation may also focus on the generalization of specific linguistic skills such as word retrieval, gestural production, or writing to everyday communication situations.

A model for evaluating discourse can be useful for both assessment and planning intervention in Area 9. Chapman and Ulatowska (1992) described discourse as involving an interaction between cognition and language and detailed the components of discourse production. Superstructure refers to elements such as setting (characters, time, place), complicating action (sequence of events), and resolution. The global meaning or semantic content is termed *macrostructure*. It is closely tied to cognition and to a lesser degree, linguistic performance. Tasks that have been suggested to address this aspect of discourse are summarizing the story, selecting the main idea/gist, identifying the main hero, formulating a title, and deriving a lesson/moral. As the complexity and degree of abstraction are increased with these activities, the stage is also set for incorporating more linguistically complex sentence forms.

The ability of the speaker to maintain coherence or a unified theme depends not only on the macro- but also on the microstructure components of discourse (Hough & Pierce, 1994). Microstructure coherence deals with the conceptual links that are established between sentences or propositions. Appropriate use of pronouns (with corresponding referents), articles, and ellipsis (a sentence construction that is incomplete but the intent is understood) signal that the speaker is aware of when information is novel or has in some way already been communicated to the listener. Coherence is also aided by inclusion of cohesive ties between sentences, such as in co-reference and anaphora.

When developing a hierarchy for discourse production, many variables can be altered depending on the particular profile of the patient. One might initiate treatment with tasks that require identification of the components of the superstructure, in relation to a particular topic. Practice in identifying the main concepts can be followed by development of accuracy and completeness of information. Nicholas and Brookshire (1995a) determined that the presence, completeness, and accuracy of main concepts in connected speech were related to severity of aphasia. Patients with less severe aphasia were generally found to have fewer absent main concepts and more accurate/complete main concepts than those with more severe aphasia when a variety of speech samples were studied. When analyzing speech samples for number of words spoken per minute and percent of words that are correct information units (CIUs), Brookshire and Nicholas (1994) concluded that it is important to elicit samples from different forms of discourse and that a total sample of 300 to 400 words leads to more reliable interpretation.

The difficulty level can further be increased with requiring the sequencing of information and establishment of coherence at the macro- and microstructure levels. Specific instruction in the use of pronouns and other devices for maintaining cohesion may be needed. When constructing tasks to improve grammatical form or word-retrieval skills in discourse, the context might be altered to promote greater opportunities for practice. Patients have been shown to demonstrate varying degrees of grammatical complexity in relation to the type of discourse involved. Expository discourse (related to a particular topic, as in picture description), procedural discourse (consisting of steps, conceptually or chronologically associated), and narrative discourse (information about an event; story retelling) have been compared (Li et al., 1996). The most complex grammar was elicited through picture description, followed by the procedural discourse task and then the story retelling condition. In contrast, however, a significantly higher percentage of content words was found with story retelling as compared to expository and procedural discourse, suggesting that the patients were conveying the informational load through lexical rather than grammatical avenues.

Topic familiarity in some instances may play a role with grammatical complexity in discourse production. When provided with less familiar topics, grammatical complexity can increase for procedural discourse but appears to have no similar effect for story retelling (Williams et al., 1994). In this study, the number of content words increased with both procedural discourse and story retelling conditions involving familiar topics. Listener familiarity evidenced no impact on discourse production.

Picture description and procedural discourse tasks involving less familiar topics might be chosen when the emphasis on discourse production is to improve grammatical form. On the other hand, story retelling and procedural discourse tasks incorporating familiar topics could be presented when one is attempting to elicit a greater number of content words.

Because the interplay between cognition and language is particularly evident in discourse, some of the mental operations (Chapey, 1994) associated with language processing and production are considered in this section. Convergent thinking or the development of logical conclusions based on information provided is involved in such tasks as explaining similarities and differences between concepts, retelling stories, describing procedures, making inferences, and organizing ideas in a logical order for expression. Divergent thinking demands the production of alternatives from given information, with an emphasis on quantity, elaboration, and originality. In discourse, this skill might be reflected by producing alternate perspectives, presenting a variety of ideas, predicting different outcomes or solutions, and changing the direction of one's responses. A hierarchy of tasks could be constructed addressing all of these parameters, in addition to varying the degree of abstractness and familiarity of the stimuli.

Chapey also highlights the role of evaluative thinking or judgment. Some aspects included in discourse are selecting the best word to fit the situation, determining an appropriate metaphor, idiom, or proverb, and judging what can and cannot be said in various contexts with different communication partners.

The processing and production of figurative language are integral to discourse. In addressing these aspects of communication, however, several factors must be considered. The ability to provide correct idiom interpretation has been correlated with years of formal education and auditory comprehension skills (Tompkins et al., 1992). Accurate explanation of proverbs also tends to be related to educational level and age (Nippold et al., 1997), with highly educated non–brain-damaged subjects performing better than their peers in all age groups. Performance has been shown to peek at 20 years and declines significantly after 70 years of age. Those with higher verbal ability demonstrate less of a decline with age than those with lower verbal ability. In examining proverb interpretation and explanation abilities in patients with fluent aphasia and relatively high auditory comprehension skills, comprehension of proverbs proves relatively intact (Chapman et al.,

1997). This performance is in contrast to the subjects' significantly impaired performance in providing explanations for both familiar and unfamiliar proverbs. Interpretation and explanation of idioms and proverbs can be used as a higher-level cognitive-linguistic task, with patients experiencing problems with conveying information of a more abstract nature. In selecting stimuli, however, age, educational background, and familiarity with the stimuli must be considered.

Finally, strategies may be introduced to facilitate self-evaluation such as monitoring for inclusion of and appropriate sequencing of relevant details and checking for redundancy and tangential or off-topic remarks. The use of written stimuli can be particularly beneficial in this area, either by having the patient write his or her narrative, when possible, or having the clinician transcribe it for review and editing.

Case Study

L.P. is a 44-year-old engineer who underwent a craniotomy with resection of a left frontal glioma. The Western Aphasia Battery, the Auditory Comprehension Test for Sentences, and the Boston Naming Test were administered. A nonfluent aphasia was exhibited, with oral speech limited to sentence fragments and frequent word-retrieval problems. Auditory and reading comprehension were both mildly impaired. Written output paralleled spoken speech.

Along with activities targeting other areas, word retrieval was chosen for treatment. Probing revealed that L.P. was 80% successful in naming pictured objects characterized by monosyllabic word forms, using Grade 1 and Grade 2 vocabulary levels. Polysyllabic nouns were named spontaneously, with 50% accuracy at these grade levels. No successful responses were elicited when pictured actions were presented.

Subsequent testing determined that the most effective cues for L.P. were presentation of the initial phoneme, description of physical and/or functional properties, and provision of the situational context (that is, the situation in which the item may be found). Because the clinician believed that phonemic cuing would be a difficult process to transfer from the clinician to the patient, use of description and situational contexts was emphasized.

In the first stage of the treatment hierarchy, specific training in the area of providing physical and functional descriptions and identifying situational contexts for pictured polysyllabic objects at a Grade 1 to a Grade 3 level was provided. Written prompts were used on individual cards to remind the patient of the various physical and functional attributes. For example, the phrases, "What color?" "What size?" "What shape?" and "What material?" were printed on one card, and on another, the question "What is it used for?" was printed. Once L.P. achieved a 70% success rate in providing the required information, another series of stimuli at the same difficulty level was presented. In this activity, the patient, by providing descriptions and situational contexts, was required to help the clinician identify pictured objects hidden from her view.

When the provision of the cues became more automatic for L.P., confrontation naming tasks were used, in which he provided needed cues only when naming was not spontaneous. To limit the patient's reliance on the clinician, the pictured items were again seen only by L.P. Difficulty levels were also systematically increased by introducing advanced vocabulary grade levels and other grammatical form classes (e.g., verbs, adjectives). Practice with implementing self-cuing strategies was also provided in various conversational activities. When treatment was discontinued, L.P. was a highly functional communicator, encountering word-finding problems primarily beyond a Grade 6 vocabulary level. His self-cuing strategies usually proved successful in assisting him to retrieve the intended word.

Sample Activities

Level 1

Stimuli: Grades 1 to 3 polysyllabic pictured objects; printed cue cards: "What color?" "What size?" "What shape?" "What material?" and "What is it used for?"

Procedure: The patient is required to provide oral responses to information requested on the cue cards.

Level 2

Stimuli: Grades 1 to 3 polysyllabic pictured objects; printed cue cards: "What color?" "What size?" "What shape?" "What material?" and "What is it used for?"

Procedure: The pictures are hidden from the clinician's view. The patient provides information prompted by the cue cards to enable the clinician to guess the identity of the pictures.

Level 3

Stimuli: Grades 1 to 3 polysyllabic pictured objects; printed cue cards: "What color?" "What size?" "What shape?" "What material?" and "What is it used for?"

Procedure: The pictures are hidden from the clinician's view. The patient first attempts to name the object spontaneously. If unsuccessful, he or she provides the information prompted by the cue cards to facilitate self-retrieval or identification by the clinician.

Graphic Expression

General Considerations

Graphic expression refers to the written output of communication through the use of graphemes (letters) or drawing. Writing is frequently the most severely affected modality in aphasia. Varying patterns of writing problems or agraphia have been described in the literature, along with a number of classification systems (Benson, 1979; Ellis, 1982; Margolin, 1984; Goodglass, 1993).

Some patients may experience writing abnormalities because of motor problems related to hand paresis/paralysis. Their writing is characterized by poorly formed letters, sometimes severe enough to make writing illegible. Often, written output is more successful with block printing. With apractic agraphia, difficulty in selecting the appropriate grapheme motor pattern is observed, although improved performance is found with copying. Other elements include intact oral spelling, normal sensory/motor function in the hand used for writing, and the ability to spell with anagrams. An accompanying limb apraxia is often found in the early stage (Alexander et al., 1992a). Spatial agraphia typically associated with a nondominant hemisphere lesion is characterized by problems with written orientation on the page and difficulties with positioning of letters in relation to each other and production of repetitive strokes in forming letters.

In addition to graphomotor deficits, written problems can be classified as aphasic agraphia because of their relationship to particular aphasic syndromes (Goodglass, 1993). Many of their characteristics mirror those found in oral speech production, such as failure to include written verb inflections observed in those with Broca's aphasia.

Selective forms of agraphia include agraphia with alexia, in which patients are unable to retrieve the graphic form of letter strings and sometimes even individual letters. Pure agraphia occurs in relative isolation of other language impairments. Varying symptomatology and localization have been noted. Signs may include inability to write words as compared to individual letters and intact oral spelling. Phonological agraphia has been described as a disorder in which phoneme-to-grapheme conversion is disrupted, with patients experiencing difficulty writing unfamiliar words and pseudowords (Alexander et al., 1992b; Margolin, 1984; Shallice, 1981). Problems manifested in phonological agraphia can overlap with those in deep agraphia. Patients are presumed to be unable to use phoneme-to-grapheme correspondence rules and whole-word phonology (Goodglass, 1993). As a result, semantic substitutions are produced and in some instances derivational errors have been reported. As with deep dyslexia, concrete nouns are generally more successfully written than abstract nouns and verbs.

The premorbid skills and interests of the patient will again dictate the degree to which the graphic expression modality will be incorporated into or perhaps be the sole focus of treatment. In some instances, writing can be facilitative for oral naming or can be targeted simultaneously when sentence or discourse formulation skills are being developed.

The final portion of this section will briefly address the use of drawing in aphasia. This channel for expression might be considered a compensatory form of communication, with varying degrees of success reported in its implementation.

Graphomotor Access

Areas 1 and 2 focus on establishing graphic and graphemic motor patterns, with Area 3 stressing the recall of highly overlearned grapheme motor patterns. In Area 1, tracing and/or copying nonverbal material, two- and three-dimensional representations of nonverbal material are used. Task difficulty may be increased by altering the complexity of the designs in producing geometric forms and objects. Letters, numbers, and words are introduced in Area 2, tracing and/or copying verbal material. Activities are designed to address such problems as incorrect letter elements, inappropriate spatial positioning, rotation of letters/elements, and repetition of elements/letters. Some patients have demonstrated better ability to print in upper case letters than to write in cursive script (Goodglass, 1993; Hanley & Peters, 1996) so this variable might also be included in designing tasks or considering response variables. Single items may be practiced followed by those in a series, for example, letters and numbers. In Area 3, writing familiar material, highly overlearned stimuli are incorporated, such as the patient's name, address, and telephone number.

Word Orthography

Areas 4 and 5, written spelling and naming, may include activities such as writing to dictation, oral spelling, and written naming. A hierarchy can be established by selection of vocabulary across several dimensions. Word frequency, imageability, concreteness, emotionality, and grammatical class may influence the accuracy of the patient's performance. When a part-of-speech effect is observed, spelling of nouns is more readily available than verbs, followed by adjectives, and grammatical functors (Goodglass, 1993).

Length is an important variable to alter as shorter words occasion fewer errors than longer ones (Friederici et al., 1981). Stimuli containing the most regular expression of phoneme-to-grapheme correspondence rules are easier than those in which letter combinations are a less frequent realization of sounds (e.g., /f/ in telephone) (Friederici et al., 1981). Although order of difficulty varies among patients and the types of aphasia, use of double vowels, double consonants, and regular versus irregular spelling may be incorporated into a treatment hierarchy. Words containing suffixes may prove more difficult for patients (Langmore & Canter, 1983), as well as may the production of homonyms and homophones. It is proposed that written word production

is accomplished through the orthographic output lexicon (Kay et al., 1996). Information is sent from the semantic and/or phonological output system depending on the task at hand. In addition, there is a mechanism for phoneme-to-grapheme conversion to account for one's ability to transcribe dictated nonwords. Once the graphemic representation has been accessed, it is held temporarily in the orthographic output buffer until the graphemes are converted into allographs, or letter shapes.

Success in improving written performance has been described using two different approaches (Carlomagno et al., 1991). In one method, semantic and visual cues were used to stimulate writing through the lexical route, and in the other, nonword writing from dictation, along with presentation of phonological cues, was employed to enhance the nonlexical phoneme-to-grapheme correspondence. Both methods may be beneficial depending on the underlying nature of the symptoms.

Treatment directed at addressing the various forms of writing disorders stemming from breakdowns within the various levels of the orthographic output model has been described (Hillis, 1992). With a patient demonstrating deficits within the semantic system, therapy was designed to teach semantic distinctions. Generalization of improved written naming to untrained items was found within the same semantic category. Another successful approach, with a different patient, involved implementation of a cuing hierarchy for written naming incorporating scrambled anagrams and initial letter cues.

Problems arising from the graphemic output lexicon in the context of intact phoneme-to-grapheme conversion (PGC) skills may result in errors that are phonologically plausible (Hillis, 1992). In this instance, treatment targeting production of homophones could be beneficial. If disruption to the PGC mechanism is invoked with an intact orthographic output lexicon spelling of nonwords is troublesome. Hillis reported on successful outcomes with tasks designed to develop the PGC system, using cuing hierarchies. In one example, self-cuing was established for a patient with verbal apraxia and in another, written monitoring of semantic errors was facilitated. Although the goals of addressing the impaired PGC system were different in these patients, systematic approaches to treating the disorder affected positive functional changes in other areas.

Text

Grammatical structures are first introduced in Area 6, written formulation, where material at the phrase, sentence, and paragraph levels may be used. Sentence complexity and length may be altered, along with topic familiarity. Many of the same variables found to influence oral expression can be incorporated into this area and developed simultaneously. At the paragraph level, a hierarchy can be established dealing with the structure of the text (Labov, cited in Freedman-Stern et al., 1984), such that task requirements might include mention of time, place, participants, complicating action, and result/resolution. Once the patient is successful in including these obligatory elements, optional ones, for example, coda/moral of the story, may be required. Instruction in the use of cohesive devices, such as anaphoric reference, relative clauses, and temporal ordering, can be systematically approached, perhaps initially through identifying their application in reading comprehension activities, followed by their incorporation in written output.

Writing complex material is included in Area 7. In addition to the variables stated above, a response hierarchy which addresses the purpose and complexity of the text can be established. A possible progression from easy to difficult is narrative, letter, and expository (Freedman-Stern et al., 1984). This aspect of treatment requires a highly individualistic application given the diversity of uses writing may have in patients' day-to-day activities.

Case Study

B.C. is a 64-year-old self-employed business consultant. A left-hemisphere stroke resulted in an infarct involving the white matter in the region of the superior temporal lobe and angular gyrus, with extension into the white matter in the left corona radiata. The Western Aphasia Battery, the Auditory Comprehension Test for Sentences, and the Boston Naming Test were administered. A fluent aphasia, characterized by moderately impaired auditory comprehension, with paraphasic speech production, anomia, mildly impaired reading comprehension, and agraphia were revealed.

At the time of initial testing, B.C. successfully wrote his name, but not his address. Only a portion of the alphabet and numbers to 20 were correctly written. Writing single words to dictation resulted in no correct responses. Letter substitutions and additions made words, for the most part, unidentifiable. Over the course of the next 2 weeks, however, spontaneous improvement was noted, such that short sentence formulation was possible, with word-finding problems identical to those in oral speech.

Spelling errors were found mainly at the ends of words, where letter substitutions were noted. Irregularly spelled words occasioned the most errors. Further probing revealed that written naming was 50% successful, using Grades 7 and 8 polysyllabic irregularly spelled words. Oral naming, followed by oral spelling, proved to be effective cues for B.C. to write the word correctly.

B.C. identified graphic expression to be an important focus in treatment. His daily work activities relied heavily on written skills, particularly related to correspondence.

As oral naming activities were being used in treatment, Area 5, written naming, was simultaneously developed. Once B.C. was able to write stimuli at the Grade 7 and 8 levels successfully, including polysyllabic, regularly spelled nouns, the difficulty level was increased by using nouns with irregular spelling, followed by other word classes, such as adjectives and verbs. Eventually, the vocabulary level was altered, along with grammatical form class, word length, and degree of imageability. Written naming activities were later incorporated into Area 7, writing complex material, in preparation for the patient's eventual return to work.

Sample Activities

Level 1

Stimuli: Grades 7 and 8 polysyllabic regularly spelled nouns.

Procedure: A written sentence is presented with the stimulus word omitted. The patient orally provides the word, spells it aloud, and finally writes it.

Level 2

Stimuli: Grades 7 and 8 polysyllabic, irregularly spelled nouns.

Procedure: A written sentence is presented with the stimulus word omitted. The patient orally provides the word, spells it aloud, and finally writes it.

Level 3

Stimuli: Grades 7 and 8 polysyllabic, regularly spelled verbs.

Procedure: A written sentence is presented with the stimulus word omitted. The patient orally provides the word, spells it aloud, and finally writes it.

Compensatory Communication

"Back to the Drawing Board" is an approach that was designed as a tool for communication by patients severely limited in their oral expression abilities (Morgan & Helm-Estabrooks, cited in Helm-Estabrooks & Albert, 1991). Uncaptioned cartoons are presented for copying from memory until the patient is able to produce triple-panel sequences. The clinician provides coaching to elicit drawings that are recognizable with productions including main ideas and essential details. In the later phase of treatment, practice in conveying information to significant others is incorporated.

Lyon (1995) views drawing as an augmentative form of communication, not as a replacement for language, for those who have retained inner thought. A highly interactive approach within a meaningful context is essential. Hypothetical situations are posed, with the patient encouraged to

TABLE 27–1

Entry and Exit Criteria for Aphasic Subjects[a]

Criterion Variable	
	Entry Criteria
Age	18 to 85 yr
Education	Literacy by history
Etiology	Infarcts
	Stable intracerebral hemorrhages
	Excluded hemorrhages due to
	AV malformation
	Subarachnoid hemorrhage
	Aneurysm
	Single unilateral strokes
	TIAs (5 days or less) excluded
Medical status	Excluded unstable medical illnesses interfering with testing or survival
Sensory status	Passed hearing screening for age appropriateness
	Blind patients (defined clinically) excluded
	Tactile dysfunction not excluded
Time post-onset	2 to 4 weeks post-stroke
Language severity	Native speakers of English or competent bilinguals for whom treatment in English was appropriate
	Severe language barrier or accent excluded
	Exit Criteria
Language recovery	WAB LQ of 94.0 or above
Death	Subject died
Second stroke	Neurological deficit persisting longer than 5 days
Prolonged illness	Absence or illness longer than 3 weeks' duration
Geographical relocation	Subject moved
Voluntary withdrawal	Subject did not wish further treatment and/or tests
Termination of project	Data collection terminated at end of funding period

[a] From Shewan, C.M., and Bandur, D.L. (1986). *Treatment of aphasia: A language-oriented approach* (p. 246). Austin, TX: Pro-Ed.

respond through drawing. The clinician aids in correcting or expanding portions that may be unidentifiable through questions and/or adding features to the drawings. As skills are developed, more complex topics are introduced, along with strategies to reflect different time periods. Involving significant others in communication exchanges through drawing and teaching them to interpret and probe for more information are viewed as key components in this treatment approach.

The development of drawing in LOT may provide an avenue of communication for those unable to access more conventional means. Some patients may encounter success in combining drawing with their limited written output to facilitate meaningful oral output. Because drawings of patients with aphasia may be initially simplistic (Lyon, 1995), implementing a treatment hierarchy to improve the complexity of both the drawings and their communicative intents could be advantageous.

EFFICACY STUDY

The LOT subjects for whom the efficacy data are reported here were part of a larger project designed to study the efficacy of three different types of aphasia treatment. LOT subjects were drawn from a population in London, Ontario, and the surrounding southwestern Ontario region in Canada. Table 27–1 shows the entry criteria met by all subjects. Only adult subjects were included, that is, individuals between the ages of 18 and 85 years. The upper cutoff of 85 years was used to eliminate subjects who were at high risk of not being available for a 1-year treatment period, the treatment duration provided in the study. Only literate subjects and those with a single, unilateral stroke, whose symptoms had lasted at least 5 days, were included in the sample.

Subjects who had a medical condition that interfered with testing or survival were eliminated, as were subjects with hearing impairment or blindness. Subjects were included if they were referred and tested within 2 to 4 weeks post-stroke. Native speakers of English and competent bilinguals for whom treatment in English was appropriate were included. Subjects who achieved an initial Western Aphasia Battery (WAB) aphasia quotient (AQ) score of less than 93.8, the cutoff score defining normal performance, were included in the study.

Random assignment to treatment type resulted in 28 subjects being assigned to LOT. To avoid an imbalance for severity or type of aphasia, assignment was stratified for these variables. Because patients with hemorrhagic strokes appeared to behave differently from those with an etiology of ischemic stroke, the subject with a hemorrhagic stroke was excluded from data analysis.

Demographic Data of LOT Subjects

Age of the subjects with aphasia ranged from 28 to 82 years, with a mean age of 62.3 years (Table 27–2). Education ranged from 4 to 21 years of formal education, with a mean of 9.85 years. (In Ontario, 9 years represents completion of the first year of high school.) Socioeconomic status was measured using the Blishen Scale (Blishen & McRoberts, 1976), which rates 500 occupations based on income and education. The

TABLE 27–2

Demographic Data for 27 LOT Subjects[a]

Age (Years)	
Mean	62.33
Median	63.0
Range	28–82
Education (Years)	
Mean	9.85
Median	9.0
Range	4–21
Socioeconomic Status	
Mean	38.92
Sex	
Male	17
Female	10
Handedness	
Right	25
Left	1
Ambidextrous	1
Language	
English	22
Polyglot	5
Etiology	
Infarction	27

[a]From Shewan, C.M., and Bandur, D.L. (1986). *Treatment of aphasia: A language-oriented approach* (p. 249). Austin, TX: Pro-Ed.

mean rating of 38.92 was similar to the mean for a group of 60 older normal subjects gathered in the area (Shewan & Henderson, 1988). This suggested that the socioeconomic status of the LOT group was similar to that of the general older population. The LOT group was composed of 17 male subjects and 10 female subjects. This ratio of 1.7:1.0 was similar to ratios in other literature reports (Abu-Zeid et al., 1975; Kurtzke, 1976). Most subjects were right-handed, with one left-handed and one ambidextrous person in the group. All subjects received treatment in English. For 22 subjects, English was their only language; 5 subjects spoke two or more languages, one of which was English.

Methods and Procedures

All LOT subjects met entry criteria (Table 27–1) and were tested at periodic intervals by trained, reliable test administrators who were independent of the clinicians providing treatment in the study. Tests occurred 2 to 4 weeks post-stroke (Entry Test) and at 3 months, 6 months, and 12 months after the first test. A follow-up test at 6 months after termination of treatment was also completed for as many subjects as possible.

The test battery included the Western Aphasia Battery (Kertesz & Poole, 1974), the Auditory Comprehension Test for Sentences (ACTS) (Shewan, 1979), Raven's Coloured Progressive Matrices (RCPM) (Raven, 1956), and a neurological examination, with site and side of lesion confirmed by computerized tomographic (CT) scan or isotope brain scan. Twenty-six subjects had left-sided lesions, and 1 had a right-sided lesion. Seventeen subjects showed some hemiplegia, 8 were hemianoptic, and 11 demonstrated some hemisensory loss.

Speech and language treatment was initiated as soon after administration of the Entry Test as possible and always within 7 weeks post-onset of aphasia. Treatment was controlled for both duration and intensity. Subjects received treatment for 1 year unless they exited from the study prior to that time (for exit criteria, see Table 27–1). Intensity of treatment was controlled by providing three 1-hour sessions weekly. LOT subjects received a mean of 55.3 sessions, with a range of 1 to 118 sessions. Only subjects who received at least 3 months of treatment were included in the efficacy evaluation. Six subjects were lost to follow-up: One died, two relocated geographically, and three withdrew voluntarily.

Treatment was provided by trained speech-language pathologists. Each clinician was trained by C.M. Shewan, the developer of LOT. Prior to providing LOT in the study, each clinician demonstrated the competence to plan LOT. Competence was assessed by having each clinician design a 1-month LOT patient treatment plan, which passed evaluation by CMS and an independent, external evaluator. At 6-month intervals, each clinician was evaluated by a second independent, external evaluator to ensure that LOT was the treatment type being provided.

Efficacy Data

The efficacy of LOT was demonstrated by comparing the LOT subjects with a no-treatment control (NTC) group. The NTC group contained 22 subjects with aphasia who did not wish to or could not attend treatment. The NTC group was comparable with the LOT group for age, education, socioeconomic status, handedness, language, and etiology. Unlike the LOT group, however, the NTC group contained an equal number of men (n = 11) and women (n = 11).

Whether LOT resulted in significantly greater language gains than no treatment was examined using analysis of covariance, controlling for initial severity of language impairment. The dependent variable in the comparison was the final test Language Quotient (LQ) score (LQLAST) on the WAB for each subject. The LQ score is a composite of the WAB oral and written language tests (Shewan, 1986). Initial severity was controlled through covarying for initial WAB LQ score (LQENTRY), because the LQ score was designed to be a measure of severity of language impairment, which, in turn, is known to affect language outcome. LOT had significant positive effects compared with no treatment ($P < .02$) (Table 27–3) when the Entry Test and the Last Test were compared. The estimate of the difference between LOT and NTC group means, after adjusting for entry score and educational level, was 11.50, with a standard error of 4.71. When age and sex, variables that could possibly influence outcome results, were added as concomitant variables in the analysis of covariance, the results remained essentially the same.

To control for the effects of spontaneous recovery, additional analyses of covariance were performed comparing

LQTEST 2 (3 months after the Entry Test) with LQLAST. Again, controlling for initial severity, the analysis of covariance indicated the gains for the LOT group were significantly greater than those for the NTC group ($P < .02$) (Table 27–3).

The number of subjects within each aphasia type was too small to permit statistical comparisons among groups. However, tracking the LQ scores over the course of treatment and through follow-up showed some interesting recovery curves. Because the number of subjects who contributed to the mean LQ score at each test could be different, as a result of subjects exiting from the group, the subjects were grouped according to the number of tests they received and were followed accordingly in streams (Figure 27–4). When the entire LOT group was considered, gains in the streams were greatest within the first 3 months of treatment, although substantial gains were noted at each test thereafter, and the gains were maintained for the most part for 6 months following treatment. The LQ mean at Test 5 (follow-up) was only 1.4 points lower than at Test 4 (treatment termination).

Type of Aphasia

For subjects with global aphasia, gains were greatest in the first 3 months, although gains were substantial in the second 3 months as well. After this time, LQ scores plateaued. For the three subjects with follow-up tests, the gains from treatment were maintained. As seen in Figure 27–4, although those with global aphasia did make notable gains, they both started and ended with lower LQ scores than did those with the other types of aphasia.

The subjects with Broca's aphasia made gains throughout the treatment period. As with other groups, the largest gains were in the first 3 months. At follow-up, scores were slightly lower than at the end of treatment (2.4 points).

The group of subjects with Wernicke's aphasia contained only four subjects, who made substantial gains in the first 3 months of treatment. Because scores for only one subject were available beyond that point, no generalizations can be made. This subject did make gains in all treatment periods and showed a slight decline during the 6-month follow-up period.

Subjects with anomic aphasia, as other groups, made their greatest gains in the first 3 months, although gains were also substantial during the next 3-month treatment period. The single subject remaining beyond that time made additional gains in the 6- to 12-month period, although no scores at follow-up were available. Overall, gains for the subjects with anomia were nearly 20 LQ points, and, in general, they were less severely impaired than the subjects with Broca's, Wernicke's, or global aphasia.

Individuals with conduction aphasia were among the less severely impaired subjects, as might be expected. In concert with other groups, they made the greatest gains in the first 3 months of treatment. The two subjects remaining at

TABLE 27–3

Summary of Analyses of Covariance for LQ Outcome Measure for LOT and NTC Groups[a]

	LQ	
ρ	Estimate of Adjusted Mean Difference	Standard Error
	Entry—Last Test	
≤.02	11.50	4.75
	Entry—Test 2	
≤.43	3.93	4.90
	Test 2—Last Test	
≤.02	5.86	2.19

[a] Adapted from Shewan, C.M., and Bandur, D.L. (1986). *Treatment of aphasia: A language-oriented approach* (p. 254). Austin, TX: Pro-Ed.

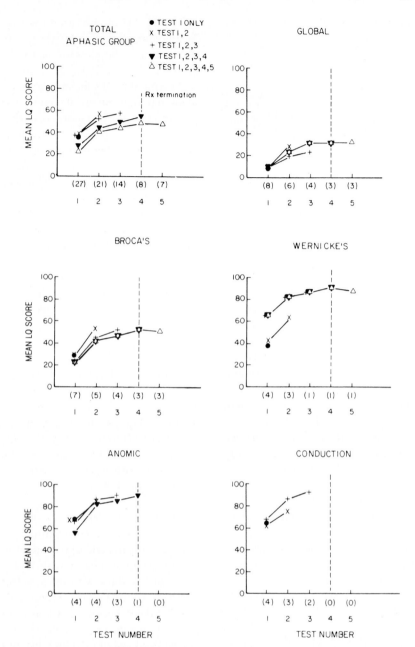

Figure 27–4. Mean LQ scores at Tests 1, 2, 3, 4, and 5 for the total LOT group and the five types of aphasia: global, Broca's, Wernicke's, anomic, and conduction. Patients have been grouped into streams according to the number of tests received. The numbers in parentheses refer to the number of patients included at each test. Termination of treatment (Rx termination) is represented with a dashed line. Test 5 is a follow-up test 6 months after treatment terminated.

Test 3 (6-month test) were approaching complete recovery (LQ > 94). No scores were available beyond this point.

Severity of Aphasia

The subjects with aphasia were separated into mild, moderate, and severe groups on the basis of the initial test battery, and subjects in these groups were followed in streams, similar to the analysis for type of aphasia (Figure 27–5). The group with mild aphasia made visible gains throughout the treatment period, averaging 24.8 LQ points. The greatest gains occurred in the first 3 months of treatment. The single subject with aphasia remaining for the follow-up test showed only a slight decline from the termination of treatment.

Subjects with moderate aphasia showed the greatest LQ gains in the first 3-month period (at least 20 LQ points on

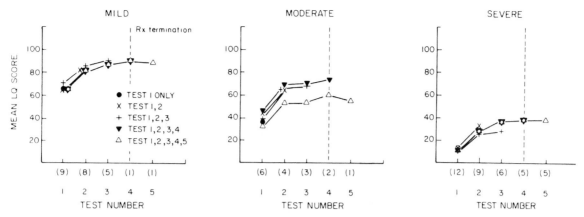

Figure 27–5. Mean LQ scores at Tests 1, 2, 3, 4, and 5 for the mild, moderate, and severe groups. Patients have been grouped into streams according to the number of tests received. The numbers in parentheses refer to the number of patients included at each test. Termination of treatment (Rx termination) is represented with a dashed line. Test 5 is a follow-up test 6 months after treatment terminated.

average). Scores stabilized for the next 3 months and increased again for the 6- to 12-month treatment period. The mean overall gain for the group was 33.8 LQ points. The one subject available at follow-up showed a moderate decline in the LQ score from the termination of treatment.

The group with severe aphasia, despite obtaining the lowest scores overall, did improve an average of 24.8 points on the LQ. Although greatest in the first 3 months, gains were also seen in the second 3-month treatment period, after which scores leveled off. These gains were maintained at the follow-up test.

FUTURE TRENDS

At times, clinicians dedicated to working with individuals with aphasia may feel overwhelmed by the complexity of the problems presented and experience feelings of helplessness at not being able to provide immediate solutions. Economic constraints pose further pressures, demanding evidence that functional changes are occurring. As a result, there is a drive to implement therapy that is "functional," interpreted by some to mean a "quick fix"; the problem being that there is typically no "quick fix" in aphasia treatment. Currently, there are hundreds of workbooks and programs available for treating the symptoms of aphasia. With the workplace having become increasingly fast paced, there is the lure of reaching for pre-designed tasks in hopes that they will somehow meet the needs of our patients. The challenge is in recognizing that over the long run, time is not saved and motivation is not maintained if tasks are ineffectual and/or frustrating for the patient.

Language-Oriented Treatment is based on the premise that improved function evolves from addressing the underlying nature of the problems, not just the symptoms. As we develop a greater understanding of normal language processing and its relationship to the impairments in aphasia, LOT will continue to evolve. This approach does, however, require time up-front in probing, analyzing, and developing hierarchies and treatment materials that actually fit the problems. Further advancements can be made by clinicians sharing information on the approaches and procedures that have proven to be effective for clearly specified problems. Publication of more workbooks and computerized programs based on these principles could serve as a rich, practical source of information for clinicians.

KEY POINTS

1. Aphasia represents an impairment in the processes for understanding and producing language.
2. Language-Oriented Treatment (LOT) is a psycholinguistic approach to intervention, applying research information about normal language processing and the impairments associated with aphasia.
3. Implementation of LOT requires a careful analysis of the nature of the underlying deficits in order to select a content of treatment that is customized for the patient.
4. The patient and significant others play central roles in determining treatment goals, activities, and expectations.
5. LOT is organized according to content reflecting potential areas of focus within five language modalities.
6. Activities incorporate a hierarchy of difficulty levels, within and across areas, based on the analysis of strengths and deficits.
7. Treatment approaches that have proven beneficial in large and small group investigations, as well as in

single case studies, are incorporated when applicable to a particular patient.

8. LOT was proven efficacious in a full-scale clinical trial, incorporating a no-treatment control group.

9. Through systematic treatment of the underlying deficits, functional improvements in language can result from a Language-Oriented Treatment approach.

References

Abu-Zeid, H.A.H., Choi, N.W., & Nelson, N.A. (1975). Epidemiologic features of cerebrovascular disease in Manitoba: Incidence by age, sex and residence, with etiologic implications. *Canadian Medical Association Journal, 113*, 379–384.

Aftonomos, L.B., Steele, R.D., & Wertz, R.T. (1997). Promoting recovery in chronic aphasia with an interactive technology. *Archives of Physical Medicine and Rehabilitation, 78*, 841–846.

Albert, M. (1998). Treatment of aphasia. *Archives of Neurology, 55*, 1417–1419.

Alexander, M.P., Fischer, R.S., & Friedman, R. (1992a). Lesion localization in apractic agraphia. *Archives of Neurology, 49*, 246–251.

Alexander, M.P., Friedman, R.B., Loverso, F., & Fischer, R. (1992b). Lesion localization in phonological agraphia. *Brain and Language, 43*, 83–95.

Arguin, M. & Bub, D. (1994). Pure alexia: Attempted rehabilitation and its implications for interpretation of the deficit. *Brain and Language, 47*, 233–268.

Aronson, M., Shatin, L., & Cook, J. (1956). Sociopsychotherapeutic approach to the treatment of aphasia. *Journal of Speech and Hearing Disorders, 21*, 325–364.

Backus, O. (1952). The use of a group structure in speech therapy. *Journal of Speech and Hearing Disorders, 17*, 116–122.

Basso, A., Capitani, E., & Vignolo, L.A. (1979). Influence of rehabilitation on language skills in aphasia patients: A controlled study. *Archives of Neurology, 36*, 190–196.

Basso, A., Faglioni, P., & Vignolo, L.A. (1975). Études controlés de la réeducation du language dans l'aphasie: Comparaison entre aphasiques traites et nontraites. *Revue Neurologique, 131*, 607–614.

Beeson, P.M., Holland, A.L., & Murray, L.L. (1997). Naming famous people: An examination of tip-of-the-tongue phenomena in aphasia and Alzheimer's disease. *Aphasiology, 11*, 323–336.

Benson, D.F. (1979). *Aphasia, alexia, and agraphia.* New York: Churchill Livingstone.

Benson, D.F. & Geschwind, N. (1969). The alexias. In P.J. Vinken & G. Bruyn (eds.), *Handbook of clinical neurology, Vol. 4.* Amsterdam: North Holland Publishing.

Benton, A.L., Smith, K.C., & Lang, M. (1972). Stimulus characteristics and object naming in aphasic patients. *Journal of Communication Disorders, 5*, 19–24.

Berndt, R.S., Mitchum, C.C., Haendiges, A., & Sandson, J. (1997). Verb retrieval in aphasia. *Brain and Language, 56*, 68–106.

Bisiach, E. (1966). Perceptual factors in the pathogenesis of anomia. *Cortex, 2*, 90–95.

Blackman, N. (1950). Group psychotherapy with aphasics. *Journal of Nervous and Mental Disorders, 111*, 154–163.

Blackman, N. & Tureen, L.L. (1948). Aphasia-psychosomatic approach in rehabilitation. *Transactions of the American Neurology Association, 73*, 193–196.

Blishen, B.R. & McRoberts, H.A. (1976). A revised socioeconomic index for occupations in Canada. *Canadian Review of Sociology and Anthropology, 13*, 71–73.

Boles, L. (1998). Conducting conversation: A case study using the spouse in aphasia treatment. *Neurophysiology and Neurogenic Speech and Language Disorders (Newsletter), September*, 24–30.

Boller, F. & Green, E. (1972). Comprehension in severe aphasia. *Cortex, 8*, 382–394.

Breedin, S., Saffron, E., & Schwartz, M. (1998). Semantic factors in verb retrieval: An effect of complexity. *Brain and Language, 63*, 1–31.

Brindley, P., Copeland, M., Demain, C., & Martyn, P. (1989). A comparison of the speech of ten chronic Broca's aphasics following intensive and non-intensive periods of therapy. *Aphasiology, 3*, 695–707.

Brookshire, R.H. & Nicholas, L.E. (1994). Speech sample size and test-retest stability of connected speech measures for adults with aphasia. *Journal of Speech, Language, and Hearing Research, 37*, 399–407.

Broida, H. (1977). Language therapy effects in long term aphasia. *Archives of Physical Medicine and Rehabilitation, 58*, 248–253.

Burbaum, L.J. & Coslett, H.B. (1996). Deep dyslexic phenomena in a letter-by-letter reader. *Brain and Language, 54*, 136–167.

Buck, R. & Duffy, R.J. (1980). Nonverbal communication of affect in brain-damaged patients. *Cortex, 16*, 351–362.

Burgio, F. & Basso, A. (1997). Memory and aphasia. *Neuropsychologia, 35*, 759–766.

Byng, S. (1992). Testing the tried: Replicating sentence-processing therapy for agrammatic Broca's aphasia. *Clinical Communication Disorders, 2*, 34–42.

Byng, S. & Black, M. (1995). What makes a therapy? Some parameters of therapeutic intervention in aphasia. *European Journal of Disorders of Communication, 30*, 303–316.

Byng, S., Nickels, L., & Black, M. (1994). Replicating therapy for mapping deficits in agrammatism: Remapping the deficit? *Aphasiology, 8*, 315–341.

Cannito, M.P., Hough, M., Vogel, S., & Pierce, R.S. (1996). Contextual influences on auditory comprehension of reversible passive sentences in aphasia. *Aphasiology, 10*, 235–251.

Caplan, D., Waters, G., & Hildebrandt, N. (1997). Determinants of sentence comprehension in aphasic patients in sentence picture matching tasks. *Journal of Speech, Language, and Hearing Research, 40*, 542–555.

Carlomagno, S., Colombo, A., Casadio, P., Emanuella, S., & Rassano, C. (1991). Cognitive approaches to writing rehabilitation in aphasics: Evaluation of two treatment strategies. *Aphasiology, 5(4–5)*, 355–360.

Chang, A. & MacKenzie, A. (1998). State self-esteem following stroke. *Stroke, 29*, 2325–2328.

Chapey, R. (1994). Cognitive intervention: Stimulation of cognition, memory, convergent thinking, divergent thinking and evaluative thinking. In R. Chapey (ed.), *Language intervention strategies in adult aphasia* (pp. 220–246). Baltimore, MD: Williams & Wilkins.

Chapman, S.B. & Ulatowska, H.K. (1989). Discourse in aphasia: Integration deficits in processing reference. *Brain and Language, 36,* 651–669.

Chapman, S.B. & Ulatowska, H.K. (1992). Methodology for discourse management in the treatment of aphasia. *Clinical Communication Disorders, 2,* 64–81.

Chapman, S.B., Ulatowska, H.K., Franklin, L.R., Shobe, A.E., Thompson, J.L., & Mc Intire, D.D. (1997). Proverb interpretation in fluent aphasia and Alzheimer's disease: Implications beyond abstract thinking. *Aphasiology, 11,* 337–350.

Cherney, L.R., Merbitz, C.T., & Grip, J.C. (1986). Efficacy of oral reading in aphasia treatment outcome. *Rehabilitation Literature, 47(5–6),* 112–118.

Coelho, C.A. (1990). Acquisition and generalization of simple manual sign grammars by aphasic subjects. *Journal of Communication Disorders, 23,* 383–400.

Coelho, C.A. & Duffy, R.J. (1986). Effects on iconicity, motoric complexity, and linguistic function on sign acquisition in severe aphasia. *Perceptual and Motor Skills, 63,* 519–530.

Coelho, C.A. & Duffy, R.J. (1987). The relationship of the acquisition of manual signs to severity of aphasias: A training study. *Brain and Language, 31,* 328–345.

Correia, L., Brookshire, R.H., & Nicholas, L.E. (1990). Aphasic and non-brain-damaged adults' descriptions of aphasic test pictures and gender biased pictures. *Journal of Speech and Hearing Disorders, 55,* 713–720.

Coslett, H.B., Saffran, E.M., Greenbaum, S., & Schwartz, H. (1993). Reading in pure alexia. *Brain, 116,* 21–37.

Dabul, B. & Hanson, W.R. (1975, October). The amount of language improvement in adult aphasics related to early and late treatment. Paper presented at the annual convention of the American Speech, Language, and Hearing Association, Washington, DC.

Daniloff, J.K., Noll, J.D., Fristoe, M., & Lloyd, L.L. (1982). Gestural recognition in patients with aphasia. *Journal of Speech and Hearing Disorders, 47,* 43–49.

Darley, F.L. (1982). *Aphasia.* Philadelphia, PA: WB Saunders.

David, R., Enderby, P., & Bainton, D. (1982). Treatment of acquired aphasia: Speech therapists and volunteers compared. *Journal of Neurology, Neurosurgery, and Psychiatry, 45,* 957–961.

Davis, G.A. & Wilcox, M.J. (1981). Incorporating parameters of natural conversation in aphasia treatment. In R. Chapey (ed.), *Language intervention strategies in adult aphasia.* Baltimore, MD: Williams & Wilkins.

De Renzi, E. & Lucchelli, F. (1994). Are semantic systems separately represented in the brain? The case of living category impairment. *Cortex, 30,* 3–25.

Deal, J.L. & Deal, L.A. (1978). Efficacy of aphasia rehabilitation: Preliminary results. In R.H. Brookshire (ed.), *Clinical aphasiology conference proceedings* (pp. 66–77). Minneapolis, MN: BRK.

Duffy, R., Watt, J., & Duffy, J.R. (1994). Testing causal theories of pantomimic deficits in aphasia using path analysis. *Aphasiology, 8,* 361–379.

Easterbrook, A., Brown, B.B., & Perera, K. (1982). A comparison of the speech of adult aphasic subjects in spontaneous and structured interactions. *British Journal of Disorders of Communication, 17,* 93–107.

Eisenson, J. (1949). Prognostic factors related to language rehabilitation in aphasic patients. *Journal of Speech Disorders, 14,* 262–264.

Eisenson, J. (1984). *Adult aphasia* (2nd ed.). Englewood Cliffs, NJ: Prentice-Hall.

Ellis, A.W. (1982). Spelling and writing (and reading and speaking). In A.W. Ellis (ed.), *Normality and pathology in cognitive functions.* London: Academic Press.

Ferguson, A. (1998). Conversational turn-taking and repair in fluent aphasia. *Aphasiology, 12,* 1007–1031.

Franz, S.I. (1906). The reeducation of an aphasic. *Journal of Philosophy, Psychology and Scientific Methods, 2,* 589–597.

Franz, S.I. (1924). Studies in re-education: The aphasics. *Journal of Comparative Psychology, 4,* 349–429.

Frazier, C.H. & Ingham, D. (1920). A review of the effects of gunshot wounds of the head. *Archives of Neurology and Psychiatry, 3,* 17–40.

Freedman-Stern R., Ulatowska, H.K., Baker, T., & Delacoste, C. (1984). Description of written language in aphasia: A case study. *Brain and Language, 22,* 181–205.

Friederici, A.D., Schonle, P.W., & Goodglass, H. (1981). Mechanisms underlying writing and speech in aphasia. *Brain and Language, 13,* 212–222.

Friedman, R. (1995). Two types of phonological alexia. *Cortex, 31,* 397–403.

Gardner, H. & Winner, E. (1978). A study of repetition in aphasic patients. *Brain and Language, 6,* 168–178.

Gardner, H. & Zurif, E. (1976). Critical reading of words and phrases in aphasia. *Brain and Language, 3,* 173–190.

Germani, M.J. & Pierce, R.S. (1992). Contextual influences in reading comprehension in aphasia. *Brain and Language, 42,* 308–319.

Glosser, G., Wiener, M., & Kaplan, E. (1986). Communicative gestures in aphasia. *Brain and Language, 27,* 345–359.

Goodglass, H. (1968). Studies on the grammar of aphasics. In S. Rosenberg & J. Koplin (eds.), *Developments in applied psycholinguistic research* (pp. 77–208). New York: Macmillan.

Goodglass, H. (1975). Phonological factors in aphasia. In R.H. Brookshire (ed.), *Clinical aphasiology conference proceedings* (pp. 132–144). Minneapolis, MN: BRK.

Goodglass, H. (1976). Agrammatism. In H. Whitaker & H.A. Whitaker (eds.), *Studies in neurolinguistics, Vol. 1* (pp. 237–260). New York: Academic Press.

Goodglass, H. (1993). *Understanding aphasia.* San Diego, CA: Academic Press.

Goodglass, H. (1998). Stages of lexical retrieval. *Aphasiology, 12,* 287–298.

Goodglass, H. & Berko, J. (1960). Aphasia and inflectional morphology in English. *Journal of Speech and Hearing Research, 10,* 257–262.

Goodglass, H. & Kaplan, E. (1972). *The assessment of aphasia and related disorders.* Philadelphia, PA: Lea & Febiger.

Goodglass, H. & Kaplan, E. (1983). *The assessment of aphasia and related disorders* (2nd ed.). Philadelphia, PA: Lea & Febiger.

Goodglass, H., Klein, B., Carey, P.W., & Jones, K.J. (1966). Specific semantic word categories in aphasia. *Cortex, 2,* 74–89.

Goodglass, H. & Wingfield, A. (1993). Selective preservation of a lexical category in aphasia: Dissociations in comprehension of body parts and geographical place names following focal brain lesion. *Memory, I(4),* 313–328.

Green, E. & Boller, F. (1974). Features of auditory comprehension in severely impaired aphasics. *Cortex, 10,* 133C145.

Hagen, C. (1973). Communication abilities in hemiplegia: Effect of speech therapy. *Archives of Physical Medicine and Rehabilitation, 54,* 454–463.

Hanley, J.R. & Peters, S. (1996). A dissociation between the ability to print and write cursively in lower-case letters. *Cortex, 32,* 737–745.

Helm, N.A. & Barresi, B. (1980). Voluntary control of involuntary utterances: A treatment approach for severe aphasia. In R. Brookshire (ed.), *Clinical aphasiology: conference proceedings.* Minneapolis, MN: BRK.

Helm-Estabrooks, N. (1981). *Helm Elicited Language Program for Syntax Simulation.* Austin, TX: Exceptional Resources.

Helm-Estabrooks, N. (1983). Approaches to treating subcortical aphasias. In W. Perkins (ed.), *Current therapy of communication disorders* (pp. 97–103). New York: Thieme-Stratton.

Helm-Estabrooks, N. (1988). The application of neurobehavioral research to aphasia rehabilitation. *Aphasiology, 2,* 303–308.

Helm-Estabrooks, N. (1998). A cognitive approach to treatment of an aphasic patient. In N. Helm-Estabrooks & A.L. Holland (eds.), *Approaches to the treatment of aphasia.* San Diego, CA: Singular Publishing Group.

Helm-Estabrooks, N. & Albert, M. (1991). *Manual of aphasia therapy.* Austin, TX: Pro-Ed.

Helm-Estabrooks, N., Fitzpatrick, P., & Barresi, B. (1982). Visual action therapy for global aphasia. *Journal of Speech and Hearing Disorders, 44,* 385–389.

Helm-Estabrooks, N., Ramsberger, G., Brownell, H., & Albert, M. (1989b). Distal versus proximal movement in limb apraxia (Abstract). *Journal of Clinical and Experimental Neuropsychology, 7,* 608.

Henri, B. (1973). A longitudinal investigation of patterns of language recovery in eight aphasic patients. Unpublished doctoral dissertation, Northwestern University, Evanston, IL.

Herrmann, M., Reichle, T., Lucius-Hoene, G., Wallesch, C.-W., & Johannsen-Horbach, H. (1988). Nonverbal communication as a compensatory strategy for severely nonfluent aphasics? A quantitative approach. *Brain and Language, 33,* 41–54.

Hillis, A. (1992). Facilitating written production. *Clinical Communication Disorders, 2,* 19–33.

Holland, A. (1991). Pragmatic aspects of intervention in aphasia. *Journal of Neurolinguistics, 6,* 197–211.

Holland, A.L., Fromm, D.S., De Ruyter, F., & Stein, M. (1996). Treatment efficacy: Aphasia. *Journal of Speech, Language, and Hearing Research, 39,* S27–S36.

Holland, A.L. & Wertz, R.T. (1988). Measuring aphasia treatment effects: Large-group, small-group, and single-subject designs. In F. Plum (ed.), *Language, communication, and the brain.* New York: Raven Press.

Hough, M.S. & Pierce, R.S. (1994). Pragmatics and treatment. In R.Chapey (ed.), *Language intervention strategies in adult aphasia* (pp. 246–268). Baltimore, MD: Williams & Wilkins.

Howard, D., Best, W., Bruce, C., & Gatehouse, C. (1995). Operativity and animacy effects in aphasic naming. *European Journal of Disorders of Communication, 30,* 286–302.

Huntley, R.A., Pindzola, R., & Werdner, W. (1986). The effectiveness of simultaneous cues on naming disturbance in aphasia. *Journal of Communication Disorders, 19,* 261–270.

Katz, R. & Wertz, R.T. (1997). The efficacy of computer-provided reading treatment for chronic aphasic adults. *Journal of Speech, Language, and Hearing Research, 40,* 493–507.

Kay, J., Lesser, R., & Coltheart, M. (1996). Psycholinguistic Assessments of Language Processing in Aphasia (PALPA): An introduction. *Aphasiology, 10,* 159–179.

Kellar, L.A. (1978). Stress and syntax in aphasia. Paper presented at the Academy of Aphasia, Chicago, IL.

Kertesz, A. & Poole, E. (1974). The aphasia quotient: The taxonomic approach to measurement of aphasic disability. *Canadian Journal of Neurological Sciences, 1,* 7–16.

Kurtzke, J.F. (1976). An introduction to the epidemiology of cerebrovascular disease. In P. Scheinberg (ed.), *Cerebrovascular diseases: Tenth Princeton Conference.* New York: Raven Press.

Langmore, S.E. & Canter, G.J. (1983). Written spelling deficit of Broca's aphasics. *Brain and Language, 18,* 293–314.

Le Dorze, G. & Brassard, C. (1995). A description of the consequences of aphasia on aphasic persons and their relatives and friends, based on the WHO model of chronic diseases. *Aphasiology, 9,* 239–255.

Lecours, A.R. (1999). Frank Benson's teachings of acquired disorders of written language (with addenda). *Aphasiology, 13,* 21–40.

Li, E.C., Kitselman, K., Dusatko, D., & Spinelli, C. (1988). The efficacy of PACE in remediation of naming deficits. *Journal of Communication Disorders, 21,* 491–503.

Li, E.C., Volpe, A.D., Ritterman, S., & Williams, S.E. (1996). Variations in grammatic complexity across three types of discourse. *Journal of Speech-Language Pathology and Audiology, 30,* 180–186.

Li, E.C. & Williams, S.E. (1989). The efficacy of two types of cues in aphasic patients. *Aphasiology, 3(7),* 619–626.

Li, E.C. & Williams, S.E. (1990). The effects of grammatic class and cue type on cueing responsiveness in aphasia. *Brain and Language, 38,* 48–60.

Lott, S.L., Friedman, R.B., & Linebaugh, C.W. (1994). Rationale and efficacy of a tactile-kinaesthetic treatment for alexia. *Aphasiology, 8,* 181–195.

Ludlow, C.L. (1973). The recovery of syntax in aphasia: An analysis of syntactic structures used in connected speech during the initial recovery period. Unpublished doctoral dissertation, New York University.

Lyon, J.G. (1995). Drawing: Its value as a communication aid for adults with aphasia. *Aphasiology, 9,* 33–50.

Margolin, D.I. (1984). The neuropsychology of writing and spelling: Semantic, phonological, motor and perceptual processes. *Quarterly Journal of Experimental Psychology, 36A,* 459–489.

Marshall, J. (1995). The mapping hypothesis and aphasia therapy. *Aphasiology, 9,* 517–539.

Marshall, J., Robson, J., Pring, T., & Chiat, S. (1998). Why does monitoring fail in jargon aphasia? Comprehension, judgment and therapy evidence. *Brain and Language, 63,* 79–107.

Mc Call, D., Cox, D.M., Shelton, J.R., & Weinrich, M. (1997). The influence of syntactic and semantic information on picture-naming performance in aphasic persons. *Aphasiology, 11,* 581–600.

McCleary, C. & Hirst, W. (1986). Semantic classification in aphasia: A study of basic superordinate and functional relations. *Brain and Language, 27*, 199–209.

Meikle, M., Wechsler E., Tupper, A., Benenson, M., Butler, J., Mulhally, D. & Stern, G. (1979). Comparative trial of volunteer and professional treatments of dysphasia after stroke. *British Medical Journal, 2*, 87–89.

Mills, C.K. (1904). Treatment of aphasia by training. *Journal of American Medical Association, 43*, 1940–1949.

Mitchum, C.C. & Berndt, R.S. (1995). The cognitive neuropsychological approach to treatment of language disorders. *Neuropsychological Rehabilitation, 5*, 1–16.

Murray, L. (1999). Attention and aphasia: Theory, research, and clinical implications (Review). *Aphasiology, 13*, 91–111.

Naeser, M.A., Baker, E.H., Palumbo, C., Nicholas, M., Alexander, M.P., Samaraweera, R., Prete, M.N., Hodge, S.M., & Weissman, T. (1998). Lesion site patterns in severe, nonverbal aphasia to predict outcome with a computer-assisted treatment program. *Archives of Neurology, 55*, 1438–1448.

Netsu, R. & Marguardt, T.P. (1984). Pantomime in aphasia: Effects of stimulus characteristics. *Journal of Communication Disorders, 17*, 37–46.

Nickels, L. (1995). Reading too little into reading?: Strategies in the rehabilitation of acquired dyslexia. *European Journal of Disorders of Communication, 30*, 37–50.

Nicholas, L.E. & Brookshire, R.H. (1995a). Presence, completeness, and accuracy of main concepts in the connected speech of non-brain-damaged adults and adults with aphasia. *Journal of Speech, Language, and Hearing Research, 38*, 145–156.

Nicholas, L.E. & Brookshire, R.H. (1995b). Comprehension of spoken narrative discourse by adults with aphasia, right-hemisphere brain damage or traumatic brain damage. *American Journal of Speech-Language Pathology, 4*, 69–81.

Nippold, M.A., Uhden, L.D., & Schwarz, I.E. (1997). Proverb explanation through the lifespan: A developmental study of adolescents and adults. *Journal of Speech, Language, and Hearing Research, 40*, 245–253.

Pashek, G.V. & Brookshire, R.H. (1980). Effects of rate of speech and linguistic stress on auditory paragraph comprehension of aphasic individuals. In R.H. Brookshire (ed.), *Clinical aphasiology conference proceedings* (pp. 64–65) (Abstract). Minneapolis, MN: BRK.

Perkins, L. (1995). Applying conversation analysis to aphasia: Clinical implications and analytic issues. *European Journal of Disorders of Communication, 30*, 372–383.

Petheram, B. (1996). Exploring the home-based use of microcomputers in aphasia therapy. *Aphasiology, 10*, 267–282.

Pierce, R.S. (1988). Influence of prior and subsequent context on comprehension in aphasia. *Aphasiology, 2(6)*, 577–582.

Pierce, R. & Grogan, S. (1992). Improving listening comprehension of narratives. *Clinical Communication Disorders, 2*, 54–63.

Pierce, R.S., Jarecki, J., & Cannito, M. (1990). Single word comprehension in aphasia: Influence of array size, picture relatedness and situational context. *Aphasiology, 4(2)*, 155–156.

Poeck, K, Huber, W., & Willmes, K. (1989). Outcome of intensive language treatment in aphasia. *Journal of Speech and Hearing Disorders, 54*, 471–478.

Porch, B.E. (1967). *Porch Index of Communicative Ability*. Palo Alto, CA: Consulting Psychologists Press.

Prins, R.S., Snow, C.E., & Wagenaar, E. (1978). Recovery from aphasia: Spontaneous speech versus language comprehension. *Brain and Language, 6*, 192–211.

Ramsberger, G. (1996). Repetition of emotional and nonemotional words in aphasia. *Journal of Medical Speech-Language Pathology, 4*, 1–12.

Rao, P.L. (1994). Use of amer-ind code by persons with aphasia. In R. Chapey (ed.), *Language intervention strategies in adult aphasia* (pp. 359–367). Baltimore, MD: Williams & Wilkins.

Raven, J. (1956). *Coloured Progressive Matrices: Sets A, A, B* (Revised Order). London: Lewis and Company.

Sarno, M.T. (1997). Quality of life in aphasia in the first post-stroke year. *Aphasiology, 11*, 665–679.

Sarno, M.T., Silverman, M., & Sands, E.S. (1970). Speech therapy and language recovery in severe aphasia. *Journal of Speech and Hearing Research, 13*, 607–623.

Schlanger, P.H. & Freemann, R. (1979). Pantomime therapy with aphasics. *Aphasia-Apraxia-Agnosia, 1*, 34–39.

Schonle, P.W. (1988). Compound noun stimulation: An intensive treatment approach to severe aphasia. *Aphasiology, 2(3–4)*, 401–404.

Schuell, H., Jenkins, J.J., & Jimenez-Pabon, E. (1964). *Aphasia in adults: Diagnosis, prognosis, and treatment*. New York: Harper & Row.

Schwartz, M.F., Saffran, E.M., Fink, R.B., Myers, J.L., & Martin, N. (1994). Mapping therapy: A treatment programme for agrammatism. *Aphasiology, 8*, 19–54.

Scott, C. & Byng, S. (1989). Computer assisted remediation of homophone comprehension disorder in surface dyslexia. *Aphasiology, 3(3)*, 301–320.

Sefer, J.W. (1973). A case study demonstrating the value of aphasia therapy. *British Journal of Disorders of Communication, 8*, 99–104.

Shallice, T. (1981). Phonological agraphia and the lexical route in writing. *Brain, 104*, 413–429.

Shewan, C.M. (1977). *Procedures manual for speech and language training: Language-Oriented Therapy (LOT)*. Unpublished manuscript. The University of Western Ontario, London, Ontario.

Shewan, C.M. (1979). *Auditory Comprehension Test For Sentences (ACTS)*. Menomonee, WI: Biolinguistics Clinical Institutes.

Shewan, C.M. (1980). Verbal dyspraxia and its treatment. *Human Communication, 5*, 3–12.

Shewan, C.M. (1986). The Language Quotient (LQ): A new measure for the Western Aphasia Battery. *Journal of Communication Disorders, 19*, 427–439.

Shewan, C.M. & Bandur, D.L. (1986). *Treatment of aphasia: A language-oriented approach*. Austin, TX: Pro-Ed.

Shewan, C.M. & Henderson, V.L. (1988). Analysis of spontaneous language in the older normal population. *Journal of Communication Disorders, 21*, 139–154.

Shewan, C.M. & Kertesz, A. (1984). Effects of speech and language treatment on recovery from aphasia. *Brain and Language, 23*, 272–299.

Silverberg, N., Vigliocco, G., Insaluco, D., & Garrett, M. (1998). When reading a sentence is easier than reading a >little=word: The role of production processes in deep dyslexics reading aloud. *Aphasiology, 12*, 335–356.

Skelly, M. (1979). *Amer-Ind gestural code*. New York: Elsevier.

Smith, A., Champoux, R., Leri, J., London, R., & Muraski, A. (1972). Diagnosis, intelligence and rehabilitation of chronic aphasics. University of Michigan, Department of Physical Medicine and Rehabilitation. Social and Rehabilitation Service (Grant No. 14-P-55198/5-01).

Springer, L., Glindemann, R., Huber, W., & Willmes, K. (1991). How efficacious is PACE-therapy when 'Language Systematic Training' is incorporated? *Aphasiology*, 5, 391–399.

Stimley, M.A. & Noll, J.D. (1991). The effects of semantic and phonemic prestimulation cues in picture naming in aphasia. *Brain and Language*, 41, 496–509.

Thomas, C.A. & Jackson, S.T. (1997). The validity of reading comprehension therapy materials. *Journal of Communication Disorders*, 30, 231–243.

Thompson, C.K. & Shapiro, L.P. (1995). Training sentence production in agrammatism: Implications for normal and disordered language. *Brain and Language*, 50, 201–224.

Tompkins, C.A., Boada, R., McGarry, K. (1992). The access and processing of familiar idioms by brain-damaged and normally aging adults. *Journal of Speech, Language, and Hearing Research*, 35, 626–637.

Tuomainen, J. & Laine, M. (1991). Multiple oral reading technique in rehabilitation of pure alexia. *Aphasiology*, 5(4–5), 401–409.

Tyler, L.K., Moss, H.E., & Jennings, F. (1995). Abstract word deficits in aphasia: Evidence from semantic priming. *Neuropsychology*, 9, 354–363.

Van Demark, A.A., Lemmer, E.C.J., & Drake, M.L. (1982). Measurement of reading comprehension in aphasia with the RCBA. *Journal of Speech and Hearing Disorders*, 47, 288–291.

Vignolo, L.A. (1964). Evolution of aphasia and language rehabilitation: A retrospective exploratory study. *Cortex*, 1, 344–367.

Wallace, G.L. & Canter, G.J. (1985). Effects of personally relevant language materials on the performance of severely aphasic individuals. *Journal of Speech and Hearing Disorders*, 50, 385–390.

Wang, L. & Goodglass, H. (1992). Pantomime, praxis, and aphasia. *Brain and Language*, 42, 402–418.

Webb, W. & Love, R. (1994). Treatment of acquired reading disorders. In R. Chapey (ed.), *Language intervention strategies in adult aphasia* (pp. 446–457). Baltimore, MD: Williams & Wilkins.

Weinrich, M., McCall, D., Weber, C., Thomas, K., & Thornburg, L. (1995). Training on an iconic communication system for severe aphasia can improve natural language production. *Aphasiology*, 9, 343–364.

Weinrich, M., Shelton, J.R., Cox, D.M., & McCall, D. (1997a). Remediating production of tense morphology improves verb retrieval in chronic aphasia. *Brain and Language*, 58, 23–45.

Weinrich, M., Shelton, J.R., McCall, D., & Cox, D.M. (1997b). Generalization from single sentence to multisentence production in severely aphasic patients. *Brain and Language*, 58, 327–352.

Weisenburg, T. & McBride, K.E. (1935). *Aphasia*. New York: Hafner.

Wepman, J.M. (1951). *Recovery from aphasia*. New York: Ronald Press.

Wertz, R.T., Collins, M., Weiss, D., Brookshire, R.H., Friden, T., Kurtzke, J.F., & Pierce, J. (1978). Preliminary report on a comparison of individual and group treatment. Paper presented at the annual meeting of the American Association for the Advancement of Science, Washington, DC.

Wertz, R.T., Collins, M., Weiss, D., Kurtzke, J.F., Frident, T., Brookshire, R.H., Pierce, J., Holtzapple, P., Hubbard, D.J., Porch, B.E., West, J.A., Davis, L., Matovitch, V., Morley, C.K., & Resurrection, E. (1981). Veterans Administration cooperative study on aphasia: A comparison of individual and group treatment. *Journal of Speech and Hearing Research*, 24, 580–594.

Wertz, R.T., Weiss, D.G., Aten, J.L., Brookshire, R.H., Garcia-Bunuel, Holland, A.H., Kurtzke, J.F., LaPointe, L.L., Milianti, F.J., Brannegan, R., Greenbaum, H., Marshall, P.C., Vogel, D., Carter, J., Barnes, N.S., & Goodman, R. (1986). Comparison of clinic, home, and deferred language treatment for aphasia. *Archives of Neurology*, 43, 653–658.

Whitney, J.L. & Goldstein, H. (1989). Using self-monitoring to reduce disfluencies in speakers with mild aphasia. *Journal of Speech and Hearing Disorders*, 54, 576–586.

Williams, S.E., Li, E.C., Volpe, A.D., & Ritterman, S. (1994). The influence of topic and listener familiarity on aphasic discourse. *Journal of Communication Disorders*, 27, 207–222.

Zurif, E.B. & Caramazza, A. (1976). Psycholinguistic structures in aphasia. In H. Whitaker & H.A. Whitaker (eds.), *Studies in neurolinguistics, Vol. 1*. New York: Academic Press.

Zurif, E.B., Caramazza, A., & Myerson, R. (1972). Grammatical judgments of agrammatic aphasics. *Neuropsychologia*, 10, 405–417.

Zurif, E.B., Green, E., Caramazza, A., & Goodenough, C. (1976). Grammatical intuitions of aphasic patients: Sensitivity to functors. *Cortex*, 12, 182–186.

APPENDIX 27–1

MODALITY: _____

AREA: _____

GOAL: _____

LOT GOALS

CLIENT: _____

CLINICIAN: _____

Level	Stimulus	Presentation Method	Cuing Provided	Criterion For Correct Response	Response Method	Additional Responses

APPENDIX 27–2

MODALITY: _____

AREA: _____

LOT DATA RECORD

CLIENT: _____

CLINICIAN: _____

Session No.	Date	Time Spent (minutes)	Difficulty Level	No. of Items	DATA and COMMENTS

Chapter 28

Treatment of Aphasia Subsequent to the Porch Index of Communicative Ability (PICA)

Bruce E. Porch

Before initiating treatment, and at various critical points during the therapeutic process, the clinician must answer a series of critical questions about the conduct of that treatment. The issues of major concern are how the brain lesion has affected the communicative ability of the patient; whether those deficits are treatable; what modalities, tasks, and stimuli should be used in treatment; what behavior should be reinforced; and when should treatment be terminated. Traditionally, answers to these problems are evolved empirically during treatment through trial-and-error methods or are arbitrarily decided on because of the clinician's bias for certain techniques and methods. In recent years, there is a growing tendency among clinicians who use the Porch Index of Communicative Ability (PICA) (Porch, 1981) to rely on the test results to help with the therapeutic decision making.

The discussion that follows will consider some of these treatment issues and will illustrate how PICA test results and PICA theory can assist the clinician in therapy planning. Much of this material is drawn from basic and advanced training courses that are designed to prepare the clinician for the use of the test. Therefore, although it is hoped that the concepts presented here are useful to a general audience, the full application of some of these methods will necessarily be limited to PICA-trained people who have demonstrated accuracy in the use of the multidimensional scoring system.

OBJECTIVES

The major objective of this chapter is to demonstrate that the nature of response behavior is indicative of the status of the brain's circuits and systems. The following main arguments are presented to help the clinician appreciate the importance of this concept to the understanding of brain function and to the development of viable aphasia treatment plans.

- The brain survives best when its circuits and systems function quickly and easily and it stores information that is accurate. When these circuits and systems are damaged, information is processed more slowly and inefficiently, more circuits are required to do simpler tasks, and information is treated as tentative and not stored.
- The patient's response behavior reflects these changes in the brain circuitry's reduced efficiency. Since response changes such as delayed responses, self-corrections, and requests for repetition of the stimulus signal significant changes within the brain systems, the use of plus-minus scoring in testing or treatment is not appropriate and multidimensional scoring or some other method of observing small behavioral changes is necessary clinically.
- Treatment planning based on this model is, therefore, directed at assisting the patient to achieve easy, immediate responses on progressively more difficult tasks.
- Decisions about the patient's potential for change due to treatment should be made on the basis of a psychometric sampling of the patient processing.

A SYSTEMS ANALYSIS APPROACH TO APHASIA TREATMENT

Fundamental to understanding the brain, why it does what it does in both normal and damaged states, and how to treat it, is the principle of the brain as survival mechanism. The ways the brain processes information, reacts to stimuli, and responds to damage are all biased by the ultimate effect of that moment on its capacity to survive. This principle pervades every aspect of treatment and must be used by the clinician to anticipate what must be done and what must be avoided while treating the patient.

A second principle essential to the development of an appropriate sequence of treatment is that all of the systems of the brain and their components are intimately interrelated, and that no part of a system can be affected positively or negatively without affecting all systems. A brief look at a hypothetical brain circuit might illustrate the practical

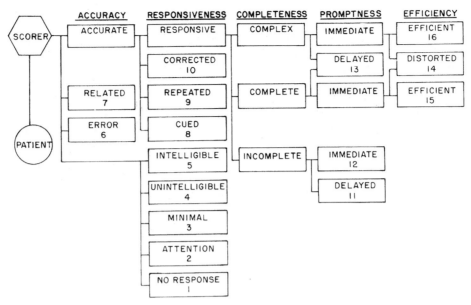

Figure 28–1. Multidimensional binary choice scoring system.

implications of these two principles and serve as an introduction to PICA theory applied to treatment.

At the simplest level, a brain circuit may be viewed as being made up of a series of modules each of which processes data from the previous module and then sends the processed information on to the next module in the circuit. Each module has the capacity to enhance the information, reject it as inaccurate, or to mark it as a survival message. For example, the auditory processing circuit theorized in Figure 28–1 shows three levels of modules between the input of each bit of raw data to the circuit and the output of the circuit to other circuits or integrators. When the input pathway sends basic data from the input transducers such as the ears, or from other circuits, to the feature detection modules, the data are stored temporarily in processing storage (PS). The module then scans its data banks or operational storage (OS) to determine if the raw data have been processed before, and if there is some information about the data that can further define the data, especially in terms of its significance to survival. This information is moved to the comparator (Cmp) to verify that the retrieved data explain or define the raw data stored in processing storage. If the comparator finds a good match between the input data and the retrieved data, it allows the combined product to be sent on to the next module in the circuit, which, in this simple circuit, is "pattern recognition." After storing the output of the features module in its processing storage, this next module scans its operational storage to see if the features coming in have a pattern that was previously processed as valid information. It then compares the retrieved information from its storage, compares it with the input data in processing storage, and if it matches, sends it to the signal processing module to determine if the recognized patterns have a specific significance, especially to survival. If

the significance of the patterns is established, the processed information may now be sent on to other circuits, or integrators that combine information from multiple circuits.

The storage units in this model are conceived of as an access core that defines the nature of the information stored around it, and each core has a surround made up of data and subcores and subsurrounds, all of which share a common relationship to the access core. The more important information is to survival, and the more frequently it is used, the closer it is to the core or subcore and, therefore, the more retrievable it is since it requires less switching to reach it. Another interesting characteristic of these storage units, operational and permanent cores and surrounds, is that they tend not to store tentative or nonverified information. Processing storage and a general persistence in the circuit will maintain data temporarily. Only when a bit of data is processed immediately and accurately is it considered appropriate for operational, long-term storage. Usually, operational storage is achieved through processing a data bit enough times to verify it is accurate and useable, or when the data bit has high impact, in terms of survival, where it must be remembered after one exposure to it, and trial and error learning is not conducive to survival. If a caveman with friends was walking down a path lined with bushes and a saber-toothed tiger jumped out and devoured one of the group, it would be important to remember that path and those bushes after one exposure rather than repeating the walk and watching his friends disappear over the next few days!

Returning to Figure 28–1, note that there are feedback loops for each module that communicate with all of the previous modules. These loops may be used when a module finds it does not have sufficient information to complete the processing of a data bit sent to it, and therefore needs the previous module to send more data. These feedback loops can also inform the previous module(s) that the information being processed is the first in a series that is well known and there is no need to process the rest of the series. This frees the previous modules for processing new and less familiar data, and this reduces the circuitry necessary to process familiar data to a minimum. Thus, circuitry reduction results in more efficient, faster processing of familiar data and allows the circuit to use its energy on more complex, unique, or "danger" kinds of data. The immature brain uses many circuits to carry out relatively simple tasks. The mature brain reduces the number of circuits necessary to carry out a task to a minimum. The damaged brain is less efficient and must once again use its circuits to cope with less complex tasks and is challenged by previously easy tasks. It is the goal of treatment to restore circuitry efficiency.

A final important observation has to do with the interconnectedness of the brain's circuits and systems and why damage has such widespread implications in the brain. If in our theoretical circuit the processing storage in the pattern recognition module fails to function, the raw data enter the module, scanning in memory occurs, and then the comparator attempts to match the retrieved information with the original input data. However, nothing is stored in processing storage and comparison is impossible. The comparator must then request that the input data be sent again from the previous module, or it must rescan memory in an attempt to verify the information. The comparator's other options are to simply stop functioning, or to assume that the retrieved information is accurate and send it on to the next module. While all this is going on in the pattern recognition module, the features recognition module is waiting to send the next bit of data forward, and the signal processing module is waiting for the patterns module to send it some data. The entire circuit is locked up because one small part of one module is broken. And further, previous circuits are waiting for this circuit to accept information and succeeding circuits are waiting for the output of this circuit. The entire system is affected and this system is interlocked with all other systems.

In summary, this systems analysis model that we will be applying to aphasia treatment suggests that the brain is made up of complex, interlocked, interrelated modules and circuits that are survival biased. Survival is facilitated by maximizing the efficiency of these circuits by permanently storing only verified information that is not tentative. The efficiency of a circuit is further increased by circuitry reduction that allows fewer modules or fewer circuits to be necessary to quickly process accurate and familiar data entering the system. The clinical caution here is that both operational storage and circuitry reduction do not occur if any aspect of processing is not easy and immediate. What constitutes "easy and immediate" brings us to a consideration of the patients' response behavior and why the use of plus-minus scoring during aphasia treatment is both impractical and unproductive.

Multidimensional Scoring

The circuitry within the brain defies direct observation and therefore the clinician must infer what is going on in a system by carefully observing the patient's response behavior during a treatment task. There is a wide range of behavior possible in a response to a given stimulus and task, depending upon how the involved circuits are able to process the data. Several examples of response behavior to follow will illustrate this and will show how PICA multidimensional scoring (shown in underlined scores) is used to quantify behavior.

Returning to the theoretical circuit described earlier, when data move through each of the modules of a circuit easily and immediately, and produce an accurate well-produced output from the circuit, those data are permanently stored in operational storage, and circuitry reduction may occur for those data. Use of the multidimensional, binary choice PICA scoring system shown in Figure 28–2 would score such responses as accurate, responsive, complete, prompt, and efficient, *15*. During treatment it is these *15* type responses that are the target behavior the clinician strives for on every response.

In contrast to an "easy" response, a patient might retrieve inaccurate or incomplete information when scanning operational storage. When the retrieved information is sent to the comparator, the discrepancy between this retrieved information and what is stored in processing storage is noted. This necessitates looping back to operational storage to retrieve a better match. When the comparator finds the second information is accurate, it sends it on to the next module for processing. Such double looping appears behaviorally as a brief hesitancy or processing delay, *13*, but is significant clinically because that bit of information is still considered as tentative by the circuit and therefore is not stored in operational storage (Aaronson, 1974). It still requires total, not reduced, circuitry for its processing. This is why any response other than an easy, accurate, immediate response, *15*, means further treatment is necessary on that item.

Let us examine this double-looping example for other types of behavior that could have resulted. After double looping, a damaged comparator might accept incorrect information from storage and send it on to the next module. If this incorrect information produces an error response but the

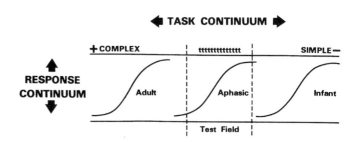

Figure 28–2. Task and response continua.

response reenters the circuit and is recognized as being inaccurate and is then changed to be accurate, the clinician observes this use of an external comparator as a self-correction, *10*. If the comparator recognized that the stored information in that module was inadequate it might feed back to earlier modules or to sensory transducers a request for additional information about the data bit, *8*, or for the same data to be sent through again, *9*. If such information is not available earlier in the circuit, the comparator might just send the erroneous information on to produce an incorrect response, *6*, or the comparator might stop all processing and accept that it cannot produce a response, and the patient rejects the item saying, "I don't know," *5*.

Although this scoring system was developed for sensitively and reliably quantifying subtle changes in a patient's test behavior it has proven to be equally vital in documenting the response characteristics during treatment. A final benefit of multidimensional scoring is that it forces the clinician to be sensitive to small but important changes in behavior.

Internal Consistency of Tasks

The PICA is designed so that all of the subtests revolve around 10 common objects. This has the psychometric advantage of holding content constant across subtests and therefore making it possible to compare the patient's skill across modalities and tasks. It also produces subtests that have very high internal consistency, with all of the items on a subtest being relatively equally difficult for the patient. Under these conditions, it is possible to detect patterns of response that are normally obscured by conventional aphasia tests that begin with easy items and get progressively more difficult.

Table 28–1 shows how having stimuli that are relatively equally difficult will reveal various types of processing problems during testing or treatment. In this simple example we see the scores for three different patients on a task involving 10 relatively equally difficult items. Patient A rejects the first item but is able to respond to the next few items after the stimulus is repeated or cued or after a significant delay. Eventually he begins to respond at normal levels and receives scores of 15s. With Patient A it is apparent that he had trouble tuning into the task and adjusting his system to perform adequately during the first part of the task, but he eventually reached fully operational levels. Patient B starts out with no difficulty but gradually has decreasing scores and tunes out on the task, suggesting that he lacks the ability to keep his system locked into the task or to handle cumulative noise that might build up during the task. Patient C has a performance that is very homogeneous and shows no variation from item to item.

We see in the bottom row of Table 28–1 that all three patients got a mean score of 11.0, indicating that they are all functioning at about the same communicative level on

| TABLE 28–1 |

Examples of Patterns of Response

Stimuli	Patient		
	A	**B**	**C**
Cat	5	15	11
Dog	8	15	11
Boy	9	15	11
Apple	10	15	11
Cup	13	15	11
Shoe	15	13	11
Car	15	10	11
Soup	15	9	11
Ball	15	8	11
Pie	15	5	11
Mean score	11.0	11.0	11.0

this task. However, it is clear that the type of processing difficulties that each manifests is quite different. In addition, patients A and B demonstrate several fully operational responses, suggesting that their circuits have the capacity to carry out the task once the processing problems are resolved. Patient C, although he got all of the 10 items correct on a plus-minus basis, shows no ability to do the task at operational levels, and his system is indicating that, at least at this point in time, it is performing the task as well as it can.

Because the PICA has high internal consistency, it is able to give some indication about these types of processing problems, and it indicates potential levels of ability that a patient may have on a given task (Disimoni et al., 1983). These same principles can be employed in treatment if the clinician will take the time to ensure that the stimulus items used on the task are relatively equally difficult.

DESIGNING A PLAN OF TREATMENT

Once the clinician has gained a thorough familiarity with the patient and his or her history, has completed comprehensive testing, and has found that the patient's condition is no longer changing dramatically from day to day, treatment planning can be initiated. The usual sequence of considerations at this point is to determine if the patient is a suitable candidate for treatment, to choose the tasks and stimuli to be used during treatment, to decide on which types of behavior will be reinforced on each task and, finally, to determine when treatment should be terminated.

Selecting Patients for Treatment

Determining whether a patient is treatable is a relatively new concern, arising in recent years as treatment became more expensive and available funding for treatment became scarce. During the 1960s, Schuell and coworkers (1964) did some work on prognosis that assigned post-recovery, stabilized patients to one of five major or two minor prognostic groups. More recently, in an effort to develop earlier predictions, Porch and coworkers (1974, 1980) have described other prognostic studies that attempted to develop more accurate predictions of eventual recovery levels; however, these studies employing multiple discriminate analysis have not yet been validated for clinical use.

Perhaps the most widely used clinical method currently is the high-overall-prediction (HOAP) method (Porch, 1970) that was developed during the late 1960s as an interim approach to prediction but that proved to be reasonably accurate and simple to use and therefore has persisted for three decades. In this method, it was theorized that the capacity of the patient's total communicative system was indicated by the highest scores or peak abilities. Therefore, the clinician could estimate the maximum potential for communication by using the average of the nine highest subtest scores achieved on the PICA or by using the highest modality score, whichever was the greatest. Appropriate tables or graphs enable the clinician to convert these scores into an estimate of the eventual outcome level and thereby make appropriate plans regarding treatment of the patient. Because this HOAP method may be applied as early as 1 month post-onset in most cases, and because it takes into consideration the normal recovery stages, the clinician is in a better position to select the patients who are most treatable and to counsel families and physicians regarding the eventual recovery levels (Porch & Callaghan, 1981).

For clinicians who use the PICA to test their patients early in the recovery process, there is another prognostic indicator, the acceleration rate of recovery. This is determined by subtracting the 1-month post-onset PICA Overall percentile from the 2-month post-onset Overall percentile. Patients who improve more than 12 percentile points during this period tend to exceed the HOAP target percentile by the time they reach 6 months post-onset. Those with slower early recovery tend to not reach the early PICA predictions.

Estimating treatment potential is equally important later in the course of recovery. Eventually, the patient's condition seems to stabilize and the clinician must decide whether to continue treatment. Once again, PICA scores are helpful in several ways in making this decision. First, discrepancies between the patient's overall score and the high modality score indicate the amount of potential change that remains. Second, after the patient is past the acute stage, it is expected that when he or she is at maximum recovery his or her subtest percentiles will be approximately equal and, therefore, differences between the nine highest subtest percentiles and the nine lowest subtest percentiles will also suggest a range of possible change or the lack of it.

These same principles hold true within subtests. The PICA scoring system provides 16 scores for any given response, and it is therefore possible for a patient to obtain a wide range of item scores. As a patient undergoes treatment for aphasia, the intrasubtest variability of scores gradually reduces until all of the item scores within the subtests are quite homogeneous, indicating that there are no peaks or depressions of ability on the task. This homogeneity suggests that the patient, at least at that point in time, is functioning at near maximum ability on that particular task. The circuits necessary to carry that task are consistently performing at their highest current potential levels of efficiency; there are no low responses that might be brought up to the patient's average level, and there are no higher scores that might serve as a target level toward which to strive. When the patient demonstrates homogeneity in all modalities on the PICA, his or her brain is indicating that it is performing communicatively and cybernetically near its maximum potential level of functioning and that further treatment of the processing problems may not be fruitful. At that point, the clinician may evolve new treatment goals to maximize the patient's use of his or her functional systems, to modify the patient's environment to facilitate his/her communication, and to educate the people in his/her environment about the status of the patient's abilities and deficits and how to assist that patient.

In summary, an ideal treatment candidate is a cooperative patient whose medical condition is stable, who has a predicted overall percentile significantly above his or her present overall score, and who exhibits variation on item scores within subtests in some modalities.

Selecting Treatment Tasks

Before the discussion on treatment can continue, it is necessary to introduce some concepts and terminology related to PICA theory. As we see in Figure 28–2, we may visualize a continuum of communicative tasks ranging from the most simple vegetative communicative processes to the most complex learned processes. The ordinate represents the response continuum ranging at the top from the most complex levels of responses to the bottom of the continuum where the patient fails to attend or give any type of response.

The PICA samples a test field somewhere in the middle of the task continuum. The tasks that were sampled range from relatively simple tasks in which only the most involved patients have difficulty, to moderately challenging tasks in which even mild patients demonstrate some processing problems. The standard PICA test battery samples 18 points in the test field and establishes the subject's capacity to carry out tasks of varying difficulty.

The PICA tests have demonstrated that the interaction between the task and the response continua is best depicted by a sigmoidal function curve. If one were to test a normal subject longitudinally from infancy to adult levels of communication, this sigmoidal function curve would move from right to left on the task continuum and finally stabilize at some fairly high level of communicative ability. When a normal brain is damaged, its circuits are less efficient, it must use more circuits to carry out simpler tasks (the reverse of circuitry reduction), and it treats more entering data as tentative and therefore does not store it easily in operation storage. Because of these changes, the sigmoidal function curve shifts negatively to the right. The PICA locates the position of that response curve on the task continuum and, as indicated above, predicts how far positively that curve can be shifted with treatment.

Returning to our premise that aphasia represents a reduction in the processing efficiency of the brain, we can see that the sigmoidal function curve depicts the individual's processing abilities on a series of tasks ranked according to their difficulty level. The highest part of the curve on the right represents processing ability that is fully operational, and so the patient carries out these tasks accurately, immediately, efficiently, and without requiring additional information in order to understand the task. The middle or fulcrum of the curve shows those tasks on which the patient is responding accurately, but only if he/she receives additional information in the form of repeats, cues, or self-corrections, or if he/she takes additional processing time to carry out the task. The bottom of the curve represents those tasks on which the patient is responding inaccurately, demonstrating that the processing necessary to carry out those tasks is beyond his/her capacity at that time.

Using this schema, the problem of task and modality selection is greatly simplified for the clinician, since the patient's system indicates precisely those tasks that need immediate attention. Once the PICA has been administered and the results plotted to indicate the patient's response curve, it is quite apparent which tasks are already operational and do not require treatment, which tasks are on the fulcrum of the curve and should be treated, and which tasks are beyond the capacity of the patient's system at this time and should be excluded from the treatment format.

The reader should not confuse the concept of the fulcrum of the curve with the earlier suggestion that tasks on which the patient has the greatest item variability have the most potential for change and, therefore, that these tasks should be chosen for treatment. While it is true that tasks on which the patient has a large variety of scores, including high target scores and low scores that may be improved, have good potential for eventual change, such a task is too far down the curve. Attempts at treating it produce some errors, suggesting that the circuits involved are getting insufficient information to perform the task or that more efficiency in the circuit needs to be developed by using tasks more within the capacity of the circuits, that is, farther up the curve. In general,

errors during treatment usually suggest that the task selected is too difficult at this point in time, or that the stimuli have been poorly chosen.

Selecting Treatment Stimuli

After the tasks in various modalities have been selected from the fulcrum of the curve, it is then necessary to select appropriate treatment stimuli to serve as vehicles for resolving the patient's processing problems on those tasks. Although it is common practice for clinicians to select stimuli on some a priori basis and then proceed with treatment, expecting the patient to do as well with whatever stimuli is selected is dangerous because it does not take into consideration the specific type of processing problem the patient has. Stimuli that are too difficult and overdrive the patient's system, or those that are too "noisy" and interfere with processing, not only may reduce the amount of positive results from treatment but may actually produce problems rather than resolve them.

The danger of using inappropriate stimuli can be obviated by testing their appropriateness on selected tasks. The PICA score sheet may have already indicated to the clinician that the patient has more difficulty on certain types of stimuli such as polysyllabic words, words with consonant blends, or words that are too short to provide adequate clues for decoding. This type of information might be used in assisting in the selection of the repertoire of stimuli that the clinician plans to use for the treatment tasks. However, it is still important to verify the selected stimuli under the actual treatment conditions.

Stimulus verification is done through the use of PICA scoring, since the classic plus-minus scoring is relatively insensitive to processing disorders. Having selected 20 or 30 stimuli that seem appropriate for the task, the clinician then explains to the patient what the task is and what he or she is expected to do. It is also useful to explain to the patient that the clinician will be scoring the responses so as to determine which stimuli will be the best to use in subsequent treatment sessions. Each stimulus, which has been listed on a treatment score sheet, is presented in order and the patient's responses are scored for later analysis. After all of the stimuli have been presented once, it is usually informative to present them again after a brief rest period to see how consistent the patient's processing is on each stimulus.

Table 28–2 shows how a few stimuli might be scored during a stimulus verification session. The clinician has selected some common nouns for treatment stimuli and has presented the list twice. In addition to the specific item scores the patient received, some other more general observations may be made about these two trials. First, the patient tends to improve slightly on the second trial, demonstrating that he has a good potential for improving after repeated trials. Second,

TABLE 28–2

Verification of Treatment Stimuli

Stimuli	Trial	
	First	Second
Apple	8	9
Hammer	13	15
Shoe	10	13
Cup	6	6
Baseball	15	15
Hat	9	9
Bicycle	15	15
Car	7	10
Window	13	13
Bus	9	10

it appears that the patient does somewhat better on polysyllabic words, thus suggesting that his auditory system may not be able to decode short stimuli rapidly enough and that the longer duration and increased information in longer words makes it easier to process them. Finally, it does not appear that there are any orderly changes as one scans down the column of scores on either trial. It is not unusual to find some patients whose scores gradually increase during a trial, suggesting that it takes several items for them to make the necessary adjustments to carry out the task. Other patients may start out a given trial with high scores and then suddenly have decreasing scores as the trial proceeds, indicating that they are unable to lock their system into the task and they gradually tune out on the succeeding stimuli. In the example in Table 28–2, these types of trends are not seen, and therefore the variation in scores is probably attributable to the stimuli themselves.

Having made these general observations, the clinician is now ready to decide on which stimuli he or she will use in subsequent treatment sessions. The first rule here is to drop out any stimuli on which the patient received errors, scores 7 or below. The fact that the patient got error scores on one of the trials on those stimuli indicates that they are either too noisy or too difficult to be used in treatment and can only interfere with processing and progress. Too often the inexperienced clinician will attempt to "teach" these words to the patient but instead ends up putting more noise into his or her system along with practice errors. A second consequence of using error-type responses is that not only do you prohibit the facilitation of good switching on these stimuli, but the effect spreads to other stimuli on the list and it creates a spread of poor processing to other stimuli in the treatment trial (Brookshire, 1976). When a clinician is treating the processing problems of the patient, no given stimulus can be considered as sacred, and whenever

one presents a problem it should be dropped out of the program.

This concept of dropping error items or stimuli should also be incorporated into the stimulus verification process, since items that are too difficult may have an interaction effect on other items. It is generally a good policy when running such trials to eliminate any error items from second and third trials to rule out possible interactions. In addition, the items that produce errors should be carefully analyzed for characteristics that are in contrast with items that invariably elicit 15-level responses. Such an analysis will give the clinician important information about what variables affect the circuits involved and what type of stimuli should be avoided in treatment.

It should be apparent that plus-minus scoring is too gross to yield meaningful information about the patient's system and that PICA scoring should be used if possible. However, clinicians who are not trained in PICA methods may achieve similar results by sorting stimuli into three categories: "easy"—items that the patient has responded to accurately, without effort or delay in a manner that might be referred to as "normal"; "medium"—items that are responded to accurately but only after processing delays, self-corrections, or repeats of the stimuli, or after cues or additional information are given; and "hard"—items that yield error responses. When using this system it is customary to designate the type of response as E, M, or H, or 3, 2, and 1, or the stimuli may be sorted into three separate piles if card-type stimuli are used.

At this point, after all of the sorting and analyzing of stimuli is complete, it would seem that the selection of tasks and stimuli is complete and the actual treatment might begin, but one more preliminary step is quite informative. Having selected a treatment task on which the patient gets 9- to 15-type scores (easy and medium responses), the clinician, instead of simply presenting the task multiple times to eventually achieve all "easy" responses, should manipulate some single variable of the task in a way that will immediately produce higher scores. If a particular manipulation does in fact improve responses, the clinician has discovered an important factor about the patient's system and what helps it to function successfully. By the same token, if the manipulation produces lower scores, evidence is obtained as to what variables have negative effects on the system. No change in responses as a result of the manipulation signifies that that variable is not a relevant factor in the patient's performance of the task.

A simple auditory task might illustrate how one carries out this probe technique. The clinician has selected a task that involves placing six pictures of common things in front of the patient and having him point to the one named. The clinician on the initial presentation obtained three easy responses (15s), a correct response after a repeat of the stimulus (9), a self-correction, and a delayed response (13). The question now is how may the task be modified to produce all easy-type responses immediately? There are several possibilities—reduce the number of items from six to four to simplify the task and reduce visual loading; use a carrier phrase before the noun ("Point to the") to negate rise-time problems; add the printed word for the noun ("Car") to the picture to add visual information to assist the auditory system; give an arousal signal ("Ready?...Car") for system activation or attention problems; and so on.

Gradually, as various modifications of the task succeed, the patient is able to come to all easy responses until he or she finally achieves all 15s. During the process the clinician learns what factors make the patient's processing more or less efficient, information that will assist in this and future therapy tasks. In addition, possible tasks for subsequent treatment have also been documented. As the original probe task that started out down the curve was manipulated, it gradually moved up the curve until it reached the all-15 level. With each change the clinician documented the location of the various modifications of the task on the curve during this upward movement. Therefore, the clinician may, by working in reverse order down the curve, move from one task to the next in that sequence documented during the probe. As each task is raised to the all-easy level, the circuits under treatment become available for assisting the processing of other tasks down the curve and the entire response curve moves toward the more complex end of the task continuum.

Treatment Format

Once the tasks and the stimuli have been selected for treatment, the clinician is now ready to organize them into a treatment format that is designed to present a consistent presentation of tasks that will facilitate the patient responding at the all-15 level. That is, it is the goal of the clinician and the patient working as a team to have the patient eventually respond to every stimulus on the task without requiring cues, repeats, self-corrections, or significant delays. Not only is this type of treatment designed to be error free, but as much as possible it tries to facilitate the patient's responses so that they are produced easily and without any processing difficulty.

All of these principles discussed thus far are roughly what is meant by "treating on the fulcrum of the curve." Processes in which the patient demonstrates delays and self-corrections are tentative processes that break down when used in more complex tasks used farther down the curve. If these minor processing problems are cleared up and the patient reaches the all-15 level in carrying out the processes, then these become available farther down the curve and all of the more complex processes can take advantage of the now normal, simpler processes. This phenomenon may, in part, explain why so many times we see tasks improving in the clinic that have not been treated directly during the therapeutic process. This schema also

makes it clear why it is so inappropriate to treat tasks too far down the response curve because we are expecting the patient to carry out complex processes that require other basic processes that are not yet available to him or her.

When setting up the sequence of presentation of treatment activities, it must be realized that the goal of treatment is to assist the patient in mastering noisy, inadequate circuits and switching. Because sudden changes in tasks, target behavior, or methods of reinforcement invariably produce distraction and noise in the patient's communicative system, it is advisable to establish an orderly and fairly fixed format of treatment. If patients can anticipate the treatment events and if they have time to make leisurely transitions from task to task, they will maintain a more efficient, quieter system.

A useful format for ensuring adequate stimulation of the patient's system without producing noise or overload might be summarized as follows:

1. Adjustment period (clearing out)
2. General activation (warmer upper)
3. Consolidation (old stuff)
4. Modification (new stuff)
5. Consolidation (old stuff)
6. Modification (new stuff)
7. Conclusion (winder upper)

Adjustment Period: Checking and Clearing Out Circuits

The adjustment period that initiates the treatment session is a brief but important time. After the patient enters the room and sits down at the treatment table, the clinician greets him/her and simply asks a broad, nondirective question such as "How's everything?" "What's new?" This is designed to give the patient the opportunity to clear out his system and to tell the clinician about any special occurrences, problems, or questions that may have arisen since the last session. It also gives him/her an opportunity to try out in a free-speech situation some of the processes that he/she has been working on previously. The clinician, on the other hand, is trying to observe several things about the patient.

First, it should be noted if there is a significant difference between how the patient currently appears compared with how he or she appeared in previous sessions. If he/she is markedly improved, it may be necessary to redesign the treatment session or to retest the patient to determine his/her new level of functioning. If he/she is functioning poorly compared with previous sessions, it may be necessary to probe into the cause of the problem or to discuss the matter with the family to see if there has been an exacerbation of the patient's medical problem. Sometimes the patient has less serious problems such as headache, shoulder pain, or some psychological or social issue that produces a depression in his/her ability and may make it necessary to be somewhat less adventurous in the treatment session on that day. Finally, while the patient is gradually adjusting his/her system to the room and to the clinician and is getting prepared for more difficult treatment tasks, the clinician is carefully noting the quality of the patient's communication and observing how much carryover there is from those processes that are being attacked during treatment to a spontaneous speech situation.

General Activation: Turning On and Warming Up Systems

Once it is certain that the patient is functioning adequately and that he/she has cleared his/her storage systems in preparation for treatment, the clinician can begin to focus the patient's attention on treatment-type tasks. For this purpose, a task is selected from the highest or consolidated part of the patient's response curve. This fairly easy, all-15-type task is for activating the patient's communicative systems and warming them up and for furnishing the patient with a gradual transition into the more difficult tasks. This activation period also will provide the clinician with a second check on the patient's general level of functioning on that day, and it gets the patient off to a successful start in his/her treatment session.

When initiating treatment with a new patient, information about what might be suitable warm-up tasks might be obtained from the PICA score sheet if one looks at the all-15 items on the easiest subtests. In the case of the patient who has been treated for a period of time, the clinician may elect tasks that at one time were on the fulcrum of the curve but that eventually became fully operational. Selecting these old tasks serves to verify that the patient is maintaining skills that were worked on formerly.

If, after a short period of general activation, the patient seems to be responding easily to simpler processing tasks, the clinician is ready to move on to the next step in treatment.

Just as in testing, where making a definite and clear transition in between tasks is important, the change between one step in treatment to the next should be made obvious to the patient so that he/she can clear out his/her system and make the necessary switching adjustments for the new task. This is done by giving the patient a general positive reinforcement for his/her efforts on the previous task and then suggesting that the patient just relax for a moment while the clinician makes notes about what has occurred in the session to that point. Then the clinician announces to the patient that they are going to be doing something different. The clinician should explain what the task will be and what the patient is expected to do, and then the first item of that task should be demonstrated for the patient. When it is apparent that the patient understands the task, the task should then be started with the demonstration item so that the patient's system is gently eased into the task. Generally, following this type of transition will minimize the amount of noise in the patient's system and greatly reduce his/her anxiety and fatigue.

Consolidation: Pushing for All "Easy" Responses on Old Stuff

Having moved through the adjustment and activation steps, the patient and clinician now are ready to begin the first of several treatment modules. A treatment module is a series of tasks directed at a given modality or process. Depending on how many steps there are in each module and how much time the total program takes, there may be two or three modules in a 1-hour treatment session. For instance, the first module might be devoted to consolidating and modifying auditory processing, and the clinician may then move on to the second module for consolidating and modifying verbal processing and, finally, turn to work on reading or writing as a third module.

A module is usually begun with a task that the clinician is trying to consolidate and make fully operational. This is a task quite high on the fulcrum of the curve, which on the first presentation has occasional delays in it but by the second or third presentation is all 15s. If, in a given session, it is found that this task is done at the all-15 level on the first presentation, the clinician might consider using that task as a warm-up in the future. If, on the other hand, the patient has continuing difficulty and cannot get to the all-15 level even after several presentations, it generally means that he/she is not ready to go on to new tasks in that module. If, after a few presentations, the patient is able to get all 15s, the clinician should do the task several times to consolidate those 15s and then prepare to move on to the next step in the module.

Modification: Moving Down the Curve to New Tasks

As the patient approaches the point where he or she is fully operational on a given task, it is then appropriate to think about modifying that task slightly so that it involves some new aspect of switching or storage. For instance, if, on an auditory task that requires the patient to point to one of four pictures after the clinician says the noun, the task might be modified by using six pictures, by having the patient point to two pictures instead of one, or by not allowing the patient to see the pictures while the clinician is saying the noun. Any of these changes probably would produce an increase in the number of delays or self-corrections that the patient might have on the task. The goal then would be to increase his/her performance until he/she achieves all 15s on the new task. If the clinician makes what is considered a small modification in the task and the patient begins to make errors or requires multiple repeats and cues before he/she gets a correct response, the modification is larger than expected, and the task should move more in the direction of the consolidation task.

If the patient does fairly well with the new material and seems to understand it after several trials, he/she should be given a brief rest period in preparation for the next module. Usually, shifting to a new modality means a shifting to new stimuli and treatment materials, but, once again, the transition should be verbalized to help the patient readjust his/her system for the new task. This same general procedure is then followed beginning with old material in the modality that needs to be consolidated and then, if appropriate, moving on to some new modifications of the task to increase the patient's processing capabilities.

Conclusion: A Positive Wind Up to the Treatment Session

The final step in the treatment format should involve a fairly easy task at the all-15 level. The patient and the clinician have moved through a variety of fairly arduous tasks during the previous hour and have just completed a relatively new modification task that has been somewhat difficult, and concluding the treatment session on that note would be psychologically undesirable. Therefore, the clinician should select a task from the easy, consolidated part of the curve, which will assure winding up the session on a successful note. The clinician may also use this final step as a verification that the patient is maintaining his/her skills on one of the earlier treated processes. It is also a nice technique to use wind-up tasks from one day's session for a warm-up task on the next day's session. This helps the patient get back to the same point that he/she was at during the previous session, and it reduces intersession regression.

To summarize this section on the treatment format, the tasks are selected and sequenced in such a way as to maximize the efficiency of the patient's communicative systems and to minimize noise. Treatment of a given process or modality is begun with tasks selected from the consolidated, all-15 part of the curve to prepare those circuits for the more difficult tasks. Next, slightly more difficult tasks are selected from the fulcrum of the curve, and these are worked on until the patient eventually reaches the all-15 level. At that point, these newly consolidated processes are available for use on other tasks and, therefore, the patient's response curve moves positively toward the predicted target level.

TREATMENT PRINCIPLES

Patient-Clinician Team

Implicit in the treatment method being described here is the involvement of the patient in the conduct of the treatment process. The patient should understand that the clinician is not trying to teach the patient words but rather is attempting to return him/her to "easy" processing, free of self-corrections, repeats, and delays. The patient must be taught what this behavior feels like. It is sometimes helpful in teaching what is meant by "easy" processing to present the task using all "medium" items first, and then to repeat the task with all "easy" items so that the patient can get the feel of the contrast between the two levels of performance. Once this distinction is clear to the patient, he/she must also be

taught to advise the clinician when a response is tentative or slightly off target so that it can be consolidated. In this sense the two people become a team in which the patient relies on the clinician to assist in selecting the tasks and stimuli and the patient keeps the clinician informed as to the impact of those items on his/her system.

Setting Treatment Priorities

The establishment of the specific modalities and processes to be treated is facilitated by careful examination of the PICA score sheet. All-15 tasks are selected for warm-up and wind-up tasks, the 13–15 level tasks should be treated, and the 9–13 level tasks, when slightly simplified, may soon be appropriate as modification tasks in the format.

In general, it is best to first treat processing problems that are not stimulus related. This includes difficulty in shifting tasks, tuning in, cumulative noise, and tuning out. These problems are diagnosed when a series of homogeneous items are presented on a task and the patient always has trouble (repeats, self-corrections, or delays) with the first few items or tunes out the last few, regardless of the order of stimulus presentation. When these temporal problems occur, a specific program may be designed to overcome them. For instance, the goal of eliminating tuning out might be achieved by discussing the problem with the patient and then presenting stimuli that generally elicit 15-type responses. At first, only a few stimuli are used, and these are worked on until the patient achieves all 15s. The number is then gradually increased until the patient can keep his/her system locked in to the task for a full complement of stimuli.

If the patient has problems that are more random or are stimulus related, those problems are overcome by getting the circuits necessary for the task to the 15 level and then processing multiple times at that level. The circuits for the task are facilitated and they will store processing information once the 15 level is achieved. Therefore, as treatment proceeds, those items on which the patient scored below 15 should be repeated until 15 is achieved and then repeated some more so that the circuit can sense what 15 processing entails and store that information.

Very often, clinicians move through a series of stimuli and score responses without repeating items enough for success to occur. This is essentially testing rather than treating because the patient's circuits never have the opportunity to experience the target behavior and achieve fully operational circuits. It is probably more beneficial to move lower scores to 15s and practice the 15s if stable improvement is desired.

Criteria for Shifting Tasks

By this point in the discussion, it should be apparent that plus-minus scoring is completely inadequate for carrying out this type of treatment and that a more detailed type of scoring such as a PICA scoring system must be used. Second, the clinician must mentally score every response of every task in order to decide whether he or she should repeat the item or move on to the next one. Some clinicians like to write down every score for every response during the session so that they have a running account of exactly what happened in the patient's system. In that way they can make the correct adjustments in the program, and they can document the patient's change very precisely over time. Another approach is to record the scores on the first presentation of the task to establish a baseline and then to work on the task for a period of time, and then rescore to measure change. Still other clinicians, who plan their treatment for a longer period of time and change the format less frequently, prefer to score the responses at the beginning of the treatment week and then rescore them at the end of the week to see what changes have taken place. Specific application of PICA scoring has been described by Bollinger and Stout (1974) in their discussion on response-contingent small-step treatment; by LaPointe (1974), who gives examples of PICA scoring as used in Base 10 Program Stimulation; and by Brookshire (1973) in his general consideration of aphasia treatment.

Some of the major differences between these types of programs and the PICA program described here are the criteria for selecting tasks and stimuli and the criteria for shifting to new tasks or terminating tasks. Many programs suggest an 80% or 90% correct criterion as an indication that the patient is ready to go on to more difficult tasks. This is undoubtedly too low, since this would allow the patient to have repeats, self-corrections, or delays on every item and still meet the criterion. Even a standard of 95%, 13s (delays), or better allows the patient to have significant problems with 5% of the items. When this amount of interference in processing occurs, the information being processed is probably considered by the system as being tentative, and, therefore, it is not stored for long-term use. This in turn means that the process being treated is not fully consolidated and is not available for use on tasks farther down the curve.

PICA theory, therefore, suggests that the target for changing or terminating tasks is all-15 responses. This may seem overly idealistic, but it is in fact realistic and essential. Such a goal is attainable because the tasks and the stimuli used have been carefully chosen and verified through the patient's system.

The second reason that all-15 responses are an appropriate treatment goal is that this type of processing seems to transfer better and is more resistant to regression. Unless a task is fully consolidated, it will tend to deteriorate in a normal life situation or in a more difficult treatment task. Cued (8) to self-corrected (10) responses often become errors, and delayed responses (13) shift to lower, more tentative scores. For this reason, transfer of these skills rarely occurs because

they are not operational. Conversely, if the patient develops a good awareness of what "easy" responses are and achieves them on all of the items on the task, transfer can be maximized and regression can be prevented.

FUTURE TRENDS

The treatment methods based on PICA test results and multidimensional scoring described in this chapter offer several advantages over less structured approaches. In starting treatment, the clinician and the patient are offered a specific target level of overall communicative ability to work toward, and this can be computed quite early in the course of recovery. The treatment, once initiated, focuses on modalities and processes that the patient's own communicative systems have indicated are appropriate to modify at that point in time; and the exact difficulty levels of the tasks, the stimuli, and the target behavior are prescribed and verified by the level of multidimensional scores the patient achieves. All of this evolves naturally out of a treatment format that maximizes the patient's processing efficiency while minimizing the possibility that the clinician is misdesigning the treatment. Finally, the predictive formulas and the measures of intrasubtest variability indicate when the patient is at last functioning at his or her highest possible levels so that plans for terminating treatment may be made.

In contrast to these advantages, the PICA approach to treatment has disadvantages, in that it requires special training to see the behavior in detail and to convert that behavior into scores; it requires a great deal of preparation and planning at every stage of treatment; it necessitates a considerable amount of book work to record and analyze all of the response scores; and, because of its emphasis on cybernetics rather than content, it is structured, and therefore gives the clinician less freedom to experiment during the treatment session.

KEY POINTS

1. An efficient brain processes information quickly and accurately and only stores information that it can trust for survival.
2. The inefficient brain must use its circuits for simpler tasks and it does the tasks less quickly and efficiently.
3. This reduced processing efficiency is evident in the response behavior of the individual.
4. The clinician must be able to discern and document all the behaviors that distinguish an easy, immediate response, the goal of treatment, from less efficient responses.
5. Multidimensional scoring, or some other method that distinguishes easy responses from less efficient responses, is necessary in aphasia treatment since both the patient and the clinician must make these distinctions.

Plus-minus scoring fails to make these distinctions and is not useful in treatment.

6. Treatment should focus on those tasks and stimuli on which the patient produces accurate but not easy responses. Error responses suggest that that item, task, or stimulus is beyond the capacity of the patient's circuits at that time and is not appropriate now.

7. Once tasks and stimuli that are appropriate for the patient's circuits and systems have been selected, a format of treatment should be organized to maximize the probability that the patient will achieve easy responses on items that previously were tentative.

8. Decisions about the reasonableness of treating or continuing to treat a patient should be made on a psychometric basis which samples the patient's processing potential.

References

Aaronson, D. (1974). Stimulus factors and listening strategies in auditory memory: A theoretical analysis. *Cognitive Psychology, 6,* 108–132.

Bollinger, R. & Stout, C.E. (1974). Response contingent small step treatment. In B.E. Porch (ed.), *Clinical asphasiology conference proceedings.* Albuquerque, NM: VA Hospital.

Brookshire, R.H. (1973). An introduction to aphasia. Minneapolis, MN: BRK.

Brookshire, R.H. (1976). Effects of task difficulty on sentence comprehension performance of aphasic subjects. *Journal of Communication Disorders, 9,* 167–173.

Disimoni, F.G., Keith, R.L., & Darley, F.L. (1983). "Tuning in" and "tuning out": Performance of aphasic patients on ordering PICA subtests. *Journal of Communication Disorders, 16,* 31–40.

LaPointe, L.L. (1974). Base 10 "programmed-stimulation": Task specification, scoring, and plotting performance in aphasia therapy. In B.E. Porch (ed.), *Clinical aphasiology conference proceedings.* Albuquerque, NM: VA Hospital.

McNeil, M.R. (1979). The Porch Index of Communicative Ability. In F.L. Darley (ed.), *Evaluation of appraisal techniques in speech and language pathology.* Cambridge, MA: Addison-Wesley.

Porch, B.E. (1981). The Porch Index of Communicative Ability. Palo Alto, CA: Consulting Psychologists Press.

Porch, B.E. (1970). PICA interpretation: Recovery and treatment (video training tape). Albuquerque, NM: VA Hospital.

Porch, B.E. (1971). Multidimensional scoring in aphasia testing. *Journal of Speech and Hearing Research, 14,* 777–792.

Porch, B.E. & Callaghan, S. (1981). Making predictions about recovery: Is there HOAP? In R.H. Brookshire (ed.), *Clinical aphasiology conference proceedings.* Minneapolis, MN: BRK.

Porch, B.E., Wertz, R.T., & Collins, M. (1974). Statistical and clinical procedures for predicting recovery from aphasia. In B.E. Porch (ed.), *Clinical aphasiology conference proceedings.* Albuquerque, NM: VA Hospital.

Porch, B.E., Collins, M., Wertz, R.T., & Friden, T.P. (1980). Statistical prediction of change in aphasia. *Journal of Speech and Hearing Research, 23,* 312–321.

Schuell, H., Jenkins, J., & Jiminez-Pabon, E. (1964). *Aphasia in adults.* New York, Harper & Row.

Chapter 29

Augmentative and Alternative Communication for Persons with Aphasia

Karen Hux, Nancy Manasse, Amy Weiss, and David R. Beukelman

OBJECTIVES

After completion of this chapter, individuals will be able to identify components of a conversation and how those components relate to persons with aphasia; identify communication patterns of elderly persons; determine the impact of augmentative and alternative communication techniques and strategies on the treatment of persons with aphasia; explain differences between replacing, supplementing, and scaffolding natural speech; and list various AAC techniques and strategies that persons with varying severities of aphasia can utilize.

IMPACT OF APHASIA ON COMMUNICATIVE INTERACTIONS

Nearly 1 out of every 275 adults in the United States has aphasia (National Aphasia Association, 1987). Although differences exist in the incidence of aphasia among people with different constellations of risk factors, aphasia occurs with approximately equal frequency among people of various educational and socioeconomic backgrounds (National Aphasia Association, 1998). What is unique about the population of persons with aphasia is their age; specifically, the vast majority of people who acquire aphasia do so as elderly adults, after a lifetime of using natural speech to communicate successfully and efficiently.

This factor of age is an important consideration when speech-language pathologists implement augmentative and alternative communication (AAC) strategies, techniques, or devices with people with aphasia. Because most stroke survivors are over 60 years of age, awareness of (a) the overall contour of conversations among elderly adults and (b) the communication patterns of elderly adults is important.

These details influence speech-language pathologists' efforts to support the communication attempts—through both natural speech and AAC techniques—of persons with aphasia and will be considered in the following sections.

CONTOUR OF A CONVERSATION

Overall, the structure of conversations among elderly adults is quite similar to that of younger adults. Conversations typically consist of segments including greetings, small talk, sharing of new information, and wrap-up and farewell statements. Despite this overall similarity, small differences within conversation segments exist between elderly and young adults. In addition, the presence of aphasia may disrupt some or all phases of conversation, and, hence, aphasia has an important impact on social interactions. The contour of a conversation and the changes that occur in conversational segments as people age are important considerations when designing and implementing AAC intervention programs for people with aphasia.

Greetings

The usual contour of a conversation begins with a rather generic greeting that contains little specific information but signals awareness of another person's presence, communicates a speaker's intent to be friendly, and provides a bid to engage in conversation. Although the purpose of the greeting is quite similar across ages, the form of the greeting changes depending upon the speaker's age. A website maintained by the authors (*http://aac.unl.edu*) provides an extensive list of vocabulary—including greetings—used by persons of different ages. A review of that list reveals that elderly adults use somewhat different utterances for greetings than young adults. For example, a common greeting used by elderly adults is, "Hello. How are you feeling today?" whereas young adults would be more likely to greet another person by simply saying, "Hi."

For people with aphasia, greetings remain an important means of connecting with others. Although communication challenges often make people with aphasia apprehensive about initiating conversations, they are more likely to attempt such interactions if they have access to greeting phrases similar to those used prior to stroke. The simple act of greeting others in socially acceptable ways can be an important step in a stroke survivor's return to community and social interactions, because it signals to others that the person with aphasia is still capable intellectually and aware of surrounding events and people.

Small Talk

Small talk is conversation that requests or shares generic information about participants. It typically follows a greeting, and consists of phrases such as, "How are you?" "How's your family?" or "What do you think about the weather?" An important function of small talk is determination of whether a listener wants to engage in further communication. At this point, the communication participants may shift to sharing new information or may terminate the conversation with appropriate wrap-up and goodbye phrases.

Providing people with aphasia with access to small talk questions and answers is relatively easy because of their standard form. As such, small talk can extend greetings into simple conversations. As with greetings, providing people with aphasia with the tools to engage in small talk can serve as an important signal to potential communication partners that, although the individual has a communication challenge, he/she remains an active participant in society. The willingness of an adult with aphasia to engage in small talk is at least somewhat dependent on whether he/she has access to phrases that match those used by peers.

Information Sharing

Information sharing may take a variety of forms, with question-and-answer exchanges and storytelling being the most common. Question-and-answer exchanges center on topics of mutual interest to both communication participants, and one person often serves as the "expert" on a given subject. Storytelling may use one or more of a variety of types of stories to share information (Schank, 1990). *First person* stories relate incidents that have occurred to the speaker personally. *Second person* stories are those that the speaker has learned by reading or listening to others and need to be acknowledged as coming from other sources. *Official stories* are used to teach lessons or explain phenomena and may be simplified or refined to highlight certain points. Families, schools, and religious groups often use official stories to communicate cultural standards. Finally, *fantasy stories* are those that are "made up" by the speaker. Although fantasy stories are relatively common in the conversations of preschool children, they occur infrequently in the communication interactions of elderly adults.

Information sharing is one of the most challenging conversational segments for people with aphasia because of its reliance on conveying information that is novel to the listener and because of the need to retrieve specific words and syntactic structures while simultaneously selecting, organizing, and sequencing information in a way that is meaningful for a listener. However, the same information and stories can serve as conversation topics for multiple listeners. Thus, once a functional information sharing system is established, maintaining it is simply a matter of periodically updating the available information.

Wrap-up and Farewell Statements

Following a period of information sharing, most conversations contain wrap-up phrases that prepare for a final farewell statement. Wrap-up phrases include comments such as, "Nice talking with you," "We should talk again sometime," or "I have to go now." Farewell statements include phrases such as, "Goodbye," or "See you later." Again, the phrases used for wrap-up and farewell purposes differ among adults of different ages and, for people with aphasia, need to match those used prior to stroke and preferred by their peers.

COMMUNICATION PATTERNS OF ELDERLY PERSONS

Elderly individuals display somewhat different communication patterns than young or middle-aged adults. In the past, researchers (e.g., Goodglass, 1980; Kynette & Kemper, 1986; Riegel & Riegel, 1964; Ulatowska et al., 1985) have made direct comparisons between the communicative performances of elderly and young adults and have concluded that older persons have slower word recall, more ambiguous noun usage, reduced variability in production of verb tenses and syntactical structures, and smaller active vocabularies than younger adults. This information provides a negative picture or "profile of deficit" about the communication skills of elderly adults. More recently, some researchers have adopted a more positive perspective for viewing the communication patterns of elderly adults and have begun attributing observed differences across the age span to variations in social roles and the contexts in which people live and interact. These variations affect the amount of interaction time that people spend engaging in "small talk" and storytelling, the time-frame to which people relate conversations, and the people and activities to which references are made during conversations. Because most people with aphasia are elderly adults, subtle differences in communication patterns among people of various ages are important considerations when designing and implementing AAC strategies.

Small Talk

Generic small talk refers to phrases that can be used with a variety of different communication partners because they do not contain or refer to specific shared information. For example, "How are you?" is a generic small talk phrase, but, "How is your hip?" is not, because it contains individual-specific, shared information.

The use of "small talk" differs between young and elderly adults. Forty percent of the utterances produced by young adults (i.e., 20 to 30 years of age) is generic small talk, whereas 31% of the utterances of adults between 65 and 74 years of age and 26% of the utterances of adults over 74 years of age fit this category (King et al., 1995; Lasker et al., 1996). Thus, with advancing age, people decrease the proportion of generic small talk in their communicative interactions; simultaneously, they increase their use of storytelling and narratives.

Storytelling (Narration)

Research has shown that storytelling or narration serves a variety of interaction purposes including instruction, entertainment, transfer of cultural traditions, and establishment of cohort relationships with other individuals. Elderly adults, in particular, tell stories to transfer cultural traditions and to instruct younger individuals (Coleman, 1986). Elderly adults engage in storytelling to establish social membership with peers. With advancing age, friendship begins to assume greater personal importance, perhaps because, of all the bonds that can hold a group of people together, the strongest is the bond of common experience (Vischer, 1967).

Having a communication disorder undoubtedly prevents elderly adults from engaging in much of the extended conversation for which they are well known. In addition, people with aphasia may have limited opportunities to meet and interact with peers outside the home, thus further affecting their roles as storytellers or narrators.

Time-Frame

Elderly persons tend to refer to the past nearly as often as they refer to the present and much more frequently than they refer to the future. This differs from the communication patterns of young adults. Furthermore, Stuart et al. (1993) found that differences in time-frame referencing exist even among elderly adults split into two groups of "young-old" (65 to 74 years) and "old-old" (75 to 85 years) individuals. These researchers reported that "young-old" individuals referred to the future 13% of the time, the present 48% of the time, and the past 39% of the time; old-old individuals referred both to the present and the past about 45% of the time and the future 10% of the time.

People and Activities

Another difference in the communication patterns of young and elderly adults concerns the individuals and activities about whom people talk. According to Stuart et al. (1993), about 28% of the utterances of women between 65 and 74 years of age refer to family members and 13% refer to friends. However, women between 75 and 85 years of age tend to refer to family members less frequently than they refer to friends. Thus, a remarkable shift in conversational emphasis occurs for women as they age. This shift may relate to the tendency for women to outlive their spouses and for a woman's children to become increasingly involved in raising families of their own rather than interacting with elderly parents.

Also, a substantial percentage of utterances produced by elderly adults refer to specific activities. Stuart (1991) reported that 6% of all utterances produced by elderly men and women referred to games (as compared to 8% referring to food, 6% referring to household relationships, 5% referring to work, and 4% referring to family life). Thus, games and game playing represent an important aspect of the communication of elderly persons.

ROLES OF AAC AND APHASIA

Traditional speech-language intervention has focused on improving the speaking ability of persons with aphasia so that they can resume their previous conversational roles. However, for many people with aphasia, complete restoration of natural speech is not possible. In these instances, AAC strategies can serve to enhance the communication participation of individuals with aphasia by replacing, supplementing, or scaffolding residual natural speech and providing a means of repairing disrupted communication.

Replacing Natural Speech

Many speech-language pathologists view AAC primarily as a replacement for natural speech. As a group, many tend to incorporate AAC strategies only when individuals fail to regain the ability to convey even the most basic messages through natural speech. This view has prompted clinicians to attempt AAC interventions only when individuals have severe or profound aphasia, and clinicians tend to delay introducing AAC strategies and techniques until the end of intervention nears and it becomes obvious that the restoration of natural speech will not be successful. Hence, although replacing natural speech with AAC strategies requires extensive training and practice by the individual with aphasia, speech-language pathologists often provide little opportunity for such training and practice during the acute rehabilitation period. Given this scenario, the existence of few reports documenting successful AAC replacement interventions for persons with aphasia is not surprising. The future success of AAC replacement efforts will depend on clinicians recognizing when such intervention is appropriate, introducing systems early, and providing extended training of speakers and listeners.

Supplementing Natural Speech

Greater success has occurred when speech-language pathologists have viewed the implementation of AAC strategies as a supplement to natural speech rather than a replacement for it. In these situations, natural speech may be adequate to meet certain types of communication needs, but the person with aphasia experiences communication breakdowns during other situations.

Garrett and Beukelman (1989) have written extensively about an individual with aphasia who used AAC strategies to supplement his natural speech. Although natural speech was adequate to handle many small talk exchanges, this person enjoyed telling stories and engaging people in extensive interactions for which his natural speech was not sufficient. To permit this type of storytelling interaction, his speech-language pathologist and his daughter—who served as his AAC facilitator—developed a communication book that contained numerous narratives. One of his favorites outlined the important events of his life with dates and relevant content about other people involved. Frequently, the individual engaged unfamiliar listeners in conversations by using natural speech to manage small talk interactions and using his communication book to communicate detailed information about himself. He would do this by pointing to statements about his life history and encouraging his listener to read the statements aloud. Then, he would make small talk about the identified events and, when finished, move on to a new item. When interacting with more familiar listeners, this individual used another portion of his communication book to relate narratives about his stroke and rehabilitation, his love for racetrack betting, his involvement in World War II, and his various work experiences. He also used and maintained a remnant book containing newspaper clippings, pictures, and agendas from meetings to convey information about current events that were important to him. Overall, the use of AAC techniques to supplement limited natural speech allowed this man to engage others in extended conversations.

Another example of using AAC strategies to supplement natural speech occurs when people with aphasia wish to participate in activities that require production of specific utterances. An example of this type of communication demand occurs during game-playing activities. As reported earlier, elderly persons often engage in game-playing activities, and persons with aphasia may retain the procedural ability to play common games—especially ones they knew well prior to stroke. However, people with aphasia may struggle with the communication demands of these games. In these cases, AAC systems designed to support specific activities can provide

a means to enhance the level of participation possible. For example, AAC systems can provide a means for people with aphasia to make statements such as, "Your turn," "I'm out," "Your deal," and "My turn."

Scaffolding Natural Speech

In addition to replacement and supplementation strategies, AAC can serve to scaffold natural speech. In this way, the listener does not interact with the AAC system itself, but, rather, the speaker with aphasia utilizes AAC strategies to compensate for his/her impairment.

An excellent example of using AAC strategies to scaffold natural speech was a man who acquired aphasia from a fall. Despite an extensive period of speech-language therapy, a deficiency in word-retrieval persisted. To compensate for this word-retrieval problem, the man would place three small notebooks in front of him at the initiation of a conversation. One of the books contained legal and medical information; the second contained a listing of places and individuals' names organized by geographic location; the third book was a collection of words that were particularly difficult for him to retrieve. As he spoke, he used the books to scaffold his recall and production of specific names, places, and events.

In addition to the three books, this man carried a plastic envelope of remnants from his life to assist in his telling of stories and narratives. The remnants included stories cut from the newspaper, bulletins from church, programs from plays, and a menu from his favorite restaurant. Some of these remnants had been in his envelope for a long time, but he changed others on a regular basis. Again, his strategy was to use the remnants to support his retrieval of specific words and scaffold his communication about recent life events. He did not routinely invite his listener to view the materials. Hence, although this individual used natural speech exclusively as his mode of communication, he relied on AAC strategies to support and scaffold his communication attempts.

AAC TECHNIQUES ACROSS THE APHASIA SEVERITY RANGE

As stated earlier, the traditional approach to treating persons with aphasia has focused on restoring natural speech, and clinicians have reserved the use of AAC strategies and devices predominantly for individuals with severe or profound aphasia. This tendency may reflect restrictions resulting from past funding policies for AAC equipment; however, these policies are currently undergoing revision, and availability of future resources is hard to predict. Changes in funding policies may prompt clinicians to initiate the use of AAC techniques and strategies earlier in the rehabilitation process. The authors of this chapter believe that AAC encompasses a wide range of strategies and techniques that can be used by people across the spectrum of aphasia severity in conjunction with residual natural speech. In fact, in the broadest sense, even normal speakers, without disability, utilize techniques in addition to speech during communication interactions, and, thus, are AAC users.

Speakers without Disabilities

Nondisabled individuals typically convey communicative intents through a combination of speech and nonverbal signals. The speech signal often carries the majority of the message burden, with nonverbal signals such as simple gestures or drawings acting as supplements or reinforcements. This distribution of message burden may shift, however, depending on speaker or environmental variations. For example, in noisy environments, speakers may find they need to use more gestures to convey a message than they typically use in quiet environments. When doing this, speakers are decreasing their reliance on natural speech and increasing their use of AAC strategies.

The Lindblom (1990) model of communication mutuality is an effective way to examine the relation between the amount of information conveyed through speech and through AAC techniques—that is, techniques other than natural speech. Figure 29–1 shows the Lindblom model as it might describe an adult speaker without communication disability. The vertical axis represents information provided to the listener through speech only. The bottom range designates conveyance of little information via speech and the top range designates conveyance of much information via speech. The horizontal dimension represents information provided from augmentative communication techniques. The left side indicates a low amount of information transfer and the right side indicates a high amount of information transfer through AAC techniques. Most individuals without disabilities rely primarily on the speech signal to communicate their intents and rely only minimally on means other than speech—such as gesturing, writing, or pointing to relevant objects—to convey information. Hence, a major contribution is represented on the vertical axis of the Lindblom model and a minor contribution is represented on the horizontal axis.

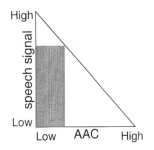

Figure 29–2. Lindblom (1990) model for a speaker with mild expressive aphasia. © David R. Beukelman, 1999

Speakers with Mild Aphasia

Figure 29–2 illustrates the communication burden shared by natural speech and AAC strategies for an individual with mild aphasia. As with nondisabled speakers, people with mild aphasia typically rely on natural speech to communicate much of their information. However, many people with mild aphasia experience anomia and have communication breakdowns because of an inability to retrieve highly specific information such as a person's name, a place, or a medication name. As a compensatory strategy, a person with anomia might rely on a word list to facilitate word retrieval. When used as prompts to cue the individual with aphasia, word lists are examples of an AAC strategy to scaffold natural speech. If the person with aphasia still cannot retrieve a specific word and shows the word list to a listener for him/her to read, it shifts from a scaffolding to a supplemental AAC technique. In either case, the person with mild aphasia conveys much information through the speech signal; however, he/she is likely to depend more on AAC techniques and strategies to support natural speech than is a nondisabled speaker.

Speakers with Moderate Aphasia

Figure 29–3 illustrates the typical relation between using natural speech and using AAC strategies for individuals with moderate aphasia. The greater degree of language impairment demonstrated by people with moderate aphasia limits their successful and effective communication of daily needs through natural speech. In this situation, AAC strategies can support residual speech and enable delivery of more comprehensive messages. At times, this additional information may supplement natural speech and, at other times, may entirely replace natural speech. Examples of AAC strategies

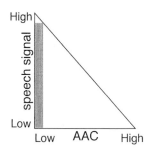

Figure 29–1. Lindblom (1990) model for an adult speaker without communication disability. © David R. Beukelman, 1999

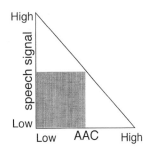

Figure 29–3. Lindblom (1990) model for a speaker with moderate expressive aphasia. © David R. Beukelman, 1999

commonly found to be beneficial to people with moderate aphasia include using gestures, pointing to items in a remnant book, writing individual letters or words, and drawing pictures. However, no one technique must be used by all individuals, and there is no limit to the number of techniques that may be successful for individual people with moderate aphasia; different situations, speakers, and listeners require the use of different strategies. Descriptions of specific AAC strategies and techniques that may be beneficial to people with moderate aphasia are provided in the next section of this chapter.

Speakers with Severe Aphasia

Expressive Impairment

Figure 29–4 illustrates the Lindblom model for a person with a severe expressive communication disorder. People with severe expressive aphasia are likely to communicate very little using natural speech; instead, they rely heavily on AAC strategies and techniques to communicate their intents. They can use many of the same techniques that benefit persons with moderate aphasia but will differ in their purpose for using the techniques and in the amount of assistance required from listeners. Although some individuals with severe expressive aphasia may be independent in using certain AAC techniques, others are likely to require a great deal of assistance from communication partners.

As an example of how AAC techniques can facilitate communication, consider the reliance that people with severe expressive aphasia typically have on others to set conversational topics. Using certain AAC strategies can greatly reduce this reliance. For example, one man with severe expressive aphasia organized his den at home so that important activities of his life were illustrated in different "centers" (Beukelman et al., 1985). One center displayed project books from his earlier work as an interior designer; the books contained photos and samples of tile, wallpaper, and paint from completed designs. Another center in the den dealt with family issues. A third center contained a VCR and a collection of videotapes of favorite sporting events. To engage someone in conversation, this man would lead a visitor to a certain area of his den, thereby establishing a topic of conversation. After exhausting one topic, he would introduce a new one by leading

his visitor to another section of the room. Hence, by using physical space in his den as an AAC device, this individual retained an ability to set conversational topics despite his severe expressive aphasia.

Many different types of AAC techniques and strategies can serve to supplement or replace the speech of persons with severe expressive aphasia. The most commonly implemented strategies include using picture or photograph books, referring to maps, and drawing simple pictures or diagrams. These and other techniques may require extensive partner support to be effective. For example, the written choice communication strategy described in detail by Garrett and Beukelman (1992) and Garrett et al. (1998) requires a communication partner to generate and write down potential topics of conversation and response options to verbal queries; the person with aphasia then selects the desired response by pointing.

Garrett and Beukelman (1989) provide another example of the importance of communication partners in their description of a man who selected the content of communication interactions from a book of personal, written narratives but depended almost entirely on his communication partner to produce speech. To initiate a conversation, this man would open the book and select one of the narratives (e.g., my life story, how I got my name, horse racing, what's happened to me lately). He would then position the book in front of his listener and point to an opening statement informing the listener to read the first paragraph aloud. Using one of his few stereotypic phrases to affirm, negate, indicate humor, or encourage the listener to relate a story about a similar experience, the person with aphasia would contribute to and encourage continued conversation.

Clinical examples such as these illustrate the importance of educating and training communication partners in AAC strategies and techniques. Adult children of people with aphasia often make excellent communication partners and may be available to attend intervention sessions as needed. Of course, clinicians do not have control over who serves as a communication partner to a person with aphasia or who is available for training (Garrett & Beukelman, 1992). However, once trained, one communication partner can educate other friends and family members in the use of specific AAC strategies and techniques that best facilitate communicative interactions.

Receptive Impairment

Most people with severe expressive aphasia have substantial receptive impairment as well. Figure 29–5 uses the Lindblom model to illustrate the relation between natural speech and AAC usage for individuals with severe comprehension impairments. In this case, AAC strategies and techniques serve to augment comprehension rather than expression, and the individual with aphasia assumes the role of listener.

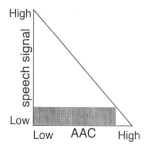

Figure 29–4. Lindblom (1990) model for a speaker with severe expressive aphasia. © David R. Beukelman, 1999

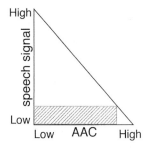

Figure 29–5. Lindblom (1990) model for a person with severe receptive aphasia. © David R. Beukelman, 1999

When conversing with a person with impaired receptive language, a speaker can facilitate comprehension through several augmentative techniques. For example, the speaker can point to pictures, maps, or objects, use gestures, or draw simple pictures or diagrams to help a person with aphasia grasp a topic of conversation. After establishing the topic, the speaker can provide further support by writing key words or drawing or pointing to additional pictures as he/she talks that focus attention on specific content information about people, places, and ideas.

Drawing is an AAC technique that can enhance both comprehension and expression. As explained by Lyon and Helm-Estabrooks (1987), drawing provides a dual means of supporting conversation because both communication participants—the person with aphasia and the partner—can contribute. When the person with aphasia assumes the role of listener, the partner can draw simple pictures or diagrams to supplement comprehension; when the roles reverse, the person with aphasia can use and add to the drawing to express his thoughts or opinions. Consider a conversation about the purchase of an automobile as an example of how drawing can play this dual role. The conversation might start with both individuals looking at pictures of cars. Then, the communication partner might draw certain feature options such as wheel covers, radios, sunroofs, and striping. Initially, these drawings could support the comprehension of the individual with aphasia. However, further in the conversation, the person with aphasia could use these same drawings to communicate a preference or opinion about the upcoming purchase.

ATTITUDES TOWARD AAC USE

Viewing AAC techniques as a natural part of communicative interactions—those generated both by disabled and nondisabled speakers—eliminates some of the stigma associated with using substitutions for natural speech. The extent to which some people with aphasia may need to rely on AAC strategies and techniques, however, raises concerns about the acceptability of these procedures to other people. In particular, the attitudes of peers and family members of people with aphasia need consideration. In addition, the attitudes of speech-language pathologists and other professionals are of interest, because the approval and support of these

people can influence strongly a person's willingness to adopt, implement, and continue using specific techniques.

Lasker (1997) examined the attitudes of three groups of communication partners who listened to a person with aphasia tell stories using unaided natural speech, a communication notebook, and a digitized speech output device. The three groups of communication partners were adult peers who had little or no experience conversing with individuals with aphasia, speech-language pathologists, and family members of people with aphasia. Using Likert scale ratings, Lasker found that all three communication partner groups rated the speaker most competent, most effective, and most understandable when he was using the AAC digitized speech output device and least competent, least effective, and least understandable when he was using unaided natural speech. In addition, all three partner groups reported the greatest anticipated comfort communicating with and the most willingness to interact with the person with aphasia when he was using the digitized speech output system. These results provide strong support for the notion that AAC strategies and techniques can greatly facilitate the ability of people with aphasia to convey information and be effective communicators.

However, concerns about AAC use and differences in the attitudes of the three communication partner groups emerged when Lasker (1997) asked them to rank-order their preferences of storytelling systems if they were the communication partner of a person with aphasia. Sixty percent of the adult peers selected the digitized speech device as the most preferred storytelling system; however, only 33.3% of the speech-language pathologists and 36.7% of the family members selected this communication mode as their most preferred system. Instead, both groups preferred natural speech (speech pathologists—46.7%; family members—43.3%). Even more striking differences were evident when comparing the least preferred systems: 76.7% of the adult peers, 16.7% of the speech-language pathologists, and 33.3% of the family members rated natural speech as their least preferred storytelling system. A clear distinction was evident in how people viewed the storytelling effectiveness of a person with aphasia who used an AAC device and their personal desire to be a communication partner with such a person.

Through qualitative analysis procedures, Lasker determined that a possible reason for these discrepant findings was the belief of speech-language pathologists and family members that, with additional training and effort, the person with aphasia could communicate successfully without the use of AAC devices. In contrast, the adult peers made no such assumption and reported acute discomfort when witnessing the person with aphasia struggle to communicate. In addition, the communication partner groups speculated that they would differ in their acceptance of various communication modes based on their familiarity and relationship with the individual with aphasia. When communicating with a family member or close friend, partners expressed a desire and willingness to be patient as the individual struggled to communicate with natural speech; however, with a stranger, partners preferred the rapid and efficient communicative interactions provided by AAC strategies and devices.

Clinicians need to be aware of differing attitudes toward AAC use by potential communication partners of people with aphasia. Differences exist dependent on the severity of the aphasia, the relationship between the person with aphasia and the communication partner, and the purpose of the communicative interaction. The roles of AAC facilitators include assessing the expectations and acceptance of AAC strategies and techniques by people with aphasia and their communication partners and educating clients and family members about the potential benefits and limitations of using specific strategies and techniques.

SPECIFIC AAC TECHNIQUES

AAC facilitators can assist people with aphasia to represent messages through a variety of techniques such as using gestures, drawing pictures, pointing to photos, or using electronic equipment. The use of these and other AAC techniques will vary depending upon the severity of aphasia and the contexts in which individuals find themselves. This section provides descriptions of many AAC strategies and techniques that people with aphasia can use to replace, supplement, or scaffold natural speech. One person may find that several of the techniques are helpful depending on the communication situation. Also, people with aphasia may need varying amounts of assistance from communication partners to use various strategies successfully.

Written Choice Communication

Written choice communication (Garrett & Beukelman, 1992) is a technique based on the notion that people with aphasia comprehend better when information is presented through multiple modalities rather than a single modality. To perform written choice communication, a communication partner and a person with aphasia decide a topic of conversation that is of mutual interest. Then, the communication partner asks a question related to that topic and generates word choices as possible response options. The communication partner says each word choice aloud while writing it in large block letters. The individual with aphasia points to the word choice that indicates his/her response or preference. The communication partner can then comment on the response and ask another question relating to the same topic. Questioning and responding continues until the topic is exhausted.

Many variations on the written choice communication strategy are possible. For example, the number of choices provided by the communication partner can vary depending

on aphasia severity. A person with severe receptive and expressive aphasia may need response options limited to two or three words; in contrast, a person with relatively good comprehension but severely limited expressive abilities may handle multiple response choices.

Another variation of written choice communication concerns the number of modalities used. Although traditional written choice communication uses simultaneous presentation of information through written and spoken modalities, research by Lasker et al. (1997) has shown that some people with aphasia do not need both modalities to have successful communication exchanges. For example, some people with aphasia can provide accurate responses when options are said aloud and are accompanied by written numbers rather than words. In this case, the person with aphasia points to the number that corresponds to the desired response.

Yet another variation of the written choice communication strategy is to use it in conjunction with other AAC strategies such as rating scales. The use of rating scales as an AAC technique will be described later in this section.

Gestures

When behaviors such as facial expressions, eye movements, body positions, and arm or hand movements convey specific messages, they are referred to as gestures. People use gestures to indicate wants and needs (e.g., raising a curved hand to the mouth to indicate a desire to drink); to convey feelings, likes, and dislikes (e.g., wrinkling the nose to indicate dislike or displeasure); and to give directives to others (e.g., pointing to a chair to instruct someone to sit down). People use gestures to replace or to supplement natural speech.

Persons with severe aphasia often attempt to incorporate numerous gestures as an immediate compensation for their communication challenges. When others can easily interpret these gestures, speech-language pathologists need to encourage their use as a simple and socially accepted means of supplementing spoken language. At other times, however, the attempts of people with severe aphasia to use gestures confuse rather than assist listeners in understanding messages. Physical limitations and challenges comprehending common events may alter a person's ability to gesture in a manner that is understood by communication partners. When a person with aphasia uses gestures in idiosyncratic ways, developing a gesture dictionary for communication partners may be helpful (Beukelman & Mirenda, 1998).

Remnant Books

A remnant book is a collection of items or mementos that are important to an individual and that reflect recent life experiences. Remnants that people with aphasia might want to collect include items such as a speeding ticket given to a spouse, programs from athletic events, price tags from newly purchased clothing, racing forms from the track, and swatches of fabric from recent sewing projects. These remnants can be used in a variety of ways, with one of the most common being presentation of a remnant to establish a topic of conversation. For example, an individual may point to a church bulletin to initiate a conversation about church. Remnant books for people with aphasia need frequent updating to remain current and useful.

Electronic Communication Devices for Expression

Electronic communication devices provide a voice output option for those who cannot express themselves through speech. Detailed descriptions of these devices are provided elsewhere (Beukelman & Mirenda, 1998; Glennan & DeCoste, 1997) and will not be summarized here. In general, these devices support two general types of expression: message retrieval and message formulation.

Some electronic communication devices provide a means for storing and retrieving with a single activation an entire phrase, sentence, or narrative. This message retrieval strategy allows for efficient communication of messages that must be spoken promptly or are lengthy. For persons with severe aphasia, these messages are usually pre-stored by someone with normal language capabilities and retrieved by selection of a graphic symbol, photograph, word, or short phrase that represents the message. Typically, persons with aphasia do not use message retrieval strategies to communicate all of their messages but, rather, to support specific communication functions such as small talk, requests for assistance, warnings, and stories. They use other strategies such as drawing, referring to remnant books, gesturing, and using residual natural speech to communicate other message functions.

In addition to message retrieval strategies, some electronic communication devices support message formulation through letter-by-letter spelling or word-by-word strategies. Although message formulation strategies have been used extensively by persons with physical disabilities, the cognitive-linguistic demands of message formulation strategies exceed the capability of many persons with aphasia.

Drawing for Expression

Some individuals with aphasia can supplement their natural speech with drawing. For example, drawing a sketch of a situation can serve to establish a topic or guide a conversation. Drawing a map can communicate information about location, such as where a child lives or the destination of a recent trip. Still other drawings can assist in resolving communication breakdowns by conveying preferences regarding decisions.

Often, people with aphasia have never before attempted drawing as a supplement to natural speech (Lyon, 1995); although it is available to speakers without disabilities,

many do not feel comfortable with their artistic ability and, hence, choose not to use drawing as a frequent means of supporting communication attempts. For the person with aphasia, normal concerns about limited artistic ability may be compounded by concerns about having to use the nondominant hand. Because of these insecurities, clinicians and family members need to be especially encouraging when asking people with aphasia to attempt drawing. Once they conquer their initial reservations, many individuals with aphasia find that simple, stereotypic drawings can provide substantial support to their communication attempts.

Partner Drawing

A communication partner can use drawing to supplement verbal or printed information given to a person with aphasia. In these instances, the communication partner draws a simple picture or sketch to establish a topic of conversation or to relate information about specific details. Drawing provides an additional modality for conveying information to the person with aphasia, thus facilitating overall comprehension. In addition, as a conversation continues, both the communication partner and the person with aphasia can add to or alter the original picture to convey additional information or preferences.

Another use for partner drawing is in conjunction with other AAC methods. For example, drawing can serve as an alternative modality to printed words when engaging in written choice communication interactions. Specifically, some people with aphasia may be more successful using the written choice communication strategy when their communication partners draw pictures rather than write single words or phrases as response options.

Communication Book (Generic)

A generic communication book is a beneficial system for people with aphasia who have limited expressive capabilities or who require extensive assistance with word finding. Typical sections of a generic communication book include wants/needs (e.g., bathroom, drink, chair), feelings (e.g., sad, tired, hungry), clothing (e.g., robe, shoes, pants), and locations (doctor's office, restaurant, home). Symbols, pictures, and/or words represent the individual items within each category. The person with aphasia can use the book either to respond to questions or to initiate conversations by turning to the appropriate section and pointing to the desired symbol.

Communication Book (Personalized)

Personalized communication books are extensions of generic communication books. A person with limited expressive capabilities or word-finding challenges can use the book to assist in conveying messages. The personalized communication book is usually developed over an extended period of time either during or following rehabilitation. In addition to the sections included in a generic communication book, a personalized book contains sections related to specific aspects of an individual's life. For example, a personalized communication book might include a section entitled, "About me," that provides important personal information such as date of birth, current address and phone number, educational and work history, date of marriage, children's and grandchildren's names and ages, date of retirement, etc. Other sections might include favorite places to visit or shop, names of special friends and family members, and information about a favorite hobby or leisure activity. Again, symbols, pictures, and/or words can represent the individual items in each category, and the person with aphasia either responds to questions or initiates conversations by turning to the appropriate section in the book and pointing to the desired symbol. Clinicians need to train family members and other communication partners to ask specific questions of people with aphasia and to assist them in locating information in the book.

Family or caregiver input is essential when developing a personalized communication system to ensure inclusion of important and accurate information. Many times, family members enjoy participating in the construction and arrangement of pages included in the book. Although many pages do not require revision, some will need routine updating.

Alphabet Board

A standard alphabet board can supplement communication attempts in a number of ways. For example, a person who has aphasia and an accompanying motor speech disorder affecting intelligibility can use it to point to the first letter of each word he/she says. This serves to assist a listener in comprehending. When necessary, the person with aphasia can provide the listener with the first several letters of a word or an entire word to facilitate comprehension. Another use of alphabet boards is to assist with the retrieval of specific words during anomic episodes. Sometimes an individual can retrieve the first letter of a word despite difficulty recalling the entire word. Having the first letter may provide the listener with sufficient information to guess the intended word and, thereby, resolve a communication breakdown. Similarly, during instances of anomia, a communication partner may determine the intended word and assist the person with aphasia to retrieve it by pointing to the first letter on an alphabet display. Alphabet board supplementation is too difficult for many persons with severe aphasia.

Word Dictionary

A word dictionary is a small book containing printed words that a person with aphasia has difficulty recalling or saying.

It may serve as a self-cuing device, or the person with aphasia can show a word to a communication partner for him/her to read. Because a word dictionary contains printed words that the person with aphasia must read, it is most appropriate for the people with mild or moderate aphasia. People with aphasia use this technique most successfully when referring to frequently occurring topics of conversation. In addition, most people with aphasia appear to have more success using word dictionaries that are organized topically rather than alphabetically. Some people with aphasia prefer to implement self-cuing dictionaries with inexpensive AAC devices so that they can cue themselves with a spoken message or word.

Picture/Photo Dictionary

A picture/photo dictionary is similar to a word dictionary; however, instead of printed words, the book contains picture communication symbols or photographs to represent words that the person has difficulty expressing. As with word dictionaries, a person with aphasia can use a picture dictionary for self-cuing, or he/she can show pictures to a communication partner to facilitate communication. Because picture dictionaries do not require reading ability, people across the severity continuum of aphasia can benefit from their use. Clinicians or family members can modify the complexity of the book by limiting or expanding the number of pictures included on each page and the number of pages in the entire book. A person with mild aphasia who has difficulty reading printed words can use picture/photo dictionaries to aid with retrieving specific words, while a person with severe aphasia may depend on a picture/photo dictionary to communicate greetings, needs, and basic thoughts.

Instruction Card for Listeners

Instruction cards can provide communication partners with information about how best to facilitate interactions with a person with aphasia. The cards typically describe specific procedures for assisting with communication interactions. For example, a card might begin with a statement such as, "I have had a stroke. I would like to talk to you, but I cannot speak. We can converse if you..." (Garrett & Beukelman, 1992). Highly specific instructions would follow to assist the partner in facilitating communication. Instruction cards often describe other AAC techniques or strategies that the person with aphasia finds helpful to initiate or maintain conversations or to resolve communication breakdowns. For example, an instruction card might provide directions for using written choice communication. Because they are highly personalized, instruction cards are helpful to people with varying severities of aphasia; however, people with relatively mild forms of aphasia may need cards only in unfamiliar or stressful situations in which anxiety increases the occurrence of expressive language challenges.

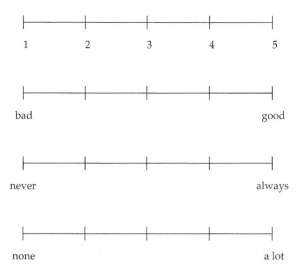

Figure 29–6. Sample rating scales.

Rating Scales

Rating scales allow people with aphasia to assign values to opinions. Typically, the endpoints of scales are labeled with numbers or single words indicating the spectrum of possible responses; intermediate points may or may not be labeled depending on the situation and the skills of the person with aphasia. Figure 29–6 provides several examples of rating scales that may allow people with aphasia to express opinions about a variety of topics. Even individuals with very severe expressive challenges may understand the notion of rating scales and find them an effective means of conveying opinions.

Eye Gaze

Eye gaze is a technique that allows people with severe expressive aphasia and accompanying severe physical limitations to indicate preferences. To implement the technique, a communication partner places a selection set of two or more objects, pictures, photographs, or words within view of the person with aphasia. By maintaining prolonged eye gaze at the desired response, the person with aphasia can indicate a preference. Successful use of the technique is highly dependent on the skill of the communication partner in selecting appropriate and meaningful topics and response options.

Summary

A single communication strategy rarely satisfies the wide range of communication needs left unmet by the residual natural speech of persons with severe aphasia. To be successful communicators, most people with aphasia must use a combination of strategies that vary depending on the communicative function, the interactional situation, and the listener. Hence, communication intervention for people with aphasia

must focus on the development of skills to support a variety of communication strategies. Initially, an intervention team needs to complete a multidimensional assessment to evaluate the speech and language strengths and challenges of an individual that will contribute to his/her overall communicative effectiveness and ability to master new communication strategies. Then, the team must develop and administer intervention services to persons with aphasia, family members, and other important listeners that will facilitate successful communication interactions.

FUTURE TRENDS

The field of AAC is relatively young, and it has evolved by focusing sequentially on the communication needs of various groups of individuals with severe communication challenges. Beginning about 30 years ago, AAC professionals focused on developing technology, intervention strategies, and financial supports to meet the needs of people with primary physical disabilities. Next, AAC professionals focused on the needs of persons with developmental disabilities who displayed cognitive as well as physical disabilities. During the past decade, technology and intervention strategies have been developed specifically for persons with cognitive challenges. Only recently have AAC professionals begun to focus attention on developing communication alternatives for persons with aphasia. With continued attention to the population of people with aphasia, the following developments within the AAC field should occur:

1. Professionals will learn to incorporate multiple communication strategies into the intervention programs of persons with moderate to severe aphasia rather than focusing almost exclusively on the restoration of natural speech and then turning to AAC strategies as a last resort.
2. Professionals will develop assessment procedures to reveal the residual skills and capabilities of persons with aphasia so that they can implement communication systems that take advantage of remaining strengths.
3. Professionals will develop AAC technology that accommodates to the residual strength profiles of persons with aphasia.
4. Speech-language pathologists, family members, and peers of people with aphasia will develop acceptance of various AAC strategies.
5. Professionals will develop service delivery models and financial supports to permit long-term interventions for adults with aphasia who make use of AAC strategies.

CONCLUSION

All individuals, disabled or not, use certain techniques that help them to be effective communicators. Although an individual may know a variety of strategies, he/she is unlikely to use them all in every communication situation. The speaker may begin a communication attempt by using specific techniques that have been successful in the past. If, however, feedback indicates the listener is not correctly understanding the message, the speaker can make modifications to aid comprehension. As an example, consider the communication style of a university professor conducting a chemistry lecture. Although he may have been successful in the past in teaching the lesson through lecture only, the same lesson may be confusing to a new group of students. When he realizes that students are not understanding his message, the professor may supplement his original lecture with drawings or written notes that further illustrate the concepts he is describing.

A similar situation is present for the person with aphasia. In treatment, clinicians can introduce a variety of strategies to replace, supplement, or scaffold communication attempts. Different situations may result in the need for a single AAC strategy or for a combination of two or more AAC strategies. In addition, the level of assistance needed to use a strategy effectively will vary with the degree of severity of aphasia. The person with mild aphasia may require no assistance; the person with moderate aphasia may need only occasional help; and the person with severe aphasia may be highly dependent on a communication partner for successful implementation of one or more AAC techniques.

It is critical, then, that treatment include not only the person with aphasia, but also family, caregivers, or others who play an active role in the person's daily living. All persons involved must be aware of the techniques that are most successful for a particular person in specific situations, the procedures for implementing various techniques, and the cues needed to encourage the person with aphasia to initiate use of the strategy.

Approximately 70% of individuals who survive a stroke causing aphasia report feeling that people avoid them because of their communication challenges (National Aphasia Association, 1987). Although many of these individuals will receive intervention services from speech-language pathologists, about 72% will never return to work (National Aphasia Association, 1987), at least in part because of their communication difficulties. The responsibility of speech-language pathologists is to minimize as much as possible the negative impact of aphasia on individuals' lives. AAC strategies, techniques, and devices need to be included as components of intervention programs aimed at improving the functional communication of people with aphasia across the severity continuum and in a variety of settings.

KEY POINTS

1. Contour of a conversation
2. Communication patterns of elderly and young adults
3. Challenges of people with aphasia related to conversational segments
4. Role of AAC and aphasia
5. Differences between replacing, supplementing, and scaffolding natural speech
6. Use of AAC strategies and techniques during communicative intents
7. Use of AAC strategies and techniques with persons with mild, moderate, and severe aphasia
8. Use of AAC strategies and techniques to augment comprehension
9. Specific AAC strategies and techniques
10. Amount of assistance required when using AAC strategies and techniques based on severity of aphasia
11. Importance of teaching family members and caregivers

Questions for Reflection

1. Why is the contour of a conversation important when considering AAC intervention programs for people with aphasia?
2. How do the aspects of a conversation and communication patterns of elderly adults and young adults differ?
3. Which component of the conversational segment is the most challenging for persons with aphasia? Why?
4. How do the communication impairments affect typical communication patterns in persons with aphasia?
5. What is the role of AAC and aphasia?
6. Describe the difference between replacing natural speech, supplementing natural speech, and scaffolding natural speech.
7. Describe how a speaker without a communication disorder uses AAC strategies during communicative intents.
8. How do speakers with mild aphasia utilize AAC strategies and techniques? Is the primary purpose to scaffold, supplement, or replace?
9. How do speakers with moderate aphasia utilize AAC strategies and techniques? Is the primary purpose to scaffold, supplement, or replace?
10. How do speakers with severe aphasia utilize AAC strategies and techniques? Is the primary purpose to scaffold, supplement, or replace?
11. Give an example of how AAC can augment comprehension.
12. What are some of the specific AAC techniques discussed in the chapter?
13. How does the severity of aphasia affect the amount of assistance needed to use various AAC strategies and techniques?

14. Why should family members and caretakers of people with aphasia learn AAC strategies/techniques?

References

Beukelman, D. & Mirenda, M. (1998). Augmentative communication: Management of children and adults with severe communication disorders (2nd ed.). Baltimore, MD: Paul H. Brookes.

Beukelman, D., Yorkston, K., & Dowden, P. (1985). *Communication augmentation: A casebook of clinical management.* Austin, TX: Pro-Ed.

Coleman, P. (1986). *Aging and reminiscence processes.* New York: Houghton Mifflin.

Garrett, K.L. & Beukelman, D.R. (1992). Augmentative communication approaches for persons with severe aphasia. In K. Yorkston (ed.), *Augmentative communication in the medical setting* (pp. 245–321). Tucson, AZ: Communication Skill Builders.

Garrett, K.L. & Beukelman, D.R. (1989). A comprehensive augmentative communication system for an adult with Broca's aphasia. *Augmentative and Alternative Communication, 5,* 55–61.

Garrett, K.L., Beukelman, D.R., & Mirenda, M. (1998). Adults with severe aphasia. In D. Beukelman & P. Mirenda (eds.). *Augmentative communication: Management of children and adults with severe communication disorders* (2nd ed.) (pp. 465–500). Baltimore, MD: Paul H. Brookes.

Glennan, S. & DeCoste, D. (1997). *Handbook of augmentative and alternative communication.* San Diego, CA: Singular Publishing Group.

Goodglass, H. (1980). Naming disorders in aphasia and aging. In L. Obler & M. Albert (eds.), *Language and communication in the elderly: Clinical, therapeutic, and experimental issues* (pp. 37–45). Lexington, MA: Lexington Books.

King, J., Spoeneman, T., Stuart, S., & Beukelman, D. (1995). Small talk in adult conversations. *Augmentative and Alternative Communication, 11,* 260–264.

Kynette, D., & Kemper, S. (1986). Aging and the loss of grammatical forms: A cross-sectional study of language performance. *Language and Communication, 6,* 65–72.

Lasker, J. (1997). Effects of storytelling mode on partners' communicative ratings of an adult with aphasia (Doctoral dissertation, University of Nebraska—Lincoln, 1997). *Dissertation Abstracts International,* 59-02B, 0627.

Lasker, J., Ball, L., Beukelman, D., Bringewatt, J., Stuart, S., & Marvin, C. (1996). Small talk across the lifespan: AAC vocabulary selection. Presentation at the American Speech-Language-Hearing Association conference, Seattle, WA.

Lasker, J., Hux, K., Garrett, K., Moncrief, E., & Eischeid, T. (1997). Variations on the written choice communication strategy for individuals with severe aphasia. *Augmentative and Alternative Communication, 13,* 108–116.

Lindblom, B. (1990). On the communication process: Speaker-listener interaction and the development of speech. *Augmentative and Alternative Communication, 6,* 220–230.

Lyon, J. (1995). Drawing: Its value as a communication aid for adults with aphasia. *Aphasiology, 9,* 33–94.

Lyon, J., & Helm-Estabrooks, N. (1987). Drawing: Its communication significance for expressively restricted aphasic adults. *Topics in Language Disorders, 8,* 61–71.

National Aphasia Association (1987). The impact of aphasia on patient and family: Results of a needs survey. New York: National Aphasia Association.

National Aphasia Association (1998). Aphasia fact sheet [On-line]. Available: *http://www.aphasia.org/NAAfactsheet.html.*

Riegel, K. & Riegel, R. (1964). Changes in associative behavior during later years of life: A cross-sectional analysis. *Vita Humana, 7,* 1–32.

Schank, R. (1990). *Tell me a story: A new look at real and artificial memory.* New York: Charles Scribner & Sons.

Stuart, S. (1991). Topic and vocabulary use patterns of elderly men and women of two age cohorts. Doctoral dissertation, University of Nebraska-Lincoln, Lincoln, NE.

Stuart, S., Vanderhoof-Bilyeau, D., & Beukelman, D.R. (1993). Topic and vocabulary use patterns of elderly women. *Augmentative and Alternative Communication, 9,* 95–110.

Ulatowska, H.K., Cannito, M.P., Hayashi, M.M., & Fleming, S.G. (1985). *The aging brain: Communication in the elderly.* San Diego, CA: College Hill Press.

Vischer, A. (1967). *On growing old.* Boston: Houghton Mifflin.

Chapter 30

Use of Amer-Ind Code by Persons with Severe Aphasia

Paul R. Rao

OBJECTIVES

As a result of reviewing and understanding this chapter, the reader will be able to define Amer-Ind Code and describe the populations it has been used with; describe the three main uses of Amer-Ind Code in the neurogenic population; identify the overall transparency of Amer-Ind Code to the layperson; list at least five techniques that enhance Amer-Ind Code transmission; list at least ten Amer-Ind Code signals that rank high both in terms of degree of transparency and ADL relevance for persons with severe aphasia; outline the prognostic factors that might indicate a patient is a viable candidate for using Amer-Ind Code; describe an Amer-Ind Code treatment hierarchy; list at least two techniques that facilitate generalization of the use of Amer-Ind Code by persons with severe aphasia; and apply Amer-Ind Code to PACE therapy for both individual and group therapy.

OVERVIEW OF APHASIA AS A CONDITION THAT REDUCES SOCIETAL PARTICIPATION

Not being able to speak isn't the same as having nothing to say.

Anonymous

Aphasia has been defined as "an acquired impairment of the cognitive system for comprehending and formulating language, leaving other cognitive capacities relatively intact" (Davis, 1993 p. 10). Persons with severe aphasia are among the most likely candidates for a nonverbal approach to functional communication. Collins (1997) provides an operational definition of the most severe variety of aphasia as a "severe, acquired impairment of communicative ability, which crosses all language modalities, usually with no single communicative modality substantially better than any other. In addition, visual, nonverbal problem-solving abilities, as well as other cognitive skills, are often severely depressed and are usually compatible with language performances" (p. 134). This chapter will concentrate on persons with severe aphasia for whom traditional approaches of aphasia treatment may not have been beneficial or productive.

Another way of operationalizing the "functional issues" with severe communication impairment is to place this discussion within the framework of the World Health Organization's Revised Model of Consequences of Pathology (Lux, 1998): "Impairment (dysfunction at the organ level), activity (functional consequences of impairment that affect performance of daily tasks), and participation (social disadvantage resulting from an impairment or a disability)." Hence, in this context, severe aphasia would be an impairment that results in a disruption of language activity and a consequent reduction in the ability to participate in communication activities.

A definition of *participation* is "the nature and extent of a person's involvement in life's situations in relation to Impairments, Activities, Health Conditions, and Contextual Factors," (Lux, 1998) representing a "limitation of choice." It is precisely in this area of "choice" that the rehabilitation professional must attempt to maximize communication options. The following three macro approaches to aphasia rehabilitation may be employed to meet this challenge:

- *Enhance functional capacity* by assisting the person with severe aphasia to change behavior through functional communication treatment.
- *Reduce demands of the environment* by removing noise in the system (e.g., turning off the TV) and optimizing transmission of signals (e.g., having action pictures in a communication book available).
- *Provide assistive devices and/or alternative methods* by determining the menu of core needs and abilities, then training the person with severe aphasia in the use of alternative communication options to convey wants and needs (the use of Amer-Ind Code is an example of this approach).

NATURE OF LANGUAGE AND COMMUNICATION

Although the terms "language" and "communication" are frequently employed interchangeably, for the purposes of this chapter it is essential to distinguish them. Language and communication are not synonymous. Indeed, according to Holland (1975), adults with aphasia are better communicators than they are language users. She adds that "every aphasia therapist has experienced moments of superb communication with patients whose language was either minimal or unintelligible" (p. 4). Oral or manual language is a code with structured properties characterized by a set of rules for producing and comprehending spoken or signed messages. Functional communication, as defined by the ASHA Advisory Panel (ASHA, 1990), is "the ability to receive a message or to convey a message, regardless of the mode, to communicate effectively and independently in a given environment." While spoken language usually serves as the primary means for communication, the communication process also makes use of a variety of other tools such as intonation, facial expression, eye movements, and body gestures, including motions of the hand and the head. When language is used to communicate, language and communication may be said to overlap. However, when the language-impaired adult attempts to communicate, the differences between language and communication become clearly evident. This dissociation between language and communication is noted by Holland (1975): "It is usually suprasegmental, gestural, and contextual cues that are most heavily relied upon by the aphasics we have observed" (p. 4). This chapter will focus on Amer-Ind Code, a form of gestural communication that has been used as a functional communication tool to meet needs when language no longer works. See Rao (1997) for a comprehensive and current review of functional communication assessment and outcomes in persons with neurogenic communication disorders.

AMER-IND CODE: A NONLANGUAGE GESTURAL SYSTEM

Amer-Ind Code is based on Native American Hand Talk. According to Skelly-Hakanson et al. (1982), Hand Talk was developed thousands of years ago to provide communication among Native American tribes with widely different linguistic systems. In establishing the Amer-Ind Code adaptation, Skelly (1979) has deleted the more culturally specific of the historical signs as well as those deemed inappropriate for clinical use. Novel signals were created (e.g., drive) and several historical signals were modified before the system was standardized by Skelly (1981a) over the past decade. Amer-Ind Code is primarily a demonstrable, expressive system that was designed to meet the functional daily needs of adult surgical patients such as those with normal cognitive abilities who have had a laryngectomy (Skelly et al., 1975). Since signals represent concepts rather than words, Amer-Ind Code signals are discussed in terms of a repertoire instead of a vocabulary. Each concept may stand for several English words, since Amer-Ind Code does not follow a signal-for-word translation. Hence, the current clinically tested signal repertoire of 236 labels has an English vocabulary equivalent of nearly 2500 words. Of the 236 concept labels, 131 are normally executed by one hand and the remaining 105 signals are normally produced with two hands. The latter signals were adapted for one-hand execution for use with individuals who do not have both hands available for signaling, such as hemiplegic stroke patients.

The advantages of Amer-Ind Code are that it is concrete, pictographic, highly transparent, easily learned, and telegraphic, and it does not make use of functors or grammar (Rao & Horner, 1980). Amer-Ind Code is recognized cross-culturally, since its iconic basis provides a concrete representation of the referent object. The Amer-Ind Code repertoire is said to be universally recognizable, similar to the international road signs. Hence, when a signaler indicates thumbs down with a frown, the viewer recognizes the message as "bad." This "guessability" factor has been referred to as the signal's transparency. Brookshire (1997) notes that most Amer-Ind Code signals are comprehensible to message recipients without extensive training. He suggests that "a major problem with most other sign systems and languages is that the signs are not comprehensible to message recipients without training, so that patients who use them cannot communicate with untrained persons." (p. 434)

The transparency of Amer-Ind Code is an important research and clinical issue. Skelly (1979) and her colleagues completed several projects to document signal transmission, with the resultant claim that the corpus of Amer-Ind Code signals is between 80% and 88% "guessable" to naive viewers. More recent evidence suggests that Amer-Ind Code may be more accurately described as approximately 50% transparent to naive viewers (Daniloff et al., 1983; Kirschner et al., 1979). Doherty et al. (1985) described a mean transparency of 60% for 50 selected Amer-Ind Code signals. Campbell and Jackson (1995) also found one-hand Amer-Ind Code signals to be at 60% transparency to unfamiliar viewers. Although this transparency factor is much less than Skelly reports, it remains significantly more transparent than the 10% to 30% reported for American Sign Language (ASL) signs (Griffith et al., 1981). This latter form of gestural communication is often confused with Amer-Ind Code. ASL is the manual language of the deaf and is distinct from nonlanguage gestural systems such as Amer-Ind Code. One who does not know ASL would require each ASL symbol to be translated into his or her own language in order to understand what the message is. Griffith et al. (1981) reported that normal viewers

Section IV □ Traditional Approaches to Language Intervention: Specialized Interventions for Aphasic Patients

found ASL to be only 20% transparent. However, one who has never encountered Amer-Ind Code before would not require the Code to be translated, because of the aforementioned iconicity and transparency (Daniloff et al., 1983). Kirschner et al. (1979) have demonstrated that Amer-Ind Code is easier to learn in a brief period of time and is retained more easily than ASL signs. Even within ASL signs, the role of iconicity in sign language learning has been found to be a crucial factor in sign recognition and retention. Lieberth and Gamble (1991) found that "iconicity may play an important role in the selection of an initial lexicon for the non-verbal client. Iconic signs may be learned more easily and quickly and retained longer than non-iconic signs" (p. 90). (See also Lloyd et al. [1985] for a comprehensive discussion of iconicity in sign acquisition.)

Amer-Ind Code's superior gestural transparency and retention, in conjunction with its relative ease of production, has prompted several investigators to suggest that iconic, simple signals are the easiest ones to teach individuals with a severe communication impairment (Coelho, 1990, 1991; Duncan & Silverman, 1978; Fristoe & Lloyd, 1980; Lloyd & Daniloff, 1983; Rao & Horner, 1980; Skelly, 1979). Davis (1993) concludes that many persons with aphasia do not have a pantomime recognition deficit and it is usually mild if they do have it (p. 82). If this intuitive clinical hypothesis is accurate, Amer-Ind Code would indeed be an appropriate gestural system to facilitate functional communication in brain-injured adults.

Amer-Ind Code Populations

Amer-Ind Code has been used successfully with the following four populations (Skelly, 1979):

1. Linguistically intact, for example, after glossectomy or patients on voice rest
2. Linguistically delayed, for example, developmentally delayed
3. Linguistically disordered, for example, persons with aphasia
4. Linguistically intact with a phonological or motor speech disorder, for example, persons with verbal apraxia or anarthria

Amer-Ind Code Validation Studies

The ability for adults with aphasia to recognize Amer-Ind Code signals was first studied by Daniloff et al. (1982). This study examined the relationship between the impairment of Amer-Ind Code recognition and the severity of aphasia and primary language skills. Administration of an Amer-Ind Recognition Test to 15 subjects with aphasia resulted in all subjects performing equally well, regardless of their aphasia severity classification. These data contrast markedly with the school that studied pantomime rather than Amer-Ind Code.

Duffy and Duffy (1981), who studied pantomime rather than Amer-Ind Code, concluded that there is a clear and significant association between gesture recognition and production and language under the umbrella term "asymbolia." According to these authors, "Aphasia is best understood as a general impairment of symbolic communication that includes nonverbal as well as verbal deficits."

This line of research was further investigated by Coelho and Duffy (1987) when they studied the relationship between successful acquisition of manual signs (n = 37, 23 of which were Amer-Ind Code signals) and degree of aphasia severity in 12 subjects with chronic, varying degrees of severe aphasia. This study demonstrated a clear and significant relationship between aphasia severity and success in the acquisition and generalization of manual signs. Results also suggest that there may be a threshold of aphasia severity below which acquisition of manual signs is negligible (e.g., a PICA below the 35th percentile). The apparent discrepancy between intact (Daniloff et al., 1982) and impaired gestural recognition (Duffy & Duffy, 1981) was investigated by Rao (1985), who found no differences between normal persons and brain-injured subjects on the Amer-Ind Recognition Test (n = 50 Amer-Ind Code signals), but a significant difference on Amer-Ind imitation (subject imitating examiner's 50 signals) and production tasks (subject demonstrating object usage of 10 pictured items).

Beyond the transparency issues between Amer-Ind Code and ASL that were discussed earlier, several studies also examined other contrasting issues between these two distinct gestural systems. Daniloff et al. (1986) examined Amer-Ind Code versus ASL recognition and imitation in aphasia and found that Amer-Ind Code signals were consistently easier to recognize and imitate than matched ASL signs. In another study, Guilford et al. (1982) explored the acquisition and use of Amer-Ind Code versus ASL. Their eight adult subjects with aphasia received 2 hours of instruction for 4 weeks on 20 signs from each system. Results indicated that there was no difference in the subjects' ease of acquisition between the sign systems. However, this study defined "acquisition and use" as the ability to produce a sign on command. It must be cautioned that this ability does not ensure that the patient will be able to use these signs spontaneously to meet activities of daily living (ADL) needs. Finally Daniloff and Vegara (1984) studied the motoric constraints for Amer-Ind Code formation versus ASL. They compared the 236 Amer-Ind Code signals and their ASL counterparts. It was found that ASL signs were indeed more complex than Amer-Ind Code signals, since ASL requires the use of two hands rather than one, involves a greater variety of hand shapes, requires more overall movement, and necessitates a greater number of changes in hand orientation during production. In sum, Amer-Ind Code has generally been found to be superior to ASL in terms of the recognition, imitation, and production of the two systems by adults with aphasia.

Amer-Ind Code Selection Considerations

Prior to selection of Amer-Ind Code for use with a communicatively impaired individual, the clinician must decide if the patient's skills are appropriate for such a system and if the system has the potential for meeting the patient's functional communication needs. Yorkston and Dowden (1984) concluded that appropriate selection of a gestural system is dependent on the clinician's understanding of the characteristics of each system, "specifically the symbolic load, motoric complexity, and communicative function of the system." Musselwhite and St. Louis (1988) list many other factors that must be considered in matching an unaided signal or symbol system to an individual with a severe communication impairment. These other factors include cognitive abilities, size of vocabulary, grammatical structure of system, and ease of learning (transparency, availability of communication partners, and availability of support methods and training). Analyzing these potent factors and considering the above validation studies, it may be concluded that, at least for severely impaired adults with aphasia, Amer-Ind Code is superior to ASL in achieving functional communication.

USES OF AMER-IND CODE BY PERSONS WITH APHASIA

Amer-Ind Code has three potential applications for the person with aphasia: (a) as an alternative means of communication, (b) as a facilitator of verbalization, and (c) as a deblocker of other language modalities. In 1979, Skelly reported on six earlier projects summarizing the use of Amer-Ind Code by 161 adults with aphasia. The results of these projects, although fairly positive, were often flawed by poor subject controls, no therapy control, and haphazard designs. Christopoulou and Bonvillian (1985) provide a comprehensive literature review regarding the use of sign language, pantomime, and gestural processing in persons with aphasia. They concluded that many individuals with aphasia who fail to regain spoken language skills may retain the ability to acquire aspects of a manual communication system. "Overall, the aphasia subjects appeared to be less impaired in their visuomotor processing than in their auditory-vocal processing. The results, however, are not definitive enough to resolve the long standing debate as to whether or not a central deficit is present aphasia" (Christopoulou & Bonvillian, 1985). Several case studies are presented below to highlight the various uses of Amer-Ind Code with adults with aphasia.

Alternative Means of Communication

Heilman et al. (1979) reported on a patient with global aphasia following a left cerebrovascular accident (CVA). The patient was trained to communicate effectively with Amer-Ind Code. He learned 100 signals and was able to sequence them in a series of three or more. This study supports the impression that Amer-Ind Code can be used successfully with severe, even global, aphasics for meeting their daily needs. Rao et al. (1980) reported on the use of Amer-Ind code by four adults with severe aphasia who had no functional expressive language skills. Two subjects who had plateaued in traditional treatment were enrolled in an Amer-Ind Code program. The remaining two subjects were enrolled in both traditional and code programs concurrently on the commencement of their rehabilitation program. All subjects made progress as reported by the patient's significant other and supported by the clinician's impression, though pre- and post-aphasia test results did not reflect significant change. It was suggested that pre- and post-measures that tap linguistic skills do not appear to be the best indicators of a patient's communication progress using Amer-Ind Code. As Skelly (1977) pointed out in an early Amer-Ind workshop, "Just as we do not measure apples with a ruler, so we should not measure use of the code with a language measure."

Case Study

J.C., who presented with severe Broca's aphasia following a left CVA, was enrolled in a 6-month Amer-Ind Code treatment program. His admission Aphasia Quotient (AQ) on the Western Aphasia Battery (WAB) (Kertesz, 1980) was 17.4, and his discharge AQ was 27.10. However, perhaps more reflective of J.C.'s excellent attainment of functional communication skills was his discharge score of 129/136 on the Communication Abilities of Daily Living (CADL) (Holland, 1980). In addition, he demonstrated a 94% acquisition level of the Amer-Ind Code core repertoire on command and on written word stimulation. The patient served as a nonverbal volunteer at a VA Medical Center for 5 years after the conclusion of treatment, as a superior patient escort, demonstrating the merits of Amer-Ind Code on a daily basis.

Finally, R.J., a 72-year-old male with jargon aphasia, demonstrated the efficacy of aphasia treatment in general and a combined graphic and gestural approach specifically. R.J. presented with global aphasia as a result of a CVA in 1985. He had a 2-year history of aphasia treatment without notable results, followed by a 3-year hiatus from any form of therapy. At the request of the patient's daughter, a speech-language pathology (SLP) re-evaluation was conducted nearly 5 years post-onset and more than 3 years after the termination of any form of communication intervention. R.J. served as his own control in a single-subject experimental design examining the efficacy of a novel, intensive treatment regimen commenced 5 years post-onset. Treatment effects and/or spontaneous recovery were clearly absent as extraneous variables. Initially, R.J.'s aphasia was so severe and his language so perseverative that no formal testing could be administered.

Following 10 weeks of aphasia treatment that focused on gesture and drawing as expressive modalities, R.J. was discharged home. The patient's initial and final functional communication status was rated using the ASHA Functional Communication Measures (Larkins, 1987), in which 0 = totally dependent and 7 = totally independent. The results were as follows:

Functional Communication Measures	Admission Status	Goal	Discharge Status
Comprehension of spoken language	3	5	4
Comprehension of written language	2	5	4
Comprehension of nonspoken language	4	6	6
Production of spoken language	2	4	3
Production of written language	2	4	3
Production of nonspoken language	4	6	5

Results of Treatment

At discharge, R.J. had demonstrated:

1. Functional repertoire of 30 Amer-Ind Code signals
2. 90% accuracy on WAB (Kertesz, 1980) Word Reading subtest
3. 90% accuracy on WAB (Kertesz, 1980) Yes/No Questions subtest
4. The ability to draw ADL needs with a high degree of transparency

Customer Satisfaction

R.J.'s daughter corresponded 3 months post-discharge with the following testimonial:

This is to keep you abreast of how dad has sustained his progress since working with you. He has initiated "letters" to his son in California who writes to him every week. He also has written to me several times and enclosed a bird's-eye view drawing of his neighborhood with the streets labeled correctly and the route of his daily walk marked in red. His salutation and signature are correct, but the words in the text of the letter are copied randomly from books. Nevertheless, they are extremely heartwarming to receive and make us feel more connected to him. He is able to negotiate his medication with housekeepers and

relatives now. As you know, most of his medication was withdrawn, and so now he sometimes feels pain from his arthritis. Previously he would have panic attacks if he noticed any change of medication routine. Now he is able to trust that he is communicating, both sending and receiving accurately enough to adjust his own pain medication. At his son's wedding in Chicago, his brothers and sisters-in-law noted that he seemed more relaxed, happy, and healthy. *He indeed gestured and drew pictures for them and clearly indicated that he was happy with the results of his hospitalization.* I game him a VCR when he left here. He now indicates to his housekeeper through drawing that he wants a National Geographic, opera, or drama video rented for him. He also communicated with a drawing to my aunt that he needed a new razor. I can't tell you how full of gratitude my heart is toward you and everyone who worked with us at the hospital. Bless you and thank you.

Sincerely, K.J.

Conclusion

Results of R.J.'s 6-week SLP treatment regimen highlight significant receptive and expressive gains that were documented by formal tests, functional outcome measures, a consumer satisfaction measure, and periodic patient and family correspondence. Efficacy issues as well as significant implications for using unconventional treatment approaches with persons exhibiting chronic, severe aphasia were outlined in this case study. It is worth noting that the entire inpatient and outpatient stays were preauthorized, paid, and well documented. Can one put a dollar value on a 72-year-old individual, 5 years post–left CVA, who finally began to live life more fully as a result of rehabilitation? The customers (the patient, the daughter, and the payor) appeared to be quite satisfied with the outcome.

Facilitator of Verbalization

Skelly et al. (1974) reported on the effects of Amer-Ind Code as a facilitator of verbalization for apraxic patients without aphasia. She noted that all six patients had mastered 50 signals within the first 6 months and were able to interpret over 200 signals. In addition, Skelly reported an increase in verbal output when speech was accompanied by gesture. This increase of verbal output was confirmed by an increase in verbal scores on the Porch Index of Communicative Ability (PICA) (Porch, 1967). Skelly concluded that Amer-Ind Code was an effective facilitator of verbalization in nonlanguage-impaired patients with verbal apraxia. Rosenbek et al. (1989) "assume that verbal expression can be improved by the appropriate pairing of performances or with the systematic use of unique sensory inputs" (p. 218).

(See Rosenbek et al. (1989) for a detailed description of an Amer-Ind Code training program that was designed to facilitate verbalization. The three-step program consists of sign selection, training, and combining gesture with speech.) Dowden et al. (1982) attempted to answer the question, "Does Amer-Ind Code facilitate aphasic-apraxic verbal communication?" Using only two severely aphasic/apraxic subjects, they attempted to replicate the earlier study by Skelly et al. (1974). Unfortunately, their results fail to replicate the earlier Skelly study, since they found no measurable change from baseline on the PICA overall or on the verbal percentile following either training or maintenance. What they did find, however, was that one of their two subjects demonstrated a sharp decrease in the proportion of verbal responses and a marked increase in the proportion of nonverbal and combined responses on the CADL (Holland, 1980) following completion of the Amer-Ind Code treatment regimen.

Kearns et al. (1982) subsequently isolated the effects of gestural training in verbal production. They systematically trained two nonfluent subjects to produce individual iconic gestures and examined the facilitation effects of training on the subjects' ability to name trained items. The results of this study demonstrated that verbal production was not enhanced by gestural training alone. Improved naming was documented, however, once gestural training was accompanied by verbal production training. Hardin and Thompson (1983) replicated these findings and demonstrated that combined gestural-verbal training enhanced naming to a greater degree than either verbal training or gestural training done separately. In Hanlon et al. (1990), an Amer-Ind Code gesture was paired with naming in a comparison of Broca's, Wernicke's, and other types of aphasia. Naming was better with gesture only for nonfluent subjects.

In a related study, the use of gesture to augment verbal communication in conversation has also been reported in a case of chronic conduction aphasia once verbal improvement had ceased (Simmons & Zorthian, 1979). In a follow-up report, Simmons-Mackie (1997) notes that gesture has proven to be a useful channel with some conduction aphasia patients. "Initial practice of gestures without encouraging simultaneous verbal responses often reduces useless or empty verbiage. When used to facilitate verbal output, gestures seem to help direct the listener's and speaker's attention to the specific idea to be communicated" (p. 87).

Deblocker of Other Language Modalities

Snead and Solomon (1977) found that some patients with global aphasia comprehended more when Amer-Ind Code was employed. They therefore suggested that Amer-Ind Code should be incorporated in diagnostic and treatment strategies to increase the likelihood of "gaining entry into each global aphasic." Gesture has been included as part of a cuing hierarchy in testing (Porch, 1967) and as a language facilitator in treatment (Rao & Horner, 1978). (See section Efficacy and Prognosis in this chapter for a fuller description of the latter case.)

AMER-IND CODE TREATMENT

Core Lexicon

The selection of an initial Amer-Ind Code signal repertoire for adults with severe aphasia (Rao et al., 1980) was based on:

1. Ease of production
2. ADL relevance to a veteran population
3. High transparency

The Amer-Ind Code limited repertoire consisted of five sets of 10 signals that met the above selection criteria. It is suggested that clinicians consider each patient's unique ADL needs and motoric constraints and also consult the transparency data by Daniloff et al. (1983) and the Amer-Ind recognition data by Rao (1985) before arriving at a decision regarding a core Amer-Ind Code repertoire (consult also Lloyd & Daniloff [1983]). Sample contrasting needs that were included in the core lexicon were hot and cold, eat and drink, shave and comb, and yes and no. Rao (1985) found near-perfect performance of the left CVA patients with aphasia (n = 12 patients) on the Amer-Ind Recognition Test (n = 50 signals).

The fact that subjects with aphasia (Rao, 1985) were able to recognize Amer-Ind Code signals—even with difficult foils (motor, semantic, and semantic/motor)—as well as were normals underlines the obvious dissociation between language and signal processing. The following eight Amer-Ind Code signals were recognized by all normals, left CVAs, and right CVAs on the Amer-Ind Recognition Test: drink, glasses, fight, telephone, sleep, time, cold, and dive (Rao, 1985). Hence, an initial core of treatment signals should include ADL-type needs such as drink, sleep, cold, and time. Amer-Ind Code is an iconic signal system that appears to be well suited for use with adults with aphasia whose sign system is disordered, but whose signal system is intact. (See Appendix 30-1 for a partial listing of Amer-Ind Code signals and corresponding transparency levels.)

Treatment Suggestions

Skelly (1981b) has highlighted six procedures that enhance Amer-Ind Code signal transmission and comprehension:

1. *Slow down.* According to Skelly, 70% of problems of transmission are due to speed of signaling.
2. *Additive signal(s).* Generally, the fewer the signals, the better, though on occasion, more signals may be called for to convey a message.
3. *Alternative signal(s).* Patient and clinician should be able to signal a message in at least two different ways.

4. *Negative contrast*. Employ the negative to rephrase a message (e.g., mad not = happy).
5. *Questions*. In the event of a confused message, the receiver should clarify the message by signaling who, what, where, etc.
6. *Reality testing*. Set up a "mock" interaction with a patient and a trained Amer-Ind Code receiver to work out what the patient's real ADL needs are, such as buying medicine or getting a haircut.

Two customized Amer-Ind Code treatment approaches that were particularly effective in the previously described case of R.J. can be described as *communicating opposites* and *name tag cues*. In the case of *communicating opposites*, the clinician attempted to obtain generalization of gesture by using simple oppositional gestures—e.g., stop and go in a conversational group therapy session. When transitioning from a communication book to gesture, the clinician video-taped R.J. responding and then using gestures in a very limited but functional context. The stimuli that were selected were simple activities that one would encounter in a greeting such as hello, goodbye, come, go, stop, sit, and stand. The clinician would first model and verbalize, hello, and then expect/coach R.J. to reciprocate with a gesture for hello. Therapy would then proceed with the SLP coaching/verbalizing/modeling "come" and the opposite concept "go." The patient quickly picked up the nonverbal game/task of controlling the SLP's behavior by signaling "stop" and "go" or "sit" and "stand." Replaying the turn-taking on video was a startlingly positive awakening for R.J. that indeed his gestures were transparent and that for the first time in 5 years, he could actually control/direct another's behavior by the movement of his hand. A core group of simple gestures were functionally used in context with two positive results: (1) the means (gesture) met an end (modified SLP's behavior) … Amer-Ind Code actually worked, and (2) R.J. began swiftly generalizing the signals to other contexts without external cues or coaching. Come or hi or sit and stop quickly became part of R.J.'s repertoire. In the *name tag cue* scenario, the SLP communicated with the patient, team, and patient's daughter what the "gesture for the day" would be and then labeled same on a name tag that the patient wore on the left side of his person. Thus, on a given day, R.J. was to focus on and the team was to assist in generalization of one concept, e.g., drink. All who encountered R.J. on that given day would see the label "drink" and thus realize that "drink" was the gesture for the day that was to be elicited as part of each therapy session or visit. By the end of week 2, R.J. had over 10 "core gestures" that he had demonstrated functional use in a variety of contexts. This core list was included on another name tag on the opposite breast of his shirt, so that all team members and his daughter could, at a glance, know what R.J. could be expected to "know" and "use" to communicate his daily wants and needs. The rationale for this approach is that the team or other potential receivers of R.J.'s message reap

immediate benefit from knowing what they can safely elicit from R.J. in terms of gestures in a given context. Clearly, success begets success and practice makes permanent. The small external cue such as the gesture for the day labeled on a name tag paid huge dividends in facilitating frequent, successful communication with a variety of viewers. The *name tag cue* concept was no longer necessary when R.J. was discharged home and to out-patient therapy. In fact, by the time R.J. went home to his daughter, he was already moving toward a combination of gesture and drawing to communicate 100% of his needs.

Amer-Ind Code Treatment Hierarchy

Once the clinician has selected Amer-Ind Code as a treatment modality, the clinician then must determine where to begin. Periodically, one may see a person with global aphasia who not only is nonverbal but also is nonstimulable for using hand gestures. This nonstimulable, nonverbal patient would not yet be a good Amer-Ind Code candidate. Helm-Estabrooks et al. (1982) developed a treatment program to get just such a patient ready for a gestural treatment program. Their visual action therapy (VAT) is a method designed to train persons with global aphasia to produce symbolic hand gestures for hidden items. VAT employs a hierarchically structured, tri-level program that ranges from tracing eight objects with the hand, such as a hammer and a razor, to producing pantomimed gestures for absent objects. According to Helm-Estabrooks et al. (1982), VAT is a means to an end, and not an end unto itself. Once the patient has demonstrated the ability to produce simple hand gestures, VAT may be discontinued and the Amer-Ind Code treatment hierarchy initiated.

Rao et al. (1980) developed a treatment hierarchy for training persons with aphasia in the use of Amer-Ind Code. The hierarchy moves along the following task continuum:

1. *Demonstration*. The clinician demonstrates the use of gestures in functional communication situations before and after the treatment session to validate the code's communication value as well as its acceptability.
2. *Recognition*. The concept that "recognition precedes production" is probably valid in a gestural training program as well as in a verbal one. Can the patient point to an object from an array, once the function of a given object is demonstrated?
3. *Imitation*. The patient imitates selected gestures under various stimulus conditions.
4. *Replication*. Remember, practice makes permanent. The patient gestures a signal without a model in response to either a spoken or written command.
5. *Consolidation*. Review and refine recognition, imitation, and replication of signals. Begin use of signals with the patient in a natural communication environment outside of the clinic, stressing the use of the patient's core repertoire.

6. *Retrieval.* The patient is required to demonstrate/use the core repertoire in context and without a model.

7. *Initiation.* The patient initiates basic messages during gestural communication with the clinician or a significant other.

Collins (1997) offers a similar 10-step program designed to strengthen the gestural response in persons with global aphasia. A unique aspect of the Collins approach is the use of enforced delay in 3 of the 10 steps—e.g., "step 4, client imitates gesture after enforced delay" (p. 144).

A potentially useful training paradigm at the consolidation stage is a matrix approach introduced by Tonkovich and Loverso (1982). They trained four adults with chronic aphasia using various pairs of signals in a 4 x 8 matrix (four verbs and eight nouns), and found that each subject was able to acquire novel gestures in a relatively short period of time and to maintain these gestures over time. This last stage, generalization, is indeed the most difficult to achieve and the most critical one for independent functional communication. The crux of the training complaints with severely aphasic patients is that clinicians may establish gestural recognition and imitation and some use in therapy, but there is little or no carryover to functional communication situations. Coelho (1990) did find that moderately to severely aphasic subjects can acquire single manual signs and a variety of basic combinations. The key was severity—that is, those subjects who acquired the most signs were the least impaired. Generalization was attainable, but subjects required additional "extraclinical" training to become proficient in the use of signs to convey a message. This finding is consistent with that of Coelho (1991), who concluded that propositional use of manual signs by aphasic subjects rarely follows a routine of simple acquisition and generalization of signs to untrained settings. This crucial step *does not occur* without additional training in natural communication situations. The case of R.J. presented previously illustrates the following training strategies that proved invaluable in fostering generalization.

- *Address other nonverbals:* Prior to addressing a gesture for a given stimulus, facial expression, tone of voice, and other nonverbals were prompted. On presentation of a picture of ice cream, a smile and "mmm" sound preceded the gesture for eat or hungry.

- *Involve consumer in signal selection:* The original repertoire of 50 was "cut down" to 30 by the patient, who wished to delete gestural signals he did not need and signals for referents that he could either point to or draw just as easily or did not need.

- *Build in environmental support:* R.J.'s primary communication partners were oriented to Amer-Ind Code and were instructed to encourage R.J.'s use of gesture. Staff who were so oriented were housekeeping, nursing, dietary, the unit manager, and the receptionist for each therapy area.

- *Encourage risk taking:* Much preparatory time was spent fostering more and varied responses to a given stimulus. The patient was constantly advised that the absence of *any* response or initiative guarantees the absence of communication.

Amer-Ind Code Scale of Progress

The Amer-Ind Scale of Progress (Table 30–1) describes 10 levels of increasing competence in the use of Amer-Ind Code signals (Skelly, 1979). Skelly recommends that the scale be followed in training patients to use the signals, because it is believed that signal recognition, execution, and retrieval lead to self-initiation and propositional use. The highest levels include gestural facilitation of verbalization and, finally, verbalization with some gestural support. Hence, the scale of

TABLE 30–1

Amer-Ind Scale of Progress[a]

Level	Label	Description	Use
X	Transfer	Verbal more than 50%	
IX	Facilitation	Verbal less than 50%	Facilitation of verbalization
VIII	Propositional	Equivalence	
VII	Conversational	At least three interchanges	Alternative means of communication
VI	Initiation	One interchange	
V	Transition	Wavers between IV and VI	
IV	Retrieval		
III	Replication	Long-term memory—no model	
II	Imitation	Short-term memory Model present	
I	Recognition	Appropriate behavioral response to clinician's signal	Deblocker of other language modalities

[a] Adapted from Skelly, M. (1979). *Amer-Ind Gestural Code based on Universal American Indian Hand Talk.* New York: Elsevier.

TABLE 30-2

Deblocking via Gesture[a]

Auditory vs. Gesture Recognition		
Listen (object name)	—Point	60%
Watch gesture	—Point	100%
Point vs. Gesture Response		
Listen	—Point	60%
Listen	—Gesture	100%
Deblocking via Gesture		
Listen—then—gesture—then	—Point	90%

[a] From Rao, P. & Homer, J. (1978). Gesture as a deblocking modality in a severe aphasic patient. In R. Brookshire (ed.), *Clinical aphasiology conference proceedings.* Minneapolis, MN: BRK.

progress is a task continuum, the goal of which is achievement of any of the three potential uses of the Code with adults with aphasia.

The Amer-Ind Scale of Progress should be regarded as a treatment barometer that can be used to document progress in the use of Amer-Ind Code over time. It can also be used to determine which use of the Code is most appropriate for the patient, and which level is ultimately attainable.

EFFICACY AND PROGNOSIS

The crucial question in discussing a novel approach to aphasia treatment is, "Does it work?" Aphasiologists are concerned not only about whether aphasia therapy is efficacious but also about whether specific approaches are efficacious. The following case (Rao & Horner, 1978) supports the impression that not only does aphasia therapy work, but Amer-Ind Code in particular works. In this case, gesture was used to deblock listening, reading, and speech through a systematic pairing procedure (Table 30–2).

Case Study

P.J. is a right-handed 38-year-old male with a B.S. degree who was self-employed. He presented with aphasia following left-hemisphere surgery for aneurysm repair. The patient awakened from surgery "with a profound right hemiplegia and was mute." He was initially evaluated at 6 months post-onset (*with no history of speech treatment*), at which time he was described as profoundly aphasic, receptively and expressively. There was a paucity of speech overall; speech was spontaneously neologistic with poor imitation. Before Amer-Ind Code Treatment, the most striking residual ability was in the *gestural modality*. He recognized gestures, and he spontaneously produced gestures.

P.J. was provided an intense Amer-Ind Code treatment program, and within 8 months learned 80 Amer-Ind Code signals.

During training and stabilization of Amer-Ind Code, a deblocking program was conducted. That is, gesture by the clinician and by the patient was systematically paired on "both" receptive tasks of listening and reading and expressive tasks of imitation and naming. To summarize this case (see Table 30–3), prior to the Amer-Ind plus Traditional treatment course, *gesture was relatively spared both receptively and expressively.* Treatment involved systematic pairing of gesture with auditory stimuli and gesture with printed words (on the input side) and systematic pairing of gesture with verbal imitation and naming performances (on the output side).

Post-treatment status found input and output modalities to be significantly improved. It was thought that this was due to the increased automaticity of transcoding processes effected through gestural deblocking procedures. Using Amer-Ind Code signals, alone or in combination with speech, P.J. was a functional communicator at 18 months post-onset. Specifically, this means that P.J. could get his message across by using gesture expressively in three ways: gesture alone, a contemporaneous gesture-verbal combination, or a sequence of gestures followed by verbals.

Possible Prognostic Indicators for Amer-Ind Code Treatment

A tentative list of prognostic variables includes the following: residual language ability, visual recognition and reasoning ability, learning ability, modality preference (Is this patient willing to use gesture in place of, or accompanying, speech?), limb praxis, motivation, and acceptance.

Pretreatment abilities specifically pertinent to Amer-Ind Code, and perhaps the most salient prognostic indicators, include gesture recognition and gesture production, including object use, imitation, and spontaneous use. Horner (1980) summarized the Amer-Ind Code prognostic issue by noting that a patient is a good Amer-Ind Code treatment candidate if:

1. A preference for the verbal modality can be shifted to a preference for gestures.
2. Gestural recognition is preserved.
3. Manual/limb praxis is preserved in the presence of severe oral-verbal apraxia.
4. Manifest limb apraxia is predominantly ideomotor rather than ideational.
5. Manifest limb apraxia is mild or moderate rather than severe in degree, and perseveration is minimal or absent.
6. Dependence on real object and/or imitative cues for gestural production can be resolved rather quickly.

7. Transient cues are as effective as static cues in eliciting gestures.
8. Gestures can be stimulated with a broad range of stimulus types and methods rather than idiosyncratic cues.
9. Impulsivity can be controlled.
10. Most important, the patient demonstrates an ability to learn elicited or responsive gestures after trial therapy, and evidence for generalization across setting, however rudimentary, is observed.

APPLICATIONS OF AMER-IND CODE TO PACE THERAPY

G.G. is one of three subjects reported on by Rao and Koller (1982). He was 35 months post-onset before he was referred for a speech and language evaluation. As Table 30–4 reveals, the patient's biomedical background was fairly unremarkable, except for the fact that he had no prior history of speech treatment. Table 30–5 presents pertinent speech and language data that corroborate the initial diagnosis of moderate to severe Broca's aphasia and severe oral apraxia. Initially, Amer-Ind Code was employed with G.G. However, since G.G. rejected Amer-Ind Code as a sole means of communication, an attempt was made to incorporate the principles of Promoting Aphasic's Communicative Effectiveness (PACE) (Wilcox & Davis, 1981) into the treatment program. In general, PACE's multimodality approach incorporates the natural rules of communication.

TABLE 30–3

Receptive-Expressive Language Deblocking via Gesture[a]

PRETREATMENT		POST-TREATMENT	
Input	Output	Input	Output
GST	GST	AUD	GST
		VIS	VBL

TREATMENT	
Input	Output
GST + AUD + (VIS)	GST + VBL

[a] From Rao, P. & Homer, J. (1978). Gesture as a deblocking modality in a severe aphasic patient. In R. Brookshire (ed.), *Clinical aphasiology conference proceedings*. Minneapolis, MN: BRK.
GST = gesture, AUD = auditory, VIS = visual, VBL = verbal.

TABLE 30–4

Patient G.G.: Biographical and Medical Data

Biographical	Medical
Age: 56	Date of onset: 10-24-76
Sex: Male	Type of CVA: Left cerebral thrombosis
Education: High school	Sequelae: Aphasia and right hemiplegia
Marital status: Married, 8 children	Perception: Moderate high-frequency sensorineural hearing loss bilaterally; wears corrective lenses
Handedness: Dextral	
Environment: Home	
Occupation: Retired lumber inspector	Earlier medical history: Myocardial infarction (1972)

TABLE 30–5

Patient G.G.: Initial Speech and Language Findings (September, 1979)[a]

		Oral	Limb
ALPS (max 10):	Listening = 5.5; Talking = 1		
	Reading = 4.5; Writing = 5.5		
BDAE (auditory):	Word Discrimination = 64.5/72		
	Body Part Identification = 18/20		
	Commands = 14/15		
	Complex Ideational = 2/12		
PPVT (max = 50):	89		
Ceiling:	115		
TACL (max = 101):	82		
YES/NO (max = 20):	19		
Boston Naming Test (max = 85):	7		
Apraxia Battery (max = 4):	Imitation	2.3	3.6
	Command	0.7	2.3
Initial Diagnosis:	Moderate to severe Broca's aphasia and severe oral apraxia		

[a] ALPS = Aphasia Language Performance Scales; BDAE = Boston Diagnostic Aphasia Examination; PPVT = Peabody Picture Vocabulary Test; TACL = Test of Auditory Comprehension of Language.

Figure 30–1 indicates the greater flexibility in the patient's responsorium as a result of treatment incorporating the principles of PACE. Specifically, at treatment Session 1, the patient described pictures employing graphic or written responses 100% of the time. By Session 5, roughly half of the responses were graphic, one-third were gestural, and one-tenth were verbal. By Session 10, approximately 20% of the responses were graphic (writing a key word or drawing an action picture), 50% were gestural (Amer-Ind Code), and 30% were verbal (telegraphic but intelligible spoken descriptors). Hence, although overall

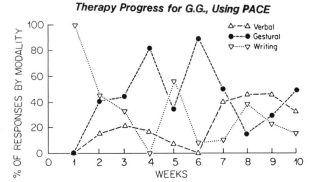

Figure 30–1. Flexibility in patient response as a result of treatment incorporating the principles of PACE.

communication accuracy may not have changed, G.G. did achieve greater communicative flexibility and success. (His spouse and 11 children verified that G.G. was a more effective communicator with more means to communicate.) His *participation* in society was maximized by increasing his options.

Although both Amer-Ind Code and PACE have essentially an expressive communication bent, Table 30–6 reveals a significant pre- and post-treatment change on the Boston Diagnostic Aphasia Examination's (Goodglass & Kaplan, 1972) complex ideational subtest (from 2/12 to 9/12). Also worthy of note on follow-up were the results of the Aphasia Language Performance Scales (Keenan & Brassell, 1975), wherein a nearly equal performance on each scale was obtained following an aggressive, multimodal therapy regimen. The discharge diagnosis of moderate Broca's aphasia was consistent with the clinician and family report that G.G. had improved considerably in these overall functional communication skills. In G.G.'s case, Amer-Ind Code played a definite, although ancillary, role in PACE therapy. Rather than resorting to simple pantomime as part of PACE therapy, Amer-Ind Code was used because of its well-documented high transparency (Daniloff et al., 1983) and ease of production (Daniloff & Vegara, 1984). Within the context of PACE therapy, it became obvious that the standardized corpus of Amer-Ind Code enhanced the efficiency and transparency of messages sent and received by the patient.

FUTURE TRENDS

Amer-Ind Code has a bright future in aphasiology in the current, rationed healthcare environment where "low-tech" methods and tools become the expedient option for getting to effective, functional communication fast! This chapter has reviewed the various uses of the Code with persons with aphasia and concluded that the Amer-Ind Code approach appears to be singularly beneficial with persons with severe aphasia. Future study should focus on clarifying the candidacy issue

TABLE 30–6

Patient G.G.: Pre-, Post-, Follow-Up Data[a]

	Pre	Post	Follow-Up
ALPS (max = 10)			
Listening	5.5	8.5	6
Talking	1	2.5	6
Reading	4.5	7	6
Writing	5.5	6	4.5
TACL (max = 101)	82	91	97
YES/NO Battery (max = 10)			
PPVT (max = 150)	89	103	95
Ceiling	115	114	127
BDAE Complex Ideational	2	9	9
(max = 12)			
Apraxia Battery (max = 4)			
Oral: Imitation	2.3	3.0	DNT
Command	.7	2.7	DNT
Limb: Imitation	3.6	4.0	DNT
Command	2.3	3.0	DNT

Final Diagnosis: Moderate Broca's aphasia and mild oral apraxia

[a] ALPS = Aphasia Language Performance Scales; BDAE = Boston Diagnostic Aphasia Examination; PPVT = Peabody Picture Vocabulary Test; TACL = Test of Auditory Comprehension of Language.

even further. Are persons with Broca's aphasia better candidates than those with Wernicke's aphasia for the various uses of the Code? Is there a certain BDAE or CADL profile that suggests that Amer-Ind Code might be warranted? What level of the Skelly (1979) Scale of Progress predicts ultimate attainment and use of the Code? These questions must be answered if clinicians are to make an informed decision on when and why to use the Amer-Ind Code.

Once the candidacy issue has been resolved, several treatment issues must be clarified. The first treatment priority is to involve the significant other in Amer-Ind Code treatment. Future case studies should include reports on the family's recognition and use of the Code in concert with the patient. If the patient and the family are trained to "think action" then the family and the patient will be more efficient in their "interactions." Once the patient and family are gesturally oriented, should the clinician avoid the use of language in treatment? There is controversy on this issue even among long-time Amer-Ind Code users. Skelly (1981b) strongly encourages a nonvocal approach with severe and global aphasics, while Rao et al. (1980) have noted improved auditory comprehension when employing a "talk and hand talk" approach to Amer-Ind Code. Tomorrow's clinicians deserve to know the optimal mode of signal presentation. The future will also see discussion of the following issues:

• How many sessions of therapy in how many weeks to achieve a functional outcome?

- Benefits of programmed video gestural practice vs traditional instruction
- Refined lexicon prioritized in terms of easiest to hardest to teach
- Group versus individual aphasia treatment
- Homogeneous group treatment (aphasia) vs. a mixed group (variety of nonverbal patients in a conversational group)
- Amer-Ind Code plus Talking Pictures
- Action Amer-Ind Code Pictures versus Amer-Ind Code itself

These, as well as many other issues, will require much time and effort to resolve. However, based on its efficacy and popularity in many nations, it is not unreasonable to expect that Amer-Ind Code will become the International Code of aphasiologists.

KEY POINTS

1. Amer-Ind Code is an adaptation of American Indian Hand-Talk. Amer-Ind Code consists of 250 signals representing over 2500 words. In the case of one-handed adaptations of Amer-Ind Code, 136 signals can be easily signaled using one hand.
2. Amer-Ind Code for persons with aphasia has three main uses: as an alternative means of communication, as a facilitator of verbalization, and as a deblocker of other modalities.
3. The main goal of the SLP in managing a person with the impairment of aphasia is to increase the patient's active *participation* in society. The SLP does this by *enhancing the patient's functional capacity, by reducing the demands of the environment*, and *by providing assistive devices and/or alternative methods*.
4. Amer-Ind Code has been used successfully with the following four populations: linguistically intact, delayed, disordered, or intact with a phonological or motor speech disorder.
5. Amer-Ind Code has been found to be more transparent/guessable than ASL. Conservative estimates are that Amer-Ind Code signals are 60% transparent.
6. Selection of an Amer-Ind Code signal repertoire for persons with severe aphasia is based on ease of production, ADL relevance to the consumer, and high degree of transparency.
7. Skelly (1981b) highlighted six procedures that enhance Amer-Ind Code signal transmission and comprehension: slow down, the fewer signals the better, be able to signal a concept more than just one way, use negative contrast—e.g. not happy/mad, use questions to clarify the message, and do reality testing.
8. Rao suggests two simple therapy approaches to facilitate generalization of gestures into functional contexts: communicating opposites in role play and name

tag cues. In addition, Rao stresses the need to address other nonverbals, involve the consumer in the signal selection, build in environmental support, and encourage at least giving it a try!
9. Rao (1980) described a simple, seven-step task continuum of Amer-Ind Code acquisition beginning with demonstration and recognition and ending with retrieval and initiation.
10. Skelly's (1979) Amer-Ind Code Scale of Progress describes 10 levels of increasing competence in the use of Amer-Ind Code signals from simple recognition of gestures to transfer to the verbal mode when the patient is verbal more than 50% of the time.
11. Horner (1980) cited at least 10 prognostic indicators for acquisition of Amer-Ind Code, the most critical being the patient's demonstrated ability to learn.
12. PACE therapy (Wilcox & Davis,1981) was reported to be the most appropriate therapeutic approach used for eliciting gestures for functional communication. Patients should be encouraged to rely on a multimodal approach to communication including the use of drawing, gesture, tone of voice, writing, and talking.

REVIEW QUESTIONS

- Why is it logical to suggest that Amer-Ind Code might be a more appropriate nonverbal option for persons with severe aphasia instead of ASL?
- List the 10 most appropriate starter signals for a person with severe aphasia based on transparency data and basic ADL needs.
- Describe at least two techniques that have reportedly been successful in facilitating rapid generalization of the use of Amer-Ind Code by persons with severe aphasia.
- Describe, with a rationale, what assessment tools might be suitable when determining whether a given person with aphasia might be a suitable candidate for Amer-Ind Code treatment.
- Based on your experience with aphasia, why has a gestural approach NOT worked and what could you have done differently to make it work?
- There exist at least three suggested "task continua" for teaching Amer-Ind Code to persons with severe aphasia. Based on your readings and experience, what are the most natural and appropriate steps for introducing gesture to a person with severe aphasia admitted to an acute rehabilitation unit/hospital?
- In the current healthcare environment, what is the role of the family in becoming extenders for the patient needing to communicate nonverbally?
- If the patient is considered a "good" Amer-Ind Code candidate, but refuses any attempt to produce gestures, what

steps might you take to coach or motivate the patient to consider gesture as a viable communication option?
• Describe a research design that would assist aphasiology in providing additional data on the efficacy of gestural communication.

▶   *Acknowledgment*–Dr. Rao wishes to acknowledge the two hospitals where this work was conducted (the Ft. Howard VA Medical Center and the National Rehabilitation Hospital) and the patients who were studied, particularly G.G., J.C., P.J., and R.J.

References

American Speech-Language-Hearing Association. (1990). Functional Communication Scales for Adults Project: Advisory Report. Rockville, MD: ASHA.

Brookshire, R. (1997). *Introduction to neurogenic communication disorders* (5th ed.). St. Louis, MO: Mosby.

Cambell, C.R. & Jackson, S.T. (1995). Transparency of one-handed Amer-Ind hand signals to nonfamiliar viewers. *Journal of Speech and Hearing Research, 38,* 1284–1289.

Christopoulou, C. & Bonvillian, J.D. (1985). Sign language, pantomime, and gestural processing in aphasic persons. *Journal of Communication Disorders, 18,* 1–20.

Coelho, C.A. (1990). Acquisition and generalization of simple manual sign grammars by aphasic subjects. *Journal of Communication Disorders, 23,* 383–400.

Coelho, C.A. (1991). Manual sign acquisition and use in two aphasic subjects. In T. Prescott (ed.), *Clinical aphasiology conference proceedings (Vol. 19).* Austin, TX: Pro-Ed.

Coelho, C.A. & Duffy, R.J. (1987). The relationship of the acquisition of manual signs to severity of aphasia: A training study. *Brain and Language, 31,* 328–345.

Collins, M.J. (1997). Global aphasia. In L.L. LaPointe (ed.), *Aphasia and related neurogenic language disorders* (2nd. ed.). New York: Thieme.

Daniloff, J., Frattelli, G., Hoffman, P.R., & Daniloff, R.G. (1986). Amer-Ind versus ASL: Recognition and imitation in aphasic subjects. *Brain and Language, 28,* 95–113.

Daniloff, J., Lloyd, L., & Fristoe, M. (1983). Amer-Ind transparency. *Journal of Speech and Hearing Disorders, 48,* 103–110.

Daniloff, J., Noll, J.D., Fristoe, M., & Lloyd, L. (1982). Gesture, recognition in patients with aphasia. *Journal of Speech and Hearing Disorders, 47,* 43–49.

Daniloff, J. & Vegara, D. (1984). Comparison between the motoric constraint for Amer-Ind and ASL sign formation. *Journal of Speech and Hearing Research, 27,* 76–88.

Davis, G.A. (1993). *A survey of adult aphasia* (2nd. ed.). Englewood Cliffs, NJ: Prentice-Hall.

Doherty, J.E., Daniloff, J.K., & Lloyd, L.L. (1985). The effect of categorical presentation on Amer-Ind transparency. *Augmentative and Alternative Communication, 1,* 10–16.

Dowden, P.A., Marshall, R.C., & Tomkins, C.A. (1982). Amer-Ind as a communicative facilitator of aphasic and apraxic patients. In R. Brookshire (ed.), *Clinical aphasiology conference proceedings.* Minneapolis, MN: BRK.

Duffy, R.J. & Duffy, J.R. (1981). Three studies of deficits in pantomimic recognition in aphasia. *Journal of Speech and Hearing Research, 46,* 70–84.

Duncan, J.L. & Silverman, F.H. (1978). Impact of learning Amer-Ind sign language on mentally retarded children. In J.R. Andrews & M.S. Burns (eds.), *Remediation of language disorders.* Evanston, IL: Institute for Continuing Professional Education.

Fristoe, M. & Lloyd, L. (1980). Planning an initial lexicon for persons with severe communication impairment. *Journal of Speech and Hearing Disorders, 45,* 170–180.

Goodglass, H. & Kaplan, E. (1972). *Assessment of aphasia and related disorders.* Philadelphia, PA: Lea & Febiger.

Griffith, P.L., Robinson, J.H., & Panagos, J.M. (1981). Perception of iconicity in ASL by hearing and deaf subjects. *Journal of Speech and Hearing Disorders, 46,* 405–412.

Guilford, A.M., Scheuerle, J., & Shirek, P.G. (1982). Manual communication skills in aphasia. *Archives of Physical Medicine and Rehabilitation, 63,* 601–604.

Hanlon, R.E., Brown, J.W., & Gerstman, L.J. (1990). Enhancement of naming in nonfluent aphasia through gesture. *Brain and Language, 38,* 298–314.

Hardin, R. & Thompson, C.K. (1983). Facilitation of verbal labeling in adult aphasia by gestural, verbal, or verbal plus gestural training. In R. Brookshire (ed.), *Clinical aphasiology conference proceedings.* Minneapolis, MN: BRK.

Heilman, K.M., Rothi, L., Campanella, D., & Wolfson, S. (1979). Wernicke's and global aphasia without alexia. *Archives of Neurology, 36,* 129–133.

Helm-Estabrooks, N., Fitzpatrick, P., & Barresi, B. (1982). Visual action therapy for global aphasia. *Journal of Speech and Hearing Disorders, 47,* 385–389.

Holland, A. (1975). Aphasics as communicators: A model and its implications. Paper presented at the Annual Convention of the American Speech-Language-Hearing Association, Washington, DC.

Holland, A. (1980). *Communicative abilities of daily living.* Baltimore, MD: University Park Press.

Horner, J. (1980). Amer-Ind candidacy. Paper presented at a George Washington University Medical Center Neuropathology Symposium, Washington, DC.

Kearns, K., Simmons, N., & Sisterhen, J. (1982). Gestural sign (Amer-Ind) as a facilitator of verbalization in patients with aphasia. In R. Brookshire (ed.), *Clinical aphasiology conference proceedings,* Minneapolis, MN: BRK.

Keenan, J.S. & Brassell, E.G. (1975). *Aphasia Language Performance Scales.* Murfreesboro, TN: Pinnacle Press.

Kertesz, A. (1980). *Western Aphasia Battery.* London, Ontario: University of Western Ontario.

Kirschner, A., Algozzine, B., & Abbott, T.B. (1979). Manual communication systems: A comparison and its implications. *Education and Training in the Mentally Retarded, 14,* 5–10.

Larkins, P. (1987). *Program evaluation system.* Rockville, MD: American Speech-Language-Hearing Association.

Lieberth, A.K. & Gamble, M.E. (1991). The role of iconicity in sign language learning by hearing adults. *Journal of Communication Disorders, 24,* 89–99.

Lloyd, L.L. & Daniloff, J. (1983). Issues in using Amer-Ind Code with retarded persons. In T.M. Gallagher & C.A. Prutting (eds.), *Pragmatic assessment and intervention issues in language.* San Diego, CA: College Hill Press.

Lloyd, L.L., Loeding, B., & Doherty, J.E. (1985). Role of iconicity in sign acquisition: A response to Orlansky & Bonvillian (1984). *Journal of Speech and Hearing Disorders, 50,* 299–301.

Lux, J. (1999). Towards a common language for functioning and disablement: ICIDH-2 (The international classification of impairments, activities and participation). *Special Interest Division Newsletter, 9,* #1, 8–10. Rockville, MD: ASHA.

Musselwhite, C.R. & St. Louis, K.W. (1988). *Communication programming for persons with severe handicaps* (3rd ed.). Boston: College Hill Press.

Porch, B. (1967). *Porch Index of Communicative Ability.* Palo Alto, CA: Consulting Psychologists Press.

Rao, P. (1997). Functional communication assessment and outcomes. In B. Shadden & M.A. Toner (eds.), *Aging and communication.* Austin, TX: Pro-Ed.

Rao, P. (1985). An investigation into the neuropsychological basis of gesture. Ph.D. dissertation, College Park, MD, University of Maryland.

Rao, P., Basil, A.G., Koller, J.M., Fullerton, B., Diener, S., & Burton, P. (1980). The use of Amer-Ind Code by severe aphasic adults. In M. Burns & J. Andrews (eds.), *Neuropathologies of speech and language diagnosis and treatment: Selected papers.* Evanston, IL: Institute for Continuing Professional Education.

Rao, P. & Horner, J. (1978). Gesture as a deblocking modality in a severe aphasic patient. In R. Brookshire (ed.), *Clinical aphasiology conference proceedings.* Minneapolis, MN: BRK.

Rao, P. & Horner, J. (1980). Non-verbal strategies for functional communication by aphasic adults. In M. Burns & J. Andrews (eds.), *Neuropathologies of speech and language diagnosis and treatment: Selected papers.* Evanston, IL: Institute for Continuing Professional Education.

Rao, P. & Koller, J. (1982). A total communication approach to aphasia treatment in three chronic aphasic adults. Paper presented at the Semi-Annual Conference of the International Neuropsychological Society, Pittsburgh, PA.

Rosenbek, J., LaPointe, L.L., & Wertz, R.T. (1989). *Aphasia: A clinical approach.* Austin, TX: Pro-Ed.

Simmons-Mackie, N. (1997). Conduction aphasia. In L.L. LaPointe (ed.), *Aphasia and related neurogenic language disorders.* (2nd. ed.). New York: Thieme.

Simmons, N. & Zorthian, A. (1979). Use of symbolic gestures in a case of fluent aphasia. In R. Brookshire (ed.), *Clinical aphasiology conference proceedings.* Minneapolis, MN: BRK.

Skelly, M. (1977). Amer-Ind Code Basic Workshop, sponsored by the Washington Hospital Center, Washington, DC.

Skelly, M. (1979). *Amer-Ind gestural code based on universal American Indian hand talk.* New York: Elsevier.

Skelly, M. (1981a). *Amer-Ind Code repertoire* (videocassette). St. Louis, MO: Auditec.

Skelly, M. (1981b). Amer-Ind Code Presentors Workshop, sponsored by the St. Louis Speech and Hearing Center, St. Louis, MO.

Skelly, M., Schinsky, L., Smith, R., Donaldson, R., & Griffin, J. (1974). American Indian sign (Amerind) as a facilitator of verbalization for the oral-verbal apraxic. *Journal of Speech and Hearing Disorders, 39,* 445–456.

Skelly, M., Schinsky, L., Smith, R., Donaldson, R., & Griffin, P. (1975). American Indian sign: Gestural communication for the speechless. *Archives of Physical Medicine and Rehabilitation, 56,* 156–160.

Skelly-Hakanson, M., Wollner, B., Bornhemer, K., & Drollinger, K. (1982). Questions and answers about the code. *AMICIL Newsletter, 1.* Wales, WI: Somed.

Snead, N.S. & Solomon, S.J. (1977). The effects of various stimulus modalities on global aphasics-phrase reception. Paper presented at the Annual Convention of the American Speech-Language-Hearing Association, Chicago, IL.

Tonkovich, J. & Loverso, F. (1982). A training matrix approach for gestural acquisition by the agrammatic patient. In R. Brookshire (ed.), *Clinical aphasiology conference proceedings.* Minneapolis, MN: BRK.

Wilcox, M.J. & Davis, A.J. (1981). Incorporating parameters of natural conversation in aphasia treatment. In R. Chapey (ed.), *Language intervention strategies in adult aphasia.* Baltimore, MD: Williams & Wilkins.

Yorkston, K. & Dowden, P.A. (1984). Non-speech language and communication systems. In A. Holland (ed.), *Language disorders in adults.* San Diego, CA: College Hill Press.

APPENDIX 30-1
Amer-Ind Code Signals (n = 38) with 90% or Better Transparency Using Either Liberal or Conservative Scoring[a,b]

100% (n = 15)	97.5%–90% (n = 23)
Bird	Automobile
Cry	Break
Cold	Telephone
Drink	Yes
No	Glasses
Pour	Pen
Quiet	Stir
Scissors	Dive
Swim	Nailfile
Toothbrush	Dig
Come	Pain
Fight	Comb
Ball	Grab
Sleep	Wash
Book	Stop
	Time
	Write
	Ring
	Good-bye
	Mirror
	Look
	Laugh
	Think

[a] Listed in rank order from 100% to 90%.
[b] From Daniloff, J., Lloyd, L., & Fristoe, M. (1983). Amer-Ind transparency. *Journal of Speech and Hearing Disorders, 48,* 103–110.

Chapter 31

Melodic Intonation Therapy

Robert W. Sparks

Numerous studies have indicated that an unimpaired right cerebral hemisphere is dominant for music in right-handed persons. This explains why aphasic persons can sing the melody of a familiar song. However, their accurate emission of the words of the song is of greater interest because of its contrast with their inability to communicate the most basic needs. This preserved skill also includes recitation of prayers, some social gesture phrases, and premorbid use of profanity. Jackson (1931) classified such utterances as nonpropositional language because they do not involve encoding of a message that contains specific information. He theorized that such utterances are processed in an undamaged so-called nondominant hemisphere of an aphasic. Today we can produce no better word to describe such language, although we no longer label the right hemisphere as being a nondominant one. Indeed, research indicates that the right hemisphere is involved in processing the prosody of propositional language.

Sparks et al. (1974) reviewed some of the literature on right-hemisphere processing of the prosodic elements of speech. Their analysis suggests that in normal right-handed persons and many left-handed persons the right hemisphere functions in a tandem relationship with the left hemisphere for both encoding and emission of propositional language. However, the final integrative process takes place in the temporal lobe of the left hemisphere. Reorganization of this interhemispheric process with increased participation of the right hemisphere probably occurs only when recovery is slow and incomplete. Of equal importance in this reorganization are preserved interhemispheral pathways for language. Indeed, Gordon (1972) states that a long period may be involved in increasing the function of the right hemisphere. The reader is referred to Code's discussion of the role of the right hemisphere in the treatment of aphasia. The probability that this is increased by melodic intonation therapy (MIT) is even more likely when we consider the right hemisphere's dominance for music. Studies of adult aphasia that have described language performance from a phonological model have included Blumstein (1973), Martin and Rigrodsky (1979), and Whitaker (1970).

The intentions of the authors of this chapter are to instruct the clinician in the technique of melodic intonation, describe the verbal behavior of both good candidates and poor candidates for MIT, discuss the administration of the MIT hierarchy, offer suggestions for involving the families of the aphasics who are selected for exposure to this language intervention strategy, and suggest future trends in further development of MIT.

Melodic intonation therapy involves singing. The specific techniques we call intonation are described in some detail later in the chapter. This type of singing is an ancient form dating back at least to the Judeo-Christian period. It is distinct from other forms of singing in that each intoned utterance is based on the melody pattern, the rhythm, and the points of stress in the spoken model. Use of an intoned utterance that resembles a familiar song may produce disastrous results, therapeutically speaking. The familiar melody will stimulate recall of the nonpropositional words of that song.

PRINCIPLES OF LANGUAGE THERAPY AFFECTING MIT

Objectives of MIT

The original intention for developing MIT for severely nonfluent aphasics was to achieve at least a basic recovery of ability to use some language accurately. Good candidates demonstrate extreme paucity of speech and show concern about such an incapacity. Reasonable priorities of therapeutic purpose for such patients would relegate the quality of articulation and syntax to secondary consideration. Emphasis on the linguistic or semantic aspects of verbal utterances for these aphasics is the primary goal of MIT. However, some clinicians are using the technique as a more phonological intervention for verbal apraxia. A review of our physiological model implies that the right hemisphere controls prosody. This, then, justifies the use of MIT for the phonological defects of such patients.

Speech Pathology Principles Applied to MIT

The Examination

A preference as to standardized aphasia examinations that are used to evaluate a potential candidate for MIT is not an issue. Sparks (1978) has presented guidelines for supplementary parastandardized examination of aphasics that make it possible to investigate more specific language skills in addition to those sampled in standardized examination batteries. In any event, MIT depends on evidence from the examination that the aphasic candidate has a distinct potential for some recovery of language.

Eight Principles of Language Therapy Involved in MIT

1. The first principle is concerned with gradual progression of the length and difficulty of the tasks in the therapeutic hierarchy. Such progression involves the type of linguistic material used, a gradual withdrawal of participation by the clinician in the purely repetition tasks, and reduction of reliance on melodic intonation in the last level of the MIT hierarchy.

2. The second principle, one endorsed by Schuell et al. (1964), maintains that direct attempts to correct the aphasic's verbal errors fail because he cannot recall the specific nature of his errors. Attempts to correct errors accomplish little and may do some harm if they detract from the smooth progression of the hierarchy. The severely handicapped aphasic who is considered to be a candidate seldom can effectively correct his verbal errors by retrial. Such retrials often result in a perseverated repetition of the error, which thus reinforces it. MIT attempts to achieve correct responses by means of a second trial that involves the technique of "backup." Specifically, when the aphasic fails a step, he is immediately guided through a repetition of the previous step and then a second attempt of the step that he failed. He may or may not be aware of the purpose of this procedure, but it is not drawn to his attention. A second backup retrial is never attempted if failure occurs again.

3. The third principle maintains that repetition is a highly effective therapeutic device. It serves as the core of MIT. Actually, repetition involves a rather complex process. The fact that normal persons can repeat familiar or simple sentences more efficiently than more difficult sentences suggests that a process of decoding the stimulus and then reencoding it for emission is involved. Accurate repetition deteriorates in longer units. However, the paraphrased repetition of the longer sentence does not alter the meaning. The stimulus has been accurately received and decoded, but some word substitutions have been used for the restatement. Perhaps the most difficult repetition task involves unknown words of another language or nonsense syllables. In this task, the usual decode-encode process is less efficient. As stated previously, the use of repetition in MIT gradually decreases as the level of difficulty of tasks increases.

4. The fourth principle is concerned with latencies of response. One such control is use of latency between completion of stimulus presentation by the clinician and permission for response by the aphasic so that the complete stimulus is received and decoded. Another use of latency is between the completion of one sentence-item progression in the hierarchy and the beginning of the next.

5. The fifth principle is avoidance of practice effect by using the same material or carrier phrases repeatedly. This is often tedious and not therapeutically effective. A well-constructed program of intervention will include many useful high-probability utterances that trigger recall of premorbid language skills. Language that is alien to the aphasic should not be used. Therefore, enough variety of meaningful material is encouraged for MIT so that no utterance is used more often than every ninth or tenth session of therapy.

6. The sixth principle maintains that the clinician should pay scrupulous attention to the purpose and semantic value of each of his or her verbal utterances. For example, exuberant reinforcements within a sequence of steps are disruptive. A smile of encouragement will serve just as well or better. This is not an indictment of a warm, holistic approach to therapeutic intervention in general. However, clinicians should practice restraint during MIT.

7. The seventh principle maintains that written or pictorial materials should not be used as added stimuli. We believe that the presumption that such material is supportive to the auditory stimulus is very suspect. Our premise is that these materials actually distract rather than support the MIT therapeutic process. This is particularly true for good candidates for MIT who have auditory comprehension that permits them to understand and retain spoken stimuli in a variety of contexts. Aphasics with severe auditory deficits may respond better to auditory stimuli when they are accompanied by pictures. However, such patients are not candidates for MIT.

8. The eighth principle pertains to the frequency of therapy sessions. Treatment sessions twice daily are essential for the aphasic with severe impairment of language. Where restrictions of time, resources, or transportation are involved, the training of family members to function as assistants in the MIT program may be very effective.

CANDIDACY FOR MIT

Assessment of the efficacy of MIT has proved that no single language intervention strategy for aphasia is a panacea.

Indeed, MIT is effective for only a portion of the aphasic population. This then implies a need for careful evaluation of each aphasic who is being considered for exposure to this method. Chapter 3 of this text describes computed tomography (CT) scan findings of cortical and subcortical lesions as predictions of candidacy for MIT. Such studies contribute much. Language profiles of both good and poor candidates are presented here as guides for selection. Emphasis is placed on auditory comprehension, several aspects of verbal expression, and nonlanguage behavior.

The Good Candidate

Auditory Comprehension

Examination of auditory comprehension indicates that the good candidate's understanding and retention of spoken language is essentially normal in a variety of contexts. It is simplistic to presume that the process of monitoring one's own verbal utterances is solely through auditory feedback. Actually, kinesthetic feedback probably alerts us to phonological or semantic errors immediately before the auditory feedback has commenced. In any event, evidence of preserved self-criticism in the good candidate is important.

Verbal Language

The clinical impression of the good candidate is that of an aphasic with a marked paucity of any kind of verbal output. In other words, he or she is a nonfluent aphasic. This is accompanied by demonstration of frustration and despondency concerning his or her language impairment. A curious and enigmatic perseveration of a neologistic utterance has been observed in some aphasics who have subsequently responded well to MIT. It is enigmatic because it is similar to the stereotypical jargon utterances of some global aphasics. However, there are two points of difference. Good candidates will modify the prosody of the utterance so that it reflects their intention to make a declarative, interrogative, or forceful imperative statement. Second, they will be annoyed by the meaningless morphology of the utterance. With the exception of such stereotyped jargon utterances, little speech is initiated except for an occasional single substantive word that is always an appropriate communication.

Phonological performance by the good candidate who has no language impairment other than speech production includes effortful but indistinct speech that is interrupted by pauses for attempted initiation of each utterance and attempts to correct himself or herself. Speech is phonologically distorted. When the articulation is analyzed, a systematic reorganization of sound patterns may seem to occur.

A summary of results of the examination of verbal expression produces a profile of the good candidate as follows:

1. Almost no responses occur in confrontation naming, responsive naming, word and phrase repetition, or sentence completion. However, an occasional response will be poorly articulated but accurate enough to indicate correct encoding of the target word.
2. Effort at self-correction is often vigorous. This is to be expected in aphasics who are acutely aware of making errors in their verbal output. Unfortunately, the product is usually not improved by this effort.

Nonverbal Behavior

Good candidates are often reasonably depressed, but they are almost always emotionally stable with a mature response to counseling by the clinician. They manifest a strong desire to enter into intensive efforts to rehabilitate their speech, and they accept MIT.

Concurrent Abnormalities

The good candidate usually demonstrates a significant buccofacial apraxia and has a hemiplegia that is more severe in the arm than in the leg.

Language Profile After MIT

A diagnosis of "classical" this or "classical" that is usually careless, but it is tempting to describe the verbal output of the post-MIT aphasic as having evolved into that of a classical Broca's aphasic. Some of the aphasic's utterances continue to be poorly articulated and agrammatical but telegraphically appropriate. An example is, "home—weekend—Saturday and Sunday. Hospital—you;—Monday." Considering the graduate's almost total inability to communicate prior to the therapy, this telegram is a triumph.

Further Improvement After MIT

The question as to whether achieved language improvement will be retained by the aphasic following successful MIT produces some concern for clinicians. Fortunately, follow-up examinations of MIT graduates have shown that not only do they maintain their new competency but they continue to improve in their own home environment. Syntactic substance begins to appear in their verbal output. MIT graduates and their families should be advised that a review of the final steps of the hierarchy will be beneficial in the continuing improvement. The clinician should discuss the extent of the family's participation and be available as a continuing consultant.

The Poor Candidate

Three aphasic syndromes are not responsive to the present form of MIT. These three types of aphasia are Wernicke's, transcortical, and global. The labels are not as important as brief reviews of the verbal behavior involved in each of the three types. They all are clearly distinct from the profile of the good candidate that has been presented.

Wernicke's Aphasia

Achieving therapeutic success with Wernicke's aphasics is a very difficult and challenging task. Concerted effort by some speech pathologists to produce more effective language therapy for persons with this type of aphasia is essential. The following characteristics of the Wernicke's aphasic are in marked contrast to those of the good candidate:

1. Auditory comprehension is poor and variable. Wernicke's aphasics show no evidence of being aware that they fail to be understood. As a matter of fact, they usually reject language therapy, and their reaction to MIT is either explosive or one of amused condescension.
2. Verbal utterances are overly fluent, syntactically normal, and clearly articulated. However, they include abundant paraphasic errors for the substantive words, and the end result is bizarre and meaningless.
3. The Wernicke's aphasic is often emotionally unstable, often hostile, but sometimes extremely cordial. The application of MIT techniques to patients with Wernicke's aphasia has produced poor results. Wernicke's aphasics accurately duplicate intonation patterns, including the melody, rhythm, and points of stress. This is in contrast to their replacement of the words in the stimulus model with their own paraphasic jargon.

Transcortical Aphasia

The aphasic demonstrating this profile may be similar in some ways to the good candidate and in other ways to the person with Wernicke's aphasia. The important feature of this form of aphasia is an isolated skill at accurately repeating long phrases and sentences, seemingly without the normal decoding process mentioned earlier. The aphasic performs perfectly in MIT, but there is no carryover to improved functional language. Investigation of repetition skill as a candidacy factor would suggest that ability to repeat even single words may be a negative prognostic factor for MIT candidacy.

Global Aphasia

The history of language therapy for persons with global aphasia indicates that such therapy has been unsuccessful in improving their functional verbal language. This was pointed out by Albert and Helm-Estabrook (1988), by Sarno et al. (1970), and by Schuell et al. (1964). MIT is no more effective than other language therapy in reestablishing any useful verbal communication.

MELODIC INTONATION

Sparks and Holland (1976) briefly describe the difference between songs and melodic intonation. Specifically, songs have distinct melodies. In contrast, melodic intonation is based solely on the spoken prosody of verbal utterances. The latter uses a vocal range that is limited to three or four whole notes. This is all that is necessary to achieve an adequate variety of melodic patterns. The range is about the same as that of the melodic line of speech.

This limited range of sung notes is comfortable for the untrained voice of adults. It is important to point out the necessity of avoiding melodic intonation patterns that are similar to those of long-lasting popular songs.

The Form of Melodic Intonation

Melodic intonation is based on three elements of spoken prosody: the melodic line or variation of pitch in the spoken phrase or sentence, the tempo and rhythm of the utterance, and the points of stress for emphasis. Certainty as to the appropriateness of the intonation pattern is essential in MIT. The need for this appropriateness becomes essential in the final level of the hierarchy when intoned utterances are gradually transposed back to spoken prosody.

Some exaggeration of the three elements of a spoken prosody model occurs when that utterance is intoned. First, the tempo is lengthened to a more lyrical utterance. Second, the varying pitch of speech is reduced and stylized into a melodic pattern involving the constant pitch of intoned notes. Third, the rhythm and stress are exaggerated for purposes of emphasis. This usually involves increased loudness and elevation of intoned notes. These three modifications of spoken prosody serve as a means of emphasizing the prosodic structure of the utterance.

Acceptable Variety of Melodic Patterns and Regional Differences

There are several alternative prosody patterns for any verbal utterance. The clinician must exercise his or her judgment as to which one will be used for a phrase or sentence in any one session of language therapy. Using a different intonation pattern in a subsequent session is a means of achieving variety of stimulation. Two such variations are illustrated in Figure 31–1 and will be discussed.

Regional differences of speech prosody are sometimes quite pronounced. This is not a matter of concern if the clinician and the aphasic come from and are in the same region. However, the emigration of a clinician from one prosodically distinct area to another implies that he or she must make an adjustment when MIT is involved. Samples of regional differences are presented in Figure 31–2 and will be discussed.

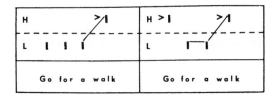

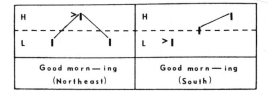

Figure 31–3. Regional differences in patterns of spoken prosody for one sentence.

Figure 31–1. Prosodic patterns of speech. H indicates higher pitch. L indicates lower pitch. A single-syllable word is indicated by a single vertical bar. Vertical bars that are connected represent multisyllabic words or clusters of words. An arrow preceding a vertical bar indicates stress on that word or syllable.

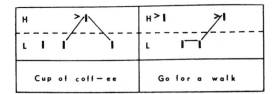

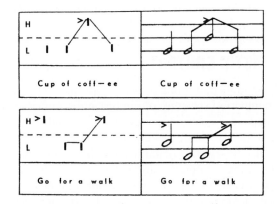

Figure 31–2. Two equally acceptable spoken prosody patterns. H indicates higher pitch. L indicates lower pitch. A single-syllable word is indicated by a single vertical bar. Vertical bars that are connected represent multisyllabic words or clusters of words. An arrow preceding a vertical bar indicates stress on that word or syllable.

Figure 31–4. Transposition of spoken prosody models to melodic intonation. Key of C in treble cleff is used for illustration. No attempt is made to present accurate musical tempo.

Plotting Spoken Prosody Patterns

Two illustrations of the method of graphically plotting verbal utterances along with an explanation of the plotting technique are presented in Figure 31–1. This method, an adaptation of the one developed at the Kodaly Musical Training Institute and presented by Knighton (1973), will be used in all subsequent illustrations.

In the first phrase, "cup of coffee," the utterance starts on a lower pitch for "cup," but the substantive importance of the word places it alone. This is followed by the cluster of words, "of coffee." Emphasis stress is on the first syllable of "coffee" along with the higher pitch that such stress produces. The last syllable of this declarative phrase has the customary drop in pitch. In the second illustration, "Go for a walk," there is stress on "go" with accompanying higher pitch, then a drop in pitch for the two functor words in the cluster, then a return to the higher pitch along with stress for the substantive word, "walk."

Figure 31–2 plots the difference of two variations for the phrase "Go for a walk." The first is as illustrated in Figure 31–1. The second illustrates a model where the word "for" is detached from the rest of the cluster that follows. This may be desirable as the aphasic improves and the clinician thinks that therapy should begin to attack absence of functor or relational words in the patient's speech.

In Figure 31–3, a comparison of prosody for the social gesture utterance "good morning" shows a rise-fall melody

pattern of the northeastern parts of the United States and a gradually rising inflectional pattern of at least some parts of the South.

Transposing Speech to Intonation

Illustrations of the transposition of plotted speech prosody models into melodic intonation are presented in Figure 31–4, using those phrases illustrated in Figure 31–1. The placing of the notes on a musical staff in these illustrations does not imply that ability to read music is a prerequisite to administering MIT, although such skill is an advantage. The primary purpose here is to duplicate graphically the pattern of spoken prosody that has served as the model. Considerable musical license has been taken, and musicians are requested not to take issue. For those who are interested, however, the key of C is used in the illustrations so that variations of sung note combinations may be demonstrated.

Sprechgesang

The fading of melodic intonation and a return to spoken prosody occurs in the fourth level of the MIT hierarchy. It is a technique that lies halfway between speech and singing. It is used in choral reading but more lyrically by Schoenberg in his Ode to Napoleon and Pierrot Luraire. Schoenberg defined the technique as sprechgesang, or "spoken song."

The exaggerated tempo, rhythm, and points of stress in sprechgesang are the same as in the intoned model. However, the more variable pitch of speech replaces the more constant pitch of intoned notes. The utterance is lyrical but spoken rather than sung.

The senior author lays claim to the use of this art form as a bridging technique in the MIT hierarchy after having heard a performance of Ode to Napoleon by the Boston Symphony Orchestra in 1973. He will furnish a cassette sample of sprechgesang on request provided the request is accompanied by phrases to be illustrated and a cassette.

LINGUISTIC CONTENT

The importance of a linguistically sophisticated control of the grammatical structure of phrases and sentences used in MIT depends largely on the severity of the individual aphasic's inability to communicate and the usefulness of the verbal material. The selection of phrases and short sentences should be high-priority communication. This involves investigation of basic aspects of the aphasic's premorbid milieu that may be used, and then some creativity on the part of the clinician to produce stimulating material. In other words, all material should be egocentric for the individual aphasic. This should be the case in all therapy for the traumatized aphasic, but it is of particular importance as a counterbalance in MIT, where the technique is so atypical of normal verbal behavior. Information about such things as basic family routines, family relationships and customs, personal needs, and personal likes and dislikes will suggest an abundance of material of both universal and individual appeal. Clusters of sentences that have a spherical relationship add an even greater significance. This is illustrated in Figure 31–5, which presents four three-item themes as an illustration of thematic relationship of therapy material along with further illustration of melodic intonation plotting. Additional illustration of the thematic arrangement of material presented by Sparks and Holland (1976) is included here with the permission of the senior author of that article:

3. Look at the sports page 6. Time to go to bed.

Sample Material for Level II
1. twelve o'clock   6. apple pie
2. time for lunch   7. glass of milk
3. bowl of soup   8. I am sleepy
4. salt and pepper   9. take a nap
5. ham sandwich

Sample Material for Levels III and IV
1. Sit down in a chair.   6. I am very tired.
2. Read the newspaper.   7. It is getting late.
3. Look at the sports page.   8. Time to go to bed.
4. Turn on the TV.   9. It is ten o'clock.
5. Go for a walk.

Meaningful stimulus items for the aphemic candidate who has no impairment other than phonological errors should, in addition to being meaningful for the individual patient, focus on facilitating more intelligible speech. The creative clinician will meet with the candidate and family and explain the importance of gaining information about specific linguistic preferences the patient used in his or her premorbid speech. Therapeutic concern for consistent phonological errors makes it more difficult to select meaningful material. Table 31–1 illustrates the use of phonological patterns in selecting stimulus materials.

MELODIC INTONATION HIERARCHY

The hierarchy of MIT is highly structured for gradual progression of difficulty. Therefore, it is presented in explicit detail because attention to every specification has contributed to its success. We are sympathetic with those clinicians who prefer less structured language intervention strategies, and we assure them that their reservations about using hierarchies is understood. Sparks and Holland (1976) referred to the dilemma of presenting a hierarchy in a way that is too detailed and seemingly dogmatic for some clinicians and perhaps not explicit enough for others. The presentation here will include a description of the technique of intoning, a detailed and illustrated discussion of the four levels of the hierarchy, and a suggested method of scoring each MIT session.

Specific Aspects of the Technique

Discussion of the hierarchy will be made more explicit by first describing the several techniques that are involved.

Use of Verbal Cuing

Phonemic cues, along with their important visual components, are used in the second level of the program and to a

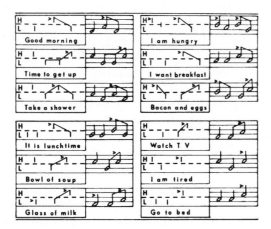

Figure 31–5. Four thematic three-item illustrations of melodic intonation material using the same figure legend presented in Figure 31–1.

TABLE 31–1

Sample Phonological Patterns for MIT Stimuli

	Facilitation of Velar Production	
cup of coffee	corn on the cob	piece of cake
calico cat	good cookie	call a cab
make music	big lake	can of coke
	Facilitation of Cluster Production	
ask the man	pass the salt	small price
stamp please	go back home	last street
deep snow fall	spare room	sports coat
	Facilitation of Syllable Sequencing	
build a snowman	light the Christmas trees	more ice cubes
it's a democracy	open the refrigerator	fix the machine
read it in the paper	time for breakfast	play the music box

lesser extent in the subsequent levels. The use of such cues is limited to assisting aphasics in initiation of their responses when it is apparent that they are having difficulty. It is never used as a means of repeating the task for purposes of correcting errors in the aphasic's responses.

Backups and Patient's Failures

A means of attempting indirect correction of errors, called "backups" is used in the third and fourth levels of the program. If the aphasic's response in any step is considered not to be adequate, the clinician has the aphasic repeat the preceding step and then attempt the failed step again. This second trial is often effective in producing the correct response without distracting the patient or making him or her directly aware of the error. As illustrated, if the third step of a level is failed, the second is repeated and the third is then attempted again. If the fourth is failed, the third is repeated as a backup, and so forth. If the aphasic again repeats the error or produces a different one after a backup sequence, the clinician terminates any further effort with that sentence-item and proceeds to the first step of the level with a new sentence. This is consistent with the concept that overt attempts to correct errors are not useful with the type of aphasic who is a candidate for MIT.

Hand Tapping and Control by Hand Signals

It is recommended that the clinician seat himself/herself across the table from the aphasic so that his/her participation is visible to the aphasic and the aphasic's performance is clearly visible to him/her. The clinician grasps the patient's left hand so that he/she can engage it in tapping out the rhythm of the stimulus as it is presented, and then the rhythm of the responses. Many subjects begin to exercise some control of the hand tapping. This should be encouraged provided it is accurate. The clinician's participation may then be faded to that of monitoring the accuracy while continuing to hold the aphasic's hand. Hand tapping has proved to be an important and effective supportive stimulus. It has a cuing value that often seems as effective as the verbal component it accompanies.

The clinician's use of his or her left hand as a means of controlling onset of the aphasic's responses is recommended as a nonverbal and nondistracting means of exercising such control. Held up, the left hand advises the aphasic to remain silent and listen. Dropped with a finger pointed at the aphasic, it signals him/her to respond. This method is useful in enforcing latency if it is used consistently. The clinician may feel like a traffic officer and may wish he or she could develop a means of also using his or her feet.

Unison Repetition and Fading Participation by the Clinician

An early step in all the levels of the hierarchy involves clinician-aphasic unison repetition of the stimulus that the clinician has just presented. The clinician fades his/her participation, first the audible and then the visible component, so that the aphasic is repeating the sentence "solo." It is often necessary for the clinician to rejoin the aphasic when it is evident that he/she is not quite ready to proceed in the repetition on his/her own.

Adapting to the Aphasic's Modification of Melody Patterns

The clinician should be prepared to change the key of the melody to that of the aphasic's inadvertent modification. Attempts to correct such modifications is an unnecessary distraction. Rather, accurate repetition of the verbal material is the primary goal. Modification of the rhythm or number of intoned syllables, however, cannot be permitted because of their effect on the substance of the sentence.

MIT Session Scoring

The best way of judging the effectiveness of any highly structured form of language therapy for aphasia is to use or develop an objective system of scoring each therapy session. This principle is recommended for MIT as a means of measuring the efficiency of the method for producing steady improvement by any one aphasic. The method suggested here involves a two-point score for an accurate response that has not required a phonemic cue to initiate a response or a backup, a one-point score for an accurate response achieved with cuing or after a backup, and a reduction of the maximum possible score for any sentence-item if steps have not been completed.

The Hierarchy of MIT

The discussion of each of the four levels of the MIT hierarchy will include a fully detailed description, and Table 31–5 will provide a quick reference. A second table for each level presents a sample therapy session that includes management of errors and scoring, and a review of the types of errors most frequently encountered.

Level I

The first level is a one-step preliminary means of establishing a set for holding hands and, as far as the aphasic may see it, singing odd little nothings. The melodies are those that are used for intoning phrases and sentences. They should increase in length and complexity of melody and stress points as the aphasic adapts to the technique. Our good candidate can usually be introduced to the idea by a simple description of the process and its purpose. The clinician hums a melody twice while hand tapping the rhythm-tempo-stress pattern with the aphasic. Humming is suggested rather than a vowel of "la-la" because of its less distinct phonemic quality. Melody patterns similar to those illustrated in Figure 31–5 should be used. Second, the clinician signals the aphasic to join him/her in unison humming of the melody along with the hand tapping. The patient may use a more phonemic verbal utterance when he/she joins in with the clinician. This is acceptable in this first nonverbal level. When the clinician thinks the aphasic is ready for a solo effort, he/she fades his/her vocal participation but continues hand tapping with the aphasic. When the aphasic has completed his unaccompanied repetition, the clinician reinforces the performance by saying "good" and proceeding to the next melody pattern. No scoring takes place in Level I. The time required to complete this first level varies from 15 minutes for some aphasics to two therapy sessions for others. In any event, moving to the second level occurs as soon as the aphasic is comfortable in the set of intoning, hand tapping, and complying with the hand-signal controls of the clinician.

Level II

At Level II, linguistic material is added to the type of intonation patterns introduced in the first level. Each of the four steps in the level is presented in detail below. The model presented by Sparks and Holland (1976) had five steps. The present model has combined the first two steps of that model. The use of phonemic cuing is indicated when applicable. Scoring involves two points for a response from the aphasic that does not require a cue to initiate it, and one point if the response is acceptable when initiated by a cue from the clinician. Hand tapping by the clinician and the aphasic occurs in all stimuli and responses.

Step 1

The clinician hums the melody-tempo-stress intonation pattern that is to be used with the sentence while hand tapping it with the aphasic, then repeats it with the sentence added. He/she pauses briefly and then repeats it. Then he/she signals the aphasic to join him/her in unison repetition of the intoned sentence. If the aphasic's performance is acceptable, the clinician proceeds to Step 2. If the aphasic's performance is not acceptable, the clinician pauses for several seconds to produce decay of the strength of the stimulus and then proceeds to the next sentence. The maximum score for an acceptable performance by the aphasic is one point.

Step 2

After a brief pause, the clinician and the aphasic begin a unison intoning of the same sentence along with hand tapping. The clinician then fades his/her verbal participation in the manner described earlier but continues to hand tap the rhythm stress pattern with the aphasic. An acceptable performance implies progression in the third step, and the maximum score is again one point. An unacceptable performance terminates further progression; the clinician pauses for several seconds and then proceeds to the next sentence to be attempted.

Step 3

The aphasic is signaled to listen. Then the clinician presents the same intoned sentence. This is accompanied by the hand tapping. Then the aphasic is signaled to repeat it, unaccompanied by the clinician except for his/her participation in the hand tapping. If the aphasic has difficulty initiating the repetition, the clinician gives a phonemic cue for the first phoneme of the sentence. Again, this is accompanied by the hand tapping and, hopefully, the aphasic will respond to the cue accurately. If this third step is completed without cuing, the score is two points. If it is unacceptable only after cuing for initiation, the score is one point. Failure to initiate the utterance after one cuing effort or failure to produce it accurately enough to be acceptable terminates progression to the fourth step. After a suitable pause, the clinician proceeds to the next sentence.

Step 4

In the final step of the second level, the clinician, without hand tapping, intones the question, "What did you say?" immediately after successful completion of the third step. He/she then signals the aphasic to repeat the intoned sentence. Cuing along with the hand tapping is offered once if the aphasic is having difficulty initiating the repetition. Occasionally, the aphasic may modify the sentence slightly by omitting a functor word or by a slight paraphrase of the sentence. This may be acceptable to the clinician. We maintain that any appropriate near-target response is evidence of progress. Scoring is the same as that of the third step. Two points are given for an acceptable uncued response; only one point is given when a cue was necessary for initiation. The aphasic is reinforced if he/she successfully completes the four steps for the sentence.

Level II Accomplishment

The aphasic who succeeds in Level II has acquired the skill of repeating intoned sentences immediately after hearing the model, and then in response to a question. The latter is more difficult because the question not only acts as a masking intrusion but also initiates the process of reencoding the stimulus for responsive speech. Attention to this becomes progressively more active in the subsequent levels.

The Most Common Errors Occurring in Level II

First, the aphasic may be so surprised by his/her solo repetition when the clinician fades his/her participation that he/she will falter. The clinician should be generous in reentering the unison repetition as much as he/she considers it useful in producing improvement of the aphasic's performance. Second, increasing repetition skill may disclose significant evidence of poor articulation, and this will continue throughout the MIT program for that aphasic. As stated previously, we give greater priority to increasing linguistic skill.

Sample MIT Session and Scoring for Level II

A brief five-item therapy session and its scoring is presented in Table 31–2 to illustrate management of errors in the aphasic's performance.

Level III

The third level is actually a liaison between the aphasic's recovery of ability to repeat during participation in Level II and the return to speech prosody and responsive speech in the fourth level. Latency of permitted responses and less specific questions in the last step begin to put more stress on the encoding of responsive speech. In this level, phonemic cuing by the clinician is replaced by the backup system already discussed. In addition to their use as an aid for initiation of responses, backups are also used as an indirect means of correcting an error in a response. As in cuing, only one backup and retrial of a failed step is permitted if the hierarchy is followed without modification. Again, the Sparks and Holland (1976) hierarchy has been modified by combining their first and second steps into one. The detailed description of this third level follows.

Step 1

The clinician presents the intoned sentence with the usual hand tapping once, then signals the aphasic to join in unison intoning and hand tapping the sentence. As the aphasic shows evidence that he/she can continue, the clinician fades his/her verbal participation, returning briefly if necessary and then fading again until the aphasic can continue alone. The maximum score is one point for acceptable performance, and the clinician proceeds to Step 2. It would be unusual for the aphasic to fail this step, but if he/she does the progression for that sentence is discontinued.

Step 2

The clinician intones the same sentence once with the usual patient-clinician hand tapping. The aphasic's response will be intoned repetition, but delay in his/her response of 1 or 2 seconds is imposed by a hand signal from the clinician; then he/she signals him/her to repeat the intoned sentence. Failure involves an immediate backup to Step 1, unison intoning with clinician fading, and then retrial of the second step. If the step is completed without a backup, the score is two points. One point is given for an adequate response following a backup if it is necessary. Failure after one retrial terminates progression to the third step for that sentence.

Step 3

There is no hand tapping in this step. The clinician intones a question asking for a substantive response concerning some element of information in the sentence that has been presented. For instance, if the sentence used in the preceding steps was, "I want some pie," the question for Step 3 could be, "What kind of pie?" Perhaps the encouraging early indications of language recovery during MIT are the occasional appropriate but nondirected responses to the question. Such responses seem to be ahead of any other evidence of recovery in the aphasic's functional language. They please and surprise the aphasic and reward the clinician. These responses are usually uttered in normal speech prosody, and they certainly should be accepted. Failure to respond appropriately to the question implies an immediate backup to Step 2, delayed repetition, and then a retrial of Step 3. The clinician

TABLE 31–2

Sample MIT Level II Session with Step and Summation Scores

Aphasic's Performance	Scores			
	Step 1	Step 2	Step 3	Step 4
First sentence: Aphasic succeeds in all steps. Maximum scores attained.	1	1	2	2
Second sentence: Succeeds in all steps but requires a cue to initiate response in Steps 3 and 4.	1	1	1	1
Third sentence: Succeeds in Steps 1 and 2, requires a cue to initiate response in Step 3, and fails Step 4 because of an unacceptable response after backup.	1	1	1	0
Fourth sentence: Succeeds in Steps 1 and 2, requires a cue to initiate response in Step 3, and requires a backup to initiate Step 4.	1	1	1	1
Fifth sentence: Succeeds in Step 1, fails in Step 2. Progression stopped and no scores given for Steps 3 and 4.	1	0	—	—
Scores	5/5	4/5	5/8	4/6
Total:	18/24 (75%)			

should not solicit some response of his/her own choosing. Scores are the same as for Step 2: two points without a backup and one point after a backup.

Level III Accomplishment

Satisfactory completion of this third level of MIT has begun the modification of the aphasic's responses from simpler repetition that is well supported by the clinician's participation to more difficult responses involving some retrieval and a beginning of attempts at encoded responses to specific questions.

The Most Common "Errors" Occurring in Level III

Although not a verbal error, the aphasic's burgeoning confidence and enthusiasm may prompt him/her to respond before the clinician has signaled him/her to do so, particularly when delayed response is required. Because of the increasing difficulty of the tasks, the clinician must insist on compliance with his/her controls. Second, the aphasic may omit an occasional functor word. Perhaps this is an error of omission, but we believe that any improvement should be free of criticism and should not be inhibited by too much attention to syntax at this point in the progression of the hierarchy. Third, the variety of appropriate but unanticipated responses to the question in Step 3 should be praised even though they may not be what was expected. They are not errors, particularly if the questions are open-ended enough to make it possible for a variety of responses to occur.

Sample MIT Session and Scoring of Level III

As in Level II, a brief five-item therapy session and its scoring are presented in Table 31–3 to illustrate management of errors.

Level IV

In this last level, the return to normal speech prosody by way of the sprechgesang technique described earlier occurs for each sentence used, longer delays are imposed by the clinician before he/she permits the aphasic to respond, and more spontaneous and appropriate verbal intrusions by the aphasic may be expected.

Step 1

The clinician signals the aphasic to listen, then intones the sentence. He/she then pauses briefly and presents the sentence twice in sprechgesang accompanied by hand tapping with the aphasic. He/she invites the aphasic to join him/her in unison sprechgesang repetition of the sentence with continued hand tapping. Failure of the aphasic to respond appropriately calls for a backup to the clinician's solo presentation accompanied by hand tapping, then a second trial of the unison repetition. A second failure terminates further effort with that sentence. If the step is completed without a backup, the score is two points; the score is one point if a backup is necessary.

Step 2

The clinician again signals the aphasic to listen. Then he/she presents the same sentence in sprechgesang with hand tapping, delays permission for the aphasic to respond for 2 or 3 seconds, and then signals him/her to repeat it in sprechgesang with hand tapping. Failure involves an immediate backup to the first step, unison repetition in sprechgesang with hand tapping and fading participation by the clinician, and then a retrial of Step 2. If the step is completed without a backup, the score is two points; the score is one point if a backup is necessary to get an acceptable response. Failure to respond

TABLE 31–3

Sample MIT Level III Session with Step and Summation Scores

Aphasic's Performance	Scores		
	Step 1	Step 2	Step 3
First sentence: Aphasic succeeds in all steps. Maximum scores attained.	1	2	2
Second sentence: Succeeds in all steps but requires backups for Steps 2 and 3.	1	1	1
Third sentence: Succeeds in Step 1, requires a backup to initiate Step 2, succeeds in Step 3.	1	1	2
Fourth sentence: Succeeds in Step 1, requires a backup for Step 2 because of inaccurate response, fails to initiate response in Step 3 after a backup.	1	1	0
Fifth sentence: Succeeds in Step 1, fails to repeat accurately in Step 2, and fails after a backup. Progression stopped and no score may be given for Step 3.	1	0	—
Scores	5/5	5/10	5/8
Total:	15/23 (65%)		

appropriately after one backup terminates progression to the third step for that sentence.

Step 3

Hand tapping is now discontinued for the remainder of Level IV for each sentence. The clinician signals the aphasic to listen, then presents the same sentence twice but now in normal speech prosody. After delaying permission to respond for 1 or 2 seconds, the clinician signals the aphasic to repeat the sentence as presented in normal speech prosody. The length of the delay may be lengthened as the aphasic develops proficiency. Failure involves a backup to the second step; delayed repetition in sprechgesang, with hand tapping; then a retrial of Step 3. Scoring is the same: two points without a backup, one point after a backup produces an acceptable response. Failure after a backup terminates progression to the fourth step for that sentence.

Step 4

As in the last step of the third level, the clinician asks questions concerning substantive information contained in the same sentence immediately after successful completion of Step 3, but the number of such questions may be increased. Then the clinician asks questions that are more associative in nature. As illustration, the following example is given:

> Sentence: I want to watch TV.
> Sequence of questions: (a) What do you want to watch?
> (b) Who wants to? (c) When do you like to do that?
> (d) What programs do you enjoy most?

The guidelines for decisions as to what may be considered acceptable responses and when a backup should be used are less specific as this last step in the hierarchy becomes less rigidly structured. One suggested solution is to demand accurate responses to the specific questions based on material in the sentence and reward the aphasic with extra credit for appropriate responses to the less specific questions. Backups should be used only for failures to initiate responses to the specific questions or when such responses are inferior to the aphasic's current ability. Principles of suggested scoring are modified to conform to the above guidelines for acceptability of responses. If a backup is used, it will be Step 3, delayed repetition of the sentence in normal speech prosody, and then a retrial of this fourth step. Backups should be restricted to use with the first specific questions, as responses to the less specific ones are bonus items. Response to the specific questions yields two points for each one, but only one point if a backup was necessary. Response to one or more of the less specific questions would yield a single score of three points, an added bonus that is a nice reinforcement the aphasic will enjoy.

This last level of the MIT hierarchy is more permissive than the first three and demands significantly more from the aphasic because he/she has recovered enough speech to reach it. The somewhat less stringent form lends itself to transition to any other language therapies that the clinician may want to employ after completion of MIT.

Level IV Accomplishments and Post-MIT Therapy

The aphasic who has completed the MIT program has maintained the skills he/she acquired earlier in the program and has carried them over to normal speech prosody along with an ongoing recovery of ability to encode and emit at least basic verbal communication. Perhaps this recovery now exceeds or will exceed the limits of what MIT is currently designed to offer. Some clinicians may think that the goals should be expanded to help the less severely impaired aphasic whose language profile is essentially that of the good candidate but with less acute impairment. This would place the method alongside other techniques that are concerned with improving syntax, articulation, and efficiency of retrieval. MIT might be used concurrently with these techniques in post-MIT language therapy. Many of us have modified the

TABLE 31–4

Sample MIT Level IV Session with Step and Summation Scores

Aphasic's Performance	Scores			
	Step 1	Step 2	Step 3	Step 4
First sentence: Aphasic succeeds in Steps 1 and 2, requires a backup to initiate normal prosody in Step 3. Succeeds in Step 4 but no bonus because of failure on last associative question.	2	2	1	2
Second sentence: Succeeds in Step 1, requires backups for Steps 2 and 3. Succeeds with bonus in Step 4.	2	1	1	3
Third sentence: Aphasic requires a backup to succeed in Step 1 and then succeed in subsequent steps.	1	2	2	3
Fourth sentence: Succeeds in Steps 1, 2, and 3, requires a backup for Step 4, fails to answer any associative question.	2	2	2	1
Fifth sentence: Succeeds in Steps 1, 2, and 3, requires a backup for one specific question in Step 4, but answers all associative questions.	2	2	2	2
Scores	9/10	9/10	8/10	11/15
Total:	37/45 (82%)			

hierarchy for limited use after completion of the four levels. The issue could be raised as to how long language therapy should continue when the improving aphasic person reaches a point where he/she can experience some continuing recovery in his/her own milieu. However, that discussion does not belong here.

A fifth, less structured postgraduate step has been used to retire melodic intonation. Its design includes only sprechgesang and normal speech prosody repetition along with an increased emphasis on answering questions such as those used in Step 4 of the last level. It is useful to encourage the aphasic to use sprechgesang as an auto-therapy when he/she is experiencing difficulty with word finding and the phonemic structure of words. Most MIT graduates find it difficult to use the technique unless some prompting takes place before final discharge from the realm of MIT.

Sample MIT Session and Scoring for Level IV

A five-item therapy session with scoring for the fourth level is presented in Table 31–4.

Quick Reference Guide for the Hierarchy

The four levels of the MIT hierarchy are presented in Table 31–5 for the convenience of the clinician during administration of the therapy.

Concurrent Language Therapies

Because MIT involves a marked departure from normal speech, and because of its carefully planned program of progression, we recommend that no other therapy that is directed specifically to improved verbal output be used concurrently. The aphasic may easily be confused if one form demands intoning all verbal output and another uses a procedure involving normal speech prosody. The gradual transition in MIT to therapy that involves normal prosody makes it possible to transfer to other language intervention strategies easily after completion of the hierarchy. This has been discussed earlier.

Progression from One Level to the Next One

Progression from Level II to Level III or from Level III to Level IV, or from Level IV to post-MIT therapy should occur after sufficient evidence that the aphasic has developed a stable proficiency. Our hypothesis that increased participation of the right hemisphere occurs in MIT implies that a somewhat prolonged process is involved. Whether the clinician who uses MIT agrees with our hypothesis is less essential than that he or she progresses slowly to ensure maintained improvement from this method. Actually, the rate of progress made by the good candidate will be slow.

Suggested Means of Controlling Rate of Progression

We recommend that moving from one level to the next higher one should occur only after a mean score of 90% or better for 10 consecutive therapy sessions has been achieved. This may often involve some approach-retreat before the 90% mean is achieved when we consider the usual fluctuation of aphasic performance from day to day.

TABLE 31–5

Quick Reference Hierarchy Guide MIT Levels I to IV

LEVEL I
Single Step
    C (HT) Hums melody twice.
    C and **A** (U) Hum melody twice. **C** fades.
    Score and progression: No score. Proceed to next melody.

LEVEL II
Step 1
    C (HT) hums melody → intones sentence.
    C signals **A**.
    C and **A** (HT) (U) intonation of sentence.
    Score and progression:
        Acceptable—1 point. Proceed to Step 2, same sentence.
        Unacceptable—Discontinue progress for sentence.

Step 2
    C (HT) hums melody → intones same sentence.
    C signals **A**.
    C and **A** (HT) (U) intonation of sentence. **C** fades.
    Score and progression:
        Acceptable—1 point. Proceed to Step 3, same sentence.
        Unacceptable—Discontinue progression for sentence.

Step 3
    C (HT) intones same sentence → **C** signals **A**.
    C and **A** as **A** intones sentence. **C** intones sentence. **C** intones
      cue if necessary.
    Score and progression:
        Acceptable without cue—2 points. Proceed to Step 4, same sentence.
        Acceptable with cue—1 point. Proceed to Step 4, same sentence.
        Unacceptable—Discontinue progression for sentence.

Step 4
    C intones "What did you say?" → **C** signals **A**.
    A repeats intoned sentence. **C** intones cue if necessary.
    Score and progression:
        Acceptable without cue—2 points.
        Acceptable with cue—1 point.
        Proceed to Step 1 for next sentence.

LEVEL III
Step 1
    C (HT) intones sentence → **C** signals **A**.
    C and **A** (HT) (U) intonation of sentence. **C** fades.
    Score and progression:
        Acceptable—1 point. Proceed to Step 2, same sentence.
        Unacceptable—Discontinue progression for sentence.

Step 2
    C intones same sentence → **C** signals **A** to wait.
    C signals **A** after 1 or 2 seconds.
    A (HT) repeats intoned sentence.
    (B) to Step 1 if **A** fails → retrial of Step 2.
    Score and progression:
        Acceptable without (B)—2 points. Proceed to Step 3, same sentence.
        Acceptable after (B)—1 point. Proceed to Step 3, same sentence.
        Unacceptable after (B)—Discontinue progression for sentence.

continued

Quick Reference Hierarchy Guide MIT Levels I to IV

continued

Step 3
    C intones a question → C signals **A.**
    A gives an appropriate answer, intoned or spoken.
    (B) to Step 2 if **A** fails → retrial of Step 3.
    Score and progression:
        Acceptable after (B)—2 points.
        Acceptable after (B)—1 point.
        Proceed to Step 1 for next sentence.

LEVEL IV

Step 1
    C (HT) intones sentence → C signals **A** to wait.
    C (HT) presents sentence twice in *sprechgesang*.
    C signals **A.**
    C and **A** (HT) (U) *sprechgesang* of sentence.
    (B) to **C** (HT) presentation in *sprechgesang* if aphasic fails.
    Retrial of **C** and **A** (HT) (U) *sprechgesang*.
    Score and Progression:
        Acceptable *sprechgesang*—2 points. Proceed to Step 2, same sentence.
        Acceptable after (B)—1 point. Proceed to Step 2, same sentence.
        Unacceptable—Discontinue progression for sentence.

Step 2
    C (HT) presents same sentence in *sprechgesang* → **C** signals **A** to wait.
    C signals **A** after 2 or 3 seconds.
    A (HT) repeats sentence in *sprechgesang*.
    (B) to Step 1 if **A** fails → retrial of Step 2.
    Score and Progression:
        Acceptable without (B)—2 points. Proceed to Step 3, same sentence.
        Unacceptable—Discontinue progression for sentence.

Step 3
    No hand tapping.
    C presents same sentence twice in normal speech prosody.
    C signals **A** to wait 2 or 3 seconds → then signals to repeat.
    A repeats sentence in normal speech prosody.
    (B) to **C** presentation in normal speech prosody if **A** fails.
    Retrial of **A** repetition.
    Score and Progression:
        Acceptable without (B)—2 points. Proceed to Step 4, same sentence.
        Acceptable after (B)—1 point. Proceed to Step 4, same sentence.
        Unacceptable—Discontinue progression for sentence.

Step 4
    C Question about substantive content, same sentence.
    A Any appropriate response.
    (B) to Step 3 if response is unacceptable → retrial of Step 4.
    C Questions about associative information.
    A Any appropriate responses.
    Score and Progression:
        2 points without (B), substantive content, 1 point after (B).
        3 bonus points, one or more responses to associative questions.
    Proceed to next sentence.

Symbols: **A**, aphasic; **C**, clinician; (HT) hand tapping by clinician with aphasic; (B) backup; (U) unison.

Participation of the Aphasic's Family During and After Clinical MIT

Much emphasis is placed on members of the aphasic's family participating in the process of attempted rehabilitation of his language. However, participation of the family in the early period when the focus is entirely on intonation and accuracy of intonation patterns is viewed with reservations unless supervision is provided by the clinician. The family of the aphasic should be encouraged to assist in selection of useful phrases used frequently by themselves and the aphasic premorbidly. It is important that these lists be extensive to provide great variety of word orders. Experience with this selective process makes it possible for the aphasic and his/her family to offer information and vocabulary based on observations and experience in their daily activities.

The role of the family to encourage sprechgesang as a means of word-retrieval efficiency for the aphasic in the home and among selected friends is strongly recommended for words and phrases that have a high frequency of use in the household.

SUMMARY

In summary, six major elements of MIT are covered. They are as follows: certain principles of language therapy for aphasia and associated phonological disorders that have influenced the design of the MIT strategy; a discussion of the candidacy that contrasts the language profiles of good and poor candidates for this type of language intervention; a description of the technique of intoning and plotting intonation patterns; a detailed instruction of administration of the MIT hierarchy; a discussion of post-MIT strategies; and participation of members of the aphasic's family during clinical intervention and after its completion.

FUTURE TRENDS

The family of the aphasic who is receiving or has received MIT should be systematically involved as a support team. Future development of Melodic Intonation Therapy should include the development of published guidelines that the family may use. Their support is particularly essential when the aphasic is receiving less than one therapy session each day with the clinician.

Further collection of data on candidacy is essential as a means of further evidence of the efficacy of melodic intonation therapy. The contributions of careful language examination and scientific studies are of equal importance.

References

Albert, M.L. & Helm-Estabrook, N. (1988). Diagnosis and treatment of aphasia, Part II. *Journal of the American Medical Association, 259*, 1208–1209.

Blumstein, S.E. (1973). *A phonological investigation of aphasic speech.* The Hague: Mouton.

Gordon, H.W. (1972). Verbal and non-verbal cerebral processing in man for audition. Doctoral thesis, California Institute of Technology.

Jackson, H. (1931). *Selected writings of John Hughlings Jackson.* London: Hodder & Stoughton.

Knighton, K. (1973). *Beginning teaching techniques: Teaching music at beginning levels.* Wellesley, MA: Kodaly Musical Training Institute.

Martin, A.D. & Rigrodsky, (1979). An investigation of phonological impairment in aphasia, Part I. *Cortex, 10*, 318–328.

Sarno, M., Silverman, M., & Sands, E. (1970). Speech therapy and language recovery in severe aphasia. *Journal of Speech and Hearing Research, 13*, 607–623.

Schuell, H., Jenkins, H., & Jimenez-Pabon, E. (1964). *Aphasia in adults.* New York: Harper & Row.

Sparks, R. (1978). Parastandardized examination guidelines for adult aphasia. *British Journal of Disorders of Communication, 41*, 135–146.

Sparks, R., Helm, N., & Albert, M. (1974). Aphasia rehabilitation resulting from melodic intonation therapy. *Cortex, 10*, 303–316.

Sparks, R. & Holland, A. (1976). Method: Melodic intonation therapy. *Journal of Speech and Hearing Disorders, 41*, 287–297.

Whitaker, H.A. (1970). A model for neurolinguistics. Occasional Papers.

Chapter 32

Computer Applications in Aphasia Treatment

Richard C. Katz

OBJECTIVES

The purpose of this chapter is to familiarize the reader with the various applications of computers and related technology in the rehabilitation of adults with aphasia; present the strengths and limitations of computerized aphasia treatment; describe classic and recent research literature demonstrating the efficacy of computerized aphasia treatment; evaluate the effectiveness and appropriateness of treatment software for patients with aphasia; and incorporate computers and related technology when appropriate into the diagnostic and treatment process for people with aphasia.

DEFINITIONS

Computerized aphasia treatment refers to the systematic use of computers and software to improve communication skills in people with aphasia. Computers are incorporated into aphasia treatment in three fundamentally different manners:

Computer-Only Treatment (COT) software is designed to allow a patient, as part of a clinician-provided treatment program, to practice alone at the computer, without the simultaneous ("on-line") supervision or direct assistance of the clinician or others (e.g., spouse, speech pathology assistant). The clinician later reviews patient performance ("off-line") by examining task performance scores saved on disk by the program for later review, by directly observing performance using the software during a subsequent treatment session, or by measuring generalization to related, noncomputer activities or tests. Operation of the program should be familiar and intuitive for patients, particularly those that cannot read extensive instructions or other text. Since clinicians and programmers cannot anticipate every possible cue or strategy that may be helpful to every patient, intervention is frequently simplistic or nonexistent. Consequently, COT software usually consists of convergent tasks with simple,

obvious goals (e.g., drills) and represents supplementary tasks designed to reinforce or help generalize recently learned skills.

Computer-Assisted Treatment (CAT) software is presented on a computer by a clinician working at the same time ("side-by-side") with the patient. The role of the computer is limited to elements of basic task structure, such as presenting stimuli, storing responses, and summarizing performance, while the clinician provides special instruction, intervention, additional cuing, and other information to modify the activity to accommodate the patient's needs in the same way as during traditional clinician-provided treatment. This symbiotic relation between clinician and computer permits considerable flexibility, thus compensating for limitations inherent in the COT approach. In addition to treatment programs written specifically for use with clinicians, other software, such as COT, word processing, or video game programs, can be used in this manner as long as the clinician provides the patient with the additional information needed to perform the task.

Augmentative Communication Devices (ACDs) in aphasia treatment usually refer to small computers functioning as sophisticated "electronic pointing boards." Unlike the devices used by patients with severe dysarthria or other speech problems, patients with aphasia cannot simply type the words they want to say. ACDs designed for speakers with aphasia may incorporate digitized speech, text, pictures, and animation. Some allow both communication partners to use the device to exchange messages during conversations. The organization and semantic content of the ACDs can frequently be modified for each patient's particular needs and abilities. In addition to providing an alternative mode of communication, some researchers attribute improved performance on standardized tests and in "natural language" (i.e., speaking, listening, etc.) to treatment involving ACDs (Aftonomos et al., 1997).

A BRIEF HISTORY OF COMPUTERS

Computers were described by an English mathematician, Charles Babbage, almost 200 years ago, but the technology for building devices recognizable to us as computers did not exist until the 20th century. Another English mathematician,

Alan Turing (1936), described a device similar to a typewriter that utilized a "contingency table" (criteria and algorithms) to perform complex calculations that up to that point had been completed only by specially trained personnel. The concept of a machine capable of complex decision-making without human intervention was revolutionary (Turing, 1950). In the 1950s, computers were large electronic calculating machines that filled rooms with switches, vacuum tubes, and mechanical relays, and read rolls of punch tape and later, reels of electronic tape. Only banks, large corporations, and civilian and military government agencies could afford to purchase and operate these machines. Over the years, computers grew smaller, more reliable, and less expensive. "Microcomputers" were first sold in the mid-to-late 1970s to hobbyists and other technology enthusiasts who programmed the machines to perform specialized tasks, such as controlling all the lights in a house, or measuring rainfall. As computers began to show up in offices and homes, software developers saw a market for functional and entertaining programs for the general public: word processing, spreadsheet, data base, graphics, communications (modem), financial planning, will writing, etc. Today's multimedia desktop, laptop, and palm-size personal computers accessing information from the world-wide web are only the latest stage in this evolution. Looking back on the recent rapid growth—some might say, intrusion—of technology, it is understandable why many expect an imminent breakthrough that will abruptly change our lives for the better, a promise the computer industry's sales force has made since the mid-1950s. People with aphasia and their families may be particularly vulnerable to the unsubstantiated promises made by an avid computer industry intent on increasing sales. While the world rushes forward to embrace technology, those of us engaged in rehabilitation should step cautiously and apply accepted standards to determine the value of computer applications for each patient with aphasia.

LIMITATIONS OF COMPUTERIZED TREATMENT SOFTWARE

A speech-language pathologist, educated in communication theory and sufficiently experienced in the clinic and real life, can generate an infinite number of novel and relevant treatment stimuli and recognize, evaluate, and modify treatment activities in response to previously unacknowledged associations and unanticipated responses. In contrast, computer-provided treatment is based on a finite set of rules that are stated explicitly to specify actions that are likely to occur at particular points during a future treatment session. Limitations in modalities (e.g., computers cannot understand speech or writing very well) ensure that computerized treatment will be a subset of clinician-provided treatment and supplemental to treatment provided by properly trained clinicians.

Computers cannot be all things to everyone. Bolter (1984) described four properties of computers and computer programming that illustrate the limitations inherent in the application of computers to aphasia treatment: discrete, conventional, finite, and isolated.

Discrete

Because computers acknowledge and manipulate discrete (i.e., digital) units, qualitative description and decisions are difficult to make. Events must first be separated into distinct, unconnected elements before they can be acted upon by a computer. Face-to-face communication is a complex act described as our "oldest and highest bandwidth technology" (Rheingold, 1991, p. 216). Many elements of language and communication are not well deliniated or even universally recognized. In summarizing research on the perception of the meaning of words versus the message's affect for listeners during face-to-face communication, Mehrabian (1968) estimated that 55% of a message's affect (i.e., the emotional content) is communicated via facial cues, 38% is communicated vocally, but only 7% is communicated by the actual words. Although individual language tasks can be programmed, applying computer technology appropriately to aphasia rehabilitation requires appreciation for the intricacies and interdependence of elements within verbal (i.e., language) and nonverbal (e.g., kinesics, proxemics) channels of communication (Egolf & Chester, 1973; Katz et al., 1978).

Conventional

Computers apply pre-determined rules to symbols that have no effect on the rules. Regardless of the value of the symbols or the outcome of the program, the rules never change. However, although a consensus exists for some fundamental guidelines of aphasia treatment, all the rules are not known and those that are accepted may not be right under all conditions (Rosenbek, 1979). Computer-only treatment does not follow the clinical cycle of (a) administer treatment, (b) measure performance, (c) modify treatment, and (d) re-administer treatment and, therefore, is not adequately responsive to the dynamics of patient performance.

Finite

The rules and symbols that control computer-provided treatment are limited to those defined within the program. Except for the most sophisticated (i.e., "artificial intelligence") programs (e.g., Guyard et al., 1990), unforeseen problems and associations do not result in creation of new rules and symbols. Therapy presents the opposite case. Not all therapeutically relevant behaviors are identified; those that have been identified often vary in importance between patients and situations. Computer-provided learning commonly defers decisions to software designers and programmers who are not physically present during the session, but must plan in advance how to handle the intervention and code these steps into a computer program (c.f., Odor, 1988).

Isolated

Problems and their solutions presented by computers exist within the computers' own parameters, apart from the real world. Problems are stated in a way so symbols can be manipulated to solve the problem by following an *algorithm*, a finite series of steps described with adequate detail to guide the program to respond to input, answer questions, or solve problems. This lack of "world knowledge" is perhaps the most significant impedance to comprehensive computer-provided treatment. Language tasks as presented by computers essentially differ from the meaningful, pragmatic setting in which communication occurs among people. Computers, therefore, only consider problems in which all the variables and rules are known ahead of time, and can be solved in a step-by-step procedure with a finite number of steps, much like a game of chess. Learning to solve linguistic riddles on a computer program may lead to better scores on conventional aphasia tests; however, improving communication is quite another matter.

Treatment is recognized as a multilevel, interactive behavioral exchange. Not all therapeutically relevant behaviors have been identified; many that have (e.g., functionality) are influenced by internal (e.g., idiopathic) and external (e.g., environmental) factors and cannot be effectively controlled by a computer. In addition, while many basic parameters of therapy and fundamental skills of clinicians have been identified (Goldberg, 1997), all the rules are not known, and those on which we agree may not be correct (Rosenbek, 1979). For example, use of linguistic models to construct software to diagnose and treat aphasia is appealing (e.g., Guyard et al., 1990) and can ultimately teach us much about language (e.g., Fenstad, 1988) and aphasia (e.g., Wallich, 1991). However, some researchers (e.g., Katz, 1986, 1990; Kotten, 1989) believe that the pathological language behavior of people with aphasia is also influenced by a variety of other factors, including cognition (e.g., attention, vigilance, memory, resource allocation); cybernetics (e.g., slow rise time, noise buildup, intermittent imperception); behavioral factors (e.g., discriminatory stimuli, chaining, extinction); pragmatics (e.g., functionality, social status); and emotion (e.g., interest, relevance, novelty, enjoyment). No one therapeutic approach currently encompasses all known intervening variables.

If a program were written that could completely represent clinician-provided treatment, the software would be massive and exceed the capacity of modern personal computers. By reducing the scope of the problem to a size manageable for the computer, treatment software has been squeezed and shaped to imitate cognitive and language therapy in small,

trivial, and predominantly symbolic activities. Rather than emphasize state-of-the-art aphasia treatment, the resultant computerized activity highlights the technical limitations of the computer medium. Odor (1988) referred to this problem when he wrote that computer intervention defers decisions to programmers who are not physically present during the session, but must *gather and send* information only through the computer medium, *plan* in advance how to handle the learning interaction, and then *encode* these steps into a computer program. Consequently, the scope of treatment software is limited because computer programs are not powerful enough to represent every potentially relevant nuance of interaction during therapy. Odor concluded that computer-assisted instruction is often based on convergent rather than divergent theories of learning. Most computer treatment studies reported in the aphasia research literature describe convergent activities, particularly drills, in which specific responses are learned. Dean (1987) stated that the inability to incorporate divergent strategies in computer programs severely limits their value and application to treatment of aphasic patients, particularly chronic aphasic patients, for whom such treatment appears promising (Chapey et al., 1976). Divergent treatment software is becoming commercially available (e.g., *My House: Language Activities of Daily Living*), but no data exist to support efficacy. The adaptation of divergent therapy to computer-provided treatment continues to remain a challenge for contemporary software developers.

TREATMENT

The earliest applications of computers to aphasia rehabilitation owe much to behavior modification and the development of instrumental learning devices or "teaching machines" (Skinner, 1958). Some of these devices were prototypes and experimental (e.g., Keith & Darley, 1967), whereas others were commercially available and widely used, such as the *Language Master* (Keenan, 1967) and the *PAL (Programmed Assistance to Learning)* filmstrip projector (Pfau, 1974). Following the introduction of small mainframe computers ("minicomputers"), reports began to appear in professional journals describing attempts of researchers and clinicians to use computers to meet the needs of patients with aphasia. For example, Vaughn (1980) incorporated small, microprocessor-driven auditory, visual, and writing devices and minicomputers (such as the PDP-11) to provide treatment to outpatients over the telephone (telecommunicology). By the time personal computers (then called "microcomputers") were introduced in the mid-to-late 1970s, sufficient interest had grown among clinicians and researchers to develop treatment protocols for specific patients and types of problems (e.g., Schwartz, 1984).

Speed, accuracy, reliability, and ease of use are characteristics valued wherever personal computers are used, but the power of computers in rehabilitation is not simply the result of faster microprocessors or larger storage devices. Schuell et al. (1964) stated that principles of aphasia treatment should be used through our increasing repertoire of clinical techniques. The role of computers will evolve as the technology improves. There are many areas in which computers have the potential to become significant tools for treating aphasia.

Supplementary Treatment

Supplementary treatment in the form of workbooks and other activities has always been a useful option for clinicians (Dressler, 1991; Eisenson, 1973). Patients can work longer and more often on a variety of activities designed to stabilize, maintain, or generalize newly acquired skills. Contemporary commercial treatment and educational software extend controlled treatment-related language and cognitive activities beyond the confines of the treatment session if they are presented in a structured setting that incorporates important therapeutic principles and factors, such as control of stimulus characteristics and response requirements, and recording of session performance for later review. Programs can vary along a continuum according to structure and content, ranging from simple repetitive drills to interactive tasks that not only evaluate individual responses, but also measure overall performance and adjust the type and degree of intervention provided (e.g., Katz & Wertz, 1997).

Treatment Efficacy and Prognosis

Measuring the effects of intervention on aphasia is an essential part of any treatment regimen. Speech-language pathologists assess the influences of various linguistic, psychological, and physical variables on communication and task performance in order to evaluate the effectiveness of a treatment approach or activity. The computer can present treatment activities in a standard manner and routinely store performance data for later descriptive and statistical analysis, thus addressing Darley's (1972) efficacy questions. Additionally, computers can help clinicians develop local and national prognostic databases to predict with confidence that, for example, a 55-year-old Broca's aphasic adult, who 1-year post-onset is at the 50th percentile on the Porch Index of Communicative Ability (PICA) (Porch, 1981), will require between 125 and 150 trials to learn to write or print 10 functionally relevant words at the third-grade level (LaPointe, 1977). This benchmark of prognostic resolution would serve as an invaluable clinical yardstick against which the success of treatment could be measured (e.g., Matthews & LaPointe, 1981, 1983).

The widely used health care assessment tool, the *SF-36 Health Survey*, is available for downloading from the Internet at http://www.sf-36.com. Like the print version of the *F-36*, this version can be used for assessing effects from clinical trials, monitoring outcomes in clinical practice, and screening medical patients for mental health referral. It provides measures of physical functioning, bodily pain, general health, vitality, social functioning, emotional role functioning, mental health, and reported health transition. Translations of the *SF-36* are being tested in over 40 countries as part of the International Quality of Life Assessment (IQOLA) Project. The face validity of this tool is impressive for clinicians and researchers interested in investigating quality of health care across health disciplines, especially as it relates to the construct of quality of life. *SF-36* software that provides administration, scoring, and data export for research support is available.

Generalization

"Prepare for rather than pray for generalization" (Rosenbek et al., 1989, p. 138). Ultimately, the value of aphasia treatment is measured by the degree in which skills acquired in treatment are observed in real-life situations. It is imperative that the clinician actively train generalization. Computer-provided treatment is an environment very different from real-life communication. Generalization can be aided by the computer, which can administer some aspects of treatment without the familiar presence and constant conscious (and unconscious) control of the clinician. Upon reaching criteria on a computer task, a similar task should be presented without the computer, for example, writing instead of typing, or performing the actual functional activity rather than a computer simulation. Rosenbek et al. (1989) recommended a series of clinical activities to increase the likelihood of generalization. Several of the recommendations appear well suited for the computer: (a) expose each patient to numerous repetitions; (b) train a large number of items in a given category; (c) extend treatment outside of the clinic; and (d) organize treatment to maximize independence so that patients learn to use treated responses when they want to rather than when told to by the clinician. *Visual Confrontation Naming* (Parrot Software) helps to teach the patient a strategy to stimulate or compensate for word-finding problems by selecting among possible cues. Optional cues provided by the program are audible (i.e., first sound) and visual (e.g., first letter, description, multiple choice list containing the word). Ideally, patients should develop and practice their own self-cuing strategies. The CD-ROM version has over 500 target words with pictures, aiding in generalization of self-cuing strategies.

Independence and Emotional Factors

To foster independence, minimize dependency and depression, and help patients develop insight into their communication problems, patients should be able to use treatment software with minimal assistance from others. The required computer skills include turning on the computer system, selecting the treatment program from a 3.5-inch disk, hard drive, or the Internet, and following the protocol for each particular program. Patients themselves can then determine when and how often they participate in supplementary language activities. This is consistent with Wertz's (1981) statement that we should allow patients to maintain as much independence as possible and that a long-term goal of aphasia treatment is to have patients become their own best therapists. The insight patients have into *their* problems and *their* strengths can be used instead of ignored, and in this way, patients can take a more active role in their recovery.

Factors such as motivation, dependency, and quality of life are concerns that may become increasingly important to people with aphasia and their families as recovery slows and the degree of disability and its subsequent effect on life become more apparent. Under conditions of perceived helplessness and hopelessness, people frequently become depressed (Seligman, 1975) and have greater difficulty coping with and adapting to changes and problems (Coelho et al., 1974). Bengston (1973), Langer and Rodin (1976), Schulz (1976), and others have shown that giving some options and responsibilities to persons in otherwise dependent situations (e.g., the institutionalized elderly) can have a strong positive effect on their satisfaction and physical well-being. Decision-making and expression of personal preferences by each patient should be a basic part of any treatment program. Computerized activities can address this aspect of treatment by providing patients with aphasia a degree of control over the content and frequency of treatment.

Administrative Functions

Currently, computers are assisting clinicians in the performance of administrative and clinical duties, and in all likelihood will continue to do more (Hallowell & Katz, 1999). Morrison (1998a) describes an active role for computers and related technology in the evaluation of many factors essential to delivery of services and quality of care. Large-scale systems are expensive to set up and maintain, so it is essential to plan carefully and consult with information technology specialists experienced in health care before attempting to integrate technology and clinical and support staff (Morrison, 1998b). On a smaller scale, many clinicians use computers to gather, organize, and report case history information (Silverman, 1997). As is the case for many other professions, general purpose programs have useful applications for clinicians working with patients, for example, report and letter writing (word processing programs), organizing, recording, and recalling information (database programs), and organizing, calculating, and projecting values (spreadsheet programs). Innovations include the use of voice recognition in report writing to increase the speed of generating reports (Tonkovich et al., 1991) and the use of authoring systems to customize database data entry and retrieval. One of the most comprehensive systems is *Computerized Patient Records System (CPRS)*,

(Department of Veterans Affairs, 1998). CPRS enables clinicians using PCs in every VA Medical Center to access patient records not only within their own medical centers, but from other VAMCs. This ability greatly saves time and simplifies the process of retrieving and updating patient records, especially for patients who are treated at different facilities across the country.

Commericially available software provide another path to incorporating technology into administrative activities. The *Beaumont Outcome Software System (BOSS)* (Parrot) collects, coordinates, and analyzes clinical outcome assessment data as well as stores and utilizes information about clinicians, patient demographics, diagnoses, charges, and billing codes. *Chart Links* (Chart Links) is one commercially available system that is based on electronic patient medical records. It creates a record for each patient and tracks reports of each patient encounter, lab report, team report, medical diagnosis, recommended treatment, and treatment schedule. Workflow applications allow for charting, sorting, organizing, filing, report writing, and automated review of patient information. *Chart Links* is based on Lotus Notes, which allows for advantageous communication and security features. *Therapist Helper* (Therapist Helper) is another clinical practice management software program developed to facilitate patient and insurance billing transactions and accounting as well as report writing.

Recreational Activities

Many commercial recreational programs (such as arcade and adventure games) have found a limited but useful role in treatment (Lynch, 1983). Enderby (1987) discussed the possibility of computers in this role providing a path toward social and intellectual stimulation for patients with aphasia. Many educational and treatment programs use familiar game formats to minimize learning time and heighten enjoyment (e.g., Laureate Learning Systems). While recreation therapy can be a valuable service for patients, our involvement is neither urgent nor necessary. However, computer game activities, as do educational software programs, the Internet, and the world wide web, all offer patients a diversion and a way of occupying their time in a novel, distracting, entertaining, and sometimes intellectually stimulating manner which can promote and stimulate social interaction.

MODALITY CONSIDERATIONS

Face-to-face conversation (i.e., talking and listening) is our primary mode of communication. Management of auditory and verbal skills is central to the concept of aphasia rehabilitation (e.g., Schuell et al., 1964). Listening and talking are the communicative behaviors used to classify most types of aphasia (Goodglass & Kaplan, 1983; Kertesz, 1982), and are the focus of most aphasia therapy. Listening and talking, more than other language modalities, affect the likelihood of an aphasic person's successful reintegration into the community, the final demonstration of the success of therapy. For most patients, and for their families, friends, and physicians, the *perception* of recovery and treatment success is measured by improvement in listening and talking.

Contemporary treatment software offers little assistance to clinicians treating the speaking and listening problems that occur during conversation for patients with aphasia. Speech recognition is limited and unreliable for multiple speakers (as would be found in a treatment room of any clinic) and for speakers who produce variable errors, such as apraxia of speech and phonemic paraphasia. While high-quality digital speech is common on today's multimedia computer systems, programs that merely repeat object names or offer nonlinguistic visual cues are of minimal value to patients with auditory comprehension deficits.

The major contribution of computers to aphasia treatment currently appears to be in reading and writing. Computers are basically visual-motor, graphic machines. Information from the user is normally entered by typing on a keyboard; the output of the computer is displayed on the monitor screen and read by the user. This makes the computer well suited for presenting reading tasks and, through typing, writing tasks. Reading and writing skills appear to be an appropriate focus for computerized aphasia treatment for several reasons. Most aphasic patients have problems reading (Rosenbek et al., 1989) and writing (Geschwind, 1973). Reading requires minimal response from the patient. Programs for treating reading can run on standard personal computers, without expensive modification or specialized peripheral devices. Typing on the keyboard can be used to examine many aspects central to writing (Selinger et al., 1987), with the obvious exception of the mechanics of handwriting. Also, reading and writing as communicative acts are usually done alone; having greater interpersonal distance, they are in many ways less direct and responsive than speaking and listening. As such, reading and writing are appropriate *communication* (as opposed to *therapeutic*) activities for people with aphasia to practice on computers. Computerized reading and writing treatment tasks can free up valuable treatment time so that face-to-face, individual therapy can emphasize complex elements of auditory comprehension and verbal output skills that computers do not address. While the computer can provide valuable reading and writing activities (e.g., Scott & Byng, 1989), additional noncomputerized, clinician-provided reading and writing therapy should be supplied as indicated by patient performance.

STRUCTURE OF TREATMENT ACTIVITIES

There are many elements that are common to the structure of all treatment activities regardless of the underlying principles or mode of delivery, and although some are obvious, none

are trivial. An understanding of these task components is useful for describing, developing, and evaluating treatment activities for the computer.

All tasks have a *goal*, which is usually an intermediate step toward a major or long-term goal. The patient should be aware of the goal of the task, and should also be aware of the logical order or steps within the task that advance toward the goal. The clinician should provide the patient with *instructions* so that the patient knows from the beginning what is expected. The *stimuli* used and the desired *responses* should be consistent with the purpose of the task. Responses should be described and quantified using a multidimensional *scoring system* (LaPointe, 1977; Porch, 1981) whenever possible to identify and measure the occurrence of salient behaviors within the task. Care should be taken that the patient is not burdened with additional, unnecessary *response requirements* that could confound performance. Responses should be as simple as possible to reflect accurately the performance of the target behavior. *General feedback* (Stoicheff, 1960) to encourage the patient and *specific feedback* to describe the most recent response should be readily provided. The clinician should provide an *intervention* (strategy or cue) to improve performance as needed. Teaching specific responses may be the goal of some tasks; a more valuable goal commonly is to develop a task to help the patient learn an intervention (e.g., self-cue or compensatory) strategy to improve communication during actual, functional situations. Criteria for *termination* of the task should be specified to provide a target against which the patient can measure progress. Responses and performance *scores should be stored* for later review and analysis. The patient's performance and the intervention can *be evaluated* using various techniques (LaPointe, 1977; Matthews & LaPointe, 1981, 1983; McReynolds & Kearns, 1983; Prescott & McNeil, 1973). Finally, the intervention can be modified or the activity discontinued, as indicated.

MODELS FOR COMPUTER REHABILITATION

In contrast to the considerable attention afforded the arrival of new treatment programs, software developers rarely provide thorough descriptions of the treatment models influencing software evolution. As described by Wolfe (1987), early reports of computerized aphasia treatment (e.g., Katz & Nagy, 1982, 1983, 1984, 1985; Mills, 1982) provided no explicit models of rehabilitation from which the software could be evaluated. Recent studies have reversed the trend (e.g., Katz & Wertz, 1997; Loverso et al., 1985; Scott & Byng, 1989). Bracy (1986) was among the first to explicitly incorporate the work of Luria (1973, 1980) in the development of rehabilitation software. Having an explicit model facilitates the systematic development of software and provides a basis for clinicians selecting software for their patients. Three general models of rehabilitation provide clinicians with the structure to develop and evaluate software. Although they are not mutually exclusive, the models offer a basis from which the role of computers in aphasia rehabilitation can be directed and examined.

Brain-Behavior Relationships

Bracy (1986) described four theories accounting for recovery of cognitive functions, but the theory that function recovers through the retraining process (Luria, 1963, 1973) is the most closely allied to the modem concept of rehabilitation. Luria believed the return of skills involved a reorganization of brain functions so that there are new methods of performing behaviors previously executed through the structures that are now damaged ("intersystemic reorganization"). One function of computerized treatment, therefore, is to provide the patient with the direction and opportunity to retrain skills through the reorganization.

Behavior Modification

Behavior modification (operant conditioning, instrumental learning) describes the process of teaching a new behavior or eliminating an established one through the systematic application of consequences (Goldberg, 1997). The principles of behavior modification are thoroughly woven into the fabric of human behavior—simply put, people tend to do things that result in rewards and avoid behaviors that result in punishment (Skinner, 1948). [According to Skinner (1957), these principles even guide the way we communicate and use language.] The frequency of occurrence, duration (e.g., exposure time), and other parameters (e.g., size, color, loudness) of elements central to behavior modification (e.g., stimulus characteristics, reinforcement schedules) can be monitored and controlled with a computer. Many computer programs control some aspect of stimulus characteristics and provide reinforcement to patients in the form of corrective and general feedback.

Educational Models

Lepper (1985) contrasted three approaches to learning with direct application to treatment software: individualized drill and practice, educational games, and simulations. Drill and practice capitalizes on the computer's advantages in providing immediate feedback, sustained attention, data analysis, and highly individualized instruction. Educational games stimulate a person's interest through game-like activities. Educational simulations, also called *microworlds*, involve the patient in a series of problems in an imaginary environment. The contingencies between actions and outcome should lead the patient to an understanding of basic principles relevant to real-world environments. These programs assume that active, inductive, "discovery-based" learning is better for learning general skills than direct, didactic approaches, which seem to be more effective when learning highly specified information. *My House: Language Activities of Daily Living* (Laureate Learning Systems) is an example of computer software that is a "microworld" in which the patient is free to explore the total simulated environment rather than respond to specific stimuli.

TYPES OF COMPUTERIZED TREATMENT TASKS

Four major types of treatment activities are appropriate for presentation on the computer: stimulation, drill and practice, simulations, and tutorials. This list is not exhaustive, and types are not mutually exclusive; one treatment activity may have several purposes and demonstrate characteristics of more than one type, for example, stimulation and drill and practice (e.g., Seron et al., 1980).

Stimulation

As described by Schuell and her colleagues (1964), stimulation activities offer the patient numerous opportunities to respond quickly and usually correctly over a relatively long period of time for the purpose of maintaining and stabilizing the underlying processes or skills, rather than simply learning a new set of responses. The process, therefore, is the focus of the task. Stimuli are not selected primarily for informational content (e.g., interest and relevance), but for salient stimulus characteristics (e.g., length, number of critical elements, complexity, and presentation rate). Computer programs can easily be designed that contain a large database of stimuli and control these variables as a function of the patient's response accuracy. Overall accuracy and other salient response characteristics (e.g., latency) are usually displayed at the end of the task. An early example of a computer stimulation task is the auditory comprehension task described by Mills (1982).

Drill and Practice

The goal of drill and practice exercises is to teach specific information so that the patient is able to (or appears able to) function more independently. Stimuli are selected for a particular patient and goal, and so an authoring or editing mode is needed to modify stimuli and target responses. A limited number of stimuli are presented and are replaced when criterion is reached. Since response accuracy is the focus of the task, the program should present an intervention or cues to help shape the patient's response toward the target response. Drill and practice exercises, therefore, are convergent tasks because the accurate response must match the target response exactly. Results are displayed or stored on disk and show the effectiveness of the intervention. Examples of drill and practice programs are described by Katz and Nagy (1984), Katz et al. (1989), Katz and Wertz (1997), and Seron et al. (1980).

Simulations

Simulations ("microworlds") are programs that present the patient with a structured environment in which a problem or problems are presented and possible solutions are offered. Simulations may be simple, such as presenting a series of paragraphs describing stages of a problem and listing possible solutions. Complex programs more closely simulate a real-life situation by using pictures and sound. The term *virtual reality* (Rheingold, 1991) describes a totally simulated environment created through the interaction of a computer and a human along verbal and nonverbal channels. Simulations have been used in fields such as chemistry, geology, meteorology, and astrophysics to test conditions impossible to experience or to train people in situations that would otherwise be too dangerous to experience firsthand. Simulations provide the opportunity to design divergent treatment tasks that could more fully address real-life problem-solving strategies than those addressed by more traditional, convergent computer tasks, for example, by including several alternative but equally correct solutions to a problem, such as during PACE (Promoting Aphasics' Communicative Effectiveness) therapy (Davis & Wilcox, 1985). The question of whether computer simulations can improve generalization of newly acquired behavior to real-life settings remains to be tested.

Tutorials

Some authors (e.g., Eisenson, 1973) have suggested that patients with aphasia are best served by modification of their communication environment. In that respect, tutorials offer valuable information regarding communication and quality of life to the family, friends, and others who influence the aphasic patient's world. At the most fundamental level, the computer tutorial could present information commonly found in patient information pamphlets in an interactive format, with additional modules provided when needed or requested. This type of self-paced, informational program can be appropriately realized in a hypertext format, such as found on the world wide web, where a family member can navigate through text, pictures, animation, and sound, describing relevant aspects of aphasia and communication. The tutorial program could incorporate features of an *expert system*, in which detailed information is provided in response to a patient/family profile, and function as a source of information for family members in the future when new problems and questions arise.

CANDIDACY FOR THERAPY

Most patients with aphasia can benefit from the thoughtful application of appropriate treatment software used in a supplementary role. Prognostic indicators common to patients with aphasia in general will apply, e.g., etiology and site of lesion, age, time post-onset, educational level, etc. (Eisenson, 1973). Cognitive factors, like those described for patients suffering right hemisphere damage (Myers, 1999) or bilateral brain damage (Goldstein, 1942, 1948) should also be considered. While many factors influence which patients benefit most from computerized aphasia treatment, the most critical factors are severity, modality, sensory and physical impairments, independence, and self-monitoring. Severely impaired patients may be limited to simple treatment drills providing little real value or generalization, while the metacommunication needs of mildly impaired patients may not be served by complex, problem-oriented software. These patients may benefit from more direct, clinician-provided treatment. Patients with reading, writing, and, to some extent, listening, problems can practice and maintain skills and compensatory strategies learned from the clinician by using various computer programs. Hemianopsia, visual neglect, or simply changes in visual acuity can interfere with the patient's ability to view material on the computer display, while right hemiparesis can prevent a patient from easily using the computer mouse, typing on the keyboard, or even sitting comfortably in front of a computer for an extended period of time (Petheram, 1988). Many patients look forward to working with their clinicians, who they see as supportive and sympathetic, feelings they do not get from working with a computer. Others may not have sufficient initiative or discipline to maintain a treatment program without the continual watchful eye of the clinician. Perhaps most critically, patients who are unable to monitor their own performance (e.g., detect errors after feedback, modify subsequent responses, etc.) will gain little or no value from working independently on a computer.

EFFICACY OF APHASIA TREATMENT SOFTWARE

Treatment efficacy considers whether outcomes are improved as a result of a specific intervention (McGlynn, 1996). According to Rosenbek (1995), efficacy is improvement resulting from treatment applied in a rigidly controlled design when treatment and no-treatment conditions are compared. Wolfe (1987) found early reports of computerized aphasia treatment did not provide explicit models of rehabilitation from which the software could be evaluated. In an extensive review of the literature, Robinson (1990) reported that the efficacy of computerized treatment for aphasia as well as for other cognitive disorders had not been demonstrated. The research studies reviewed suffered from inappropriate experimental designs, insufficient statistical analyses, and other deficiencies. Since Robinson's critique, a number of studies have reported the effect of particular computerized interventions (e.g., Crerar et al., 1996; Katz & Wertz, 1992, 1997; Loverso et al., 1992).

According to Loverso (1987), most computer advocates focus on "appealing" features of computers, such as cost effectiveness and operational efficiency, while the real issue that demands attention from clinicians is treatment effectiveness; treatment activities must be effective before they can be efficient. Ineffective treatment programs would be damaging to the overall quality of treatment provided aphasic patients. If computerized treatment is to continue to develop and improve, it should undergo the same scientific scrutiny and systematic modification as do all other aspects of treatment.

Software, however, cannot reproduce every process and variable that occurs during treatment, and so computerized treatment in this sense will never be as efficacious as clinician provided treatment. One way clinicians increase the likelihood that software is efficacious is to develop and test their own treatment programs. Mills (1988) suggested that clinicians who program with only limited programming skills tend to produce limited programs. It is important, however, that programmers have more than a superficial understanding of treatment principles if treatment software is not to be limited in its effectiveness.

A range of support for the clinical application of computers exists in aphasiology. Dean (1987) wrote that existing computer treatment programs "are not firmly grounded in a theoretical rationale for remediation" (p. 267), thus limiting their potential. To Katz (1984, 1986) and Loverso et al. (1988), most contemporary treatment software consists of drills with no explicitly stated intervention goals; their use should be conservative and practical. Others (e.g., Bracy, 1983; Lucas, 1977; Skilbeck, 1984) have advocated the computer rather than the clinician as the primary treatment medium, and a few (e.g., Rushakoff, 1984) have described the development of clinician-independent, autonomous computerized aphasia treatment programs. Literature reviews have resulted in conflicting opinions of the efficacy of computers (e.g., Katz, 1987; Robinson, 1990). The strongest statement thus far is from Robinson (1990), who argued that research evidence is simply not available to support the use of computers for most language and cognitive problems. Robinson stated that some researchers obscured the basic issue by asking what works with whom under what conditions (see Darley, 1972), and concluded that because computers are prematurely promoted in clinical work, their routine clinical use may be causing patients more harm than good.

There is no substitute for carefully controlled, randomized studies, the documentation of which has become the scientific foundation of aphasiology. Research reported over the last 15 years incorporated increasingly sophisticated designs and greater numbers of subjects to assess efficacy of computerized aphasia treatment, from simple A-B-A designs and comparisons of pre- and post-treatment testing (Katz & Nagy, 1982, 1983, 1984, 1985; Mills, 1982) to large, randomly assigned single-subject studies (Loverso et al., 1992) and group studies incorporating several conditions (Katz & Wertz, 1992, 1997). Efficacy of computerized aphasia treatment is being addressed one study at a time.

Auditory Comprehension

Few studies have investigated the effects of computerized treatment drills on auditory comprehension problems. Until recently, high-quality digitized speech was costly and difficult to include in computer systems found in most clinics. Also, agreement on treatment approaches are few due to the varied, complex, and transient nature of auditory comprehension problems. Mills (1982) first used computer-controlled digitized speech to provide one-, two-, and three-part auditory "pointing" commands in a simple drill to a patient with chronic aphasia. Intervention was limited to repetitions of the auditory stimulus. Improvement was noted on pre- and post-treatment testing and on PICA and Token Test scores. The influence of other factors (e.g., placebo effect) should not be discounted as no withdrawal or multiple baseline single-subject research strategies were used, but the study is a good first step towards adapting auditory comprehension activities to the computer.

Verbal Output

Few researchers developed technology in an attempt to compensate for aphasic verbal output problems. Two researchers focused technology on dysnomia in different ways. Colby and his colleagues made extensive use of computers and speech synthesizers in attempts to increase verbalization and communication in autistic and other "nonspeaking" children (e.g., Colby & Kraemer, 1975; Colby & Smith, 1973). Later et al. (1981) built and programmed a small, portable microcomputer carried by a subject with dysnomia on a sling and shoulder strap combination, thus allowing the use of the device in actual communicative situations. When the subject experienced word-finding problems (Brown & Cullinan, 1981), she pushed keys in response to prompts from the computer. On a small LCD (Liquid Crystal Display) screen, the computer printed a series of questions designed to help the individual with dysnomia identify the forgotten word: for example, "Do you remember the first letter of the word?" "…the last letter?" "…any other letters?" "…any other words that go with the forgotten word?" The subject's answers were applied according to an algorithm outlined in the program, and a list of possible words was produced and displayed across the computer screen, beginning with the most "probable" words. When the patient recognized the forgotten word, she pressed a button and the word was produced via synthesized speech. [Most dysnomic patients usually can recognize the correct word and say it after a visual or auditory model (e.g., Benson, 1975).] The authors reported that the subject was cued successfully by the portable computer in real-life situations that were functional and communicatively stressful. Christinaz (personal communication) reported that the cuing algorithm subsequently generalized to noncomputer settings. Patients reported after several weeks of using the computer that they no longer required it, instead asking themselves the same series of questions previously displayed by the computer. Christinaz reasoned that the subjects had "internalized the algorithm" and now cued themselves without the need of external prompts. The frequency and success of this observation was not reported, but the implication of Christinaz's statement is certainly relevant and potentially significant. As more powerful portable computers are used as compensatory devices, acquisition and generalization of functional communication behaviors may occur if these or similar devices modeled self-cuing strategies for patients during actual communicative situations.

Van de Sandt-Koenderman (1994) described a computer program, "Multicue," that is designed to help patients with dysnomia identify and select self-cuing and compensatory strategies for word-finding problems. A picture is presented in the left upper quarter of the computer screen and the patient's goal is to type the appropriate name. If the patient does not know the name (or cannot type it), various cues can be selected (e.g., word meaning, word form, sentence completion) to help the patient retrieve the word. The goal of the program is to allow the patient to evaluate and practice several word-finding strategies, ultimately changing the process of word finding for the patient. The effectiveness of Multicue in a controlled study has not been reported.

Reading Comprehension

Early work by Katz and Nagy demonstrated various functions computers could provide when treating reading problems in patients with aphasia, although interpretation of the results must be tempered due to small sample sizes and limited research designs. Katz and Nagy (1982) described a program designed to test reading and also provide reading stimulation for aphasic patients. Five aphasic subjects ran the computer programs two to four times per week for 8 to 12 weeks. Although several subjects demonstrated improved accuracy, decreased response latency, and increased number of attempted items on some computer tasks, changes in pre- and post-treatment test performance were minimal. The following year, Katz and Nagy (1983) reported a drill and practice computer program for improving word recognition in chronic aphasic patients. The program was designed to accomplish a task difficult to undertake for a clinician and

used the advantages of a computer. The program presented 65 words that occur frequently in text and varied the rate of exposure as a function of accuracy of response. The goal of the program was to help increase and stabilize the subject's sight vocabulary, but no changes were observed on pre- and post-treatment measures for the five chronic aphasic subjects. Later et al. (1985) described a self-modifying drill and practice computerized reading program for severely impaired aphasic adults. The objective of the study was to improve functional reading, and a program was developed to teach subjects to read single words without intensive clinician involvement. The program also generated, through a printer, homework (writing activities) that corresponded to the subject's performance. Four of the five subjects demonstrated pre- to post-treatment changes on the treatment items that ranged from 16% to 54%.

Scott and Byng (1989) tested the effectiveness of a computer program designed to improve comprehension of homophones (similarly sounding words) for a 24-year-old subject who suffered traumatic head injury and underwent subsequent left temporal lobe surgery. Eight months after the accident, the subject continued to demonstrate aphasic symptoms as well as surface dyslexia and surface dysgraphia. Reading was slow and labored; she was able to understand printed words by sounding them out, presenting particular problems with homophones. The computer program, based on an information-processing model, was designed to focus on this particular aspect of the subject's reading problem. The subject demonstrated steady improvement on the 136-item treatment program, which was run 29 times over a 10-week period. The subject improved in recognition and comprehension of treated ($P < .001$) and untreated ($P < .002$) homophones used in sentences. Improvement was also demonstrated on recognition of isolated homophones that were treated ($P < .05$) and on defining isolated treated ($P < .03$) and untreated homophones ($P < .02$). Recognition of isolated untreated homophones and spelling of irregular words showed no improvement.

Katz and Wertz (1997) conducted a longitudinal group study to investigate the effects of computerized language activities and computer stimulation on language test scores for chronic aphasic adults. Fifty-five chronic aphasic subjects who were no longer receiving speech-language therapy were randomly assigned to one of three conditions: 78 hours of Computer Reading Treatment, 78 hours of Computer Stimulation ("nonlanguage" activities), or No Treatment. The Computer Reading Treatment software consisted of 29 activities, each containing eight levels of difficulty, totaling 232 different tasks. Treatment tasks required visual matching and reading comprehension skills, displayed only text (no pictures), and used a standard, match-to-sample format with two to five multiple choices. Treatment software automatically adjusted task difficulty in response to subject performance by incorporating traditional treatment procedures, such as hierarchically arranged tasks and measurement of performance on baseline and generalization stimulus sets, in conjunction with complex branching algorithms. Software used in the Computer Stimulation condition was a combination of cognitive rehabilitation software and computer games that used movement, shape, and/or color to focus on reaction time, attention span, memory, and other skills that did not overtly require language or other communication abilities. Subjects in the two computer conditions worked on the computer for 3 hours per week for 26 weeks. Clinician interaction during the two computer conditions was minimal. Subjects from all three conditions were tested using the PICA and Western Aphasia Battery (WAB) at baseline, 3 months, and 6 months. Significant improvement over the 26 weeks occurred on 5 language measures for the computer reading treatment group, on 1 language measure for the computer stimulation group, and on none of the language measures for the no-treatment group. The computer reading treatment group displayed significantly more improvement on the PICA Overall and Verbal modality percentiles and on the WAB Aphasia Quotient and Repetition subtest than did the other two groups. The results suggest that (a) computerized reading treatment can be administered with minimal assistance from a clinician, (b) improvement on the computerized reading treatment tasks generalized to noncomputer language performance, (c) improvement resulted from the language content of the software and not stimulation provided by a computer, and (d) the computerized reading treatment we provided to chronic aphasic patients was efficacious.

Writing: Typing and Spelling Words

Many reading comprehension activities are easily transferred to the computer. Writing activities, however, are less easily adapted. The most obvious problem is the inability of the common computer to evaluate handwriting and printing. The computerized writing treatment programs described in the literature substitute typing for writing during the intervention. In a comparison of writing and typing abilities of aphasic subjects, Selinger et al. (1987) examined seven subjects with left-hemisphere damage in order to assess differences between PICA graphic scores on subtests A through E using standardized PICA graphics responses, and PICA responses typed on a computer. No differences were found between scores on the PICA subtests as generated with a pencil and paper and PICA responses typed on a computer. These results suggest that the graphic language abilities of brain-damaged adults are equally represented by the two output systems.

Several investigators have incorporated complex branching algorithms in computerized writing programs to provide multilevel intervention. Seron et al. (1980) described a minicomputer/clinician combination that helped aphasic patients learn to type words to dictation. The clinician said the target word, and the subject typed a response on the computer keyboard. (The clinician had to know in advance the order of the stimuli programmed in the computer.) Intervention consisted of three levels of feedback: the number of letters in the target word; whether the letter typed was in the word; and when the correct letter was typed, whether that letter was in the correct position. The five subjects completed the program in 7 to 30 sessions. Pre- and post-treatment tests required the subjects to write a generalization set of single words to dictation. A decrease ($P < .05$) in the number of misspelled words and in the total number of errors made on the post-treatment test suggested that the computer program had improved spelling of words written by hand. Four of the five subjects maintained improved performance on a second post-treatment test administered 6 weeks later.

Katz and Nagy (1984) used complex branching steps to evaluate responses and provide patients with specific feedback in a computerized typing/handwriting confrontation/spelling task. A stimulus was randomly selected by the program, and a drawing representing the stimulus was displayed on the computer screen. The subject responded by typing on the keyboard. Feedback consisted of auditory sounds and text printed on the screen. Single and multiple cues from a hierarchy of six were selected by the program in response to the number of errors made for each of 10 stimuli. A seven-point multidimensional scoring system was used to describe performance and track the effectiveness of the various cues. Additional feedback included repetition of the successful and most recently failed cues. At the end of the computer session, pencil-and-paper copying assignments automatically generated via the computer printer were completed by the subject. Pre- and post-writing tests revealed improved spelling of the target words for seven of the eight aphasic subjects ($P < .01$).

Glisky et al. (1986) reported the ability of four memory-impaired, nonaphasic subjects to type words in response to definitions displayed on the computer screen. Cues included displaying the number of letters in the word and displaying the first and subsequent letters in the word, one at a time, as needed. Cues continued until either the patient typed the word correctly or the program displayed the entire word. All patients improved in the ability to type the target words without cues. Patients maintained their gains after a 6-week period of no treatment and demonstrated generalization to another typing task, although generalization to writing was not measured.

Katz et al. (1989) developed and tested a computer program designed to improve written confrontation naming of animals for nine aphasic subjects with minimal assistance from a clinician. The treatment program required subjects to type the names of 10 animals in response to pictures displayed on the computer monitor. If the name was typed correctly, feedback was provided and another picture was displayed. If an error was made, hierarchically arranged cues were presented and response requirements were modified. Five of the nine subjects reached criterion within six treatment sessions, and the performance of all nine subjects improved an average of 40% on the computer task ($P < .0001$). In addition, improvement was measured on noncomputerized written naming tasks, such as written confrontation naming of the treatment stimuli and written word fluency for animal names ($P < .001$). The PICA Writing modality score improved by +4.1 percentile points ($P < .05$). Improvement did not extend to PICA Overall and Reading scores. Because the goal of the program was to teach subjects the 10 names, improvement did not, nor was it expected to, generalize to written word fluency for an unrelated category. The lack of change in these latter language activities for these nine chronic aphasic subjects contrasts with their improved performance on treated words.

Deloche et al. (1993) developed software to treat oral and written modality differences in confrontation naming for two aphasic subjects, a surface dysgraphic and a conduction aphasic. The intervention focused on written naming from the keyboard. Both subjects maintained improvements 1 year following therapy.

Augmentative Communication Device

Published reports from Gardner and Gardner (1969), Premack (1970), and others involved in animal communication described success teaching nonhuman primates (e.g., chimps, apes) the use of nonverbal, language-like symbolic communication systems. These reports stimulated efforts to teach visually based, alternative communication systems to severely aphasic people (e.g., Gardner et al., 1976). Developing the concept further, Steele et al. (1987), Weinrich et al. (1989), and Steele et al. (1989) developed and tested a graphically oriented computer-based alternate communication system called the *Computer-Aided Visual Communication* system, or *C-VIC*, for chronic, global aphasic adults. C-VIC is an interactive pointing board that runs on a Macintosh computer and uses a picture-card design, or metaphor. Subjects use the mouse to select one of several pictures, called icons, each of which represents a general category. The selected icon then "opens up" to reveal pictures of the items within the selected category. After selecting the desired item, the picture is added to a sequence of other selected pictures; this "string" of pictures represents the message. The message can be read via the sequence of icons, words printed below the sequence, or, in some cases, heard through digitized speech. Much attention is given to the selection of icons. Weinrich et al. (1989) reported that concrete icons were learned and generalized faster than were abstract icons, but neither type of icon generalized well to new situations. The empirical evidence to support the efficacy of C-VIC was collected in a series of single-case studies (Steele et al., 1987; Weinrich et al., 1993; Weinrich et al., 1989). Steele et al. (1987)

noted that, although globally impaired aphasic subjects using C-VIC improve on expressive and receptive tasks, communication through more traditional modes of communication remains unchanged. However, Weinrich et al. (1995) trained two Broca's aphasic subjects in the production of locative prepositional phrases and S-V-O sentences on C-VIC and reported that their verbal ability improved considerably.

A commercial version of C-VIC, called *Lingraphica*, incorporates animation and digitized speech on a Macintosh Powerbook computer. Lingraphica is an integrated, computerized communication system that combines spoken words, printed words, pictures (icons), and text processing. Patients use a mouse device to select one of several icons, each of which represents a general category. The selected icon then "opens up" to reveal pictures of the items within the selected category. After selecting the desired item, the picture is added to a sequence of other selected pictures; this "string" of pictures represents the message which can be read via the sequence of icons, words printed below the sequence, or heard through digitized speech. Aftonomos et al. (1997) used Lingraphica with 20 subjects and reported improvement in multiple modalities for most subjects, inlcuding verbal. Clearly, further single-subject and group research utilizing standardized measurements is needed to test the effectiveness of new computer technology adapted to the communicative needs of aphasic patients. The treatment approach referred to in the study by Aftonomos et al. (1997) formed the basis of multimodal treatment for aphasia administered by speech-language pathologists using Lingraphica at *LingraphiCare* clinics.

Artificial Intelligence

Reports by Guyard et al. (1990) represent beginnings of a new stage in the development of treatment software by integrating artificial intelligence (AI) programming and computer-assisted instruction (CAI) for the rehabilitation of aphasic patients. Researchers (e.g., Barr & Geigenbaum, 1982) described this union between AI and CAI as "Intelligent CAI" (ICAI). ICAI can expand the scope, responsiveness, and flexibility of aphasia therapy software so that a computer program would determine the type, sequence, and rate of stimuli presented based on evaluation of the patient's responses. While valued in education, ICAI has met limited success in aphasia rehabilitation primarily due to two factors: the heterogeneity of the aphasic population and the complexity of aphasia therapy (Katz, 1990).

Simulations

Roth (1992) and Gadler and Zechner (1992) each described computer-simulated worlds (NeueWEGE and AUSWEGE, respectively) in which patients, guided by their clinicians, explore a microworld, making decisions, "traveling," and taking chances without any real physical or interpersonal risks. Topics of tasks are familiar and functional to patients (e.g., planning a vacation). However, no controlled study measuring efficacy has been reported. Crerar and Ellis (1995) described the "Microworld Project," a computer system based on sound neuropsychologic and psycholinguistic theory designed to treat sentence-processing impairments. Concepts such as agent, action, object, and spatial relations were manipulated to improve sentence comprehension. A series of experiments (Crerar & Ellis, 1995; Crerar et al., 1996) demonstrated improvement in chronic aphasic subjects after a relatively short duration of treatment.

Telemedicine

ASHA teleseminars and videoconferences and the Tele-rounds series sponsored by the National Center for Communication Disorders are good signs that telecommunications technology is coming of age in our own discipline (Duffy, 1998). This technology permits improved access to health services, especially for remote and underserved populations. While there are numerous potential advantages to the use of telecommunications technology to provide clinical services, many factors must be carefully evaluated, such as image quality, appropriateness of the fields of view, training requirements, user preferences, cost, and reliability and validity of diagnostic findings using such technology (Peters & Peters, 1998).

Technology has been used in the past to provide assessment and treatment for patients with communication impairments who live in remote locations. *Tele-Communicology* (Vaughn, 1980; Vaughn et al., 1987) incorporated small, microprocessor-driven auditory, visual, and writing devices placed in the homes of patients, and remote computers to provide assessment and treatment over the telephone. Wertz et al. (1987) compared the effectiveness of closed-circuit television, computer-controlled video laser disc, and traditional face-to-face interaction for providing appraisal and treatment for patients with aphasia in remote settings. Subjects in all three treatment conditions demonstrated clinically significant improvement as indexed by scores on the *Porch Index of Communicative Ability (PICA)* (Porch, 1981). No significant differences among the three conditions were observed. The results suggest that television and video laser disc over the telephone could be employed to provide services for patients who live where services do not exist. Brodin and Magnusson (1994) reported numerous studies conducted in Sweden demonstrating the feasibility of treatment provided over telephone lines for patients with aphasia in rural settings.

Duffy et al. (1997) summarized results of telemedicine evaluations of speech and language disorders in patients in a small, rural hospital and in large multidisciplinary medical practices. They concluded that telemedicine evaluations can be reliable, beneficial, and acceptable to patients with a variety of acquired speech and language disorders, both in rural settings and within large multidisciplinary medical settings. To date, there are no explicit technical or clinical national standards or guidelines for the use of telecommunications to deliver services in the field of speech-language pathology. Although Medicare does provide coverage for some telehealth services, there is no explicit provision of coverage for speech-language pathology services at this time (c.f., Goldberg, 1997).

Comparison of Traditional and Computer Mediums

Comparing the effect of similar treatment activities provided by two different mediums should improve understanding of the influence of the medium and the relative effectiveness of the treatment. Many researchers are attempting to simulate accepted testing and treatment protocols on the computer. Some researchers think that, because of speed, reliability, and relative autonomy, computers are ideally suited to administer tests to aphasic patients, who can then work at their own pace without embarrassment or fear of humiliation (e.g., Enderby, 1987). Odell et al. (1985) developed two computerized versions of the Raven Coloured Progressive Matrices (Raven, 1975). The program used high-resolution graphics and a touch screen input device to administer and analyze test performance quickly and accurately with minimal supervision from a clinician. The authors compared the two computerized versions of the Raven matrices with a traditional, clinician-controlled, paper-booklet administration of the test. The performances of 16 subjects with aphasia were essentially equivalent under all three conditions, leading the authors to conclude that the computer testing conditions did not present greater visual or cognitive demands on the subjects.

Wolfe et al. (1987) compared the real-object and computer simulation performances of non-brain-damaged and aphasic adults on another nonverbal problem-solving task, "The Towers of Hanoi" puzzle, originally administered to aphasic subjects by Prescott et al. (1984). The performance of 19 aphasic and 19 non-brain-damaged subjects was compared using two different methods of presentation: two-dimensional color computer simulation of the puzzle versus the manipulation of the actual wooden model. Non-brain-damaged subjects performed equally well under both conditions. As in the study by Odell et al. (1985), subjects with aphasia demonstrated similar performance on the task under both conditions. These same subjects, however, required more time to complete the puzzle in the computer condition than when manipulating the actual wooden model. The results suggest that while the computer medium did not affect the accuracy of performance for the subjects with aphasia, task completion took longer and was less efficient under the computer condition.

The effectiveness of closed-circuit television, computer-controlled video laser disc, and traditional face-to-face interaction for providing appraisal and treatment to patients with aphasia in remote settings, as measured by Wertz et al. (1987), was described earlier. Results suggested no significant differences among the three conditions in the diagnoses assigned to subjects; additionally, subjects in all three treatment conditions demonstrated clinically significant change (between 12 and 17 percentile points on the PICA). No significant differences in improvement among the three treatment groups were observed, indicating that patients with aphasia could benefit from treatment provided in any of the three conditions.

An excellent example of the process of demonstrating efficacy in a computerized treatment program involves 14 years of published research by Felice L. Loverso and his colleagues, who have documented a series of data-based reports describing the development and testing of a model-driven clinician-provided treatment approach, the "verb as core," from its origins as a "clinician-delivered therapy" (Loverso et al., 1979; Loverso et al., 1988) to its encoding and refinement as a computer/clinician-assisted program (Loverso et al., 1985; Loverso et al., 1988; Loverso et al., 1992).

Loverso et al. (1979, 1988), and Selinger et al. (1987) initially developed and tested a treatment protocol for aphasic patients in which verbs were presented as starting points and paired with different wh-question words to provide cues to elicit sentences in an actor-action-object framework. Thirty verbs were used at each of six modules. The hierarchy was divided into two major levels, each consisting of an initial module and two submodules that provided additional cuing for subjects unable to achieve 60% or better accuracy on the initial module. Level I presented stimulus verbs and the question words "who" or "what" to elicit an actor-action sentence. Level II elicited actor-action-object sentences by presenting stimulus verbs and the question words "who" or "what" for the actor and the question words "how," "when," "where," and "why" for the object. Subjects responded verbally and graphically. Subjects were scheduled for treatment three to five times per week. During each session, 30 stimulus verbs were presented for generation of sentences. Statistically significant improvement ($P < .05$) was demonstrated on the PICA following 3.5 months of treatment for each of the two subjects with aphasia.

Later, Loverso et al. (1985) compared the effects of the same treatment approach when treatment was provided by a clinician and when it was provided by a computer and speech synthesizer assisted by a clinician. The aphasic subject responded in the clinician-only condition by speaking and writing and in the clinician-computer condition by speaking and typing. Stimulus presentation and feedback in the clinician/computer condition was normally provided only by the computer. The clinician intervened only if the patient's typed response was correct but the spoken response was in error. The subject improved on the task under both conditions but took longer to reach criteria under the computer and clinician-assisted condition. Based on the subject's improvement, both on the treatment task and on "clinically meaningful" changes on successive administrations of the PICA ($P < .01$), the authors concluded that their listening, reading, and typing activities under the clinician/computer condition had a positive influence on the patient's language performance. They suggested that, although still in the early stages of development, aphasia treatment administered by computers is practical and has the capacity for success. Loverso et al. (1988) replicated the study by Loverso et al. (1985) with five fluent and five confluent aphasic subjects for the purpose of examining whether treatment provided under the computer/clinician condition was as collective as that provide by a clinician alone when treating various types and severities of aphasia using their cuing-verb-treatment technique. The 10 subjects required 28% more sessions ($P < .05$) to reach criteria under the computer/clinician condition than under the clinician-only condition. Fluent subjects required 24% more sessions and nonfluent subjects required 33% more sessions under the computer/clinician conditions than under the clinician-only condition. Of the 10 subjects, 8 showed significant improvement ($P < .05$) on the PICA Overall percentile measure, on the Verbal modality measure, and on the Graphic modality measure. All subjects maintained gains after a maintenance phase of 1 month post-treatment or longer. Similar results were reported following a replication of the study using 20 subjects (Loverso et al., 1992).

EXAMPLES OF COMMERCIALLY AVAILABLE SOFTWARE

Auditory Comprehension

Although developed primarily for children, three programs from Laureate Learning Systems, *My House*, *My Town*, and, to a lesser extent, *My School*, are good examples of software that can be used to provide stimulation treatment for adults with aphasia. For example, in *My House*, rooms within a house can be viewed, along with many items typically found in the rooms. For example, the bedroom contains a bed, end table, lamp, bureau, closet, clothes, etc. A natural-sounding, digitized voice identifies the target item by name or function (pre-selected by the clinician). After the patient uses the mouse (or touch screen if available) to designate an item, the program indicates accuracy visually and/or auditorally. Text (name or function) can also be displayed, as selected by the clinician. The program provides repetitions when requested by the patient and options for repetitions and nonlinguistic (visual) cues following incorrect responses to help the patient complete the item successfully. Items are drawn with color and charm.

Direction Following Plus (Parrot) is a program that requires patients to move items on a screen with the keyboard or mouse in response to auditory or written commands. The publisher reports that over 500,000 novel verbal items can be generated. Item difficulty may be manipulated in terms of number of items shown on the screen; shape, size, and color of items; and the number of steps in the commands. Both Laureate and Parrot offer a number of programs that produce high-quality digital speech.

Verbal Output

Technology has been more readily adapted to motor speech problems than to the complex and less completely understood language formulation problems of adults with aphasia. However, some recent programs show promise. *Visual Confrontation Naming* (Parrot) helps to teach the patient a strategy to stimulate or compensate for word-finding problems by selecting among possible cues. Cues may be audible (i.e., first sound) or visual (e.g., first letter, description, multiple choice list containing the word). Ideally, patients should develop self-cuing strategies using the most successful cue. The CD-ROM version has over 500 target words with pictures. *Verbal Picture Naming Plus* (Parrot) recognizes spoken words by using sophisticated speech recognition technology. The patient is prompted to name a picture displayed by the computer. The computer evaluates the verbal response and, if incorrect, prompts the patient to repeat the word after it is verbally presented. While the task requirements for patients are not unusual, clinicians may wish to determine for themselves whether or not the voice recognition software is sufficiently accurate for the needs of each patient. Also, be aware that speech recognition software designed for some versions of Windows (e.g., Windows 95/98) may not work for others (e.g., Windows NT).

Aphasia Tutor 0: Sights 'n Sounds (Bungalow) is a word repetition task that displays a word or picture while presenting the word using digitized speech. The patient's repetition is recorded and both the computer model and patient's response are played back for comparison. The software provides over 400 words and clinicians can add their own words (in the "Professional version").

Reading Comprehension

Treatment of reading problems using computers appears to be particularly appropriate when considering the nature of patients, activities, interventions, and computers. Most people with aphasia, even mild, residual aphasia, report problems understanding long or complex text. As reading is a task in which we typically engage alone, it is socially appropriate to practice alone. Reading requires minimal responses by the patient, thus simplifying software development. These programs can run on minimally configured, less expensive systems.

Multimedia Reading Comprehension Plus (Parrot) presents three-page, large-type short stories. The patient controls two types of cues: words can be defined or "read aloud" by the computer using digitized speech. Patients can also select a vocabulary test or a story comprehension test. *Aphasia Tutor* (levels 1–4) (Bungalow) provides reading exercises to improve reading comprehension, allowing for progression from letters to words to sentences to paragraphs. It also includes a module allowing for "practical reading" of items such as newspapers, product labels, and bills. *Direction Following Plus* (described previously) (Parrot) allows for written command functions that would be appropriate for reading comprehension goals. For patients who drive or hope to drive again, *Traffic Sign Tutor* (Bungalow) may complement functional reading as well as symbolic comprehension goals. This program allows for interactive practice with traffic sign recognition and responding to written hypothetical driving scenarios.

Writing: Typing and Spelling

Computers are also an appropriate medium for treating writing disorders, a common and persistent problem in aphasia. Like reading, writing tasks are usually done alone. While it is unexpected for computers to improve the mechanics of writing, they can provide tasks designed to improve other components of written language, such as spelling and grammar. For spelling of single words, *Picture Naming Plus* (Parrot) requires the patient to type the name of a photographic-quality picture displayed on the monitor. The program recognizes alternate names of items (e.g., couch, sofa, davenport). Options allow the clinician to accept responses that are incorrect, but recognizable, such as letter reversals. Word processing software, such as Word (Microsoft), offers many features that could assist mildly impaired patients, such as spelling check, grammar check, thesaurus, templates, and the "Assistant," which automatically provides guidance when writing letters or performing other common functions.

Brubaker on Disk: Database of Customized Language and Cognitive Exercises (Parrot) contains over 1500 exercises that can be arranged and printed to create personalized activities or workbooks for patients to complete during treatment sessions or as homework. The clinician uses a mouse to select among different language and cognitive tasks, difficulty levels, response types, print size, and type face. The program uses the choices to select exercises from a large database. The clinician then reviews on screen the selected exercises and prints what he or she wants to include in a personalized workbook.

Cognitive Problems

Treatment efficacy for computerized cognitive retraining is less clearly documented than for speech and language treatment (Robinson, 1990), but researchers are striving to better assess efficacy. Two multilevel computerized cognitive treatment programs that are shared among professionals in neuropsychology and speech-language pathology are

Captain's Log and *PSSCogReHab*. *Captain's Log* (BrainTrain) includes 33 separate computer programs that focus on visual/motor, conceptual, and numeric skills as well as attention. It allows for tracking of performance across several sessions, and includes reaction time measures and analyses of error responses. *PSSCogReHab* (Psychological) includes a set of eight software packages with treatment activities focused on attention, executive skills, visuospatial and memory skills, and problem solving. Many other programs are designed to help treat specific problems. For example, *Listening Skills Plus* (Parrot) uses digitized speech to present one- to five-part instructions (involving color, size, and shape). Responses are indicated by pointing with the mouse. Clinicians may also build their software libraries by subscribing to the *Journal of Cognitive Rehabilitation* (Psychological). Each monthly issue includes a 3.5-inch disk that contains *Soft Tools*, a treatment program (frequently, a "game") designed for the PC to focus on a different cognitive problem, such as memory or visuospatial skills.

Additionally, many devices are designed to help patients with cognitive impairments cope with complex daily activities. Electronic scheduling and reminding devices and computerized calendars (c.f., Herrmann et al., 1996) are increasingly affordable for integration into cognitive rehabilitation programs. *PocketCoach* (Parrot) is a portable voice recorder designed to help patients with cognitive problems complete complex, real-life tasks. Using his or her own voice, the clinician records a series of instructions or steps into the device. The patient plays back the steps, one at a time, until the task is completed. *MoneyCoach* (Parrot) runs on a multimedia PC and helps patients develop shopping lists, write checks, and maintain their budgets.

Augmentative Communication Device

Lingraphica as a compensatory device was described earlier. Steele and his colleagues recently have re-directed their efforts. As LingraphiCARE America, they have begun to establish a network of specialized "Language Care Centers" for the treatment of adults with aphasia by combining the use of Lingraphica technology with standardized clinical treatment strategies and a growing patient database containing demographics and outcome measures. Although preliminary outcome data have been reported (Aftonomos et al., 1997), further single-subject and group research utilizing standardized measurements is needed.

Another example of an ACD device is the DynaVox 2c, a lightweight (about 6 pounds) system designed for children and adults. The device utilizes a color display and text-to-speech conversion. It has built-in infrared environment control capabilities that permit the user to easily transmit files between the DynaVox and a desktop PC. Infrared capability also permits control of televisions, VCRs, and other appliances, providing more independence for the user. DynaVox software utilizes symbol and word prediction capability and a searchable "concept tagged" vocabulary list, enabling faster programming and automatically generated "pages" or screens of associated pictures and words.

FUTURE TRENDS

The computer can become a very powerful clinical tool by incorporating what we know about aphasia treatment, and technology. New multimedia PCs are common, providing better platforms for treatment software focusing on auditory comprehension and verbal output problems. Improved speech recognition, a goal for the entire computer industry, can result in an entirely new generation of treatment programs and ACDs. Replacing traditional, static, still images with dynamic digital video segments in treatment software increases interest and relevance for many patients. Affordable digital still and video cameras increase the ease with which software can be individualized for each patient's needs and interests. Palm-size PCs will influence the development of ACDs and computers in rehabilitation in the same manner laptop computers did just a few years ago. Eisenson (1973) suggested clinicians consider changes in the environment of patients with aphasia in order to maximize their communicative potential. Technology is helping us do that.

The most influential element, though, is not technological, but clinical. In all computerized aphasia treatment studies cited in this chapter, clinicians selected and tested the patients, designed the treatment plans, designed and modified the treatment tasks, trained the patients to use the computers, and measured treatment efficacy. Computers, programmers, publishers, or researchers are not responsible for treatment effectiveness; clinicians are. As treatment cannot be effectively "prescribed" like medicine, software should be viewed as supplementary treatment, with the clinician providing critical intervention as indicated by performance and other considerations. The role of computers and treatment software, like all tools, should extend the abilities of the clinician, allowing clinicians to intervene when skills, experience, and flexibility are required. Rather than emphasize what computers can or cannot do better than clinicians, our focus should be on an intelligent division of labor between computers and clinicians, a combination that can do more than either alone. The real danger comes from a failure to appreciate the scope and depth of clinical work. An autonomous, robotic therapist, representing the knowledge and experience of a competent aphasia clinician, is some fantasy dreamed up by people who focus too much on the *costs* of care and not enough on the *efficacy* of care. Until we can describe to others precisely how to treat specific problems in individual patients, it is unreasonable, unethical, and a misrepresentation of the complexity of aphasia therapy to assume that at this time a machine can perform the functions of a clinician.

The true value of computers in the rehabilitation of aphasia continues to be studied. Just like the question of efficacy itself in aphasia rehabilitation (Darley, 1972; Fitz-Gibbon, 1986; Howard, 1986) the effectiveness of computer use in aphasia treatment cannot be answered with a simple "yes" or "no." Much more work is needed. Treatment software may always be an imperfect reflection of clinician-provided therapy, but by improving the software, clinicians and programmers will learn more about how and why treatment works. In the best tradition of scientific and rehabilitative efforts, aphasiologists can work together to shape this new tool of technology for the development of their professions and the benefit of all patients.

KEY POINTS

1. What is believed about aphasia and treatment should be reflected in treatment software and not diminished by the limitations of computers.
2. Four properties of computers and computer programming that illustrate the limitations inherent in the application of computers to aphasia treatment are discrete (quantity rather than quality), conventional (pre-applied, unchanging rules), finite (cannot anticipate every possibility), and isolated (artificial rather than real world).
3. Major areas in which computers have the potential to become significant tools for treating patients with aphasia include providing supplemental treatment, measuring efficacy, making prognoses, helping generalization, fostering independence and a more active role in treatment, providing recreational activities, and performing administrative functions.
4. Contemporary multimedia computers are ideal for providing auditory stimulation, reading treatment, and, to a lesser extent, writing treatment (through typing).
5. Speech recognition software has improved in recent years, but is still inadequate for most clinical applications in aphasia due to poor ability to understand (a) multiple, different speakers and (b) speakers with variable phonologic errors (as in aphasic paraphasias and apraxia of speech).
6. Clinicians should assess the following components of any treatment software considered for use with patients with aphasia: goal, instructions, stimulus characteristics, response requirements, scoring system, general feedback, specific ("corrective") feedback, type and degree of intervention, criteria for termination, and scores stored for later analysis.
7. Treatment software, like all treatment activities, should be based on a treatment model or models.

Three basic models are brain-behavior relationships, behavior modification, and educational models.
8. Four basic types of treatment software include stimulation, drill and practice, simulation, and tutorial.
9. Treatment efficacy refers to whether or not outcomes are improved as a result of a specific intervention.
10. A large body of research published in peer-reviewed journals demonstrates the effectiveness of aphasia treatment and computerized aphasia treatment for various populations of people with aphasia.
11. The value of aphasia treatment is measured by the degree in which skills acquired in treatment are observed in real-life situations. Generalization can be aided by the computer, which can administer some aspects of treatment without the familiar presence and constant conscious (and unconscious) control of the clinician.
12. Success of treatment for adults with chronic aphasia depends more on their acceptance of their residual disabilities and their social re-integration than on periodic but minimal gains in language tasks. Technology can assist patients with aphasia in these goals (a) by helping them gain new language skills, (b) by modifying and helping them gain control of their environment, and (c) by providing them with options to improve their communication and quality of life.

Questions and Tasks

1. Review treatment programs in your clinic. Evaluate the programs as though they were clinician-provided treatment activities. How do they measure up to the treatment you provide your patients?
2. Critically review treatment programs described in commercial catalogs. Are expectations stated or implied that seem a little too good to be true? Do the tasks seem worthwhile as treatment activities or supplementary activities?
3. Under what circumstances could a person with aphasia improve talking, listening, reading, and/or writing by using an ACD?
4. What are some of the major limitations of computer-provided treatment? How can you, as a clinician, overcome these limitations with your patients?
5. What would you like to see computers do in aphasia treatment? Describe a program that helps a clinician improve a patient's reading comprehension.
6. Design a computer program based on a favorite or familiar treatment activity. Incorporate options that allow the clinician to modify task requirements for patients with different types or severities of aphasia.

CLINICAL EXAMPLES

Example 1: Auditory Comprehension

MODALITY:	listening
DESIGN:	stimulation
GOALS:	to maintain accuracy, self-monitoring, and attention as response time decreases
TASK:	using digitized speech, the computer states the name (or function) of an item in a complex scene containing several functionally related items displayed on the monitor. The patient selects the correct item with the mouse.
SOFTWARE:	*My House* (Laureate Learning Systems)
PROCEDURE:	The clinician selects a response time (e.g., 10 seconds) which permits the patient to respond to all items with 100% accuracy. Response time is reduced for subsequent trials until the patient begins to make errors.
INTERVENTION:	Keep response time at the level when errors first occurred. Reduce the number of items to two, and identify those two to the patient before beginning ("The computer is going to ask you to point to only this one or that one."). When 100% accurate for three consecutive trials, increase number of items to three, four, etc., until all items are presented.
SCORING:	1 point per correctly selected item

Example 2: Writing/Printing Personal ID Information

MODALITY:	writing (typing)
DESIGN:	drill and practice
GOAL:	to improve the ability to write or print personal information for a chronic, severely impaired, predominantly nonverbal patient with aphasia using a typing drill
TASK:	type name, address, and telephone number in response to a diminishing set of cues
SOFTWARE:	word processor
PROCEDURE:	The clinician creates a series of word processing documents with diminishing cues, e.g., Document 1 has the intact model for simple copying, Document 2 has every third letter or number missing, Document 3 has every other word missing, etc. (The diminishing cues can take any form thought useful by the clinician.) From either the word processing program or from within a Windows (or Macintosh) folder, the patient selects the document containing the level of cuing needed to successfully type the personal information. The patient can save the file or the "autosave" option invoked for later review of performance by the clinician. To aid in generalization, the documents are printed and the patient practices writing (printing) at home directly on the same pages.
INTERVENTION:	The clinician dictates error items to the patient. If errors persist, the clinician provides models or other cues as needed.
SCORING:	Number of correctly spelled words, legible words, etc.

References

Aftonomos, L.B., Steele, R.D., & Wertz, R.T. (1997). Promoting recovery in chronic aphasia with an interactive technology. *Archives of Physical Medicine, 78* (August), 841–846.

Barr, A. & Geigenbaum, E.A. (eds.) (1982). *The handbook of artificial intelligence.* Stanford, CA: HeurisTech Press.

Bengston, V.L. (1973). Self-determination: A social psychologic perspective on helping the aged. *Geriatrics, 28*(12), 1118–1130.

Benson, D.F. (1975). Disorders of verbal expression. In D.F. Benson & D. Blumer (eds.), *Psychiatric aspects of neurologic disease* (pp. 121–137). New York: Grune & Stratton.

Bolter, J.D. (1984). *Turing's man: Western culture in the computer age.* Chapel Hill, NC: University of North Carolina Press.

Bracy, O.L. (1983). Computer based cognitive rehabilitation. *Cognitive Rehabilitation, 1*(1), 7–8, 18–19.

Bracy, O.L. (1986). Cognitive rehabilitation: A process approach. *Cognitive Rehabilitation, 4,* 10–17.

Brodin & Magnusson, (1994).

Brown, C.S. & Cullinan, W.L. (1981). Word-retrieval difficulty and dysfluent speech in adult anomic speakers. *Journal of Speech and Hearing Research, 24,* 358–365.

Chapey, R., Rigrodsky, S., & Morrison, E. (1976). Divergent semantic behavior in aphasia. *Journal of Speech and Hearing Research, 19,* 664–677.

Coelho, G.V., Hamburg, D.A., & Adams, J.E. (1974). *Coping and adaptation.* New York: Basic Books.

Colby, K.M., Christinaz, D., Parkison, R.C., Graham, S., & Karpf, C. (1981). A word-finding computer program with a dynamic lexical-semantic memory for patients with anomia using an intelligent speech prosthesis. *Brain and Language, 14,* 272–281.

Colby, K.M. & Kraemer, H.C. (1975). An objective measurement of nonspeaking children's performance with a computer-controlled program for the stimulation of language behavior. *Journal of Autism and Childhood Schizophrenia, 5*(2), 139–146.

Colby, K.M. & Smith, D.C. (1973). Computers in the treatment of nonspeaking autistic children. In J.H. Masserman (ed.), *Current psychiatric therapies, Vol. 11* (pp. 1–17). New York: Grune & Stratton.

Crerar, M.A. & Ellis, A.W. (1995). Computer-based therapy for aphasia: Towards second generation clinical tools. In C. Code & D. Müller (eds.), *Treatment of aphasia: From theory to practice* (pp. 223–250). London: Whurr.

Crerar, M.A., Ellis, A.W., & Dean, E.C. (1996). Remediation of sentence processing deficits in aphasia using a computer-based microworld. *Brain and Language, 52,* 229–275.

Darley, F.L. (1972). The efficacy of language rehabilitation in aphasia. *Journal of Speech and Hearing Research, 37,* 3–21.

Davis, G.A. & Wilcox, M.J. (1985). *Adult aphasia rehabilitation: Applied pragmatics.* Austin, TX: Pro-Ed.

Dean, E.C. (1987). Microcomputers and aphasia. *Aphasiology, 1*(3), 267–270.

Delouche, G., Dordain, M., & Kremin, H. (1993). Rehabilitation of confrontational naming in aphasia: Relations between oral and written modalities. *Aphasiology, 7,* 201–216.

Dressler, R.A. (1991). Beyond workbooks: the computer as a treatment supplement. Poster session presented at the American Speech-Language-Hearing Association Annual Convention, Atlanta, GA.

Duffy, J.R. (1998, June). Telehealth practice applications. 1998 ASHA Leadership Inservice Delivery Conference, Tucson, AZ.

Duffy, J.R., Werven, G.W., & Aronson, A.E. (1997). Telemedicine and the diagnosis of speech and language disorders. *Mayo Clinic Proceedings, 72,* 1116–1122.

Egolf, D.B. & Chester, S.L. (1973). Nonverbal communication and the disorders of speech and language. *ASHA, 15,* 511–518.

Eisenson, J. (1973). *Adult aphasia.* New York: Appleton-Century-Crofts.

Enderby, P. (1987). Microcomputers in assessment, rehabilitation and recreation. *Aphasiology, 1*(2), 151–166.

Fenstad, J.E. (1988). Language and computations. In R. Herken (ed.), *The universal Turing machine: A half-century survey* (pp. 327–348). New York: Oxford University Press.

Fitz-Gibbon, C.T. (1986). In defense of randomized controlled trials, with suggestions about the possible use of meta-analysis. *British Journal of Disorders of Communication, 21,* 117–124.

Gadler, H.P. & Zechner, K. (1992). AUSWEGE—WEGE in Osterreich [AUSWEGE-WEGE in Austria]. In V.M. Roth (ed.), *Computer in der Sprachtherapie* [Computers in speech-language therapy] (pp. 147–160). Tubingen Germany: Gunter Narr Verlag.

Gardner, R. & Gardner, B. (1969). Teaching sign language to a chimpanzee. *Science, 165,* 664–672.

Gardner, H., Zurif, E., Berry, T., & Baker, E. (1976). Visual communication in aphasia. *Neuropsychologia, 14,* 275–292.

Geschwind, N. (1973). Writing and its disorders. Paper presented at the Second Pan-American Congress of Audition and Language, Lima, Peru.

Glisky, E.L., Schlacter, D.L., & Tuving, E. (1986). Learning and retention of computer-related vocabulary in memory-impaired patients: Method of vanishing cues. *Journal of Clinical and Experimental Neuropsychology, 8*(3), 292–312.

Goldberg, S.A. (1997). *Clinical skills for speech-language pathologists.* San Diego, CA: Singular.

Goldstein, K. (1942). *After-affects of brain injury in war.* New York: Grune & Stratton.

Goldstein, K. (1948). *Language and language disturbances.* New York: Grune & Stratton.

Goodglass, H. & Kaplan, E. (1983). *Boston Diagnostic Aphasia Examination.* Philadelphia: Lea & Febiger.

Guyard, H., Masson, V., & Quiniou, R. (1990). Computer-based aphasia treatment meets artificial intelligence. *Aphasiology, 4*(6), 599–613.

Hallowell, B. & Katz, R.C. (1999). Technological applications in the assessment of acquired neurogenic communication and swallowing disorders in adults. *Seminars in Speech, Language and Hearing, 20*(2), 149–167.

Herrmann, D., Yoder, C.Y., Wells, J., & Raybeck, D. (1996). Portable electronic scheduling/reminding devices. *Cognitive Technology, 1,* 19–24.

Howard, D. (1986). Beyond randomized controlled trials: The case for effective case studies of the effects of treatment in aphasia. *British Journal of Disorders of Communication, 21,* 89–102.

Katz, R.C. (1984). Using microcomputers in the diagnosis and treatment of chronic aphasic adults. *Seminars in Speech, Language and Hearing, 5*(1), 11–22.

Katz, R.C. (1986). *Aphasia treatment and microcomputers.* New York: Taylor & Francis.

Katz, R.C. (1987). Efficacy of aphasia treatment using microcomputers. *Aphasiology, 1*(2), 141–150.

Katz, R.C. (1990). Intelligent computerized treatment or artificial aphasia therapy. *Aphasiology, 4*(6), 621–624.

Katz, R.C., LaPointe, L.L., & Markel, N.N. (1978). Coverbal behavior and aphasic speakers. In Brookshire, R.H. (ed.), *Clinical aphasiology: 1978 Conference proceedings* (pp. 164–173). Minneapolis, MN: BRK.

Katz, R.C. & Nagy, V.T. (1982). A computerized treatment system for chronic aphasic adults. In R.H. Brookshire (ed.), *Clinical aphasiology: 1982 Conference proceedings* (pp. 153–160). Minneapolis, MN: BRK.

Katz, R.C. & Nagy, V.T. (1983). A computerized approach for improving word recognition in chronic aphasic patients. In R.H. Brookshire (ed.), *Clinical aphasiology: 1983 Conference proceedings* (pp. 65–72). Minneapolis, MN: BRK.

Katz, R.C. & Nagy, V.T. (1984). An intelligent computer-based task for chronic aphasic patients. In R.H. Brookshire (ed.), *Clinical aphasiology: 1984 Conference proceedings* (pp. 159–165). Minneapolis, MN: BRK.

Katz, R.C. & Nagy, V.T. (1985). A self-modifying computerized reading program for severely-impaired aphasic adults. In R.H.Brookshire (ed.), *Clinical aphasiology: 1985 Conference proceedings* (pp. 184–188). Minneapolis, MN: BRK.

Katz, R.C. & Wertz, R.T. (1992). Computerized hierarchical reading treatment in aphasia. *Aphasiology, 6,* 165–177.

Katz, R.C. & Wertz, R.T. (1997). The efficacy of computer-provided reading treatment for chronic aphasic adults. *Journal of Speech, Language and Hearing Research, 40*(3), 493–507.

Katz, R.C., Wertz, R.T., Davidoff, M., Schubitowski, Y.D., & Devitt, E.W. (1989). A computer program to improve written confrontation naming in aphasia. In T.E. Prescott (ed.), *Clinical aphasiology: 1988 Conference proceedings* (pp. 321–338). Austin, TX: Pro-Ed.

Keenan, J.S. (1967). *A language rehabilitation program—aphasia.* Chicago: Bell & Howell.

Keith, R.L. & Darley, F.L. (1967). The use of a special electric board in rehabilitation of the aphasic patient. *Journal of Speech and Hearing Disorders, 32*(2), 148–153.

Kertesz, A. (1982). *Western Aphasia Battery.* New York: Grune & Stratton.

Kotten, A. (1989). Aphasia treatment: A multidimensional process. In E. Perecman (ed.), *Integrating theory and practice in neuropsychology* (pp. 293–315). Hillsdale, NJ: Lawrence Erlbaum.

Langer, E.J. & Rodin, J. (1976). The effect of choice and enhanced personal responsibility for the aged: A field experiment in an institutional setting. *Journal of Personality and Social Psychology, 34,* 191–198.

LaPointe, L.L. (1977). Base-10 programmed stimulation: Task specification, scoring and plotting performance in aphasia therapy. *Journal of Speech and Hearing Disorders, 42,* 90–105.

Lepper, M.R. (1985). Microcomputers in education: Motivational and social issues. *American Psychologist, 40,* 1–18.

Loverso, F.L. (1987). Unfounded expectations: Computers in rehabilitation. *Aphasiology, 1*(2), 157–160.

Loverso, F.L., Prescott, T.E., & Selinger, M. (1988). Cueing verbs: A treatment strategy for aphasic adults. *Journal of Rehabilitation Research and Development, 25,* 47–60.

Loverso, F.L., Prescott, T.E., & Selinger, M. (1992). Microcomputer treatment applications in aphasiology. *Aphasiology, 6*(2), 155–163.

Loverso, F.L., Prescott, T.E., Selinger, M., & Riley, L. (1988). Comparison of two modes of aphasia treatment: Clinician and computer-clinician assisted. In T.E. Prescott (ed.), *Clinical aphasiology, Vol. 18* (pp. 297–319). Austin, TX: Pro-Ed.

Loverso, F.L., Prescott, T.E., Selinger, M., Wheeler, K.M., & Smith, R.D. (1985). The application of microcomputers for the treatment of aphasic adults. In R.H. Brookshire (ed.), *Clinical aphasiology: 1985 Conference proceedings* (pp. 189–195). Minneapolis, MN: BRK.

Loverso, F.L., Selinger, M., & Prescott, T.E. (1979). Application of verbing strategies to aphasia treatment. In R.H. Brookshire (ed.), *Clinical aphasiology: 1979 Conference proceedings* (pp. 229–238). Minneapolis, MN: BRK.

Lucas, R.W. (1977). A study of patients' attitudes to computer interrogation. *International Journal of Man-Machine Studies, 9,* 69–86.

Luria, A.R. (1963). *Restoration of function after brain injury.* New York: Macmillan.

Luria, A.R. (1973). *The working brain.* New York: Basic Books.

Luria, A.R. (1980). *Higher cortical functions in man* (2nd ed.). New York: Basic Books.

Lynch, W.J. (1983). Cognitive retraining using microcomputer games and commercially-available software. *Cognitive Rehabilitation, 1,* 19–22.

Matthews, B.A.J. & LaPointe, L.L. (1981). Determining rate of change and predicting performance levels in aphasia therapy.

In R.H. Brookshire (ed.), *Clinical aphasiology: 1981 Conference proceedings* (pp. 17–25). Minneapolis, MN: BRK.

Matthews, B.A.J. & LaPointe, L.L. (1983). Slope and variability of performance on selected aphasia treatment tasks. In R.H. Brookshire (ed.), *Clinical aphasiology: 1983 Conference proceedings* (pp. 113–120). Minneapolis, MN: BRK.

McGlynn, E.A. (1996). Domains of study and methodological challenges. In L.I. Sederer & B. Dickey (eds.), *Outcomes assessment in clinical practice* (pp. 19–24). Baltimore, MD: Williams & Wilkins.

McReynolds, L.V. & Kearns, K.P. (1983). *Single-subject experimental designs in communicative disorders.* Baltimore, MD: University Park Press.

Mehrabian, A. (1968). Communication without words. *Psychology Today, 2,* 52–55.

Mills, R.H. (1982). Microcomputerized auditory comprehension training. In R.H. Brookshire (ed.), *Clinical aphasiology: 1982 Conference proceedings* (pp. 147–152). Minneapolis, MN: BRK.

Mills, R.H. (1988). Book review (*Aphasia treatment and microcomputers*). *Journal of Computer Users in Speech and Hearing, 41*(1), 40–41.

Morrison, M.H. (1998a). Information technology for medical rehabilitation, Part 1: An overview. In E.A. Dobrzykowski (ed.), *Essential readings in rehabilitation outcomes measurements: Application, methodology, and technology* (pp. 255–257). Gaithersburg, MD: Aspen.

Morrison, M.H. (1998b). Information technology for medical rehabilitation, Part 2: Requirements. In E.A. Dobrzykowski (ed.), *Essential readings in rehabilitation outcomes measurements: Application, methodology, and technology* (pp. 258–261). Gaithersburg, MD: Aspen.

Myers, P.S. (1999). *Right hemisphere damage.* San Diego, CA: Singular.

Odell, K., Collins, M., Dirkx, T., & Kelso, D. (1985). A computerized version of the Coloured Progressive Matrices. In R.H. Brookshire (ed.), *Clinical aphasiology: 1985 Conference proceedings* (pp. 47–56). Minneapolis, MN: BRK.

Odor, J.P. (1988). Student models in machine-mediated learning. *Journal of Mental Deficiency Research, 32,* 247–256.

Peters, L.J. & Peters, D.P. (1998). Telehealth part II: A total system approach. *ASHA, 40*(2).

Petheram, B. (1988). Enabling stroke victims to interact with a minicomputer—comparison of input devices. *International Disabilities Studies, 10*(2), 73–80.

Pfau, G.S. (1974). *Instruction manual for the General Electric/project LIFE program: Programmed Assistance to Learning (PAL).* Ballston Lake, NY: Instructional Industries.

Porch, B.E. (1981). *Porch Index of Communicative Ability, Vol. 1: Administration, scoring and interpretation* (3rd ed.). Palo Alto, CA: Consulting Psychologists Press.

Premack, D. (1970). The education of Sarah: A chimp learns the language. *Psychology Today, 4,* 55–58.

Prescott, T.E., Loverso, F.L., & Selinger, M. (1984). Differences between normals and left brain damaged (aphasic) subjects on a nonverbal problem solving task. In R.H. Brookshire (ed.), *Clinical aphasiology: 1984 Conference proceedings* (pp. 235–240). Minneapolis, MN: BRK.

Prescott, T.E. & McNeil, M.R. (1973). Measuring the effects of treatment of aphasia. Paper presented at the Third Conference on Clinical Aphasiology, Albuquerque, NM.

Raven, J.C. (1975). *Coloured Progressive Matrices*. Los Angeles, CA: Western Psychologic Services.

Rheingold, H. (1991). *Virtual reality*. New York: Summit Books.

Robinson, I. (1990). Does computerized cognitive rehabilitation work? A review. *Aphasiology*, 4(4), 381–405.

Rosenbek, J.C. (1979). Wrinkled feet. In R.H. Brookshire (ed.), *Clinical aphasiology: 1979 Conference proceedings* (pp. 163–176). Minneapolis, MN: BRK.

Rosenbek, J.C. (1995). Efficacy in dysphagia. *Dysphagia*, 10, 263–267.

Rosenbek, J.C., LaPointe, L.L. & Wertz, R.T. (1989). *Aphasia: A clinical approach*. Austin, TX: Pro-Ed.

Roth, V.M. (1992). SICH-ÄUSSERNDES Verstehen NeueWEGE [Understanding SICH-ÄUSSERNDES: NeueWEGE]. In V.M. Roth (ed.), *Computer in der Sprachtherapie* [Computers in speech-language therapy] (pp. 187–214). Tubingen: Gunter Narr Verlag.

Rushakoff, G.E. (1984). Clinical applications in communication disorders. In A.H. Schwartz (ed.), *Handbook of microcomputer applications in communication disorders* (pp. 148–171). San Diego, CA: College Hill Press.

Schuell, H., Jenkins, J.J., & Jiménez-Pabón, E. (1964). *Aphasia in adults*. New York: Harper & Row.

Schulz, R. (1976). Effects of control and predictability, on the physical well being of the institutionalized aged. *Journal of Personality and Social Psychology*, 33, 563–573.

Schwartz, A.H. (1984). *Handbook of microcomputer applications in communication disorders*. San Diego, CA: College-Hill Press.

Scott, C. & Byng, S. (1989). Computer-assisted remediation of a homophone comprehension disorder in surface dyslexia. *Aphasiology*, 3(3), 301–320.

Seligman, M. (1975). *Helplessness: On depression, development and death*. San Francisco, CA: Freeman.

Selinger, M., Prescott, T.E., & Katz, R.C. (1987). Handwritten versus typed responses on PICA graphic subtests. In R.H. Brookshire (ed.), *Clinical aphasiology: 1987 Conference proceedings* (pp. 136–142). Minneapolis, MN: BRK.

Selinger, M., Prescott, T.E., Loverso, F.L., & Fuller, K. (1987). Below the 50th percentile: Application of the verb as core model. In R.H. Brookshire (ed.), *Clinical aphasiology: 1987 Conference proceedings* (pp. 55-63). Minneapolis, MN: BRK.

Seron, X., Deloche, G., Moulard, G., & Rouselle, M. (1980). A computer-based therapy for the treatment of aphasic subjects with writing disorders. *Journal of Speech and Hearing Disorders*, 45, 45–58.

Silverman, F.H. (1997). *Computer applications for augmenting the management of speech, language, and hearing disorders*. Boston: Allyn & Bacon.

Skilbeck, C. (1984). Computer assistance in the management of memory and cognitive impairment. In B.A. Wilson & N. Moffat (ed.), *Clinical management of memory problems*. Rockville, MD: Aspen Publications.

Skinner, B.F. (1948). *Walden two*. New York: Macmillan.

Skinner, B.F. (1958). Teaching machines. *Science*, 128, 969–977.

Skinner, B.F. (1957). *Verbal behavior*. New York: Appleton-Century-Crofts.

Steele, R.D., Weinrich, M., Kleczewska, M.K., Wertz, R.T., & Carlson, G.S. (1987). Evaluating performance of severely aphasic patients on a computer-aided visual communication system. In R.H. Brookshire (ed.), *Clinical aphasiology: 1987 Conference proceedings* (pp. 46–54). Minneapolis, MN: BRK.

Steele, R.D., Weinrich, M., Wertz, R.T., Kleczewska, M.K., & Carlson, G.S. (1989). Computer-based visual communication in aphasia. *Neuropsychologia*, 27, 409–427.

Stoicheff, M.L. (1960). Motivating instructions and language performance of dysphasic subjects. *Journal of Speech and Hearing Research*, 3, 75–85.

Tonkovich, J.D., Horowitz, D.M., Kawahigashi, J.N., Krainen, G.H., & Kronick, D. (1991). An application of voice recognition technology for clinical documentation. Computer poster session presented at the 1991 American Speech-Language-Hearing Association Annual Convention, Atlanta, GA.

Turing, A.M. (1936). On computable numbers, with an application to the Entscheidungs problem. *Proceedings of the London Mathematical Society*, 42(2), 230–265.

Turing, A.M. (1950). Computing machinery and intelligence. *Mind*, 59(236), 433–460.

Van de Sandt-Koenderman, M. (1994). *Multicue, a computer program for word finding in aphasia, 1. International Congress Language-Therapy-Computers*. Graz, Austria: University of Graz.

Vaughn, G.R. (1980, August). REMATE (Remote Machine Assisted Treatment and Evaluation): Communication outreach innovative health care delivery system for persons with communicative disorders workshop. Birmingham, AL: Veterans Administration Medical Center.

Vaughn, G.R., Amster, W.W., Bess, J.C., Gilbert, D.J., Kearns, K.P., Rudd, A.K., Tidwell, A.A., & Ozley, C.F. (1987). Efficacy of remote treatment of aphasia by TEL-Communicology. *Journal of Rehabilitative Research and Development*, 25(1), 446–447.

Wallich, P. (1991, October). Digital dyslexia: Neural network mimics the effects of stroke. *Scientific American*, (p. 36).

Weinrich, M., McCall, D., Shoosmith, L., Thomas, K., Katzenberger, K., & Weber, C. (1993). Locative prepositional phrases in severe aphasia. *Brain and Language*, 45, 21–45.

Weinrich, M., McCall, D., Weber, C., Thomas, K., & Thornburg, L. (1995). Training on an iconic communication system for severe aphasia can improve natural language production. *Aphasiology*, 9, 343–364.

Weinrich, M., Steele, R.D., Kleczewska, M., Carlson, G.S., Baker, E., & Wertz, R.T. (1989). Representation of "verbs" in a computerized visual communication system. *Aphasiology*, 3(6), 501–512.

Wertz, R.T. (1981). Aphasia management: The speech pathologist's role. *Seminars in Speech, Language and Hearing*, 2, 315–331.

Wertz, R.T., Dronkers, N.F., Knight, R.T., Shenaut, G.K., & Deal, J.L. (1987). Rehabilitation of neurogenic communication disorders in remote settings. *Journal of Rehabilitative Research and Development*, 25(1), 432–433.

Wolfe, G.R. (1987). Microcomputers and treatment of aphasia. *Aphasiology*, 1(2), 165–170.

Wolfe, G.R., Davidoff, M., & Katz, R.C. (1987). Nonverbal problem-solving in aphasic and non-aphasic subjects with computer presented and actual stimuli. In R.H. Brookshire (ed.), *Clinical aphasiology: 1987 Conference proceedings* (pp. 243–248). Minneapolis, MN: BRK.

APPENDIX 32–1
Sources for Software and Other Relevant Technology

Avaaz Innovations
258 Beckley Lane
P.O. Box 1055
Dublin, OH 43017-6055
614-932-0757
www.avaaz.com

BrainTrain
727 Twin Ridge Lane
Richmond, VA 23235
800-822-0538

Bungalow Software
5390 NE Stanchion Ct.
Hillsboro, OR 97124
800-891-9937
www.BungalowSoftware.com

Chart Links
74 Forbes Avenue
New Haven, CT 06512
203-469-0707
www.chartlinks.com

Clinician Magician
P.O. Box 426
Bedford, NY 10506
800-434-1886

Communication Skill Builders/
The Psychological Corporation
555 Academic Court
San Antonio, TX 78204-2498
800-211-8378
800-232-1223

Don Johnston
1000 N Rand Rd, Bldg 115
P.O. Box 639
Wauconda, IL 60084-0639
800-999-4660
www.donjohnston.com

Gus Communications
1006 Lonetree Court
Bellingham, WA 98226
360-715-8580
www.gusinc.com

IBM
New Orchard Road
Armonk, NY 10504
800-426-4968
www.ibm.com

Interactive Learning Materials
150 Croton Lake Road
P.O. Box S
Katonah, NY 10536
(914) 232-4682

Laureate Learning Systems, Inc.
110 East Spring Street
Winooski, VT 05404-1898
800-562-6801
www.llsys.com

The Learning Company
One Athenaeum Street
Cambridge, MA 02142
617-494-5700
www.learningco.com

LingraphiCARE America
3460 Washington Drive
Suite 109
St. Paul, MN 55122
888-274-2742
www.languagecarecenter.com

Madenta Communications Inc.
9411A-20 Avenue
Edmonton, Alberta
Canada, T6N 1E5
403-450-8926
www.madenta.com

Mayer-Johnson Co.
P.O. Box 1579
Solana Beach, CA 92075-1579
800-588-4548
www.mayer-johnson.com/

Medical Software Products
6415 Oak Hill Drive
Granite Bay, CA 95746-8909
916-797-2363
www.medsoftware.com

Microsoft
One Microsoft Way
Redmond, WA 98052-6399
425-882-8080
www.microsoft.com/ms.htm

Parrot Software
P.O. Box 250755
West Bloomfield, MI 48325
800-PARROT-1
www.parrotsoftware.com/index.html

Prentke Romich Company
1022 Heyl Road
Wooster, OH 44691
800-262-1984
www.prentrom.com/

Pro-Ed
8700 Shoal Creek
Austin, TX 78758-6897
512-451-3246
www.proed.com

Psychological Software Services
6555 Carrollton Avenue
Indianapolis, IN 46220
317-257-9672
www.inetdirect.net/pss

Roger Wagner Publishing
1050 Pioneer Way, Suite P
El Cajon, CA 92020
(800) HYPERSTUDIO
www.hyperstudio.com

Sentient Systems Technology
888-697-7332
www.sentient-sys.com

Sunburst Communications
101 Castleton Street
Pleasantville, NY 10570
800-321-7511
www.nysunburst.com

SPSS
444 North Michigan Avenue
Chicago, IL 60611
312-329-2400
www.spss.com

Therapist Helper Brand Software
500 West Cummings Park
Suite 1950
Woburn, MA 01801
800-3-HELPER
www.helper.com

APPENDIX 32–2
Websites of Interest

Academy of Aphasia
cortex.neurology.umab.edu/~academy

Academy of Neurologic Communication Disorders and Sciences (ANCDS)
www.duq.edu/ancds/

American Stroke Association (American Heart Association)
http://www.americanheart.org/catalog/Stroke_catpage30.html

American Medical Association (AMA) Insight: Atlas of the Human Body
http://www.ama-assn.org/insight/gen_hlth/atlas/atlas.htm

American Speech-Language-Hearing Association (ASHA)
www.asha.org

Brain Injury Associations, Inc.
www.biausa.org

CenterNet Homepage (National Center for Neurogenic Communication Disorders at the University of Arizona)
www.cnet.shs.arizona.edu

Communication Disorders and Sciences Home Page (resource center by Judith Kuster)
www.mankato.msus.edu/dept/comdis/kuster2/welcome.html

Mayo Clinic: Division of Cerebrovascular Diseases (Stroke Education)
http://www.mayo.edu/cerebro/education/stroke.html

Mayo Clinic: Speech After Stroke
http://www.mayohealth.org/mayo/9608/htm/speech.htm

National Aphasia Association (NAA)
www.aphasia.org

National Audiology and Speech Pathology Program, Department of Veterans Affairs Medical Centers
www.washington/med/va/gov/audio-speech/index.htm

National Institutes of Health (NIH)
www.nih.gov

National Institute of Neurologic Diseases and Stroke (NINDS)
http://www.ninds.nih.gov/healinfo/disorder/stroke/strokehp.htm

National Resource Center for Traumatic Brain Injury
www.neuro.pmr.vcu.edu

National Stroke Association
www.stroke.org

Neurology Web Forums at Massachusetts General Hospital
http://neuro-www.mgh.harvard.edu/forum/

Speechweb
http://www.speedline.ca/johnv/

Virtual Hospital: Stroke and Brain Attack
http://www.vh.org/Providers/ClinGuide/Stroke/Index.html

Washington University School of Medicine: Stroke Center
http://www.neuro.wustl.edu/stroke/

Section V

Therapy for Associated Neuropathologies of Speech and Language Related Functions

Chapter 33

Communication Disorders Associated with Traumatic Brain Injury

Mark Ylvisaker, Shirley F. Szekeres, and Timothy Feeney

OBJECTIVES

Upon completion of this chapter, the reader will be able to describe epidemiological trends related to traumatic brain injury (TBI), articulate the critical incidence-to-prevalence ratio; describe central themes in the pathophysiology of TBI, including diffuse axonal injury (DAI) and surface injuries related to irregular surfaces on the floor of the skull; describe risk factors for TBI and the relation between preinjury factors and long-term outcome; describe central tendencies in long-term outcome from the perspectives of communication, cognition, executive functions, and behavior; describe central themes in two competing approaches to rehabilitation for individuals with chronic cognitive, communication, and behavioral impairment after TBI; offer several rationales for a contextualized, everyday routine-based approach to intervention; describe procedures associated with ongoing, contextualized, collaborative hypothesis testing assessment and give a rationale for this approach to assessment for planning intervention. The reader will also be able to describe executive function routines and give illustrations for individuals at varied stages of recovery; create functional, individualized cognitive rehabilitation plans; distinguish between antecedent-focused and consequence-focused behavior management and offer a rationale for antecedent-focused approaches for individuals with TBI; create functional intervention plans designed to teach positive communication alternatives to negative behavior; and offer several rationales for collaborating with everyday people as well as describe effective ways to create such collaborative relationships.

In this chapter, we offer a functional and highly contextualized perspective on assessment and intervention for individuals with chronic cognitive and behavioral impairments, which underlie the most common and most debilitating communication-related disabilities after TBI, damage to the brain caused by external forces acting on the skull. The perspective is based on (1) our combined 60 years of clinical experience in the field, (2) current theory and research in cognitive neuroscience, (3) a considerable body of efficacy research in related disability fields, and (4) a growing body of efficacy literature in TBI rehabilitation. The importance of the approach to cognitive rehabilitation described in this chapter is underscored by recent pessimistic reviews of the effectiveness of restorative, decontextualized cognitive exercises, possibly combined with neuropharmacologic management.

The length of this chapter is dictated by our attempt to address many critical themes associated with an increasingly important disability group for specialists in cognitive and communication disorders. Because readers tend to use this textbook as an ongoing resource, we have included a large number of tables, figures, and appendices designed to organize and summarize large quantities of information for easy access. The chapter is divided into eight sections:

1. Epidemiology
2. Pathophysiology
3. Disability associated with TBI, including frequently used measures of disability, considerations associated with prediction of outcome, stages of improvement, and commonly occurring communication consequences of TBI
4. Framework for everyday, routine-based intervention, including theoretical, neuropsychological, and economic rationales
5. Functional assessment for planning intervention
6. Intervention for cognitive and executive function disorders associated with TBI
7. Intervention for behavioral and psychosocial disorders associated with TBI

8. Collaboration among professional clinicians, the person with disability, and the everyday people in that person's life.

Throughout the chapter, we highlight the role of the executive system because of its vulnerability following frontal lobe injury and its significance in relation to successful outcome in the domains of rehabilitation discussed in this chapter. In other publications, we have developed these themes in greater detail than is possible here (e.g., Feeney & Ylvisaker, 1995, 1997; Szekeres et al., 1987; Ylvisaker & Feeney, 1996, 1998a,b, 2000a,b; Ylvisaker et al., 1998a,c,d, 1999).

EPIDEMIOLOGY OF TBI

Incidence and Prevalence

Kraus (1993) estimated that in the United States in 1993, TBI resulted in 75,000 deaths, 366,000 hospitalizations, and a total of close to 2,000,000 injuries requiring some degree of medical attention (a rate of 145/100,000 persons per year). Approximately 80% of those hospitalized with TBI have mild injuries, with an expectation of excellent recovery in most, but not all cases (Kraus & Nourjah, 1988). Many more cases of mild injury are uncounted because they do not seek medical attention or because their brain injury is masked by more pressing medical concerns (e.g., high spinal cord injury).

Comparison of pre-1990 with post-1990 data indicates an apparent reduction in incidence over the past two decades (AHCPR, 1999; CDC, 1997, 1999; Thurman & Guerrero, 1999a,b), suggesting that the commonly reported statistics of roughly 500,000 TBI hospitalizations per year in the United States and over 75,000 deaths may now be overestimates. However, a declining TBI hospitalization rate may reflect changes in admissions standards rather than a reduction in incidence of TBI (Thurman & Guerrero, 1999b). Furthermore, even the most optimistic *incidence* trends should not obscure frank recognition of the growing numbers of individuals living, often for several decades, with TBI-related disability requiring some degree of ongoing professional support and societal accommodation. Each year, an estimated 50,000 to 80,000 people in the United States are added to the prevalence total of those with some degree of persistent disability associated with TBI, yielding a somewhat speculative prevalence estimate of 5.3 million Americans in 1999 (CDC, 1999). Because of the relative youth of most individuals with TBI, prevalence-to-incidence ratios are much higher than is the case with neurogenic disorders associated with aging. Direct medical costs (acute hospitalization and rehabilitation) have been estimated at $48.3 billion per year, not including the enormous financial and psychological costs associated with ongoing support and reduced employability (AHCPR, 1999).

Risk Factors

The incidence of TBI is highest among young people, with 15- to 24-year-old males being most vulnerable. Secondary peaks have been identified in people over 65 and children age 5 and younger (CDC, 1997; Kraus et al., 1990). With the introduction of TBI as an educational disability category (IDEA, Federal Register, 1991), children have received increasing attention in the clinical and education literatures. In contrast, elderly individuals, who are also at risk for TBI and for relatively severe consequences of the injury, continue to be under-represented in the literature (Goldstein & Levin, 1995; Payne, 1999).

Several risk factors in addition to age have been identified. Overall, males have twice the rate of TBI as females, with this ratio even higher (3 or 4 to 1) for the highest risk group of older adolescents and young adults (Kraus, 1993). Clinicians often characterize this highest risk group as including adolescent and young adult males from lower socioeconomic groups whose preinjury lives may have been characterized by some degree of risk-taking behavior, poor academic and vocational achievement, and greater than average use of alcohol and recreational drugs. Supporting this stereotype, incidence studies have suggested that TBI appears to be especially common in lower socioeconomic groups, among people with less than a high school education, and among those with a history of poor academic performance (Fife et al., 1986; Haas et al., 1987; Sosin et al., 1996). Alcohol is often a contributing factor in the occurrence of TBI, strongly associated with both motor vehicle–related injuries and falls in both young adults and the elderly (Hartshorne et al., 1997; Kraus, 1993; Santora et al., 1994; U.S. Department of Transportation, 1995). Previous TBI increases the risk of subsequent TBI threefold (Annegers et al., 1980; Gerberich et al., 1983). Prior TBI may also increase the *consequences* of subsequent TBI (Collins et al., 1999; Gronwall & Wrightson, 1975).

However, not all epidemiological reports are consistent with the stereotype. For example, in two Australian studies, Tate (1998) failed to find a high rate of pretrauma social maladjustment in her cohort and, more surprisingly, found that such maladjustment, when present, appeared not to have a pronounced effect on outcome. In contrast to Tate, our experience with several hundred young adults referred for neurobehavioral support as a result of behavior-related community reintegration problems suggests that preinjury factors play a significant role in outcome, with preinjury developmental and adjustment problems often exacerbated by the injury (Ylvisaker & Feeney, 2000a).

With respect to cause of injury, transportation-related events account for about 50% of cases of TBI (CDC, 1997), followed by falls (slightly over 20% of the total, but much higher in young children and the elderly), assaults (about 20%), and finally, sports-related injuries and other causes. Tragically, abuse is a major factor in infants and the elderly. Consideration of the causes of TBI reveals that it is a largely preventable epidemic. With concerted efforts to improve automobile safety, reduce alcohol-impaired driving, enhance safety measures in sports, and eliminate child and elder abuse, the epidemiology of TBI could be dramatically changed.

PATHOPHYSIOLOGY OF TBI

TBI refers to damage to the brain caused by external forces. Traumatic brain injuries can be open, involving penetration of the dural covering of the brain, or closed. Penetrating missile injuries, in which focal damage is related to the site of penetration and trajectory of the missile, are more strongly associated with aphasia than is closed head injury (CHI) (Newcombe, 1969). CHI generally refers to brain injuries in which the primary mechanism of damage is a blunt blow to the head, or rapid changes of skull motion, both associated with acceleration/deceleration forces acting on the brain (Levin et al., 1982). In special education discussions of students with brain injury, acquired brain injury (ABI) is often used to identify an even broader pathophysiologic category, including stroke, tumor, anoxia, toxic encephalopathy,

meningitis, encephalitis, and other causes of noncongenital brain impairment. Federal education law, PL 101–476 (Individuals with Disabilities Education Act, 1990; amended 1997), defined TBI in relation to external causes, but some state departments of education use TBI as a synonym for ABI.

Primary Impact Damage

Primary and secondary injuries associated with TBI are summarized in Figures 33–1 and 33–2 (information taken from Alexander, 1987; Katz, 1992; Pang, 1985; Young, 1999). Contact of a moving skull with a stationary surface may cause skull distortion and fracture, and is traditionally thought to be responsible for *coup* (site of contact) and *contrecoup* (opposite side) brain contusion and cavitation injury (Figure 33–3). Neurobehavioral deficits associated with lesions that vary with the site of impact cannot explain central tendencies within the population as a whole. It is rather damage associated with differential tissue movements within the skull, both brain-skull and brain-brain movements created by inertial forces (especially rotational inertia), that often

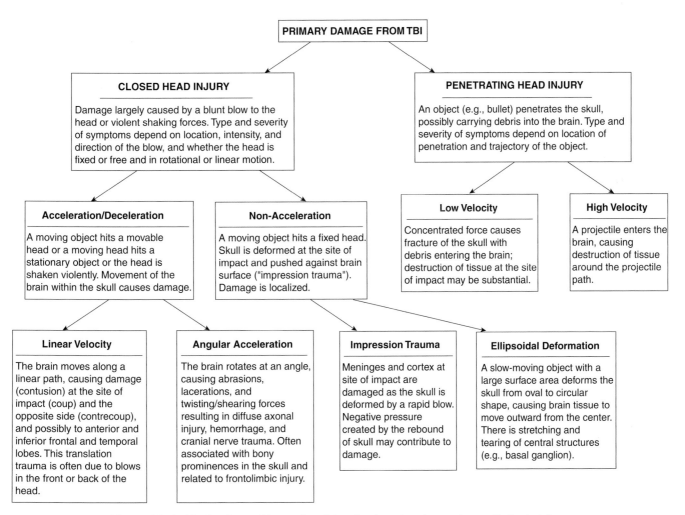

Figure 33–1. Mechanisms of immediate injury in closed and open traumatic brain injury.

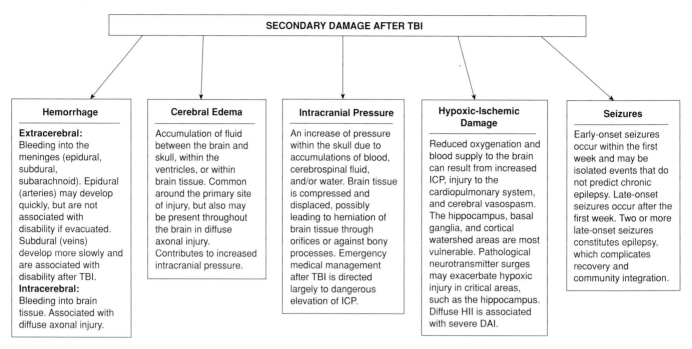

Figure 33–2. Pathologic events that often follow severe TBI and contribute to impairment.

play the greatest role in determining outcome and best explain population commonalities. This type of injury is possible even in the absence of a blow to the head if the skull is accelerated and/or decelerated rapidly (e.g., shaken baby syndrome) (Gennarelli et al., 1982).

In severe CHI, brain-skull differential movement in the area of bony prominences within the skull can cause surface

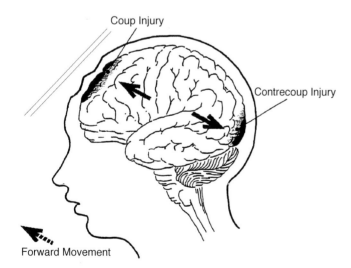

Figure 33–3. Representation of coup injury (i.e., contusion and cavitation at the site of impact) and contrecoup injury (i.e., contusion and cavitation at the opposite side of the brain). (Adapted with permission from Walker, W. & the North Carolina State Board of Education [1997]. *Best practices in assessment and programming for students with traumatic brain injury.* Raleigh, NC: State Board of Education.)

contusion and laceration as well as deeper shearing of axons (DAI) and blood vessels (subdural and intracerebral hematoma). Regardless of site of impact in high-speed CHI, focal contusion as well as axon shearing is often concentrated within anterior and inferior frontal and temporal lobe structures bilaterally because of their adjacency to sharp, irregular surfaces inside the skull (Alexander, 1987; Courville, 1937; Katz, 1992) (Figures 33–4 and 33–5). Damage to these areas explains many of the commonly observed neurobehavioral symptoms that negatively affect communication after CHI, including (a) depressed executive control over cognitive and communicative functions (prefrontal damage), (b) impaired social perception and social reactivity (prefrontal and frontolimbic damage, particularly right hemisphere), and (c) generally reduced behavioral self-regulation (prefrontal, frontolimbic, and anterior temporal lobe damage). Diffuse neuronal shearing is also often concentrated in the brain stem and corpus callosum, contributing to initial coma and subsequent arousal/attentional deficits and slowed mental processing (Adams et al., 1982). The relative infrequency of specific aphasic syndromes in CHI is in part a consequence of the smooth interior surface of the skull adjacent to the traditional perisylvian language centers in the brain.

Secondary Damage

Secondary damage in TBI is associated with slowly developing hemorrhages and localized or widespread swelling and edema, both of which contribute to increased intracranial

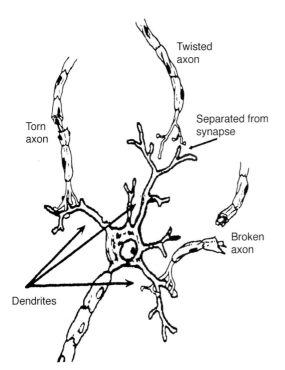

Figure 33–4. Diffuse axonal injury: twisting, tearing, and breaking of axons associated with primary impact damage in traumatic brain injury.

pressure, which can be acutely life threatening, and contribute to morbidity in those who survive. In addition, hypoxic-ischemic injury and pathologic neurotransmitter surges, both common secondary consequences of severe TBI, often pick out specific vulnerable structures, notably the hippocampus bilaterally, thereby contributing to memory and new learning problems after the injury (Katz, 1992). This is an especially ominous consequence for young people who face substantial new learning challenges in school and on

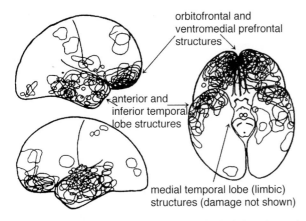

Figure 33–5. Contusions after traumatic brain injury, based on 40 consecutive cases, clearly depicts the tendency for maximum pathology in the orbitofrontal and temporal regions. (Reprinted from Courville, J. [1937]. *Pathology of the central nervous system.* Mountain View, CA: Pacific Publishers.)

the job. Tragically, the vast majority of individuals with TBI are children, adolescents, and young adults. Post-traumatic seizures, including both early-onset (within the first week) and late-onset (appearing after the first week) seizures, can also complicate recovery and become a major concern if epilepsy persists.

DISABILITY FOLLOWING TBI

There are predictable inconsistencies in the published descriptions of disability following TBI. Because of the extended period of neurologic improvement, the time post-injury at which consequences of the injury are assessed influences the description of central tendencies in the population. Variation in the severity mix from study to study adds to variation in this outcome picture. Furthermore, as increasingly valid language and cognitive assessments have become available (e.g., sensitive analysis of extended discourse versus aphasia batteries developed for a different clinical population), increasing numbers of individuals with TBI have been shown to have language and more general cognitive processing difficulties. Finally, because of the variable associations among impairment, disability, and handicap, different outcome profiles inevitably emerge depending on which domain is assessed.

Impairment, Disability (Activity) and Handicap (Participation)

Throughout the chapter, we use the World Health Organization framework of impairment, disability, and handicap (WHO, 1980). This language is currently under revision, substituting the positive terms *activity* for disability, and *participation* for handicap (ICIDH-2: WHO, 1998). However, the underlying concepts remain the same. Impairment refers to the loss or abnormality of underlying physiological or psychological processes, directly tied to the injury (e.g., slowed processing, loss of organizing schemata, disruption of phonological or grammatical systems, hemiplegia). Disability (or activity reduction), which may or may not be associated with the impairment, refers to reduced ability to successfully perform activities that are important in the individual's life (e.g., difficulty maintaining a conversation, problems comprehending written text, difficulty remaining focused and organized at work, impulsive or aggressive interaction under stress). Handicap (or reduced participation) refers to the individual's potential social losses as a result of the disability, including loss of work, educational opportunity, friends, living situation, avocational pursuits, social status, community mobility, and the like.

Many of the changes in neurologic rehabilitation over the past two decades have been associated with an increasing emphasis on functional activities (disability-oriented intervention) and supports for social, educational, vocational, and avocational participation (handicap-oriented intervention), in contrast to the primary focus on impairment, characteristic of traditional rehabilitation. Clearly, the relationships among impairment, disability, and handicap are complex and relative to individuals and their contexts in life. For example, the same underlying impairment can result in dramatically different types and degrees of disability and handicap in different individuals with varying activity and environmental demands, compensatory strategies, emotional adjustment, and social/educational/vocational supports. Furthermore, as we argue later in this chapter, intervention that begins as handicap- or participation-oriented can ultimately result in reduced disability and impairment as the individual practices supported compensatory procedures until they become habitual and automatic aspects of information processing.

Measures of Injury and Disability Severity

Several rating scales have enjoyed increasing popularity as measures of initial severity of injury, of ongoing improvement, and of chronic disability. These scales are not intended to be used for planning interventions for specific individuals. Sensitive individualized assessments are needed for this purpose. Furthermore, rating scales are rarely sufficient to measure the effectiveness of intervention in individual cases. For that purpose, there is no substitute for objective documentation of achievement of individualized functional objectives directly related to important personal life goals.

However, general rating scales have become part of the *lingua franca* of medical rehabilitation, are useful in capturing severity of injury and disability in general terms, and are often used in epidemiologic and program evaluation studies. Table 33–1 includes descriptions of commonly used scales. Many other functional scales have been developed in recent years, attesting to the shortcomings of impairment-oriented tests for measuring functional disability after TBI. These include the Patient Competency Rating Scale (Prigatano & Altman, 1990), Mayo-Portland Adaptability Inventory (Malec & Thompson, 1994), Neurobehavioral Functioning Inventory (Kreutzer et al., 1996), Supervision Rating Scale (Boake, 1996), and BIRCO-39 Scales (Powell et al., 1998).

Prediction of Outcome

Many studies suggest a general "dose-response" relation between injury severity and long-term outcome (Katz & Alexander, 1994). However, most studies correlating injury severity and outcome after TBI use broad severity categories (e.g., four or five grades of severity, based on Glasgow Coma Scale [GCS] score, duration of coma, or duration of post-traumatic amnesia, possibly combined with focal neurologic signs) and broad outcome categories (e.g., the five grades of outcome defined by the Glasgow Outcome Scale). Although useful for epidemiological purposes, these studies must be interpreted cautiously by rehabilitation clinicians. First, in correlation studies there are always individuals who deviate sharply from the general population relationships (Ponsford et al., 1995); it is often these exceptional individuals and their families with whom clinicians interact in their everyday clinical practice. Second, within broad severity of injury and outcome categories, there is substantial individual variation, rendering specific predictions hazardous and leaving room for optimism regarding the potential effectiveness of intervention efforts. For example, two individuals in the good outcome category can be extremely different with respect to (a) their level of success measured in relation to preinjury success, (b) the effort required to maintain that level of functioning, (c) the level of supports they require and associated caregiver burden, and (d) their subjective level of satisfaction and adjustment to life after the injury. Because of these sources of variability, intervention that fails to change a person's outcome category may, nevertheless, be very effective for the individual and caregivers alike.

Patterns and Stages of "Recovery"

In the heading, the word *recovery* is in quotation marks because it is a frequent source of miscommunication. In ordinary language, to recover is to return to normal. In contrast, rehabilitation professionals typically use the word to refer to gradual improvement, without intending to suggest that improvement will continue until a full recovery is achieved. Indeed, full recovery is rare following TBI with coma of 1 week or more. Therefore, *improvement* may be a better choice of words to communicate what professionals often intend with *recovery* (Kay & Lezak, 1990).

Most individuals with severe TBI experience a large number of distinct stages or levels of cognitive and self-regulatory functioning over the course of their spontaneous neurologic improvement and rehabilitation. In many cases, improvement is characterized by a stairstep pattern rather than a smooth recovery curve, commonly observed following ischemic stroke (Brookshire, 1997). Furthermore, spontaneous neurologic improvement can continue for many months and, in some cases, for years (at decreasing rates of improvement) after severe TBI.

The popular Rancho Los Amigos Hospital Levels of Cognitive Functioning (RLA: see Table 33–1) organizes cognitive and behavioral recovery into eight relatively distinct levels. An understanding of typical levels of improvement helps treatment staff, family members, and individuals with TBI place in perspective behaviors that would otherwise be distressing (e.g., agitation associated with Level IV) and organize their rehabilitative efforts effectively. For purposes of discussing broadly different focuses of assessment and intervention, and importantly, different levels and types of support provided to the patient by rehabilitation staff and families, we have collapsed the eight Rancho levels into three broadly distinct stages of improvement (Szekeres et al., 1985). However, any discussion of stages must be sensitive

TABLE 33–1

Assessments Commonly Used to Measure Injury Severity and Associated Disability

Assessment Procedure	Description
Glasgow Coma Scale (Teasdale & Jennett, 1974)	A 3-category (eye opening, motor response, verbal response), 15-point scale commonly used to measure the initial severity of TBI. Scores of 8 or lower within the first several hours after injury typically classified as severe injuries, 11–12 as moderate, and 13–15 as mild.
Duration of Coma	Generally based on time from injury to eye opening and resumption of normal sleep-wake cycles. Measured in minutes or hours for mild to moderate injuries and in days, weeks, or months for severe injuries. Sometimes used more informally to refer to the period of significantly altered consciousness.
Duration of Post-Traumatic Amnesia	Based on time from injury to resumption of orientation and integration of day-to-day memories. Very hard to establish with precision in severe cases.
Galveston Orientation and Amnesia Test (GOAT) (Levin et al., 1979)	A 10-question test of orientation to person, place, and time and of memory for recent, post-injury events as well as for most recent preinjury events.
Glasgow Outcome Scale (Jennett & Bond, 1975)	A 5-category global outcome scale: death, persistent vegetative state, severe disability (conscious, but disabled and dependent), moderate disability (disabled but independent), and good recovery (relatively normal life, but possibly with ongoing minor impairment).
Rancho Los Amigos Levels of Cognitive Functioning (Hagen, 1981)	An 8-level scale of cognitive recovery, based on observation of responsiveness, purposeful activity, orientation, memory, self-regulation, spontaneity, independence. Levels: no response, generalized response, localized response, confused-agitated, confused-nonagitated, confused-appropriate, automatic-appropriate, and purposeful-appropriate.
Disability Rating Scale (Rappaport et al., 1982)	A rating scale developed to track improvement of people with TBI from coma to community. Includes subscales for impairment (similar to GCS), disability (cognitive ability for feeding, toileting, and grooming), and handicap (level of community functioning and employability).
Functional Assessment Measure (FIM + FAM) (Hall, 1992)	A rating scale that adds 12 domains for disability rating to the 12 domains of the older Functional Independence Measure (FIM). The additional items, added specifically for individuals with brain injury, include swallowing, reading, writing, orientation, attention, safety judgment, emotional status, and adjustment to limitations.
ASHA-FACS (Frattali et al., 1995)	A rating scale designed to assess functional communication with greater precision than is possible with most general disability rating tools.
Communication Effectiveness Survey (Beukelman, 1998)	A survey designed to assess functional communication in natural contexts.
Community Integration Questionnaire (Willer et al., 1994)	A 15-item questionnaire designed to assess home and social integration and productivity in the following domains: household activities, shopping, errands, and leisure activities.

to the varied patterns and rates of improvement experienced by specific individuals and also to the many small changes in functioning, required supports, and appropriate expectations that are more properly represented as a continuum than as a series of qualitatively different stages.

Early Stage (RLA Levels 2–3)

These levels begin with the first generalized responses to environmental stimuli and end with stimulus-specific responses (e.g., visual tracking, localizing to sound), recognition of some common objects through appropriate use of the object (if motorically capable), and comprehension of some simple commands in context. From a cognitive perspective,

this is often called the sensory or coma stimulation stage of rehabilitation, currently a controversial and hotly debated field of intervention. Zasler et al. (1991) presented a useful review of these themes and a conservative approach to coma management. From the perspective of performance of everyday activities, individuals at this stage require intensive levels of support.

Middle Stage (RLA Levels 4–6)

These levels begin with heightened alertness and increased activity combined with some degree of confusion and disorientation, which may include agitated behavior unrelated to environmental provocation. The middle stage ends with a reduction in confusion, which is manifested by adequate orientation and behavior that is generally goal directed in a familiar environment. Most individuals experience gradual improvement in focused attention and episodic (autobiographical) memory, but memory impairment may remain a residual deficit. Behavior, including social communication, may continue to be impulsive; lack of initiation is an alternative possibility. Most individuals have difficulty organizing complex tasks, including discourse tasks, and planning how to achieve their goals.

During this stage, individuals require moderate, but systematically decreasing levels of support to succeed at everyday tasks. The rehabilitation (or home) environment as well as group and individual therapy sessions are simplified, structured, focused, and rich in external compensatory supports so as to reduce confusion, facilitate improved and increasingly independent performance of functional activities (including relevant social, educational, and vocational activities), and promote adaptive behavior and a progressively increasing ability to process information and communicate effectively.

Late Stage (RLA Levels 7, 8, and Beyond)

These levels begin with an adequate, though perhaps superficial and fragile orientation to important aspects of life and end with the individual's ultimate level of neurologic improvement, which may or may not include cognitive and communicative impairments that are functionally disabling. Environmental supports are gradually withdrawn for purposes of helping individuals become maximally independent and learn how to compensate for and adjust to their residual deficits. It is also the stage of refinement of skills with a focus on effective information processing and social communication in real-world settings and with real-life demands (e.g., school, work, and social life). There is no specific upper limit to learning, compensation, and adjustment that can be facilitated by creative clinicians and thereby substantially improve real-world success.

Sequence of Service Settings

Severe TBI is typically associated with many service settings and sets of service providers. Emergency medical services are routinely administered at the site of the injury and during transport to a trauma center. Emergency room care is largely devoted to managing life-threatening increases in intracranial pressure (ICP) as well as treatment for other injuries (e.g., orthopedic injuries, internal organ injuries) that frequently accompany TBI. Following initial stabilization, patients are transferred to the intensive care unit for ongoing management of critical intracranial dynamics. Stabilization of ICP is often followed by transfer to the hospital's neurologic care floor and the beginning of early rehabilitation. Speech-language pathologists may be members of the early rehabilitation team, often focusing their efforts on

resumption of oral feeding, development of simple communication systems, and family education and support.

In the event of slow recovery, patients may be transferred to a rehabilitation unit or free-standing rehabilitation hospital for intensive acute rehabilitation. When cognitive, behavioral, physical, and general medical needs reach a level at which the person can be cared for in a less restrictive setting, the individual is discharged to home—and often ongoing outpatient or community support services—or to a community reintegration post-acute rehabilitation facility. Individuals with ongoing intense medical needs (e.g., respirator-dependent patients) or severe and unchanging cognitive impairment (e.g., persistent unresponsiveness) may be discharged to a long-term care nursing facility, with the possibility of resuming aggressive rehabilitation if signs of neurologic improvement are noted.

Individuals with concussion (i.e., traumatically induced alteration in mental status not necessarily resulting in loss of consciousness) or mild TBI (i.e., brief loss of consciousness or initial GCS score of 13–15) may be examined in a physician's office, observed in a hospital emergency room, admitted briefly, or not come to the attention of medical professionals at all. In most cases, mild TBI is associated with full recovery within a few days to a few weeks. However, persistent serious disability is possible, requiring professional support and possible work accommodations. Individuals with a history of previous concussion or other neurologic vulnerability (e.g., learning disabilities, neurologic impairment associated with aging) are at increased risk for persistent symptoms (Collins et al., 1999; Gronwall & Wrightson, 1975; Rimel et al., 1981).

Long-Term Communication-Related Outcome

Earlier, we stated that the relation between injury severity and outcome is at best very general. Many factors interact to determine a person's ultimate level of impairment; ability to perform activities of daily living; ability to maintain desired levels of participation in social, educational, vocational, and avocational pursuits; level of personal satisfaction with life after the injury; and level of support required from everyday people in the environment. In addition to the injury itself, these factors include preinjury and postinjury variables summarized in Figures 33–6 and 33–7.

Given preinjury variability (33–6) and the variety of pathophysiologic mechanisms in TBI (see Figures 33–1 and 33–2), some of which are related to site of impact, it is understandable that there are no consistent outcome profiles with respect to communication. Constellations of communication-related strengths and weaknesses potentially associated with TBI are extremely varied, depending on the nature, location, and severity of the injury, as well as characteristics of the individual who is injured and post-trauma supports. Indeed, many professionals consider TBI to be at best misleading as a disability category because it is actually an *etiology* category,

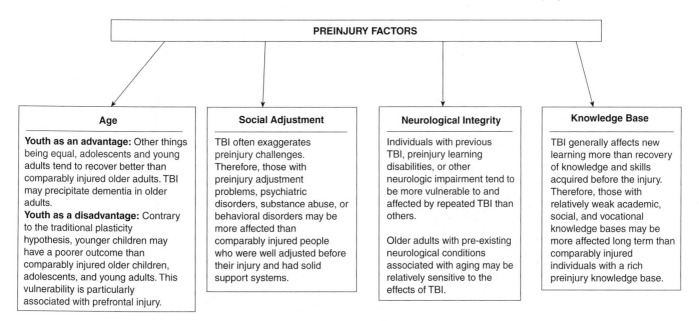

Figure 33–6. Factors that are often present prior to TBI and that may contribute to outcome.

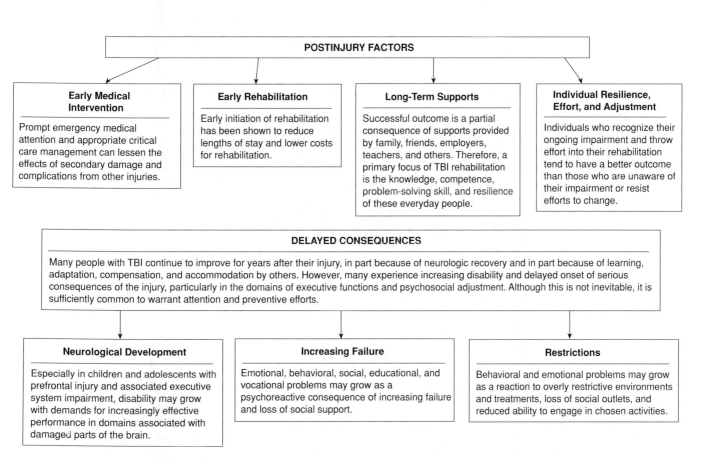

Figure 33–7. Factors that occur after TBI and that contribute to outcome.

identifying a potential cause of varied disabilities, not the disability itself. In this respect, TBI is comparable to stroke or perinatal asphyxia, neurologic events that may or may not produce varied disabilities. Therefore, clinicians should not only expect great diversity within this group, but also substantial overlap between TBI and other categories of adult neurogenic communication disorder, such as aphasia, dementia, and the so-called right hemisphere syndrome.

As indicated in Figures 33–6 and 33–7, heterogeneity within the population is increased by diversity in pretraumatic intelligence, educational and vocational levels, age, personality, and coping styles as well as by variation in posttraumatic environments, support systems, and emotional and behavioral reactions of the individual. Despite many commonalities among survivors of severe TBI (described below), these considerations underscore the importance of customizing assessment procedures and intervention goals and methods for this diverse clinical population.

Infrequency of Aphasia

Although symptoms of aphasia are often present early in recovery and, in some cases, specific language impairment does persist, aphasia defined in terms of the classical syndromes is relatively uncommon after TBI in adults (Heilman et al., 1971; Sarno, 1980, 1984; Sarno et al., 1986) and children (Chapman, 1997; Ylvisaker, 1993). Anomia, which can be associated with a wide variety of brain lesions, is often reported to be the primary residual aphasic symptom in the absence of general cognitive disruption (Heilman et al., 1971; Levin et al., 1981; Sarno, 1980, 1984; Thomsen, 1975). Generalized and persistent expressive and receptive language impairment is generally associated with widespread diffuse injury that also produces global cognitive deficits (Levin et al., 1981). If aphasia is present, clinicians should apply the assessment and intervention frameworks presented elsewhere in this text.

Nonaphasic Communication Disorders: Executive Functions, Cognition, Behavior, and Communication

Communication challenges following TBI are most often "nonaphasic" in nature, that is, they co-exist with intelligible speech, reasonably fluent and grammatical expressive language, and comprehension adequate to support everyday interaction. Depending upon the severity of injury, stage of recovery, and particular focus of research, the characteristic communication profiles following TBI have been variously referred to as "the language of confusion" (early in recovery, Halpern et al., 1973), "nonaphasic language disturbances" (Prigatano, 1986; Prigatano et al., 1985), "cognitive-language disturbances" (Hagen, 1981), and "subclinical aphasia" (Sarno, 1980, 1984). Sarno (1984) found that, although a distinct minority of a consecutive series of 69 severely injured individuals admitted to an inpatient rehabilitation facility could be diagnosed with aphasia, *all* of the patients were found to have some combination of

language deficits that were not apparent in everyday interaction. These included impaired confrontation naming, word fluency, and comprehension of complex oral commands. She did not evaluate their interactive competence with increasing cognitive and social demands, factors that clinicians, teachers, family members, and recent investigators often identify as major contributors to communication breakdowns after TBI.

The overlapping collections of communication deficits highlighted by these investigators have been grouped by the American Speech, Language, and Hearing Association under the heading "cognitive-communicative impairment" (ASHA, 1988) and are all associated with frontolimbic damage, the most common damage in CHI. These impairments are included in Table 33–2, which also includes lists of impairments under three additional headings: executive system, cognitive, and psychosocial/behavioral impairments. In important respects, these four lists are descriptions of the same underlying impairments, using four distinct professional frameworks. The extent of overlap in deficit domains underscores the importance of professionals from different clinical fields collaborating in their approach to assessment and intervention.

Pathophysiological Bases: Frontolimbic Injury

Prefrontal or frontolimbic structures are most vulnerable in CHI (Adams et al., 1980; Levin et al., 1991; Mendelsohn et al., 1992; Varney & Menefee, 1993). Although it is certainly possible to escape frontolimbic injury in TBI, its frequency and profound impact on communicative effectiveness combine to give it and its general neurobehavioral correlate, executive system dysfunction, an important heuristic role in organizing intervention planning (Ylvisaker, 1992). In recent years, investigators have increasingly differentiated varied frontal and limbic functions, and have loosened to some degree the connection between frontal lobe functions and executive functions (Stuss, 1999a,b). However, the most common communication-related themes after TBI continue to be associated with frontolimbic injury.

Indeed, all of the symptoms listed in Table 33–2 are associated with damage to the frontal lobes, limbic structures, and/or the critical axonal connections between prefrontal and limbic structures (Alexander et al., 1989; Stuss & Benson, 1986). For example, both right and left hemisphere prefrontal structures are associated with self-regulation (initiation, inhibition, direction) of behavior, including communication behavior; with organization of language into coherent discourse; and with control over attentional and memory processes to make them useful in daily life. Both left and right hemisphere orbital frontal damage has been associated with personality changes, including disinhibition, volatility, and verbal "dysdecorum" (Alexander et al., 1989). Right frontal lobe damage has been associated with more specific pragmatic deficits, such as (1) decreased ability to *produce* appropriate paralinguistic accompaniments

---

TABLE 33–2

Vulnerable Frontolimbic Structures and Frequently Associated Impairments

Frontolimbic Injury and Executive System Impairment
- reduced awarness of personal strengths and weaknesses
- difficulty setting realistic goals
- difficulty planning and organizing behavior to achieve the goals
- impaired ability to initiate action needed to achieve the goals
- difficulty inhibiting behavior incompatible with achieving the goals
- difficulty self-monitoring and self-evaluating
- difficulty thinking and acting strategically, and solving real-world problems in a flexible and efficient manner
- general inflexibility and concreteness in thinking, talking, and acting

Frontolimbic Injury and Cognitive-Communication Impairment
- disorganized, poorly controlled discourse or paucity of discourse (spoken and written)
- inefficient comprehension of language related to increasing amounts of information to be processed (spoken or written) and to rate of speech
- imprecise language and word-retrieval problems
- difficulty understanding and expressing abstract and indirect language
- difficulty reading social cues, interpreting speaker intent, and flexibly adjusting interactive styles to meet situational demands in varied social contexts
- awkward or inappropriate communication in stressful social contexts
- impaired verbal learning

Frontolimbic Injury and Cognitive Impairment
- reduced internal control over all cognitive functions (e.g., attentional, perceptual, memory, organizational, and reasoning processes)
- impaired working memory
- impaired declarative and explicit memory (encoding and retrieval)
- disorganized behavior related to impaired organizing schemes (managerial knowledge frames, such as scripts, themes, schemas, mental models)
- impaired reasoning
- concrete thinking
- difficulty generalizing

Frontolimbic Injury and Psychosocial/Behavioral Impairment
- disinhibited, socially inappropriate, and possibly aggressive behavior
- impaired initiation or paucity of behavior
- inefficient learning from consequences
- perseverative behavior; rigid, infexible behavior
- impaired social perception and interpretation

Adapted with permission from Ylvisaker et al. (1999).

to speech, including gesture and facial expression as well as prosody in speech; (2) decreased ability to *comprehend* prosodic features in the speech of others and to interpret indirect pragmatic intents, including humor, sarcasm, metaphor, and other indirect meanings; and (3) inattention to context, including social context, resulting in socially inappropriate behavior (Alexander et al., 1989; Shammi & Stuss, 1999; Stuss & Alexander, in press).

Damage to the hippocampus and surrounding limbic tissue is associated with impaired declarative and explicit memory (roughly, memory for facts rather than procedures combined with a subjective sense that one possesses the memory) (Schacter, 1996; Squire, 1992). Because of the extreme vulnerability of the hippocampus to postinjury anoxia, new learning problems are very common after TBI, despite

potentially good recovery of pretraumatically acquired and effectively stored knowledge and skills. Damage to other limbic structures and frontolimbic connections contribute to the transient or persistent difficulty with the emotional and behavioral self-regulation commonly seen after TBI (Izard, 1992; Ledoux, 1991, 1996).

Discourse Impairment

Discourse impairment (i.e., difficulty organizing language over more than one utterance or sentence) has probably received more attention than other communication-related deficits in the recent TBI research literature. Both adults and children with TBI have been found to be impaired relative to controls on many measures of interactive (conversational) and noninteractive (monologic) discourse (Biddle et al., 1996; Chapman, 1997; Chapman et al., 1995, 1997; Coelho et al., 1991; Dennis, 1991, 1992; Dennis & Barnes, 1990; Dennis et al., 1996; Dennis & Lovett, 1990; Ehrlich, 1988; Groher, 1990; Hagen, 1981; Hartley, 1995; Hartley & Jenson, 1991; Liles et al., 1989; McDonald, 1992a,b, 1993; McDonald & Pearce, 1998; Mentis & Prutting, 1991; Pearce et al., 1998; Sarno et al., 1986; Togher et al., 1997; Turkstra & Holland, 1998; Ylvisaker, 1992, 1993).

Discourse impairment in the presence of adequate vocabulary, grammar, and motor speech ability can often be understood as a language consequence of more general cognitive disruption, that is, the loss or inaccessibility of the knowledge structures needed to organize thought units across multiple utterances (sometimes referred to as ideational apraxia). Alternatively, discourse impairment may be a consequence of failure to select and implement the appropriate organizing schemas when they are needed (sometimes referred to as frontal apraxia), or to maintain directed attention to the organizing scheme in a conversation or monologue, and monitor success of the communication. The latter phenomenon is sometimes referred to as impairment of the supervisory attentional system, which is the component of the executive system responsible for controlling behavior-regulating schemas in nonroutine contexts (Shallice, 1982). In most cases, discourse impairment after TBI represents a failure of executive control over cognitive and linguistic organizing processes rather than a linguistic impairment per se (Schwartz, 1995; Schwartz et al., 1993).

In the intervention section of this chapter, we focus on organizational functioning in part because of its important relation to these common discourse impairments. According to many cognitive theories, the same cognitive macrostructures or managerial knowledge units (e.g., scripts, themes, schemas, plans, mental models) that guide organized thinking, remembering, reasoning, and acting also guide organized talking, writing, and comprehension of lengthy discourse. According to one leading neuropsychological theory, such managerial knowledge units are stored in prefrontal parts of the cortex, explaining the frequency of organizational impairment in TBI (Grafman, 1995; Grafman et al., 1993). Thus, discourse is one of the critical points of intersection between language and cognition, mandating an informed cognitive focus in intervention and collaboration among professionals who address the cognitive dimensions of behavior.

Communication Disability Related to Memory/Retrieval Impairment

Memory deficits are among the most commonly reported problems after TBI. *Encoding* of new information into memory is often impaired, either as a result of damage to the vulnerable hippocampal system responsible for consolidating new declarative memories, or of damage to the frontal lobes (especially left hemisphere), resulting in poorly focused attention and/or shallow, nonstrategic organization and elaboration of information as it is initially being processed (Anderson et al., 1988; Brazzeli et al., 1994; Cabeza & Nyberg, 1997; Gluck & Myers, 1995; Schacter, 1996; Squire et al., 1993). Encoding new memories for facts and events (declarative memory) is often more severely impaired than for procedures (procedural memory); similarly, memories stored with some awareness of the memory (explicit memory) are often more vulnerable than those stored without such awareness (implicit memory) (Ewert et al., 1989; Schacter, 1996). *Storage* over time is less commonly impaired in TBI; once information is adequately processed and encoded, it is unlikely to decay rapidly, as is the case in degenerative diseases such as Alzheimer's.

Retrieval may be impaired in TBI as a result of posterior damage that reduces the number of retrieval routes in the networks of neural connections that compose the storage system (Buschke & Fuld, 1974). More commonly, however, word and information retrieval is impaired as a result of frontal lobe injury, which can result in nonstrategic searches of memory (Petrides, 1995; Schacter, 1996) and degraded managerial knowledge units used to direct those searches (Grafman, 1995). For example, when looking for car keys, people characteristically focus their search around organized routines of everyday life. Similar organizational schemas are used to guide internal searches of memory, which are therefore rendered ineffective in the presence of degraded schemas. Recent PET scan investigations of explicit retrieval of information have isolated important contributions of left lateral prefrontal cortex, right anterior frontal-polar cortex, and anterior cingulate gyrus (Buckner et al., 1995). Retrieval of episodic memories is differentially impaired by right frontal lobe damage, even if encoding of that same information may have made greater use of left frontal lobe systems (Schacter, 1996; Tulving et al., 1994).

These memory problems affect communication in a variety of ways. Inefficient information and word retrieval slows interaction and can be socially distracting. Failure to recall information can result in tedious repetition in conversation and embarrassing social breakdowns. Impaired verbal learning has an obvious negative impact on return to school or to a job that requires new learning, possibly resulting in failure that may lead to social withdrawal. Impaired prospective memory without effective compensation creates substantial everyday difficulties as the individual misses appointments or other scheduled activities, forgets medication, and the like.

Communication Disability Associated with Psychosocial and Behavioral Impairment

Any combination of the deficits listed in Table 33–2 can substantially affect life after TBI. However, it is often the communication-related personality and psychosocial changes that most profoundly influence the individual's social, vocational, familial, and academic reintegration. For example, families routinely report that it is easier to adjust to physical disability in a loved one than to personality changes manifested in stressful and unsatisfying communication; employers often highlight communication-related obstacles to maintenance of employment; and teachers frequently identify social and behavioral changes as most problematic in school re-entry (Bond, 1990; Brooks et al., 1987; Brooks & McKinlay, 1983; Brooks et al., 1987; Brown et al., 1981; Filley et al., 1987; Fletcher et al., 1995; Hall et al., 1994; Jacobs, 1993; Klonoff et al., 1986; Lezak, 1986, 1987; Livingston & Brooks, 1988; McKinlay et al., 1981; Morton & Wehman, 1995; Petterson, 1991; Prigatano, 1986; Thomsen, 1974, 1984, 1987; Weddell et al., 1980).

Personality changes frequently highlighted in the TBI literature include irritability, impatience, frequent loss of temper, emotional volatility, egocentrism, impulsiveness, anxiety, depression, loss of social contact, lack of interests, and reduced initiation. Blumer and Benson (1975) summarized the inhibition-related and initiation-related personality changes associated with frontal lobe injury with the labels pseudopsychopathic and pseudodepressed personalities respectively. For communication specialists, these psychosocial and behavioral themes are typically grouped under the heading, pragmatics of language.

Variability in Performance

Teachers, family members, work supervisors, and others often emphasize a frustrating inconsistency in performance in describing people with TBI. An uncharitable but common interpretation of this variability is that the person is unmotivated or excessively moody. Although these characteristics may be present, neuropsychological investigations have found relatively extreme variability in performance to be associated with frontal lobe injury, particularly injury to the right frontal lobes (Stuss, 1999b; Stuss et al., 1994). Variability is increased with increasing task demands and with aging. This inconsistency in performance is one of several reasons for caution in interpreting standardized tests with this population (see below).

FRAMEWORK FOR COGNITIVE AND PSYCHOSOCIAL INTERVENTION

Our goal in this section is to explain and offer a rationale for an approach to intervention that deviates in important ways from standard approaches to medical rehabilitation for individuals with severe TBI. In addition, we offer operational definitions of cognition and executive functions, two of the primary targets of intervention for individuals with TBI. Later in the chapter, we offer procedural detail in two

overlapping domains: (1) cognitive and executive system intervention and (2) behavioral and psychosocial intervention.

Appendix 33-1 contrasts central tendencies in two generally different approaches to communication, behavioral, and cognitive rehabilitation for people with TBI. We have labeled these approaches *conventional* and *functional*, with the caveat that any approach to rehabilitation that is successful as measured by real-world indices is functional. Therefore, the appropriateness of these labels depends in part on relatively disappointing results of TBI efficacy research conducted within the traditional or conventional paradigm (Carney et al., 1999, in press; Park et al., 1999, in press; Thoene, 1996) and on the accumulation of supporting research conducted within the functional paradigm (Feeney et al., in press). What we refer to as the conventional approach has a long history in medical speech-language pathology (and other fields), featuring restorative services offered in medical settings and dominated by massed practice of hierarchically organized decontextualized cognitive training exercises. In this section we explain the general approach referred to as "functional" in Appendix 33-1.

Positive, Everyday, Routine-Based Intervention

Central to the functional approach outlined in Appendix 33-1 is the concept of positive, supported, everyday routines of action and interaction. From a behavioral perspective, a routine is a behavior chain in which each link—each discrete behavior—is a discriminative stimulus for the next link and a conditioned reinforcer for the previous link (Halle & Spradlin, 1993). The goal of intervention, from this perspective, is to help people acquire flexible and situationally successful behavior chains (defined by stimulus and response *classes*) that include observable as well as internal (cognitive and emotional) behaviors as links in the chains—that is, successful routines of everyday life.

From a cognitive perspective, a routine is a concrete structured event complex (SEC, Grafman et al., 1993), which, at a more general level, becomes a script, which is an organized internal (mental) representation of a type of event complex that includes the people, places, associated objects, associated language, and their organization. Everyday routines and scripts are those that occur in the course of everyday social, familial, vocational, recreational, and educational life and involve everyday communication partners, including family members, friends, work supervisors, and teachers. The organized knowledge that enables one to be oriented and behave successfully in a variety of restaurants, from McDonald's to fine restaurants, is an example of a fairly general script. From a cognitive perspective, a primary goal of rehabilitation is to help people with TBI acquire and apply appropriate scripts and other general knowledge structures (or managerial knowledge units, Grafman et al., 1993) to guide successful thinking, remembering, problem solving, decision making, talking, and acting in social context.

We highlight the word *routine* for several reasons. First, routine suggests *habit*—behavior that does not require effortful deliberation or planning. With frontal lobe injury and associated executive function impairment, habitual behavior is often relatively unaffected, whereas behavior that requires a novel plan for unfamiliar circumstances may be severely impaired (Stuss & Benson, 1986). Later in this chapter, we suggest that executive functions themselves, including planning, organizing, and problem solving, can become routine with extensive coached practice of executive function routines within everyday action contexts. Second, routine suggests normal activities of life, motivating clinicians to move beyond commercial therapy materials, generic therapy activities, and exclusively clinical intervention settings, capitalizing rather on the activities that are routine for the individual and using everyday communication partners as

collaborators in intervention. Countless studies of generalization and maintenance of learned behaviors with many disability groups support the conclusion that adequate performance of targeted skills in a treatment setting—even after mastery of the skill using personally meaningful activities—is no guarantee of ongoing use of the skill in the routines of everyday life.

Supports (Scaffolding)

Within an everyday, routine-based approach to intervention, the technical term *support* designates a pivotal concept, connected with a Vygotskyan approach to cognitive and behavioral intervention, discussed later. To say that routines of action or interaction are positive and supported is to say that people with disability are provided with the supports or "scaffolding" (Wood et al., 1976) they need to be successful. Table 33–3 lists examples of supports commonly used to

---

TABLE 33–3

Antecedent Procedures for Supporting Individuals with Cognitive and Behavioral Impairment

Supported Cognition
1. Ensure do-ability of tasks; eliminate unreasonable demands
2. Create facilitative work/study environment
3. Ensure orientation to setting and task; use clear, facilitative instructions
4. Induce positive internal setting events (see section on behavioral intervention) before cognitively demanding tasks
   - positive behavioral momentum (see section on behavioral intervention)
   - choice and control
   - rest, relaxation, absence of pain
5. Establish well-rehearsed routines and scripts
6. Use advance organizers (e.g., organizationally clear graphic organizers) for complex tasks
7. Use appropriate cognitive prosthetics, as needed (e.g., memory aids, electronic pager/reminder systems, organization aids, attention aids)
8. Use collaboration to complete difficult tasks (e.g., cooperative work/learning groups; buddy system)
9. Ensure that communication partners use elaborative and collaborative conversational competencies (see later in this chapter)
10. Ensure that communication partners use supportive cognitive scripts (see later in this chapter)
11. Desensitize the individual to events and tasks that cause anxiety
12. Help the individual manage cognitive antecedents

Supported Behavioral Self-Regulation
1. Eliminate unreasonable provocation, including unreasonable demands
2. Ensure orientation to setting and task
3. Ensure do-ability of tasks
4. Induce positive internal setting events before stressful tasks
   - positive behavioral momentum
   - choice and control
   - rest, relaxation, absence of pain
5. Teach positive communication alternatives to negative behavior
6. Establish alternative scripts to negative behavior (e.g., give individual a positive role that requires responsible behavior)
7. Ensure that the individual has positive, meaningful roles to play and goals to achieve
8. Desensitize the individual to events that cause anxiety
9. Help the individual manage behavioral antecedents (e.g., avoid overly stressful tasks; create scripts for potentially negative interactions; alert friends and supervisors to how they might help during a stressful experience)

Adapted with permission from Ylvisaker & Feeney (1998a).

Progression of Intervention Within a Functional Everyday Approach to Rehabilitation

Step 1. Identify successful and unsuccessful routines of everyday life: What is working and what is not working?
Step 2. Identify what changes (including changes in the environment, in the behavior of others, and in the individual's own behavior) hold the potential to transform negative, unsuccessful routines into positive, successful routines and build repertoires of positive behavior.
Step 3. Identify how those changes in everyday routines can be motivating for the individual and for critical everyday people in that environment.
Step 4. Implement whatever supports are necessary for intensive practice of positive routines in real-world contexts.
Step 5. Systematically withdraw supports and expand contexts as it becomes possible to do so.

Reproduced with permission from Ylvisaker et al. (1999).

facilitate success with cognitively demanding tasks ("supported cognition," Ylvisaker & Feeney, 1996) and with behaviorally stressful tasks ("supported behavioral self-regulation"). In both cases, supports can be understood using the more familiar model of supported employment, wherein workers with disability are enabled to perform otherwise difficult work tasks because they have the help of a job coach or designated peer, use customized equipment and strategies to compensate for their disability, and/or rely on other environmental supports. Supported employment has enjoyed considerable success with adults with TBI (Curl et al., 1996; Wehman et al., 1993, 1995) and is one of the few areas of TBI rehabilitation found by a recent systematic evidence review to have a solid research base (NIH, 1999).

Progression of Intervention

Table 33–4 outlines a progression of intervention consistent with a contextualized, everyday, routine-based approach to cognitive, psychosocial, and communication rehabilitation. First, staff and everyday people (ideally including the person with disability) collaborate to identify what is and is not working in the everyday routines of life. Second, the same group of collaborators identifies what changes in everyday routines could result quickly in reduction of handicap (i.e., increases in participation) and, in the longer run, in reduction of disability (i.e., improved performance of functional activities) and ultimately in reduction of the underlying impairment. Systematic hypothesis testing (described in the next section) is often required to identify the source of the manifest problem and therefore to identify the most useful and positive changes in everyday routines.

Third, the same stakeholders collaborate to identify the supports needed for positive changes in everyday routines and ways to motivate these changes for the person with disability and for others in the environment. Often, this stage requires considerable creativity and flexibility. There exists no rehabilitation textbook that can prescribe the unique combinations of supports that are often needed in people's real-world contexts or that can show how these changes in everyday routines can be motivating for everyone involved.

Fourth, systems of support are implemented so that everyday routines of action and interaction are successful, and important skills, possibly including compensatory skills, can be practiced extensively in real-world contexts. Finally, levels of support are systematically reduced as the individual becomes more successful at everyday tasks and/or habituates the use of compensatory procedures; at the same time, contexts of successful action and interaction are systematically increased. Later in this section, we illustrate how the process of modification and reduction of supports applies across the continuum of recovery after severe TBI.

This contextualized, everyday, routine-based approach to rehabilitation reverses the traditional "first impairment, then disability, then handicap" hierarchy in rehabilitation. Table 33–5 outlines this reversal. Within traditional rehabilitation, the initial goal has generally been to eliminate or reduce the underlying impairment with decontextualized exercises or medical interventions. If these efforts are insufficiently successful, the intervention has tended to shift to attempts to equip the individual with compensatory behaviors to overcome the ongoing disability. Finally, in the event of insufficiently successful disability-oriented interventions, the focus shifts to attempts to reduce the individual's handicap and support social participation by simplifying tasks or modifying the environment and increasing the support behaviors of others in the environment. This traditional approach is often most efficient in the case of physical restoration and in other domains as well, if there is reason to believe that decontextualized, restorative interventions are effective. However, research and clinical experience give little reason for such optimism in the case of individuals with significant chronic cognitive and psychosocial impairment after TBI.

Reversing the traditional hierarchy does *not* imply abandoning the goal of reducing the individual's underlying impairment. Rather, impairment is potentially reduced as a result of internalizing habits of action and interaction that may have originated as deliberate compensations for chronic impairment. For example, a person who uses a graphic

TABLE 33-5

Two Perspectives on the Relations Between Impairment-Oriented, Disability Activity-Oriented, and Handicap Participation-Oriented Interventions for People with Chronic Cognitive, Communication, and Behavioral Impairment After Brain Injury

I. THE TRADITION IN REHABILITATION:

First: Attempt to eliminate the individual's underlying *impairment* with impairment-oriented treatments.
- medical treatments (e.g., neuropharmacology, surgery)
- impairment-oriented exercises

Second: Attempt to reduce functional *disability* (i.e., improve performance of daily activities) if impairment-oriented treatment is insufficiently successful.
- practice with compensatory procedures
- extensive practice of specific functional activities

Third: Attempt to reduce social, vocational, and/or educational *handicap* (i.e., increase participation) if impairment- and disability-oriented interventions are insufficiently successful.
- modification of tasks, routines, and the environments in which they take place
- modification of the behavior of other people in the environment

II. AN ALTERNATIVE PERSPECTIVE:

First: Reduce *handicap* (i.e., increase participation) by modifying everyday routines, including the support provided by everyday people in the environment.

Second: Potentially decrease *disability* (i.e., improve performance of daily activities) by including functional compensatory procedures in the individual's everyday routines and ensuring intensive contextualized practice in the use of those compensatory procedures.

Third: Potentially reduce the *impairment* by ensuring that the individual practices compensatory procedures—in increasingly varied contexts—to the point at which they are internalized and become components of his or her automatic cognitive or self-regulatory mechanism.

Reproduced with permission from Ylvisaker et al. (1999).

organizer to succeed in complex vocational planning tasks or discourse tasks may internalize the organizer so that it becomes an automatically applied knowledge structure, thereby reducing the original underlying impairment. Ylvisaker and Feeney have presented several case illustrations in which impairment reduction was a long-term outcome of intervention that began with handicap- and disability-oriented supports for successful performance of everyday activities (Ylvisaker & Feeney, 1998a, 2000a; Ylvisaker et al., 1999).

Rationale for a Contextualized, Everyday, Routine-Based Approach to Cognitive and Psychosocial Rehabilitation

Theoretical Support

For many years, our work in cognitive and behavioral rehabilitation for children and adults with TBI has been guided in part by the theoretical formulations of the great Russian psychologist, Lev Vygotsky. Over the past 20 years, his work has enjoyed a striking renaissance in many applied fields, including educational psychology (e.g., Brown et al., 1990), reading instruction (e.g., Palinscar & Brown, 1989), early childhood education (e.g., Bodrova & Leong, 1996; Berk & Winsler, 1995), special education (e.g., Evans, 1993; Ashman & Conway, 1989), child language disorders (e.g., Schneider & Watkins, 1996; Westby, 1994), and other professions. In

light of Vygotsky's life-long influence on the work of his influential colleague, Alexander Luria (Luria, 1979), it is rather surprising that relatively little attention has been paid to Vygotsky's work in adult neurologic rehabilitation (Ylvisaker & Feeney, 1998a).

According to Vygotsky, internal cognitive and self-regulatory functions, beyond those that are instinctive or purely sensorimotor, are derived in childhood from internalization of interaction with others who are more competent, that is, of social-communication routines. "Higher mental functions evolve through social interactions with adults; they are gradually internalized as the child becomes more and more proficient and needs less and less cuing and other support from the adult" (Vygotsky, 1981). Thus, cognitive processes like remembering, organizing, and problem solving, as well as self-regulatory processes like self-instructing, first exist as supported *interpsychological* processes—as interaction between a child or other "apprentice-in-thinking" and a more mature thinker. Gradually, the processes are internalized and become internal or *intrapsychological* processes. Within cognitive and psychosocial rehabilitation, clinicians and other everyday communication partners play a role comparable to expert-parents in relation to apprentice-children with the goal of equipping the client with the cognitive, communication, and self-regulatory skills needed for success in his or her chosen contexts of life.

TABLE 33–6

Features of Teaching Tasks: Traditional Training Model Versus Vygotskyan Apprenticeship Model

TRADITIONAL TRAINING MODEL

Context
- Training takes place outside of a natural setting.
- Performance of the learner is demanded by the trainer.
- Performance is solo, not social.
- Tasks and components of tasks are hierarchically organized.

Task Structure
- The trainer requests performance of a specific task.
- The trainer may model performance.
- The learner performs.
- If the performance is adequate, the learner is reinforced.
- If the performace is inadequate, the trainer either
  - requests a hierarchically easier task;
  - reduces the difficulty of the task;
  - provides needed cues, prompts, shaping procedures.
- When performance is adequate, repeated practice is required to habituate the learned behavior.
- Systematic transfer procedures are then applied.

VYGOTSKYAN APPRENTICESHIP MODEL

Context
- Learning (ideally) takes place in a natural setting for the behavior or skill that is to be learned.
- Learning takes place within the context of projects designed to achieve a meaningful goal.
- Performance is not demanded from the learner; rather, the task is completed collaboratively.
- Completion of the task is social, not solo.
- The learner is not expected to fail; the collaborator is available to contribute whatever the learner cannot contribute to successful completion of the task.
- Tasks are not necessarily organized hierarchically; the learner can learn aspects of difficult tasks by participating with a collaborator.

Task Structure
- The teacher (facilitator, collaborator) introduces a task and engages the learner in guided observation (not necessarily task specific).
- The teacher engages the learner in collaborative, functional, goal-oriented, project-oriented work.
- The learner contributes what he or she can contribute.
- The teacher coaches (including suggestions, modeling, brainstorming, cues, feedback, and encouragement) and continues to collaborate as the learner accomplishes more components of the task.
- As the learner improves, supports are systematically withdrawn, or the task is made more difficult, or both.
- The teacher continues to provide ongoing incidental coaching.
- Transfer is guaranteed because it is part of the contextualized teaching process from the beginning.

Reproduced with permission from Ylvisaker & Feeney (1998a).

The apprenticeship metaphor, which is often used to capture the spirit of Vygotsky's theories (Rogoff, 1990), helps in translating a developmental theory into operational terms in adult rehabilitation. Table 33–6 contrasts two importantly different approaches to teaching: the traditional behavioral training model and a Vygotskyan apprenticeship model. The latter underpins interventions described later in this chapter.

Neuropsychological Support

A Rehabilitation Dilemma and Its Resolution

Ylvisaker and Feeney (1998a) borrowed from the work of Antonio Damasio in building neuropsychological support for an everyday, routine-based approach to rehabilitation after TBI. In his classic book *Descartes Error* (1994), Damasio sketched an apparently destructive dilemma associated with frontolimbic injury. To be successful in everyday activities, it appears that one must either (1) make good decisions, based on careful consideration of the information available and memory for past successes and failures (the "high reason" approach) or (2) act on the basis of learned behaviors derived from one's personal history of reinforcement (the operant or "somatic marker" approach). Unfortunately, frontolimbic injury jeopardizes both routes to successful action.

Success via high reason presupposes reasonable planning skill, adequate space in working memory for consideration of many relevant factors, adequate explicit memory for past actions and their consequences, reasonable ability to inhibit impulsive action, and an ability to flexibly transfer learning from one context to another. People with significant frontolimbic injury tend to be impaired in all of these cognitive functions.

Success via learning from consequences presupposes reasonable intactness of the neural circuits that are responsible for connecting two types of memory—memory for the factual aspects of past behavior and for the "somatic markers" or feeling states associated with the consequences of those behaviors. Without such connections in memory (however unconscious they may be), past rewards and punishments lack the power to drive future decision making and behavior. Extensive investigations of adults with frontal lobe injury have convinced Damasio and his colleagues that ventromedial prefrontal lesions, which are very common in closed head injury, weaken the ability to connect these two types of memory, resulting in the common clinical profile of people who respond immediately to rewards and punishments, but whose behavior in the long run is inefficiently shaped by the organized arrangement of such consequences (Damasio et al., 1990, 1991).

Some clinicians respond to this dilemma by suggesting (a) that consequences must be much more extreme than is commonly necessary or (b) that individuals with significant frontolimbic injury may require a substantial degree of external control indefinitely. In our view, escaping through the horns of the dilemma requires the development of contextually relevant cognitive, communication, and behavioral habits, acquired with the help of antecedent-focused apprenticeship procedures (see Tables 33–3 and 33–6 for operational definitions) rather than relying on consequences to shape behavior, as is done in traditional training models of intervention and traditional behavior management. In the section on behavioral and psychosocial rehabilitation (below) we return to this theme of relative inefficiency in learning from consequences.

Procedural Memory, Implicit Memory, and Errorless Learning

The practice of teaching habits (routines) of thought, communication, and social conduct using antecedent supports is additionally bolstered by recent findings in the areas of implicit and procedural memory and errorless learning. Significant damage to the hippocampus and parahippocampal structures (common in TBI) typically impairs declarative memory (i.e., remembering *that* such and such is the case) and explicit memory (i.e., having a subjective sense that one possesses the memory), but may leave procedural memory (i.e., remembering *how to do* something) and implicit memory (i.e., possessing a memory trace that influences future behavior, but lacking a subjective sense that one remembers) relatively intact (Bachman, 1992; Izard, 1992; Pascual-Leone et al., 1995; Schacter, 1996; Squire, 1992).

In their now classic studies, Glisky and Schacter have found that people with apparently dense amnesia after brain injury are still capable of procedural learning (Glisky & Schacter, 1988, 1989). Similarly, Shum and colleagues (1996) found that subjects with TBI performed relatively poorly on explicit memory tasks, but comparable to controls on implicit memory tasks. In their "good guy/bad guy" experiments, Tranel and Damasio (1993) found that individuals with severe amnesia associated with damage to parahippocampal structures nevertheless create implicitly stored affective memories about people they have had positive or negative experiences with, despite no explicit memories for those people.

In the presence of such neuropsychological profiles, common in varying degrees after TBI, Barbara Wilson and her colleagues have found errorless learning procedures to be a critical component of rehabilitation (Wilson & Evans, 1996; Wilson et al., 1994). When people with *severe* explicit and declarative memory impairment make errors and experience a rush of embarrassment or anger when those errors are corrected, they are likely to store the erroneous response, but not associated with an awareness of the response *as an error*. Thus, the erroneous memory influences future behavior in an insidious manner. That is, people who seem to have severe memory impairment may encode and store some memories effectively, particularly when associated with strong emotional reactions. Under these circumstances, clinicians must ensure that the information being processed and the behaviors being rehearsed are the correct information and desired behaviors. These neuropsychological considerations have revived a decades-old tradition of errorless learning in animal training and in developmental disabilities, and serve as an additional buttress for a supported, everyday, routine approach to rehabilitation for people with significant cognitive impairment after TBI.

Empirical Support: Generalization and Maintenance

Decades of experimental studies of generalization and maintenance offer yet another support for a richly contextualized, everyday, routine-based approach to intervention. Many investigators in behavioral, cognitive, and educational psychology have amassed large quantities of evidence that yields the following heuristic principle: *Behaviors or skills acquired in a laboratory or training context are unlikely to transfer to functional application contexts and be maintained over time without heroic efforts to facilitate that transfer and maintenance* (Horner et al., 1988; Martin & Pear, 1996; Morris, 1992; Singley & Anderson, 1989). Recognition of the impact of this principle has led to the development and validation of increasingly contextualized interventions in many clinical fields, including vocational rehabilitation (e.g., Wehman et al., 1993, 1995), special education (e.g., Giangreco et al., 1993), strategy intervention for students with and without specific disability (e.g., Pressley, 1995), behavioral intervention (e.g., Carr et al.,

1994; Carr et al., 1997; Kennedy, 1994; Koegel et al., 1997; Reichle & Wacker, 1993), and language and social skills intervention (e.g., Fey, 1986; Koegel & Koegel, 1995; MacDonald, 1989; Walker et al., 1994; Wiener & Harris, 1998).

In our judgment, the use of decontextualized cognitive retraining exercises (popular in the 1980s in TBI rehabilitation and still used by some practitioners) is insensitive to this important principle. Isolating components of cognition (e.g., selective attention, working memory, sequential or categorical organization, deductive reasoning) and engaging people in massed learning trials with tasks largely unrelated to functional application tasks falls squarely in the tradition of decontextualized cognitive training that has been found relatively ineffective with many disability groups, including mental retardation (Mann, 1979), learning disabilities (Kavale & Mattson, 1983), and TBI (Carney et al., 1999), as well as with people with normal cognition (Singley & Anderson, 1989). More than 100 years ago, William James made the same observation in connection with memory training: "the retention of particular things" can be improved with practice, but not "general physiological retentiveness" (James, 1890, p. 665).

Economic Support: Managed Care and the Demand for Efficient Rehabilitation

A fourth category of support for an everyday routine-based approach to rehabilitation is provided by the fierce economic realities that have come to play a prominent role in rehabilitation planning. Managed care and cutbacks in federal supports for rehabilitation have dramatically shortened lengths of inpatient rehabilitation stay and reduced access to outpatient services (AHCPR, 1999; Johnson, 1999). Some funders routinely deny reimbursement for interventions, such as cognitive rehabilitation, that are said to have an inadequate research base. At the same time, funders increasingly demand improved functional outcomes in return for their limited support for rehabilitation (Henri & Hallowell, 1999; Schmidt, 1997).

Meanwhile, the prevalence of TBI-related disability continues to increase because of the population's relative youth at the time of injury. For example, in New York State over the past 4 years, we have served over 325 young adults with a history of TBI and ongoing difficulty with community reintegration, often many years after their injury. This community support program was designed specifically for individuals with serious chronic cognitive and behavioral impairment after TBI.

Under these stressful economic circumstances, it is critical for rehabilitation specialists to creatively design ways to accomplish more with less, to achieve positive outcomes with fewer resources. Inviting specialists to intensify their collaboration with everyday people (e.g., family members, direct care staff, job coaches, and others) so that long-term rehabilitation can be provided in large part in the context of the everyday routines of life represents a positive response to the crisis of funding for rehabilitation. Feeney and colleagues (in press) presented cost-effectiveness data supporting this approach for individuals with behavioral impairment after TBI.

The Role of Individual and Group Therapy Within an Everyday Rehabilitation Framework

In highlighting the importance of context and the role of supported routines of everyday life as the core of rehabilitation for individuals with chronic cognitive, psychosocial, and communication impairment after TBI, we do not wish to suggest that there is no role for individual and group therapy. First, many of the traditional roles played by speech-language pathologists in relation to swallowing, motor speech, and aphasic deficits are appropriate and necessary for some individuals with TBI. Second, the meaning of *context* is not restricted to setting. Clinicians can contextualize therapy sessions with personally meaningful activities and materials (e.g., academic texts and tasks for a college student) and also people (e.g., including family members in communication therapy sessions).

Third, individual and group therapy sessions can be used to brainstorm about and explore the usefulness of alternative strategies and supports (Step 2 of everyday intervention, Table 33–4). Having identified what works and what doesn't work under controlled conditions, plans can be implemented for contextualized practice in the routines of everyday life, possibly supported by everyday people and possibly self-managed. Fourth, the intimacy of individual therapy sessions is often necessary to address the sensitive issue of self-awareness of ongoing impairment. Finally, individual or group sessions are a useful venue for the motivational and supportive interaction needed by individuals who struggle to maintain the level of effort needed to be successful after their injury (Step 3 of everyday intervention, Table 33–4). *Having highlighted the potential value of therapy sessions, however, we wish to stress the goal of transforming every hour of reimbursed therapy into several hours of well-conceived rehabilitation by virtue of effective alliances with everyday people and creative use of the routines of everyday life.*

Cognition and Executive Functions as Intervention Targets

Cognition: An Intervention-Relevant Operational Definition

Because of the complexity of cognition and the relationships among its components, as well as the variety of theoretical descriptions of cognition and its development in childhood (e.g., Ashcraft, 1994; Barsalou, 1992; Dodd & White, 1980; Flavell et al., 1993; Siegler, 1991), the

TABLE 33–7

Aspects of Cognition

Component Systems

Working memory (system for holding and acting on information in consciousness)
- Structural capacity (7±2 units of information) versus functional capacity (information organized for efficient processing)
- Phonological, visuospatial, and other holding spaces versus supervisory control system

Knowledge base (system for long-term storage of information, rules, schemas, word meanings, and other memories)
- Episodic (autobiographical) versus semantic memory
- Declarative (remembering that . . .) versus procedural (remembering how to . . .) memory
- Explicit (including awareness of the memory) versus implicit (no awareness) memory
- Remote memory (memory for preinjury events, associated with retrograde amnesia) versus recent memory (memory for post-injury events, associated with anterograde amnesia)

Executive system (system for initiating, directing, and regulating all cognitive processes)

Response system (system for expressing knowledge, including speech, writing, and other modalities)

Component Processes

Attention
- Arousal and alertness
- Preparing attention
- Maintaining/sustaining attention
- Selecting a focus of attention (concentrating attention)
- Suppressing/filtering distractions
- Shifting/switching attention
- Dividing/sharing attention

Perception

Memory and Learning
- Encoding (placing items in memory), storage (holding memories over time), and retrieval (retrieving items from memory)
- Involuntary (memory as a byproduct of functional activity) versus deliberate (effortful or strategic) memory
- Retrospective (memory for the past) versus prospective (memory for appointments and other future events) memory
- Verbal versus nonverbal memory
- Sensory modality-specific (e.g., auditory versus verbal) memory

Organization
- Feature identification
- Organization by categories
- Organization by temporal sequences
- Organization by analysis into parts
- Organization by integration into wholes, main ideas, themes, and scripts

Reasoning
- Deductive (formal inference) versus inductive (inference from experience) reasoning
- Analogical reasoning (drawing indirect inferences from experience, perceiving relationships)
- Evaluative reasoning (value judgments)
- Convergent (identifying main ideas and themes) versus divergent (exploring possibilities) thinking

Functional Integrative Performance

Efficiency of Information Processing
- Rate of performance
- Amount accomplished

Scope of Processing, including settings and knowledge domains in which processing is efficient

Manner of Processing, including impulsive/reflective, dependent/independent, rigid/flexible, active/passive processing

Level, developmental, academic, linguistic, or vocational level at which information can be processed

construction of a coherent and manageable framework for cognitive-communication intervention becomes a major challenge. However, just such a framework is critical because it helps clinicians to avoid a haphazard and inefficient "workbook" approach to treatment, facilitates communication among professionals and between clinicians and clients, promotes systematic observation and program evaluation, and serves as a source of intervention principles and procedures.

Table 33–7 presents a scheme for organizing descriptions of behavior from a cognitive perspective. The scheme is based generally on information-processing theories of cognition, wherein cognition is viewed broadly as the processing of information for particular purposes and within specific mental structures and environmental constraints (Dodd & White, 1980). In our clinical work, we have found it productive to describe cognitive functioning and recovery in terms of three general aspects of cognition: processes, systems, and functional-integrative performance. Each of the processes and systems relates in identifiable ways to language and communication.

Profiles of cognitive impairment after TBI can be varied and complex, requiring thorough exploration with formal neuropsychological assessments and, more importantly, for treatment purposes and contextualized hypothesis testing, described later. Treatment decisions are further driven by decisions about relationships among cognitive processes and systems. For example, a person with TBI may process information slowly, appear inattentive, forget easily, evidence disorganized thinking and behavior, misperceive social cues, respond impulsively, and appear to have lost social and vocational knowledge. These may be separate impairments, but more likely, at least some are related. For example, problems with memory, organization, and social perception may all be secondary to attentional impairment. Alternatively, difficulty attending and slowed processing may be due in part to loss of organizing schemes and preinjury knowledge, which may also reduce memory efficiency. Hypothesis testing with alternative support strategies helps answer these questions, which are often left unanswered by comprehensive neuropsychological assessment.

An understanding of cognition from a developmental perspective (Flavell et al., 1993; Siegler, 1991) is useful in avoiding common pitfalls in cognitive rehabilitation for adults. Clinicians who believe that cognitive processes are serially ordered in development are naturally inclined to embrace a hierarchical progression in rehabilitation, addressing components of attention first, then perhaps perception, then perhaps organization and memory, and finally executive control over cognitive processes. This model is inconsistent with the essential interrelations among components of cognition that dominate cognitive development in children, and very likely yields an inefficient approach to intervention.

Executive Functions: An Intervention-Relevant Operational Definition

In Table 33–7, the executive system is included as a component of cognition. In this limited and "cold" sense of the term (Denckla, 1996), executive functions direct and regulate cognitive processes. Thus, people with frontal lobe injury may perform well on tests of intelligence and may appear to attend, perceive, organize, learn, and reason adequately under highly structured and externally directed conditions, but because of executive system impairment, fail to use their cognitive processes effectively under real-world conditions.

In discussions of TBI and frontal lobe injury, executive functions are often highlighted for separate consideration in their role as planner, initiator, and regulator of all aspects of behavior, not just cognitive processes. Understood most generally, the executive system includes those mental functions involved in formulating goals, planning how to achieve them, carrying out the plans, and revising those plans in response to feedback (Lezak, 1982; Luria, 1966). In this broad sense, the same set of control functions directs all deliberate, nonroutine behavior, including cognitive behavior (e.g., paying attention in the presence of distractions), communication behavior (e.g., planning an effective way to express a complex or sensitive thought), social behavior (e.g., inhibiting aggressive behavior when provoked), academic behavior (e.g., studying for an exam), and vocational behavior (e.g., planning a day at work to complete a large number of assigned tasks). In this broad and "hot" sense of the term, executive functions are similar to the functions involved in *self-determination* as that term has been used in recent discussions in the field of developmental disabilities (Wehmeyer & Schwartz, 1997).

Table 33–8 offers a functional operational definition of the executive system, based in part on analysis of the characteristics (beyond intellectual, linguistic, and motor skills) that

---

TABLE 33–8

A Functional Operational Definition of the Executive System

1. Awareness of strengths and limitations, and associated understanding of the difficulty level of tasks
2. Based on this awareness, an ability to
   - Set reasonable goals
   - Plan and organize behavior designed to achieve the goals
   - Initiate behavior toward achieving goals
   - Inhibit behavior incompatible with achieving those goals
   - Monitor and evaluate performance in relation to the goals
   - Flexibly revise plans and strategically solve problems in the event of difficulty or failure
3. Ability to assume a nonegocentric perspective
4. Ability to think abstractly and transfer skills from training to application contexts

enable successful people to be successful—to make efficient real-world use of the abilities and knowledge that they possess.

In discussions of neuropsychological rehabilitation, executive functions are often characterized as high on a hierarchy of cognitive functions and therefore an inappropriate target for intervention until late in recovery after most aspects of cognition have undergone substantial recovery. Unfortunately, this hierarchical view is insensitive to developmental studies of both animals (Goldman, 1971) and human children (Bjorkland, 1990; Welsh & Pennington, 1988). Recent work in developmental cognitive psychology strongly suggests a developmental course for executive functions characterized by early onset of development (in infancy), slow maturation of functions (continuing through the adolescent years), dynamic interaction with other aspects of cognitive, linguistic, and social development, and modifiability of development with experience and training (Bjorklund, 1990; Tranel et al.,

1995; Welsh & Pennington, 1988). Indeed, one of the most popular and successful curricula for preschoolers with and without disability, the High Scope Curriculum, organizes preschool activities around a simple executive function Goal-Plan-Do-Review routine (Schweinhart & Weikart, 1993). Recognizing the profound importance of executive functions for success in life and with these developmental themes as background, we introduce executive functions as a rehabilitation target relatively early in recovery, along with all other aspects of cognition (see Table 33–11 later in the chapter).

Summary

Table 33–9 summarizes ways in which an everyday, routine-based approach to rehabilitation addresses chronic obstacles to social success after TBI. Obstacles are grouped under the headings of executive functions, cognition, and behavior. Some of the solutions are elaborated later in the chapter.

TABLE 33–9

Rationale for an Everyday, Routine-Based Approach to Intervention for Individuals with TBI

FROM THE PERSPECTIVE OF EXECUTIVE FUNCTIONS

A. *Threat to Social Success:* Difficulty making good decisions based on thoughtful consideration of consequences and other relevant factors
Possible Solution: Provide needed supports in everyday routines, stopping short of a degree of support that creates learned helplessness or oppositional behavior.

B. *Threat to Social Success:* Reduced inhibition
Possible Solutions: (1) Create everyday routines that include ample antecedent supports, such as positive setting events and avoidance of identified triggers. (2) Help the individual self-manage antecedents.

C. *Threat to Social Success:* Reduced initiation
Possible Solution: Create everyday routines that include initiation supports, such as initiation scripts, initiation cues (e.g., alarm watch), and peer support for initiation.

FROM THE PERSPECTIVE OF COGNITION

A. *Threat to Social Success:* Impaired working memory
Possible Solutions: (1) Practice positive everyday routines so that they come to be elicited by everyday environmental cues, obviating the need for complex thought processes. (2) Create prosthetic reminder systems (e.g., pager systems). (3) Create positive metaphors that package several pieces of information into one thought unit.

B. *Threat to Social Success:* Impaired explicit and strategic memory; difficulty remembering past successes and failures
Possible Solution: Proceduralize positive contextualized routines using implicit versus explicit memory processes, procedural versus declarative memory systems, and involuntary versus strategic or effortful learning tasks.

C. *Threat to Social Success:* Reduced organizational skills
Possible Solution: Create positive everyday routines that include external organizers, possibly including graphic advance organizers.

D. *Threat to Social Success:* Difficulty transferring newly acquired skills from training to application contexts
Possible Solution: Facilitate acquisition of social competencies in the context of everyday social interaction.

FROM THE PERSPECTIVE OF BEHAVIOR MANAGEMENT

A. *Threat to Social Success:* Inefficiency in learning from consequences
Possible Solution: Build repertoires of positive behaviors using antecedent supports versus relying on consequences to shape positive behaviors.

B. *Threat to Social Success:* Oppositional behavior
Possible Solutions: (1) As much as possible, work within the individual's world of meaning and personal goals. (2) Tie interventions to positive personal metaphors or life narratives.

Reproduced with permission from Ylvisaker & Feeney (2000a).

ASSESSMENT FOR PLANNING FUNCTIONAL CONTEXTUALIZED INTERVENTION

Cognitive and communication assessments may be conducted for several distinct purposes, including (a) diagnosing a disorder, (b) formulating a prognosis, (c) generating epidemiologic information, (d) preparing for legal testimony, (e) acquiring services or funding, (f) developing an intervention plan, and (g) monitoring the results of intervention. Specific assessment procedures may be valid for some but not all purposes of assessment. For example, a standardized aphasia battery may be useful in diagnosing a specific language impairment, but offer little help in identifying the associated disability (i.e., degree of difficulty performing activities of everyday life) or handicap (i.e., reduction in social participation) associated with that impairment or in offering the most fruitful approach to reducing the individual's impairment, disability, or handicap.

In recent years, several standardized tests have been developed for use with adults with TBI, including *Scales of Cognitive-Linguistic Abilities for Traumatic Head Injury* (Adamovich & Henderson, 1992), the *Ross Information Processing Assessment* (RIPA-2; Ross-Swain, 1996), *Brief Test of Head Injury (BTHI)* (Helm-Estabrooks & Hotz, 1991), and others. Brookshire (1997) discusses these and other standardized tests in common clinical use. Standardized assessments, discussed elsewhere in this text, can serve a variety of useful purposes.

In this chapter, however, we have chosen to restrict our discussion to assessment for purposes of planning, monitoring, and modifying individualized intervention. Functional intervention is often directed at reducing disability by improving compensatory behavior in specific functional contexts of activity or at reducing handicap (i.e., increasing participation) by modifying the environment or improving the support behaviors of others. In these cases, standardized office-bound assessments are not particularly helpful.

In Table 33–10 we present categories of assessments, grouped under the headings impairment, disability (activity), and handicap (participation). This scheme for classifying

---

TABLE 33–10

Approaches to Communication Assessment for People with TBI

Impairment-Oriented Assessment

Purpose:	For diagnosis: to identify underlying neuropsychological, including linguistic and motor, strengths and weaknesses
Static:	• Standardized neuropsychological tests and test batteries
	• Standardized aphasia tests and test batteries
	• Standardized motor speech tests
Dynamic:	Process assessment: to identify what intact neuropsychological processes explain successful performance and what affected processes explain unsuccessful performance, using systematic hypothesis-testing modifications of test items (Kaplan, 1988)

Disability (Activity)-Oriented Assessment

Purposes:	• For diagnosis: to identify possible effects of neuropsychological impairments on real-world performance of functional activities
	• For treatment planning: to identify everyday activities that require intervention and to identify strategies that may improve performance
Static:	• Customized: Observation of performance of functional tasks of everyday life
	• Standardized: Functional scales (e.g., ASHA FACS; FIM; DRS)
Dynamic:	Experimentation with strategies and supports that hold the potential to improve performance of daily activities (OCCHTA)

Handicap (Participation)-Oriented Assessment

Purposes:	For treatment planning:
	• To identify limitations on educational, vocational, social, or familial participation;
	• To identify environmental modification strategies that may enhance participation;
	• To identify strengths and needs of everyday communication partners (e.g., family members, friends, job supervisors, teachers) relative to their ability to serve as supports for the individual with ongoing disability;
	• To identify changes in the behavior of communication partners that may enhance successful participation
Static:	• Standardized: Quality of life inventories
	• Customized: Observation of and interviews regarding level of participation and level of success in social, familial, academic, and vocational pursuits and roles
Dynamic:	Contextualized experimentation with environmental supports and with potentially helpful changes in the behavior of others (OCCHTA)

assessment procedures may help clinicians avoid the common pitfall of attempting to achieve an assessment goal by administering a type of assessment designed for other purposes. Furthermore, static versus dynamic assessments are contrasted. Whereas static assessment is often used for diagnosis, classification, and outcome monitoring, dynamic assessment is designed to identify intervention and support procedures that hold greatest rehabilitation promise for the individual.

Functional, Collaborative, Contextualized, Hypothesis-Testing Assessment for Planning Intervention

Elsewhere we have described and illustrated an experimental approach to assessment that is consistent with the functional, everyday approach to intervention described in this chapter (Ylvisaker & Gioia, 1998; Ylvisaker & Feeney, 1998a). In the case of individuals with complex impairment and disability in the domains addressed in this chapter, assessment *for purposes of planning intervention* is ongoing, contextualized, collaborative, and based on careful tests of hypotheses. This approach to assessment has its historical roots in Vygotsky's dynamic assessment (Vygotsky, 1978), elaborated by Feuerstein (1979) and more recently by many practitioners in educational psychology (e.g., Palinscar et al., 1994), special education, speech-language pathology, and other fields. Behavioral psychologists have a long history of assessment by means of experimental analysis of variables that potentially influence behavior (Iwata et al., 1990; Kern et al., 1994). Our goal in this section is restricted to presenting a brief rationale for this type of assessment and an outline of the steps of functional, hypothesis-testing assessment (see Ylvisaker et al., 1999).

Rationale

Why Ongoing?

Following severe TBI, individuals can continue spontaneous neurological recovery for months and in some cases years. This by itself mandates ongoing assessment. In addition, changes in environmental and task demands, in the individual's ability levels and psychoreactive responses, and in the skill levels of everyday people in the environment all contribute to ongoing unpredictability in evolving outcome, inviting ongoing assessment to ensure that services and supports are maximally effective.

Why Contextualized?

The ecological validity of office-bound standardized tests of cognitive and communication functioning for individuals with TBI (or, more specifically, frontal lobe injury) has been challenged by the results of many neuropsychological studies

(Benton, 1991; Bigler, 1988; Crépeau et al., 1997; Dennis, 1991; Dywan & Segalowitz, 1996; Eslinger & Damasio, 1985; Grattan & Eslinger, 1991; Mateer & Williams, 1991; Stelling et al., 1986; Stuss & Benson, 1986; Stuss & Buckle, 1992; Varney & Menefee, 1993; Welsh et al., 1991). Some individuals with executive function impairment perform better on standardized tests than one would expect based on real-world performance, because the tests are externally structured and impose few demands in the areas of goal setting, task identification, initiation, self-monitoring, or real-world strategic thinking. Others perform surprisingly poorly on standardized tests because the tasks are novel and the familiar stimulus cues of everyday life are not present to support performance. In either case, tests must be supplemented by effective use of real-world contexts in functional assessment.

Why Collaborative?

Collaboration increases the number of observations that can be made, the number of real-world contexts that can be explored, and the number of functional experiments that can be performed. In addition, when many people collaborate in assessment, the likelihood is increased that these same people will collaborate in implementing the intervention plan that results from the assessment. Participation in collaborative assessment is also an ideal way for everyday people to learn about the realities associated with the disability. Finally, asking professional colleagues, aides, family members, and others to become collaborators in assessment is a profound statement of respect and therefore contributes to team building.

Why Tests of Hypotheses?

Many capacities, processes, and skills are involved in most human behavior. Therefore, if a person has trouble with a task, there are typically scores of potential explanations for that difficulty. Similarly, when a person succeeds, that success may be a product of varied strategies (Kaplan, 1988). If specialists in rehabilitation do not know why people succeed when they succeed or what underlying impairment explains failure when they fail, they are not in a position to create a meaningful, appropriately targeted intervention program. Therefore, alternative hypotheses must be tested.

Assessment Process

Collaboratively Identify the Problem

In some cases, there is little difficulty identifying the functional problem that calls out for intervention. In other cases, it is not so easy. For example, one and the same behavioral issue may be identified by one person as defiance, by another as withdrawal, and by others as lack of initiation or laziness. In these cases, it is critical to agree to a neutral description of the problem behavior before proceeding.

Collaboratively Formulate Hypotheses

Hypotheses may be derived from neurodiagnostic information, from neuropsychological or other testing, from clinical experience with similar individuals, or from real-world interaction with the person whose intervention plan is being developed. Typically, teams of professionals and others have little difficulty generating possible explanations for the person's behavior or proposing intervention plans. It may not be as easy to label one's favored explanation a hypothesis and subject it to testing along with other hypotheses. However, this is precisely the process that enables teams to move beyond conflict over treatment plans and to identify interventions that have a demonstrable effect.

Collaboratively Select Hypotheses to Test

Some hypotheses may be easier to test than others; some may have greater face validity than others; some may have more interesting implications for intervention than others; some may be embraced by more members of the team than others. Selecting hypotheses to test and the order in which to test them requires balancing these considerations.

Collaboratively Test Hypotheses

In some cases, several hypotheses can be tested within a short period of time and possibly within a controlled assessment setting. In other cases, the process extends for weeks and mandates exploration in several real-world settings. In some cases, hypothesis testing is designed to explore the impact of hypothesized variables one at a time. In other cases in which the issue to be explored is serious (e.g., aggressive behavior), requiring immediate attention, it may be desirable to combine hypotheses, that is, experiment with a multi-faceted intervention. If the complex hypothesis is confirmed (i.e., the intervention is successful), it may not be possible to know which individual hypotheses were confirmed and in what combination, but at least the clinical problem is solved. Feeney and Ylvisaker (1995) presented three single-subject experimental designs that fit this description.

Collaboratively Interpret the Results and Formulate an Intervention Plan

In many cases, the test is in effect a trial intervention. If the trial intervention works well, then the treatment plan may follow in a relatively automatic manner. In other cases, the treatment plan may be an elaboration of the initial experiments. When people have chronic disability in executive system, cognitive, communication, and behavioral domains, intervention often takes the form of supportive modifications of everyday routines, modifications that were identified as positive by means of hypothesis testing (Ylvisaker & Feeney, 1998a).

Contextualized, Experimental Assessment in the Early and Middle Stages of Recovery

Early in neurologic recovery, contextualized experimental assessment from the perspective of cognition, communication, and behavior is designed in part to identify the conditions under which the individual is maximally alert, externally focused, and responsive to environmental stimuli. Variables that need to be explored include time of day; the sensory environment (e.g., lighting, auditory stimuli, tactile responsiveness, and the like); responses to positioning, movement (e.g., rocking), and temperature (e.g., warm bath); levels of medication; and differential responses to people and their communication styles. The goal of this systematic exploration is to maximize the amount of time the individual spends at the highest levels of responsiveness, to minimize stimulation that is associated with pathologic responses or withdrawal, and to encourage basic levels of communication (e.g., reaching for desired objects, pushing undesired objects away). In addition, staff explore ways in which the individual can be supported to participate in activities of everyday life (e.g., self-care, turning on and off lights, controlling sources of stimulation like tape-recorded music). Once appropriate supports are identified, family members and nursing staff are encouraged to engage the individual frequently in meaningful activities of everyday life, even if it appears that there is little response at the time.

During the middle stage of recovery, contextualized experimental assessment from the perspective of cognition, communication, and behavior is largely designed to identify the environmental and task supports needed to perform adaptively on activities of daily living as well as personally meaningful communication, educational, vocational, recreational, and social tasks. The supports and scaffolding highlighted later in this chapter (Table 33–11) are often the variables manipulated experimentally to identify the nature of the disability and the supports useful in handicap (participation)-and disability (activity)-oriented intervention (see Table 33–11).

Illustration of Contextualized, Collaborative Hypothesis Testing

Sue incurred severe TBI at age 35 in a motor vehicle crash. In addition to diffuse injury, neurodiagnostic imaging revealed significant left hemisphere frontotemporal damage. Prior to her injury, Sue was employed as a laborer in a large factory. She had a history of marital conflict and her two children had been removed from her home as a result of neglect and suspected abuse.

At the time of our involvement, Sue was 47 years old and had been a resident of a nursing home for 12 years. She had been diagnosed with serious cognitive-language impairment (including anomia, circumlocution, and wandering, tangential discourse), disorganized behavior in all

TABLE 33–11

Illustration of Functional, Contextualized Cognitive Rehabilitation Through the Continuum of Recovery: Organization, Memory, Language, and Executive Functions

Client: Tom is a 30-year-old married father of two, with a pretrauma avocational and vocational interest in baseball cards. He collected cards and traded them at shows and on the Internet. Residual impairment in the areas of executive functions (e.g., self-awareness, planning, organizing, self-monitoring), memory, and organization of language were associated with frontolimbic injury.
Long-Term Goal: The client will manage his baseball card collection and resume trading with minimal assistance.
Facilitators: Therapists, family members, direct care staff, friends

Early Stages (Maximal Support)	Middle Stages (Moderate Support)	Late Stages (Relative Independence; Support as Needed)
Cognitive-Language Goals: • Increase alertness and arousal • Improve external focus • Increase recognition of objects and people • Increase engagement in overlearned activities • Improve basic communication: comprehension of simple, everyday language; expression of basic wants, needs, and reactions	**Cognitive-Language Goals:** • Increase duration of attention; ability to shift attention from object to object and activity to activity; ability to filter out distractions • Improve perceptual scanning abilities • Use organizing schemes, including external organizers, to complete functional tasks • Use a prosthetic log/memory system to aid orientation, organization, memory, and self-management • Improve organization of spoken and written discourse, with external supports • Improve awareness of needs and strategies to compensate for deficits	**Cognitive-Language Goals:** • Improve awareness of self as a thinker, learner, communicator, and self-manager • Increase independent use of strategies to compensate for ongoing cognitive deficits • Improve organization of discourse with decreasing use of external organizers • Improve comprehension of vocabulary and extended texts related to vocational and avocational interests • Improve independent goal setting, planning, initiating, and self-evaluating • Increase independent creation, implementation, review, and revision of compensatory strategies
Meaningful Activities/Everyday Routines: • Turn pages of a baseball card album or collector book • Move cards in and out of album sleeves • Stack cards as others look at them • Find particular cards on the page • Help find all the cards from a team • On request, hand the cards to visitors to see • Place cards into rows for viewing • **Transfer Activities:** With support, participate in self-care activities and other activities of daily living • With prompts, activate switches to control electronic devices (e.g., TV, tape recorder) • Review family picture albums • Look at greeting cards	**Meaningful Activities/Everyday Routines:** • Organize cards by team or value • Write names of players on each team • Show and describe cards to others, including children • Read/write short narratives or biographical sketches about players; describe players to others (e.g., in group therapy) • Determine value of cards and list prices • Role play selling cards at a show; determine costs for purchase of various combinations of cards • Explain features of card trading to peers in group therpy; prepare script in advance with the help of a graphic organizer • **Transfer Activities:** Use graphic organizers and written reminders for other tasks (e.g., activities of daily living on the nursing unit, writing letters to family members) • Plan menus, prepare own lunch • Organize narratives and descriptions of experiences to offer visitors	**Meaningful Activities/Everyday Routines:** • Use sales books and the Internet to determine availability and cost of cards • Purchase and organize new cards in the collection • Keep financial records • Read and write articles about baseball card collecting • Create organized displays for card shows • Set up a display at a card show • Interact with visitors at a card show • Help his children with their collections • **Transfer Activities:** Assist other individuals with TBI at an earlier stage of recovery or with greater disability • Work with his children in the use of organizing systems for their homework • Develop strategies and organizers for other demanding activities (e.g., banking, shopping) • Continue to use Goal-Plan-Do-Review format for major life activities

continued

Illustration of Functional, Contextualized Cognitive Rehabilitation Through the Continuum of Recovery: Organization, Memory, Language, and Executive Functions

continued

- Play simple card games with children
- Write letters, thank you cards
- Use Goal-Plan-Do-Review format in all therapies, including physical therapies

Facilitator Expectations and Mediation:

- Facilitator is responsible for modifying the environment and stimulus presentation to fit Tom's response potential.
- Facilitator treats Tom's actions, even if accidental, as meaningful and makes them seem appropriate to the situation (e.g., touching a card is interpreted as a request).
- Facilitator associates simple language with actions (e.g., "Let's see if we can find a Yankee; no, that's a Dodger").
- **Scaffolding:** Facilitator may be required to perform all components of the task, but collaboratively engages Tom in any way possible (e.g., hand-over-hand joint performance of the task).

Facilitator Expectations and Mediation:

- Facilitator ensures that the environment is appropriate for efficient information processing.
- Facilitator gradually turns over more components of tasks to Tom.
- Facilitator changes prompts from physical (e.g., hand-over-hand) to verbal (simple instructions) to graphic (e.g., graphic organizers such as price sheets, inventory sheets, discourse guides for narrative and biographical sketches, feature analysis guide for organizing full descriptions and practicing organized word retrieval).
- Facilitator begins all activities with identification of the goal and formulation of a plan (e.g., use of an organizer); monitors progress ("Let's make sure we're getting the job done right"); ends all sessions with review of achievement ("Did you finish? How'd you do?") and usefulness of supports (e.g., "Did this organizer help?"); and helps Tom record important information in a memory book for future reference.
- Facilitator highlights improvements and the value of the supports that are used, helping Tom gain greater insight into his strengths and needs.
- **Scaffolding:** In addition to cues and organizers, the facilitator uses verbal mediation to highlight the important aspects of each component of the task, routinely reviews the goal, plan, and progress, models organized thinking, makes connections to related activities.

Facilitator Expectations and Mediation:

- Tom increasingly assumes responsibility for creating organizing systems to accomplish home and work tasks; facilitator (e.g., therapist, Tom's wife) may simply play a monitoring role.
- Tom assumes responsibility for independent use of memory aids; facilitator engages Tom in brainstorming if systems fail.
- Tom assumes responsibility for independent use of organizing systems (e.g., graphic organizers; prepared scripts) to communicate (speak and write) in an organized manner; facilitator provides feedback.
- Tom assumes primary responsibility for self-management (e.g., sets goals, makes plans, initiates work, evaluates self and products, chooses strategic compensations); facilitator encourages daily use of executive function routines and brainstorms with Tom about strategies.
- **Scaffolding:** Facilitator plays an ongoing role as coach (if necessary), consultant, and source of emotional support. As a consultant, the facilitator helps Tom identify barriers to success (e.g., inattention to scheduled responsibilities, reading comprehension problems, disorganized record keeping, gaps in his knowledge base) and develop customized strategies to overcome them.

Log/Journal/Memory Book

Facilitators keep a log of Tom's significant experiences and progress. The system is used in part to help facilitators identify factors that promote improved cognitive and adaptive functioning, and to communicate with one another. Facilitators review the log with Tom with the ultimate goal of improving recall of daily events and establishing a routine of review.

Log/Journal/Memory Book

Tom gradually assumes greater responsibility for management of the log/ memory book system. He begins to write his own entries, with guidance. The book plays a meaningful role in helping Tom stay oriented, know his schedule, plan activities, remember important events, and keep track of goals and assignments. Photographs of staff, well-organized schedules, and graphic organizers for important tasks are included in the book.

Log/Journal/Memory Book

Tom has primary responsibility for upkeep and use of the book, which may become more like a traditional day planner to organize daily events and facilitate memory. An outline of needs and strategies may continue to be included. An electronic pager system and/or computer memory system may be used.

domains of life, episodic and semantic memory impairment, reduced anger control, and physically aggressive behavior. With newly available community support funding through a Medicaid waiver program, she was placed in a supported apartment and given a job in a developmental disabilities sheltered workshop. In the social environment of that work setting, Sue's aggression escalated.

Local staff proposed that she be returned to the nursing home until she demonstrated the communication and anger management skills and positive attitude needed to live and work in the community. Sue's opposing view, which she offered in emotionally strong language, was that she would do fine if she had a meaningful life, including work in a "real" work setting. The staff insisted that she must first demonstrate work and interpersonal skills in a sheltered setting. With considerable encouragement, staff were convinced to treat Sue's proposal as a testable hypothesis. With the approval of her preinjury boss, she was placed in her old job with detailed, negotiated plans for asking for help when needed and for anticipating and dealing with frustration. Relevant employees in the factory were oriented to Sue's cognitive and communication deficits and given scripts to negotiate routine, work-related interaction. A job coach was used for less than a month. Four years later, Sue continues to be successful in her nonsupported job and community living, an achievement made possible in part by framing alternative recommendations (those of staff versus Sue) as hypotheses to be tested collaboratively and using real-world routines as the context for those tests.

COGNITIVE AND EXECUTIVE FUNCTION INTERVENTION

Decontextualized Cognitive Retraining

In the early period of program development for survivors of severe TBI, cognitive rehabilitation was understood by many practitioners as an enterprise that involved (a) hierarchical organization of cognitive processes and subprocesses (e.g., attention is more basic than organization; maintaining attention is more basic than shifting attention, etc.), (b) creation of cognitive exercises that targeted specific aspects of cognition in a hierarchical manner, and (c) efficient delivery of exercises, using massed learning trials outside of the context of functional application of the cognitive processes being trained (Ben-Yishay & Diller, 1983; Ben-Yishay et al., 1987; Sohlberg & Mateer, 1987). In the 1970s, customized retraining devices were designed for the delivery of cognitive exercises. In the 1980s, these devices were largely replaced by cognitive retraining software.

These early developments in TBI rehabilitation were remarkably similar in theory and practice to unsuccessful 19th century attempts to cure mental retardation with hierarchically organized cognitive exercises and also to largely unsuccessful efforts in the 1950s, 60s, and 70s to cure

learning disabilities with similar decontextualized cognitive exercises (Mann, 1979). In both of these older fields of intervention, decontextualized cognitive training exercises have largely given way to contextualized efforts to improve cognitive processing within the context of meaningful academic, social, vocational, and other daily activities. Similarly, studies demonstrating the limited effectiveness of attention process retraining (Park et al., 1999, in press; Ponsford, 1990), memory retraining (Schacter & Glisky, 1986; Thoene, 1996), and other types of decontextualized cognitive retraining for people with severe TBI have increasingly encouraged clinicians to emphasize contextualized approaches (Carney et al., 1999), although decontextualized retraining exercises still have their proponents (e.g., Mateer & Mapou, 1996).

Functional and Contextualized Cognitive Rehabilitation

General Executive System Routine

Ylvisaker et al. (1998) described a variety of interventions that address specific components of executive functioning. However, specific interventions are ideally integrated within a general Goal-Plan-Do-Review routine. As a rule, successful people facing important decisions (a) make choices about what they wish to accomplish, (b) set reasonable goals for themselves (based on their understanding of their strengths and limitations), (c) create intelligent plans for achieving their goals (possibly predicting their level of success), (d) act on the plans, and (e) review their performance, profiting from the feedback they receive (what worked and what did not work) (Meichenbaum & Biemiller, 1998). Often, these processes operate in a relatively automatic manner (Bargh & Chartrand, 1999). These same self-regulatory processes can and should become routine for people with disability, from preschoolers through adults. Clearly, people with significant executive function impairment require considerable support from others to engage in these intellectual processes and ultimately make them habitual. However, it is precisely such habits that are the goal of executive function intervention.

Figure 33–8 presents a guide for addressing the executive components of any task. With relevant modifications (e.g., simplifying the routine for people with substantial impairment), this general schema can be used to incrementally improve everyday routines of self-regulation. To remind individuals with disability and their caregivers to use the routine, we frequently post brightly colored reminders with the words, GOAL-PLAN-DO-REVIEW, and help family members, staff, and the person with TBI to become comfortable with simple, conversational use of the routine. Focusing intervention on the routines of everyday life is consistent with the efficacy literature in related fields, such as social skills intervention with varied populations (McIntosh et al., 1991; Wiener & Harris, 1998; Zaragoza et al., 1991), cognitive strategy intervention for students with learning impairment (Meichenbaum & Beimiller, 1998; Pressley, 1995), and cognitive rehabilitation for individuals

GOAL

What do I want to accomplish?

PLAN

How am I going to accomplish my goal?

Materials/equipment	Steps/assignments
1.	1.
2.	2.
3.	3.
4.	4.
5.	5.

PREDICT

How well will I do? How much will I get done?

CHOOSE

DO

Problems arise?	Formulate solutions!
1.	1.
2.	2.
3.	3.

REVIEW

HOW DID I DO?

Self rating:

1 2 3 4 5 6 7 8 9 10

Other rating (teacher, therapist, peer, family member)

1 2 3 4 5 6 7 8 9 10

WHAT WORKED?	WHAT DIDN'T WORK?
1.	1.
2.	2.
3.	3.

What will I try differently next time?

Figure 33–8. Guide for explicitly teaching or highlighting the executive components of any task. This form can be simplified to Goal-Plan-Do-Review for ease of remembering. (Reproduced with permission from Ylvisaker et al. [1998]).

with TBI (Carney et al., 1999), intervention domains in which decontextualized training routinely fails at the level of generalization and maintenance. Furthermore, similar systematic efforts to help students with disabilities internalize everyday routines of executive functioning (commonly referred to as "self-determination" in the developmental disabilities literature) have recently been shown to be effective in special education settings (Wehmeyer et al., 2000).

Individuals with frontal lobe impairment are often characterized as having significant difficulty with conscious control of behavior, whereas automatic behavior is said to remain relatively intact. It would seem, then, that interventions focused on conscious self-regulation would be poorly conceived for such people. However, there exists evidence that conscious intentions are especially helpful for frontal lobe patients, at least under experimental conditions (Gollwitzer, 1999). More to the point, the interventions described in this article are designed to create *habits* of self-regulatory cognitive

activity within natural contexts of action and interaction, thereby reducing the need for effortful, conscious self-regulation.

Functional Approaches to Cognitive Processes and Systems Through the Continuum of Recovery

In Table 33–11 we present a plan for improving cognitive functioning for a specific individual who improved slowly after TBI and retained residual cognitive impairment. The focus of intervention in this case included organization, memory, language, and general executive functions, although any aspect of cognition could be targeted within this everyday, routine-based framework. The table includes appropriate goals, activities, and daily routines within which the intervention plan was implemented (including transfer activities), and a description of the types of mediation and support used at each phase. We use the term "facilitator" to refer to people who have regular interaction with the person with disability (e.g., family members, direct care staff, therapists, teachers, job coaches, friends, coworkers, and others) and who are therefore in a position to use everyday activities and routines of life to facilitate improved cognitive functioning. Table 33–11 also suggests evolving uses for a log or memory book system over the continuum of recovery.

Clearly, specific activities and routines as well as specific intervention emphasis within the broad domain of cognition vary from individual to individual. Our goal in offering the detailed intervention plan in Table 33–11 is to encourage clinicians to similarly apply in an individualized manner the intervention framework described earlier to specific individuals, integrating their goals, interests, needs, support systems, and routines of life.

Compensatory Strategies and Strategic Behavior

In the general five-step template for functional, everyday, routine-based intervention (Table 33–4) and also in the description of Tom's cognitive intervention (Table 33–11), we highlighted the use of compensatory procedures. Compensatory strategies are procedures—sometimes unconventional—that an individual deliberately uses to achieve goals that cannot be achieved without such special effort. Although the ultimate goal of intervention is habituation ("routinization") of the procedures so that their use need not consume limited attentional resources, we emphasize the word "deliberate" in order to distinguish this sense of "strategy" from the general notion of organized behavior (which is often referred to as a strategy even if not deliberate) and also from instructional or treatment strategies, which are procedures used by therapists and teachers.

Strategies designed to compensate for cognitive deficits may involve the use of *external aids* (e.g., memory book, printed reminders, maps, task guide, alarm watch, electronic organizer, pager system). Alternatively, a person might compensate using *overt behavior* (e.g., requesting clarification or repetition) or *covert behavior* (e.g., self-reminders, mental rehearsal or elaboration, structured thinking procedures). Appendix 33-2 includes a large number (by no means exhaustive) of strategic procedures that appropriately selected individuals can use to compensate for selected cognitive and communicative deficits.

Compensatory strategies may be used temporarily in the case of transient impairment. Alternatively, they may be used indefinitely to reduce the functional disability of people with chronic impairment. Compensatory procedures may require effort initially, but with sufficient practice become a routine component of the individual's automatic processing system, thereby possibly reducing the underlying impairment. Unfortunately, the parts of the brain associated with strategic thinking and behavior (i.e., the frontal lobes) are particularly vulnerable in TBI. Therefore, intervention designed to equip individuals with strategic procedures for overcoming obstacles is at the same time extremely important and extremely tricky.

It is tempting to conceive of strategy intervention as no different from other teaching, that is, the clinician identifies the client's needs, selects an appropriate strategy, selects appropriate teaching procedures, teaches the strategy, and monitors and evaluates the outcome. The client's role is, then, to follow the clinician's lead and acquire the strategic procedure. However, if strategies are what strategic people do, then this model of teaching must be thought of as **antistrategic strategy intervention**, because all of the truly strategic, problem-solving behavior is assumed by the clinician. In denying the client the right to participate in the strategic aspects of strategy learning, the clinician might inadvertently contribute to the client's learned helplessness—that is, passive reliance on others to solve critical problems posed by cognitive and communicative weakness. Furthermore, not only does this model of teaching fail to promote truly strategic behavior, it also has been found to fail the litmus tests of generalization and maintenance when applied to a variety of populations of impaired learners (Flavell et al., 1993; Meichenbaum & Beimuller, 1998; Pressley, 1995; Pressley & Associates, 1990).

There is clinical wisdom, therefore, in following Pressley's advice to structure strategy intervention around a model of a good strategy user (Pressley et al., 1989). Such a model serves not only to identify a variety of diverse goals that may be components of this intervention; it also helps to separate reasonable from risky candidates for strategy intervention. Truly strategic people have the following characteristics:

- They have goals to which strategies are relevant;
- They know that their performance needs to be enhanced, that strategies enhance performance, and that they are capable of using strategies;
- They know when, where, and why to use specific strategic procedures;

- They monitor and evaluate the effectiveness of their performance so that being strategic is its own reward;
- They know a number of strategic procedures, can select the procedure most relevant to a particular challenge, and can flexibly modify it as needed or create new procedures;
- They use strategic procedures frequently so that they become relatively automatic and require little effort or planning;
- They have adequate "space" in working memory so that they can think about the task at hand and strategic procedures at the same time;
- They are not so impulsive that they habitually act before considering a strategic maneuver;
- They are not so anxious that they neglect strategic behavior because of their focus on fear of failure;
- They have the support of teachers, employers, and family members to use strategies;
- They know enough about the subject at hand that they can meaningfully use strategies to learn more.

Ideal candidates for strategy intervention are individuals who have specific goals, are aware of their needs, have sufficient metacognitive maturity to think about thinking, communicating, and other cognitive issues, are disposed to strategic behavior (e.g., like to play games of strategy), have adequate attentional resources, are motivated, have reasonable self-control, and live in supportive environments. College students returning to school after a mild-to-moderate injury often fall into this category. At the other extreme, individuals who are extremely weak in many of these dimensions may require considerable support to use all but the most simple external aid strategies (e.g., printed schedules, maps). For most people with TBI, strategy intervention includes attempts to improve functioning in a variety of domains (outlined above) that are related to strategic behavior.

Selection of the areas for compensation and of specific strategic procedures must involve active engagement of the client, which frequently includes a tension between his or her natural strategic inclinations and the judgment of the clinician. Brainstorming and experimentation with alternative strategies (described in Table 33–12) helps to resolve this tension. The ultimate test of the appropriateness of the strategy is spontaneous use and improved performance in natural settings. Intervention will inevitably fail if clients do not see the usefulness of the strategy relative to their goals or if the strategy does not fit the individual's overall style of learning, interacting, and coping. For example, it is quixotic at best to expect a shy and generally noninteractive person to enthusiastically adopt an input control strategy that requires him or her to request that speakers slow down or clarify and simplify their language. Variables to be reviewed in negotiating the selection of strategies include whether the procedure is used spontaneously; whether its degree of complexity and abstractness fits the client's cognitive level; how difficult the

TABLE 33–12

Teaching Compensatory Strategies

Note: These components of intervention are not necessarily hierarchical or mutually exclusive.

Component I: General Strategic Thinking

A. Metacognitive-Awareness

  Goals: Clients will discriminate effective from ineffective performance; become increasingly aware of their strengths and needs; recognize implications of their deficits

  Rationale: Given the frequency of frontolimbic and right hemisphere damage in TBI, self-awareness is frequently compromised. Individuals are unlikely to acquire and use procedures designed to compensate for problems that they do not recognize as problems.

  Procedures:

    1. **Objective:** Improve the client's perception of successful versus unsuccessful task performance.

      Procedures: Illustrate successful and unsuccessful performance of a functional task through role play or on videotape. With the client, analyze the performances in sufficient detail that the client can identify the features that account for successful versus unsuccessful performance.

    2. **Objective:** Improve the client's ability to perceive functional impairments.

      Procedures: Individually, request that the client make note of specific deficits of other clients in the program or of individuals observed on tape. Discuss these observations. Planned peer teaching is useful. Discuss the effects of TBI on cognitive and social functioning. If appropriate, read and discuss literature on the effects of TBI.

    3. **Objective:** Improve the client's awareness of his or her own strengths and weaknesses.

      Procedures: Videotape the client in activities designed to reveal strong and weak areas of functioning. (Alternatively, use role play.) Review the tapes (beginning with strong performance), first without commentary, subsequently inviting comments about what was done well and what needs improvement. Gradually turn over to the client the responsibility for stopping the tape when problems are noted. Note: Considerable desensitizing may be needed before video self-viewing is possible.

    4. **Objective:** Improve the client's understanding of the relation between deficits and long-term goals.

      Procedures: Discuss in concrete detail the individual's long-term goals and expectations. Jointly create a list of specific skills and resources needed to achieve these goals. Jointly identify the skills that are present and those that are weak relative to this goal.

    Note: These metacognitive discoveries are facilitated if the activities are personally meaningful and intimately connected to the client's goals.

B. Value of Being Strategic

  Goal: Clients will recognize the importance of being strategic and will identify the characteristics of strategic people.

  Rationale: Since the ultimate goal of this intervention is to promote strategic thinking and strategic behavior in general—not simply to teach specific strategic behaviors as routines—it is important that the client understand what it is to be strategic and that these are valuable attributes.

  Procedures:

    1. **Objective:** Improve the client's understanding of strategy.

      Procedures: Using games, sports, or other relevant models, clarify the concept of strategy as something that one does to achieve goals when there are obstacles.

    2. **Objective:** Heighten the client's appreciation of strategic behavior.

      Procedures: Together with the client, identify several individuals who are known to be very strategic (e.g., sports heroes, military heroes). Discuss why they are considered heroic. Clinicians should also clearly model their own strategic behavior and discuss the value of their own strategies.

    3. **Objective:** Improve the client's understanding of the behaviors that are part of being strategic.

      Procedures: Using models relevant to the client (e.g., military, sports, or business analogies), brainstorm about the characteristics of people who are known to be very strategic. Include: high level of motivation and initiative, ability to identify and clarify obstacles to goals; ability to plan procedures to overcome obstacles; ability to monitor and evaluate performance; willingness to engage in ongoing problem solving.

Component II: Selecting Specific Strategic Procedures

  Goal: Clients will identify specific procedures useful in overcoming important personal obstacles.

  Rationale: It is important that clients participate in the selection of strategic procedures that they will use and that the procedures be truly useful in achieving their goals.

  Procedures:

    1. Use group brainstorming procedures to identify possible strategies.

continued

Teaching Compensatory Strategies
continued

---

2. Use "product monitoring" tasks to test the value of strategies: Have the client perform a task with and without the strategy or with a variety of different strategies. Objectively compare the results. (Video analysis may be useful here.)
3. Have advanced clients demonstrate the value of certain procedures or offer testimonials.
4. Discuss the widespread use of compensatory procedures (lists, memos, tape recorders, and so forth) by people who do not have brain injury.

Component III: Teaching Specific Strategies
Note: If the discovery procedures in Component II (e.g., brainstorming and product monitoring) are effective, there may be little need for specific teaching procedures.

Procedures:
A. **Modeling:** The steps in the strategy can be modeled by the therapist or by a peer, or by means of videotape or other media. Modeling is initially accompanied by overt verbalization of the strategy by the model. The client then rehearses the strategy with gradually decreasing cues and self-talk.
B. **Direct Instruction:** The carefully programmed behavioral teaching procedures of direct instruction can be used to teach strategies. However, if this is the only approach used, it is likely that the best result will be the acquisition of a learned sequence of behaviors (which may be a desirable outcome), without positive movement in the direction of becoming a strategic person.
C. **Functional Practice:** However the strategy is acquired, it must be frequently rehearsed in natural settings using functional activities.

Component IV: Generalization and Maintenance
Generalization of strategic behavior beyond the context of training is a combined consequence of the perceived utility of the strategy for the individual, the inherent generalizability and utility of the strategy, widespread environmental support for strategic behavior and thinking, intensive practice in a variety of real-world contexts, and specific teaching procedures designed to enhance generalization.

Note 1: Generalization includes generalized use of specific strategies as well as strategic behavior in general.

Note 2: Generalization may not be a separate phase if the acquisition stage takes place in the context of functional activities and natural settings. This is particularly important for very concrete people.

Note 3: Generalization may be a relatively unimportant phase of intervention if the individual has acquired a strategic attitude and actively seeks occasions for transfer.

Note 4: Some individuals may need environmental reminders indefinitely to use their strategic procedures.

1. **Objective:** Improve the client's discrimination of situations that require or do not require a given strategy.
   Procedures: Use videotaped scenes or role-playing to illustrate the correct use of a strategy in an appropriate situation, inappropriate use of the strategy, and failure to use the strategy when appropriate. Discuss the conditions that require the strategy. Use short videotaped scenes to train the client in efficient and accurate judgments as to whether a strategy is appropriate in a context.
2. **Objective:** Increase the client's spontaneous use of strategies in varied situations.
   Procedures: Include family members, work supervisors, and teachers in strategy intervention to (1) provide varied opportunities for the use of specific strategies and of strategic behavior in general, (2) reinforce the client's use of strategies, and (3) model strategic behavior themselves. Ask clients to keep a log in which they record their successes and failures in strategy use. Make generalization an explicit goal.
3. **Objective:** Increase the client's acceptance of strategic behavior.
   Procedures: Ensure that the client is successful using strategies. Promote emotional acceptance of strategic behavior by using whatever motivating procedures work (e.g., personal images or metaphors, testimonials, and the like).

Modified with permission from Haarbauer-Krupa, J., Henry, K., Szekeres, S., & Ylvisaker, M. (1985). Cognitive rehabilitation therapy: Late stages of recovery. In M. Ylvisaker (ed.), *Head injury rehabilitation: Children and adolescents* (pp. 318–319). Austin, TX: Pro-Ed.

procedure is to use relative to its pay-off; whether it fits the client's profile of neuropsychological strengths; whether it fits the client's personality; and whether it specifically addresses obstacles to the individual's concrete goals.

In Table 33–12 we outline intervention procedures that we have found useful in working with individuals with TBI. The three components are very roughly sequential, but should not be considered mutually exclusive or hierarchical. For example, attempts to promote improved awareness of strengths and weaknesses (part of Component I) often continue throughout a client's entire rehabilitation program. In

addition, work on generalization (Component III) should begin early, before a procedure is habituated in a clinical setting.

In summary, our experience in helping individuals with TBI to become increasingly strategic underscores the importance of the following principles of strategy intervention: (1) Intervention should be embedded in natural, meaningful activities and settings, with strategic procedures specifically related to the client's goals. (2) The individual should be maximally engaged in experimenting with strategies, using the general Goal-Plan-Do-Review format, selecting the strategies to use, and monitoring their effectiveness.

(3) Intervention should be intensive and long term. (4) Goals should be modest. (5) Other things being equal, simple, low-technology options are often preferable to complicated, high-technology options; external supports (e.g., graphic organizers for complex tasks) are often preferable to internal elaboration and organization strategies. (6) The environment as a whole should be supportive of and promote strategic thinking and strategic behavior. In the absence of sensitivity to these principles, strategic compensations for cognitive impairment are unlikely to be maintained over time (Wilson & Watson, 1996). There are increasing numbers of reports in the TBI literature regarding the effectiveness of compensatory strategy intervention (Carney et al., 1999), but a much larger evidence base in educational psychology (reviewed by Pressley & Associates, 1990), which Pressley (1993) has attempted to apply to the field of cognitive intervention after TBI. Meichenbaum (1993) discussed the application of a related set of intervention procedures, cognitive behavior modification, to TBI rehabilitation.

BEHAVIORAL AND PSYCHOSOCIAL REHABILITATION

Importance of Behavioral and Psychosocial Issues

In the earlier section on outcome, we highlighted the frequency of personality changes, behavior problems, and associated social interactive weakness after TBI. Difficulties in this domain may be a result of the injury, but are often complicated by preinjury challenges and postinjury social, academic, and vocational failure and consequent adjustment problems. Our work with several hundred adolescents and young adults with chronic school and work problems and general community reintegration difficulty suggests that behavioral and psychosocial themes are often at the core of these problems, although in most cases complex patterns of interaction exist between cognitive and behavioral consequences of the injury.

Furthermore, costs associated with failure of rehabilitation and community support efforts are staggering. In recent years, we have served over 325 young adults through a New York State community support project for individuals with TBI, some degree of chronic behavioral impairment, and demonstrated lack of success in community reintegration using standard services and supports. Conservative Department of Health estimates of the cost of serving these individuals, based on expenses for the year prior to their introduction to the program, exceed $30,000,000 annually. Because most of the people served by the program were more than 5 years post-injury at the time of referral and had failed in previous rehabilitation attempts, the state had projected enormous lifetime costs for this population.

Speech-language pathologists have a natural role in this domain of service delivery under the headings *pragmatics of language* and *teaching positive communication alternatives to*

challenging behavior. Pragmatics has a long history within the profession, and is addressed in detail elsewhere in this text. The role of speech-language pathologists in behavior management may be somewhat more controversial, but is included in ASHA's scope of practice and has become commonplace in many settings in which individuals with developmental disabilities are served (Carr et al., 1994; Reichle & Wacker, 1993; Reichle & Johnston, 1993). In this section, we outline and offer a rationale for a positive, antecedent-focused approach to challenging behavior, present a collaborative and contextualized approach to teaching positive communication alternatives, and provide some suggestions for dealing with difficult motivational issues that often block successful implementation of intervention plans.

Concerns About Traditional Consequence-Based Behavior Management

Traditional operant applications of applied behavior analysis, dating back to Skinner's early work (Skinner, 1938), have explained behavior as a consequence of both antecedents and consequences, but placed the major burden on manipulation of consequences in teaching new behaviors or modifying undesirable behavior. Within this tradition, behavior plans are largely reactive, specifying positive consequences for desirable behavior and negative or no consequences for undesirable behavior. Furthermore, to the extent that antecedents are targeted in behavior management, it has largely been the immediate antecedents (e.g., the trainer's commands, cues, and prompts; environmental stressors at the time of the behavior). An enormous literature and impressive technology of behavior change has evolved within this tradition. Furthermore, there are reports documenting some success with traditional consequence management applied to both adults (e.g., Alderman & Ward, 1991; Pace & Ivancic, 1994; Wood, 1987, 1990) and children with TBI (e.g., Slifer et al., 1995, 1996).

Unfortunately, clinicians who work with individuals with frontal lobe impairment, whether congenital (e.g., ADHD) or acquired (e.g., TBI), often report a frustrating lack of success or at best inefficiency in their implementation of primarily consequence-oriented behavior modification programs (Barkley, 1987; Hallowell & Ratey, 1994). This inefficiency has been documented in the frontal lobe research literature, which offers at least four potential explanations, summarized in Table 33–13. Damasio and colleagues (Bechera et al., 1994, 1996; Damasio, 1994; Damasio et al., 1991) have suggested that favorable or unfavorable consequences of behavior can influence future behavior only if *somatic markers*, or feeling states, are associated with the stored representation of the original behavior. Their neuropsychological investigations indicate that ventromedial prefrontal cortex is critical to the laying down of somatic markers, explaining the inefficiency of consequence-oriented behavior management in many people with closed

TABLE 33–13

Possible Explanations for Inefficiency of Consequence-Oriented Behavior Management in TBI Rehabilitation

Hypothesis	Discussion
Somatic Marker Hypothesis (Damasio, 1994)	Because of the high frequency of ventromedial prefrontal injury in TBI, attachment of somatic markers (feeling states associated with rewards and punishments) to stored representations of past experiences is inefficient. According to this theory, somatic marker storage is critical to learning from consequences and is weak in individuals with ventromedial prefrontal damage.
Disinhibition Hypothesis (Rolls et al., 1994)	Because of the high frequency of orbitofrontal injury in TBI, impulsiveness is a common impairment. People who are impulsive, like young children, are capable of learning from consequences, but immediate impulses easily overwhelm learned behaviors on the occasion of action.
Working Memory Hypothesis (Alderman, 1996)	Because of the relative frequency of dorsolateral prefrontal injury in TBI, reduced working memory is a common impairment. Alderman found a correlation between impaired working memory and difficulty learning from consequences, perhaps suggesting that reasonably adequate working memory is needed for correct selection of learned responses.
Initiation Hypothesis (Stuss & Benson, 1986)	Because of the relative frequency of dorsal (especially dorsomesial) prefrontal injury in TBI, some individuals lack organically-based initiation/activation capacity to act in situations in which they have learned the correct behavior and are adequately motivated to act.
Infantilization and Oppositionality Hypothesis (Ylvisaker & Feeney, 1998a)	Because many people with TBI, especially adolescents and young adults, react negatively to others' attempts to manage their behavior with consequences, traditional behavior management systems may be counterproductive. The common complaint is that reward and punishment systems are childlike or that external manipulation beyond their control and approval is in general offensive to them.

head injury, given its high frequency of ventral prefrontal damage.

Rolls and colleagues (1994) highlighted *impulsiveness*, associated with orbitofrontal lesions, as a hypothesis capable of explaining maintenance of behaviors that have resulted in a history of seriously punishing consequences. Alderman (1996) concluded that weakness in the central executive component of *working memory* may explain the failure of many individuals with frontal lobe injury to respond to traditional operant training techniques, including reinforcement, extinction, and time-out intervention. In some cases, reduced *initiation/activation*, associated with dorsal (especially dorsomesial) prefrontal injury, may explain failure to act despite possession of the appropriate learned response (Stuss & Benson, 1986). In individual cases, a satisfactory explanation of the inefficiency of traditional behavior management may include a combination of these four phenomena, possibly exacerbated by *oppositionality*, which may grow in response to ineffective consequence-oriented management (Ylvisaker & Feeney, 2000a). For our purposes, the research literature at least directs clinicians to focus their attention on both immediate and remote antecedents of behavior.

Positive, Antecedent-Focused Behavior Management

In Table 33–14 we outline alternative approaches to the role of *antecedent* manipulation in behavior management (based on Carr et al., 1998). Historically, the narrow "molecular" approach co-existed with a primary focus on consequences.

Until recently, relatively little attention has been paid to remote events (e.g., an unpleasant interaction earlier in the day) or internal states of the individual (e.g., anger due to loss of friends; anxiety over lost skills; frustration associated with an unsatisfying job or no meaningful role in life) as potentially modifiable antecedents that increase or decrease the likelihood of certain behaviors.

In the 1990s, momentum has grown within the field of applied behavior analysis favoring an approach to teaching and supporting individuals with challenging behavior that places greatest emphasis on manipulation of antecedents, including immediate and remote as well as observable and unobservable antecedents (the "molar" approach in Table 33–14). Although most of the research and clinical discussions within this new tradition address behavioral issues associated with developmental disabilities (Carr et al., 1999), application of antecedent technologies has entered the experimental and clinical literatures in TBI rehabilitation (Feeney & Ylvisaker, 1995, 1997; Jacobs, 1993; Ylvisaker & Feeney, 1996, 1998a, 2000a; Zencius et al., 1989). Furthermore, the molar approach to antecedent-focused behavior management is completely consistent with the theoretical and procedural discussion of positive, everyday, routine-based intervention, presented earlier.

Building Positive, Everyday, Behavioral and Communication Routines

Earlier, we offered a rationale for a positive, everyday, routine-based approach to rehabilitation, equally applicable

TABLE 33–14

Behavior Management Via Control of Antecedents: Alternative Approaches

MOLECULAR APPROACH TO ANTECEDENT CONTROL: THE TRADITION IN APPLIED BEHAVIOR ANALYSIS

Antecedents: Discrete measurable stimuli that precede a behavior and increase or decrease its likelihood of occurrence (e.g., a specific instruction, cue, warning, promise)

Assessment: To identify these antecedents for purposes of control (a-b-c analysis, including active experimentation with antecedents), often in controlled settings (i.e., analog assessment)

Intervention: To increase or decrease specific behaviors by manipulating the specific immediate antecedents related to the behavior (e.g., eliminate triggers, modify antecedents, fade antecedents in or out)

MOLAR APPROACH TO ANTECEDENT CONTROL: LATE 90s

Antecedents: Broad, potentially continuous, often hard-to-measure variables that may increase or decrease the likelihood of occurrence of positive or negative behavior

- internal states (e.g., illness)
- living arrangements
- social relationships
- education (e.g., placement, demands, level of success)
- work (e.g., placement, demands, level of success, perceived meaningfulness)
- leisure (frequency and quality of enjoyable activities)
- the relation between the person's needs, competencies, and environmental demands
- self-perception, including implicit metaphors that guide thinking and behavior

Assessment:

- To identify the background antecedents or nonimmediate "setting events" that may be related to positive or negative behaviors, generally in natural settings
- To assess the "goodness of fit" between the person's needs, competencies, and social, educational, and vocational demands

Intervention:

Primary Purpose: To influence major background setting events and conditions with the goal of helping the individual to create a satisfying lifestyle

- may be most efficiently met by educating and training everyday communication partners and in other ways creating a "best fit" between the individual and his or her living, work, social, and/or educational environments and activities

Secondary Purpose: To indirectly increase desirable and decrease undesirable behaviors

Based on Carr et al. (1998); reproduced with permission from Ylvisaker & Feeney (2000a).

to intervention for individuals with chronic cognitive, behavioral, and communication impairment. Behavior management within this approach can be divided into two overlapping efforts: preventing negative behaviors and building repertoires of positive communication routines.

Preventing Negative Behavior with Antecedent Manipulations

Part 2 of Table 33–3 in the Framework section of this chapter lists several categories of antecedent procedures designed in part to avoid negative behavioral routines and increase the likelihood that positive behaviors will become habitual. Critical to antecedent management is the concept of *setting events*, which are potentially remote occurrences or conditions that increase or decrease the likelihood of a behavior and determine whether a specific behavioral intervention will be effective (Baer et al., 1987). Because the concept of setting event is unfamiliar to some rehabilitation specialists and bears meaning that is not transparent (e.g., "event" is not restricted to temporally discrete occurrences, but can include

internal states and conditions), we include in Table 33–15 a list of positive and negative setting events that can be used as a checklist in working with individuals with difficult behavior after TBI.

Attention to setting events is particularly critical in working with people with acquired brain injury because of the cumulative negative effect on behavior of chronic discomfort, restrictions on activities and choices, limited control over major life events, frequent changes in living situation and routines, and, perhaps most critically, failure to achieve goals consistent with preinjury expectations and aspirations. A background of negative setting events lowers behavioral thresholds that may already be low as a result of the injury (Figure 33–9). Conversely, a background of positive setting events elevates those thresholds and increases the likelihood that the individual will become productively engaged in difficult tasks (Figure 33–10). The developmental disabilities behavioral literature is rich in reports of experiments demonstrating the positive effects on behavior of inducing positive setting events, including creating positive

TABLE 33–15

Categories and Examples of Setting Events That Potentially Influence Behavior

INTERNAL STATES OF THE INDIVIDUAL
- **Neurologic States**
  positive setting events: normal neurology
  negative setting events: overactivity of the limbic regions; seizures; neurotransmitter disruption; decreased cerebral blood flow
- **Other Physiologic States**
  positive setting events: rest, relaxation, satiation, appropriate levels of medication
  negative setting events: pain, illness, hunger, overmedication, undermedication, motor deficits, sensory deficits
- **Cognitive States**
  positive setting events: orientation to task, familiarity with routine, adequate recall of relevant events, adequate recognition of things and people
  negative setting events: confusion, disorientation, frustration, inadequate recall and recognition
- **Emotional States**
  positive setting events: sense of accomplishment, success, achievement, acceptance by others, respect from others, meaningful role, sense of self consistent with life circumstances, feeling in control
  negative setting events: anxiety, anger, depression, sense of loss and failure
- **Perception of Task Meaningfulness and Difficulty**
  positive setting events: belief that assigned tasks are meaningful and can be accomplished
  negative setting events: belief that assigned tasks are meaningless, infantilizing, or impossible

EXTERNAL EVENTS AND CONDITIONS
- **Living Arrangement**
  positive setting events: living in a self-selected environment without excessive restrictions
  negative setting events: living in an excessively restrictive setting; living at home with parents after having lived independently
- **Presence or Absence of Specific People**
  positive setting events: presence of preferred people, reciprocal friendships
  negative setting events: absence of preferred people, loss of friends, presence of nonpreferred people
- **Recent History of Interaction**
  positive setting events: recent positive and pleasurable interactions
  negative setting events: recent conflict or disrespectful interactions
- **Other Environmental Stressors**
  positive setting events: appropriate and desirable environmental stimulation
  negative setting events: irritating environmental stimulation (e.g., ambient noise, improper lighting, other distractors)
- **Time of Day**
  positive setting events: alertness, best time of day relative to the individual's natural cycles
  negative setting events: bad time of day relative to the individual's natural cycles

Reproduced with permission from Ylvisaker & Feeney (1998a).

behavioral momentum before introducing difficult tasks (Carr et al., 1997; Fowler, 1996; Kennedy et al., 1995; Mace et al., 1988, 1990; Mace et al., 1997) and offering choice and control (Bannerman et al., 1990; Brown et al., 1993; Dunlap et al., 1994; Harchik et al., 1993). Harchik and colleagues (1993) reviewed over 100 experimental reports in the developmental disabilities literature and concluded that increasing an individual's opportunities for choice and control decreases challenging behavior, increases participation, and increases subjective reports of satisfaction derived from that participation.

The Role of Consequences

In emphasizing antecedents in behavior management for people with TBI, we do not wish to recommend inattention to consequences. First, many people with TBI escape fronto-limbic injury entirely and can therefore be expected to be as efficient at learning from consequences as are their un-injured peers. Furthermore, the frontolimbic threats to efficiency of consequence-oriented behavior management come in degrees and may not be serious in individual cases. Third, the positive, everyday routines that antecedent supports are designed to facilitate are positive in part because they result in extrinsic or intrinsic rewards for the person. Fourth, the possibility of serious punishment (e.g., jail) may serve as motivation for participation in the development of antecedent-supported routines. Finally, even those who are inefficient at learning from consequences benefit from a positive culture in which there is ample noncontingent reinforcement, successful performance is greeted with encouragement and praise, and failure and negative behavior elicit efforts to help

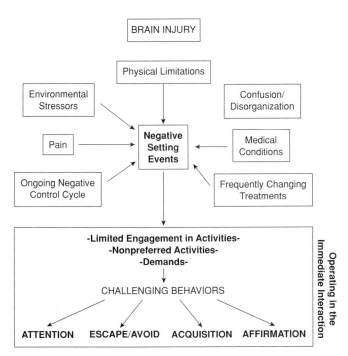

Figure 33–9. Relationship between negative setting events and challenging behavior. (Modified from Feeney & Ylvisaker [1997].)

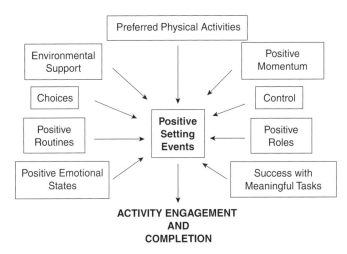

Figure 33–10. Relationship between positive setting events and positive behavior. (Modified from Feeney & Ylvisaker [1997]).

the person succeed rather than punishment that may breed anger and additional failure.

With the goal of helping people succeed in the real world, rewards and punishments should be as *natural* and *logically related* to the individual's behavior as possible. For example, a good grade is a natural and logical consequence of effective preparation for a test; a raise or promotion is a natural and logical consequence of hard work on the job; an enjoyable social interaction is a natural and logical consequence of socially appropriate initiation. On the punishment side, cleaning one's room is a natural and logical consequence of "trashing" the room during a tantrum; receiving a poor grade is a natural and logical consequence of failing to prepare for an exam. In contrast, the following contingent responses are not related in a natural and logical way to the behavior and therefore not likely to help shape enduring positive behaviors: "Nice talking, John," "I liked the way you responded to Jeremy; I'll give you a point for that," and "That's not an appropriate way to request cigarettes; you will not be allowed to go on the outing tonight."

Token economies, which are popular components of consequence-oriented behavioral programs, often fail to promote understanding of natural and logical relationships in the world. For example, if an appropriate conversational bid from a person known for sexual acting out is rewarded with a token that can be exchanged later for a cigarette, the natural connection between appropriate conversational openers and subsequent satisfying conversations is violated. Furthermore,

liberal use of extrinsic rewards can create dependence on such rewards and interfere with internally driven motivation, a finding that has been replicated many times in many contexts over the past 30 years (Deci, 1995). Finally, our experience suggests that many oppositional young people become increasingly oppositional in an environment that they perceive as dominated by arbitrary authority figures arbitrarily dispensing rewards and punishments that are not personally meaningful.

Building Repertoires of Positive Behaviors and Communication Routines

Social skills include general competencies (e.g., self-control), personal attributes (e.g., concern for others), and situationally relative social behaviors (e.g., communication scripts appropriate for the workplace, classroom interaction, church groups, bar room conversations, and others) that enable a person to be socially successful in selected settings. Social skills intervention, a component of which is pragmatics training, has generally been understood as an effort to equip individuals with knowledge of social rules, roles, and routines along with the communication competencies that are components of those routines. Training often takes place in social skills groups guided by a curriculum that specifies the social competencies needed by the group members and the types of modeling and role playing that are used to teach and rehearse the skills. Many structured social skills training programs have been developed for individuals representing varied age groups and types of disability (e.g., Goldstein et al., 1980; Sheinker & Sheinker, 1988; Waksman et al., 1989; Walker et al., 1988a,b).

Partly because of the logistical ease with which such group social skills training can be implemented in rehabilitation hospitals and outpatient clinics, social skills or pragmatics groups enjoy considerable popularity in TBI rehabilitation. There is limited evidence that social skills training of this sort can be somewhat effective with some adolescents and young adults with TBI, particularly if there is an emphasis on self-monitoring (Braunling-McMorrow et al., 1986; Brotherton et al., 1988; Gajar et al., 1984; Johnson & Newton, 1987). Furthermore, with ongoing changes in life circumstances and chronic impairment of learning efficiency, young people with TBI may be candidates for deliberate teaching of new social routines with each transition to new situations (e.g., employment) in which they face novel social demands.

However, concerns about the usefulness of decontextualized role play–based social skills training arise at several levels. First, many people with TBI retain the knowledge of social rules, roles, and routines that social skills training is designed to teach. Areas of the cortex in which such knowledge is believed to be stored are not particularly vulnerable in TBI. *Production* deficiencies, rather than *knowledge* deficiencies, tend to be common in TBI and such deficiencies are inadequately addressed with reliance on decontextualized role-play exercises.

Second, the combination of inhibition, initiation, planning, and working memory impairment common in TBI lends itself to intervention designed to create positive habits of interaction in the social contexts in which the skills in question are needed. Creation of positive habits of interaction requires individualized selection of teaching targets and extensive coached practice in context. Finally, reviews of research on effectiveness of decontextualized, role play–based social skills training are not promising, even in the case of disability groups for which such training would seem to be well conceived, including students with learning disorders (McIntosh et al., 1991; Wiener & Harris, 1998) and behavioral disorders (Zaragoza et al., 1991). In most cases, decontextualized training is capable of modifying social behaviors in the training setting, but with minimal evidence of generalization to important social settings of everyday life, maintenance over time, or positive influence on the social ratings offered by everyday communication partners.

Teaching Positive Communication Alternatives to Challenging Behavior

Behavior management and social skills training come together in the process of helping people with challenging behavior substitute a socially acceptable mode of communication for behavior that is unsuccessful or considered inappropriate in their social contexts. As an organized approach to behavior management, positive communication training has its roots in work with individuals with mental retardation, autism, and other developmental disabilities (Bird et al., 1989; Carr & Durand, 1985; Carr et al., 1994; Donnellan

et al., 1984; Doss & Reichle, 1989; Reichle & Wacker, 1993). Functional analysis of problem behavior in those groups typically indicates that the behavior serves a communication function, often expressing an intention to *gain access* to a desired activity, person, thing, or place, or to *escape* an activity, person, demand, or place. Organized procedures for assessing the communication value of challenging behavior (e.g., Durand & Crimmins, 1992) and for teaching positive alternatives are available in the developmental disabilities literature, along with evidence of the effectiveness of these efforts.

In Table 33–16 we present a summary of the communication approach to behavior management, including the premises underlying the approach, considerations in assessment, preteaching activities, categories of teaching procedure, and, finally, obstacles to success, along with suggestions for overcoming the obstacles. Elsewhere we have discussed and illustrated this approach to behavior management for individuals with TBI in greater detail (Feeney & Ylvisaker, 1995, 1997; Ylvisaker & Feeney, 1994, 1998a; Ylvisaker et al., 1999; Ylvisaker et al., 1998).

We have used the approach outlined in Table 33–16 with a large number of children and adults with challenging behavior after TBI. In some cases, particularly people with significant cognitive, behavioral, and possibly also motor impairment, the messages communicated in problematic ways were relatively simple to decipher (e.g., a desire to escape demands) and the intervention process was not unlike that described in the developmental disabilities literature. In other cases, particularly people with relatively good cognitive and motor recovery, but complex behavioral and emotional profiles both before and after their injuries, the messages delivered in challenging ways were more complex and the process of intervention involved a higher level of collaboration with the individual. In these cases, motivation and negotiation (discussed in the next section) are central to the intervention.

Motivation, Metaphor, and Collaboration with the Person with Disability

In the case of adolescents and young adults struggling unsuccessfully to reestablish preinjury activities and levels of success, aggression, withdrawal, sexual acting out, and other forms of challenging behavior often communicate messages like the following:

- "You just treated me disrespectfully and I won't take it!"
- "I know I can't do this and it's driving me crazy, but it's just too hard to ask for help!"
- "I find you very attractive and I would like to spend time with you."

Because loss of friends, difficulty maintaining work, and increasingly stressful family interaction may be the result of

---

TABLE 33–16

Behavior as Communication: Teaching Positive Communication Alternatives to Challenging Behavior

Premises

1. All behaviors (potentially) communicate something to someone. One cannot not communicate, although not all communication is intentional.
2. There are few truly maladaptive behaviors; most apparently maladaptive behaviors (e.g., aggression, self-injury, withdrawal) achieve a social, communication goal.
3. The messages communicated with challenging behavior can often be understood as communicating the individual's need to escape (e.g., escape a task, person, place, or activity), to access/acquire (e.g., access a task, person, place, activity, thing, form of stimulation, or attention from others), or to protest (e.g., protest restrictions on behavior or disrespectful interaction).
4. The behavior of communication partners is a critical part of the context of behavior (antecedent conditions and consequences that potentially elicit and maintain types of behavior) and must figure prominently in intervention efforts.
5. Clearly defined communication routines of everyday life, supported by well-trained everyday communication partners, are the ideal context within which communication and behavior goals are optimally achieved.
6. Communication specialists and behavior specialists play essentially the same role in helping individuals with communication-related behavior problems.

Assessment

1. Collaboratively identify and describe the unacceptable behavior and the contexts in which it occurs.
2. Collaboratively interpret the meaning of the challenging behavior
   a. Systematic, passive observation: what are the stimuli and responses that trigger and maintain the undesirable behavior in varied everyday contexts?
   b. Systematic, active experimentation with hypotheses regarding the meaning/purpose of the challenging behavior (e.g., if communication partners routinely reward verbal requests for a desirable activity, does the challenging behavior disappear? If so, the meaning/purpose of the challenging was probably: "I want that activity!"). (See also Durand & Crimmins, 1992, and the discussion of collaborative, contextualized, hypothesis-testing assessment earlier in this chapter.)
3. Collaboratively explore potential positive alternatives to the challenging behavior.

Preteaching

1. Collaboratively decide under what circumstances the individual will be allowed to control tasks and settings with positive communication (e.g., escape undesirable tasks, people, settings; gain access to desirable tasks, people, settings).
2. Collaboratively select a positive communication alternative to the negative behavior. Ideally, the communication alternative should have the following characteristics:
   - Easy to produce: if the alternative is harder for the individual to produce than the behavior it is intended to replace, it is unlikely to be adopted.
   - Satisfying: the positive communication alternative should fit the person's personality and communication milieu.
   - Effective: the alternative must be at least as effective for the individual as the negative behavior it is replacing.
   - Promptable: there is an advantage to physically promptable communication alternatives (e.g., signing, gesturing, pointing to a picture on a board) versus those that are not promptable (e.g., talking) in the initial stages of teaching, but this is often not possible.
   - Interpretable: the communication must be interpretable by all relevant communication partners.

Teaching the Positive Communication Alternative

1. Collaboratively ensure many successful positive communication routines daily (i.e., successful, rewarded use of the positive communication alternative) throughout the day and in a variety of contexts.
   a. Naturally occurring opportunities.
   b. Contrived opportunities.
2. Initially attempt to achieve a high ratio of positive communication alternatives to challenging behavior (e.g., 10:1), with prompts and other supports as necessary.
3. Gradually reduce prompts and other supports.
4. Gradually re-introduce normal demands.
   a. This may require explicit teaching of the difference between choice and no-choice situations.
   b. This may require considerable focus on antecedent supports (e.g., positive behavioral momentum, other positive setting events) to ensure that the individual does not revert to challenging behavior during stressful tasks.
5. Monitor and modify as necessary.

Obstacles to Teaching Communication Alternatives

1. **Staff insularity:** The success of this teaching depends on all or most everyday communication partners being generally consistent in their communication with the person with challenging behavior.

continued

Behavior as Communication: Teaching Positive Communication Alternatives to Challenging Behavior
continued

Possible Solutions:
a. Try to include everybody in the initial functional assessment of behavior.
b. Negotiate the behavior plan so that all relevant people agree that the plan is reasonable and do-able.

2. **Concern about contributing to the behavior problem:** Many staff and family members are concerned that rewarding positive escape or access-motivated behavior will give the individual too much control.
Possible Solutions:
a. Point out research and experience that shows that this natural fear is unfounded if the teaching is implemented correctly.
b. Emphasize that normal demands will be reintroduced once the challenging behavior is substantially eliminated.

3. **Concern that some activities are mandatory, others forbidden:**
Possible Solutions:
a. Try to achieve agreement about those activities that are *mandatory* and therefore cannot be escaped (e.g., taking medication) and those that are *forbidden* and therefore cannot be chosen (e.g., harming others, interacting with dangerous materials, placing oneself at risk).
b. Try to help all everyday communication partners agree that improving behavior and communication is a high priority at this time, necessitating considerable control by the individual using positive communication alternatives.

4. **No-choice times heavily outweigh choice times:** It is unlikely that the individual will change old communication habits in the absence of a large number of meaningful, successful, rewarded learning trials with the positive alternative.
Possible Solutions:
a. Create—artificially if necessary—a large number of choice occasions so that the individual has many opportunities to practice and be rewarded for the positive communication alternative.

5. **Behavior management is somebody else's job:** Some people believe that behavior problems should be dealt with by behavior specialists and not by others.
Possible Solutions:
a. Ensure that all relevant communication partners are involved in identifying the need for behavior change, in implementing the functional analysis of behavior, and in modifying everyday routines of communication so that the individual has many opportunities to practice positive communication alternatives.

6. **Difficulty with timing:**
Possible Solutions:
a. Ensure that communication partners know that they must respond to the positive communication alternative promptly—knowing that if they wait, the individual is likely to revert to the challenging behavior—and will likely be unintentionally rewarded for the challenging behavior.

7. **Concern about power/authority roles:** Some adults, particularly those who are personally insecure, resist creating the impression that a client or student or employee is in a position of power or authority over them.
Possible Solutions:
1. Work with resistive staff to help them understand that this teaching strategy ultimately gives them more, not less authority.
2. Help everybody understand the importance of substituting positive for negative communication and that this may require giving the individual a sense of power with positive communication.
3. Help everybody understand that normal expectations will be re-instituted once the challenging behavior is under adequate control.

negative communication behavior, intervention designed to substitute positive alternatives can be critical to social, vocational, and familial success. However, proud and oppositional adolescents and young adults, particularly those from cultural backgrounds in which communication is often somewhat unrefined, are most *unlikely* to accept alternatives like the following:

• "Excuse me, but I think we need to spend some quality time working on our relationship because I find your attitude unacceptable."
• "Since my accident I have a hard time doing even simple things. I need a lot of help. Please help me."

• "Is there any chance we could spend some time talking? I would like to get to know you better."

In our experience, the most critical component of intervention is the negotiation that leads to communication scripts or a general communication style that enables the person to be successful in chosen educational, vocational, and social contexts, and is at the same time consistent with his or her sense of self (Step 3 of the intervention sequence outlined in Table 33–4). Often, this negotiation is facilitated by collaborative identification of a positive role model or metaphor that can help the individual overcome emotional barriers to positive communication alternatives to negative behavior.

Compelling metaphors have the added advantage that they combine into one thought unit a set of social behaviors or scripts otherwise difficult to remember when considered separately, particularly under stress. Thus, for one young adult with a post-injury history of aggressive behavior and multiple psychiatric hospitalizations and incarcerations, calling up the image of Clint Eastwood when stressed yielded a compelling image of self-control and also a script that included a very few words designed to extricate himself from potentially volatile situations. The Clint Eastwood metaphor at the same time motivated positive, self-regulated behavior and compensated for reduced space in working memory. Functioning in this manner, effective metaphors are components of the "implicational code" or organized set of emotional beliefs as those concepts have recently emerged in new interpretations of cognitive psychotherapy (Teasdale, 1997).

Ylvisaker and Feeney (2000a,b) explored the facilitating role played by positive metaphors for individuals with cognitive impairment and oppositional behavior following TBI. They illustrated this role by describing their intervention for a fiercely oppositional adolescent who had been in serious trouble with the law and who had threatened several staff members in his residential program. His initial resistance to any intervention was overcome by hiring him as a consultant to develop a training video about oppositionality. In his capacity as a paid consultant, he revealed that his overriding goal in interacting with authority figures and many peers was to avoid being a "suck up" (his term). The only "nonsuck-up" role with which he was familiar was that of a fiercely oppositional and defiant bulldog, which he played effectively (and which routinely got him into serious trouble). He agreed to refer to this role with a vulgar metaphor (to cast it in a negative light) and worked with the clinicians to identify a third way of acting, that of "winners"—successful people who are not suck ups, but who do what needs to be done to achieve their goals. He then agreed to practice negotiating many everyday social interactions in three ways: as a suck up, as his traditional defiant self, and as a winner. These interactions were videotaped (as part of developing the training program) and he reviewed the tapes as part of his responsibilities as a consultant to the project and as part of his communication therapy.

During his contextualized practice, a social skills coach (speech-language pathology intern) mediated his experience with discussion of which of these three interactive styles were comfortable for him (predictably, the suck-up style was never comfortable) and which were successful (the defiant style was never successful). Success and adequate comfort came to be associated with a wide range of positive ("winner") interactive behaviors. Social cues could then be reduced to one positive reminder—"You can be a winner"—as opposed to the top-down admonitions that he had routinely interpreted as nagging and to which he had routinely reacted

with oppositional behavior. Perhaps more importantly, success came to be associated with a conviction that "winner behavior" was his route to freedom, a good job, and other personally significant goals. This metaphorical transformation at least brought him onto the playing field of successful social interaction, which he continued to practice with considerable success.

Other metaphors described by Ylvisaker and Feeney (2000) and used successfully in TBI rehabilitation include the following:

1. *Social skills as basketball plays*: A former basketball player whose impulsiveness had led to substance abuse and serious trouble with the authorities came to agree that he needed "to be like Mike (Michael Jordan) and use *set plays* rather than running around the court like a crazy kid." Social skills training then became a process of defining successful *plays*, putting them in his *play book*, and videotaping him engaged in these plays so that he could review the *game films* as part of routinizing the plays. Social cues for this extremely disinhibited person were then reduced to the nonthreatening "What's the play?" and "Is this play in the play book?" as opposed to the cues (i.e., nagging) that staff had previously used and that had routinely elicited oppositional behavior.

2. *Requests for clarification as journalistic behavior*: A well-educated young woman with a commitment to feminism before her injury overcame her reluctance to asking communication partners for clarification of their message (and increasing social withdrawal) once she associated these requests for clarification with the journalistic practices of her heroine, the well-known feminist and journalist Gloria Steinem.

3. *Cognitive prostheses as common workplace practices*: A young man who before his injury had been a truck driver at a gravel pit overcame his resistance to compensatory procedures, such as a small memory notebook, when he connected these strategies with the common practice at his former job site of having unused trucks and drivers available for emergency purposes if the others broke down.

4. *Risk-taking behavior as red-card violations in soccer*: A former soccer player, who had been arrested twice on drug charges after his injury, began to work hard on his recovery after formulating the following metaphorical insight, "I want to play the game, but I have a yellow card. The next time, it's a red card and I'm off the field. But my teammates will still be playing—and playing at a disadvantage because I got myself thrown out of the game. I can play and enjoy playing and win, but I've got to pay attention to the rules."

5. *Ignoring provocation as cool behavior*: A young adult who before his injury was a drug user and dealer in New York City was placed in a developmental disabilities workshop

as part of his community reintegration plan. John routinely reacted with physical and verbal aggression when coworkers irritated him at work. His resistance to ignoring these provocations was overcome after discussion of his hero, the rap musician LL Cool J, who not only delivers firey lyrics in his performances, but also is a successful and self-controlled business man and family man. Ignoring provocation at work came to be seen not as weakness, but as an aspect of the strength of LL Cool J.

In a self-advocacy videotape that we helped John (illustration #5) produce and that he asked his work supervisor to watch, he explained that it was difficult to overcome instincts and communication styles fashioned during his years on the streets. He described his efforts to resist impulsive aggressive responses and to use the behavior that he had chosen as a substitute (a somewhat sarcastic dismissive comment, followed by turning away). He ended his video with a plea to the supervisor, "Please, let me be me." Subsequently, this supervisor used a subtle written cue ("Cool J") at the first sign of John's loss of control, resulting in his successful effort to regain control because of its association with his positive self-metaphor.

People will be who they are. It is not the job of communication specialists to force individuals to communicate in ways that are foreign to their understanding of who they are, but rather to help them communicate in ways that contribute to the achievement of meaningful goals in their lives, consistent with the needs of others. That this aspect of communication intervention enters the domain of self-discovery and self-acceptance counseling should not frighten away communication specialists inadequately trained as counselors, but rather cause them to redouble their collaboration with other rehabilitation professionals. Through such collaborative efforts, including collaboration with colleagues, the person with disability, and everyday people in the environment, functional intervention is allowed to take root in the real world, facilitated by positive alliances among all relevant stakeholders. These intervention themes are further elaborated by Ylvisaker and Feeney (2000b).

COLLABORATION WITH EVERYDAY PEOPLE THROUGHOUT RECOVERY

In this chapter, we have placed major emphasis on the role played by everyday people (family members, direct care staff, teachers, work supervisors, coworkers, friends, and others) in the long-term rehabilitation of individuals with chronic cognitive, communication, and behavioral impairment after TBI. This emphasis is motivated in part by the economic realities governing neurologic rehabilitation at the turn of the century, but also by enduring principles of sound, appropriately contextualized intervention. Rehabilitation within this framework mandates effective collaborative alliances with

everyday people. In Appendix 33-3 we list reasons for such alliances, along with obstacles to establishing collaborative alliances, strategies for overcoming the obstacles, characteristics of effective everyday coaches/facilitators, and training and support options.

In medical rehabilitation, there exist many obstacles to the creation of such collaborative alliances. Appendix 33-3 lists some of these obstacles and offers a menu of strategies to overcome them. In our experience, managers in rehabilitation facilities play a critical role in supporting a culture of rehabilitation that values alliances with everyday people. In such facilities, therapists' schedules are creatively designed so that they have natural opportunities to interact collaboratively with one another, nursing staff (in an inpatient facility), assistant-level staff, and family members. In addition, training opportunities and materials (e.g., peer coaching, customized training videos) are available for orientation of staff who did not learn collaborative principles and procedures in their professional training programs.

Appendix 33-3 includes a list of characteristics of people who are effective in their role as everyday coach and facilitator for people with chronic impairment after TBI. Some family members, therapists, direct care staff, work supervisors, and others have these characteristics in abundance. Others need considerable help to play their role effectively. Appendix 33-3 concludes with a list of procedures that can be used to put everyday people in a position to play this role. Traditional training procedures (e.g., brief inservices for direct care staff, family conferences) are notoriously insufficient. Situational coaching and support are typically necessary to change behavior (just as clinical practicum experiences are critical for clinicians in training). Strong support systems are critical for people whose resilience and optimism become severely strained. Specific scripts may be needed by those people who are not by nature flexible or enthusiastic problem solvers, but who need to create everyday routines of flexibility and effective problem solving. Because of their expertise in communication, speech-language pathologists often play a central role in developing interaction scripts and in general staff and family training. Ylvisaker and Feeney (1998a,b) explored these themes in greater detail.

Communication Partner Conversational Support Competencies

Speech-language pathologists are often called on to train direct care staff and others in interactive competencies needed to communicate effectively with patients in neurologic rehabilitation settings (Ylvisaker et al., 1993a). It is less common, however, for communication partner training to be considered a critical component of cognitive rehabilitation. Recent research in developmental cognitive psychology has emphasized the role of parent-child conversations about the past in facilitating children's development of thought organization and autobiographical memory (Fivush, 1991; Fivush & Fromhoff, 1988; Fivush & Reese, 1992; Haden et al., 1997; Hudson, 1990; McCabe & Peterson, 1991; Nelson, 1992; Reese & Fivush, 1993; Reese et al., 1993). The evolving view is that parents who interact frequently with their preschool children in a collaborative, elaborative, and socially enjoyable way have children who develop internal cognitive organization and autobiographical memory more effectively than comparable children whose parents interact with them less frequently or in a way that is not similarly supportive. Although these interactions can focus on a variety of topics, developmental investigations in this area have largely targeted parent-child interaction while jointly talking about events that they have experienced together, that is, socially co-constructed narratives about the past.

In Appendix 33-4, we attempt to capture the competencies associated with a cognitively facilitative style under two general headings: *collaboration* and *elaboration*. That is, conversation partners who are effective in facilitating cognitive growth in children or people with cognitive impairment tend to *participate with* them in conversation rather than *demand performance from* them; in addition, facilitators use conversational procedures to help their conversation partner understand how things, people, and events in the world are organized, that is, they gradually clarify the many ways in which things in the world go together. In effect, within this Vygotskyan framework, facilitative conversationalists, whether parents, teachers, therapists, aides, or others, are able to teach their partner how to think and how to organize their thoughts while at the same time enjoying pleasant conversations about topics of mutual interest.

We have used the competencies listed in Appendix 33-4 in the training of family members and staff serving children and adults with cognitive impairment after TBI. In addition to enhancing the cognitive value of everyday interaction, these competencies often have the effect of reducing tension between people with TBI and staff members. In our experience, many well-meaning people interact with adults with cognitive impairment in an inquisitorial and nonelaborative manner, a style of interaction that tends to elicit negative behavioral responses and that is the opposite of facilitative from a cognitive perspective. An additional component of staff communication training, associated with an everyday, routine-based approach to intervention, is the development of scripts that promote problem solving and flexibility in individuals who are otherwise rigid and disorganized in their approach to everyday problems. Appendix 33-4 concludes with examples of such scripts.

Self-Advocacy Videotapes

As part of a general focus on collaboration and executive functions in rehabilitation, it is useful to engage individuals with TBI, working collaboratively with staff and family members, in the production of a videotape that has as its primary purpose to orient and train future (or current) staff in how to teach, help, coach, and otherwise work with the person. This can be a project for the last 2 or 3 weeks of the inpatient rehabilitation program or at any time when such a training vehicle may be useful. The person with disability is engaged in a meaningful and important project that has a concrete and very legitimate goal—to help others understand his or her strengths and needs, and become oriented to the teaching or support procedures that are most helpful.

There are several secondary purposes for this project, including consolidation of collaborative alliances through product-oriented efforts. Furthermore, this process helps the person with disability, family members, and other relevant everyday people gain insight into post-injury issues. Their learning is often enhanced when important information and procedures are processed *in order to teach someone else*. A general protocol (that can and should be modified to meet the needs of specific individuals and situations) and its rationale are presented in Table 33–17.

CLINICAL DECISION MAKING IN THE FACE OF INCOMPLETE EVIDENCE

Throughout the chapter we have cited key pieces of experimental literature and general reviews of the efficacy literature in TBI rehabilitation and, importantly, in closely related fields of intervention. In our view, serious consideration of this literature, combined with clinical experience in many practice settings, supports the general approach to intervention described in this chapter. However, at this time, there is insufficient evidence from well-designed clinical trials with large numbers of subjects to draw strong conclusions. Therefore, clinicians must make responsible clinical judgments in the absence of accepted standards of practice.

In domains of impairment in which the need for clinical services is undeniable, but published experimental guidance is at best incomplete, responsible clinicians make decisions about intervention for specific individuals with disability based on informed consideration of the following factors:

- Is the proposed intervention supported by any intervention outcome studies with subjects with TBI who possess the same impairments and needs as the client?
- Is the proposed intervention supported by intervention outcome studies with related populations (e.g., learning disabilities, developmental disabilities, ADHD, behavioral disorders)?
- Is the proposed intervention supported by trial intervention with the client?
- Is the proposed intervention supported by extensive clinical experience with clients with TBI?

- Is the proposed intervention supported by theory, including neuropsychological, cognitive, behavioral, pedagogical, and other theories?
- Is the proposed intervention supported by negotiation with the client and relevant stakeholders in the client's life?
- Is the proposed intervention consistent with known constraints, including expertise of service providers, availability of support personnel, time to complete the intervention, and adequate resources?
- Can the proposed intervention be judged to be preferable to known alternatives—in relation to predicted functional outcome for the client—based on the previous considerations?
- Is the proposed intervention humane, morally justifiable, and consistent with the scope of practice and relevant licensing laws governing the provider of services?

In our experience with several hundred children, adolescents, and adults with chronic disability after TBI—disability in the territory in which communication, cognition, executive functions, and behavior overlap and interact—the approach outlined and illustrated in this chapter requires creative effort, but can be effective and functional, based on all of these considerations. Furthermore, data from our work with the New York State Department of Health TBI Medicaid Waiver Program demonstrates the cost effectiveness of this approach (Feeney et al., in press).

FUTURE TRENDS

At the beginning of the 21st century, managed care and associated reductions in funding for rehabilitation have become thoroughly established as dominant themes in adult neurogenic rehabilitation. Inpatient lengths of stay have decreased dramatically over the past 15 years and funding for traditional outpatient therapies has also been substantially reduced (AHCPR, 1999). The staggering cost of catastrophic neurologic rehabilitation, estimated in 1993 to be approximately $4 billion a year and increasing at a rate of 15% a year (Cope & O'Lear, 1993), has motivated draconian cost-cutting measures. Even as they cut funding, funders of services increasingly demand meaningful evidence of improved functional outcomes. Clinicians attempting to meet the challenge of having a greater effect with fewer resources have attempted to create efficiencies in the form of increased use of group therapy and indirect therapy using adequately trained support staff, volunteers, family members, and others. There is reason to believe that these trends will continue.

We anticipate that professionals in brain injury rehabilitation will increasingly look to other disability groups for insights into the provision of effective community-based services and supports. Community-based service delivery models have a longer (although not uniformly successful) history in developmental disabilities, mental health, and spinal cord injury than in brain injury rehabilitation. More generally, professionals serving other populations of people with chronic cognitive, communication, and behavioral impairment may offer wisdom regarding the process of contextualizing and "demedicalizing" long-term services and supports.

Although driven by economic forces, some of the new directions in service delivery may simply be good practice finally come of age. Following severe TBI, even the best combination of medical and other clinically based interventions generally leave survivors with some degree of impairment and associated disability. Because a majority of these people are relatively young, the ongoing impairments affect social life, work, family life, and community living in dynamic and evolving ways. Therefore, we believe that demands will continue to increase for community-based services and supports, including appropriate supported housing and work, recreational possibilities, behavioral services, and family supports. Cognitive, behavioral, and communication competence plays a critical role in real-world success in these domains. Therefore, specialists trained in community-based cognitive, behavioral, and communication intervention will likely be in increasing demand.

In our experience, delivery of services and supports becomes increasingly challenging years after the injury, particularly if the person with TBI has experienced considerable failure in attempting community reintegration and, possibly, has made unfortunate choices, such as abuse of alcohol and drugs, to escape the pain of ongoing failure. We expect that more states will recognize the combined rehabilitative, humanistic, and budgetary advantages of long-term community support services, like those provided through the New York State TBI Medicaid Waiver Program, for individuals with TBI who are particularly difficult to serve (Ylvisaker, 1999; Feeney et al., in press). Potentially lifelong supports through community support agencies, including the services of professionals with expertise in cognition, communication, and behavior, will be found cheaper and more effective than periodic crisis services (e.g., psychiatric hospitalization, jail). Communication specialists will need to be comfortable delivering services within teams that necessarily include the person with disability, and in nonstandard venues like the workplace, private residences, and other community settings. Furthermore, specialists in rehabilitation will increasingly deliver their services indirectly through everyday people in the life of the person with disability.

Reports from animal laboratories regarding the potential usefulness of neuropharmacologic agents in the treatment of individuals with TBI continue to be promising. However, despite the trumpeting of this promise for at least two decades, "there are currently no drugs available that are of demonstrated benefit in promoting cognitive and motor recovery from TBI …" (NIH, 1999, p. 269). Clinicians are well advised to remain alert to developments in this field and to ensure that significantly impaired individuals receive needed

TABLE 33–17

Transitional/Self-Advocacy Video: Rationale and Procedures

GOALS:

Primary Goal: To produce a videotape that can be used to orient and train people (e.g., school staff, employers, family members, home health aides, others) who may need to be trained in how to teach, interact with, or otherwise support the person with disability.

Important Associated Goals:
The individuals with disability will:
- gain a sense of empowerment.
- gain progressively more insight into his or her strengths and needs.
- progressively become more strategic in his or her thinking about himself/herself and his/her rehabilitation and school careers.

Family members will:
- gain a sense of empowerment.
- gain progressively more insight into the individual's strengths and needs, and will share their insights with staff.
- gain an appreciation of the importance of executive functions and the individual's participation in goal setting, planning, and strategic thinking.

Staff will:
- strengthen their collaborative relationships with other team members (including family members) as they work together to produce the video.
- gain greater appreciation for the perspective of the individual with disability and family members.

PROCEDURES (subject to considerable variation in individual cases)
1. Several weeks before a substantial transition (e.g., discharge from inpatient rehabilitation, return to work or school), staff, individual with disability, and family members hold a **planning meeting.** The purposes of this meeting are:
   a. To decide what **content** would be most important to demonstrate on video. This could include:
      - **Physical** strengths, weaknesses, and intervention/support issues (e.g., seating, positioning, mobility, dressing, eating)
      - **Cognitive** strengths, weaknesses, and intervention/support issues (e.g., types of advance organizers needed; types of environmental or materials modifications needed due to attentional, perceptual, or other processing problems; types of cues and prompts needed)
      - **Communication** strengths, weaknesses, and intervention/support issues (e.g., use of an augmentative communication system; demonstration of partner communication styles that facilitate comprehension)
      - **Behavioral/Social** strengths, weaknesses, and intervention/support issues (e.g., procedures for preventing behavior problems; ways to diffuse behavioral outbursts; ways to facilitate peer interaction)

      It is critical that **strengths** be highlighted and that the **goals of the individual with disability and family members** be highlighted.
   b. To decide what **format and scripts** would be most effective in demonstrating critical points.
      1. It is often effective to show the individual (1) succeeding at a task that he or she is good at; (2) failing at an important but difficult task when appropriate procedures, modifications, or equipment are **not** in place, and then (3) succeeding when they are in place.
      2. It is often effective to communicate content by means of a **conversation** between individual with disability and staff or between staff and family members, as opposed to simply videoing a "talking head."
      3. It is ideal to video the individual's own orientation to and commentary about the video segments and then edit these into the tape as orientation for the viewer. This videoing can be made after the person has watched the other segments.
   c. To decide **who should play what role** in the video. If possible, the person with disability should play a leading role (possibly with considerable support). If the person is extremely impaired, family members can play a leading role.
   d. To work out **logistics** of videoing and editing.

   The individual and family members may be more or less involved in this planning, depending on many factors.
2. During the following weeks, the planning of video demonstrations can be included in therapy sessions. For example, development of scripts can be part of speech-language therapy sessions; development of presentation of strengths and needs can be part of counseling sessions; development of physical demonstrations can be part of PT, OT, ST, and other therapies.
3. The actual videotaping may be no more than a camera in a therapy session capturing an important demonstration. If other individuals are present, they must have signed releases. The video may or may not be edited, depending on the skills of staff and time available.

ADVANTAGES OF THIS TRANSITIONAL/SELF-ADVOCACY ROUTINE
Beyond the obvious goal of orienting future staff and caregivers, transitional, self-advocacy videos serve a number of purposes:

continued

Transitional/Self-Advocacy Video: Rationale and Procedures
continued

1. **Incidental Learning: Individual with Disability:** People acquire important information about themselves and about their rehabilitation program by being engaged in a fun, product-oriented activity.
2. **Incidental Learning: Staff:** Staff members acquire important information about the person with disability, the family, and their own program by being engaged in a fun, product-oriented activity.
3. **Incidental Learning: Family Members:** Family members acquire important information about the individual and the intervention program by being engaged in a fun, product-oriented activity.
4. **Efficient Cross-Training:** Staff currently working with the person may learn important things from other staff or from family members without the stigma associated with being singled out for remedial instruction.
5. **Development of a Shared Conceptual Framework:** The intervention team refines its own shared conceptual framework by being engaged in a fun, product-oriented activity.
6. **Fun:** Producing this video can be fun.
7. **Permanent Record:** If this practice becomes routine, the person with disability and family will have an invaluable permanent record of the recovery process.
8. **Customer Satisfaction:** In general, people with disability and family members are pleased when staff accord them the respect that is implicit in this activity. Indeed, this can be a vehicle for overcoming an adversarial relationship if that exists.

Modified with permission from Ylvisaker et al. (1998c). Cognitive rehabilitation: Executive functions. In M. Ylvisaker (ed.), *Traumatic brain injury rehabilitation: Children and adolescents* (Rev. Ed.) (pp. 221–269). Boston: Butterworth-Heinemann.

evaluations from a physician with expertise in TBI pharmacology. However, hopefulness must be muted by the realistic expectation that into the foreseeable future, the greatest effects for individuals with chronic impairment will be derived from a combination of contextualized behavioral interventions and environmental supports.

KEY POINTS

1. Because most individuals with severe TBI are relatively young and therefore live for several decades with ongoing impairment, the *prevalence* of TBI is high and the costs to society are extraordinary.
2. Although virtually any combination of preserved and impaired functions is technically possible after TBI, there are central tendencies within the population, associated in large part with damage to the vulnerable frontal lobes, limbic structures, and neural connections among these regions.
3. TBI does not randomly select its victims. Disproportionately large numbers of people with TBI are adolescents or young adults, and in many cases had preinjury predisposing factors, including weak academic and vocational histories, risk-taking behavior, and, possibly, substance abuse.
4. Among the common consequences of TBI is weak executive control over behavior, including cognition, communication, and social behavior generally.
5. Historically, the dominant intervention approach in medical rehabilitation has been characterized by a focus on reducing the underlying impairment with decontextualized exercises administered by specialists in specialized treatment settings. An alternative approach that has gained increasing acceptance focuses flexibly on impairment, disability, or handicap—often starting with the handicap (or threat to participation); involves contextualized practice of successful everyday, routines; and is supported in large part by everyday people.
6. Contextualized, everyday, routine-based intervention has its rationale in the special needs of people with frontal lobe injury, in recent developments in learning theory, and in the economic realities of neurologic rehabilitation.
7. Contextualized, everyday, routine-based intervention is associated with an approach to assessment that is ongoing, contextualized, and collaborative, and that involves the testing of intervention hypotheses.
8. At the center of executive system intervention is the concept of an executive function routine, wherein the individual with disability contributes as much as possible to identifying goals and potential obstacles to achieving the goals, creating plans for achieving the goals, reviewing the usefulness of the plans, and reflecting on what works and what does not work for that person in attempting to achieve his or her goals.
9. Functional, individualized cognitive rehabilitation plans are centered around goals and activities important to the individual, with varied cognitive impairments and disabilities targeted within the context of these activities in an attempt to improve cognitive functioning routinely.
10. For reasons that are in part neuropsychological and in part psychological, behavior plans for individuals

with TBI should be largely antecedent focused, understanding antecedents broadly to include both immediate and remote setting events.

11. Communication/behavior plans for individuals with TBI often focus on teaching positive communication alternatives to negative behavior. Positive communication scripts must be integrated into the individual's sense of personal identity, which may have to be revised after the injury.

12. Helping individuals with TBI overcome their handicaps (i.e., increase their participation in chosen life activities), reduce their disabilities (i.e., improve performance of activities of everyday life), and ultimately reduce their impairments (i.e., improve neurologically mediated processing) frequently requires massive amounts of supported practice in the routines of everyday life. Ensuring adequate amounts of practice, in turn, requires that specialists collaborate with everyday people who become the primary facilitators of improved performance.

REVIEW QUESTIONS, THOUGHT QUESTIONS, TASKS

1. Explain the difference between incidence and prevalence. Explain why TBI is associated with extraordinary societal costs.

2. Why are the frontal lobes especially vulnerable in TBI? List and explain common communication-related impairments associated with frontal lobe injury.

3. What are the most important reasons for contextualizing assessment for individuals with TBI?

4. List and explain several possible hypotheses that could explain why a specific individual with TBI speaks very little and only when spoken to. How would you test the hypotheses?

5. List and explain several possible hypotheses that could explain why a young adult with TBI becomes verbally aggressive when reminded to perform a routine task. How would you test the hypotheses?

6. List and explain several possible hypotheses that could explain why a specific individual with TBI speaks in a way that is disorganized, tangential, and verbose. How would you test the hypotheses?

7. What are the most important reasons for contextualizing intervention for individuals with TBI?

8. Describe differences in executive function routines for people in the middle and late stages of recovery from TBI.

9. What is meant by "supported cognition" and why is it important?

10. What are the most important reasons for focusing on antecedents in TBI behavior management?

11. Why is it important for speech-language pathologists to be included on behavior management teams?

12. Describe strategies for maximizing the effects that can be obtained from shrinking resources available for long-term rehabilitation.

References

Adamovich, B.B. & Henderson, J. (1992). *Scales of cognitive ability for traumatic head injury*. Chicago: Applied Symbolix.

Adams, J.H., Graham, D.I., Scott, G., Parker, L.S., & Doyle, D. (1980). Brain damage in fatal non-missile head injury. *Journal of Clinical Pathology, 33,* 1132–1145.

Adams, J.H., Graham, D.I., Murray, L.S., & Scott, G. (1982). Diffuse axonal injury due to non-missile head injury in humans: An analysis of 45 cases. *Annals of Neurology, 12,* 557–563.

Alexander, M. (1987). Syndromes in the rehabilitation and outcome of closed head injury. In H.S. Levin, J. Grafman, and H.M. Eisenberg (eds.), *Neurobehavioral recovery from head injury* (pp. 192–205). New York: Oxford.

Alexander, M.P., Benson, D.F., & Stuss, D.T. (1989). Frontal lobes and language. *Brain and Language, 37,* 656–691.

AHCPR (1999). Rehabilitation for traumatic brain injury: Evidence report/technology assessment Number 2 (Agency for Health Care Policy and Research Publication No. 99-E006).

Alderman, N. (1996). Central executive deficit and response to operant conditioning methods. *Neuropsychological Rehabilitation, 6,* 161–186.

Alderman, N. & Ward, A. (1991). Behavioral treatment of the dysexecutive syndrome: Reduction of repetitive speech using response cost and cognitive overlearning. *Neuropsychological Rehabilitation, 1,* 65–80.

American Speech-Language-Hearing Association (ASHA) (1988, March). The role of speech-language pathologists in the identification, diagnosis, and treatment of individuals with cognitive-communicative impairments. *ASHA, 30,* 79.

Anderson, S.W., Damasio, H., Tranel, D., & Damasio, A.R. (1988). Neuropsychological correlates of bilateral frontal lobe lesions in humans. *Society for Neuroscience, 14,* 1288.

Annegers, J.F., Grabow, J.D., Kurland, L.T., & Laws, E.R. (1980). The incidence, causes, and secular trends of head trauma in Olmsted County, Minnesota, 1935–1974. *Neurology, 30,* 912–919.

Ashcraft, M. (1994). *Human memory and cognition.* Reading MA: Addison-Wesley, Longman.

Ashman, A.F. & Conway, R.N.F. (1989). *Cognitive strategies for special education.* London: Routledge.

Bachman, D.L. (1992). The diagnosis and management of common neurologic sequelae of closed head injury. *Journal of Head Trauma Rehabilitation, 7,* 50–59.

Baer, D.M., Wolf, M.M., & Risley, T.R. (1987). Some still current dimensions of applied behavior analysis. *Journal of Applied Behavior Analysis, 20,* 313–327.

Bannerman, D.J., Sheldon, J.B., Sherman, J.A., & Harchik, A.E. (1990). Balancing the right to habilitation with the right to personal liberties: The rights of people with developmental disabilities to eat too many doughnuts and take a nap. *Journal of Applied Behavior Analysis, 23,* 79–89.

Bargh, J.A. & Chartrand, T.L. (1999). The unbearable automaticity of being. *American Psychologist, 54,* 462–479.

Barkley, R.A. (1987). *Defiant children: A clinician's manual for parent training.* New York: The Guilford Press.

Barsalou, L.W. (1992). *Cognitive psychology: An overview for cognitive scientists.* Hillsdale, NJ: Lawrence Erlbaum.

Bechara, A., Damasio, A.R., Damasio, H., & Anderson, S.W. (1994). Insensitivity to future consequences following damage to the human prefrontal cortex. *Cognition, 50,* 7–12.

Bechara, A., Tranel, D., Damasio, H., & Damasio, A. (1996). Failure to respond autonomically to anticipated future outcomes following damage to prefrontal cortex. *Cerebral Cortex, 6,* 215–225.

Benton, A. (1991). Prefrontal injury and behavior in children. *Developmental Neuropsychology, 7*(3), 275–281.

Ben-Yishay, Y. & Diller, L. (1983). Cognitive remediation. In M. Rosenthal, E. Griffith, M. Bond, & J.D. Miller (eds.), *Rehabilitation of the head injured adult* (pp. 367–380). Philadelphia: F.A. Davis.

Ben-Yishay, Y., Piasetsky, E.B., & Rattok, J. (1987). A systematic method for ameliorating disorders in basic attention. In M.J. Meier, A.L. Benton, & L. Diller (eds.), *Neuropsychological rehabilitation* (pp. 165–181). New York: Churchill Living-stone.

Berk, L.E. & Winsler, A. (1995). Scaffolding children's learning: Vygotsky and early childhood education. *NAEYC Research and Practice Series, 7.* Washington, DC: National Association for the Education of Young Children.

Beukelman, D.R. (1998). Communication Effectiveness Survey. In Beukelman, D.R., Mathy, P., & Yorkston, K. (1998). Outcomes measurement in motor speech disorders. In C.M. Frattali (ed.), *Measuring outcomes in speech-language pathology* (pp. 334–353). New York: Thieme.

Biddle, K.R., McCabe, A., & Bliss, L.S. (1996). Narrative skills following traumatic brain injury in children and adults. *Journal of Communication Disorders, 29*(6), 447–470.

Bigler, E.D. (1988). Frontal lobe damage and neuropsychological assessment. *Archives of Clinical Neuropsychology, 3,* 279–297.

Bird, F., Dores, P.A., Moniz, D., & Robinson, J. (1989). Reducing severe aggressive and self-injurious behaviors with functional communication training: Direct, collateral, and generalized results. *American Journal of Mental Retardation, 94,* 37–48.

Bjorklund, D.F. (1990). *Children's strategies: Contemporary views of cognitive development.* Hillsdale, NJ: Lawrence Erlbaum.

Blumer, D. & Benson, F. (1975). Personality changes with frontal and temporal lobe lesions. In D.F. Benson & D. Blumer (eds.), *Psychiatric aspects of neurologic disease* (pp. 151–170). New York: Grune & Stratton.

Boake, C. (1996). Supervision Rating Scale: A measure of functional outcome from brain injury. *Archives of Physical Medicine and Rehabilitation, 77,* 765–772.

Bodrova, E. & Leong, D.J. (1996). *Tools of the mind: The Vygotskyan approach to early childhood education.* Englewood Cliffs, NJ: Prentice-Hall.

Bond, M. (1990). Standardized methods of assessing and predicting outcome. In M. Rosenthal, E.R. Griffith, M.R. Bond, & J.D. Miller (eds.), *Rehabilitation of the adult and child with traumatic brain injury.* Philadelphia: F.A. Davis.

Braunling-McMorrow, D., Lloyd, K., & Fralish, K. (1986). Teaching social skills to head injured adults. *Journal of Rehabilitation, 52,* 39–44.

Brazzeli, M., Colombo, N. DellaSala, S., & Spinnler, H. (1994). Spared and impaired cognitive abilities after bilateral frontal lobe damage. *Cortex, 30,* 27–51.

Brooks, D.N., Campsie, L., Symington, C., Beattie, A., Bryden, J., & McKinley, W. (1987). The effects of severe head injury upon patient and relative within seven years of injury. *Journal of Head Trauma Rehabilitation, 2,* 1–13.

Brooks, D.N. & McKinlay, W. (1983). Personality and behavioral change after severe blunt head injury—a relative's view. *Journal of Neurology, Neurosurgery, and Psychiatry, 46,* 336–344.

Brookshire, R.H. (1997). *Introduction to neurogenic communication disorders* (5th ed.). St. Louis, MO: Mosby.

Brotherton, F.A., Thomas, L.L., Wisotzek, I.E., & Milan, M.A. (1988). Social skills training in the rehabilitation of patients with traumatic closed head injury. *Archives of Physical Medicine and Rehabilitation, 69,* 827–832.

Brown, A.L., Campione, J.C., Weber, L.S., & McGilly, K. (1992). *Interactive learning environments: A new look at assessment and instruction.* Berkeley, CA: University of California, Commission on Testing and Public Policy.

Brown, F., Belz, P., Corsi, L., & Wenig, B. (1993). Choice diversity for people with severe disabilities. *Education and Training in Mental Retardation, 28,* 318–326.

Brown, G., Chadwick, O., Shaffer, D., Rutter, M., & Traub, M. (1981). A prospective study of children with head injuries. III. Psychiatric sequelae. *Psychological Medicine, 11,* 63–78.

Buckner, R.L., Peterson, S., Ojemann, J., Miezin, F., Squire, L., & Raichle, M. (1995). Functional anatomical studies of explicit and implicit memory. *Journal of Neuroscience, 15,* 12–29.

Buschke, H. & Fuld, P.A. (1974). Evaluating storage, retention, and retrieval in disordered memory and learning. *Neurology,* 1019–1025.

Cabeza, R. & Nyberg, L. (1997). Imaging cognition: An empirical review of PET studies with normal subjects. *Journal of Cognitive Neuroscience, 9,* 1–26.

Campione, J.C. & Brown, A.L. (1990). Guided learning and transfer. In N. Fredrickson, R. Glaser, A. Lesgold, & M. Shafto (eds.), *Diagnostic monitoring of skill and knowledge acquisition* (pp. 114–172). Hillsdale, NJ: Lawrence Erlbaum.

Carney, N., Chesnut, R.M., Maynard, H., Mann, N.C., Patterson, P., & Helfand, M. (1999). Effect of cognitive rehabilitation on outcomes for persons with traumatic brain injury: A systematic review. *Journal of Head Trauma Rehabilitation, 14,* 277–307.

Carr, E.G., Carlson, J.I., Langdon, N.A., Magito-McLaughlin, D., & Yarbrough, S.C. (1998). Two perspectives on antecedent control. In J.K. Luiselli & M.J. Cameron (eds.), *Antecedent control: Innovative approaches to behavioral support* (pp. 3–28). Baltimore, MD: Paul H. Brookes.

Carr, E.G., & Durand, V.M., (1985). Reducing behavior problems through functional communication training. *Journal of Applied Behavior Analysis, 18,* 111–126.

Carr, E.G., Horner, R.H., Turnbull, A.P., et al. (1999). *Positive behavior support for people with developmental disabilities: A research synthesis.* Washington, DC: American Association of Mental Retardation.

Carr, E.G., Levin, L., McConnachie, G., Carlson, J.I, Kemp, D.C., & Smith, C.E. (1994). *Communication-based intervention for problem behavior: A user's guide for producing positive change.* Baltimore, MD: Paul H. Brookes.

Carr, E.G., Reeve, C.E., Magito-McLaughlin, D. (1997). Contextual influences on problem behavior in people with developmental disabilities. In L.K. Koegel, R.L. Koegel, & G. Dunlap (eds.), *Positive behavioral support: Including people with difficult behavior in the community* (pp. 403–423). Baltimore, MD: Paul H. Brookes.

Centers for Disease Control (1997). Traumatic brain injury—Colorado, Missouri, Oklahoma, & Utah, 1990–1993. *MMWR, 46,* 8–11.

Chapman, S.B. (1997). Cognitive-communication abilities in children with closed head injury. *American Journal of Speech-Language Pathology, 6,* 50–58.

Chapman, S., Culhane, K., Levin, H., Harward, H., Mendelsohn, D., Ewing-Cobbs, L., Fletcher, J., & Bruce, D. (1992). Narrative discourse after closed head injury in children and adolescents. *Brain and Language, 43,* 42–65.

Chapman, S.B., Levin, H.S., Matejka, J., Harward, H.N., & Kufera, J. (1995). Discourse ability in head injured children: Consideration of linguistic, psychosocial, & cognitive factors. *Journal of Head Trauma Rehabilitation, 10,* 36–54.

Chapman, S.B., Watkins, R., Gustafson, C., Moore, S., Levin, H.S., & Kufera, J.A. (1997). Narrative discourse in children with closed head injury, children with language impairment, and typically developing children. *American Journal of Speech-Language Pathology, 6,* 66–76.

Cicerone, K.D. (1999). Commentary: The validity of cognitive rehabilitation. *Journal of Head Trauma Rehabilitation, 14,* 316–321.

Coelho, C.A., Liles, B.Z., & Duffy, R.J. (1991). Analysis of conversational discourse in head-injured clients. *Journal of Head Trauma Rehabilitation, 6,* 92–99.

Collins, M.W. et al. (1999). Relationship between concussion and neuropsychological performance in college football players. *Journal of the American Medical Association, 282*(10), 964–970.

Cope, D.N., & O'Lear, J. (1993). A clinical and economic perspective on head injury rehabilitation. *Journal of Head Trauma Rehabilitation, 8,* 1–14.

Courville, J. (1937). *Pathology of the central nervous system.* Mountain View, CA: Pacific Publishers.

Crépeau, F., Scherzer, B.P., Belleville, S., & Desmarais, G. (1997). A qualitative analysis of central executive disorders in a real-life work situation. *Neuropsychological Rehabilitation, 7*(2), 147–165.

Curl, R.M., Fraser, R.T., Cook, R.G., & Clemmons, D. (1996). Traumatic brain injury vocational rehabilitation: Preliminary findings for the coworker as trainer project. *Journal of Head Trauma Rehabilitation, 11,* 75–85.

Damasio, A.R. (1994). *Descartes error.* New York: Harper-Collins.

Damasio, A.R., Tranel, D., & Damasio, H. (1990). Individuals with sociopathic behavior caused by frontal lobe damage fail to respond automatically to socially charged stimuli. *Behavioral Brain Research, 14,* 81–94.

Damasio, A.R., Tranel, D., & Damasio, H. (1991). Somatic markers and the guidance of behavior: Theory and preliminary testing. In H.S. Levin, H.M. Eisenberg, & A.L. Benton (eds.), *Frontal lobe function and dysfunction* (pp. 217–229). New York: Oxford University Press.

Deci, E.L. (1995). *Why we do what we do: Understanding self-motivation.* New York: Penguin Books.

Denckla, M.B. (1996). Research on executive function in a neurodevelopmental context: Application of clinical measures. *Developmental Neuropsychology, 12,* 5–15.

Dennis, M. (1991). Frontal lobe function in childhood and adolescence: A heuristic for assessing attention regulation, executive control, and the intentional states important for social discourse. *Developmental Neuropsychology, 7*(3), 327–358.

Dennis, M. (1992). Word–finding in children and adolescents with a history of brain injury. *Topics in Language Disorders, 13,* 66–82.

Dennis, M. & Barnes, M. (1990). Knowing the meaning, getting the point, bridging the gap, and carrying the message: Aspects of discourse following closed head injury in childhood and adolescence. *Brain and Language, 39,* 428–446.

Dennis, M. & Barnes, M. (1994). Developmental aspects of neuropsychology. In D. Zaidel (ed.), *Handbook of perception and cognition: Neuropsychology, Vol. 15* (pp. 219–246). New York: Academic Press.

Dennis, M., Barnes, M.A., Donnelly, R.E., Wilkinson, M., & Humphreys, R.P. (1996). Appraising and managing knowledge: Metacognitive skills after childhood head injury. *Developmental Neuropsychology, 12,* 77–103.

Dennis, M., & Lovett, M. (1990). Discourse ability in children after brain damage. In Y. Joanette & H.H. Brownell (eds.), *Discourse ability and brain damage: Theoretical and empirical perspectives* (pp. 199–223). New York: Springer Verlag.

Dodd, D. & White, R.M. (1980). *Cognition: Mental structures and processes.* Boston, MA: Allyn & Bacon.

Donnellan, A.M., Mirenda, P.L., Mesaros, R.A., & Fassbender, L.L. (1984). Analyzing the communicative functions of aberrant behavior. *Journal of the Association for Persons with Severe Handicaps, 9,* 201–212.

Doss, S. & Reichle, J. (1989). Establishing communicative alternatives to the emission of socially motivated excess behavior: A review. *Journal of the Association for Persons with Severe Handicaps, 14,* 101–112.

Dunlap, G., dePerczel, M., Clarke, S., Wilson, D., Wright, S., White, R., & Gomez, A. (1994). Choice-making to promote adaptive behavior for students with emotional and behavioral challenges. *Journal of Applied Behavior Analysis, 27,* 505–518.

Durand, V.M. & Crimmins, D.B. (1992). *The Motivation Assessment Scale.* Topeka, KS: Monaco & Assoc.

Dywan, J. & Segalowitz, S.J. (1996). Self- and family-ratings of adaptive behavior after traumatic brain injury: Psychometric scores and frontally generated RRPs. *Journal of Head Trauma Rehabilitation, 11*(2), 75–79.

Ehrlich, J.S. (1988). Selective characteristics of narrative discourse in head-injured and normal adults. *Journal of Communication Disorders, 21,* 1–9.

Eslinger, P.J. & Damasio, A.R. (1985). Severe disturbance of higher cognition following bilateral frontal lobe oblation: Patient EVR. *Neurology, 35,* 1731–1741.

Evans, P. (1993). Some implications of Vygotsky's work for special education. In H. Daniels (ed.), *Charting the agenda: Education activity after Vygotsky.* London: Routledge.

Ewert, J., Levin, H.S., Watson, M.G., & Kalisky, Z. (1989). Procedural memory during posttraumatic amnesia in survivors of severe closed head injury: Implications for rehabilitation. *Archives of Neurology, 46,* 911–916.

Federal Register (1991, August). Public Law 101–476: Individuals with disabilities education act: IDEA. Department of Education.

Feeney, T.J. & Urbanczyk, B. (1994). Behavior as language. In R.C. Savage & G. Wolcott (eds.), *Educational dimensions of acquired brain injury* (pp. 277–302). Austin, TX: Pro-Ed.

Feeney, T.J. & Ylvisaker, M. (1995). Choice and routine: Antecedent behavior interventions for adolescents with severe traumatic brain injury. *Journal of Head Trauma Rehabilitation, 10,* 67–86.

Feeney, T.J. & Ylvisaker, M. (1997). Communication-based approaches to challenging behaviors after brain injury. In G.H.S. Singer, A. Glang, & B. Todis (eds.), *Traumatic brain injury: The School's response* (pp. 229–254). Baltimore, MD: Paul H. Brookes.

Feeney, T., Ylvisaker, M., Rosen, B., & Greene, P. (in press). Cost effectiveness of community supports for individuals with challenging behavior after TBI: Public policy implications. *Journal of Head Trauma Rehabilitation.*

Feuerstein, R. (1979). *The dynamic assessment of retarded performers: The learning potential assessment device, theory, instruments, and techniques.* Baltimore, MD: University Park Press.

Fey, M. (1986). *Language intervention with young children.* San Diego, CA: College-Hill Press.

Fife, D., Faich, G., Hollinshead, W., & Boynton, W. (1986). Incidence and outcome of hospital-treated head injury in Rhode Island. *American Journal of Public Health, 77,* 810–812.

Filley, C.M., Cranberg, M.D., Alexander, M.P., & Hart, E.J. (1987). Neurobehavioral outcome after closed head injury in childhood and adolescence. *Archives of Neurology, 44,* 194–198.

Fivush, R. (1991). The social construction of personal narratives. *Merrill-Palmer Quarterly, 37*(1), 59–81.

Fivush, R. & Fromhoff, F.A. (1988). Style and structure in mother-child conversations about the past. *Discourse Processes, 11,* 337–355.

Fivush, R. & Reese, E. (1992). The social construction of autobiographical memory. In M.A. Conway, D.C. Rubin, H. Spinnler, & W.A. Wagenaar (eds.), *Theoretical perspectives on autobiographical memory* (pp. 115–132). The Netherlands: Kluwer Academic Publishers.

Flavell, J.H., Miller, P.H., & Miller, S.A. (1993). *Cognitive development.* (3rd ed.). Englewood Cliffs, NJ: Prentice-Hall.

Fletcher, J.M., Levin, H.S., & Butler, I.J. (1995). Neurobehavioral effects of brain injury on children: Hydrocephalus, traumatic brain injury, and cerebral palsy. In M.C. Roberts (ed.), *Handbook of pediatric psychology* (2nd ed.) (pp. 362–383). New York: Guilford Press.

Fowler, R. (1996). Supporting students with challenging behaviors in general education settings: A review of behavioral momentum techniques and guidelines for use. *The Oregon Conference Monograph, 8,* 137–155.

Frattali, C.M., Thompson, C.K., Holland, A.L., Wohl, C.B., & Ferketic, M.M. (1995). *The American Speech-Language-Hearing Association Functional Assessment of Communication Skills for Adults (ASHA FACS).* Rockville, MD: ASHA.

Gajar, A., Schloss, P.J., Schloss, C.N., & Thompson, C.K. (1984). Effects of feedback and self-monitoring on head trauma youths'

conversation skills. *Journal of Applied Behavior Analysis, 17,* 353–358.

Gennarelli, T.A., Thibault, L.E., Adams, J.H., Graham, D.I., Thompson, C.J., & Marcincin, R.P. (1982). Diffuse axonal injury and traumatic coma in the primate. *Annals of Neurology, 12,* 564–574.

Gerberich, S.G., Priest, J.D., Boen, J.R., Staub, C.P., & Maxwell, R.E. (1983). Concussion incidences and severity in secondary school varsity football players. *American Journal of Public Health, 73,* 1370–1375.

Giangreco, M.F., Cloninger, C.J., & Iverson, V.S. (1993). *Choosing Options and Accommodations for Children (COACH): A guide to planning inclusive education.* Baltimore, MD: Paul H. Brookes.

Glisky, E.L. & Schacter, D.L. (1988). Acquisition of domain-specific knowledge in patients with organic memory disorders. *Journal of Learning Disabilities, 21,* 333–339, 351.

Glisky, E.L. & Schacter, D.L. (1989). Models and methods of memory rehabilitation. In F. Boller & J. Grafman (eds.), *Handbook of neuropsychology, Vol. 3: Sec. 5. Memory and its disorders* (pp. 233–246). Amsterdam: Elsevier.

Gluck, M.A. & Myers, C.E. (1995). Representation and association in memory: A neurocomputational view of hippocampal function. *Current Directions in Psychological Science, 4,* 23–29.

Goldman, P.S. (1971). Functional development of the prefrontal cortex early in life and the problem of neural plasticity. *Experimental Neurology, 32,* 366–387.

Goldstein, F.C. & Levin, H.S. (1995). Neurobehavioral outcome of traumatic brain injury in older adults: Initial findings. *Journal of Head Trauma Rehabilitation, 10,* 57–73.

Goldstein, A.P., Sprafkin, R.P., Gershaw, N.J., & Klein, P. (1980). *Skillstreaming the adolescent: A structured learning approach to teaching prosocial skills.* Champaign, IL: Research Press.

Gollwitzer, P.M. (1999). Implementation intentions: Strong effects of simple plans. *American Psychologist, 54,* 493–503.

Grafman, J. (1995). Similarities and distinctions among current models of prefrontal cortical functions. In J. Grafman, K.J. Holyoak, & F. Boller (eds.), *Structure and function of the human prefrontal cortex* (pp. 337–368). New York: The New York Academy of Sciences.

Grafman, J., Sirigu, A., Spector, L., & Hendler, J. (1993). Damage to the prefrontal cortex leads to decomposition of structured event complexes. *Journal of Head Trauma Rehabilitation, 8,* 73–87.

Grattan, L.M., & Eslinger, P.J. (1991). Frontal lobe damage in children and adults: A comparative review. *Developmental Neuropsychology, 7,* 283–326.

Groher, M. (1977). Language and memory disorders following closed head trauma. *Journal of Speech and Hearing Research, 20,* 212–223.

Groher, M. (1990). Communication disorders in adults. In M. Rosenthal, E. Griffith, M. Bond, & J.D. Miller (eds.), *Rehabilitation of the adult and child with traumatic brain injury* (pp. 148–162). Philadelphia: F.A. Davis.

Gronwall, D. & Wrightson, P. (1975). Cumulative effect of concussion. *Lancet, 2,* 995–997.

Haas, J., Cope, D.N., & Hall, K. (1987). Premorbid prevalence of poor academic performance in severe head injury. *Journal of Neurology, Neurosurgery, and Psychiatry, 50,* 52–56.

Haden, C.A., Haine, R.A., & Fivush, R. (1997). Developing narrative structure in parent-child reminiscing across the preschool years. *Developmental Psychology, 33,* 295–307.

Hagen, C. (1981). Language disorders secondary to closed head injury. *Topics in Language Disorders, 1,* 73–87.

Hall, K.M. (1992). Overview of functional assessment scales in brain injury rehabilitation. *NeuroRehabilitation, 2,* 98–113.

Hall, K.M., Karzmark, P., Stevens, M., Englander, J., O'Hare, P., & Wright, J. (1994). Family stressors in traumatic brain injury: A two-year follow-up. *Archives of Physical Medicine and Rehabilitation, 75,* 876–884.

Halle, J.W. & Spradlin, J.E. (1993). Identifying stimulus control of challenging behavior: Extending the analysis. In J. Reichle & D.P. Wacker (eds.), *Communicative alternative to challenging behavior: Integrating functional assessment and intervention strategies* (pp. 83–109). Baltimore: Paul H. Brookes.

Hallowell, E.M. & Ratey, J.J. (1994). *Driven to distraction.* New York: Touchstone.

Halpern, H. Darley, F.L., & Brown, J.R. (1973). Differential language and neurologic characteristics in cerebral involvement. *Journal of Speech and Hearing Disorders, 38,* 162–173.

Harchik, A.E., Sherman, J.A., & Bannerman, D.J. (1993). Choice and control: New opportunities for people with developmental disabilities. *Annals of Clinical Psychiatry, 5,* 151–162.

Hart, T. & Jacobs, H. (1993). Rehabilitation and management of behavior disturbances following frontal lobe injury. *Journal of Head Trauma Rehabilitation, 8,* 1–12.

Hartley, L.L. (1995). *Cognitive-communicative abilities following brain injury: A functional approach.* San Diego, CA: Singular Publishing Group.

Hartley, L.L. & Jensen, P.J. (1991). Narrative and procedural discourse after closed head injury. *Brain Injury, 5,* 267–285.

Hartshorne, N.J., Harruff, R.C., & Alvord, E.C. (1997). Fatal head injuries in ground-level falls. *American Journal of Medical Pathology, 18,* 258–264.

Heilman, K.M., Safran, A., & Geschwind, N. (1971). Closed head trauma and aphasia. *Journal of Neurology, Neurosurgery, and Psychiatry, 34,* 265–269.

Helm-Estabrooks, N., & Hotz, G. (1991). *Brief Test of Head Injury (BTHI).* Chicago, IL: Riverside.

Henri, B.P. & Hallowell, B. (1999). Mastering managed care: Problems and possibilities. In B. Cornett (ed.), *Clinical practice management in speech-language pathology: Principles and practicalities* (pp. 3–28). Gaithersburg, MD: Aspen.

Horner, R.H., Dunlap, G., & Koegel, R.L. (eds.) (1988). *Generalization and maintenance: Lifestyle changes in applied settings.* Baltimore, MD: Paul H. Brookes.

Hudson, J.A. (1990). The emergence of autobiographical memory in mother-child conversations. In R. Fivush & J.A. Hudson (eds.), *Knowing and remembering in young children* (pp. 166–196). New York: Cambridge University Press.

Iwata, B.A., Vollmer, T.R., & Zarcone, J.R. (1990). The experimental (functional) analysis of behavior disorders: Methodology, applications, and limitations. In A.C. Repp & N.N. Singh (eds.), *Perspectives on the use of nonaversive and aversive interventions for persons with developmental disabilities* (pp. 301–330). Sycamore, IL: Sycamore Publishing Co.

Izard, C.E. (1992). Four systems for emotion activation: Cognitive and noncognitive. *Psychological Review, 100,* 68–90.

Jacobs, H.E. (1993). *Behavior analysis guidelines and brain injury rehabilitation: People, principles, and programs.* Gaithersburg, MD: Aspen.

James, W. (1890). *Principles of psychology, Vol. 1.* New York: Dover.

Jennett, B. & Bond, M. (1975). Assessment of outcome after severe brain damage: A practical scale. *Lancet, 1,* 480–484.

Johnson, A. (1999). Speech-language pathology in health settings: A view of the future. In B. Cornett (ed.), *Clinical practice management in speech-language pathology: Principles and practicalities* (pp. 219–242). Gaithersburg, MD: Aspen.

Johnson, D.A. & Newton, A. (1987). Social adjustment and interaction after severe head injury: II. Rationale and bases for intervention. *British Journal of Clinical Psychology, 26,* 289–298.

Kaplan, E. (1988). A process approach to neuropsychological assessment. In T. Boll & B.K. Bryant (eds.), *Clinical neuropsychology and brain function: Research, measurement, and practice* (pp. 129–167). Washington, DC: American Psychological Association.

Katz, D.I. (1992). Neuropathology and neurobehavioral recovery from closed head injury. *Journal of Head Trauma Rehabilitation, 7,* 1–15.

Katz, D.I. & Alexander, M.P. (1994). Traumatic brain injury. In D.C. Good & J.R. Couch (eds.), *Handbook of neurorehabilitation* (pp. 493–549). New York: Decker.

Kavale, K. & Mattson, P. (1983). "One jumped off the balance beam": Meta-analysis of perceptual-motor training. *Journal of Learning Disabilities, 16,* 165–173.

Kay, T. & Lezak, M. (1990). The nature of head injury. In D.W. Corthell (ed.), *Traumatic brain injury and vocational rehabilitation* (pp. 21–65). Menomonie, WI: University of Wisconsin, Stout.

Kennedy, C.H. (1994). Manipulating antecedent conditions to alter the stimulus control of problem behavior. *Journal of Applied Behavior Analysis, 27,* 161–170.

Kennedy, C.H., Itkonen, T., & Lindquist, K. (1995). Comparing interspersed requests and social comments for increasing student compliance. *Journal of Applied Behavior Analysis, 28,* 97–98.

Kern, L., Childs, K.E., Dunlap, G., Clarke, S., & Falk, G.D. (1994). Using assessment based curricular intervention to improve the classroom behavior of a student with emotional and behavioral challenges. *Journal of Applied Behavior Analysis, 27,* 7–19.

Klonoff, P.S., Costa, L.D., & Snow, W.G. (1986). Predictors and indicators of quality of life in patients with closed-head injury. *Journal of Clinical and Experimental Neuropsychology, 8,* 469–485.

Koegel, R. & Koegel, L.K. (1995). *Teaching children with autism: Strategies for initiating positive interactions and improving learning opportunities.* Baltimore, MD: Paul H. Brookes.

Koegel, L.K., Koegel, R.L., & Dunlap, G. (1997). *Positive behavioral support: Including people with difficult behavior in the community.* Baltimore, MD: Paul H. Brookes.

Kraus, J.F. (1993). Epidemiology of head injury. In P.R. Cooper (ed.), *Head injury* (3rd ed.). Baltimore, MD: Williams & Wilkins.

Kraus, J.F. & Nourjah, P. (1988). The epidemiology of mild, uncomplicated brain injury. *Journal of Trauma, 28,* 1637–1643.

Kraus, J.F., Rock, A., & Hemyari, P. (1990). Brain injuries among infants, children, adolescents, and young adults. *American Journal of Diseases of Childhood, 144,* 684–691.

Kreutzer, J.S. (1999). Commentary: Cognitive rehabilitation outcomes. *Journal of Head Trauma Rehabilitation, 14*, 312–315.

Kreutzer, J.S., Marwitz, Seel, R., & Serio, C. (1996). Validation of a neurobehavioral inventory for adults with traumatic brain injury. *Archives of Physical Medicine and Rehabilitation, 77*, 116–124.

LeDoux, J.E. (1991). Emotion and the limbic system concept. *Concepts in Neuroscience, 2*, 169–199.

LeDoux, J.E. (1996). *The emotional brain*. New York: Touchstone.

Levin, H.S., Benton, A.L., & Grossman, R.G. (1982). *Neurobehavioral consequences of closed head injury*. New York: Oxford University Press.

Levin, H.S., Goldstein, F.C., Williams, D.H., & Eisenberg, H.M. (1991). The contribution of frontal lobe lesions to the neurobehavioral outcome of closed head injury. In H.S. Levin, H.M. Eisenberg, & A.L. Benton (eds.), *Frontal lobe function and dysfunction* (pp. 318–338). New York: Oxford University Press.

Levin, H.S., Grossman, R.G., Sarwar, M., & Meyers, C.A. (1981). Linguistic recovery after closed head injury. *Brain and Language, 12*, 360–374.

Levin, H.S., O'Donnell, V.M., & Grossman, R.G. (1979). The Galveston Orientation and Amnesia Test: A practical scale to assess cognition after head injury. *Journal of Nervous and Mental Diseases, 167*, 675–684.

Lezak, M. (1982). The problem of assessing executive functions. *International Journal of Psychology, 17*, 281–297.

Lezak, M. (1986). Psychological implications of traumatic brain damage for the patient's family. *Rehabilitation Psychology, 31*, 241–250.

Lezak, M. (1987). Relationships between personality disorders, social disturbances, and physical disability following traumatic brain injury. *Journal of Head Trauma Rehabilitation, 2*, 57–69.

Liles, B.J., Coelho, C.A., Duffy, R.J., & Zalagens, M.R. (1989). Effects of elicitation procedures on the narratives of normal and closed head-injured adults. *Journal of Speech and Hearing Disorders, 54*, 356–366.

Livingston, M.G. & Brooks, D.N. (1988). The burden on families of the brain injured: A review. *Journal of Head Trauma Rehabilitation, 3*, 6–15.

Luria, A.R. (1966). *Higher cortical functions in man*. New York: Basic Books.

Luria, A.R. (1970). *Traumatic aphasia: Its syndromes, psychology, and treatment*. The Hague: Mouton.

Luria, A.R. (1979). *The making of mind: A personal account of Soviet psychology*. Cambridge, MA: Harvard University Press.

Mace, F.C., Hock, M.L., Lalli, J.S., West, B.J., Belfore, P., Pinter, E., & Brown, K. (1988). Behavioral momentum in the treatment of noncompliance. *Journal of Applied Behavior Analysis, 21*, 123–132.

Mace, F.C., Lalli, J.S., Shea, M.C., Lalli, E.P., West, B.J., Roberts, M., & Nevin, J.A. (1990). The momentum of human behavior in a natural setting. *Journal of the Experimental Analysis of Behavior, 54*, 163–172.

Mace, F.C., Mauro, B.C., Boyajian, A.E., & Eckert, T.L. (1997). Effects of reinforcer quality on behavioral momentum: Coordinated applied and basic research. *Journal of Applied Behavior Analysis, 30*, 1–20.

MacDonald, J. (1989). *Becoming partners with children: From play to conversation*. Chicago, IL: Riverside.

Malec, J.F. & Thompson, J.M. (1994). Relationship of the Mayo-Portland Adaptability Inventory to functional outcome and cognitive performance measures. *Journal of Head Trauma Rehabilitation, 9*, 1–11.

Mann, L. (1979). *On the trail of process: A historical perspective on cognitive processes and their training*. New York: Grune & Stratton.

Martin, G. & Pear, J. (1996). *Behavior modification: What it is and how to do it* (5th ed.). Upper Saddle River, NJ: Prentice Hall.

Mateer, C.A. & Mapou, R.L. (1996). Understanding, evaluating, and managing attention disorders following traumatic brain injury. *Journal of Head Trauma Rehabilitation, 11*, 1–16.

Mateer, C.A. & Williams, D. (1991). Effects of frontal lobe injury in childhood. *Developmental Neuropsychology, 7*, 359–376.

McCabe, A. & Peterson, C. (1991). Getting the story: A longitudinal study of parental styles in eliciting narratives and developing narrative skills (pp. 217–253). In A. McCabe & C. Peterson (eds.), *New directions in developing narrative structure*. Hillsdale, NJ: Lawrence Erlbaum.

McDonald, S. (1992a). Communication disorders following closed head injury: New approaches to assessment and rehabilitation. *Brain Injury, 6*, 283–292.

McDonald, S. (1992b). Differential pragmatic language loss following severe closed head injury: Inability to comprehend conversational implicature. *Applied Psycholinguistics, 13*, 295–312.

McDonald, S. (1993). Pragmatic language loss following closed head injury: Inability to meet the informational needs of the listener. *Brain and Language, 44*, 28–46.

McDonald, S., & Pearce, S. (1998). Requests that overcome listener reluctance: Impairment associated with executive dysfunction in brain injury. *Brain and Language, 61*, 88–104.

McIntosh, S., Vaughn, S., & Zaragoza, N. (1991). A review of social interventions for students with learning disabilities. *Journal of Learning Disabilities, 24*, 451–458.

McKinlay, W.W., Brooks, D.N., Bond, M.R., Martinage, D.P., & Marshall, M.M. (1981). The short-term outcome of severe blunt head injury as reported by relatives of the injured persons. *Journal of Neurology, Neurosurgery, and Psychiatry, 44*, 529.

Meichenbaum, D. (1993). The "potential" contributions of cognitive behavior modification to the rehabilitation of individuals with traumatic brain injury. *Seminars in Speech and Language, 14*, 18–30.

Meichenbaum, D. & Biemiller, A. (1998). *Nurturing independent learners: Helping students take charge of their learning*. Cambridge, MA: Brookline Books.

Mendelsohn, D., Levin, H.S., Bruce, D., Lilly, M.A., Harward, H., Culhane, K., & Eisenberg, H.M. (1992). Late MRI after head injury in children: Relationship to clinical features and outcome. *Child's Nervous System, 8*, 445–452.

Mentis, M. & Prutting, C. (1987). Cohesion in the discourse of head injured and normal adults. *Journal of Speech and Hearing Research, 30*, 88–98.

Mentis, M. & Prutting, C.A. (1991). Analysis of topic as illustrated in a head-injured and a normal adult. *Journal of Speech and Hearing Research, 34*, 583–595.

Milton, S.B., Prutting, C.A., & Binder, G.M. (1984). Appraisal of communicative competence in head injured adults. In

R. Brookshire (ed.), *Clinical aphasiology conference proceedings.* Minneapolis, MN: BRK.

Milton, S.B. & Wertz, R.T. (1986). Management of persisting communication deficits in patients with traumatic brain injury. In B.P. Uzzell & Y. Gross (eds.), *Clinical neuropsychology of intervention.* Boston: Martinus Nijhoff.

Morris, E.K. (1992). The aim, progress, and evolution of behavior analysis. *The Behavior Analyst, 15,* 3–29.

Morton, V.M. & Wehman, P. (1995). Psychosocial and emotional sequelae of individuals with traumatic brain injury: A literature review and recommendations. *Brain Injury, 9,* 81–92.

Nelson, K. (1992). Emergence of autobiographical memory at age 4. *Human Development, 35*(3), 172–177.

Newcomb, F. (1969). *Missel wounds of the brain.* London: Oxford University Press.

NIH (1999). *Report of the Consensus Development Conference on the rehabilitation of persons with traumatic brain injury.* National Institutes of Health: Rockville, MD.

Oddy, M. (1984). Head injury and social adjustment. In N. Brooks (ed.), *Closed head injury: Psychological, social, and family consequences* (pp. 108–192). New York: Oxford University Press.

Oddy, M., Coughlan, T., Tyerman, A., & Jenkins, D. (1985). Social adjustment after closed head injury: A further follow-up seven years after injury. *Journal of Neurology, Neurosurgery, and Psychiatry, 48,* 565.

Pace, G.M. & Ivancic, M.T. (1994). Stimulus fading as treatment for obscenity in a brain-damaged client. *Journal of Applied Behavior Analysis, 27,* 302–305.

Palinscar, A.S. & Brown, A.L. (1989). Classroom dialogues to promote self-regulated comprehension. In J. Brophy (ed.), *Teaching for understanding and self-regulated learning, Vol. 1.* Greenwich, CT: JAI Press.

Palinscar, A.S., Brown, A.L., & Campione, J.C. (1994). Models and practices of dynamic assessment. In G.P. Wallach & K.G. Butler (eds.), *Language learning disabilities in school-age children and adolescents* (pp. 132–134). New York: Macmillan.

Pang, D. (1985). Pathophysiologic correlates of neurobehavioral syndromes following closed head injury. In M. Ylvisaker (ed.), *Head injury rehabilitation: Children and adolescents* (pp. 3–70). Newton, MA: Butterworth-Heinemann.

Park, N.W. & Ingles, J.L. (in press). Effectiveness of attention rehabilitation after an acquired brain injury: A meta-analysis. *Neuropsychology.*

Park, N.W., Proulx, G.B., & Towers, W. M. (1999). Evaluation of the Attention Process Training Programme. *Neuropsychological Rehabilitation, 9,* 135–154.

Pascual-Leone, A., Grafman, J., & Hallett, M. (1995). Procedural learning and prefrontal cortex. In J. Grafman, K.J. Holyoak, & F. Boller (eds.), *Structure and function of the human prefrontal cortex* (pp. 61–70). New York: The New York Academy of Sciences.

Payne, J.C. (1999). *Adult neurogenic language disorders: Assessment and treatment.* San Diego, CA: Singular Publishing Group.

Pearce, S., McDonald, S., & Coltheart, M. (1998). Ability to process ambiguous advertisements after frontal lobe damage. *Brain and Cognition, 38,* 150–164.

Petterson, L. (1991). Sensitivity to emotional cues and social behavior in children and adolescents after head injury. *Perceptual and Motor Skills, 73*(3 pt. 2), 1139–1150.

Petrides, M. (1995). Functional organization of the human frontal cortex for mnemonic processing. In J. Grafman, K.J. Holyoak, & F. Boller (eds.), *Structure and function of the human prefrontal cortex* (pp. 85–96). New York: The New York Academy of Sciences.

Ponsford, J. (1990). The use of computers in the rehabilitation of attention disorders. In R.L. Wood & I. Fussey (eds.), *Cognitive rehabilitation in perspective* (pp. 48–67). New York: Taylor & Francis.

Ponsford, J.L., Olver, J.H., Curren, C., & Ng, K. (1995). Prediction of employment status two years after traumatic brain injury. *Brain Injury, 9,* 11–20.

Powell, J.H., Beckers, K., & Greenwood, R.J. (1998). The measurement of progress and outcome in community rehabilitation after brain injury: A new assessment measure, the BIRCO-39 Scales. *Archives of Physical Medicine and Rehabilitation.*

Pressley, M. (1993). Teaching cognitive strategies to brain-injured clients: The good information processing perspective. *Seminars in Speech and Language, 14,* 1–16.

Pressley, M. (1995). More about the development of self-regulation: Complex, long-term, and thoroughly social. *Educational Psychology, 30,* 207–212.

Pressley, M. & Associates (1990). *Cognitive strategy instruction that really improves children's academic performance.* Cambridge, MA: Brookline Books.

Pressley, M., Borkowski, J.G., & Schneider, W. (1989). Good information processing: What is it and what education can do to promote it. *International Journal of Educational Research, 13,* 857–867.

Prigatano, G.P. (1986). *Neuropsychological rehabilitation after brain injury.* Baltimore, MD: Johns Hopkins University Press.

Prigatano, G.P. (1999). Commentary: Beyond statistics and research design. *Journal of Head Trauma Rehabilitation, 14,* 308–311.

Prigatano, G.P. & Altman, I.M. (1990). Impaired awareness of behavioral limitations after traumatic brain injury. *Archives of Physical Medicine and Rehabilitation, 71,* 1058.

Prigatano, G.P., Roueche, J.R., & Fordyce, D.J. (1985). Nonaphasic language disturbances after closed head injury. *Language Sciences, 1,* 217–229.

Rappaport, M., Hall, K.M., Hopkins, H.K., & Belleza, T., & Cope, D.N. (1982). Disability Rating Scale for severe head trauma: Coma to community. *Archives of Physical Medicine and Rehabilitation, 63,* 118–123.

Reese, E. & Fivush, G. (1993). Parental styles of talking about the past. *Developmental Psychology, 29,* 596–606.

Reese, E., Haden, C.A., & Fivush, R. (1993). Mother-child conversations about the past: Relationships of style and memory over time. *Cognitive Development, 8,* 403–430.

Reichle, J. & Johnston, S.S. (1993). Replacing challenging behavior: The role of communication intervention. *Topics in Language Disorders, 13,* 61–76.

Reichle, J. & Wacker, D.P. (eds.) (1993). *Communicative alternatives to challenging behavior.* Baltimore, MD: Paul H. Brookes.

Rimel, R.W., Giordani, B., Barth, J.T., Boll, T.J., & Jane, J.A. (1981). Disability caused by minor head injury. *Neurosurgery, 9,* 221–228.

Robinson, T.R., Smith, S.W., Miller, M.D., & Brownell, M.T. (1999). Cognitive behavior modification of hyperactivity/impulsivity and aggression: A meta-analysis of school-based studies. *Journal of Educational Psychology, 91,* 195–203.

Rogoff, B. (1990). *Apprenticeship in thinking: Cognitive development in social context.* New York: Oxford University Press.

Rolls, E.T., Hornak, J., Wade, D., & McGrath, J. (1994). Emotion-related learning in patients with social and emotional changes associated with frontal lobe damage. *Journal of Neurology, Neurosurgery, and Psychiatry, 57,* 1518–1524.

Ross-Swain, D. (1996). *Ross Information Processing Assessment* (RIPA-2). Austin, TX: Pro-Ed.

Santora, T.A., Schinco, K.A., & Trooskin, S.Z. (1994). Management of trauma in the elderly patient. *Surgical Clinics of North America, 74,* 164–186.

Sarno, M.T. (1980). The nature of verbal impairment after closed head injury. *Journal of Nervous and Mental Disease, 168,* 685–692.

Sarno, M.T. (1984). Verbal impairment after closed head injury: Report of a replication study. *Journal of Nervous and Mental Disease, 172,* 475–479.

Sarno, M.T., Buonaguro, A., & Levita, E. (1986). Characteristics of verbal impairment in closed head injured patients. *Archives of Physical Medicine and Rehabilitation, 67,* 400–405.

Schacter, D.L. (1996). *Searching for memory: The brain, the mind and the past.* New York: Basic Books.

Schacter, D.L. & Glisky, E.L. (1986). Memory remediation: Restoration, alleviation, and the acquisition of domain-specific knowledge. In B. Uzzell & Y. Gross (eds.), *Clinical neuropsychology of intervention* (pp. 257–282). Boston: Martinus Nijhoff.

Schmidt, N.D. (1997). Outcome-oriented rehabilitation: A response to managed care. *Journal of Head Trauma Rehabilitation, 12,* 44–50.

Schneider, P. & Watkins, R. (1996). Applying Vygotskyan developmental theory to language intervention. *Language, Speech, and Hearing Services in the Schools, 27,* 157–170.

Schwartz, M.F. (1995). Re-examining the role of executive functions in routine action production. In J. Grafman, K.J. Holyoak, & F. Boller (eds.), *Structure and function of the human prefrontal cortex* (pp. 321–335). New York: The New York Academy of Sciences.

Schwartz, M.F., Mayer, N.H., FitzpatrickDeSalme, E.J., & Montgomery, M.W. (1993). Cognitive theory and the study of everyday action disorders after brain damage. *Journal of Head Trauma Rehabilitation, 8(1),* 59–72.

Schweinhart, L.J. & Weikart, D.P. (1993). Success by empowerment: The High/Scope Perry preschool study through age 27. *Young Children, 49,* 54–58.

Shallice, T. (1982). Specific impairments of planning. *Philosophical Transactions of the Royal Society of London, 298,* 199–209.

Shammi, P. & Stuss, D.T. (1999). Humour appreciation: A role of the right frontal lobe. *Brain, 122,* 657–666.

Sheinker, J. & Sheinker, A. (1988). *Metacognitive approach to social skills training.* Rockville, MD: Aspen.

Shum, D., Sweeper, S., & Murray, R. (1996). Performance on verbal implicit and explicit memory tasks following traumatic brain injury. *Journal of Head Trauma Rehabilitation, 11,* 43–53.

Siegler, R. (1991). *Children's thinking.* Englewood Cliffs, NJ: Prentice Hall.

Singley, M.K. & Anderson, J.R. (1989). *Transfer of cognitive skill.* Cambridge, MA: Harvard University Press.

Skinner, B.F. (1938). *The Behavior of organisms: An experimental analysis.* New York: Appleton.

Slifer, K.J., Cataldo, M.D., Kurtz, P.F. (1995). Behavioral training during acute brain trauma rehabilitation: An empirical case study. *Brain Injury, 9,* 585–593.

Slifer, K.J., Tucker, C.L., Gerson, A.C., Cataldo, M.D., Sevier, R.C., Suter, A.H., & Kane, A.C. (1996). Operant conditioning for behavior during posttraumatic amnesia in children and adolescents with brain injury. *Journal of Head Trauma Rehabilitation, 11,* 39–50.

Sohlberg, M. & Mateer, C. (1987). *Introduction to cognitive rehabilitation: Theory and practice.* New York: Guilford Press.

Sosin, D.M., Sniezek, J.E., & Thurman, D.J. (1996). Incidence of mild and moderate brain injury in the United States, 1991. *Brain Injury, 10,* 47–54.

Squire, L.R. (1992). Memory and the hippocampus: A synthesis from findings with rats, monkeys, and humans. *Psychological Review, 99,* 195–231.

Squire, L.R., Knowlton, B., & Musen, G. (1993). The structure and organization of memory. *Annual Review in Psychology, 44,* 453–495.

Stelling, M.W., McKay, S.E., Carr, W.A., Walsh, J.W., & Bauman, R.J. (1986). Frontal lobe lesions and cognitive function in craniopharyngioma survivors. *American Journal of Diseases of Childhood, 140,* 710–714.

Stuss, D.T. (1999, October). New data on frontal functioning—localization and assessment. Workshop presented at the 20th Annual Neurorehabilitation Conference on Traumatic Brain Injury and Stroke, Boston, MA.

Stuss, D.T. (1999, October). Variability in performance and outcome after brain injury. Plenary lecture presented at the 20th Annual Neurorehabilitation Conference on Traumatic Brain Injury and Stroke, Boston, MA.

Stuss, D.T. & Alexander, M.P. (in press). Affectively burnt in: A proposed role of the right frontal lobe. In E. Tulving (ed.), *Memory, consciousness and the brain.* Oxford: Oxford University Press.

Stuss, D.T. & Benson, D.F. (1986). *The frontal lobes.* New York: Raven.

Stuss, D.T. & Buckle, L. (1992). Traumatic brain injury: Neuropsychological deficits and evaluation at different stages of recovery and in different pathologic subtypes. *Journal of Head Trauma Rehabilitation, 7,* 40–49.

Stuss, D.T., Pogue, J., Buckle, L., & Bondar, J. (1994). Characterization of stability of performance in patients with traumatic brain injury: Variability and consistency on reaction time tests. *Neuropsychology, 8,* 316–324.

Szekeres, S. (1993). Organization as an intervention target after traumatic brain injury. *Seminars in Speech and Language, 13,* 293–307.

Szekeres, S., Ylvisaker, M., & Holland, A. (1985). Cognitive rehabilitation therapy: A framework for intervention. In M. Ylvisaker (ed.), *Head injury rehabilitation: Children and adolescents.* Boston: College-Hill Press/Little, Brown.

Szekeres, S., Ylvisaker, M., & Cohen, S. (1987). A framework for cognitive rehabilitation therapy. In M. Ylvisaker & E. Gobble (eds.), *Community re-entry for head injured adults.* Boston: College-Hill Press/ Little, Brown.

Tate, R.L. (1998). It is not only the kind of injury that matters, but the kind of head: The contribution of premorbid psychosocial factors to rehabilitation outcomes after severe traumatic brain injury. *Neuropsychological Rehabilitation, 8,* 1–18.

Teasdale, J.D. (1997). The transformation of meaning: The interacting cognitive subsystems approach. In M. Power & C.R. Brewin (eds.), *The transformation of meaning in psychological therapies* (pp. 141–156). New York: John Wiley & Sons.

Teasdale, G. & Jennett, B. (1974). Assessment of coma and impaired consciousness. *Lancet, ii,* 81–84.

Thoene, A. (1996). Memory rehabilitation—recent developments and future directions. *Restorative Neurology and Neuroscience, 9,* 125–140.

Thomsen, I.V. (1974). The patient with severe head injury and his family. *Scandinavian Journal of Rehabilitation and Medicine, 6,* 180–183.

Thomsen, I.V. (1975). Evaluation and outcome of aphasia in patients with severe head trauma. *Journal of Neurology, Neurosurgery, and Psychiatry, 38,* 713–718.

Thomsen, I.V. (1984). Late outcome of very severe blunt head trauma: A 10–15 year second follow-up. *Journal of Neurology, Neurosurgery, and Psychiatry, 47,* 260–268.

Thomsen, I.V. (1987). Late psychosocial outcome in severe blunt head trauma. *Brain Injury, 1,* 131–143.

Thomsen, I.V. (1989). Do young patients have worse outcome after severe blunt head trauma? *Brain Injury, 3,* 157–162.

Thurman, D.J., & Guerrero, J. (1999a). Trends in hospitalization associated with traumatic brain injury. *Journal of the American Medical Association, 282,* 954–957.

Thurman, D.J. & Guerrero, J. (1999b). Trends in traumatic brain injury-related hospitalizations—United States, 1980–1995. In *Report of the Consensus Development Conference on the rehabilitation of persons with traumatic brain injury.* Bethesda, MD: National Institutes of Health.

Togher, L., Hand, L., & Code, C. (1997). Analysing discourse in the traumatic brain injury population: Telephone interactions with different communication partners. *Brain Injury, 11,* 169–189.

Tranel, D., Anderson, S.W., & Benton, A.I. (1995). Development of the concept of executive function and its relationship to the frontal lobes. In F. Boller & J. Grafman (eds.), *Handbook of neuropsychology* (pp. 125–148). Amsterdam: Elsevier.

Tranel, D. & Damasio, A. (1993). The covert learning of affective valence does not require structures in hippocampal system or amygdala. *Journal of Cognitive Neuroscience, 5,* 79–88.

Tulving, E., Kapur, S., Craik, F.I.M., Moscovitch, M., & Houle, S. (1994). Hemispheric encoding/retrieval asymmetry in episodic memory: Positron emission tomography findings. *Proceedings of the National Academy of Sciences, USA, 91,* 2016–2020.

Turkstra, L.S. & Holland, A.L. (1998). Assessment of syntax after adolescent brain injury: Effects of memory on test performance. *Journal of Speech, Language, and Hearing Research, 41,* 137–149.

U.S. Department of Transportation (1995). *Traffic safety facts 1994: Older population.* Washington, DC: National Highway Traffic Safety Administration.

Varney, N.R. & Menefee, L. (1993). Psychosocial and executive deficits following closed head injury: Implications for orbital frontal cortex. *Journal of Head Trauma Rehabilitation, 8,* 32–44.

Vygotsky, L.S. (1978). *Mind in society: The development of higher psychological processes* (M. Cole, V. John-Steiner, S. Scribner, & E.

Souberman, eds. & trans.). Cambridge, MA: Harvard University Press.

Vygotsky, L.S. (1981). The genesis of higher mental functions. In J.V. Wertsch (ed.), *The concept of activity in Soviet psychology* (pp. 144–189). Armonk, NY: M.E. Sharps.

Waksman, S., Messmer, C.L., & Waksman, D.D. (1989). *The Waksman Social Skills Curriculum: An assertive behavior program for adolescents.* Austin, TX: Pro-Ed.

Walker, H.M., McConnell, S.M., Holmes, D., Todis, B., Walker, J., & Golden, N. (1988a). *The Walker Social Skills Curriculum: The ACCEPTS program.* Austin, TX: Pro-Ed.

Walker, H.M., Todis, B., Holmes, D., & Horton, G. (1988b). *The Walker Social Skills Program: The ACCESS program: Adolescent curriculum for communication and effective social skills.* Austin, TX: Pro-Ed.

Walker, H.M., Schwarz, I.E., Nippold, M.A., Irvin, L.K., & Noell, J.W. (1994). Social skills in school-age children and youth: Issues and best practices in assessment and intervention. *Topics in Language Disorders, 14,* 70–82.

Weddell, R., Oddy, M., & Jenkins, D. (1980). Social adjustment after rehabilitation: A two year follow-up of patients with severe head injury. *Psychological Medicine, 10,* 257–263.

Wehman, P., Kregel, J., Sherron, P., Nguyen, S., Kreutzer, J., Fry, R., & Zasler, N. (1993). Critical factors associated with the successful supported employment of patients with severe traumatic brain injury. *Journal of Head Trauma Rehabilitation, 7,* 31–44.

Wehman, P. & Kreutzer, J.S. (1990). *Vocational rehabilitation for persons with acquired brain injury.* Rockville, MD: Aspen.

Wehman, P., West, M.D., Kregel, J., Sherron, P., & Kreutzer, J.S. (1995). Return to work for persons with severe traumatic brain injury: A data-based approach to program development. *Journal of Head Trauma Rehabilitation, 10,* 27–39.

Wehmeyer et al. (2000). Promoting causal agency: The self-determined learning model of instruction. *Exceptional Children, 66,* 439–453.

Wehmeyer, M. & Schwartz (1997). Self determination and positive adult outcomes: A follow-up study of youth with mental retardation or learning disabilities, *Exceptional Children, 4,* 245–255.

Welsh, M.C. & Pennington, B.F. (1988). Assessing frontal lobe functioning in children: Views from developmental psychology. *Developmental Neuropsychology, 4,* 199–230.

Welsh, M.C., Pennington, B.F., & Groisser, D.B. (1991). A normative-developmental study of executive function: A window on prefrontal function in children. *Developmental Neuropsychology, 7*(2), 131–149.

Westby, C.E. (1994). The effects of culture on genre, structure, and style of oral and written texts. In G.P. Wallach & K.G. Butler (eds.), *Language learning disabilities in school-age children and adolescents* (pp. 180–218). New York: Merrill.

Wiener, J. & Harris, P.J. (1998). Evaluation of an individualized, context-based social skills training program for children with learning disabilities. *Learning Disabilities Research and Practice, 12,* 40–53.

Willer, B., Ottenbacher, K.J., & Coad, M.L. (1994). The Community Integration Questionnaire. *American Journal of Physical and Medical Rehabilitation, 73,* 103–107.

Wilson, B.A. & Evans, J.J. (1996). Error-free learning in the rehabilitation of people with memory impairments. *Journal of Head Trauma Rehabilitation, 11,* 54–64.

Wilson, B.A., Baddeley, A.D., Evans, J.J., & Shiel, A. (1994). Errorless learning in the rehabilitation of memory-impaired people. *Neuropsychological Rehabilitation, 4,* 307–326.

Wilson, B. & Watson, P. (1996). A practical framework for understanding compensatory behaviour in people with organic memory impairment. *Memory, 4*(5), 465–486.

Wood, D., Bruner, J., & Ross, G. (1976). The role of tutoring in problem solving. *Journal of Child Psychology and Psychiatry, 17,* 89–100.

Wood, R. Ll. (1987). *Brain injury rehabilitation: A neurobehavioral approach.* London: Croom-Helm.

Wood, R. Ll. (1988). Management of behavior disorders in a day treatment setting. *Journal of Head Trauma Rehabilitation, 3,* 53–61.

Wood, R. Ll. (ed.) (1990). *Neurobehavioral consequences of traumatic brain injury.* London: Taylor and Francis.

World Health Organization (1980). *International classifications of impairments, diseases, and handicaps: A manual of classification relating to the consequences of diseases.* Geneva: WHO.

World Health Organization (1998). *Toward a common language for functioning and disablement: ICIDH-2, The international classification of impairments, activities, and participation.* Prefinal draft. Geneva: WHO.

Ylvisaker, M. (1992). Communication outcome following traumatic brain injury. *Seminars in Speech and Language, 13,* 239–251.

Ylvisaker, M. (1993). Communication outcome in children and adolescents with traumatic brain injury. *Neuropsychological Rehabilitation, 3,* 367–387.

Ylvisaker, M. (1999). A contextualized and routine-based approach to cognitive and behavioral rehabilitation: A historical perspective. In *Report of the NIH Consensus Development Conference on the Rehabilitation of Persons with Traumatic Brain Injury.* Bethesda, MD: National Institutes of Health.

Ylvisaker, M. & Feeney, T.J. (1994). Communication and behavior: Collaboration between speech-language pathologists and behavioral psychologists. *Topics in Language Disorders, 15,* 37–54.

Ylvisaker, M. & Feeney, T.J. (1995). Traumatic brain injury in adolescence. *Seminars in Speech and Language, 16,* 32–44.

Ylvisaker, M. & Feeney, T. (1996). Executive functions after traumatic brain injury: Supported cognition and self-advocacy. *Seminars in Speech and Language, 17,* 217–232.

Ylvisaker, M. & Feeney, T. (1998a). *Collaborative brain injury intervention: Positive everyday routines.* San Diego, CA: Singular Publishing Group.

Ylvisaker, M. & Feeney, T. (1998b). Everyday people as supports: Developing competencies through collaboration. In M. Ylvisaker (ed.), *Traumatic brain injury rehabilitation: Children and adolescents* (Rev. Ed.) (pp. 429–464). Boston: Butterworth-Heinemann.

Ylvisaker, M. & Feeney, T. (2000a). Reflections on Dobermanns, poodles, and social rehabilitation for difficult-to-serve individuals with traumatic brain injury. *Aphasiology, 14,* 407–431.

Ylvisaker, M. & Feeney, T. (2000b). Construction of identity after traumatic brain injury. *Brain Impairment, 1,* 12–28.

Ylvisaker, M., Feeney, J., & Feeney, T. (1999). An everyday approach to long-term rehabilitation after traumatic brain injury. In B. Cornett (ed.), *Clinical practice management in speech-language pathology: Principles and practicalities* (pp. 117–162). Gaithersburg, MD: Aspen.

Ylvisaker, M., Feeney, T., & Szekeres, S. (1998a). A social-environmental approach to communication and behavior. In M. Ylvisaker (ed.), *Traumatic brain injury rehabilitation: Children and adolescents* (Rev. Ed.) (pp. 271–302). Boston: Butterworth-Heinemann.

Ylvisaker, M., Feeney, T., & Urbanczyk, B. (1993a). Developing a positive rehabilitation culture for communication. In C. Durgin, N. Schmidt, & J. Freyer (eds.), *Brain injury rehabilitation: Clinical intervention and staff development techniques.* Baltimore, MD: Aspen.

Ylvisaker, M., Feeney, T.J., & Urbanczyk, B. (1993b). A social-environmental approach to communication and behavior after traumatic brain injury. *Seminars in Speech and Language, 14,* 74–87.

Ylvisaker, M. & Gioia, G. (1998). Comprehensive cognitive assessment. In M. Ylvisaker (ed.), *Traumatic brain injury rehabilitation: Children and adolescents* (Rev. Ed.) (pp. 159–179). Boston: Butterworth-Heinemann.

Ylvisaker, M. & Holland, A. (1985). Coaching, self-coaching, and the rehabilitation of head injury. In D. Johns (ed.), *Clinical management of neurogenic communicative disorders* (pp. 243–257). Boston: Little, Brown.

Ylvisaker, M., Sellars, C., & Edelman, L. (1998b). Rehabilitation after traumatic brain injury in preschoolers. In M. Ylvisaker (ed.), *Traumatic brain injury rehabilitation: Children and adolescents* (Rev. Ed.) (pp. 303–329). Boston: Butterworth-Heinemann.

Ylvisaker, M., Szekeres, S.F., & Feeney, T. (1998c). Cognitive rehabilitation: Executive functions. In M. Ylvisaker (ed.), *Traumatic brain injury rehabilitation: Children and adolescents* (Rev. Ed.) (pp. 221–269). Boston: Butterworth-Heinemann.

Ylvisaker, M., Szekeres, S.F., & Haarbauer-Krupa. J. (1998d). Cognitive rehabilitation: Organization, memory and language. In M. Ylvisaker (ed.), *Traumatic brain injury rehabilitation: Children and adolescents* (Rev. Ed.) (pp. 181–220). Boston: Butterworth-Heinemann.

Ylvisaker, M., Szekeres, S., Henry, K., Sullivan, D., & Wheeler, P. (1987). Topics in cognitive rehabilitation. In M. Ylvisaker & E. Gobble (eds.), *Community re-entry for head injured adults.* Boston: College Hill Press/Little, Brown.

Young, P.H. (1999, October). Anatomy and pathophysiology of traumatic brain injury and stroke. Presented at the 20th Annual Neurorehabilitation Conference on Traumatic Brain Injury and Stroke, Boston, MA.

Zaragoza, N., Vaughn, S., & McIntosh, R. (1991). Social skills interventions and children with behavior problems: A review. *Behavioral Disorders, 16,* 260–275.

Zasler, N.D., Kreutzer, J.S., & Taylor, D. (1991). Coma stimulation and coma recovery: A critical review. *NeuroRehabilitation, 1,* 33–40.

Zencius, A.H., Wesolowski, M.D., Burke, W.H., & McQuade, D. (1989). Antecedent control in the treatment of brain injured clients. *Brain Injury, 3,* 199–205.

APPENDIX 33–1
Conventional Versus Functional Approaches to Intervention After Brain Injury: Communication, Behavior, and Cognition

(Modified with permission from Ylvisaker, M. & Feeney, T. (1998). *Collaborative brain injury intervention: Positive everyday routines.* San Diego, CA: Singular Publishing Group.)

Scope of Intervention

Conventional Approach

1. *Speech-Language Pathology*: The focus is on speech and specific aspects of linguistic competence (semantics, syntax, morphology).
2. *Behavioral Psychology*: The focus is on management of specific problem behaviors in a narrow sense.
3. *Cognitive Rehabilitation*: The focus is on neuropsychological assessment and intervention that sequentially targets separate components of cognition, arranged in a hierarchy for treatment purposes.

Functional Approach

1. The focus of each profession is on helping individuals with brain injury achieve their real-world goals in real-world contexts, including academic, vocational, and social success.
2. Correctly understood, applied behavior analysis in psychology, pragmatics in speech-language pathology, and social-cognitive intervention in cognitive rehabilitation are essentially the same service, necessitating close collaboration among service providers.
3. Each profession recognizes the overarching importance of executive or self-control functions for academic, vocational, and social success.

Integration of Intervention: Collaboration

Conventional Approach

1. Cognition, communication, and behavior are targeted for assessment and intervention by separate professionals working in relative isolation.
2. Evaluation reports, including proposed goals, objectives, and plans to achieve the objectives, are produced separately by three professionals.

Functional Approach

1. Although behavioral psychologists, cognitive rehabilitation specialists (including special educators), and speech-language pathologists are recognized as possessing special and unique expertise, the important overlap in their services is explicitly acknowledged.
2. Assessments are conducted and plans for intervention are developed in an integrated manner. Ideally, reports are written as integrated, cross-disciplinary documents.
3. Individuals with disability and significant everyday people in their lives are included as contributing members of the collaborative assessment and intervention teams.

Orientation of Intervention: Deficits and Strengths

Conventional Approach: Deficit Orientation

1. The *cognitive rehabilitation specialist* attempts to remediate cognitive deficits and restore specific pre-existing cognitive skills in areas of impairment.
2. The *speech-language pathologist* attempts to remediate communication deficits and restore specific pre-existing speech and language skills in areas of impairment.
3. The *behavioral psychologist* attempts to eliminate undesirable behaviors (e.g., noncompliance, agitation, combativeness) and increase specific desirable behaviors (e.g., participation, "socially appropriate" behaviors).

Functional Approach: Strength Orientation

1. Each professional begins with existing strengths and builds upon them with (a) attempts to ensure success in functional activities at the individual's current level of capacity, (b) apprenticeship procedures (including chaining and shaping), and (c) compensatory strategies, using strengths to compensate for weaknesses.
2. Success is a goal throughout intervention, using whatever antecedent supports may be necessary to succeed at functional tasks at the individual's current level of ability.
3. Undesirable and challenging behaviors, including explicitly communicative behaviors, are never *simply* extinguished without an attempt to substitute a positive alternative that achieves the same goal.
4. Preservation and enhancement of the individual's self-esteem is a background goal for all professionals.

Service Delivery: Settings and Activities

Conventional Approach

1. The *speech-language pathologist* uses repetitive drill and practice in isolated settings that bear little resemblance to real-world communication settings (e.g., pull-out therapy). Activities in therapy settings are not necessarily related to real-world communication activities.

2. The *cognitive rehabilitation specialist* uses repetitive drill and practice in isolated settings that bear little resemblance to real-world settings (e.g., pull-out therapy using decontextualized workbook or computer exercises). Activities in therapy settings are not necessarily related to real-world activities that require the targeted cognitive skill.

3. The *behavioral psychologist* delivers targeted behavioral services on a behavior unit, in a neurobehavioral rehabilitation facility, or in a behavior classroom, with little opportunity to facilitate transfer of training to real-world settings and tasks.

Functional Approach

1. Each profession focuses on real-world needs in real-world contexts. This focus includes supports for achieving real-world goals in real-world contexts and practice of functional communication, social, and cognitive skills in real-world contexts. Specific aspects of the individual's environments and demands in those environments are considered in choosing objectives.

2. As much as possible, communication and behavioral services are delivered in meaningful social groups, in settings that resemble settings in which the skills will need to be used, and in the context of meaningful activities.

3. Pursuit of cognitive, executive function, communication, and behavioral goals is largely in the context of everyday routines, involving modification of those routines with supports that are gradually withdrawn as the individual's skills improve.

Providers of Service: Involvement of Everyday Communication Partners

Conventional Approach

1. Professionals are considered the primary agents of change in the individual with disability.

2. Each profession focuses primarily on remediation of deficits in the individual; that is, the intervention is impairment oriented.

Functional Approach

1. Each profession focuses on improvement of function within everyday routines. Therefore, everyday communication partners (e.g., family members, paraprofessional aides, supervisors, teachers, coworkers, friends) are critical deliverers of rehabilitation services and supports.

2. A primary role of rehabilitation specialists is to train and provide ongoing supports for everyday communication partners. Within a rehabilitation facility, evening and weekend staff are recognized as particularly critical to the development of a positive and therapeutically efficient rehabilitation environment.

Source of Control

Conventional Approach

1. There is near total reliance on external control of behavior. Little emphasis is placed on helping the individual to set goals and make good choices, plan how to achieve selected goals, monitor and evaluate behavior in relation to those goals,

and make strategic decisions in the face of failure. Professionals assume responsibility for most executive dimensions of behavior.

2. The individual with disability is *not* included as a member of the team of people who perform assessments, select goals and objectives, plan intervention, monitor and evaluate performance, and create strategic solutions to problems as they arise over the course of intervention.

Functional Approach

1. The ultimate goal is to ensure that the indivudual controls his or her behavior as much as possible by means of effective decision making, strategic thinking, self-regulation of behavior, and self-regulated control over environmental contingencies.

2. The individual with disability is included as a member of the team of people who perform assessments, select goals and objectives, plan intervention, monitor and evaluate performance, and create strategic solutions to problems as they arise over the course of intervention.

Intervention Procedures

Conventional Approach

1. Prescriptive behavioral objectives specify isolated targets; for example, specific language behaviors are selected for training.

2. Modification of behavior is largely a result of the manipulation of the *consequences* of behavior. Within training tasks, correct performance of the target behavior is consequated with presumably desirable objects or events; failure to use the target behavior is followed by a withholding of rewards, a cost of some kind, removal from the situation, or some other neutral or undesirable consequence.

Functional Approach

1. The goal is an acceptable *range* of behaviors (versus a specific behavior) that may vary in their effectiveness in achieving the communicative objective.

2. Modification of behavior (including cognitive and social behavior) is considered a result of manipulating the consequences as well as antecedents of the behavior, but the focus is on *antecedents*. Antecedent control procedures include creating environmental supports, avoiding triggers for negative behavior, inducing positive setting events, generating positive momentum, creating opportunities for choice and control, establishing familiar, positive routines and effective procedures for deviating from routines, providing advance organizers for difficult tasks, teaching scripts for negotiating difficult social situations, and ensuring that the individual has maximal self-management skills.

3. Contingency management (i.e., manipulation of consequences of behavior) focuses on positive consequences for desirable behavior (versus punishing consequences and "time out" for negative behavior) and on natural contingencies (versus artificial rewards).

   a. As much as possible, rewards are internally related to the action performed (e.g., when people request something

appropriately, they get it; when people initiate social interaction, they are rewarded with a pleasant interaction: when people use strategies, they succeed in their endeavors).
  b. Feedback (positive or negative) is given as much as possible by natural communication partners (e.g., peers or family members).

4. As much as possible, teaching and learning take place within an apprenticeship relationship. The teacher and the learner are jointly engaged in projects designed to achieve meaningful goals. Initially, the teacher assumes much of the responsibility for achieving the goal, but turns over responsibility to the learner/apprentice as soon as possible.

APPENDIX 33–2
Examples of Compensatory Strategies for Individuals with Cognitive Impairments

(Modified with permission from Ylvisaker, M., Szekeres, S., Henry, K., Sullivan, D., & Wheeler, P. (1987). Topics in cognitive rehabilitation. In M. Ylvisaker & E. Gobble (eds.), *Community re-entry for head injured adults* (pp. 137–220). Boston: Butterworth-Heinemann. NOTE: Please see text for suggestions and cautions about the teaching/facilitating process.

Attention and Concentration

External Aids

- Use a timer or alarm watch to focus attention for a specified period.
- Organize the work environment to reduce distractions.
- Use a written or graphic task planner, with built-in rest periods and reinforcement; move a marker along to show progress.
- Place a symbol or picture card in an obvious place in the work area as a reminder to maintain attention.
- Alternate low-interest tasks with high-interest tasks.

Internal Procedures

- Set increasingly demanding goals for self, including work time.
- Self-instruct (e.g., "Am I wandering? What am I supposed to do? What should I be doing now?). Written cue cards may be needed.

Orientation (to Time, Place, Person, and Events)

External Procedures

- *Time*: Use a watch that includes day and date.
- *Schedule*: Use a day timer or other user-friendly schedule form; use alarm watch or pager system to stay oriented to schedule.
- *Person*: Use photos of persons not readily identified (e.g., in log book).
- *Place*: Refer to customized maps or diagrams for spatial orientation; label places or routes.
- *Event*: Use a log book or journal or tape recorder to record significant information and events of the day.

Internal Procedures

- Select anchor points or events during the week and then attempt to reconstruct previous or subsequent points in time (e.g., "My birthday was yesterday—Wednesday—so today must be Thursday and I have to go to work.")
- Request time, date, and other information from others.
- Scan environment for landmarks.

Input Control/Comprehension

External Procedures

- Give feedback to speakers (e.g., "Slow down; speed up; break that down for me").
- Request repetition in another form (e.g., "Could you write that down please?").
- Request longer viewing time or repeated readings.
- Create charts or graphs to assist in comprehending complex material.
- Use a finger or index card to assist scanning and reading.
- Use symbols to mark right and left margins of written material.
- Use large-print books.
- Use books on tape; request a verbal description if reading is weak.
- Place items to be viewed in the best visual field and eliminate visual distractions.
- Turn head to compensate for visual field cut.

Internal Procedures

- Use self-questioning (e.g., "Do I understand? Do I need to ask a question? How is this meaningful to me? How does this fit with what I know?").
- Prepare self for new information by presetting with questions and building frames of relevant background information.
- Attempt to summarize and explain information to oneself; check with speaker or source.
- Use a study guide for complex material (e.g., SQ3R: survey, question, read, recite, review).
- Impose organization using diagrams or other advance organizers (see below).

Memory

External Procedures

- *Retrospective Memory*: Use a log book, journal, tape recorder, or computerized information storage system to record significant information and events of the day.
- *Prospective Memory*: *Nonelectronic*: Use memos, pictures, post-it notes, calendars, graphic time lines, and the like as self-reminders. *Electronic*: E-mail self reminders. Use pager system, telememo watch, beeping watch, handheld personal information storage system.
- *Encoding*: See attention, comprehension, and organization strategies.
- Keep items in a designated place (e.g., keys). Label the places.

Internal Procedures

- See attention, comprehension, and organization strategies.
- Rehearse to-be-remembered information (covert or overt; pantomime).
- Instruct self about when and why the information will be needed.
- Relate information to personal life experiences and current knowledge.
- Use knowledge of common scripts to reconstruct to-be-remembered events.
- Use mnemonics (e.g., meaningful/novel imagery, method of loci, rhymes).
- Visualize verbal information; verbalize visuospatial information.
- At the time of retrieval, reconstruct the environment at the time of encoding.

Word Retrieval

External Procedures

- Circumlocute, describing the items in an organized way (e.g., "What kind of thing is it? What does it do? What is it used for? What are its parts? What are its attributes? Where is it found? What do I associate with it?").
- Use gestures or signs.
- Start a sentence with a carrier phrase (e.g., "I eat with a . . .").
- Attempt to write the word.

Internal Procedures

- Search lexical memory using an organized feature analysis system (e.g., "What kind of thing is it? What does it do? What is it used for? What are its parts? What are its attributes? Where is it found? What do I associate with it?").
- Attempt to cue self with phoneme cues, proceeding through the alphabet (slow, and appropriate only for items in a limited category, such as proper names).
- Create an image of the item in a scene, then attempt to describe the scene.
- Attempt to retrieve the overlearned opposite.
- Engage in free association, having an image in mind.
- Associate persons' names with physical characteristics or a known person of the same name.

Thought Organization, Task Organization, and Organized Expression

External Procedures

- Use a graphic organizer or flow chart appropriate for the task or content (e.g., *task organizer*: goal, materials needed, people and their responsibilities, sequence of steps, timeline, evaluation of results; *narrative discourse organizer*: people, places, time, initiating event, main character's response, plan, action, resolution).
- Prepare work space; assign space as task demands.
- Construct a timeline to maintain appropriate sequence of events.
- Alert others before shifting topic in conversation.
- Watch others for feedback in conversation; ask, "Am I being clear?"
- Use outlining software.

Internal Procedures

- Use a mental representation of a graphic organizer or flow chart appropriate for the task or content.
- Use knowledge scripts (e.g., discourse scripts like narrative form; event scripts like going out to eat, applying for a job, visiting a doctor).
- Note topics in conversation; self-question about the main point.
- Rehearse important comments; listen to self.
- Set limits of time or allowable sentences in any turn of conversation.

Reasoning, Problem Solving, and Judgment

External Procedures

- Ask others for advice or problem-solving guidance.
- Use others for reality checks.
- Post important social rules to follow.

Internal Procedures

- Use an organized problem-solving guide (e.g., "What exactly is the problem? What do I need to know in order to solve it? What are some possible solutions? What are the pros and cons of each? Which is best? [Following action] How'd I do?").
- Use self-questioning for alternative courses of action or consequences.
- Examine possible courses of action from at least two perspectives.
- Scan environment for cues to appropriateness of action.

Self-Monitoring and Self-Evaluating

- Post reminder: Goal-Plan-Do-Review.
- Post reminders or use alarms that mean, "Pause and review: How am I doing?"
- Place monitoring reminder cards in books, at work station, and wherever needed: "How am I doing?" or "Summarize what you have read or done."
- Set aside a review time at the end of the day or at the end of the work day.

APPENDIX 33–3
Rationale for Rehabilitation Professionals to Create Collaborative Relationships with Everyday People, Obstacles to Such Alliances, Strategies to Overcome the Obstacles, Characteristics of Everyday Facilitators, and Training/Support Options

Rationale for Collaborative Relationships with Everyday People

1. To communicate respect
2. To integrate useful insights and skills of everyday people
3. To increase the intensity, consistency, and duration of services by ensuring concordance among all relevant people
4. To enhance generalization and maintenance of treatment gains
5. To infuse reality, common sense, and functional goals into professional practice
6. To ensure appropriate services and supports over the long term as unpredictable problems are encountered (often associated with major life transitions)
7. To enhance community inclusion, by creating networks of community support. (Individuals rely more on community supports than on rehabilitation professionals over the long term.)
8. To stretch limited professional resources in an era of managed care
9. To increase the amount of available data on the basis of which intervention decisions are made

Obstacles to Collaborative Alliances with Family Members and Other Everyday People

1. Distrust; adversarial relationships based on
   - judgmental attitudes (staff or everyday people)
   - failure to respect the other's perspective
2. Professional self-perception that, as experts, they do not collaborate with everyday people
3. Insufficient access to everyday people, possibly because services are provided entirely outside of natural contexts
4. Potential barriers to learning
   - quantity and complexity of information and skills
   - family: accepting need to learn is a threat to hope
   - family: severely competing priorities: exhaustion and stress
   - time
5. Conflict of priorities between rehabilitation professionals and everyday people
6. Language barriers: vocabulary, cross-cultural barriers

Strategies to Overcome Obstacles to Alliances with Everyday People

1. Be available to interact with everyday people in contexts that facilitate collaborative activity
2. Listen actively and nonjudgmentally

3. Be respectful: "I am a guest in your home"
   - respect diversity
   - seek capacity
   - respect expertise
   - be sensitive to differences in behavior in different circumstances
   - acknowledge mistakes
   - understand grieving
   - identify effective communicator
   - ensure that everyday people are supported
4. Clarify roles and expectations
5. Collaborate in assessment (see section on collaborative assessment)
6. Use in vivo coaching—demonstrate competence in context
7. Provide training videos
   - generic videos
   - customized videos
   - collaboratively produced transitional/self-advocacy videos (see Table 33–17)

Characteristics of Effective Everyday Coach/Facilitator

1. Knowledge
2. Interactive competence
3. Competence in facilitation procedures
4. Optimism
5. Flexibility
6. Creativity
7. Problem-solving ability and enthusiasm
8. Maturity, nondefensiveness
9. Sense of humor
10. Empathy based on rich experience with the realities of the individual's life

Collaborating with Everyday People: Training and Support Options

1. Informational inservices
2. Family conferences
3. Creation of support networks
4. Decontextualized competency-based training sessions
5. Apprenticeship teaching
   - teaching in vivo
   - self-observation on video
   - collaborative formulation of scripts, including problem-solving, flexibility, and optimism scripts (see Appendix 33–4)
   - community meetings

- peer teaching and support
  - staff and family training chains
  - child peers
6. Training videos

- generic videos
- customized videos
- collaboratively produced transitional/self-advocacy videos (see Table 33–17)

APPENDIX 33–4
Communication Partner Competencies for Supporting and Improving Cognition in Individuals with Cognitive Impairment: Conversational Support Procedures to Ensure Participation (Overcome Handicap) and, with Repetition, Improve Cognitive Function (Reduce Impairment), and Illustrations of Associated Interactive Scripts

(Modified with permission from Ylvisaker, M., Sellars, C., & Edelman, L. (1998b). Rehabilitation after traumatic brain injury in preschoolers. In M. Ylvisaker (ed.), *Traumatic brain injury rehabilitation: Children and adolescents* (Rev. Ed.) (pp. 303–329). Boston: Butterworth-Heinemann.

COLLABORATION PROCEDURES

Implicit Message: "We Are Doing This Together as a Cooperative Project"

Supportive Collaborative Style	Noncollaborative Style
COLLABORATIVE INTENT	*Noncollaborative (e.g., Teaching, Testing) Intent*
☐ Shares information	☐ Demands information
☐ Uses collaborative talk (e.g., "Let's think about this")	☐ Talks as teacher or trainer
☐ Communicates understanding of partner's contribution	☐ Fails to communicate understanding of partner's contribution
☐ Invites partner to evaluate own contribution	☐ Fails to invite partner to evaluate own contribution
☐ Confirms partner's contributions	☐ Fails to confirm partner's contribution
☐ Shows enthusiasm for partner's contributions	☐ Expresses lack of enthusiasm
☐ Makes effort to establish equal leadership roles	☐ Takes leadership role, despite other's attempt to contribute
Cognitive Support	*Lack of Cognitive Support*
☐ Gives information when needed (within statements or question)	☐ Does not give information when needed; continues to quiz
☐ Makes available memory and organization supports (e.g., calendar, photos, memory book, gestures)	☐ Fails to use cognitive supports at appropriate times
☐ Gives cues in a conversational manner	☐ Fails to give necessary cues
☐ Responds to errors by giving correct information in a nonthreatening, nonpunitive manner.	☐ Corrects errors in a punishing manner
Emotional Support	*Lack of Emotional Support*
☐ Communicates respects for other's concerns, perspectives, and abilities	☐ Fails to communicate respect for other's concerns, perspectives, and abilities
☐ Explicitly acknowledges difficulty of the task (e.g., "It's hard to put all these things in order, isn't it?")	☐ Fails to acknowledge difficulty of the task

continued

COLLABORATION PROCEDURES

continued

Questions: Positive Style
☐ Questions in a nondemanding manner

☐ Questions in a supportive manner (e.g., questions include needed cues: "Do you need a wake-up call in the morning?")

Collaborative Turn-Taking
☐ Takes appropriate conversational turns

☐ Helps partner express thoughts when struggle occurs (e.g. word finding difficulties)

Questions: Negative Style
☐ Questions in a demanding manner (i.e., performance-oriented quizzing)

☐ Questions in a nonsupportive manner (e.g., questions lack needed cues: e.g., "How are you going to get that done?")

Noncollaborative Turn-Taking
☐ Interrupts in a way that disrupts partner's thought process and statements

☐ Fails to help partner when struggle occurs

ELABORATION PROCEDURES

Implicit Message: "I Am Going to Help You Organize and Extend Your Thinking"

Positive Elaborative Style	Nonelaborative Style

Elaboration of Topics
☐ Introduces/initiates topics of interest with potential for elaboration
☐ Maintains topic for many turns
☐ Contributes many pieces of information to topic
☐ Invites elaboration (e.g., "I wonder what happened . . .")

Elaborative Organization
☐ Conversationally organizes information as clearly as possible:
  ☐ sequential order of events (e.g., "First we . . ., then we . . .")
  ☐ physical causality (e.g., "The radio's not working because it got wet.")
  ☐ psychological causality (e.g., "Maybe you're avoiding it because you're scared.")
  ☐ similarity & difference (e.g., "Yes, they're similar because . . .")
  ☐ analogy & association (e.g., "That reminds me of . . . because . . .")
☐ Reviews organization of information
☐ Makes connections when topics change
☐ Makes connections among day-to-day conversational themes

Elaborative Explanation
☐ Conversationally adds explanation for events (e.g., "Maybe the fact that you were drunk at the time had something to do with it.")
☐ Invites explanations for events
☐ Invites discussion of problems and solutions (e.g., "I wonder whether we can think of a better way to handle this if it comes up again"); invites partner to address problems and solutions.
☐ Reflects on other's physical and psychological states (e.g., "You must have felt miserable about that") and invites other to reflect on his/her physical and psychological states.

Nonelaboration of Topics
☐ Introduces topics of marginal interest, with little potential for elaboration
☐ Changes topic frequently
☐ Fails to add adequate information to topic
☐ Fails to invite other to add information

Nonelaborative Organization
☐ Fails to organize information

☐ Fails to review organization of information
☐ Fails to make connections explicit when topics change
☐ Fails to make connections among day-to-day conversational themes. Meaning is vague.

Nonelaborative Explanation
☐ Offers few explanations

☐ Fails to invite explanations
☐ Does little problem solving or all of the problem solving; fails to invite partner to address problems and solutions

☐ Fails to reflect on or invite the other to reflect on other's physical or psychological states

Illustrations of Everyday Cognitive Support Scripts Designed to Improve Problem-Solving Skill and Flexibility

Problem-Solving Conversation Script

Problem arises:

Staff or Person with TBI: Identifies the problematic issue

Staff: Invites reflection about what might work (e.g., "Let's see; there's gotta be something that can be done about this.")

Person with TBI: Expresses frustration

Staff: Outlines a few possible solutions

Person with TBI: Rejects one or more

Staff: Continues review of possibilities until person with TBI chooses one to try.

Staff: Facilitates an experimental attitude, reflection about what works, what doesn't work.

Flexibility Conversation Script

Person with TBI resists an activity:

Staff: "Alright, maybe my idea wasn't such a good one. There's got to be another way to do this. Let's try your idea. (OR Let's think about it . . . . .) What are we trying to make happen here? You're trying to be successful at . . . . .? Am I right?"

OR

Person with TBI perseverates on an action or thought:

Staff: "This isn't working real well. You have another thought? (OR here's another way [or thought] . . . and another.)"

Chapter 34

Communication Disorders Associated With Right Hemisphere Damage

Penelope S. Myers

OBJECTIVES

Upon completion of this chapter, readers will be able to describe the major communication deficits associated with acquired right hemisphere damage (RHD) and apply that knowledge to clinical work; recognize the impact of deficits in arousal, orienting, vigilance, and selective attention on the communicative performance of adults with RHD; explain the potential impact of neglect on communicative ability in adults with RHD; distinguish cognitive from true affective deficits in RHD adults; describe deficits in specific prosodic parameters and recognize that prosodic production and comprehension can be impaired simultaneously or independently of one another; evaluate published and informal measures of RHD deficits; distinguish process-oriented from task-oriented treatment strategies and apply that knowledge to management of RHD deficits; and apply treatment suggestions, generate appropriate stimuli, and apply various scoring systems to their clinical work with RHD adults.

Patients with damage confined to the right hemisphere may have a variety of processing deficits, including impairments in attention, visual perception, cognition, and communication. Not all patients with right hemisphere damage (RHD) have communication impairments, but it is generally accepted that those who do are not aphasic. Their command over basic linguistic structures is usually adequate, and they may do well in superficial or straightforward conversation. Their communication problems typically become apparent in more complex communicative events in which verbal and nonverbal contextual cues must be used to assess and convey communicative intent. Before discussing their problems in detail, it might be useful to draw a very general portrait of a typical RHD patient, Mr. Smith.

An initial and fairly casual encounter with Mr. Smith may leave the visitor with an overly optimistic picture of his cognitive and communicative capacity. Questions about the weather, treatment by the hospital staff, the quality of the food, and so on will elicit responses that seem not only linguistically accurate, but appropriate as well. He may seem a bit less responsive, and may speak in a monotone, but these characteristics might easily be attributed to fatigue and to the general effects of his recent trauma. The visitor may even be cheered by Mr. Smith's occasional jocularity and blithe assurances about resuming all aspects of his former life.

During subsequent visits, however, the very factors that led to a firm belief in his full recovery seem suspect. He may deny a need for rehabilitative services, refusing to take his physical limitations seriously. His assessment of his capabilities may be at odds with his progress in simple self-care. He may be unable to groom himself properly or to figure out how to put on his shirt. He may talk about returning to work next week, yet be unable to transfer himself from bed to wheelchair. Once in his wheelchair, he may demonstrate difficulty finding his way to the nearby nurses' station, or back to his room.

He may have trouble recognizing friends and may deny that they have visited him before. In extended conversation he may seem excessively bound up in himself. He may not respect conversational rules. He may interrupt, fail to assess, and appear not to care about his listener's reaction. He may not maintain eye contact, and he may seem wholly unresponsive to the emotional tone of verbal and nonverbal messages. His tendency to personalize abstract topics, his seeming difficulty in grasping the point of a conversation, and his tendency to digress furthers the impression that he is either confused or that he operates in isolation during conversation.

His jocularity will now strike a discordant note, and he may trivialize topics and focus on tangential and unnecessary detail. Although quick to provide a response, he may take an excessive amount of time to actually answer substantive questions. He may seem verbose and disorganized. The patient's responses, then, may seem inefficient and lacking an organizational base. His ready answers may seem impulsive, produced without internal reflection.

In short, despite an apparently adequate linguistic system, many RHD patients neither respond to nor participate in communicative events as they once did. The near-universal refrain of friends and families associated with communicatively impaired RHD adults is, "He (she) can talk, but it isn't the same."

As this portrait suggests, RHD patients not only have communication impairments, but may also suffer from a variety of other cognitive impairments. Regardless of whether these deficits affect communication directly or indirectly, their potential impact on the patient must be recognized by the clinician.

NONLINGUISTIC DEFICITS

Nonlinguistic deficits associated with RHD include left-sided neglect, attentional deficits, and visuoperceptual problems. Neglect and attention can affect communication and are discussed below.

Neglect

Unilateral or hemispatial neglect is a complex disorder in which patients fail to report, respond, or orient to stimuli on the side opposite their brain lesion (the contralesional side), despite the motor and sensory capacity to do so (Heilman et al., 1983). Although it may occur with left-hemisphere damage (LHD), neglect is usually longer lasting, more severe, and more common in individuals with RHD lesions (Mesulam, 1985; Ogden, 1985). Neglect most often occurs with lesions of the *frontal, temporal,* or *parietal* cortex (Horner et al., 1989; Mesulam, 1981; 1985; Vallar, 1993; Vallar & Perani, 1986), but can occur as well with subcortical lesions, specifically in the *thalamus* (Rafal & Posner, 1987; Vallar & Perani, 1986; Watson et al., 1981) and the *basal ganglia* (Damasio et al., 1980; Ferro et al., 1987) . Neglect may occur in the visual, tactile, auditory, or olfactory senses, or in combinations thereof, but it is most commonly seen in the visual modality.

RHD patients with neglect fail to attend to left-sided input; that is, to input in contralesional space. They may not notice the phone ringing on the left side of the room, nor eat food on the left side of their trays, nor notice people on the left side of their beds. More severe manifestations of neglect may include failure to recognize their paralyzed or weakened left limbs as their own ("I'd be all right if I had my own arm"), part of a disorder called "anosognosia," which is a lack of awareness of illness. Denial of neglect and other deficits is characteristic of patients with neglect.

Patients with neglect have problems attending to stimuli not only in contralesional space, but also in middle and in ipsilesional space (i.e., the same side as their brain lesion),

(Gainotti et al., 1986). That is, they may not attend to left-sided detail anywhere in the environment.

Neglect has a motor as well as a sensory component. According to Mesulam (1981), neglect may disrupt the motor sequences (including eye movements) necessary for exploring and manipulating stimuli in contralesional space. Thus, patients with neglect may fail to perform tasks that require them to visually explore left-sided space or tasks that involve movements on both sides of the body. For example, patients with neglect may not include left-sided detail in their drawings (sometimes called "constructional apraxia"). They may not be able to dress or groom themselves properly because they fail to reach over to the contralesional side of their bodies.

Attention to visual stimuli can shift prior to actual eye movement (i.e., covert attentional shifts) (Posner, 1980; Posner et al., 1980). Patients with neglect may have difficulty shifting covert attention and disengaging attention, particularly when their attention is captured by right-sided stimuli. For example, RHD subjects canceled more lines in a cancellation task when asked to erase (rather than cancel) the lines, thus removing the attention-attracting right-sided stimuli as they progressed through the task (Mark et al., 1988). Problems disengaging attention can also occur in the auditory modality, although they may be more prominent in the visual modality (Farah et al., 1989; Robin & Rizzo, 1989). Clinicians should take into account the level of right-sided stimulation present in tasks designed to measure or alleviate left-sided neglect.

Most theories of neglect hold that it is a deficit in attention (see Bisiach et al., 1981 and Bisiach et al., 1979 for an alternative hypothesis). Many types of attention are implicated in neglect, including 1) *arousal* (Coslett et al., 1987; Heilman et al., 1978, 1984); 2) *sustained attention* (Bub et al., 1990); 3) the capacity to *disengage attention from ipsilesional space* (Heilman et al., 1985; Posner et al., 1984); and 4) *selective and directed attention* (Mesulam, 1981; Rapcsak et al., 1989).

Neglect may be one manifestation of a larger, more generalized attentional impairment (Myers, 1998). Attention has an obvious impact on cognition. For this reason, neglect can be considered an intellectual, not just a perceptual deficit. It has been found to have significant negative ramifications for the recovery of independence (Denes et al., 1982; Kinsella & Ford, 1980; Kinsella et al., 1993; Sundet et al., 1988). It may also interfere in some of the cognitive operations involved in communication (Myers & Brookshire, 1996; Rivers & Love, 1980).

Evaluation of Neglect

Professionals participating in the evaluation of neglect include physicians, occupational therapists, neuropsychologists, and speech pathologists. There are several formal tests of neglect (Weintraub & Mesulam, 1985; Wilson et al., 1987).

The presence of neglect also can be established by the informal tasks described below.

Typical paper and pencil tests of neglect include *cancellation*, *scanning*, *line bisection*, and *drawing* tasks. Cancellation tasks require patients to look at an array of stimuli (e.g., lines, letters, numbers, or shapes) that are distributed in equal numbers on the left and right across a sheet of paper (Albert, 1973). The patient is asked to cross out all occurrences of the stimuli by marking through or canceling them with a pencil. Neglect is measured by comparing the number of left-sided to the number of right-sided stimuli missed by the patient. Generalized attention deficits may be measured by the total number missed, regardless of their spatial location. Because the target stimuli do not differ from each other, this type of cancellation task is considered simple.

Complex cancellation tasks involve selective attention. The stimuli may be two or three different shapes or letters or numbers and/or different colors. The patient is asked to cancel instances of a particular target in a field of foils. For example, patients may be asked to cancel only red triangles in an array of red and blue triangles and squares. Selective attention deficits may exacerbate neglect in complex cancellation or visual search tasks and may further impair attention in non-neglect patients. Thus, a patient may not only omit left-sided stimuli, but may miss targets on the right and may miss more targets on the left in a *complex* compared to a *simple* cancellation task. By using both simple and complex cancellation tasks, the influence of selective attention on the patient's neglect can be assessed. In general, task difficulty is increased by increasing the field density, by placing targets and foils in random arrays (versus rows), and by having targets and foils differ in more than one feature, such as shape and color (Myers, 1998).

Scanning tasks require patients to scan an array of letters or numbers or objects in which instances of a target stimulus are embedded (e.g., finding all the instances of the letter "A" in a line of letters). Typically, the stimuli are arranged in horizontal lines, rather than randomly distributed on a page. Neglect is measured by the number of target stimuli missed by the subject to the left of the midline. Scanning tasks are often given to assess the influence of neglect on reading.

Line bisection tasks require patients to bisect a straight horizontal line by making a vertical mark through the center of the line. Neglect may be measured by how far to the right of center the patient's vertical line is. Line bisection helps establish the degree to which the patient's sense of space is skewed to the right. Several recent studies of line bisection have found that there is wide variability in the normal population in accuracy of line bisection, and that deviations of 6 mm to either side of the middle of a 270-mm line can be considered within normal limits. In general, the shorter the line, the more accurate patients are in judging its center (Halligan et al., 1990; Halligan & Marshall, 1988; Marshall & Halligan, 1989; Tegner et al., 1990).

The effects of neglect on reading can be measured by asking patients to read compound words, sentences, or paragraphs presented at their visual midline. The longer the material, the more likely neglect will surface in the form of left-sided omissions (e.g., "able" for "table") or inaccuracies (e.g., "tree" for "three"). A particularly sensitive test of neglect in reading requires the patient to read a paragraph in which the left margins are randomly indented from 2 to 25 spaces in (see Caplan, 1987). The unpredictability of the left margin makes this test well suited to detecting mild neglect. Scores consist of the number of words read aloud by the patient.

The effect of neglect on writing can be assessed by asking patients to write or copy sentences or a short paragraph. Patients may omit the left half of sentences and words (i.e., "house" for "greenhouse"), and their writing samples may contain excessive left-sided margins, iterations, and/or omissions of letters and words.

Finally, patients may be asked to draw from memory or copy symmetrical objects such as a flower, a man, or a geometric form. Neglect is measured by comparing the number of left-sided details to those included on the right in the patient's rendition (see Myers, 1998 for a scoring method for scene-copying). Drawings may also be inspected for overall structure and integration of object parts. Typically, drawings from LHD patients are somewhat primitive, but the drawings of RHD patients may not only be primitive, but also disorganized and disconnected.

Based on results of testing neglect by line bisection, drawing from memory, copying, reading, and writing in a large RHD sample, Horner et al. (1989) reported that no single task in isolation identified neglect in all subjects. This suggests that combinations of tasks should be administered to establish the presence of neglect. Severity can be estimated by combinations of scores on the informal tests mentioned above. In scoring drawings, clinicians should note inattention to right- as well as left-sided detail as a measure of attention.

Establishing the presence of neglect helps clarify whether or not reading and writing deficits are linguistically based. It helps establish the patient's capacity to attend to stimuli in other diagnostic and therapy materials. Finally, as a reflection of a general attention deficit, neglect may signal a decrease in the patient's general level of arousal, his or her readiness to respond, and his or her ability to produce and sustain effortful, directed attention during complex communicative events.

Treatment of Neglect

Management of neglect revolves around the issue of treating the symptoms versus the cause. Treatment of symptoms attempts to compensate for neglect by external aids which are meant to encourage leftward scanning. However, verbally cuing the patient to look to the left or highlighting stimuli on the left (e.g., drawing a red line down the left margin of a printed page), rarely translates into an internal self-cue by the patient.

Examples of tasks which encourage internal self-cuing include leftward search tasks and tasks designed to stimulate unconscious perception (see Myers, 1998 and Myers, in press for specific tasks). For example, one can present a very simple leftward search task in which patients are required to find only one or two target objects (e.g., colored cubes) within specified borders. Because the number of targets is so low, patients typically continue the search until the total number is found without external reminders. Cubes can be placed on a flat board that has been divided into quadrants. One may begin such a search-and-find task with as few as two cubes of a single color. Task difficulty can be increased by changing cube placement (i.e., placing cubes to the left as well as the right of midline, then in the lower left as well as the upper left quadrant), by increasing the number of cubes, and by having target cubes differ in color from foils. This type of task has been described in detail in Myers (1998) and Myers and Mackisack (1990). The theory behind the task is that by enlisting voluntary attention without external cuing, the potential for generalization of leftward search increases. A second advantage, noted clinically, is that it appears to increase patients' general level of attention and thus may be a good introduction to therapy for cognitive and communication impairments.

Tapping into unconscious perception of left-sided details is another way to approach stimulating leftward movement of attention without external monitoring. There are numerous examples in the literature of the phenomenon of unconscious perception, the most common of which is letter substitution (versus omission) in single-word reading (e.g., reading "table" for "sable"), which demonstrates patients have processed left letters at some early level of processing. Stimuli that are contiguous such as a person on the right side of a page holding hands with someone on the left side, may also encourage movement of attention leftward such that the patient reports two people in the drawing, unconsciously perceiving them as a single object. Other tasks of this type are described in Myers (1998).

Finally, if one accepts that various types of attention are a significant factor in neglect and in RHD deficits in general, then it makes sense to work on attention directly in tasks designed to increase the level of arousal, vigilance, and selective attention capacity. Clinicians should also counsel patients about their neglect and discuss its effects on activities of daily living, including communication, and if necessary, demonstrate the problems in a way that enables patients to overcome possible denial. Families should be included in understanding the effects of these impairments on communication.

Attention Deficits

RHD patients with and without demonstrable neglect may experience attention deficits. Each type of RHD attention disorder is discussed briefly in the sections that follow.

Arousal and Orienting

RHD patients are sometimes called "hypoaroused," and studies comparing them to LHD patients suggest they are generally less attentive to external stimuli and less aroused or alert (Coslett et al., 1987; Heilman et al., 1978; Howes & Boller, 1975). Behavioral, anatomical, neurochemical, and autonomic evidence suggests that the RH plays a special role in arousal and in orienting to the external environment (see Myers, 1998). Unlike the LH, the RH appears to be able to orient attention to both right and left hemispace. There is evidence that neurotransmitter pathways supporting arousal are to some extent lateralized to the right (Oke et al., 1978; Oke et al., 1980; Posner & Peterson, 1990; Robinson, 1985; Tucker & Williamson, 1984). Physiologic correlates of arousal such as galvanic skin response (GSR) indicate that RHD subjects have significantly lower GSRs to pain and to emotional material than nonlesioned controls and aphasic subjects (Heilman et al., 1978; Morrow et al., 1981). RHD subjects have slower reaction times (RTs) in response to simple visual and auditory stimuli, such as a point of light or a simple tone, compared to LHD and non-brain-damaged (NBD) subjects (Howes & Boller, 1975; Ladavas et al., 1989; Yokoyama et al., 1987), suggesting a reduction in arousal or general attention. Finally, neglect may inhibit the scanning necessary to generate a broad-based view, so fundamental to environmental scanning, and for which the arousal and orienting systems are critical.

In functional terms, RHD patients may need more intense stimulation or more time to get ready to attend than other populations of brain-damaged patients with focal lesions, and they may not be as attuned to the environment, nor able to expand attention beyond a narrow focus. A narrowed focus of attention and poor orienting, characteristic of neglect, can reduce sensitivity to environmental cues that signal important pragmatic information.

Vigilance and Sustained Attention

Vigilance is a state of alertness in anticipation of an event. Reaction time (RT) tasks have been conceptualized as measures of general attention and/or of vigilance. Subjects must be ready to respond to stimuli that occur at unpredictable or random intervals. To measure attention adequately, RT tasks elicit many responses which requires sustained attention over long periods of time. Studies have found that the performance of RHD subjects deteriorates over time (Bub et al., 1990) and with longer interstimulus intervals (Wilkins et al., 1987).

In addition, neuroimaging studies show increased metabolic activity in the RH during vigilance tasks (Cohen et al., 1988; Deutsch et al., 1987; Pardo et al., 1991). Finally, heart rate changes in RHD patients do not follow a pattern indicating vigilant attention during vigilance tasks (Yokoyama et al., 1987).

These results support the clinical impression that some RHD patients have difficulty sustaining attention and remaining vigilant, factors that may affect their progress in therapy. Their level of attention during any demanding communicative situation can fluctuate such that they may not process crucial information even when prepared to do so (Myers, 1998).

Selective Attention

Selective attention enables one to screen out distracting stimuli and to recognize stimulus significance. It can be automatic or voluntary, and is dependent on adequate performance of the arousal, orienting, and vigilance systems. Studies of NBD adults and those with focal damage suggest that the RH is particularly important to selective attention. For example, positron emission tomography (PET) studies have found prominent activation of the right anterior cingulate gyrus (Bench et al., 1993; Pardo et al., 1990), and in the right as opposed to the left frontal cortex of NBD subjects (Deutsch et al., 1987). In a reaction time task in which targets were embedded in a field of distracters (i.e., calling for selective attention) patients with right frontal lesions performed slower and less accurately than did patients with lesions in other cortical areas (Ruff et al., 1992).

In addition, neglect increases as the selective attention demands of tasks increase (Kaplan et al., 1991; Rapcsak et al., 1989; Riddoch & Humphreys, 1987). Patients cancel fewer targets if targets must be selected out from a field of distracters. These findings support the notion that neglect is a symptom of a larger attentional deficit.

Effect of Attention Deficits on Communication

Attentional impairments have cognitive consequences that may affect all levels of experience, including communication. Attention deficits may impair the appreciation of the verbal and visual cues that specify the context within which communication takes place. Patients may be less able to shift attention, actively or covertly, during conversations. They may be less able to sustain attention to stimuli anywhere in the stimulus array, and to filter out distracters. Thus, they may not be able to attend selectively to important information during communicative events and may be overwhelmed by complex levels of discourse. Finally, attention deficits may place demands on the patient's internal resources such that as tasks become more difficult, cognitive resources are strained. These potential effects will be addressed more thoroughly in the section on extralinguistic disorders.

Evaluation and Treatment

It should be emphasized that most RHD patients will have some type of impaired attention, regardless of presence of neglect. Thus, all RHD patients should be tested for attentional deficits, and the results should be included in family counseling and taken into account in evaluating and treating RHD communication impairments. Tests of attention and treatment techniques can be found in published materials designed for traumatic brain-injury patients and in the literature on cognitive rehabilitation. Any task that requires attention to the occurrence of simple, but unpredictable stimuli may increase the capacity for vigilance (i.e., listening for a target word in a word list or monitoring a computer screen for target appearance in one of four quadrants). Selective attention may be addressed by modifying the complex cancellation tasks designed for evaluating neglect (see Myers, 1998, 1999). Additional tasks for treating attentional deficits subsequent to brain injury can be found in published materials (see Baines & Robinson, 1991; and Sohlberg & Mateer, 1986, 1987, 1989) and in computer software designed for attention training.

LINGUISTIC DEFICITS

Pure linguistic deficits are not considered a major source of RHD communication impairments. It is true that some RHD patients may make errors on straightforward expressive and receptive language tasks such as naming, word discrimination, following simple commands, word definitions, verbal fluency, and reading and writing. However, the available data suggest that the problems are relatively mild, are not characteristic of aphasia, and rarely affect communication significantly (Archibald & Wepman, 1968; Deal et al., 1979; Eisenson, 1962). In addition, visuospatial deficits, neglect, and attentional impairments have been cited as possible contaminating factors in some studies investigating linguistic disorders in RHD subjects (Adamovich & Brooks, 1981; Archibald & Wepman, 1968; Swisher & Sarno, 1969).

In general, RHD patients are able to structure sentences and paragraphs according to the rules of their language. They do not have particular problems in retrieving words, and they rarely make paraphasic errors. However, their control over linguistic structure may belie a more general problem with language use at the narrative and discourse level of communication, as discussed in the section on extralinguistic deficits.

Evaluation and Treatment

If a true linguistic problem is suspected, subtests from aphasia batteries, designed to test language in constructions that are essentially context free, are useful in assessing linguistic comprehension (e.g., following verbal commands rather than interpreting paragraphs) and expression (e.g., object naming, rather than scene description). Errors should be examined in light of visuoperceptual and attentional deficits. If the clinician feels certain that the patient has a language problem rather than, or in addition to, signs of RHD, treatment should follow the traditional approaches used in the management of aphasia. It is important to remember that language is not always lateralized to the LH, particularly in left-handed people. Thus, although extremely rare, a patient with RHD could have aphasia.

EXTRALINGUISTIC DEFICITS

Although RHD patients typically do not have aphasia, many of them do have communication disorders. Extralinguistic deficits represent the heart of RHD communication problems. The term "extralinguistic" refers to factors that affect communication but are not strictly linguistic in nature. The extralinguistic and pragmatic aspects of communication specify the context within which communication takes place and allow one to understand and convey intentions, emotional tone, and implied meaning. These aspects of communication extend communicated meaning beyond the literal or surface structure of words and sentences. Context is conveyed through an array of sensory cues such as gesture, body language, facial expression, prosodic contour, as well as through the choice and grouping of words themselves. Extralinguistic cues allow us to interpret what is meant from what is said, to understand the relative formality and emotional tone of discourse, the roles played by participants in a conversation (e.g., peer versus subordinate), and whether someone is being funny or sarcastic or serious. These same cues help us express our own intended meanings.

Some RHD patients appear to have difficulty using these cues to understand the implied meaning of complex narratives. Thus, they may miss the theme or point of a story. They may not recognize relationships among characters, their emotional state, and/or the motives behind their actions.

In conversation, RHD patients may not understand humor or the subtleties of irony. They may miss the main points a speaker is making because they focus on unimportant details and have difficulty integrating information into an overall theme. They may not attend to a speaker's facial expression, the prosodic cues that convey emotion and emphasis, or to the physical setting in which the communicative act takes place.

They may also have difficulty expressing their own intended meaning. Their speech may be inefficient, uninformative, and lack specificity. They may have problems getting to the point they are trying to make. Finally, they may have difficulty using the extralinguistic cues that convey emotion through gesture and prosody.

It is of note that we still use the term "right hemisphere communication disorders" to describe these symptoms, a label that refers to a location in the brain, rather than the nature of the problem. However, it has only been in the last 20 years that the notion of communication disorders associated with "minor" hemisphere damage gained credence. Early studies focused on describing the deficits and the conditions under which deficits may be observed. With descriptions more firmly established, studies have now begun to address underlying cause in a systematic way. By addressing

the mechanisms of the impairments, we may eventually arrive at a more appropriate term to capture the nature of the extralinguistic deficits associated with RHD. In addition, hypotheses about underlying mechanisms will move management toward treating the cause, rather than the symptoms. Certainly, impaired attentional mechanisms contribute to all levels of cognitive processing, including communication. In addition, there may be specific *semantic* deficits that have an impact on the RHD communicative impairments.

Discourse Deficits

Macrostructure Deficits

A macrostructure is the overall theme, central message, or main point of narratives, pictured scenes, situations, or discourse. RHD patients may have difficulty generating macrostructures in comprehension and expression of complex communication. They may miss the point of conversation and be unable to stick to the point or convey the gist of their own messages. They may produce fewer core concepts, have problems giving titles to or choosing a summary statement for story contents, and have difficulty extracting story morals and themes in linguistic and pictured stories (Benowitz et al., 1990; Gardner et al., 1983; Hough, 1990; Joanette et al., 1986; Lojek-Osiejuk, 1996; Mackisack et al., 1987; Moya et al., 1986; Myers & Brookshire, 1996; Rehak et al., 1992; Wapner et al., 1981).

Generating a macrostructure depends on the capacity to draw inferences or interpret information. According to Myers (1992), "an inference is a hypothesis about sensory data such that input is not only sensed, but interpreted." Inferences about individual features must be integrated within the entire context to produce the overall theme we call a macrostructure. Initial inferences are beliefs or hypotheses about sensations. Later-stage inferences are hypotheses based on those initial beliefs. Thus, a viewer might interpret a picture of a man in a purple robe, wearing a crown, and holding a scepter as a king. The conclusion that he is a king is a hypothesis about the intended meaning of the visual image.

There are many levels of inference. In the above example, organizing the visual image into the form of a human is an inference, and determining that the image is that of a man is another inference. In general, the type of communication impairments experienced by RHD patients suggests that inference breaks down at a later stage of processing, rather than at the level of translating light rays into shapes or sound waves into phonemes.

Inferences depend on at least four operations: (1) attention to individual cues; (2) selection of relevant cues; (3) integration of relevant cues with one another; and (4) association of cues with prior experience. In the above example, the color of the man's hair would be considered an irrelevant cue.

Relevant cues include the crown, the robe, and scepter, and perhaps the color purple. These combined cues create the context from which the inference of royalty is made. That is, the elements must not only be recognized, but must be sorted for relevance, and those considered relevant must be combined or integrated to create a context or pattern or meaning beyond the superficial recognition of color, form, light, and shadow. The cues also must be associated with prior experience. These operations are not necessarily ordered sequentially, but more likely occur in parallel.

In similar fashion, recognizing the intended meaning of verbal communication requires that one go beyond the superficial, literal, or referential meaning of individual words to their implied or inferred meaning. RHD patients do not have difficulty with simple or automatic inferences (Brownell et al., 1986; Lehman & Tompkins, submitted; McDonald & Wales, 1986; Myers, 1998). Problematic inference generation occurs with what McKoon & Ratcliff (1989) call "elaborative" inferences. Elaborative inferences expand or embellish information and place demands on processing resources. They are called for in situations where information is ambiguous, oblique, requires revision, or runs counter to expectations and/or world knowledge (Lehman & Tompkins, submitted; Myers, 1998).

Selection and Integration Deficits

Problems in generating an organizing principle or macrostructure for narrative discourse may be related to deficits in integrating contextual information (Hough, 1990; Wapner et al., 1981). As explained by Hough (1990) and Brownell (1988), understanding the theme or overall gist of narratives involves the extraction of meaning from individual sentences and the integration of their meaning into the context supplied by the other sentences. One must often infer the semantic links between sentences because not all the links are explicitly stated (Brownell, 1988; Joanette et al., 1986). Narrative discourse, then, requires the extraction and integration of individual units of meaning (explicit and implicit) into a larger whole. Similarly, interpreting pictured scenes or real situations involves the extraction of key individual objects and their integration with one another.

Impaired ability to extract and integrate selected bits of information can be demonstrated by patient descriptions of the familiar "cookie theft" picture from the *Boston Diagnostic Aphasia Examination* (Goodglass & Kaplan, 1983). The "cookie theft" scene depicts a series of disasters taking place in a kitchen. A mother stands distractedly washing dishes at an overflowing sink, her back to two children who are attempting to steal cookies from a high cupboard as their stool tips over. Adequate interpretation of the scene (i.e., the overall implication of disaster) requires selecting and integrating relevant cues to build elaborative inferences about individual elements upon which the overall theme or macrostructure

rests. For example, calling the woman a "mother" (versus a "woman") is an inference based on recognizing and integrating the appliances that suggest a kitchen, her apron, and the children behind her. Determining that the children are not just "reaching for cookies," but stealing them, requires the integration of the action of the boy reaching in the cookie jar with the action of the girl who has her finger to her mouth in the gesture of "shhh." RHD patients may say the boy has his hand in the jar, and the girl has her finger to her mouth without combining the two actions into the inference of "stealing."

RHD patients often begin their descriptions of this picture by discussing irrelevant detail such as the garden outside the window or the cups on the counter. This tendency suggests a problem in selecting relevant information, which further inhibits interpretation. Myers (1979) and Myers and Linebaugh (1980), for example, found RHD subjects produced significantly fewer "interpretive" or inferential individual concepts in describing the "cookie theft" picture compared to NBD controls. They noted that RHD subjects tended to list individual elements without explicitly connecting them to each other or to the central focus of the action. Much of what RHD subjects did list was irrelevant to the central theme or action.

This latter observation has been documented in several other studies. For example, Mackisack et al. (1987) found that RHD subjects labeled more than twice as many items as NBD controls when describing Norman Rockwell illustrations. Similarly, when Hough (1990) asked subjects to interpret the theme of short verbal narratives she found that RHD subjects tended to list information and "retained isolated pieces of paragraph data rather than integrating this information to deduce the meaning of the narratives" (p. 271). In a discussion of narrative discourse deficits, Brownell et al. (1986) state "Where normal listeners are concerned to weave a coherent interpretation of an entire discourse so that each component jibes with the broader reality, RHD patients are often stuck with, or are satisfied with, a limited and piecemeal understanding. . ." (p. 319).

RHD patients also demonstrate integration deficits when asked to organize printed sentences into paragraphs (Delis et al., 1983) and to name object categories (Myers & Brookshire, 1995). Deficits in such tasks support the notion that RHD patients may have difficulty integrating isolated pieces of information, although their command over basic narrative structure or framework is intact (i.e., "script knowledge") (Lojek-Osiejuk, 1996; Ostrove et al., 1990; Rehak et al., 1992).

Integration deficits also occur in perceptual impairments associated with RHD. Piecemeal processing in the visuospatial realm is thought to be a factor in "constructional apraxia." That is, a patient may know the components of an object such as a house or flower, but fail to integrate them into a coherent structure. A chimney might extend straight out from the side of a house or the petals of a flower may trail away from the stem, suggesting that the patient grasps the components, but cannot put them together. Other studies have found a relationship between difficulty organizing spatial relations and problems integrating verbal information (Benowitz et al., 1990).

Selective attention deficits may inhibit the ability to filter irrelevant information and recognize important contextual cues. Perceptual level deficits in organizing and integrating component features into coherently structured drawings may be related to impaired integration of units of narrative content and to impairments in generating a narrative macrostructure. As a result, RHD subjects may have difficulty not only comprehending externally presented extralinguistic information, but also in filtering, integrating, and organizing internal information in such a way as to generate efficient narrative expression.

Producing Informative Content

RHD patients may produce as many or more words than NBD adults, but what they say may convey less information. Studies investigating informative content have found RHD subjects' narratives contain fewer concepts, less relevant concepts, and less specific information than those of NBD subjects (Bloom et al., 1992; Cimino et al., 1991; Diggs & Basili, 1987; Joanette et al., 1986; Myers & Brookshire, 1996; Urayse et al., 1991). Conversational output of RHD patients may also suffer from reduced informative content, but not from lack of words. As one of this author's patients said, "I know the point I want to reach, but as I get there my mind, like a vacuum cleaner, sucks up every thought along the way and spews it out."

The conversational expression of some RHD patients has been described as hyperfluent and digressive; that of others as truncated and abrupt (Myers, 1998; Sherratt & Penn, 1990; Roman et al., 1987; Trupe & Hillis, 1985). Patients with unelaborated output often seem perfunctory, giving the most immediate response without reflection about or interest in its accuracy or adequacy. Excessive output, the more common tendency, is often characterized as digressive and tangential. In reviewing their RHD subjects' picture descriptions, Tompkins and Flowers (1985), for example, noted that low concept scores were overwhelmingly associated with excessive verbal output, reflecting "repetitiveness," and "irrelevant comments" (p. 529).

Tangential comments may not be off the topic altogether, but their presence signals difficulty in getting to the point the patient wants to express. For example, asked what had happened to her and why she was in the hospital, one patient responded:

"My husband saw I wasn't in bed, and he found me in the clothes that I came to the hospital in, same robe and gown and everything. And we have a very thick rug, what

they call a sculptured pattern with swirls and all that. It goes down to the base—fiber base, about two, more than two inches down deep..."

Her comments about the carpet continued. They are tangential, but related—related to the fact that although she had fallen on the floor, the cause of her hospitalization was a stroke, not the blow to her head since the carpet softened the fall. She was unable to make her point explicitly, and thus her listener was burdened with having to fill in the missing information.

Digressive and inefficient output may be related to impaired appreciation of listener needs. Rehak et al. (1992) found RHD subjects impaired in judging the effects of tangentiality on conversational partners. Their lack of sensitivity to the interference of tangential remarks seems to mirror insensitivity to their own tendencies in this direction.

Occasionally, tangential or irrelevant output appears to be a reflection of uncertainty about the intended meaning of events. Failing to infer the examiner's intended meaning when asked to describe a pictured scene, or perhaps confused by its contents, one RHD patient discussed the size and weight of the paper, its plastic coating, and the type of ink used to create the drawing without ever describing the action depicted in the picture. Sometimes, RHD patients confabulate when faced with uncertainty or nonsensical information. For example, when re-telling stories with surprise or nonsensical endings, RHD subjects have been known to make up details that would make the events more plausible (Wapner et al., 1981). This same tendency can be seen in everyday situations when patients may confabulate reasons for impaired performance.

It is possible that narratives based on visual stimuli result in lower informative content because RHD subjects have problems perceiving what is in the pictures. However, several studies of scene description have demonstrated that RHD patients do not have problems recognizing objects and people in scenes as visually complex as Norman Rockwell illustrations and that the level of inference required to interpret a scene significantly affected performance while visual complexity had no effect (Mackisack et al., 1987; Myers & Brookshire, 1996). Reduced informative content has also been found in response to verbally presented narrative passages (Cimino et al., 1991; Wapner et al., 1981).

Generating Alternative Meanings

It often happens that we must generate different, less familiar, or alternative meanings during discourse. Sometimes this occurs because we need to accommodate new information that alters our original interpretation. Sometimes we need to call on a less familiar meaning for a word or set of words. For example, if we walk in on a conversation as someone says, "He was really flying," we might assume that they were talking about someone going at great speed. If we listen further and find it is a discussion about the Wright brothers and their first aircraft, we would have to revise our initial assumption and re-interpret the phrase to mean the person really *was* flying—in an airplane. RHD patients have been found to have difficulty producing alternate meanings *under effortful processing conditions*.

Connotative and Metaphoric Meanings

Individual words may evoke a denotative or connotative meaning. Denotative meanings are like dictionary definitions and are appropriate for words taken out of context where further interpretation is not called for. Connotative meanings refer to alternative, nonliteral, or interpretive meanings. Thus, for example, the denotative meaning of the word "lion" is "large animal that lives in Africa." Its connotative meanings may include "regal," "king of the jungle," "ferocious," or even "MGM." Metaphoric or figurative language and idiomatic phrases have two meanings—the literal face value of the words, and the metaphoric meaning. Either meaning may be called upon, depending on the context.

Studies have demonstrated RHD impairments in generating connnotative meanings for single words that are not embedded in context (Brownell et al., 1984; Brownell et al., 1990; Gardner & Denes, 1973). A number of other studies have found RHD patients impaired in appreciating both metaphoric and nonmetaphoric alternative meanings for sentences and phrases (Brownell et al., 1990; Myers & Linebaugh, 1981; Van Lancker & Kempler, 1987; Winner & Gardner, 1977) and indirect requests (Foldi, 1987; Hirst et al., 1984; Weylman et al., 1989). As Brownell et al. (1990) suggest, these impairments "may not be restricted to metaphor; rather they may be but one reflection of a more pervasive impairment affecting appreciation of different types of alternative meanings" (p. 376).

Revising Initial Interpretations

Sometimes, one must change one's original interpretation of sentences or events to accommodate new information. Revisions require generating alternative meanings. As Bihrle et al. (1986) said, "In these tasks RHD patients seem to appreciate isolated meanings, but they cannot consider the importance of relevant information for revising their initial interpretation" (p. 409).

Impaired ability to revise expectations may be a factor in RHD patients' problems in following conversations. For example, Kaplan et al. (1990) found RHD subjects were impaired in interpreting whether or not conversational remarks between two speakers were to be taken literally. Nonliteral remarks occurred when one speaker was making fun, being sarcastic, or telling a white lie. Understanding the intended meaning of these nonliteral remarks required reinterpreting them in light of previous information.

Similarly, Brownell et al. (1986) found RHD subjects impaired at interpreting the meaning of sentence pairs when misleading information was presented in the first as opposed to the second sentence, as in the example, "Barbara became too bored to finish the history book. She had already spent five years writing it." Taken in isolation, the first sentence implies that Barbara is reading a book, rather than writing one. When misleading information was presented first, RHD subjects had more difficulty than NBD subjects in revising their original interpretations to accommodate the information contained in the second sentence. Impairments in revision have even been found in a lexical task that required revising the lexical function of a single word (Schneiderman & Saddy, 1988).

Deficits in revising expectations may have a significant impact on the patient's capacity to follow the flow of events. We are continually confronted with new information that alters our original interpretations. We must revise as we participate in the twists and turns in everyday events and conversations. For the RHD patient such seemingly automatic revisions may overtax resources, so that new information is processed inadequately and entire meanings are missed.

Explanatory Theories: Activation and Suppression Deficit

It has been postulated that the intact RH is more adept at processing multiple, alternate, less familiar, more loosely connected meanings than the LH, and that the LH is more adept at automatic processing of dominant single meanings or several meanings that are tightly overlapped (Beeman, 1993; Brownell et al., 1984; Brownell et al., 1990; Burgess & Simpson, 1988; Chiarello et al., 1990). Two opposing theories have been proposed to accommodate impaired ability to manage alternative meanings and to revise initial interpretations (see Myers, 1998, for review).

The *activation theory* holds that RHD patients have difficulty in activating multiple, distant, or subordinate meanings (Beeman, 1993). It may take more effort than normal to generate alternate meanings during discourse, interfering in efficient and accurate processing.

The *suppression theory* holds that RHD patients have difficulty suppressing (versus activating) all the possible meanings for a concept. Continued activation of meanings that are not appropriate to the context interferes in the selection of the particular alternate meaning that *is* appropriate (Tompkins et al., 1997; Tompkins et al., 1996).

More studies are needed in this area to sort out which hypothesis best explains the problems RHD patients have with alternate meanings. For now, it appears probable that RHD can cause interference in the semantic processing of alternate meanings. This problem can disrupt the ability to manage complex discourse which contains ambiguities and/or requires revising initial impressions.

Summary

Problems in generating elaborative inferences, in integrating information, and in generating alternate meanings can contribute to impaired discourse processing in RHD patients. RHD patients may have problems inferring the links among sentences, integrating verbal information into an overall structure and theme, filtering unnecessary information, and revising original interpretations as new information unfolds. As a result they may fixate on irrelevant details and be vague, nonspecific, and uninformative. They may have problems selecting, integrating, and organizing information and be digressive and verbose. In some circumstances, they may not appreciate figurative and other nonliteral forms of language. Finally, they may have difficulty accommodating new, ambiguous, or seemingly conflicting information.

Evaluation of Discourse Deficits

Not every RHD patient will have communication impairments, so the primary goal in evaluation is establishing either the presence or an absence of deficits. Commercially available assessment tools (Appendix 34-1) can be used in conjunction with informal approaches described below.

Patient Interview

The purpose of the interview is to establish rapport and to obtain a sample of patients' conversational speech which can be assessed for content and structure. Establishing rapport with RHD patients is particularly crucial for several reasons. First, they may not recognize or may deny their problems. They may wonder why they are seeing a speech-language clinician when their speech sounds fine to them. Second, families often support patients' denial unwittingly by exhibiting their relief that the patient "can talk." If patients have communication problems, families may not be immediately aware of them. One way of addressing denial is to explain in the initial interview that all stroke patients are tested for communication deficits, to agree with patients that they may not have any problems, and to explain that communication consists of more than speech and language.

Another reason patients may be resistant is that they are aware of some of their deficits (perhaps they have trouble following T.V. shows and complex conversations, or have noticed problems in reading). They may be afraid to admit to these problems in the face of family relief that they can talk (and hence, "do not have communication problems"). They may fear they are mentally unbalanced or generally confused. Their fears can be allayed by clinician assurances that there may be very specific reasons that they are having difficulty which have nothing to do with their mental stability. The clinician can help patients overcome denial by demonstrating some specific problems they may have and by explaining that help is available. Explaining and demonstrating problems to the patient can decrease fear,

make problems seem more manageable, and increase insight and cooperation.

The second goal of the interview is to obtain a sample of conversational speech on audio- or videotape which can be reviewed for structure and content. Questions should address patients' orientation, their assessment of their problems, their daily activities, something about their work history or personal lives, and their plans for the future. The interview thus addresses memory, orientation, and insight. Responses can be assessed for the degree to which they observe pragmatic rules of conversation (i.e., turn taking, listener burden, etc.), and the degree to which content is informative, organized, and efficient.

Picture Description

A pictured scene that tells a story or depicts a situation can be used to elicit narrative discourse for the evaluation of macrostructure and integration deficits. Commercially available pictures that require elaborative inferences such as the "cookie theft" picture from the *Boston Diagnostic Aphasia Examination* (Goodglass & Kaplan, 1983) can be used. A picture description task enables the clinician to quickly assess patients' abilities to attend to and interpret contextual or extralinguistic information. The advantages over asking patients to retell stories are that it elicits a more spontaneous production, does not involve memory, and missed or inaccurate concepts can be pointed out by directing the patient's attention to the visually present contextual cues.

The patient's response can be scored in several ways. The number of inferential concepts generated can be compared to the number of noninferential concepts. Such a scoring system for the "cookie theft" picture has been developed (Myers, 1998). It can be adapted as clinicians see fit and used during treatment as a probe task to measure progress in therapy.

Transcribed picture descriptions can also be evaluated by techniques of discourse analysis (see Sherratt & Penn, 1990; Urayse et al., 1991) or other types of concept analysis (see Cherney & Canter, 1993; and Nicholas & Brookshire, 1993, 1995) (see Myers, 1998, for a review of the advantages and disadvantages of these scoring systems). Pragmatic rating scales can also be useful in assessing problems recognizing the limits of shared knowledge, turn-taking, topic maintenance, eye contact, and other pragmatic deficits.

Treatment of Extralinguistic Deficits

Management of extralinguistic deficits usually consists of a combination of functional or task-oriented methods and process-oriented methods (see Myers, 2000, for a review of these two methods for deficits associated with RHD). Task-oriented treatments typically attempt to retrain a specific task—usually through compensation—and address symptoms, rather than the underlying cause of deficits.

Process-oriented treatments, on the other hand, address underlying processes and attempt to stimulate recovery of function. For that reason they may have greater potential for generalization across tasks.

One way of stimulating recovery of function for many of the extralinguistic deficits associated with RHD is to work directly on attention and neglect. One should also work on increasing informative content, on generating elaborative inferences, and on generating alternate meanings and inference revisions.

Clinicians must be creative in designing tasks and evaluating their impact on communication. Specific treatment tasks that are grounded in theory can be found in Myers (1998), Myers (2000), Tompkins (1995), and Tompkins and Baumgaertner (1998). It is assumed that clinicians will use the techniques mentioned elsewhere in this book to establish cuing hierarchies and to probe patient progress. The next sections provide some general directions for designing therapy techniques for RHD discourse deficits.

Inference and Macrostructure Generation

Macrostructure tasks include asking patients to report the overall themes of pictured scenes, stories, or conversational interactions. This can be done by asking them to produce titles for pictures, headlines for news stories, or to simply state the main theme. Task difficulty depends on the complexity of the inference to be generated. The less explicit the theme, the more difficult the inference. By manipulating the level of inferential complexity, one can stimulate the process of inference generation through repeated trials at a level at which the patient is around 80% successful.

One can also guide inference generation by working on scenes or stories for which the patient was not able to arrive at an inference. In the process, the clinician attempts to train the patient to have conscious control over what was once a more automatic task. Patients can be asked to (1) label items in a scene; (2) specify the relevant or significant items; (3) point to items that are related; and (4) explain the relationships among items or some variant thereof. Obviously, to understand the significant items, one must have a sense of the overall theme in a chicken-egg conundrum. However, often the process of asking the patient to overtly specify significant items usually helps him or her come closer to the overall theme. For example, in the "cookie theft" picture, the insignificance of the bushes beyond the window and the cups and saucers on the counter to which RHD patients are often so attracted becomes clear when one asks, "what are the most important items in the picture?" Typically, patients will point to the people and the water overflowing from the sink and from there arrive at an integrated concept of the picture's meaning.

Integration tasks include asking patients to organize printed sentences into a story or pictures into a logical sequence. Stimuli can vary in number of details and in how explicit or implicit the content is.

Tasks that require patients to recognize commonalities may also improve integration skills. Patients can be asked to group pictured objects, scenes, or printed words into categories. Categories can range from concrete (foods) to more abstract themes for pictured scenes. The clinician can identify the categories, or require the patient to generate them.

At the perceptual level, integration can be addressed in tasks that require patients to arrange puzzle pieces or identify fragmented objects from their individual parts. To make such materials, one can simply photocopy large line drawings of common objects, cut them into several pieces, and rearrange and re-photocopy them.

In addition, patients can be asked to provide an opinion for open-ended questions on current topics of interest. One-minute answers can be tape recorded, transcribed, and rated according to how integrated, complete, efficient, related, and coherent the answer is. Impairments in each of these areas can then be worked on separately. Tape recording conversational interactions is a useful way to review various pragmatic deficits (e.g., topic maintenance, turn-taking).

Managing Alternative Meanings

Improving the ability to manage alternative meanings can be addressed several ways. If one subscribes to the *activation deficit* hypothesis, one can ask the patient to provide two meanings for homographs (e.g., bank, bat, choke, knot, dough) or to group sets of words according to their denotative or their connotative meanings.

If one subscribes to the *suppression deficit* theory, one can attempt to stimulate inhibition of alternate word meanings by asking patients to provide a single meaning as rapidly as possible for homographs. At the sentence level, the clinician can present a single sentence with several interpretations and ask patients to rapidly generate a continuation of the story in a second sentence. To help the patient enlist conscious control over the suppression of alternate meanings, the clinician can then provide contextual cues that lead the patient to a second or alternative meaning, followed by a discussion of why the original interpretation was no longer accurate.

Tasks designed to improve the ability to formulate revisions should also be provided. One method is to present patients with two-sentence stories, the first of which leads one to a faulty conclusion unless it is re-evaluated in light of the second sentence. For example, the sentence, "Ella grabbed her bag and rushed to the gate" might lead one to picture an airport scene until the second sentence, "Once there, she pulled out her key and unlocked it" leads to a different conclusion (Myers, 1998, p. 106) (see Bloise & Tompkins, 1993; Brownell et al., 1986; Kaplan et al., 1990, for other examples). Another type of stimulus is a brief story that ends in a statement by the main character. The final statement may be either congruent or incongruent with the preceding information (Tompkins et al., 1995). Stories can be followed by inferential questions that probe patients' abilities to revise their initial impressions of story content.

Processing Emotional Content

RHD patients may have difficulty interpreting and expressing emotional content. They may speak in a monotone, may seem unresponsive, and may appear to have little reaction to their illness. These symptoms have been referred to as the "indifference" reaction (Denny-Brown et al., 1952; Gainotti, 1972). Reduced sensitivity to emotional material coupled with reduced intensity of emotional expression ("flattened affect") and attenuated prosodic expression has led researchers to investigate possible emotional or affective disorders subsequent to RHD.

Several investigators have suggested that the right hemisphere plays a special role in processing emotional content (Bear, 1983; Borod, 1992; Silberman & Weingartner, 1986; Tucker, 1981). It is not clear whether these impairments are the result of an altered internal experience of emotion, reduced levels of arousal, cognitive interference, or some combination thereof. Evidence of an association between altered internal emotional states and site of lesion following stroke is inconclusive (Dennis et al., 1990; Folstein et al., 1977; Robinson et al., 1984; Robinson et al., 1984; Sinyor et al., 1986). In RHD patients "indifference" and "flattened affect" may be associated with reduced arousal (Heilman et al., 1978). That is, RHD patients may be less aware of and less responsive to external stimuli, including the cues that signal emotions. Cognitive processing deficits may also interfere in emotional processing. Comprehension of emotion requires generation of elaborative inferences using contextual and other extralinguistic cues that enable us to recognize emotional states of story characters and conversational partners.

It is important to remember that "flat affect," reduced responsivity, and flattened prosodic production also can be signs of depression. Other signs of depression include feelings of hopelessness, sleep disturbance, reduced concentration, loss of energy, psychomotor slowing or agitation, and significant changes in weight. Depression occurs in 30% to 60% of stroke patients in the acute phase (Andersen et al., 1994; Cummings, 1994; Icoboni et al., 1995; Ng et al., 1995; Ramasubbu & Kennedy, 1994). Obviously, if other signs of depression are present or if depression is suspected in addition to the clinical signs of RHD, a referral for psychiatric evaluation should be made.

Facial Expression Deficits

Comprehension of Facial Expression

Decreased arousal and attention may affect patients' responses to the nonverbal cues that signify emotional expression. Numerous studies have reported that RHD patients have difficulty interpreting facial expressions depicting emotions (Benowitz et al., 1983; Blonder et al., 1991; Borod et al., 1986; Bowers et al., 1985; Cancelliere & Kertesz, 1990; Cicone et al., 1980; DeKosky et al., 1980). It is uncertain whether these deficits represent an emotional disorder or a perceptual one.

Most studies investigating the interpretation of facial expression present faces in isolation without other contextual cues to specify the emotion. The expression must thus be determined by inspection and analysis of the spatial characteristics of facial features such as how close the eyebrows are, how wide are the eyes, and the degree to which the corners of the mouth are upturned, etc. This type of perceptual feature analysis depends on spatial or "metric" judgments which may be in the province of the intact right hemisphere (Kosslyn, 1987, 1988). Furthermore, individual features must be combined with one another to arrive at an accurate judgment. Thus, feature integration deficits may also play a role.

Production of Facial Expression

Even in patients without "flat affect," facial expressivity may be reduced. Studies of spontaneous facial expression have found that relative to LHD and NBD controls RHD patients had reduced spontaneous emotional facial expression in response to slides depicting emotional situations (Borod et al., 1986; Buck & Duffy, 1981). In a similar task, Mammucari et al. (1988) found no differences in emotional expression between LHD and RHD subject groups, both of which had less facial expression than NBD controls. The effects of facial paresis were not controlled for in the above studies.

Reduced comprehension of emotional stimuli may be a factor in reduced spontaneous facial expression. In the above studies responses depended on comprehension of the stimuli as well as on the ability to translate comprehension into expression, although this variable was not analyzed.

Comprehension of Verbal Emotional Content

Comprehension of emotion has been assessed by asking patients to (1) match emotions depicted in stories with those depicted in scenes (Cicone et al., 1980); (2) answer questions in response to pictured stories that are neutral or emotional (Bloom et al., 1992); (3) identify the emotions depicted in pictured scenes (Cancelliere & Kertesz, 1990); and (4) identify the emotions depicted in sentences that describe emotions (Blonder et al., 1991). RHD patients are impaired relative to NBD controls in many of these tasks.

Evidence that a cognitive as opposed to an emotional deficit is responsible for these findings comes from a closer inspection of the tasks by which "emotional" deficits are elicited. Determining the emotional valance of situations, expressions, and narratives requires generation of elaborative inferences. For example, "He went into the house" is inferentially less complex than "He stole into the house."

Most studies documenting problems in inferring emotions from stimuli have not included comparable tasks designed to test subjects' capacity to infer nonemotional or neutral content (i.e., Dekosky et al., 1980; Benowitz et al., 1983; Blonder et al., 1991; Cancelliere & Ketesz, 1990; Cicone et al., 1980). Studies that have done so have produced mixed results. Thus, it is difficult to know if the findings relate to emotional content independent of inferential complexity.

Verbal Expression of Emotional Content

Most studies of the verbal expression of emotional content involve a comprehension task, making it hard to know if subjects' impairments are based on failure to comprehend or to express emotions or both. Cimino et al. (1991) circumvented this problem by investigating the spontaneous verbal expression of emotional content. They asked RHD and NBD subjects to recall episodes from their own lives in response to a cue word. Cue words were emotional or neutral. Not surprisingly, RHD responses were rated as less specific than those of NBD subjects regardless of type of cue word. Although the emotional cue words produced higher emotionality ratings than neutral cues for both groups, the RHD patients' reports were significantly less emotional than were the NBD subjects'.

Summary

RHD patients may have problems both in interpreting and in expressing emotional content. However, it is not clear that they have an affective disorder per se. Studies investigating emotional status following stroke have produced conflicting results. Emotional "indifference" may be a component of a more general attention deficit that reduces responsiveness to the external environment. Reduced responsivity may impair the appreciation of the extralinguistic cues from which one can infer the emotional valence of situations and narratives. In addition, perceptual impairments in spatial judgment and feature integration may contribute to impaired ability to identify emotional facial expression.

Prosodic Processing

The prosodic features of speech convey both emotional and linguistic information. Alterations in pitch, volume, duration of utterances, and in duration of pause time between words create intonational patterns that add extralinguistic information to linguistic content. Linguistic prosody disambiguates word and sentence types, distinguishing noun phrases from compound nouns (e.g., "green house" from "greenhouse"), interrogative from declarative sentences, and clarifies meaning through the use of stress ("Joe loves *Ella*," versus "*Joe* loves Ella."). Emotional prosody captures not only emotional states, but intents such as sarcasm and irony. RHD patients may be impaired in their appreciation and expression of these prosodic features of speech.

Initial investigations of prosodic disturbances suggested that the deficits were the outcome of an emotional disorder,

and terms such as "auditory affective agnosia" were used to describe the problem (Heilman et al., 1975). Recent research investigating the complicated array of phenomena that may contribute to impaired prosodic processing suggests that prosodic deficits are not the result of an emotional disturbance.

Prosodic Comprehension

Most studies investigating comprehension of prosody have used a paradigm in which subjects listen to neutral sentences expressed with an emotional overlay and identify the mood conveyed by the speaker. These studies have found that RHD subjects are more impaired than LHD subjects in identifying and discriminating emotional prosody (Heilman et al., 1975; Tucker et al., 1977). RHD subjects have also been found impaired in discriminating emotions when speech was filtered so that prosodic features remained while words did not (Denes et al., 1984; Heilman et al., 1984; Laland et al., 1992; Tompkins & Flowers, 1985).

RHD prosodic comprehension impairments can also occur in the linguistic, propositional aspects of speech (Bryan, 1989a; Heilman et al., 1984; Weintraub et al., 1981). Interestingly, even in a study on discriminating emotional prosody, Tompkins and Flowers (1985) found that most of the RHD subjects' errors occurred on discriminating nonemotional stimuli.

The cause of impaired prosodic comprehension is uncertain, but because it extends to nonemotional, linguistic prosody, it is unlikely the result of an affective disorder. It may be the result of a perceptual deficit in detecting changes in tonal patterns. It has been found that pitch perception may be selectively impaired subsequent to RHD (Chobor & Brown, 1987; Robin et al., 1990; Sidtis & Feldman, 1990; Sidtis & Volpe, 1988; Tompkins & Flowers, 1985; Tompkins, 1991a). The RH is thought to be more adept at processing nontemporal properties of spectral information, pitch, and harmonic structure, whereas the LH is specialized for processing temporal order, sequence, sound duration, and intervals between sound (Carmon & Nachson, 1971; Chobor & Brown, 1987; Robin et al., 1990). In a series of psychoacoustic tasks Robin et al. (1990) found that RHD was more closely associated with impaired pitch discrimination and matching than with impaired temporal processing (i.e., discriminating auditory gaps between stimuli). They concluded that RHD deficits in prosodic comprehension may be "related to an inability to perceive frequency-related information rather than a higher level disability in assigning a meaningful representation to a normal acoustic trace" (p. 552).

Impaired attention may be another factor in prosodic comprehension deficits. The tasks used to assess prosodic comprehension make particular demands on attention. In many studies subjects must listen to sentences but dissociate meaning from tone, forcing them to divide their attention in the performance of a rather unnatural task. Considering that neglect is associated with attention deficits, it is interesting to note that RHD subjects with neglect have difficulty with such tasks (Heilman et al., 1975; Tucker et al., 1977; Tompkins & Flowers, 1985), yet those without neglect may not (Schlanger et al., 1976).

Prosodic judgments by RHD subjects may improve when the task becomes less difficult. Tompkins (1991b) found that increased semantic redundancy in the form of a word suggesting a given emotion improved accuracy of LHD, RHD, and NBD subjects in judging the mood conveyed in a short paragraph. The redundancy also improved RHD subjects' prosodic judgments of neutral sentences that followed the paragraphs.

The extent to which patients suffer from difficulty in prosodic comprehension in everyday conversation is not clear. Laboratory investigation of prosodic deficits attempt to control the variables that operate in natural conversation. RHD subjects are impaired in tasks designed to assess comprehension of prosody when it is devoid of linguistic content, and in tasks in which prosody is incongruent with linguistic content. These tasks force patients to select and detect relevant features, to attend to two things at once, and to ignore one thing while attending to another. Thus, it is uncertain whether or not prosodic impairments in the laboratory reflect true deficits in processing prosodic aspects of conversations. It is likely, however, that some RHD patients may not be able to mount the resources to attend to these important extralinguistic cues and that they may have problems specifically in pitch perception. The severity of the deficit may vary with the level of redundancy of contextual information specifying the intended meaning of the speaker.

Prosodic Production

Prosodic production ability, both emotional and linguistic, has been tested by asking subjects to repeat or read neutral sentences with a specified emotional tone, to imitate the prosodic production of a speaker, and to spontaneously produce emphatic stress. Prosodic productions have been analyzed perceptually and acoustically. The findings from these studies, particularly those using acoustic analysis, have been mixed. RHD patients who have prosodic production deficits tend to rely less on pitch variation and more on shifts in intensity or volume to signal emotions, and tend to use consistent duration and pause time, giving a robotic quality to their speech (Myers, 1998). In mild cases of prosodic production impairments, the patient may sound fatigued. In more severe cases, they may sound mechanical and stilted.

Although patients generally do not have problems producing emphatic stress to distinguish nouns phrases from compound nouns, they may use fewer of the cues available to signal contrastive stress. In sentence production, they tend not to vary intersyllabic pause time as much as much as NBD adults to produce emphatic stress (Behrens, 1988), but these deficits are extremely mild. Acoustic analyses of the speech wave suggest that RHD patients may have a fast rate, reduced acoustic contrast, and reduced energy in frequencies above 500 Hz (Kent & Rosenbek, 1988). In general, it appears that damage to the RH can result in reduced use of pitch variation and increased use of intensity to convey emphatic emotional stress (Colsher et al., 1986; Ross et al., 1988; Ryalls, 1986). Of note, pitch variation is one of the most critical prosodic features used to distinguish emotional tone (Shapiro & Danly, 1985; Van Lancker & Sidtis, 1992). Thus, attenuated pitch variation has the potential to have a negative impact on the production of emotional prosody.

RHD patients with prosodic production impairments may complain of difficulty getting emotional tone into their speech (Ross & Mesulam, 1979; Ryalls et al., 1987). A patient recently seen by this author stated that she tried to get more inflection into her speech, but that it required "a lot of concentration" and was often ineffective. Patients in the Ryalls et al. study reported a sense of reduced volume and pitch range and that their voices sometimes felt "hoarse" and "strangled." These findings combined with problems in voluntary control over prosody suggest that impaired prosodic production subsequent to RHD may be in part a motor execution disorder (i.e., a form of dysarthria).

Summary

Prosodic comprehension and production deficits may occur subsequent to RHD. Prosodic comprehension impairments are not restricted to emotional prosody, and may include linguistic prosodic deficits. Whether or not prosodic comprehension deficits found in the laboratory translate into similar deficits in natural conversations is not clear. Prosodic comprehension deficits may be related to impaired pitch perception and/or to attentional deficits in response to tasks designed to isolate prosodic from linguistic information.

Prosodic production impairments may also exist in some RHD patients. Clinical impressions of impaired prosody have been difficult to quantify. Patients tend to be aware of, but unable to correct these deficits. It is possible that dysarthria plays a role in prosodic production of some RHD patients, although this possibility has not been formally addressed in studies of prosodic disturbance.

Evaluation

Emotional prosodic comprehension can be assessed by asking patients to identify the emotion conveyed in prerecorded sentences with neutral content. For example, a tape of sentences such as "The boy came home" can be read with a prosodic contour conveying anger, sadness, or happiness, and patients can be asked to identify the emotion contained in the phrase. For linguistic prosody, patients can be asked to match a spoken word to one of a set of two that vary in stress placement (e.g., "hot dog" versus "hotdog").

Prosodic production can be difficult to assess. Patients can be asked to produce or imitate prosodic contour that distinguishes words or phrases from one another either in mood or in emphatic stress. Productions should be tape recorded and played for judges (e.g., other staff) who try to identify the emotion the patient was attempting to express. This method can be cumbersome. Acoustic measures are more objective, but may not be available to clinicians, and there is uncertainty about which acoustic measures are best.

Treatment

Treatment for prosodic deficits may not be a priority in patient management if the patient has other extralinguistic deficits. However, prosodic impairment can occur in patients with few other RHD problems, and it may interfere in their resumption of their daily lives and work. Retraining conscious control over prosodic production in drills similar to the tasks presented for evaluation may help. Clinicians should remember that such training is not like accent reduction therapy. Though aware of their deficit, patients may not have the voluntary control over their production or the ability to improve, particularly if the effort required diverts resources from other types of extralinguistic processing. If the patient is free of other impairments, such training may be worth the attempt. In addition, patients and family members should be counseled about the problem and the patient can be trained to more explicitly state the emotion they are trying to convey in everyday conversations.

KEY POINTS

1. Neglect can occur across modalities, in ipsilesional as well as in contralesional space. As an attentional deficit, neglect may affect cognitive processing, and hence communicative ability, as well as recovery of independence.
2. Attentional deficits associated with RHD include hypoarousal and deficits in orienting, vigilance, maintenance, and selective attention. These deficits may have a significant negative impact on the cognitive processes that contribute to the pragmatic and extralinguistic aspects of communication.
3. Basic linguistic performance (e.g., word retrieval, sentence structure) is rarely affected by unilateral RHD.
4. RHD discourse impairments tend to be cognitively based and include deficits in generating a macrostructure, integrating information, disambiguating information, and drawing complex inferences based on contextual cues. These deficits may result in reduced levels of informative content in patient productions and reduced sensitivity to shades of meaning in communicative comprehension.
5. RHD may include pragmatic deficits in recognizing speaker intentions, understanding the internal motivations of others, and following conversational conventions.
6. RHD may affect the capacity to process alternative meanings in discourse, a capacity for which the intact RH is thought to be dominant.
7. RHD may reduce sensitivity to emotional content and can affect the ability to express emotion in facial expression, body language, gesture, and written and spoken discourse.
8. Assessment should consist of an initial screening that includes an interview, tests of neglect, and a discourse sample, followed by further testing using informal and/or formal measures.
9. Patient management should include task-oriented (i.e., functional) and process-oriented treatment approaches as well as patient and family counseling.
10. Treatment for discourse deficits should include tasks to reduce neglect and attentional deficits, as well as tasks to stimulate integration abilities, increase ability to process alternate meanings, generate inferences, and improve the use of contextual cues.

FUTURE TRENDS

It is hoped that the description of deficits and the framework in which they have been placed in this chapter will encourage clinicians to design innovative therapy techniques. Future directions for research include (1) furthering our understanding of the connections between nonlinguistic and extralinguistic deficits; (2) development of better assessment measures; (3) studies on prognosis and recovery patterns subsequent to RHD; (4) studies on the efficacy of treatment techniques that include increasing our knowledge of the cues that facilitate performance; and (5) studies that address the mechanisms underlying discourse deficits.

References

Adamovich, B.L. & Brooks, R.L. (1981). A diagnostic protocol to assess the communication deficits of patients with right hemisphere damage. In R.H. Brookshire (ed.), *Clinical aphasiology: Conference proceedings* (pp. 244–253). Minneapolis, MN: BRK.

Albert, M.L. (1973). A simple test of visual neglect. *Neurology, 23,* 658–664.

Andersen, G., Vestergaard, K., Riis, J.O., & Lauritzen, L. (1994). Incidence of post-stroke depression during the first year in a large unselected stroke population determined using a valid standardized rating scale. *Acta Psychiatria Scandinavia, 90,* 190–195.

Archibald, T.M. & Wepman, J.M. (1968). Language disturbances and nonverbal cognitive performance in eight patients following injury to the right hemisphere. *Brain, 91,* 117–130.

Baines, K.A. & Robinson, R.L. (1991). *Exercises for right*

hemisphere rehabilitation: Attentional processing and visual reorganization. Austin, TX: Pro-Ed.

Bear, D.M. (1983). Hemispheric specialization and the neurology of emotion. *Archives of Neurology, 40,* 195–202.

Beeman, M. (1993). Semantic processing in the right hemisphere may contribute to drawing inferences from discourse. *Brain and Language, 44,* 80–120.

Behrens, S.J. (1988). The role of the right hemisphere in the production of linguistic stress. *Brain and Language, 33,* 104–127.

Bench, C.J., Frith, C.D., Grasby, P.M., Friston, K.J., Paulesu, E., Frackowiak, R.S.J., & Dolan, R.J. (1993). Investigations of the functional anatomy of attention using the Stroop Test. *Neuropsychologia, 31,* 907–922.

Benowitz, L.I., Bear, D.M., Rosenthal, R., Mesulam, M.M., Zaidel, E., & Sperry, R.W. (1983). Hemispheric specialization in nonverbal communication. *Cortex, 19,* 5–11.

Benowitz, L.I., Moya, K.L., & Levine, D.N. (1990). Impaired verbal reasoning and constructional apraxia in subjects with right hemisphere damage. *Neuropsychologia, 28,* 231.

Bihrle, A.M., Brownell, H.H., & Powelson, J. (1986). Comprehension of humorous and nonhumorous materials by left and right brain-damaged patients. *Brain and Cognition, 5,* 399–411.

Bisiach, E., Capitani, E., Luzzatti, C., & Perani, D. (1981). Brain and the conscious representation of outside reality. *Neuropsychologia, 19,* 543–551.

Bisiach, E., Luzzatti, C., & Perani, D. (1979). Unilateral neglect, representational schema and consciousness. *Brain, 102,* 609–618.

Bloise, C.G.R. & Tompkins, C.A. (1993). Right brain damage and inference revision revisited. *Clinical Aphasiology, 21,* 145–155.

Blonder, L.X., Bowers, D., & Heilman, K.M. (1991). The role of the right hemisphere in emotional communication. *Brain, 114,* 1115–1127.

Bloom, R.L., Borod, J.C., Obler, L.K., & Gerstman, L.J. (1992). Impact of emotional content on discourse production in patients with unilateral brain damage. *Brain and Language, 42,* 153–164.

Borod, J. (1992). Interhemispheric and intrahemispheric control of emotion: A focus on unilateral brain damage. *Journal of Consulting and Clinical Psychology, 60,* 339–348.

Borod, J.C., Koff, E., Lorch, M.P., & Nicholas, M. (1986). The expression and perception of facial emotion in brain-damaged patients. *Neuropsychologia, 24,* 169–180.

Bowers, D., Bauer, R.M., Coslett, H.B., & Heilman, K.M. (1985). Processing of faces by patients with unilateral hemisphere lesions. *Brain and Cognition, 4,* 258–272.

Brownell, H.H. (1988). The neuropsychology of narrative comprehension. *Aphasiology, 2,* 247–250.

Brownell, H.H., Potter, H.H., Bihrle, A.M., & Gardner, H. (1986). Inference deficits in right brain-damaged patients. *Brain and Language, 27,* 310–321.

Brownell, H.H., Potter, H.H., Michelow, D., & Gardner, H. (1984). Sensitivity to lexical denotation and connotation in brain damaged patients: A double dissociation? *Brain and Language, 22,* 253–265.

Brownell, H.H., Simpson, T.L., Bihrle, A.M., Potter, H.H., & Gardner, H. (1990). Appreciation of metaphoric alternative word meanings by left and right brain-damaged patients. *Neuropsychologia, 28,* 375–383.

Bub, D., Audet, T., & Lecours, A.R. (1990). Re-evaluating the effect of unilateral brain damage on simple reaction time to auditory stimulation. *Cortex, 26,* 227–237.

Buck, R. & Duffy, R.J. (1981). Nonverbal communication of affect in brain-damaged patients. *Cortex, 6,* 351–362.

Burgess, C. & Simpson, G.B. (1988). Cerebral hemispheric mechanisms in the retrieval of ambiguous word meanings. *Brain and Language, 33,* 86–103.

Cancelliere, A.E.B. & Kertesz, A. (1990). Lesion localization in acquired deficits of emotional expression and comprehension. *Brain and Cognition, 13,* 133–147.

Caplan, B. (1987). Assessment of unilateral neglect: A new reading test. *Journal of Clinical and Experimental Neuropsychology, 9,* 359–364.

Carmon, A. & Nachson, I. (1971). Effect of unilateral brain damage on perception of temporal order. *Cortex, 7,* 410–418.

Cherney, L.R. & Canter, G.J. (1993). Informational content in the discourse of patients with probable Alzheimer's disease and patients with right brain damage. *Clinical Aphasiology, 21,* 123–133.

Chiarello, C., Burgess, C., Richards, L., & Pollock, A. (1990). Semantic and associative priming in the cerebral hemispheres: Some words do, some words don't. . .sometimes, in some places. *Brain and Language, 38,* 75–104.

Chobor, K.L. & Brown, J.W. (1987). Phoneme and timbre monitoring in left and right cerebrovascular accident patients. *Brain and Language, 30,* 278–284.

Cicone, M., Wapner, W., & Gardner, H. (1980). Sensitivity to emotional expressions and situations in organic patients. *Cortex, 16,* 145–158.

Cimino, C.R., Verfaellie, M., Bowers, D., & Heilman, K.M. (1991). Autobiographical memory: Influence of right hemisphere damage on emotionality and specificity. *Brain and Cognition, 15,* 106–118.

Cohen, , R.M., Semple, W.E., Gross, M., Holcomb, H.J., Dowling, S.M., & Nordahl, S. (1988). Functional localization of sustained attention. *Neuropsychiatry, Neuropsychology, and Behavioral Neurology, 1,* 3–20.

Colsher, P.L., Cooper, W.E., & Graff-Radford, N. (1987). Intonational variability in the speech of right-hemisphere damaged patients. *Brain and Language, 32,* 379–383.

Coslett, H.B., Bowers, D., & Heilman, K.M. (1987). Reduction in cerebral activation after right hemisphere stroke. *Neurology, 37,* 957–962.

Cummings, J.L. (1994). Depression in neurological disease. *Psychiatric Annals, 24,* 525–531.

Damasio, A.R., Damasio, H., & Chui, H.C. (1980). Neglect following damage to frontal lobe or basal ganglia. *Neuropsychologia, 18,* 128–132.

Deal, J., Deal, L., Wertz, R.W., Kitselman, K., & Dwyer, C. (1979). Right hemisphere PICA percentiles: Some speculations about aphasia. In R.H. Brookshire (ed.), *Clinical aphasiology: Conference proceedings* (pp. 30–37). Minneapolis, MN: BRK.

Denes, G., Semenza, C., Stoppa, E., & Lis, A. (1982). Unilateral spatial neglect and recovery from hemiplegia. *Brain, 105,* 543–552.

Denes, G., Caldognetto, E.M., Semenza, C., Vagges, K., & Zettin, M. (1984). Discrimination and identification of emotions in human voice by brain-damaged subjects. *Acta Neurologica Scandinavia, 69,* 154–162.

Deutsch, G., Papanicolaou, A.C., Bourbon, T., & Eisenberg, H.M.

(1987). Cerebral blood flow evidence of right cerebral activation in attention demanding tasks. *International Journal of Neuroscience, 36,* 23–28.

DeKosky, S.T., Heilman, K.M., Bowers, D., & Valenstein, E. (1980). Recognition and discrimination of emotional faces and pictures. *Brain and Language, 9,* 206–214.

Delis, D., Wapner, W., Gardner, H., & Moses, J. (1983). The contribution of the right hemisphere to the organization of paragraphs. *Cortex, 19,* 43–50.

Denny-Brown, D., Myers, J.S., & Horenstein, S. (1952). The significance of perceptual rivalry resulting from parietal lesion. *Brain, 75,* 433–471.

Diggs, C. & Basili, A.G. (1987). Verbal expression of right cerebrovascular accident patients: Convergent and divergent language. *Brain and Language, 30,* 130–146.

Eisenson, J. (1962). Language and intellectual modifications associated with right cerebral damage. *Language and Speech, 5,* 49–53.

Farah, M.J., Wong, A.B., Monheit, M.A., & Morrow, L.A. (1989). Parietal lobe mechanisms of spatial attention: Modality-specific or supramodal? *Neuropsychologia, 27,* 461–470.

Ferro, J.M., Kertesz, A., & Black, S.E. (1987). Subcortical neglect: Quantification, anatomy, and recovery. *Neurology, 37,* 1487–1492.

Foldi, N.S. (1987). Appreciation of pragmatic interpretation of indirect commands: Comparison of right and left hemisphere brain-damaged patients. *Brain and Language, 31,* 88–108.

Folstein, M.R., Maiberger, R., & McHugh, P.R. (1977). Mood disorder as a specific complication of stroke. *Journal of Neurology, Neurosurgery, and Psychiatry, 40,* 1018–1020.

Gainotti, G. (1972). Emotional behavior and hemispheric side of lesion. *Cortex, 8,* 41–55.

Gainotti, G., D'Erme, P., Monteleone, D., & Silveri, M.C. (1986). Mechanisms of unilateral spatial neglect in relation to laterality of cerebral lesions. *Brain, 109,* 599–612.

Gardner, H., Brownell, H.H., Wapner, W., & Michelow, D. (1983). Missing the point: The role of the right hemisphere in the processing of complex linguistic materials. In E. Perecman (ed.), *Cognitive processing in the right hemisphere* (pp. 169–191). New York: Academic Press.

Gardner, H. & Denes, G. (1973). Connotative judgments by aphasic patients on a pictorial adaptation of the semantic differential. *Cortex, 9,* 183–196.

Goodglass, H. & Kaplan, E. (1983). *The Boston Diagnostic Aphasia Examination.* Philadelphia: Lea & Febiger.

Halligan, P.W., Manning, L., & Marshall, J.C. (1990). Individual variation in line bisection: A study of four patients with right hemisphere damage and normal controls. *Neuropsychologia, 28,* 1043–1051.

Halligan, P.W. & Marshall, J.C. (1988). How long is a piece of string? A study of line bisection in a case of visual neglect. *Cortex, 24,* 321–328.

Heilman, K.M., Bowers, D., Coslett, H.B., Whelan, H., & Watson, R.T. (1985). Directional hypokinesia: Prolonged reaction times for leftward movements in patients with right hemisphere lesions and neglect. *Neurology, 35,* 855–859.

Heilman, K.M., Bowers, D., Speedie, L., & Coslett, H.B. (1984). Comprehension of affective and nonaffective prosody. *Neurology, 34,* 917–921.

Heilman, K.M., Scholes, R., & Watson, R.T. (1975). Auditory affective agnosia. *Journal of Neurology, Neurosurgery, and Psychiatry, 38,* 69–72.

Heilman, K.M., Schwartz, H.D., & Watson, R.T. (1978). Hypoarousal in patients with the neglect syndrome and emotional indifference. *Neurology, 28,* 229–232.

Heilman, K.M., Valenstein, E., & Watson, R.T. (1984). Neglect and related disorders. *Seminars in Neurology, 4,* 209–219.

Heilman, K.M., Watson, R.T., Valenstein, E., & Damasio, A. (1983). Localization of lesions in neglect. In A. Kertesz (ed.), *Localization in neuropsychology* (pp. 471–492). New York: Academic.

Hirst, W., LeDoux, J., & Stein, S. (1984). Constraints on the processing of indirect speech acts: Evidence from aphasiology. *Brain and Language, 23,* 26–33.

Hough, M. (1990). Narrative comprehension in adults with right and left hemisphere brain-damage: Theme organization. *Brain and Language, 38,* 253–277.

Horner, J., Massey, E.W., Woodruff, W.W., Chase, K.N., & Dawson, D.V. (1989). Task-dependent neglect: Computed tomography size and locus correlations. *Journal of Neurological Rehabilitation, 3,* 7–13.

Howes, D. & Boller, F. (1975). Simple reaction time: Evidence for focal impairment from lesions in the right hemisphere. *Brain, 98,* 317–332.

Iacoboni, M., Padovani, Padovani, A., DiPiero, V., & Lenzi, G.L. (1995). Post-stroke depression: Relationships with morphological damage and cognition over time. *International Journal of Neurological Science, 16,* 209–216.

Joanette, Y., Goulet, P., Ska, B., & Nespoulous, J.-L. (1986). Informative content of narrative discourse in right-brain-damaged right-handers. *Brain and Language, 29,* 81–105.

Kaplan, J., Brownell, H.H., Jacobs, J.R., & Gardner, H. (1990). The effects of right hemisphere damage on the pragmatic interpretation of conversational remarks. *Brain and Language, 38,* 315–333.

Kaplan, R.F., Verfaillie, M., Meadows, M.E., Caplan, L.R., Peasin, M.S., & de Witt, D. (1991). Changing attentional demands in left hemispatial neglect. *Archives of Neurology, 48,* 1263–1266.

Kent, R.D. & Rosenbek, J.C. (1982). Prosodic disturbance and neurologic lesion. *Brain and Language, 15,* 259–291.

Kinsella, G. & Ford, B. (1980). Acute recovery patterns in stroke. *Medical Journal of Australia, 2,* 663–666.

Kinsella, G., Olver, J., Ng, K., Packer, S., & Stark, R. (1993). Analysis of the syndrome of unilateral neglect. *Cortex, 29,* 135–140.

Kosslyn, S.M. (1987). Seeing and imagining in the cerebral hemispheres: A computational approach. *Psychological Review, 94,* 148–175.

Kosslyn, S.M. (1988). Aspects of a cognitive neuroscience of mental imagery. *Science, 240,* 1621–1626.

Ladavas, E., Del Pesce, M., & Provinciali, L. (1989). Unilateral attention deficits and hemispheric asymmetries in the control of visual attention. *Neuropsychologia, 27,* 353–366.

Lalande, S., Braun, C.M.J., Carlebois, N., & Whitaker, H.A. (1992). Effects of right and left hemisphere cerebro-vascular lesions on discrimination of prosodic and semantic aspects of affect in sentences. *Brain and Language, 42,* 165–186.

Lehman, M.T. & Tompkins, C.A. (submitted). Inferencing in adults with right hemisphere brain damage: An analysis of conflicting results. *Aphasiology.*

Lojek-Osiejuk, E. (1996). Knowledge of scripts reflected in

discourse of aphasics and right-brain-damaged patients. *Brain and Language, 53,* 58–80.

McDonald, S. & Wales, R. (1986). An investigation of the ability to process inferences in language following right hemisphere brain damage. *Brain and Language, 29,* 68–80.

McKoon, G. & Ratcliff, R. (1989). Semantic associations and elaborative inference. *Journal of Experimental Psychology: Learning, Memory, and Cognition, 15,* 326–338.

Mackisack, E.L., Myers, P.S., & Duffy, J.R. (1987). Verbosity and labeling behavior: The performance of right hemisphere and non-brain-damaged adults on an inferential picture description task. In R.H. Brookshire (ed.), *Clinical aphasiology Vol. 17* (pp. 143–151). Minneapolis, MN: BRK.

Mammucari, A., Caltagrione, C., Ekman, P., Friesen, W., Gianotti, G., Pizzamiglio, L., & Zoccolotti, P. (1988). Spontaneous facial expression of emotions in brain-damaged patients. *Cortex, 24,* 521–533.

Mark, V.W., Kooistra, C.A., & Heilman, K.M. (1988). Hemispatial neglect affected by non-neglected stimuli. *Neurology, 38,* 1207–1211.

Marshall, J.C. & Halligan, P.W. (1989). When right goes left: An investigation of line bisection in a case of visual neglect. *Cortex, 25,* 503–515.

Mesulam, M.-M. (1981). A cortical network for directed attention and unilateral neglect. *Annals of Neurology, 10,* 307–325.

Mesulam, M.-M. (1985). Attention, confusional states, and neglect. In M. Mesulam (ed.), *Principles of behavioral neurology* (pp. 125–168). Philadelphia: F.A. Davis.

Morrow, L., Vrtunsk, P.B., Kim, Y., & Boller, F. (1981). Arousal responses to emotional stimuli and laterality of lesion. *Neuropsychologia, 19,* 65–71.

Myers, P.S. (1979). Profiles of communication deficits in patients with right cerebral hemisphere damage. In R.H. Brookshire (ed.), *Clinical aphasiology: Conference proceedings* (pp. 38–46). Minneapolis, MN: BRK.

Myers, P.S. (1998). *Right hemisphere damage: Disorders of communication and cognition.* San Diego, CA: Singular Publishing Group.

Myers, P.S. (2000). Process-oriented treatment of right hemisphere communication disorders. *Seminars in Speech and Language, 20,* 319–334.

Myers, P.S. & Brookshire, R.H. (1995). Effects of noun type on naming performance of right-hemisphere-damaged and non-brain-damaged adults. *Clinical Aphasiology, 23,* 195–206.

Myers, P.S. & Brookshire, R.H. (1996). Effect of visual and inferential variables on scene descriptions by right-hemisphere-damaged and non-brain-damaged adults. *Journal of Speech and Hearing Research, 39,* 870–880.

Myers, P.S. & Linebaugh, C.W. (1980, November). The perception of contextually conveyed relationships by right brain-damaged patients. Paper presented to the American Speech-Language-Hearing Association Convention, Detroit, MI.

Myers, P.S. & Linebaugh, C.W. (1981). Comprehension of idiomatic expressions by right-hemisphere-damaged adults. In R.H. Brookshire (ed.), *Clinical aphasiology: Conference proceedings* (pp. 254–261). Minneapolis, MN: BRK.

Myers, P.S. & Mackisack, E.L. (1990). Right hemisphere syndrome, in L.L. LaPointe (ed.), *Aphasia and related neurogenic language disorders* (pp. 177–195). New York: Thieme.

Ng, K.C., Chan, K.L., & Straughan, P.T. (1995). A study of post-stroke depression in a rehabilitative center. *Acta Psychiatrica Scandanavia, 92,* 75–79.

Nicholas, L.E. & Brookshire, R.H. (1993). A system for quantifying the informativeness and efficiency of the connected speech of adults with aphasia. *Journal of Speech and Hearing Research, 36,* 338–350.

Nicholas, L.E. & Brookshire, R.H. (1995). Presence, completeness, and accuracy of main concepts in the connected speech of non-brain-damaged adults and adults with aphasia. *Journal of Speech and Hearing Research, 38,* 145–157.

Ogden, J.A. (1985). Anterior-posterior interhemispheric differences in the loci of lesions producing visual hemineglect. *Brain and Cognition, 4,* 59–75.

Oke, A., Keller, R., Medford, I., & Adams, R. (1978). Lateralization of norepinephrine in human thalamus. *Science, 200,* 1411–1413.

Oke, A., Lewis, R., & Adams, R.N. (1980). Hemispheric asymmetry of norepinephrine distribution in rat thalamus. *Brain Research, 188,* 269–272.

Ostrove, J.M., Simpson, T., & Gardner, H. (1990). Beyond scripts: A note on the capacity of right hemisphere-damaged patients to process social and emotional content. *Brain and Cognition, 12,* 144–154.

Pardo, J.V., Fox, P.T., & Raichle, M.E. (1991). Localization of a human system for sustained attention by positron emission tomography. *Nature, 349,* 61–64.

Pardo, J.V., Pardo, P.J., Janer, K.W., & Raichle, M.E. (1990). The anterior cingulate cortex mediates processing selection in the Stroop attentional conflict paradigm. *Proceedings of the National Academy of Science, USA, 87,* 256–259.

Posner, M.I. (1980). Orienting of attention. *Quarterly Journal of Experimental Psychology, 32,* 3–25.

Posner, M.I. & Petersen, S.E. (1990). The attention system of the human brain. *Annual Review of Neuroscience, 13,* 25–42.

Posner, M.I., Snyder, C.R., & Davidson, B.J. (1980). Attention and the detection of signals. *Journal of Experimental Psychology: General, 109,* 160–174.

Posner, M.I., Walker, J.A., Friedrich, F.J., & Raphal, R.D. (1984). Effects of parietal lobe injury on convert orienting of visual attention. *Journal of Neuroscience, 4,* 1863–1864.

Ramasubbu, R. & Kennedy, S.H. (1994). Factors complicating the diagnosis of depression in cerebrovascular disease Part I: Phenomenological and nosological issues. *Canadian Journal of Psychiatry, 39,* 596–607.

Rafal, R.D. & Posner, M.E. (1987). Deficits in human visual spatial attention following thalamic lesions. *Proceedings of the National Academy of Science, USA, 84,* 7349–7353.

Rapcsak, S.Z., Verfaellie, M., Fleet, W.S., & Heilman, K.M. (1989). Selective attention in hemispatial neglect. *Archives of Neurology, 46,* 178–182.

Rehak, A., Kaplan, J.A., & Gardner, H. (1992). Sensitivity to conversational deviance in right-hemisphere-damaged patients. *Brain and Language, 42,* 203–217.

Rehak, A., Kaplan, J.A., Weylman, S.T., Kelly, B., Brownell, H.H. (1992). Story processing in right-hemisphere-brain damaged patients. *Brain and Language, 42,* 320–336.

Riddoch, M.J. & Humphreys, G.W. (1987). Perceptual action systems in unilateral neglect. In M. Jeannerod (ed.), *Neurophysiological and neuropsychological aspects of spatial neglect* (pp. 151–181). Amsterdam: Elsevier.

Rivers, D.L. & Love, R.J. (1980). Language performance on visual processing tasks in right hemisphere lesion cases. *Brain and Language, 10,* 348–366.

Robin, D.A. & Rizzo, M. (1989). The effect of focal cerebral lesions on intramodal and cross modal orienting of attention. In T. Prescott (ed.), *Clinical aphasiology, Vol. 18* (pp. 61–74). Austin, Texas: Pro-Ed.

Robin, D.A., Tranel, D., & Damasio, H. (1990). Auditory perception of temporal and spectral events in patients with focal left and right cerebral lesions. *Brain and Language, 39,* 539–555.

Robinson, R.G. (1985). Lateralized behavioral and neurochemical consequences of unilateral brain injury in rats. In S.G. Glick (ed.), *Cerebral lateralization in nonhuman species* (pp. 135–156). Orlando, FL: Academic Press.

Robinson, R.G., Kubos, K.L., Starr, L.B., Rao, K., & Price, T.R. (1984). Mood disorders in stroke patients: Importance of location of lesion. *Brain, 107,* 81–93.

Robinson, R.G., Starr, L.B., Lipsey, J.R., Rao, K., & Price, T.R. (1984). A two-year longitudinal study of post-stroke mood disorders: Dynamic changes in associated variables over the first six months of follow-up. *Stroke, 15,* 510–517.

Roman, M., Brownell, H.H., Potter, H.H., Seibold, M.S., & Gardner, H. (1987). Script knowledge in right hemisphere-damaged and normal elderly adults. *Brain and Language, 31,* 151–170.

Ross, E.D., Edmondson, J.A., Seibert, G.B., & Homan, R.W. (1988). Acoustic analysis of affective measures of prosody during right-sided Wada test: A within-subjects verification of the right hemisphere's role in language. *Brain and Language, 33,* 128–145.

Ross, E.D. & Mesulam, M.-M. (1979). Dominant language functions of the right hemisphere? Prosody and emotional gesturing. *Archives of Neurology, 36,* 561–569.

Ruff, R.M., Nieman, H., Allen, C.C., Farrow, C.E., & Wylie, T. (1992). The Ruff 2 and 7 selective attention test: A neuropsychological application. *Perceptual and Motor Skills, 75,* 1311–1319.

Ryalls, R. (1986). What constitutes a primary disturbance of speech prosody? A reply to Shapiro and Danly. *Brain and Language, 29,* 183–187.

Ryalls, R., Joanette, Y., & Feldman, L. (1987). An acoustic comparison of normal and right-hemsiphere-damaged speech prosody. *Cortex, 23,* 685–694.

Schneiderman, E.I. & Saddy, J.D. (1988). A linguistic deficit resulting from right-hemisphere damage. *Brain and Language, 34,* 38–53.

Schlanger, B.B., Schlanger, P., & Gerstman, L.J. (1976). The perception of emotionally toned sentences by right hemisphere-damaged and aphasic subjects. *Brain and Language, 3,* 396–403.

Shapiro, B.E. & Danly, M. (1985). The role of the right hemisphere in the control of speech prosody in propositional and affective contexts. *Brain and Language, 25,* 19–36.

Sherratt, S.M. & Penn, C. (1990). Discourse in a right-hemisphere brain-damaged subject. *Aphasiology, 4,* 539–560.

Silberman, E.K. & Weingartner, H. (1986). Hemispheric lateralization of functions related to emotion. *Brain and Cognition, 5,* 322–353.

Sinyor, D., Jacques, P., Kaloupek, D.G., Becker, R., Goldenberg, M., & Coopersmith, H. (1986). Poststroke depression and lesion location: An attempted replication. *Brain, l09,* 537–546.

Sohlberg, M.M. & Mateer, C.A. (1986). *Attention Process Training (APT).* Pyyallup, WA: Association for Neuropsychological Research and Development.

Sohlberg, M.M. & Mateer, C.A. (1987). Effectiveness of an attention training program. *Journal of Clinical and Experimental Neuropsychology, 9,* 117–130.

Sohlberg, M.M. & Mateer, C.A. (1989). *Introduction to cognitive rehabilitation.* New York: Guilford Press.

Swisher, L.P. & Sarno, M.T. (1969). Token test scores of three matched patient groups: Left brain-damaged, right brain-damaged without aphasia, and non-brain-damaged. *Cortex, 5,* 264–273.

Tegner, R., Levander, M., & Caneman, G. (1990). Apparent right neglect in patients with left visual neglect. *Cortex, 26,* 455–458.

Tompkins, C.A. (1991a). Automatic and effortful processing of emotional intonation after right or left hemisphere brain damage. *Journal of Speech and Hearing Research, 34,* 820–830.

Tompkins, C.A. (1991b). Redundancy enhances emotional inferencing by right- and left-hemisphere-damaged adults. *Journal of Speech and Hearing Research, 34,* 1142–1149.

Tompkins, C.A. (1995). *Right hemisphere communication disorders: Theory and management.* San Diego, CA: Singular Publishing Group.

Tompkins, C.A. & Baumgaertner, A. (1998). Clinical value of online measures for adults with right hemisphere brain damage. *American Journal of Speech-Language Pathology, 7,* 68–74.

Tompkins, C.A., Baumgaertner, A., Lehman, M.T., & Fossett, T.R.D. (1997). Suppression and discourse comprehension in right brain-damaged adults: A preliminary report. *Aphasiology, 11,* 505–520.

Tompkins, C.A., Bloise, C.G.R., Timko, M.L., & Baumgaertner, A. (1994). Working memory and inference revision in brain-damaged and normally aging adults. *Journal of Speech and Hearing Research, 37,* 896–912.

Tompkins, C.A. & Flowers, C.R. (1985). Perception of emotional intonation by brain-damaged adults: The influence of task processing levels. *Journal of Speech and Hearing Research, 28,* 527–538.

Tompkins, C.A., Lehman, M.T., Baumgaertner, A., Fossett, T.R.D., & Vance, J.E. (1996). Suppression and discourse comprehension in right brain-damaged adults: Inferential ambiguity processing. *Brain and Language, 55,* 172–175.

Trupe, E.H. & Hillis, A. (1985). Paucity vs. verbosity: Another analysis of right hemisphere communication deficits. In R.H. Brookshire (ed.), *Clinical aphasiology, Vol. 15* (pp. 83–96). Minneapolis, MN: BRK.

Tucker, D.M. (1981). Lateral brain function, emotion, and conceptualization. *Psychological Bulletin, 89,* 19–46.

Tucker, D.M. & Williamson, P.A. (1984). Asymmetric neuronal control systems in human self-regulation. *Psychological Review, 91,* 185–215.

Tucker, D.M., Watson, R.T., & Heilman, K.M. (1977). Discrimination and evocation of affectively intoned speech in patients with right parietal disease. *Neurology, 27,* 947–950.

Urayse, D., Duffy, R.J., & Liles, B.Z. (1991). Analysis and description of narrative discourse in right-hemisphere-damaged adults: A comparison with neurologically normal and left-hemisphere-damaged aphasic adults. In T. Prescott (ed.), *Clinical aphasiology, Vol. 19* (pp. 125–138). Austin, TX: Pro-Ed.

Vallar, G. (1993). The anatomical basis of spatial hemi-neglect in humans. In I.H. Robertson & J.C. Marshall (eds.), *Unilateral neglect: Clinical and experimental studies.* Hillsdale, NJ: Lawrence Erlbaum.

Vallar, G. & Perani, D. (1986). The anatomy of unilateral neglect after right-hemisphere stroke lesions: A clinical/CT-scan correlation study in man. *Neuropsychologia, 24,* 609–622.

Van Lancker, D.R. & Kempler, D. (1987). Comprehension of familiar phrases by left- but not by right hemisphere damaged patients. *Brain and Language, 32,* 265–277.

Van Lancker, D.R. & Sidtis, J.J. (1992). The identification of affective prosodic stimuli by left and right-hemisphere damaged subjects: All errors are not created equal. *Journal of Speech and Hearing Research, 35,* 963–970.

Wapner, W., Hamby, S., & Gardner, H. (1981). The role of the right hemisphere in the appreciation of complex linguistic materials. *Brain and Language, 14,* 15–33.

Watson, R.T., Valenstein, E., & Heilman, K.M. (1981). Thalamic neglect. *Archives of Neurology, 38,* 501–506.

Weintraub, S. & Mesulam, M.-M. (1985). Verbal and nonverbal cancellation test. Philadelphia: F.A. Davis.

Weintraub, S., Mesulam, M.M., & Kramer, L. (1981). Disturbances in prosody: A right-hemisphere contribution to language. *Archives of Neurology, 38,* 742–744.

Weylman, S.T., Brownell, H.H., Roman, M., & Gardner, H. (1989). Appreciation of indirect requests by left- and right-brain-damaged patients: The effects of verbal context and conventionality of wording. *Brain and Language, 36,* 580–591.

Wilkins, A.M., Shallice, T., & McCarthy, R. (1987). Frontal lesions and sustained attention. *Neuropsychologia, 25,* 359–365.

Wilson, B., Cockburn, J., & Halligan, P. (1993). The behavioral inattention test. Gaylord, MI: Northern Speech Services.

Winner, E. & Gardner, H. (1977). The comprehension of metaphor in brain damaged patients. *Brain, 100,* 719–727.

Yokoyama, K., Jennings, R., Ackles, Pl, Hood, B.S., & Boller, F. (1987). Lack of heart rate changes during an attention-demanding task after right hemisphere lesions. *Neurology, 37,* 624–630.

APPENDIX 34–1
PUBLISHED ASSESSMENT INSTRUMENTS FOR RHD DISCOURSE DEFICITS

- **ASSESSMENT OF LANGUAGE-RELATED FUNCTIONAL ACTIVITIES**
K. Baines, H. McMartin Heeringa, & A. Martin (1999)
Available from: Pro-Ed
8700 Shoal Creek Boulevard
Austin, TX 78757-6897

- **MINI INVENTORY OF RIGHT BRAIN INJURY (MIRBI)**
Pimental, P.A. & Kinsbury, N.A. (1989)
Available from: Pro-Ed
8700 Shoal Creek Boulevard
Austin, TX 78758-6897

- **REHABILITATION INSTITUTE OF CHICAGO CLINICAL MANAGEMENT OF RIGHT HEMISPHERE DYSFUNCTION (RICE) (2nd Edition).**
Halper, A., Cherney, L.R., & Burns, M.S. (1996)
Available from: Aspen Publications
P.O. Box 6018
Gaithersburg, MD 20877

- **RIGHT HEMISPHERE LANGUAGE BATTERY (RHLB) (2nd Edition)**
Bryan, K.L. (1995)
Available from: Whurr Publishers, Ltd.
19b Compton Terrace
London N1 2UN, England

- **THE BURNS BRIEF INVENTORY OF COMMUNICATION AND COGNITION**
Burns, M. (1997).
Available from: Psychological Corporation
555 Academic Court
San Antonio, TX 78204
1-800-211-8378

Chapter 35

Management of Neurogenic Communication Disorders Associated with Dementia

Tammy Hopper and Kathryn A. Bayles

OBJECTIVES

After reading this chapter, the reader will be able to define the dementia syndrome and commonly associated diseases; describe memory and the pattern of spared and preserved memory functions in dementia; explain the effects of memory impairment on linguistic-communication abilities of dementia patients; discuss assessment of dementia patients; and design treatment programs based on principles of dementia management.

Older Americans comprise the fastest growing segment of the population, and will continue to grow faster than any other age group during the next several decades (ASHA, 1999). In 1993, the percentage of the United States population 65 years of age and older was 12.7, and is projected to increase to 16.4% by the year 2020 (ASHA, 1999). This tremendous growth in the number of elderly people translates to an increased incidence and prevalence of individuals with dementia. One in 10 people over 65 have dementia of the Alzheimer type, and 50% of those over 85 have the diagnosis. The National Alzheimer's Association reports that 4 million people currently have Alzheimer disease, the leading cause of dementia, and estimate that 14 million individuals will have the disease by the middle of the twenty-first century, unless a cure or effective prevention is found.

Understanding the pathogenesis of Alzheimer disease and other diseases that cause dementia, and developing pharmacological and behavioral strategies for improving quality of life for affected individuals are national research priorities. The cognitive-communicative difficulties experienced by dementia patients, and the contribution of these deficits to diminished quality of life, necessitate speech-language pathology services. In this chapter, the syndrome of dementia

will be defined, common dementing illnesses described, effects of dementia on communication specified, and principles for improving the communicative functioning of dementia patients presented. The chapter will conclude with examples and empirical evidence of behavioral treatment programs that promote clinically significant changes in individuals with dementia.

THE DEMENTIA SYNDROME

Dementia is a clinical syndrome defined by deterioration of memory and at least one other cognitive function that is severe enough to interfere with daily life activities. The *Diagnostic and Statistical Manual of Mental Disorders* (4th edition) (DSM-IV; American Psychiatric Association, 1994) specifies certain criteria that must be met for a diagnosis of dementia. Specifically, a patient must have multiple cognitive deficits that include both (1) evidence of short- and long-term memory impairment, and (2) at least one of the following conditions: aphasia, apraxia, agnosia, impaired executive functioning. These deficits must result in significant problems with employment and social functioning and not occur exclusively with delirium. Dementia is associated with many diseases, infections, trauma, and toxins, and although many cases of dementia are reversible, speech-language pathologists primarily deal with patients who have irreversible dementia caused by degenerative neurological disease.

Individuals with dementia are referred to speech-language pathologists because of impairments in communicative functioning. These deficits are a direct result of deterioration in higher cognitive processes, most notably memory. Therefore, understanding memory systems, and their neuroanatomy, is necessary to understanding why and how communicative functioning is affected in individuals with dementing diseases.

MEMORY

Memory can be defined as stored representations and the processes of encoding, consolidation, and retrieval through which knowledge is acquired and manipulated (Bayles & Tomoeda, 1997). Memory is not a unitary phenomenon, but is better characterized as comprising multiple systems. Although the systems are inter-related, some degree of modularity exists. For example, patients with neurological disease or injury that affects specific brain regions may demonstrate relative preservation of one type of memory, whereas another memory system is severely impaired. The idea of memory systems is not without controversy; however, the distinction between short- and long-term memory systems is generally accepted.

Short-term or working memory is the system responsible for activating and retrieving information, holding information in consciousness, and focusing attention (Baddeley, 1986), and is thought to be subserved by the dorsolateral prefrontal cortex. Working memory is described as comprising a central executive control system, and two "slave" or buffer systems: the phonological loop and the visual-spatial scratchpad (Baddeley & Hitch, 1974). In Baddeley's model, the central executive system functions to integrate sensory input, coordinate and allocate processing resources, and plan and control actions. The phonological loop and the visual-spatial scratchpad are buffers for acoustic and visual information, respectively. Working memory not only integrates sensory information from the environment, but also is involved in processing of information retrieved from long-term memory.

Long-term memory can be conceptualized as being declarative or nondeclarative (Squire, 1994). Declarative memory is memory for factual information, and comprises semantic, lexical, and episodic subsystems. Semantic memory refers to general conceptual knowledge, whereas lexical memory comprises knowledge for words. Tulving (1983) defines episodic memory as an individual's autobiographical memory, encoded in a temporal/spatial context. Declarative memory is routinely assessed using explicit memory tasks that require recall or recognition of past episodes or specific facts (Schacter & Tulving, 1994). Declarative memory is dependent upon the hippocampus and adjacent structures and connections of the medial temporal lobe, as well as areas of prefrontal cortex that are active during encoding and retrieval (Schacter, 1996). Patients with damage to these neuroanatomical areas have difficulty with explicit memory. However, implicit memory expression may be preserved.

Implicit memory is the "unintentional or nonconscious use of previously acquired information" (Schacter & Tulving, 1994, p. 12). For example, patients with dementia may be unable to consciously recall a previous learning episode in which several words were practiced. However, if given the first few letters or stem of the practiced word, the practiced word may come to mind. This exemplifies how knowledge gained in the training sessions is expressed through improved performance rather than conscious recollection (Squire, 1994). This facilitated performance, following exposure to a related stimulus, is referred to as positive "priming" and is inferred from decreased response time and/or increased response accuracy. The fact of positive priming suggests that, in patients with Alzheimer disease (AD), semantic memory is not lost nor as impaired as was previously thought. Earlier reports of semantic memory loss may reflect deficits in the ability to access semantic memory during effortful, cognitively demanding tasks. The occurrence of priming in individuals with deficits in explicit memory suggests that priming depends on different neuroanatomical and functional systems than those that support explicit memory (Butters et al., 1990; Schacter & Tulving, 1994).

Nondeclarative memory consists of verbal and motor procedural memory subsystems, reflexes, and habit memory (Squire, 1994). Procedural motor memory refers to knowledge for motor procedures, like playing tennis or shoveling snow. Importantly, learning of procedures may not require conscious recollection of previous study episodes. Rather, motor learning can be implicit, and is demonstrated by behavioral change rather than explicit recall (Squire, 1994). The anatomical systems underlying procedural memory are the basal ganglia, cerebellum, and other neuromotor regions and connections.

The vulnerability of declarative and nondeclarative memory systems varies by disease. Those diseases that primarily affect cortical structures are more likely to produce declarative memory deficits. Diseases that primarily affect subcortical structures and the basal ganglia produce nondeclarative memory impairments. The memory and language profiles of four common diseases associated with progressive dementia will be presented in the following section (Table 35–1).

ALZHEIMER DISEASE

The most common cause of irreversible dementia is Alzheimer disease. Katzman (1998) states that 70% of cases of dementia are caused by AD; however, only 55% of those are "pure" AD, with the other 15% being caused by a combination of AD and another neurological disease. The criteria for diagnosis of AD are specified in the DSM-IV (American Psychiatric Association, 1994) and include gradual onset of cognitive deficits that progressively worsen and are not due to other central nervous system etiologies, systemic conditions, or substance-induced conditions. Neither do they result from a psychiatric disorder such as schizophrenia or depression.

Neuropathological and neurochemical changes play a role in the development of AD (Figure 35–1). Neuropathological changes are characterized by neurofibrillary tangles and neuritic plaques that are widely, although not uniformly, distributed (Tomlinson, 1977), predominantly in the temporal and frontal lobes, the hippocampus, and adjacent areas. The denser the distribution of morphological changes, the more severe the dementia. In parieto-occipital areas changes are

TABLE 35–1

Common Etiologies of Irreversible Dementia and Associated Cognitive Profiles

Alzheimer disease	• Early stage deficits in episodic and working memory • Later stage impairments in semantic memory • Relatively spared procedural memory in early to middle stages of disease
Vascular disease	• Cognitive signs and symptoms are heterogeneous depending on lesion distribution • Cortical lesions are associated with amnesia, visuospatial deficits, and aphasia • Subcortical lesions (common in the periventricular white matter and basal ganglia) are associated with impairments of memory, attention, and motor function
Lewy Body disease	• Fluctuating presentation of cognitive symptoms • Procedural memory and learning deficits may occur with subcortical pathology • Declarative memory systems may be impaired with cortical pathology
Parkinson disease	• Procedural memory impairment • Declarative memory deficits when cortical lesions exist

less apparent and are least common in inferior frontal and inferior occipital gyri (Tomlinson, 1982).

Neurofibrillary tangles, the most characteristic morphological change, are intracellular deposits that occur when fibers within the neuron become twisted in a helical fashion. Scientists have provided evidence to suggest that these paired helical filaments are composed of the protein tau in an abnormally phosphorylated state (Goedert, 1993). Neurofibrillary lesions develop in predictable stages in the brain of the individual with AD. The first nerve cells to develop these lesions are located in the trans-entorhinal cortex and become apparent in entorhinal, hippocampal, basal forebrain, and cortical association regions as the disease progresses (Goedert, 1993). The well-documented nature of the development of neurofibrillary lesions provides investigators with a useful marker for staging the neuropathology of AD.

The development of extracellular deposits, called neuritic plaques, is more idiosyncratic, typically first appearing in cortical areas of the frontal, temporal, and occipital lobes (Goedert, 1993). Neuritic plaques are aggregations of neurons with an amyloid core surrounded by a ring of granular material. It is not clear how amyloid deposition is related to AD: it may be an inert by-product of neuronal death, or a causative agent in neuronal degeneration (Goldman & Côté, 1991).

General overall neuronal atrophy also is present in the brains of individuals with AD, and is seen in areas that have plaque and tangle pathology (Goldman & Côté, 1991). Neuronal degeneration in AD is marked by a loss of synapses and "presynaptic marker proteins" in the neocortex and hippocampus (Goldman & Côté, 1991). Taken together, these neuropathological changes interfere with axonal transport and cause synaptic dysfunction. Neurochemical deficiencies, specifically in the cholinergic system, also contribute to the disruption of nerve transmission at the cellular level.

The cholinergic system is a neuronal network that transmits nerve impulses through acetylcholine. Enzymes necessary for the manufacture of acetylcholine, choline acetyltransferase, and acetylcholinesterase have been found to be reduced by 80% in AD patients (Bowen et al., 1981; Davies, 1983). Curiously, reduction is marked in those brain areas with the greatest concentration of neuritic plaques and neurofibrillary tangles. Of interest to scientists is the connection between cortical changes and subcortical nuclei containing cholinergic neurons, particularly the nucleus basalis of Meynert (Coyle et al., 1983). This nucleus is a major component of the substantia innominata located beneath the globus pallidus. In AD patients, extensive reduction of cholinergic neurons has occurred within the nucleus basalis, a finding that has led researchers to theorize a relation between lack of cortical cholinergic input and the development of neuritic plaques and neurofibrillary tangles. Consistent with the cholinergic hypothesis is the observation that drugs that interfere with acetylcholine can produce memory impairment and confusion in normal individuals (Drachman & Leavitt, 1974; Goldman & Côté, 1991). In addition to the loss of acetylcholine, reductions are apparent in other neurochemicals, among them dopamine and serotonin.

Although specific causative factors of AD have not been determined, certain risk factors have been identified (Salmon & Bondi, 1997). Besides age, which is the most important risk factor, a genetic contribution to the development of late-onset AD recently has been discovered. Apolipoprotein E (ApoE), a protein involved in cholesterol transport, is associated with an increased risk of AD. The gene for ApoE is found on Chromosome 19 and exists in three common allelic forms in humans: ApoE-2, ApoE-3, and ApoE-4 (National Institute on Aging/Alzheimer's Association Working Group, 1996). Individuals having one or two alleles for the e4 form are at a greater risk for developing AD than those who do not have the e4 allele (Honig, 1997), and the e4 form

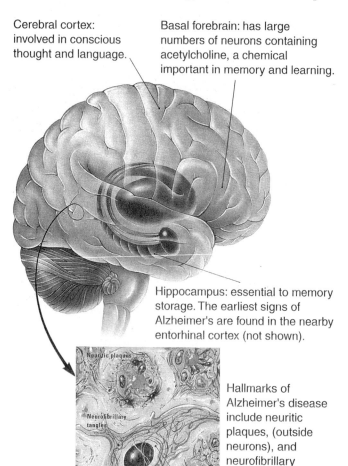

Cerebral cortex: involved in conscious thought and language.

Basal forebrain: has large numbers of neurons containing acetylcholine, a chemical important in memory and learning.

Hippocampus: essential to memory storage. The earliest signs of Alzheimer's are found in the nearby entorhinal cortex (not shown).

Neuritic plaques

Neurofibrillary tangles

Neuron

Hallmarks of Alzheimer's disease include neuritic plaques, (outside neurons), and neurofibrillary tangles, (inside neurons).

Figure 35–1. Neuropathological changes associated with Alzheimer disease. Nerve cells (neurons) in several regions of the brain are affected. Illustration by Lydia Kibiuk. Reprinted with permission from Alzheimer's disease: Unraveling the mystery. NIH Publication #96-3782. National Institutes of Health, 1995.

has been found to exist about three times more frequently in AD patients than among age-matched controls (National Institute on Aging/Alzheimer's Association Working Group, 1996). Despite the genetic risk factor of ApoE-4 presence, late-onset AD is not characterized as an "inherited" disorder. Only a small proportion of AD cases are transmitted by autosomal dominant inheritance (Honig, 1997).

Memory Deficits of AD Patients

The neuropathology of AD is distributed in areas of the brain important to episodic memory. Not surprisingly, therefore, the most reported initial symptom is difficulty remembering recent events. Individuals with early AD consistently perform poorly on tests of episodic memory, such as verbal recall tasks, which are useful for early differential diagnosis.

Working memory also is impaired in AD. Deficits in verbal and visuospatial span tasks have been reported (Spinnler et al., 1988), and AD patients have demonstrated diminished performance on tasks of central executive function (e.g., dual task performance) compared to control subjects (Baddeley et al., 1991).

As dementia severity increases semantic memory also is affected. AD patients have particular difficulty on tasks that require the use of conceptual information, such as naming, category knowledge, attribute knowledge, and verbal fluency (Bayles & Kaszniak, 1987). However, the exact nature of the breakdown in semantic memory is debatable. Some researchers have argued that it occurs from the "bottom up," with knowledge of attributes of objects being lost before generic categorical knowledge (Martin & Fedio, 1983; Warrington, 1975). Evidence from this hypothesis comes from the misnamings of AD patients who often give the name of another item in the same category, such as "orange" for "lemon." The argument is that AD patients lose knowledge of the attributes that distinguish "orange" from "lemon," but retain the categorical knowledge that they are "fruit." Several investigators have challenged the "bottom-up" deterioration theory (Cox et al., 1996; Nebes & Brady, 1988), showing that AD patients are as likely to give attributes as category information when asked to define words.

Other evidence for relative preservation of semantic memory comes from the literature on priming. As mentioned earlier, priming occurs when a response is facilitated by previous exposure to a related stimulus. Some researchers have found that AD patients benefit from priming (Nebes, 1994; Nebes et al., 1984; Nebes et al., 1986), although others report negative effects (Salmon et al., 1988). Nevertheless, the presence of positive priming supports the notion of gross preservation of semantic memory in some patients with mild to moderate AD.

Other types of memory that may be spared in AD include nondeclarative types of memory such as procedural memory. On implicit memory tasks of motor learning, AD patients in the mild-to-moderate stages have been shown to improve in performance over time (Heindel et al., 1989). These types of memory are preserved relative to declarative memory because the basal ganglia, cerebellum, and other neuromotor areas are relatively spared throughout much of the course of the disease.

VASCULAR DISEASE

Patients with dementia, subsequent to multiple infarctions, form a much less homogeneous population than AD patients, and are thought to account for a large proportion of dementia cases. Vascular disease (VaD) commonly co-occurs with AD and, until recently, has been reported to be the second leading cause of dementia, occurring either alone or in conjunction with AD (McKeith et al., 1996). Patients with VaD typically have a history of hypertension, previous strokes, abrupt onset of mental change with stepwise deterioration, and focal neurological signs (Hachinski et al., 1975).

VaD is most commonly caused by thrombolic or embolic strokes, although hemorrhagic disorders also can result in VaD (McPherson & Cummings, 1997). The term *vascular dementia* has replaced the older term, *multi-infarct dementia*, in the DSM-IV (American Psychiatric Association, 1994). Multi-infarct dementia is considered to be a syndrome of VaD, along with strategic infarct dementia, and small vessel disorders (McPherson & Cummings, 1997).

Cognitive signs and symptoms associated with VaD are heterogeneous and depend on the distribution and type of lesions involved. When the major infarctions are cortical, patients may exhibit amnesia, visuospatial deficits, and aphasia. Major subcortical infarctions, frequently in the periventricular white matter and basal ganglia, are associated with memory impairment, motor deficits, sometimes attentional dysfunction, and personality changes (McPherson & Cummings, 1997). VaD patients may be confused with Lewy body or Parkinson disease patients because of the presence of extrapyramidal signs.

LEWY BODY DISEASE

Lewy body disease (LBD) is an increasingly recognized cause of dementia. In fact, McKeith and colleagues (1996) report that LBD now may be the second leading cause of dementia. Although LBD commonly co-occurs with AD, and is considered by some researchers to occur most often as a variant of AD (LBV of AD), others report that it is neuropathologically distinct from AD (Cercy & Bylsma, 1997) and can occur in isolation.

The neuropathology of LBD is marked by protein deposits in neuronal cell bodies. These cellular inclusions are called Lewy bodies and are distributed in the neocortex of frontal and temporal lobes, and in the basal ganglia (Katzman, 1998). The primary behavioral signs of a patient with the LBV of AD include fluctuating presentation of cognitive symptoms, and at least one of the following signs: visual and/or auditory hallucinations with paranoid delusions, mild extrapyramidal features, repeated unexplained falls, and/or clouding of consciousness (McKeith et al., 1996). Although few reports exist of the neuropsychological sequalae associated with LBD, it is reasonable to expect patients to demonstrate impairments in procedural memory and learning, because of neuropathology in the basal ganglia, and in declarative memory systems when Lewy bodies extend to cortical areas.

PARKINSON DISEASE

Idiopathic Parkinson disease (PD) accounts for most cases of Parkinsonism. The classic signs of rigidity, resting tremor,

and bradykinesia are consequent to deterioration of dopaminergic neurons in the basal ganglia. The basal ganglia are important in the control of movement, and dopamine is a neurotransmitter involved in the initiation of movement. As a result of decreased levels of dopamine, PD patients have difficulty initiating movement and commonly exhibit a slow, shuffling gait, flexed posture, and an inexpressive masklike face. Morphological changes, such as the presence of Lewy bodies, also are present in the majority of PD patients and are considered a highly characteristic feature of the disease (Bondi & Troster, 1997).

Dementia is relatively uncommon among PD patients, occurring in only 10 to 20% of cases, according to most estimates (Tison et al., 1995). In those patients who do have dementia, AD-like neurodegenerative changes have been found (Hakim & Mathieson, 1979). Several investigators suggest there may be two forms of PD: a motor disorder without dementia in which changes are limited to subcortical structures and a motor disorder with dementia because of both cortical and subcortical changes (Boller et al., 1979; Garron et al., 1972; Lieberman et al., 1979). Both demented and nondemented PD patients have been shown to be impaired on tasks involving new procedural learning as a result of neuropathology in the basal ganglia (Saint-Cyr et al., 1988).

EFFECTS OF MEMORY DEFICITS ON COMMUNICATION ABILITY OF DEMENTIA PATIENTS

Because of memory impairments, dementia patients have considerable difficulty with linguistic communication. Early in the disease, AD patients become repetitious and forget what they have heard or read. Over time, the discourse of AD patients becomes impoverished and fragmented (Tomoeda & Bayles, 1993), and is characterized by a lack of coherence (Ripich & Terrill, 1988), tangentiality (Obler, 1983), and perseverations (Hier et al., 1985). The ability to formulate ideas and express them orally and in writing diminishes (Bayles & Kaszniak, 1987). Comprehension of language also is impaired because memory for what was recently seen or heard fades rapidly. Nonetheless, phonology and syntax are relatively preserved into the advanced stages of the disease. The following discourse samples are from an AD patient who was followed for several years. His responses to the same stimulus picture reveal the disease effects on linguistic communication. The devastation of semantic content and verbal output is apparent. Note, however, the relative preservation of grammar.

Sample 1—Year 1

Examiner (E): Now I'd like you to look at that picture there.

Subject (S):   Too many children.

E: Yes, I'd like you to tell me everything you can about that. Describe what's happening in the picture.

S: Well, here's a man reading something. It's happening, but he's not looking at the reading. See he's looking someplace else, and he's he's talking to these beautiful ladies here, and also reading his own paper beside. And here's his little boy. Isn't he cute?

E: Describe what's happening there.

S: Well the father's gotten a little tired of reading all this, see, so he's just getting rid of that, one at a time as they march past him going to their own reading or whatever else they do. (laugh) That's real good. And he has his own great big, great great big newpaper. And then he has a few down here like this. Two feet for all that. That's a cute thing right there. (laughing)

E: Okay, do you want to say anything else about that?

S: No, I don't think anything needs to be seen on it.

E: Okay, great.

S: There's a man that thinks maybe something else might be, but he's left everything alone except his newspaper. So everything is all right with him. Don't you think?

E: Yeah.

S: He's he's keeping some of the papers with his teeth. (laughs)

E: All right, thanks.

Sample 2—Year 2

E: Describe what's going on in this picture, and say what you would like to about that.

S: Well, they look like the pictures that uh don't want to be pick-picketed or or made made up into an odd creature in in the meantime.

E: Is there anything else that you want to say about that?

S: Yes, they do. They they they they they actually look so actable that it makes you want to run away for some reason or other. But um they have their their special aqualelge over. The way people take uh take uh an (actoba) that they don't even know anything about. But they just don't try to bother with these other people who have their.

E: Okay, great, thank you.

Sample 3—Year 3

E: Tell me about this picture. What can you tell me about that picture?

S: Yes. Mmhm. It must be a ah, ah, somebody that really thought themselves really gone and close way.

E: What's happening in this picture?

S: No.

E: What's happening in this picture?

S: Well, there's that's something that we'd be supplied with it, but usually goes away with a.

E: Okay. good.

ASSESSMENT

Clinicians need to evaluate for the presence of dementia and its effect on communication skills. To detect dementia, the clinician will benefit from case history information about any neuropsychological changes. Interviewing the primary caregiver, usually the spouse, is advantageous. As part of a longitudinal study of the effects of AD on language, the primary caregivers of 99 AD patients were interviewed about early linguistic and nonlinguistic symptomatology (Bayles, 1991). Caregivers commonly reported memory deficits, word-finding problems, difficulty with finances, and trouble writing letters as antedating the medical diagnosis of the disease.

Identifying the presence of dementia demands consideration of whether current behavior is congruent with the individual's premorbid intellectual ability. For example, an individual whose clinical performance on intellectual tasks was average, but who was a Phi Beta Kappa in college, would be suspect. Such an individual would be expected to perform above average. Premorbid intelligence can be estimated using demographic information (Barona et al., 1984; Wilson et al., 1979). Because dementia patients are older, hearing and visual problems may exist and can confound the dementia diagnosis. Polypharmacy also can confound the diagnosis because many drugs affect mental status.

Another condition that can cause the performance of the individual to mimic dementia is depression, often referred to as pseudodementia. Consider screening for depression using one of the many depression scales, such as the *Hamilton Rating Scale* (Hamilton, 1960), and the *Beck Depression Inventory* (Beck et al., 1961). The *Hamilton Rating Scale* is an interview-based rating scale composed of a 17-item inventory of symptoms, both physical and psychological, which are rated for severity by one or two clinicians. The *Beck Depression Inventory* is a self-report instrument comprising 21 items, and has been used extensively in research and screening applications with elderly adults (Gallagher et al., 1983; Miller & Seligman, 1973).

As mentioned previously, AD and vascular disease commonly co-occur in dementia patients, making it important to consider the possibility of vascular disease in the patients suspected of having dementia. The *Hachinski Ischemic Scale* (Hachinski et al., 1975) is widely used to identify individuals with symptoms typically associated with vascular disease and stroke. The scale comprises 13 features associated with vascular disease and stroke, such as history of hypertension, focal neurological signs, and abrupt onset. Each feature is evaluated and points are accumulated for those present. Individuals who have seven or more points are considered at risk for vascular disease.

Summary of Assessment Measures

Screening
  Story Retelling Subtest, Arizona Battery for Communication Disorders of Dementia (Bayles & Tomoeda, 1993)
  FAS Verbal Fluency Test (Borkowski et al., 1967)

Staging Severity
  Mini-Mental State Examination (MMSE; Folstein et al., 1975)
  Global Deterioration Scale (GDS; Reisberg et al., 1982)

Comprehensive Assessment of Cognitive-Communicative Functioning
  The Arizona Battery for Communication Disorders of Dementia (ABCD; Bayles & Tomoeda, 1993)
  The Functional Linguistic Communication Inventory (FLCI; Bayles & Tomoeda, 1994)

Neuropsychological Tests Sensitive to Dementia

The neuropsychological test most sensitive to early dementia is the episodic memory test. However, because dementia is by definition the loss of multiple cognitive abilities, neuropsychologists typically evaluate attention, problem-solving, reasoning and other intellectual functions in addition to memory. It is beyond the scope of this chapter to review all of the neuropsychological tests used with dementia patients. Instead, the focus will be on measures of cognitive-linguistic function that can be used to screen for dementia, stage dementia severity, and comprehensively evaluate the communicative abilities of dementia patients (Table 35–2).

Screening Tests

Tasks most sensitive to the dementia syndrome are those that are active, nonautomatic, or generative, or ones that depend on logical reasoning. Active nonautomatic tasks require the patient's mental and linguistic involvement in a creative way, such as in retelling a story or generating names of items in a category.

The Story Retelling subtest of the *Arizona Battery for Communication Disorders of Dementia* (ABCD; Bayles & Tomoeda, 1993) is an effective screening tool. In this test, subjects are asked to tell a short story immediately after hearing it and later after an imposed delay. The subtest takes about 5 minutes to administer, and has high sensitivity (i.e., correctly classifies adults who have dementia as having dementia) and specificity (i.e., correctly classifies adults who are not demented as being nondemented) (Bayles & Tomoeda, 1993). The scores of individuals with mild and moderate AD and the scores of nondemented and demented patients with PD are shown in Table 35–3. Note that moderate AD patients remember nothing about the story in the delayed condition.

Generative naming or verbal fluency tests also have been demonstrated to be sensitive to the presence of dementia (Chertkow & Bub, 1990; Ober et al., 1986). When individuals have to conceive of and produce, either in writing or orally, a series of related ideas or examples of objects in a category, they are performing a generative task. The two most common types of fluency tasks are semantic and letter tests.

Mean Scores and Standard Deviations of Normal Elders (NC), Mild and Moderate Alzheimer Disease (AD) Patients and, Parkinson Disease Patients With and Without Dementia on Story Retelling in the Immediate and Delayed Conditions

	Old NC	Mild AD	Mod AD	NPD*	DPD*
Story Retelling Immediate	14.0 (2.3)	7.3 (4.1)	2.6 (3.0)	13.8 (2.5)	7.3 (4.1)
Story Retelling Delayed	12.4 (4.5)	1.0 (2.6)	0.0 (0.0)	12.9 (3.9)	4.1 (6.3)

*NPD = nondemented Parkinson disease; DPD = demented Parkinson disease.
Reprinted with permission from Bayles KA and Tomoeda, CK: *Improving function in dementia and other cognitive linguistic disorders.* Tucson, AZ: Canyonlands Publishing Inc., 1997.

Semantic verbal fluency requires that individuals produce words in a specific category, such as animals. The *Boston Diagnostic Aphasia Examination* (Goodglass & Kaplan, 1983), and the *Arizona Battery for Communication Disorders of Dementia* (Bayles & Tomoeda, 1993) both contain semantic verbal fluency tests. Letter fluency tasks involve the production of words that begin with a target letter. An example of a letter task is the *FAS Verbal Fluency Test* or the *Controlled Oral Word Association Test* (Borkowski et al., 1967), in which an individual must think of as many words as possible beginning with the letters F, A, and S in 1 minute. AD patients have been reported to be deficient in performing on both types of verbal fluency tests, likely because of frontal lobe damage. PD patients and patients with LBD also are reported to be deficient on generative naming tasks (Salmon et al., 1996; Bayles et al., 1993). Because verbal fluency performance involves recruitment of multiple memory systems, it is an extremely sensitive indicator of the cognitive impairments of dementia patients (Azuma & Bayles, 1997).

Staging Severity

The *Mini-Mental State Examination* (MMSE; Folstein et al., 1975) is a widely used measure for staging dementia severity and often is used as a screening instrument. The MMSE comprises 11 items related to orientation, attention, calculation, language, memory, and visuospatial construction, and takes 5 to 10 minutes to administer. Although education may influence examinee performance, reliability and validity of the measure for assessing mental status have been reported to be high (Farber et al., 1988; Foreman, 1987).

The *Global Deterioration Scale* (GDS; Reisberg et al., 1982) is an observation scale used solely for staging dementia severity. It is composed of seven stages that include detailed descriptions of functional deficits typical of individuals at each stage of disease severity. An extension of the GDS, the *Functional Assessment Staging Scale* (FAST; Reisberg et al., 1985), was developed to better characterize the functional abilities (e.g., dressing, communication) of individuals in the more severe stages of cognitive decline.

Comprehensive Evaluation of Communicative Functioning

Although individual tests are appropriate for domain-specific assessment, a comprehensive evaluation of language and communication abilities is best accomplished with a battery of tests. A battery for testing the communicative functions of dementia patients must contain measures of the effects of intellectual deterioration, particularly memory deficits, on linguistic communication.

Pragmatic and semantic skills are more vulnerable to deficits in higher cognitive functions than are phonological and syntactic skills. This is understandable because the content of language and the purpose for which it is used require conscious thought, memory, and planning. The rules of phonology and syntax are finite, predictable, and typically do not require conscious attention. For this reason, measures of semantic and pragmatic reasoning should be included in a test battery for patients with dementia.

Bayles and Tomoeda (1993) designed the *Arizona Battery of Communication Disorders of Dementia* (ABCD) for the purpose of quantifying the communication disorders associated with mild-to-moderate dementia. The battery contains 14 subtests that yield information about five cognitive constructs: linguistic expression, linguistic comprehension, verbal episodic memory, mental status, and visuospatial construction. Raw scores are obtained from individual subtests and are converted to summary scores to allow comparisons between subtests. Summary scores can be converted to construct scores, for interconstruct comparisons, and construct scores can be summed to obtain a total score for the complete test (Bayles & Tomoeda, 1997). Validity and reliability have been reported to be high, and the test has been standardized on AD patients, PD patients, and healthy young and elderly control subjects in the United States, Great Britain (Armstrong et al., 1996), The Netherlands (Dharmaperwira-Prins et al., 1997), and Australia (Moorhouse et al., 1998).

The ABCD was designed for the mild-to-moderate dementia patient. For the more severe dementia patient, a second test battery was developed, the *Functional Linguistic Communication Inventory* (FLCI; Bayles & Tomoeda, 1994). The FLCI has 10 components that allow quantification of linguistic communication. Subtests include tasks such as greeting and naming, writing, reminiscing, comprehending signs, and gesturing. The test battery is sensitive to differences in patients with moderate, moderately severe, severe, and very severe dementia (Bayles & Tomoeda, 1994), and has established reliability and validity. Additionally, patterns of responses to test questions can be profiled to determine intra-individual communication strengths and weaknesses. These profiles are extremely useful for completing the Minimum Data Set (MDS) and developing care plans, as well as for designing individualized stimulation and activity programs for the moderate and severe dementia patient.

BEHAVIORAL TREATMENT FOR INDIVIDUALS WITH AD

The functional deficits that individuals with dementia experience in communication, activities of daily living, and quality of life result directly from the cognitive impairments that define dementia. As mentioned previously, the pattern of these impairments depends upon the distribution of the neuropathology associated with different diseases that cause dementia. In AD, certain aspects of cognitive processing remain relatively preserved, despite severe impairments in other cognitive areas. Recognition of residual capacities, in addition to diminished abilities, will provide the basis for successful interventions for dementia patients.

Principles for Successful Intervention

Bayles and Tomoeda (1997) propose several principles for improving function in AD patients. Clinicians should first reduce demands on episodic and working memory systems. Second, they should increase reliance on nondeclarative memory systems. Third, they should provide activities that strengthen lexical and conceptual associations, and fourth, provide sensory cues that evoke positive fact memory, action, and emotion.

Application of these principles to treatment can help to improve or maintain cognitive-linguistic abilities of individuals with AD. In the following section, several recent studies are reviewed in which one or more of these principles has been utilized to improve functioning of AD patients.

Spaced-Retrieval Training

Spaced-retrieval training (SRT) is increasingly being used to teach new and forgotten information and behaviors to patients with dementia. In SRT, a patient is told a piece of information and then is asked to recall that information repeatedly and systematically over time. Intervals are manipulated to facilitate production of a high number of correct responses to the stimulus question and retention of information over increasingly longer periods of time. SRT is considered to require little cognitive effort (Schacter et al., 1985) and can occur without the patient having explicit recall of the training situation. Also, because strength of association between concepts in semantic memory depends on how often they are activated, repeatedly bringing into consciousness these associations will result in their increased accessibility (Bayles & Tomoeda, 1997). Therefore, SRT involves strengthening of associations, increasing reliance on implicit memory expression (Camp et al., 1996), and reducing demands on episodic and working memory.

Clinicians are using SRT to teach individuals with dementia new information and helpful behaviors. Camp and colleagues (1996) assessed the effectiveness of SRT to teach calendar use for improving prospective memory performance. Also of interest to these investigators was whether the effects of the calendar intervention would be maintained at least 6 months after training. Treatment sessions lasted approximately 30 minutes and continued for 10 weeks. Each session started with the prompt question "How are you going to remember what to do each day?" The subject had to answer "Look at my calendar" to be correct. If the response was correct, a delay was followed by another recall trial. Intervals were increased if the subject continued

with correct responses. If a response was incorrect on any trial, the experimenter provided the correct answer and then immediately repeated the prompt question. When the subject could recall the strategy after a 1-week interval, SRT was terminated.

Once calendar training was successful, up to 5 weeks of additional therapy, one session per week, was provided to teach each patient to complete two tasks on each page of the daily calendar. In this way, the investigators were able to teach the implementation of the skill and evaluate its usefulness in aiding performance of prospective memory tasks in daily life (e.g., walk the dog, write a letter).

Results indicated that the AD patients with mild, moderate, and moderately severe dementia were able to recall the calendar strategy over a 1-week period, and some subjects used the calendar to remember to perform daily tasks. Although participants did not consistently perform tasks on each day, they showed improvement in using the calendar to carry out the majority of the noted tasks. Six-month follow-up visits showed that calendar use continued well after completion of the study.

McKitrick et al. (1992) also conducted a study in which prospective memory was targeted. Four individuals with mild-to-moderate dementia participated. Sessions were conducted once weekly, and involved teaching subjects verbal and motor responses necessary to redeem a coupon for money. SRT was used to first teach subjects a verbal response to the prompt question "What are you going to do when I come back next week?" ("Give you the [pink] coupon"). The motor response consisted of having the subject select the correct coupon and hand it to the examiner. To be successful, the subject had to hand the coupon to the experimenter at the start of the following week's session. In return, the subject was given a dollar. Different colored coupons were trained to criterion successively.

The results again showed that AD patients could learn to perform a task following intensive training. Three of the participants required only one session of therapy whereas one subject required five training sessions. Two of the subjects, who had the lowest cognitive functioning scores, actually performed better on the task than the two with higher scores. This finding suggests that level of cognitive function may not be the only predictor of performance on the SRT task and that more severe memory dysfunction does not prevent the learning of some types of factual and procedural information.

Other functional information also has been taught to dementia patients using SRT. Vanhalle et al. (1998) used SRT to teach face-name associations to a dementia patient. Although they found that the patient was affected by proactive interference (i.e., learning of previous items interfered with the learning of subsequent items), the SRT technique was successful in teaching the patient to recall caregiver names.

SRT can be implemented in the context of other activities, such as speech-language therapy sessions. To demonstrate the utility of SRT in this context, Brush and Camp (1998) conducted a study with nine participants: seven with memory deficits resulting from dementia, and two patients with memory disorders resulting from stroke. The goal was to assess the effect of SRT with memory-disordered patients of different etiologies, and to examine the application of SRT within the speech-language therapy session.

Three pieces of information were taught to each participant: the therapist's name, a personal fact that was considered important to the person (e.g., wife's birthday, room number), and a compensatory technique that was being practiced in speech-language therapy sessions (e.g., using a louder voice, describing an item when unable to name it). Successful recall of the information at the beginning of two consecutive sessions was criterion for completion of the SRT for each piece of information. The three pieces of information were taught sequentially.

Five of the subjects with dementia completed the study. All learned the three pieces of information but had varying levels of recall of the information at 4 weeks post-therapy. The two CVA patients also successfully completed the study and had consistent successful recall of the information at the 4-week follow-up probe.

Using SRT to teach compensatory strategies that enhance communication is a useful technique for speech-language pathologists. Although patients may not remember the specific episodes of learning, they may show an increase in the number of correct responses produced and exhibit a change in the trained behavior.

Capitalizing on Spared Memory Processes

Treatment approaches that draw on spared abilities, specifically procedural memory skills, have been shown to be effective when used with AD patients. Zanetti et al. (1997) assessed the effects of procedural memory stimulation on performance of activities of daily living (ADL) of mild-to-moderate AD patients. Ten AD patients were trained to perform different basic and instrumental activities of daily living, such as washing the face and using the telephone. Twenty activities were chosen for treatment and divided into two sets. Over 3 weeks, five patients were trained on the first set of 10 activities, and the other five patients were trained on activities in the second set. Training sessions were structured such that performance would be more dependent on procedural rather than episodic memory processes (Zanetti et al., 1997). Specifically, verbal cues and prompts were provided during tasks and patients were not asked to remember how to perform any task. The time it took for patients in both groups to perform the trained and untrained activities was recorded. Other outcome measures included performance on neuropsychological batteries including tests of skill learning, word-stem completion (a measure of lexical priming), and paired-associate learning (a test of episodic memory). These measures were given at the beginning and end of the treatment program.

After 3 weeks of training, patients performed the trained tasks in significantly less time than they did at baseline testing. They also showed a significant improvement in the time taken to perform untrained tasks. No significant differences between scores on neuropsychological tests administered before and after treatment were obtained, although a statistical trend for improvement by patients on the lexical priming tests was reported. Although limited by the absence of a control group of patients, these preliminary results provide evidence that ADL training that is focused on the motor or procedural aspects of tasks may be an effective technique for improving the performance of AD patients. The improvement on the untrained tasks may have resulted from generalization from trained activities, although practice effects may have contributed to improved performance.

Another technique that capitalizes on spared memory systems and that may be beneficial for promoting new learning by individuals with AD is referred to as errorless learning. Errorless learning involves minimization of the number of errors that are allowed to occur during learning trials. This approach differs from usual protocols for rehabilitation of memory and language deficits in that it does not involve "trial and error" techniques to promote learning. Baddeley and Wilson (1994) suggest that individuals with episodic memory impairment have difficulty eliminating errors made during learning trials because they cannot explicitly recall the learning experience. Therefore, these individuals continue to make the same errors on subsequent trials, rather than learning from the errors and making corrections.

The errorless learning technique has been used successfully with amnesic patients (Baddeley & Wilson, 1994; Wilson et al., 1994) and recently, the technique has been applied to memory rehabilitation with an individual with AD. Clare et al. (1999) used errorless learning principles, in conjunction with several other techniques, to teach a 72-year-old man with early AD to learn the names and faces of members at his social club. The subject learned the name-face associations, demonstrated some generalization from the pictures to real faces in the environment, and retained the information for 9 months. Although the design of the study makes it difficult to attribute the improved performance solely to reduced errors during learning trials, errorless learning principles were the core component of the instruction and clearly contributed to learning and retention of new information.

Reducing Demands on Episodic and Working Memory Systems: Using Recognition Memory

Bourgeois (1990; 1992) has improved the functioning of dementia patients by capitalizing on spared recognition memory and decreasing demands on impaired episodic and working memory systems. In 1990, she studied the effect on conversational ability of providing stimulus materials in the form of wallets with photographs. Three subjects and their spouses participated in the study. An individualized memory wallet was assembled for each AD subject, consisting of pictures of events and persons the patient could not remember. Caregivers were trained to use the memory wallets in conversation with the subjects, and data were collected on communicative behaviors that occurred when the wallets were used in conversation. When caregivers used the memory wallets in conversation, subjects made significantly more statements of fact and fewer ambiguous utterances.

In a second study, Bourgeois (1992) sought to replicate the treatment effects of the first study, and to investigate whether training the use of the wallets was necessary for patients to use them effectively. Initially, six patients with AD and their caregivers were trained to use the memory wallets in conversation. Positive treatment effects were obtained, with patients making more novel, on-topic statements and fewer ambiguous statements when wallets were used in conversation. Next, three additional subjects with AD were given memory wallets without any specific training. The experimenter served as the communication partner during this phase of the study. Two of the subjects generated more novel, on-topic utterances when the wallets were used in conversation, although the third subject's behavior was more variable. Generally, the results were positive, suggesting that the use of memory wallets improved communication even when subjects were not trained in their use.

The memory wallets used by the AD patients were stimuli that remained visible in a conversation, alleviating the demands that conversation typically places on working memory. Additionally, the photographs stimulated recognition of episodes and people in the patients' lives, reducing the reliance on free recall that usually occurs during conversations about remote and recent events. The use of pictures and sentences about familiar people and places in patients' lives may also promote positive reminiscence and emotion.

Using Sensory Stimulation to Evoke Positive Fact Memory, Action, and Emotion

Providing sensory stimulation to evoke positive fact memory, action, and emotion is an important principle in the management of AD patients. Frequently, individuals with AD in the more moderate to advanced stages are given stuffed animals as companions or decorations in their rooms. Results of several case studies and anecdotal reports support the use of such stimuli to improve the communicative function of AD patients. Bailey et al. (1992) observed improved levels of alertness, increased smiling and nodding, and decreased agitation when four patients with AD were given dolls and stuffed animals. Other researchers have noted similar outcomes (Francis & Baly, 1986; Milton & MacPhail, 1985).

In a single-subject experiment, Hopper et al. (1998) showed that using toy stimuli improved the amount and quality of language produced by four female AD patients with moderate to moderately severe dementia. In response to questions, the subjects produced more information units when toy stimuli were present than when they were absent. The results lend support to the use of tangible stimuli, individualized according to patient preferences, when attempting to improve conversation and social interaction.

Multicomponent Treatment Programs

A program that is based on several of the aforementioned treatment principles and capitalizes on the life experience of AD patients is the Montessori-based intervention developed and described by Camp et al. (1997). Montessori activities were originally developed for children and include materials and tasks that require active participation. The use of Montessori programming promotes learning through procedural memory processes, utilizes concrete everyday stimuli to facilitate action and memory, and reduces demands on episodic and working memory by using structured tasks and repetition.

Camp et al. (1997) describe intergenerational Montessori programming between individuals with dementia and children, and the positive results from a pilot study. In the study, adults and children were matched according to cognitive level, with the adult being more advanced cognitively than the child. This pairing allowed the adult to act as a mentor and teacher to the child during the Montessori activities (e.g., matching, sorting, reading aloud). The primary measure of interest was "disengagement." Disengagement was defined as time spent staring into space for at least 10 seconds or sleeping (Camp & Brush, 1998). Five-minute observation intervals were used to record data on the amount of time AD patients were disengaged. Results showed that when the adults were working with the children, no instances of disengagement were observed, in contrast to the times when adults were not working with the children and episodes of disengagement were common.

Camp and Brush (1998) also have reported on the use of Montessori-type tasks in group activities for dementia patients in skilled nursing facilities. They collected data on the amount of time individuals spent in active engagement (defined as verbal or motor activity focused on the environment), and passive engagement (defined as passively observing what is going on in the environment) during Montessori activities, and compared those instances to the time spent actively and passively engaged during regular adult day care activities. Results showed that individuals participating in the Montessori group activities were more actively engaged than those who participated in the regular programming.

Santo Pietro and Boczko (1998) also compared the effectiveness of different group therapies for AD patients. Outcomes of a multimodality group communication therapy called the "Breakfast Club" were compared to those of "standard" conversational group therapy. Four groups of five midstage AD patients participated in the Breakfast Club, 5 days per week for 12 weeks, and four matched control groups participated in short conversation groups at the same frequency and duration.

Activites in the Breakfast Club were based on facilitation of procedural memory, stimulation of positive emotions, and strengthening of associations, and included a 10-step protocol to facilitate communication. Topics related to breakfast were introduced and the group members engaged in the familiar task of choosing and preparing a breakfast. Throughout, language was elicited by the clinician who "facilitated" conversation using visual cues, semantic associations, and paired-choice questions during meal preparation, eating, and clean-up.

Individuals in the control conversation group sat at a table with a clinician who facilitated conversation by introducing a topic for discussion. Language was elicited using open-ended questions, paired choices, and key word visual prompts, and social conversation was encouraged during greeting and leave-taking.

Group differences were compared using pre/post treatment scores on the *Arizona Battery for Communication Disorders of Dementia* (ABCD; Bayles & Tomoeda, 1993), and the *Communication Outcomes of Communicative and Functional Independence Scale* (COMFI; Santo Pietro & Boczko, 1997), a caregiver rating scale with 20 items related to cognition, psychosocial behavior, communication and conversation, and meal-time independence. Also, the number of incidents of "cross-conversation" between members within a group was compared. Cross-conversation was defined as any utterance between one group member and another, and was proposed to be a measure of social awareness and communicative ability. Results showed that individuals in the Breakfast Club exhibited significantly improved language skills, improved functional independence, and increased use of cross-conversation as compared to members in the standard conversation groups who showed no improvement on any measure. Several other within-group improvements for Breakfast Club participants were noted, including changes in interest and involvement in meal-time activities.

The multifaceted approaches underlying the Montessori group activities and the Breakfast Club were effective in promoting meaningful change in the cognitive and communicative abilities of mild-to-moderate AD patients. Most investigators have favored procedures and programs that focus on relatively preserved skills and have not attempted to directly stimulate the cognitive processes impaired in dementing diseases. However, some recent research provides encouragement for cognitive stimulation programs.

Strengthening Associations Through Cognitive Stimulation

Quayhagen et al. (1995) produced preliminary evidence that suggests that intensive cognitive therapy may slow the general cognitive and behavioral decline associated with dementia. These researchers sought to determine the impact on AD patients of a home-based intervention program of active cognitive stimulation provided by family caregivers. Pairs of AD patients and their primary caregivers were assigned to experimental, placebo, and control groups. Families in the experimental group were trained to provide 60 minutes of "active" cognitive stimulation. The cognitive stimulation program consisted of memory, problem-solving, and conversation activities in which the patient had to actively participate. Memory techniques were characterized by recall and recognition tasks in the verbal and visual domains. The placebo group engaged in more "passive" interventions that were designed to match experimental interventions, yet did not require active participation by the subject. For example, patients might watch "Wheel of Fortune" in the placebo group instead of playing the game "Hangman" in the experimental group. The control group families were placed on a wait list for therapy sessions after the study was complete. Multiple behavioral and cognitive measures were used to assess intervention effects on memory, verbal fluency, problem solving, and attention. Patients in all three groups were tested at three points in time: on entrance into the study, after 12 weeks of treatment, and 6 months after completion (Quayhagen et al., 1995).

The AD patients who received the active cognitive stimulation showed no decline from pre- to post-testing on the measures of global cognitive functioning, whereas the control group declined on all measures. The placebo group declined on some measures and remained stable on others. Interestingly, the experimental group improved on some measures throughout treatment and for a period after treatment, and maintained their pre-treatment level of cognitive function on others, although their performance returned to baseline levels at the 9-month probe.

Bach et al. (1995) also compared the effects of two treatments on the function of 44 individuals with mild-to-moderate dementia. The subjects were randomly assigned to a control group and a treatment group. The control group received 24 weeks of "functional" rehabilitation, including tasks from occupational, physical, and speech therapists. The treatment group received the same functional treatment, in addition to twice-weekly small group treatment consisting of memory training, manual/creative activities, and self-management tasks. Several measures were used to assess change as a result of treatment, including cognitive tests, measures of psychosocial function, and measures of depression. The results showed that both groups had significantly higher levels of cognitive performance and a decrease in depressive symptoms after 24 weeks of treatment. However, the patients in the treatment group had significantly better scores than did the people in the functional group on measures of cognition, psychosocial functioning, subjective well-being, and depression (Bach et al., 1995).

Promoting Generalization

A primary goal of any cognitive-linguistic intervention is the generalization of treatment effects and their continuance after the intervention is discontinued. Little research has been done to determine the factors that promote generalization and maintenance of behaviors in individuals with dementia. Further, the progressive nature of dementia leads clinicians to think that generalization over time is unrealistic. However, the duration of dementia can be quite long, sometimes more than 10 years, and change in cognitive status occurs gradually. A treatment that improves function for several months can improve quality of life and reduce demands on caregivers, and therefore is worth investigating. To assess generalization and maintenance of treatment effects, consider evaluating behaviors that reflect stimulus generalization rather than response generalization.

Stimulus generalization is the occurrence of trained behaviors in nontraining conditions that include different people, situations, or materials than those used in treatment sessions (Thompson, 1989; Olswang & Bain, 1994). The trained response, or treatment behavior, generalizes to different stimulus conditions. For example, stimulus generalization is exhibited by the patient with dementia who is taught a strategy for requesting help in a treatment session with the clinician, who later asks for help outside of the treatment session, showing transfer of the trained response to an untrained context.

Response generalization is the occurrence of untrained responses or behaviors as a result of training other, related responses or behaviors (Thompson, 1989). For example, Lowell et al. (1995) taught patients with aphasia to use a semantic features diagram to aid in self-cuing and improve naming skills. Two of the three subjects used the schema to improve naming of trained items as well as to "generate semantic information regarding any word they wished to retrieve" (p. 110), thus demonstrating response generalization.

Stimulus generalization may be the more appropriate measure for documenting the effects of treatment with dementia patients, as the multiple cognitive deficits associated with dementia may prevent robust response generalization. Measurement of generalization should be focused on trained responses, such as names of family members, that can be used in different stimulus situations.

Clinicians need to program for generalization. The "train and hope" (Stokes & Baer, 1977) method, in which clinicians conduct treatment and hope for functional effects, is a commonly used, yet frequently ineffective, procedure for facilitating generalization. Stokes and Baer (1977) recommend several techniques for facilitating generalization, among them, the introduction of natural contingencies and the use of common stimuli during treatment. Introducing natural maintaining contingencies involves teaching the patient behaviors that will be reinforced in the natural environment. Choosing treatment behaviors that are functional and important to patients and caregivers increases the likelihood that these behaviors will be maintained outside of the treatment situation (Bourgeois, 1991). The use of common stimuli similarly increases the probability that the dementia patient will exhibit trained behaviors in other contexts.

Given the importance of generalization, it is highly desirable to include caregivers in the treatment. They can learn to promote generalization and provide patients with opportunities to strengthen their communication skills.

Caregiver Training Programs

Nash Koury and Lubinski (1991) have evaluated different methods of training nursing staff about how to communicate with dementia patients. These researchers investigated the effect of two training programs on nursing assistants' interactions with patients, their knowledge of geriatric communication disorders, and problem-solving skills. Program A was traditional in-service training (i.e., 1-hour lecture format) and program B involved in-service role-playing (i.e., 1-hour training with the focus on enacting situations and problem solving). One group of nursing assistants received no training.

Outcome scores on a test of knowledge of geriatric communication disorders and strategies for improving communication were compared before and after treatment. Results revealed that role-playing was more effective than lecture for promoting a change in employee behavior, although nursing assistants in the lecture group also showed improved test performance. These findings underscore the importance of staff training in creating a supportive communication environment and improved quality of care for institutionalized individuals with dementia.

Ripich (1994) developed a functional communication program for training caregivers of AD patients. The seven-step program is called FOCUSED. Each letter in the word FOCUSED refers to a strategy for improving communication: (F) functional and face-to-face, (O) orient to topic, (C) continuity of topic—concrete topics, (U) unstick any communication blocks, (S) structure with yes/no and choice questions, (E) exchange conversation—encourage interaction, and (D) direct, short, simple sentences. The FOCUSED training program is divided into six 2-hour modules designed for family and "formal" caregivers. To test its effectiveness, a pilot study was conducted. Seventeen nursing assistants completed the FOCUSED training. Knowledge of communication strategies was measured prior to and after completion of the training. The participants demonstrated increased knowledge of communicative strategies following training, and anecdotally reported increased satisfaction during interactions with AD patients (Ripich, 1994).

Functional Maintenance Therapy

The primary avenue of service delivery for speech-language pathologists who work with dementia patients in skilled nursing facilities under Medicare reimbursement policies is through functional maintenance therapy (FMT). Glickstein and Neustadt (1995) define FMT as a program for individuals with chronic conditions, who need intervention by skilled professionals. FMT typically consists of an evaluation by the rehabilitation professional, followed by the development, establishment, and short-term implementation of a treatment program. As speech-language pathologists and other rehabilitation professionals increasingly provide services to dementia patients in a consultant role, caregivers must be trained to carry out treatment prescribed by therapists. Functional maintenance therapy and other short-term treatment programs necessitate early planning and inclusion of caregivers for carry-over of treatment behaviors to the natural environment. Such an approach is preferable to one in which the planning takes place only when the patient is discharged from therapy.

An example of a functional maintenance program that was focused on functional behavior has been reported in a case study (Bayles et al., 1998) of an individual (BW) with moderately severe dementia (Mini-Mental State Examination score of 9/30) (Folstein et al., 1975). He was living at home with 24-hour care, until he fractured his hip while transferring from his chair to the bed. BW was admitted to the hospital for 3 days, and then discharged to a skilled nursing facility for short-term rehabilitation. The speech-language pathologist evaluated BW and spoke with caregivers about techniques to improve communication during transfers. Caregivers were concerned that his dementia, coupled with a moderate hearing loss, would make it impossible for them to teach him transfer strategies. The speech-language pathologist worked with the physical therapist and the family caregivers, using the spaced-retrieval training (SRT) technique, to teach a "safe transfer" maneuver. The patient was prompted with the stimulus question, "You are standing up. You go to sit down. What do you do with your hands?" which was used consistently during training. Initially, the patient responded with statements such as "put them in my pockets" or "put them on my lap." However, after only eight sessions of SRT, and correct responding in the therapy sessions, he learned to reach back with his hands and

generalized this strategy to everyday situations when cued by caregivers. This case illustrates the benefit of collaborating with caregivers to promote improved functioning after discharge from treatment.

Use of Volunteers in Treatment with Dementia

Collaborations with activities personnel and recruitment of volunteers are two other ways to extend services to AD patients following skilled treatment. Arkin (1995) provided a model for the use of volunteers with her Volunteers in Partnership (VIP) program. Mild-to-moderate dementia patients are paired with university students who assist them in performing weekly volunteer services and who provide memory and language stimulation. Volunteer activities are tailored to each patient's preferences, and include helping at daycare centers, working at animal shelters, and assisting other residents in nursing homes. Memory and language tasks are designed by the clinician, and students are trained in their implementation. Audiotaped quiz tasks (Arkin, 1992) are used to teach memory for factual information, and language is stimulated through activities such as association, picture description, solicitation by the student of opinions or advice about how to solve real-life problems, and reading short passages of text. In a pilot program, 7 of 11 patients produced more on-topic utterances in response to questions about specific topics such as President Kennedy's assassination. Eight patients produced more information units during picture description, and 3 of 4 patients, who used memory tapes, substantially increased their recall of biographical facts (Arkin, 1995). Doing volunteer work in partnership with university students not only stimulates dementia patients; it provides respite for family caregivers.

Measurement Issues

Measuring the effects of treatment for dementia patients is especially challenging because intellectual deterioration is progressive. However, as Camp et al. (1996) have noted, AD patients can demonstrate improvement on specific treatment tasks, despite exhibiting an overall decline in cognitive function. Assessment of change as a result of treatment should include three dimensions: body structures and function, personal activities, and participation in society (World Health Organization [WHO] 1999).

Evaluating change in one dimension of function will be insufficient. For example, assessing change with only pre- and post-standardized tests of memory and language will not capture the improvement that dementia patients may exhibit in conversational ability, affect and level of engagement, and skills or behaviors taught in treatment sessions. However, measures of quality-of-life, quality and quantity of communicative interactions, level of engagement and activity participation, and change in behavior may reveal the positive impact of treatment. Focusing solely on improvement in amount or degree of deficit as a means to demonstrate improvement in therapy is inadequate with patients whose impairments are progressive. Inclusion of multiple measures allows the clinician to determine treatment efficacy by providing converging evidence of behavioral change.

FUTURE TRENDS

In 1991, Bourgeois reviewed the meager literature on behavioral treatments for dementia patients. Few speech-language pathologists had published studies on the efficacy of treating dementia patients. Since 1991, however, interest in treating the communication problems of individuals with dementia has increased and results of studies to date suggest that dementia patients can improve function and maintain abilities longer when engaged in behavioral treatment. Future researchers should continue to focus on factors that influence patient performance in behavioral therapy, including stage of cognitive decline, type of dementing illness, profile of cognitive deficits, degree of caregiver support, and type of living situation.

Data are needed from large numbers of dementia patients to support treatment for individuals at different stages of decline. Generally, most of the treatment studies reported in this chapter involved participants with mild-to-moderate dementia. Treatment of individuals with moderate and moderately severe dementia should be examined in future research. Also, differences exist between institutionalized and noninstitutionalized individuals, making it difficult to extend results of working with patients who reside at home to patients living in nursing homes or assisted-living centers. Characteristics of the learning environment, particularly frequency, intensity and type of therapy, as well as the educational background and expertise of the person providing the therapy still require systematic investigation.

Speech-language pathologists can make important contributions to the well-being of individuals with dementia. With knowledge of preserved abilities and effective intervention principles, the cognitive-communication deficits of dementia patients can be minimized. Positive outcomes of behavioral treatment are promising and provide the foundation for continued investigation of effective therapeutic interventions.

KEY POINTS

1. Dementia is a syndrome associated with several different causes, the most common of which is Alzheimer disease.
2. Individuals with dementia are the fastest-growing clinical population.
3. Individuals with dementia develop multiple cognitive deficits and therefore problems communicating.

4. The distribution of neuropathology of the various dementing diseases explains the patterns of spared and impaired cognitive abilities.
5. Knowledge of these patterns is necessary to provide appropriate assessment and treatment services.
6. By capitalizing on spared memory systems and reducing demands on impaired memory systems, the functioning of dementia patients can be improved.
7. Dementia patients can learn new information and behaviors with appropriate therapeutic techniques.
8. To measure change as a result of therapy, clinicians must evaluate patient function in personal activities and societal participation, rather than focusing solely on level of cognitive impairment.

▶ *Acknowledgments*–This work was supported by the National Multipurpose Research and Training Center Grant DC-01409 from the National Institute on Deafness and Other Communication Disorders.

References

American Psychiatric Association (1994). *Diagnostic and statistical manual of mental disroders* (4th ed.). Washington, DC: APA.

American Speech-Language-Hearing Association (1999). Data snapshots: Gerontology. *ASHA Magazine*, January/February, p. 56.

Arkin, S.M. (1992). Audio-assisted memory training with early Alzheimer's patients: Two single-subject experiments. *Clinical Gerontologist, 12*(2), 77–96.

Arkin, S.M. (1995). Volunteers in partnership: A rehabilitation program for Alzheimer's patients. (J. Chitwood, Director). In C.K. Tomoeda (Producer), *Telerounds*. Tucson, AZ: The University of Arizona.

Armstrong, L., Bayles, K.A., Borthwick, S.E., & Tomoeda, C.K. (1996). Use of the Arizona battery for communication disorders of dementia in the UK. *European Journal of Disorders of Communication, 31*, 171–180.

Azuma, T. & Bayles, K.A. (1997). Memory impairments underlying language difficulties in dementia. *Topics in Language Disorders, 18*(1), 58–71.

Bach, D., Bach, M., Bohmer, F., Fruhwald, T., & Grilc, B. (1995). Reactivating occupational therapy: A method to improve cognitive performance in geriatric patients. *Age and Ageing, 24*, 222–226.

Baddeley, A. (1986). *Working memory*. Oxford, England: Oxford University Press.

Baddeley, A.D., Bressi, S., Della Sala, S., Logie, R., & Spinnler, H. (1991). The decline of working memory in Alzheimer's disease: A longitudinal study. *Brain, 114*, 2521–2547.

Baddeley, A.D. & Hitch, G. (1974). Working memory. In G.A. Bower (ed.), *The psychology of learning and motivation* (pp. 47–89). New York: Academic Press.

Baddeley, A.D. & Wilson, B.A. (1994). When implicit learning fails: Amnesia and the problem of error elimination. *Neuropsychologia*, *32*(1), 53–68.

Bailey, J., Gilbert, E., & Herweyer, S. (1992, July). To find a soul. *Nursing*, 63–64.

Barona, A., Reynolds, C., & Chastain, R. (1984). A demographically based index of premorbid intelligence for the WAIS-R. *Journal of Clinical Consulting Psychology*, *52*, 885–887.

Bayles, K.A. (1991). Alzheimer's disease symptoms: Prevalence and order of appearance. *Journal of Applied Gerontology*, *10*, 419–430.

Bayles, K.A., Trosset, M.W., Tomoeda, C.K., Montgomery, E.B., & Wilson, J. (1993). Generative naming in Parkinson disease patients. *Journal of Clinical and Experimental Neuropsychology*, *15*(4), 547–562.

Bayles, K.A., Hopper, T., Gillispie, M., Mahendra, N., Cleary, S., & Tomoeda, C.K. (1998, November). Improving the functioning of dementia patients: An emerging science. Paper presented at the annual meeting of the American Speech-Language-Hearing Association, San Antonio, TX.

Bayles, K.A. & Kaszniak, A.W. (1987). *Communication and cognition in normal aging and dementia*. Boston, MA: College-Hill Press.

Bayles, K.A. & Tomoeda, C.K. (1993). *The Arizona battery for communication disorders of dementia*. Tucson, AZ: Canyonlands Publishing.

Bayles, K.A. & Tomoeda, C.K. (1994). *The functional linguistic communication inventory*. Tucson, AZ: Canyonlands Publishing.

Bayles, K.A. & Tomoeda, C.K. (1997). *Improving function in dementia and other cognitive-linguistic disorders*. Tucson, AZ: Canyonlands Publishing.

Beck, A.T., Ward, C.H., Mendelson, M., Mock, J., & Erbaugh, J. (1961). An inventory for measuring depression. *Archives of General Psychiatry*, *4*, 53.

Boller, F., Mizutani, T., Roessmann, V., & Gambetti, P. (1979). Parkinson's disease, dementia, and Alzheimer's disease: Clinical pathological correlations. *Annals of Neurology*, *7*, 329–335.

Bondi, M.W. & Troster, A.I. (1997). Parkinson's disease: Neurobehavioral consequences of basal ganglia dysfunction. In P.D. Nussbaum (ed.), *Handbook of neuropsychology and aging*. New York: Plenum Press.

Borkowski, J.G., Benton, A.L., & Spreen, O. (1967). Word fluency and brain damage. *Neuropsychologia*, *5*, 135–140.

Bourgeois, M.S. (1990). Enhancing conversation skills in patients with Alzheimer's disease using a prosthetic memory aid. *Journal of Applied Behavior Analysis*, *23*(1), 29–42.

Bourgeois, M.S. (1991). Communication treatment for adults with dementia. *Journal of Speech and Hearing Research*, *34*(4), 831–844.

Bourgeois, M.S. (1992). Evaluating memory wallets in conversations with persons with dementia. *Journal of Speech and Hearing Research*, *35*(6), 1344–1357.

Bowen, D.M., Davison, A.N., & Sims, N. (1981). Biochemical and pathological correlates of cerebral aging and dementia. *Gerontology*, *27* 100–101.

Butters, N., Heindel, W.C., & Salmon, D.P. (1990). Dissociation of implicit memory in dementia: Neurological implications. *Bulletin of the Psychonomic Society*, *28* 359–366.

Brush, J.A. & Camp, C.J. (1998). Using spaced-retrieval as an intervention during speech-language therapy. *Clinical Gerontologist*, *19*(1), 51–64.

Camp, C.J. & Brush, J.A. (1998). Montessori-based interventions for persons with dementia. (J. Chitwood, Director). In C.K. Tomoeda (Producer), *Telerounds*. Tucson, AZ: The University of Arizona.

Camp, C.J., Foss, J.W., O'Hanlon, A.M., & Stevens, A.B. (1996). Memory intervention for persons with dementia. *Applied Cognitive Psychology*, *10*, 193–210.

Camp, C.J., Judge, K.S., Bye, C.A., fox, K.M., Bowden, J., Bell, M., Valencic, K., & Mattern, J.M. (1997). An intergenerational program for persons with dementia using Montessori methods. *The Gerontologist*, *37*(5), 688–692.

Cox, D.M., Bayles, K.A., & Trosset, M.W. (1996). Category and attribute knowledge deterioration in Alzheimer's disease. *Brain and Language*, *52*, 536–550.

Cercy, S.P. & Bylsma, F.W. (1997). Lewy bodies and progressive dementia: A critical review and meta-analysis. *Journal of the International Neuropsychological Society*, *3*, 179–194.

Chertkow, H. & Bub, D. (1990). Semantic memory loss in dementia of Alzheimer type: What do various measures measure? *Brain*, *113*, 397–417.

Clare, L., Wilson, B.A., Breen, K., & Hodges, J.R. (1999). Errorless learning of face-name associations in early Alzheimer's disease. *Neurocase*, *5*(1), 37–46.

Coyle, J.T., Price, D.L., & DeLong, M.R. (1983). Alzheimer's disease: A disorder of cortical cholinergic innervation. *Science*, *219*, 1194–1219.

Davies, P. (1983). An update on the neurochemistry of Alzheimer disease. In R. Mayeux & W.G. Rosen (eds.), *The dementias*. New York: Raven Press.

Dharmaperwira-Prins, R., Bayles, K.A., & Tomoeda, C.K. (1997). Translation and standardization of the Arizona battery for communication disorders of dementia in the Netherlands: Does the test cross language and culture boundaries. Manuscript submitted for publication.

Drachman, D.A. & Leavitt, J. (1974). Human memory and the cholinergic system: A relationship to aging. *Archives of Neurology*, *30*, 113–121.

Farber, J.F., Schmitt, F.A., & Logue, P.E. (1988). Predicting intellectual level from the Mini-Mental State Examination. *Journal of the American Geriatrics Society*, *36*, 509–510.

Folstein, M.F., Folstein, S.E., & McHugh, P.R. (1975). "Mini-Mental State": A practical method for grading the cognitive state of patients for the clinician. *Journal of Psychiatric Research*, *12*, 189–198.

Foreman, M.D. (1987). Reliability and validity of mental status questionnaires in elderly hospitalized patients. *Nursing Research*, *36*, 216–220.

Francis, G. & Baly, A. (1986). Plush animals—Do they make a difference? *Geriatric Nursing*, *74*(9), 140–143.

Gallagher, D., Breckenridge, J., Steinmetz, J., & Thompson, L. (1983). The Beck Depression Inventory and research diagnostic criteria: Congruence in an older population. *Journal of Consulting and Clinical Psychology*, *51*, 945.

Garron, D.C., Klawans, H.L., & Narin, F. (1972). Intellectual functioning of persons with idiopathic parkinsonism. *Journal of Nervous and Mental Disease*, *154*, 445–452.

Goedert, M. (1993). Tau protein and the neurofibrillary pathology of Alzheimer's disease. *TINS, 16*(1), 460–465.

Goldman, J. & Côté, L. (1991). Aging of the brain: Dementia of the Alzheimer's type. In E.R. Kandel, J.H. Schwartz, & T.M. Jessell (eds.), *Principles of neural science. (3rd ed.).* New York: Elsevier.

Goodglass, H. & Kaplan, E. (1983). *Boston diagnostic examination for aphasia.* Philadelphia: Lea & Febiger.

Glickstein, J.K. & Neustadt, G.K. (1995). *Reimbursable geriatric service delivery: A functional maintenance therapy system.* Gaithersburg, MD: Aspen.

Hachinski, V.C., Iliff, L.D., Zilhka, E., duBoulay, G.H.D., McAllister, B.L., Marxhall, J., Russell, R.W.R., & Symon, L. (1975). Cerebral blood flow in dementia. *Archives of Neurology, 32,* 632–637.

Hakim, A.M. & Mathieson, G. (1979). Dementia in Parkinson's disease: A neuropathological study. *Neurology, 29,* 1209–1214.

Hamilton, M. (1960). A rating scale for depression. *Journal of Neurological Neurosurgery and Psychiatry, 23,* 56.

Heindel, W.C., Salmon, D.P, Shults, C.W., Walicke, P.A., & Butters, N. (1989). Neuropsychological evidence for multiple implicit memory systems: A comparison of Alzheimer's, Huntington's, and Parkinson's disease patients. *Journal of Neuroscience, 9,* 582–587.

Honig, L.S. (1997). Genetics of Alzheimer's disease. *Neurophysiology and Neurogenic Speech and Language Disorders, 7*(4), 6–10.

Hopper, T., Bayles, K.A., & Tomoeda, C.K. (1998). Using toys to stimulate communicative function in individuals with Alzheimer's disease. *Journal of Medical Speech-Language Pathology, 6*(2), 73–80.

Hier, D.B., Hagenlocker, D., & Shindler, A.G. (1985). Language disintegration in dementia: Effects of etiology and severity. *Brain and Language, 25,* 117–133.

Katzman, R. (1998, May). Diagnosis and etiology of related disorders. Paper presented at the meeting of the University of California, San Diego School of Medicine, Alzheimer's Disease Research Center, San Diego, CA.

Lieberman, A., Dziatolowski, M., Kupersmith, M., Serby, M., Goodgold, A., Korein, J., & Goldstein, M. (1979). Dementia in Parkinson disease. *Annals of Neurology, 6,* 355–359.

Lowell, S., Beeson, P.M., & Holland, A.L. (1995). The efficacy of a semantic cueing procedure on naming performance of adults with aphasia. *American Journal of Speech-Language Pathology, 4*(4), 109–114.

Martin, A. & Fedio, P. (1983). Word production and comprehension in Alzheimer's disease: The breakdown of semantic knowledge. *Brain and Language, 19,* 124–141.

McKeith, I.G., Galasko, D., Kosaka, K., Perry, E.K., Dickson, D.W., Hansen, L.A., Salmon, D.P., Lowe, J., Mirra, S.S., Byrne, E.J., Lennox, G., Quinn, N.P., Edwardson, J.A., Ince, P.G., Gergeron, C., Burns, A., Miller, B.L., Lovestone, S., Collerton, D., Jansen, E.N.H., Ballard, C., de Vos, R.A.I., Wilcock, G.K., Jellinger, K.A., & Perry, R.H. (1996). Consensus guidelines for the clinical and pathologic diagnosis of dementia with Lewy bodies (DLB): Report of the consortium on DLB international workshop. *Neurology, 47,* 1113–1124.

McKitrick, L.A., Camp, C.J., & Black, F.W. (1992). Prospective memory intervention in Alzheimer's disease. *Journal of Gerontology: Psychological Sciences, 47*(5), 337–343.

McPherson, S.E. & Cummings, J.L. (1997). Vascular dementia: Clinical assessment, neuropsychological features, and treatment. In P.D. Nussbaum (ed.), *Handbook of neuropsychology and aging.* New York: Plenum Press.

Miller, W.R. & Seligman, M.E.P. (1973). Depression and the perceptions of reinforcement. *Journal of Abnormal Psychology, 82,* 62.

Milton, I. & MacPhail, J. (1985). Dolls and toy animals for hospitalized elders: Infantilizing or comforting? *Geriatric Nursing,* 204–206.

Nash Koury, L. & Lubinski, R. (1991). Effective in-service training for staff working with communication impaired patients. In R. Lubinski (ed.), *Dementia and communication.* Philadelphia, PA: BC Decker.

National Institute on Aging/Alzheimer's Association Working Group. (1996). Apolipoprotein E genotyping in Alzheimer's disease. *The Lancet, 347*(9008), 1091–1095.

Nebes, R.D. (1994). Contextual facilitation of lexical processing in Alzheimer's disease: Intralexical priming or sentence-level priming? *Journal of Clinical and Experimental Neuropsychology, 16*(4), 489–497.

Nebes, R.D., Boller, F., & Holland, A. (1986). Use of semantic context by patients with Alzheimer's disease. *Psychology and Aging, 1*(3), 261–269.

Nebes, R.D. & Brady, C.B. (1988). Integrity of semantic fields in Alzheimer's disease. *Cortex, 24,* 291–300.

Nebes, R.D., Martin, D.C., & Horn, L.C. (1984). Sparing of semantic memory in Alzheimer's disease. *Journal of Abnormal Psychology, 93*(3), 321–330.

Ober, B.A., Dronkers, N.F., Koss, E., Delis, D.C., & Friedland, R.P. (1986). Retrieval from semantic memory in Alzheimer-type dementia. *Journal of Clinical and Experimental Neuropsychology, 8,* 75–92.

Obler, L.K. (1983). Language and brain dysfunction in dementia. In S. Segalowitz (ed.), *Language functions and brain organization* (267–282). New York: Academic Press.

Olswang & Bain (1994). Data collection: Monitoring children's treatment progress. *American Journal of Speech-Language Pathology, September,* 55–65.

Quayhagen, M.P., Quayhagen, M., Corbeil, R.R., Roth, P.A., & Rodgers, J.A. (1995). A dyadic remediation program for care recipients with dementia. *Nursing Research, 44*(3), 153–159.

Reisberg, B., Ferris, S.H., deLeon, M.J., & Crook, T. (1982). The global deterioration scale (GDS): An instrument for the assessment of primary degenerative dementia (PDD). *American Journal of Psychiatry, 139,* 1.136–1.139.

Reisberg, B., Ferris, S.H., & Franssen, E. (1985). An ordinal functional assessment tool for Alzheimer's type dementia. *Hospital and Community Psychiatry, 36,* 939–944.

Ripich, D.N. & Terrell, B.Y. (1988). Patterns of discourse cohesion and coherence in Alzheimer's disease. *Journal of Speech and Hearing Disorders, 53,* 8–19.

Ripich, D.N. (1994). Functional communication training with AD patients: A caregiver training program. *Alzheimer Disease and Associated Disorders, 8*(3), 95–109.

Saint-Cyr, J.A., Taylor, A.E., & Lang, A.E. (1988). Procedural learning and neostriatal dysfunction in man. *Brain, 111,* 941–959.

Salmon, D.P. & Bondi, M.W. (1997). The neuropsychology of Alzheimer's disease. In P.D. Nussbaum (ed.), *Handbook of neuropsychology and aging.* New York: Plenum Press.

Salmon, D.P., Galasko, D., Hansen, L.A., Masliah, E., Butters, N., Thal, L.F., & Katzman, R. (1996). Neuropsychological deficits associated with diffuse Lewy body disease. *Brain and Cognition, 31,* 118–165.

Salmon, D.P., Heindel, W.C., & Butters, N. (1991). Patterns of cognitive impairment in Alzheimer's disease and other dementing disorders. In R. Lubinski (ed.), *Dementia and communication.* Philadelphia: BC Decker.

Salmon, D.P, Shimamura, A.P., Butters, N., & Smith, S. (1988). Lexical and semantic priming deficits in patients with Alzheimer's disease. *Journal of Clinical and Experimental Neuropsychology, 10,* 477–494.

Santo Pietro, M.J. & Boczko, F. (1997). *The communication outcome measure of functional independence: COMFI scale.* Vero Beach, FL: The Speech Bin.

Santo Pietro, M.J. & Boczko, F. (1998). The Breakfast Club: Results of a study examining the effectiveness of a multi-modality group communication treatment. *American Journal of Alzheimer's Disease, May/June,* 1998.

Schacter, D.L. (1996). *Searching for memory.* New York: Basic Books.

Schacter, D.L., Rich, S.A., & Stampp, M.S. (1985). Remediation of memory disorders: Experimental evaluation of the spaced-retrieval technique. *Journal of Clinical and Experimental Neuropsychology, 7,* 79–96.

Schacter, D.L. & Tulving, E. (eds.) (1994). *Memory systems 1994.* Cambridge, MA: MIT Press.

Spinnler, H., Della Salla, S., Bandera, R., & Baddeley, A.D. (1988). Dementia, aging, and the structure of human memory. *Cognitive Neuropsychology, 5,* 193–211.

Squire, L.R. (1994). Priming and multiple memory systems: Perceptual mechanisms of implicit memory. In D.L. Schacter & E. Tulving (eds.), *Memory systems 1994.* Cambridge, MA: MIT Press.

Stokes, T.F. & Baer, D.M. (1977). An implicit technology of generalization. *Journal of Applied Behavior Analysis, 10,* 349–367.

Thompson, C.K. (1989). Generalization in the treatment of aphasia. In L.V. McReynolds & J. Spradlin (eds.), *Generalization strategies in the treatment of communication disorders.* Lewiston, NY: BC Decker.

Tison, F., Dartigues, J.F., Auriacombe, S., Letenneur, I., Boller, F., & Alperovitch, A. (1995). Dementia in Parkinson's disease: A population based study in ambulatory and institutionalized individuals. *Neurology, 45,* 705–708.

Tomlinson, B.E. (1977). The pathology of dementia. In C.E. Wells (ed.), *Dementia.* Philadelphia: F.A. Davis.

Tomlinson, B.E. (1982). Plaques, tangles, and Alzheimer's disease. *Psychological Medicine, 12,* 449–459.

Tomoeda, C.K. & Bayles, K.A. (1993). Longitudinal effects of Alzheimer disease on discourse production. *Alzheimer Disease and Associated Disorders, 7*(4), 223–236.

Tulving, E. (1983). *Elements of episodic memory.* Oxford: Oxford University Press.

Vanhalle, C., Van der Linden, M., Belleville, S., & Gilbert, B. (1998). Putting names on faces: Use of a spaced-retrieval strategy in a patient with dementia of the Alzheimer type. *Neurophysiology and Neurogenic Speech and Language Disorders, 8*(4), 17–21.

Warrington, E.K. (1975). The selective impairment of semantic memory. *The Quarterly of Experimental Psychology, 27,* 635–657.

Wilson, B.A., Baddeley, A., & Evans, J., & Shiel, A. (1994). Errorless learning in the rehabilitation of memory impaired people. *Neuropsychological Rehabilitation, 4*(3), 307–326.

Wilson, R.S., Rosenbaum, G., & Brown, G. (1979). The problem of premorbid intelligence in neuropsychological assessment. *Journal of Clinical Neuropsychology, 1,* 49–53.

World Health Organization. (07/1999). *ICIDH-2: International classification of impairments, activities, and participation.* [online]. Available: http://www.who.ch/icidh

Zanetti, O., Binetti, G., Magni, E., Rozzini, L., Bianchetti, A., & Trabucchi, M. (1997). Procedural memory stimulation in Alzheimer's disease: Impact of a training program. *Acta Neurologica Scandinavica, 95,* 152–157.

Chapter 36

Nature and Treatment of Neuromotor Speech Disorders in Aphasia

Paula A. Square, Ruth E. Martin, and Arpita Bose

As early as 1825, reports of a motor speech disorder resulting from dominant hemisphere damage appeared in the literature. The motor speech disorder was caused by brain insult or diseases similar to those that caused aphasia. The speech disorder, however, had very different symptoms from aphasia (Bouillaud, 1825) in that it was thought to be one of *"articulated speech"* (e.g., Broca, 1861; Liepmann, 1913; Marie, 1906). In aphasia, verbal comprehension, reading and writing, inner language, and possibly even intellect and memory were impaired (e.g., Jackson, 1868 as cited by Head, 1915; Marie, 1906; Wernicke, 1874). These abilities seemed to be *relatively* spared in the disorder of articulated speech.

Over the last 175 years, there have been numerous other reports of speech disorders resulting from dominant hemisphere damage. The nomenclature used to describe the acquired speech disorder has been as diverse as have been the descriptions of symptoms and the pathophysiological, linguistic, and psychological constructs put forth to explain the speech errors. Disagreements regarding the site of structural lesion underlying dominant hemisphere speech impairment have also been prevalent. Square and Martin (1994) presented a summary of the myriad of historical views regarding disordered speech production because of left hemisphere brain damage. Readers are urged to consult that review for further information.

Despite the controversy and terminological confusion, several major themes regarding motor speech disorders because of dominant hemisphere damage emerge from the historical literature. First and foremost, the existence of a significant acquired motor speech disorder of sudden onset resulting from brain damage, the characteristics of which differ significantly from aphasia, continues to be widely acknowledged (Alajouanine et al., 1939; Critchley, 1952; Darley, 1968; Duffy, 1995; Schiff et al., 1983). Second, the articulatory impairment is thought to coexist with

aphasia (Marie et al., 1917; Wernicke, 1885; Schuell et al., 1964) although the disorder can also appear in a pure form (Alajouanine et al., 1939; Dejerine, 1901; Goodglass & Kaplan, 1972; Marie et al., 1917; Square et al., 1982; Schiff et al., 1983; Square-Storer & Apeldoorn, 1991). Third, there is a subgroup of patients with both disorders for whom treatment of the motor speech impairment should take precedence over the treatment of aphasia, although rehabilitation for both disorders is usually undertaken simultaneously (Darley et al., 1975; Tonkovich & Peach, 1989; Wertz et al., 1984). Fourth, the motor speech disorder, like aphasia, might result from either subcortical (e.g., Damasio et al., 1982; Dejerine, 1901; Marie, 1906; Naeser et al., 1982; Wernicke, 1885) or cortical damage (Broca, 1861). Historically, the belief was that cortical damage, especially to the left frontal lobe involving the third and sometimes the second convolution, caused the speech impairment (Lichteim, 1885; Wernicke, 1874, 1885). The notion that cortical damage to the third left frontal convolution was responsible for the motor speech disorder was also the prevailing one in the early to mid 1900s (Alajouanine et al., 1939; Darley, 1977; Denny-Brown, 1965; Goldstein, 1948; Shankweiler & Harris, 1966). Some, however, implicated left parietal cortical damage (Itoh et al., 1980; Marie et al., 1917; Square, 1995; Square et al., 1982; Square-Storer & Apeldoorn, 1991) but most speculated that the apraxia was caused by left frontal cortical damage. More recently, the insula has also been implicated (Dronkers, 1996). Fifth, the speech disorder was, and continues to be, thought of as *not* paralytic/paretic (Broca, 1861; Darley, 1968; Darley et al., 1975; Shankweiler & Harris, 1966; Wertz et al., 1984) but, instead, somewhat akin to other movement disorders such as those associated with (1) cerebellar ataxia (Broca, 1861; McNeil et al., 1989; McNeil et al., 1990); (2) lesions to or dysfunction of the extrapyramidal system (Marie et al., 1917; Schiff et al., 1983) with dystonic speech symptoms resulting (Alajouanine et al., 1939; Square & Mlcoch, 1983); and/or (3) an apraxia affecting speech production (Bay, 1962; Darley, 1968). Finally, it was hypothesized by a few French aphasiologists that the motor speech disorder might in fact be a combination of **dystonic, paretic, and apraxic components** and that each patient's speech handicap was comprised of different proportions of each component (Alajouanine et al., 1939).

In this chapter, we will argue that neuromotor speech impairments are probable in many patients with acquired brain damage that also results in aphasia. It is well known that the dominant, usually left hemisphere, is specialized for both language and motor speech control; thus, both disorders are likely to coexist. While many patients will present with a clinically significant motor speech impairment, especially those with Broca's and global aphasia, and some with conduction aphasia, others with fluent aphasia such as those classified as Wernicke's aphasics, will have a subclinical motor speech impairment (Baum et al., 1990; Vijayan & Gandour, 1995). We will provide information that demonstrates the significant role played by the dominant hemisphere in the control of motor behavior through a relevant review of the literature on the neural control of motor behavior in both nonhuman primates and humans. We will also argue that the motor speech impairments observed in individuals with damage to the dominant hemisphere are most likely heterogeneous in nature. Because of the varying nature and severity of motor speech impairments in aphasia, a framework for establishing treatment goals must be developed to diminish the effects of both the speech and language aspects of the resulting verbal production disorder. Treatment methods that have appeared in the literature will be described and an attempt will be made to explain the neurophysiological basis for the effectiveness of each.

OBJECTIVES

Our overarching goal in writing this chapter is to provide speech-language pathologists with the background information necessary to understand the significance of motor speech impairments that co-occur with aphasia, and to select appropriate management approaches based upon the state of our science. In order to achieve this goal, the following objectives were specified:

- To provide readers with an understanding of the role of left hemisphere in control of movement, specifically speech movement.
- To demonstrate, based upon functional neuroanatomy, that neuromotor speech impairments are probable in many patients with acquired brain damage that also results in aphasia, most probably because of the intimacy of neural substrates mediating linguistic and motor behaviors.
- To provide evidence from the motor physiology literature that argues for the hypothesis that motor deficits, especially motor speech deficits, that result from dominant

hemisphere damage, are likely to be heterogeneous because of different constellations of predominant symptoms.

- To provide arguments that support the hypothesis that different characteristics, such as oral posturing disorders or sequencing disorders, will predominate in different patients with neuromotor speech disorder resulting from dominant hemisphere damage.
- To provide a framework for establishing treatment goals for central neuromotor speech disorders that accompany aphasia based upon predominate characteristics of the speech and oromotor control deficit.
- To review the various facilitative techniques and the range of treatment methods that exist in the literature for the management of speech disorders that accompany aphasia and to formulate hypotheses with regard to the neurophysiological basis for the effectiveness of these treatment methods.

MOTOR SPEECH DISORDERS ACCOMPANYING APHASIA: FUNCTIONAL NEUROANATOMY

The neural control of speech production continues to be poorly understood. While local reflex circuits (for review, see Smith, 1992), brain stem centers (Grillner, 1982), subcortical nuclei of the basal ganglia, cerebellum, and thalamus (Darley et al., 1975; Kent et al., 1979; McLean et al., 1990), and a number of distinct cortical regions (Gracco & Abbs, 1987) have been implicated in speech, the functions and integration of these structures in motor speech control are unclear.

However, over the past quarter century, a number of important insights into the neural control of motor behavior have emerged which may inform our understanding of speech production. For example, anatomical fiber-tracing techniques have revealed the intricate connections between the cerebral cortex and subcortical nuclei in the primate (e.g., see Schell & Strick, 1984; Wiesendanger & Wiesendanger, 1985a,b). Application of single neuron recording techniques and intracortical microstimulation (ICMS) have elucidated the functional organization of a number of cortical motor areas (for reviews, see Asanuma, 1989; Wiesendanger & Wise, 1992), including the orofacial representation (Martin et al., 1997; Murray & Sessle, 1992 a,b). And, data from regional cerebral blood flow (rCBF) (Roland, 1981), positron emission tomography (PET) (Metter et al., 1988; Petersen et al., 1988), and functional magnetic resonance imaging studies (fMRI) (Paus et al., 1993) have contributed to our understanding of neural processing of motor functions including speech.

One of the major concepts to emerge from recent neuroanatomical and neurophysiological studies is that **the motor cortex is made up of a number of spatially separate, functionally distinct cortical motor fields** (Dum & Strick, 1991, 1993; Fink et al., 1997; He et al., 1993, 1995;

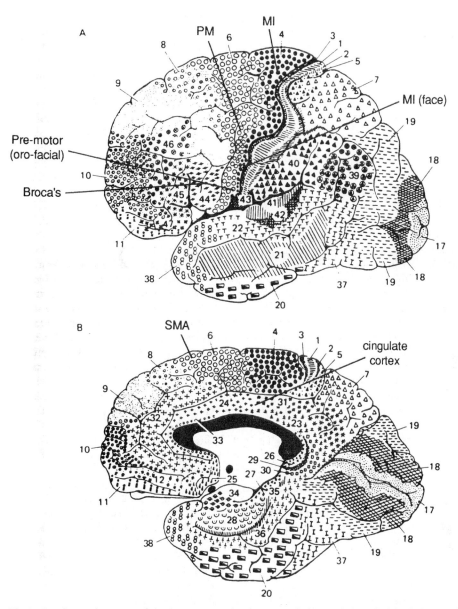

Figure 36–1. Brodmann's areas of the human cerebral cortex. A. Lateral view. B. Medial view. Cortical motor fields are also indicated. MI = primary motor cortex; SMA = supplementary motor area; PM = premotor cortex; Area 44 = Broca's area. (Adapted from Kelly, 1985; with permission).

Muakkassa & Strick, 1979; Picard & Strick, 1996; Wiesendanger & Wise, 1992). These cortical motor fields are illustrated in Figure 36–1.

The primary motor cortex, or MI (Brodmann's area 4), located immediately rostral to the central sulcus, can be distinguished from the more rostral nonprimary motor cortex (Brodmann's area 6). Indeed, it has been suggested that the primary and nonprimary cortical regions play different roles in the regulation of movement. **The nonprimary motor cortex has been implicated in the "programming" of complex volitional movements, particularly in movement preparation and sensory guidance.** In contrast, the

primary motor cortex appears to control movement execution at a lower level of specification (for discussions, see Gracco & Abbs, 1987; Wise & Strick, 1984).

The nonprimary motor areas have been further differentiated into a number of spatially separate, somatotopically organized regions. The two most prominent of these are a medial region, of which the supplementary motor area (SMA) and the cingulate cortex are major components, and a lateral region, known as the premotor cortex (PM) in man, which is analogous to the arcuate premotor area (APA) in the primate (for review, see Goldberg, 1985). Recent evidence suggests that the PM, SMA and cingulate cortex are further differentiated into several fields (Fink et al., 1997; Paus et al., 1993; Wiesendanger & Wise, 1992).

A second and related concept that has emerged in recent years is that **regions of the primary and nonprimary motor cortex are functionally linked to specific subcortical nuclei of the basal ganglia and cerebellum through a number of parallel circuits** (Asanuma et al., 1983; Schell & Strick, 1984; Wise & Strick, 1984). A common feature of these parallel circuits is that each receives inputs from a large region of cortex and projects back to a restricted cortical region.

Several such circuits involving basal ganglia and cerebellar inputs to motor cortex appear to be particularly important in motor control. The basal ganglia access the cortex through a number of segregated basal ganglia–thalamocortical circuits (for reviews, see Alexander & Crutcher, 1990; DeLong, 1990; Graybiel, 1990), one of which has been referred to as the "motor circuit" (Alexander et al., 1986). Within the motor circuit, MI, SMA, APA (PM for humans), and the somatosensory cortex each send topographic, largely nonoverlapping projections to the putamen, a region of the striatum (Alexander & Crutcher, 1990). The striatum is believed to be the 'input stage' of the basal ganglia. This topographic arrangement is maintained as the putamen projects, in turn, to portions of the globus pallidus (GP) and substantia nigra (SN). Motor portions of the GP and SN send topographic projections to specific thalamic nuclei, particularly the VLo (nucleus ventralis posterior lateralis, pars oralis), and VLm (nucleus ventralis lateralis, pars medialis). As seen in Figure 36–2, the circuit is completed through projections from VLo and VLm to the SMA (Schell & Strick, 1984). **Thus, a major output of the putamen is directed to the SMA.** Furthermore, the prefrontal, parietal, and temporal association cortices project via the caudate to parts of the GP and SN which project, in turn, to the anterior thalamic nuclei and then to the lateral precentral cortex (area 6) (for review, see Rolls & Johnstone, 1992). **Thus, a major output of the caudate is directed to the PM (area 6).**

There are two major circuits through which cerebellar output accesses the motor cortex (see Figure 36–2). One circuit originates in the caudal portions of the deep cerebellar nuclei (e.g., the dentate, interpositus, and fastigial nuclei) and projects largely to nucleus X of the thalamus in a somatotopic fashion (Asanuma et al., 1983; Schell & Strick, 1984). This is the area of thalamus which projects, in turn, to PM. **Thus, a major output of the cerebellum is directed to the PM.** A second, separate cerebello-thalamo-cortical system also has been described (Asanuma et al., 1983). This originates in the rostral parts of the deep cerebellar nuclei and projects largely to the VPLo (nucleus ventralis lateralis, pars oralis) of the thalamus. Outputs from this area of thalamus output directly to the MI. **Thus, there is a prominent cerebellar output to MI.** Regarding these parallel circuits, Schell and Strick (1984) have suggested that, **"although the SMA and**

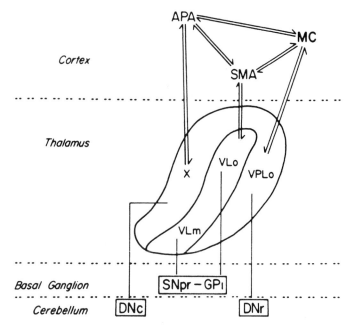

Figure 36–2. Summary of anatomical relationships between cerebellar and basal ganglia efferents and motor and premotor cortical areas. The diagram illustrates: (1) the pathway from caudal portions of the deep cerebellar nuclei (DNc) to area X and the arcuate premotor area (APA); (2) the pathways from the pars reticulata of the substantia nigra (SNpr) and the internal segment of the globus pallidus (GPi) to the thalamic nuclei and on to the supplementary motor area (SMA) and premotor cortex (PM); (3) the pathway from rostral portions of the deep cerebellar nuclei (DNr) to VPLo and the motor cortex (MC); and (4) the reciprocal connections between the MC, APA, and SMA. (Reproduced with permission from Schell & Strick, 1984, p557.)

APA are interconnected with the motor cortex, it may be important to view the three cortical areas as components of functionally distinct efferent systems which are driven by largely separate subcortical nuclei" (p. 558).

Primary Motor Area (MI)

The primary motor cortex (MI) is located anterior to the central sulcus on both the lateral and medial surfaces of the frontal hemisphere and coincides with Brodmann's area 4. It has diverse interconnections between both cortical and subcortical regions. For example, MI receives prominent cortical inputs from a number of premotor fields, including SMA, PM, Brodmann's area 44, and the cingulate cortex (Muakkassa & Strick, 1979). The basal ganglia and cerebellum gain access to MI by way of these premotor inputs (Schell & Strick, 1984). The MI also receives direct projections from regions of the primary somatosensory cortex (SI), including areas 1, 2, and 5 (Asanuma, 1989; Jones, 1987), and the presence of such inputs suggests that MI has access to sensory information which has already undergone processing at the cortical level. In addition to these indirect sensory inputs to MI from somatosensory cortex, the primary motor cortex also receives direct peripheral sensory inputs via thalamocortical fibers. MI also receives prominent cerebellar input via the VPLo of the thalamus (Schell & Strick, 1984).

The outputs from MI are equally diverse (for reviews, see Evarts, 1986; Wiesendanger, 1986). Both anatomic and physiologic data from nonhuman and human primates (Kuypers, 1958a,b; Sirisko & Sessle, 1983) have indicated that **MI neurons project directly to motoneurones.** This important finding has lead to the suggestion that MI cells represent "upper motoneurones" which exert direct effects on motoneurones. In addition, MI projects to a number of cortical and subcortical regions in a distributed fashion, including the premotor cortex, thalamic nuclei, the striatum, red nucleus, pontine nuclei, brain stem, and spinal cord dorsal and ventral horns (Wiesendanger, 1986). Wiesendanger (1986) suggested that the activation of subcortical structures by motor cortex output may provide a means by which the accuracy of an evolving movement is checked in relation to stored "algorithms" resident in subcortical nuclei.

Stimulation experiments demonstrated that the primary motor cortex is somatotopically organized (Huntley & Jones, 1991; Mitz & Wise, 1987). Stimulation studies also have shown that **lower limb, upper limb, and orofacial regions are represented in the medial, middle, and lateral regions of MI,** respectively. Disproportionately large areas are devoted to representation of the face and hand.

Electrophysiological simulation experiments have also implicated MI in the control of movements (for review, see Evarts, 1986; Wiesendanger, 1986). Results of these studies indicated that the primary motor cortex plays an important role in the execution of contralateral movement occurring primarily around a single joint with emphasis on hand and finger movements. **Evidence suggests that the predominant function of the primary motor cortex is in the execution of simple fractionated movements with emphasis on the distal musculature** (Luppino et al., 1991; Mitz & Wise, 1987). Small hand and finger movements requiring **finely graded responses** appear to be directed from this area (Evarts, 1986). In addition, single-unit recording studies show that individual neurons in the primary motor cortex are concerned with parameters of movements such as **force generation** and **modulation.** Wiesendanger (1986) suggested that there are multiple "efferent microzones" in MI that represent a given muscle or elemental movement. These efferent microzones represent the fundamental organization within the MI. The functional implication of these multiple nested representations of muscles is that they may provide a basis for the functional coupling of subsets of muscles and/or structures characteristic of complex coordinated movements (e.g., the "coordinative structure"). This organization also underlies the ability to generate a given elemental movement within the context of a variety of motor behaviors.

The MI receives direct sensory input from the primary somatosensory area (SI). Thus, it has been suggested that this is the means by which movement synergies are preprogrammed at subcortical levels and "fine-tuned" during motor execution in relation to incoming afferent information (for discussion, see Murray, 1989). Gracco and Abbs (1987) have suggested that the direct sensory inputs to MI via the thalamus and SI would be well suited for the "time-critical" processes of orofacial motor execution and suggested that they are involved preferentially in motor programming. Indeed, unilateral lesions to SI and the dorsal column of spinal cord have been suggested to result in severe motor deficits that resembled the effects of MI lesions in some respects (Asanuma & Arissian, 1984).

Lesions to MI typically result in a contralateral paresis, most pronounced distally, which recedes rapidly, leaving **lasting deficits in the ability to perform fractionated movements involving the distal musculature** (Freund, 1987), **and in the use of sets of muscles for executing certain movements** (Evarts, 1986).

Although current understanding of the primary motor cortex is based largely on studies of limb motor control, recent studies have provided insights into the functional organization of regions of MI involved in the control of orofacial motor behavior. In the monkey, the primary motor cortex controlling facial muscles (i.e., face-MI) appears to be organized in multiple efferent microzones which underlie the production of subunits of face movement (Huang et al., 1989; Murray & Sessle, 1992a). This is similar to the pattern seen in limb primary motor cortex (limb-MI). However, unlike limb-MI, which receives primarily deep afferent inputs, the predominant inputs to face-MI appear to be superficial mechanosensory afferents, suggesting the potential importance of such inputs in the generation and fine control of orofacial movements. Furthermore, a close spatial matching of afferent input and motor output has been documented for face-MI. That is, afferent inputs to face-MI neurons tend to arise from a region of the face or mouth, which responds with a twitch movement when electrical stimulation is applied to the neuronal recording site (Murray & Sessle, 1992a).

Functionally, the primate face-MI has been shown to play a role in the generation of voluntary, trained tongue movements, with some neurons showing a relation to tongue movements executed in a particular direction (Murray & Sessle, 1992b). However, primate face-MI neurons also appear to be active in relation to semi-automatic orofacial movements, such as those produced during swallowing (Martin et al., 1997). This finding suggests the possibility that face-MI plays a role in volitional as well as semi-automatic oral motor behaviors.

Usually, unilateral damage to the orofacial regions of MI is traditionally thought to result in a mild transient weakness of the contralateral tongue, lips, and lower face and transient imprecision of speech articulation (Abbs & Welt, 1985; Darely et al., 1975), but cases of persisting unilateral upper motor neuron dysarthia (UUMN), however, have recently been reported by Duffy and Folger (1986), Duffy (1995), and Hartmann and Abbs (1992).

The above description allows us to formulate three hypotheses regarding the influence of lesions to MI on motor speech control in aphasia. First, the ability to produce fractionated speech movements, e.g., use of tongue independent of jaw assistance, or independent regions of the tongue, is likely to be impaired. Second, damage of the MI results in disorders of generation and modulation of movement force. Since speech movements require finely graded minimal forces, MI damage will likely result in effortful, imprecise speech output. Third, a unilateral UMN dysarthria may coexist with aphasia if MI is lesioned.

Premotor Areas

While the size of the primary motor cortex remains constant across primate phylogeny in proportion to body weight, the premotor areas increase in size sixfold from the macque monkey to humans. The axons of neurons in the premotor areas project to the primary motor cortex, as well as to the subcortical structures and to the spinal cord. There are two principal premotor areas: the **premotor cortex,** located on the lateral surface of the hemisphere and the **supplementary motor area,** located on the superior and medial aspects of the hemisphere.

Lateral Premotor Cortex

The lateral premotor cortex (PM) is located rostral to the primary motor cortex and corresponds to Brodmann's area 6. The PM is divided into dorsal and ventral components. The cortical connections of the PM involve the primary and premotor areas, the frontal operculum, the frontal eye field, the supplementary somatosensory cortex (S2), and the anterior part of the parietal association cortex (Barbas & Pandya, 1987; Kurata, 1992). There are also connections with the visual and auditory areas (Wise, 1985) as well as reciprocal inputs from the MI (Godschalk et al., 1984; Pandya & Seltzer, 1982), and extensive cerebellar input. Schell and Strick (1984) have suggested that **cerebellar input is so great that the cerebellum drives lateral area 6.** PM also projects reciprocally to SMA, to regions surrounding the lateral fissure, the cingulate cortex (Matelli et al., 1986; Rizzolatti et al., 1998), prefrontal cortex, and basal ganglia (Pandya & Barnes, 1987).

The lateral premotor area appears to play a role in the planning and production of purposeful complex movement. Physiologic evidence also indicates that activity in lateral area 6 is related to motor acts that are initiated by the presentation of sensory cues, which include visual or somatosensory stimuli (Rizzolatti et al., 1988; Okano & Tanji, 1987). This suggests that purposeful activities under the influence of sensory guidance are processed in this motor area. Wise (1985) suggested that **the role of this area is to use sensory inputs to organize and guide motor behavior.**

Lesions of PM result in a number of sensorimotor deficits, which are generally distinct from the symptoms of SMA and MI lesions. In primates, PM lesions result in a failure to respond to contralateral sensory stimuli (for review, see Pandya & Seltzer, 1982) and, in humans, have been associated with **deficits for production of complex movements.**

Freund (1987) reported that humans with lesions to this area demonstrated a loss of kinetic melody, dissolution of context for composite movements, and disintegration of complex skilled movements. **Both the PM and SMA are also implicated for the generation of sequential motor tasks and temporal organization of movement** (Freund, 1990; Halsband et al., 1993). Freund (1990) also suggested that the motor organization in premotor cortex is bilateral and is important for acquisition and performance of skilled motor acts, including speech and writing.

Lesions of lateral PM and area 44 disrupt the coordinated movements of the lips, tongue, and jaw necessary for intraoral manipulation of food, mastication, and swallowing in nonhuman primates (Larson et al., 1980). Stimulation studies have also suggested a role for this area in orofacial function (Lund & Lamarre, 1974; Huang et al., 1989; for an extensive review see Square & Martin, 1994).

Single-neuron recording studies have also implicated lateral PM in complex oral movements. Luschei et al. (1971) found that the activity of neurons in the precentral face area, including Brodmann's areas 6 and 4, was related to a visually cued, phasic bite task. The activity of other neurons was related to the oral movements associated with ingestion, but not to the bite task. This finding leads us to question whether PM in humans has specialized neurons for speech that are distinct from those for nonspeech oromotor movements.

To our knowledge, there are no studies of the effects on speech from isolated damage to lateral area 6. More extensive damage to the inferior region of area 4 and subadjacent white matter, with extension into the rolandic operculum and insula, but sparing Broca's area (area 44) and the white matter underlying area 44, results generally in a speech deficit without accompanying aphasia (Alexander et al., 1989; Baum et al., 1990; Damasio, 1991; Lecours & Lhermitte, 1976; Pellat et al., 1991; Schiff et al., 1983; Tonkonogy & Goodglass, 1981). This speech deficit is characterized by slow rate, effortful articulatory struggle, articulatory distortions, and disrupted prosody and has been variably referred to as *aphemia* (Schiff et al., 1983), *apraxia of speech* (Darley, 1968), and *phonetic disintegration* (Lecours & Lhermitte, 1976).

Apraxia of speech has been reported to result from lesions of the lateral PM and insula, regions which also have been implicated in the control of complex orofacial movements associated with ingestion, mastication, and swallowing in the primate. Moreover, the deficits seen following such lesions in humans, including slow, effortful, struggle-like movements and disintegration of complex movement sequences, bear certain similarities to the deficits of ingestive behavior seen following lesions of similar cortical regions in primates (for discussion, see Abbs & Welt, 1985). Further, it is important to consider that the lateral PM, implicated in apraxic deficits, receives prominent cerebellar and parietal afferent inputs. The cerebellar inputs to PM may be consistent with reports that apraxia of speech shares many features with ataxic dysarthria (McNeil et al., 1989, 1990).

Supplementary Motor Area (SMA)

The supplementary motor area is located on the medial wall of the cerebral hemispheres, along the superior frontal lobule, and coincides with Brodmann's area 6. It receives both cortical and subcortical inputs and is considered to be **an area of cortical convergence** in that it receives projections from the primary and nonprimary motor cortex, cingulate cortex, and parietal and temporal cortical regions (for review, see Goldberg, 1985).

The efferent projections from SMA represent a cascading system to a number of different levels including MI bilaterally, PM, prefrontal, parietal, and cingulate cortex (Jurgens, 1985). The fact that SMA receives projections from cingulate cortex and projects to MI has been taken to support the view that SMA is part of the system that "focuses limbic outflow onto motor executive regions, thus linking intention formation to programming and execution of specific acts" (Goldberg, 1985, p. 576). Subcortically, SMA makes connections with a number of nuclei of the thalamus, basal ganglia, red nucleus, reticular formation, pontine gray matter, spinal cord, and cerebellum. It has recently been demonstrated that SMA also makes direct corticospinal projections in the primate (Dum & Strick, 1991). Based on this finding, it has been suggested that the SMA has the potential to influence movement directly, independent of MI. Thus, **outputs from SMA, PM, and MI may constitute distinct, parallel pathways through which movements are generated and controlled.**

In recent years it has been found that in monkeys, in addition to four cortical motor areas, there is a fifth motor field, the pre-SMA, which lies rostral to the SMA. In humans, it is possible that there are four cortical areas on the medial wall of the hemisphere analogous to those of monkeys—the pre-SMA, the SMA, and two of the cingulate motor areas (Picard & Strick, 1996). The **pre-SMA is considered to play more complex roles in motor control than the SMA.** The pre-SMA may receive not only basal ganglia inputs via the ventroanterior nucleus, the ventrolateral nucleus, and mediodorsal nucleus of the thalamus, but also via cerebellar input (Inase et al., 1996).

Single-neuron recording studies in awake monkeys have provided clues as to the role of the SMA in motor behavior. These investigations have shown that **SMA neurons respond preferentially in relation to sequential motor behaviors, particularly if the movements are internally generated or self-initiated** (Mushiake et al., 1991). Further, the SMA has been implicated in the sensory guidance of movement (Wise & Strick, 1984). As mentioned earlier, like the PM, the SMA has bilateral and somatotopic organization (Marsden et al., 1996). Electrical stimulation of the SMA evokes complex multi-joint movements, and has also been associated with transient arrest of ongoing motor activity (Fried et al., 1991; Penfield & Welch, 1951). These findings are consistent with the suggestion that the **SMA is involved in establishing a "preparatory state" or "motor set" which precedes the execution of complex motor sequences** (for discussions, see Kurata, 1992; Wise & Strick, 1984). Thus, the SMA participates in the planning, organization, and execution of complex movements with an emphasis on proximal and bilateral activities, and those arising from internal intent as opposed to those driven by external stimuli. **Behavioral studies suggest that the SMA may regulate the planning, sequencing, and coordination of voluntary movements, as well as bilateral execution of action** (Morecraft & Van Hoesen, 1998; Ghez, 1991).

With regard to the influence of SMA on speech, cortical electrical stimulation has been reported to evoke involuntary sustained or interrupted vocalization, speech arrest, slowing of speech, hesitations, word and syllable repetitions, speech slurring, and distortions (Penfield & Welch, 1951; Penfield & Roberts, 1959; Chauvel et al., 1985; Fried et al., 1991). Ryding et al. (1996) observed clear activation pattern in regional cerebral blood flow (rCBF) for SMA in silent speech (internal speech). Murphy et al. (1997) found that during articulation of a phrase there was bilateral activation in sensorimotor and motor cortex, together with activation in the thalamus, cerebellum, and supplementary motor area. They emphasized the bilaterality of the cerebral control of "speaking" without language processing. Interestingly, neurons in the most rostral areas of SMA, whose firing patterns are related to chewing and licking, have been reported in the primate (Chen et al., 1991).

Lesions of the left SMA and/or cingulate cortex have been shown to result initially in a transient period of mutism and akinesia (Alexander et al., 1986; Damasio & Van Hoesen, 1980; Damasio & Geschwind, 1984; Jonas, 1981), which is more pronounced with bilateral lesions (Freund, 1987). As the mutism lifts, there is a paucity of speech (and motor behavior in general) and speech is delayed due to initiation difficulty. However, speech articulation is relatively intact and there are no overt signs of aphasia (Alexander et al., 1989; Damasio & Van Hoesen, 1980; Damasio & Geschwind, 1984). Damasio and Geschwind (1984) suggest that these symptoms reflect a reduced "drive" to communicate verbally and that the underlying deficit is motoric/affective and not primarily linguistic. SMA lesions also have been reported to result in paroxysmal speech or pallilalia, characterized by sudden involuntary vocalizations such as rhythmic repetitions of syllables, words, and phrases (Alajounine et al., 1959; Jonas, 1981; Nagafuchi et al., 1991; Wallesch, 1990). Associated speech symptoms, including echolalia (Alexander et al., 1989; Jonas, 1981), "stuttering" (Jonas, 1981), hesitations, perseverations, and word-finding difficulty have been reported. SMA lesions also have been associated with reduced phonatory volume and aphonia (Jonas, 1981). Petrovici (1983) described the speech patterns of several patients with tumors of the left SMA. He labeled the disorder "aphemia" and highlighted the characteristics of blocks, reiterations, and reduced speech drive. It was concluded from the results of this study that SMA, as one of its functions, serves as a motor control center, especially with regard to the sequencing of speech behaviors.

Hypothetically, the following functions of the premotor areas are implicated for motor speech control in aphasia. First, lesions to these areas impair the ability to prepare to produce and sequence complex purposeful speech movements. Second, lesions to PM result in the loss of kinetic melody and impairment of sequencing motor elements temporally. Similarly, lesions to the SMA result in impaired organization and preparation of internally generated motor speech sequences. Third, speech initiation difficulty caused by lesions in these areas results in articulatory groping, struggle behavior, and dysfluency. Fourth, purposeful activity like speech that relies in part on sensory guidance is impaired in PM damage.

Area 44

Brodmann's area 44 is adjacent to PM area 6. It is a part of the frontal operculum and is considered to be the motor association cortex. Relatively little is known about its inputs and outputs. Abbs and Welt (1985) described area 44 as receiving projections from the posterior parietal and temporal cortical regions with output to regions adjacent to cranial motor nuclei. The output projections are less dense and more diffuse than those originating from MI, PM, and area 6. Thus, area 44 would be expected to exert less direct effects on motor execution than would PM and MI.

In 1861, Broca described the deficit of articulated speech caused by left-hemisphere damage as one in which "memory of the motor images" of words was lost. He ascribed the disorder to damage to the third frontal convolution. The third frontal convolution has since been called Broca's area. Broca's belief has been erroneously sustained, not withstanding intensive debates as to whether damage to the third frontal convolution resulted in linguistically or motorically based deficits of verbal expression. In recent years, Mohr et al. (1978) reported that the disorder of apraxia of speech resulted

from a circumscribed lesion to area 44, Broca's area, while the syndrome of aphasia resulted from larger lesions encompassing not only Broca's area but also a relatively large area surrounding area 44 and white matter deep to Broca's area.

Although area 44 has historically been acknowledged as the cortical center of articulated speech (Broca, 1861), there have been numerous lines of evidence which contradict this long-held notion. Recent studies using neuroimaging techniques such as MRI and CT imaging, have resulted in persuasive evidence that area 44 is not damaged in all cases of Broca's aphasia (Dronkers, et al., 1992; Kertez et al., 1979; Poeck et al., 1984). Further, Dronkers et al. (1992) have demonstrated that damage to Broca's area may result in chronic aphasia syndromes other than Broca's aphasia, especially anomic aphasia, without accompanying motor speech impairment. The work of Dronkers and colleagues also has indicated that area 44 is not necessarily damaged in patients with the specific diagnosis of "apraxia of speech." That is, area 44 may or may not be damaged in cases of left hemisphere motor speech impairment.

Parietal Lobe

The parietal lobe is the region of cerebrum posterior to the central sulcus and superior to the lateral sulcus. The anterior parietal lobe contains the primary somatosensory cortex. The more posterior region contains higher-order sensory areas including the parietal posterior association area and an association area of extensive polymodal convergence. The parietal lobe is characterized by a number of polysensory association areas that are believed to be critical for sensory integration of complex cognitive function (for review, see Freund, 1987).

In humans, the posterior parietal cortices include areas 5, 7, the supramarginal gyrus (area 39), and the angular gyrus (area 40). The two hemispheres are highly differentiated for function (Ghez, 1991). The left posterior parietal cortex is specialized for processing linguistic information while the right parietal cortex is specialized for processing visuospatial information.

The primary motor areas and the primary somatosensory cortices are adjacent and directly interconnected. This is the only circumstance in which primary areas are directly interconnected. This relationship allows output from the primary motor cortex to be rapidly affected by peripheral feedback that has been subjected to little cortical transformation. This synergy is essential to provide adequate and timely motor responses (Morecraft & Van Hoesen, 1998). Further, the links between the parietal and frontal lobes have been suggested to mediate the integration of sensory input in the preparation of motor acts (see Square & Martin, 1994, for discussion).

The posterior parietal lobe plays a critical role in providing the visual information for targeted limb movements and is responsible for integrating information about the state of the individual/animal with that of potential targets, i.e., **creating a context or frame of reference and the spatial coordinates for directing movements** (Ghez, 1991). Rizzolatti et al. (1998) suggested that the parietal cortex is formed by a multiplicity of areas, each of which is involved in the analysis of particular aspects of sensory information.

Lesions to the parietal posterior lobe result in severe attentional disturbances, referred to as *neglect*. Cortical neglect syndromes have been described as those in which errors locating objects in space, deficits in recognizing or performing complex gestures, and deficits in learning tasks requiring knowledge of the body in space occur (Ghez, 1991; Kupfermann, 1991; Mountcastle et al., 1975). Lesions of the parietal lobe or its junction with the temporal and occipital lobes also results in various forms of apraxias, for example, ideational, ideokinetic, tactile, and visuomotor apraxias (for review, see Freund, 1987).

Deficits of fine motor control of the hands may also result from parietal lobe damage. Freund and colleagues, in a series of studies (e.g., Pause & Freund, 1989; Pause et al., 1989) with individuals having unilateral parietal cortex lesions, demonstrated disturbance in **motor deficits concerning force control, fine movements,** manipulation with the hand contralateral to the lesion, and also **loss of the purposive nature of motor acts.** They concluded that limb motor disability as a result of damage to the parietal lobe does not lie in the loss of the kinetic memory to perform movements, but rather in the loss of their evocation by appropriate sensory stimuli.

The fundamental role that the parietal lobe plays in the regulation of motor functions has also been highlighted in a neuropsychological investigation undertaken by Ghika et al. (1998). Manual control was studied in a series of 32 patients who had suffered strokes that resulted in damage only to the parietal lobe. Ghika et al. (1998) reported that **"parietal motor syndrome"** was marked by the predominance of the following symptoms: **unilateral akinesia; limb kinetic and manipulatory apraxia; inability to maintain postures in a steady-state; sensory ataxia; and hand dystonia.** They concluded that **parietal motor syndrome probably reflects the loss of multiple sensory feedback to motor programs.**

Kimura and colleagues (Kimura, 1979, 1982; Mateer & Kimura, 1977) examined the role of parietal lobe in speech and oromotor control, and suggested that the parietal lobe is concerned more with general programming of movements. It subsequently influences the more specific motor control systems in the left frontal region. Thus, they suggested that the unit movements of speech are critically dependent on the integrity of frontal brain regions, but that the production of several sequenced units requires an intact parietal system.

In recent years, Kimura and Watson (1989) examined production of single and multiple-speech and nonspeech oral movements of aphasic patients with anterior and posterior lesions. Patients with anterior lesions were impaired in their ability to reproduce single nonverbal oral movements, and single isolated speech sounds; whereas patients with posterior lesions had difficulty only when they were required to produce multiple oral movements. Based on these findings, Kimura and Watson suggested that the region of the left hemisphere anterior to the central sulcus is critical for control at the "unit" level of movement, whereas the posterior region is involved in accurate selections of movements in multiple movement sequences.

Buckingham (1979, 1983) also addressed the role of the parietal lobe in the regulation of speech. He suggested that motor memories for speech movements are stored both in Broca's area and the parietal lobe, the latter possibly including the inferior postcentral sensory area and/or the supramarginal gyrus. Destruction of these brain regions may result in a disturbance of praxis for vocal tract musculature in the production of speech. There has been a recent report of a patient with temporoparietal hemorrhage who evidenced apraxia of phonation (Sieron et al., 1995).

Recently, Square-Storer and Apeldoorn (1991) reported one patient with bilateral parietal lobe lesions who had apraxia of speech without aphasia. This patient's speech characteristics were different from other patients in the study who also had apraxia of speech without aphasia following frontal lesion of the left hemisphere. Perceptually, the parietal lobe-lesioned patient had relatively normal prosodic contours and speech rate but evidenced frequent reattempts, trial-and-error groping for initial sounds in words, and false starts. Square et al. (1997) also proposed that left parietal regions may play a critical role in the control of speech praxis.

Insula

The insula is a small island of cortex within the cerebral hemispheres. It lies mesial to the frontal, the parietal, and the temporal lobes. The insula has been described as "one of the most mysterious regions of the brain cortex" (Habib et al., 1995).

The insula is a six-layered cortical structure with extensive cortical and subcortical interconnections with brain regions involved in emotional and purposive behavior (Mesulam & Mufson, 1982, 1985). The interconnections within brain regions including speech and language (Benette & Netsell, 1999) are reciprocal.

The human insula is covered by the opercula of the inferior frontal gyrus, the superior temporal gyrus, and the inferior parietal lobe (Augustine, 1985; Bennett & Netsell, 1999). It is formed of four to six gyri. The anterior and posterior regions of the insula are separated by the central sulcus (Augustine, 1985), which encompasses the main branch of the middle cerebral artery.

Evidence suggesting the involvement of the insula in oromotor behavior has come from both animal and human studies. For example, in the awake monkey, electrical stimulation of insula has been shown to evoke chewing-like movements (Huang et al., 1989).

In recent years, the **insula has been implicated as a region that has a significant role in speech and language behaviors.** The massive afferent and efferent connections provide an extensive network for receptive and expressive speech-language processing (Habib et al., 1995). Habib et al. (1995) suggested that the insular cortex, because of its strategic anatomical position and connections, represents a crucial element pertaining to several networks involved in verbal and nonverbal communication. Benette and Netsell (1999) noted that the insula is contiguous with Broca's area, Wernicke's area, the supramarginal gyrus, and the angular gyrus, and spans the entire length of the "language zone."

Most information regarding insular function in normal speech and language processing comes from imaging studies. The **significant role of the insula in speech praxis** has been evidenced by double dissociation, in studies by Dronkers and colleagues. Dronkers et al. (1992) and Dronkers (1996) identified a small and discrete region of the left precentral gyrus of the insula, which is important for motor planning of speech and articulation. Results of these studies showed that damage to this structure was common to all patients with apraxia of speech in their study.

Ardila et al. (1997) propose that "left anterior insula damage is often present in cases of moderate to severe Broca's aphasia, middle insula damage is frequently correlated with repetition deficits (conduction aphasia), and posterior insula damage co-occurs with word deaf features of Wernicke's aphasia" (p. 1164). Damasio and Damasio (1980) conducted a study in which CT scans of patients with conduction aphasia evidenced lesions of the insula and its underlying matter.

Benette and Netsell (1999) hypothesized the following function of the insula in speech and language behaviors. First, the insula contains multiple regions that mediate specific speech and language functions. For example, a focal lesion of the left precentral gyrus of the insula (named "Dronker's area" by Benette & Netsell) results in apraxia of speech. Second, a lesion to a particular insular region will cause permanent deficits. That is, if damage to Dronker's area does not resolve, apraxia of speech will be unremitting. Third, normal development of insula is essential for normal development of speech and language processes. Although we have gathered much evidence about insular function in recent years, its various roles in speech and language processes require further elucidation.

Internal Capsule

The internal capsule is a compact mass of neurons of corona radiata which converges near the vicinity of basal ganglia and thalamus. The internal capsule is an important region because it contains all afferent and efferent fibers that project to and from the cortex. The thalamocortical radiations are the afferent fibers of the internal capsule which arise from the thalamus and project to all regions of the cerebral cortex.

The internal capsule can be divided into three divisions: the anterior limb, the posterior limb, and the genu. The thalamocortical, corticobulbar, and corticospinal fibers are so compactly arranged in the internal capsule that a small capsular lesion can produce widespread motor deficits (Duffy, 1995). **Lesion to the genu and the posterior limb produce greater effects on speech** than lesions anywhere else in the internal capsule (Baum et al., 1990; Duffy, 1995; Metter et al., 1993). Speech is often slow with impaired articulation having the percept of dysarthric quality.

Summary and Implications for a Model of Motor Speech Disorders Accompanying Aphasia

The neuroanatomic and neurophysiologic data presented here lead to a number of conclusions that are relevant to a discussion of motor speech deficits that accompany aphasia. First, a number of areas that control motor behavior are found within the frontal and parietal lobes of the language-dominant hemisphere. Thus, the language-dominant hemisphere is also specialized for the control of human motor behavior. Many of the same areas that control motor behavior also have been implicated in language functions (Ojemann, 1988). Lesions to these areas frequently are associated with aphasia and motor speech disruption.

Second, the frequency and profound significance of coincidence of both language and motor speech control deficits are fundamental for a full appreciation of the verbal communication impairment that results in patients diagnosed as "aphasic," particularly those classified as "nonfluent aphasic," such as Broca's, global and transcortical motor, and some conduction aphasics. Both the motor and language impairments must be considered in order to administer efficient treatment for the verbal expressive disorder in aphasia.

Third, the biological substrates underlying the coincidence of language and motor speech control impairments remain a mystery. The two deficits may co-occur because of the intimacy of the neural structures that mediate linguistic and motoric functions. Alternatively, the language and motor deficits may commonly coexist because the same neural structures mediate both speech motor and language functions (Ojemann, 1988).

Fourth, the motor subsystems within the language-dominant hemisphere that mediate the control of oral and speech functions are (1) spatially and cytoarchitectonically distinct and (2) functionally heterogeneous. Thus, different lesion sites would be expected to result in qualitatively different and/or functionally heterogeneous constellations of speech deficits. The variety of constellations will be dependent on the lesion site, extent, and regional and remote metabolic effects in the brain.

Fifth, it is likely that the disorder that speech-language pathologists have clinically termed "apraxia of speech" is at the least a bi-dimensional disorder, with both a frontal and a posterior apraxia of speech existing (Buckingham, 1979, 1998; Deutch, 1984; Duffy, 1995; Luria, 1964; Square, 1995; Square-Storer & Apeldoorn, 1991; Square et al., 1997). The frontal apraxia of speech may appear distinct from the posterior apraxia of speech because it is more likely to coexist with a significant dysarthria, although the apraxic symptoms may predominate (Rosenbek & McNeil, 1991; Square-Storer & Apeldoorn, 1991). The posterior apraxia of speech, on the other hand, may be a disorder based upon dysfunction of the speech somatosensory system and/or disregulation of posterior speech praxis mechanism resulting in difficulty sequencing speech movements.

Sixth, many patients with aphasia and apraxia of speech may also have a significant dysarthria. All experienced aphasia clinicians recognize that there is often an overriding coexisting dysarthric-like quality to the speech of patients diagnosed as having apraxia of speech. Indeed, over the years, apraxia of speech often has been referred to as a dysarthric condition. While we believe that apraxia of speech and dysarthria are distinct, many patients demonstrate an effortfulness of speech production and/or overriding voice and resonance qualities that are unlikely to be wholly apraxic in nature. Further, classical notions of apraxia indicate that automatic motor function is preserved while propositional movement is not, even when the same muscle collectives are called into play. In what we have traditionally labelled as apraxic-aphasic speakers, the automatic-volitional dichotomy of motor performance is only rarely observed (e.g., Wertz et al., 1984). It might be that the automatic-volitional dichotomy is the essence of apraxia but that the "apraxia of speech" we most commonly encounter is frequently complicated by dysarthric symptoms.

The heterogenous nature of the motor speech disruption that accompanies aphasia caused by perisylvian damage to MI, SI, and PM may be explained as follows. The neurophysiologic data suggest that MI lesions impair motor execution and activation of distal musculature for fractionated movements. PM lesions, however, may result in impairments in the preparation of movement, programming of complex multiple movement sequences, kinetic melody, and use of sensory information to guide movements. Lesions to SI result in degradation of kinesthesia and/or a disregulation of praxis. As such, perisylvian lesions involving MI, PM, and SI may result in deficits of motor execution, and motor programming and somatosensory control of speech. Similarly, given the inputs of basal ganglia and cerebellum to MI via the premotor areas, deficits traditionally associated with pathology of these subcortical regions may also result in heterogenous motor speech disorders. This view is further substantiated by the results of the PET studies which have demonstrated the functional linkages between spatially remote brain regions such as cerebellar and frontal regions (Metter et al., 1988; Metter et al., 1989). Although apraxia of speech is likely to occur with frontal subcortical and cortical lesions as well as midparietal lesions, it may coexist with other neuromotor speech disruptions which are **dystonic, paretic, ataxic, and/or dysfluent,** i.e., stuttering-like, in nature. Our neurophysiological evidence thus substantiates the acoustic evidence offered by Alajouanine et al. (1939). Furthermore, we agree with the conclusion of Alajouanine et al. (1939) that the proportions and various combinations of these disorders will likely vary across individuals.

An attempt to summarize our review of the literature regarding the neurophysiological control of motor speech within a clinically relevant framework is shown in Table 36–1. Suspected primary functional effects and expected speech symptoms arising from primary lesion sites are summarized. This table represents a preliminary attempt to explain our understanding of the possible components that contribute to the "heterogeneous" impairment of articulated speech that often coexists with aphasia. From a functional perspective (column two of Table 36–1), those dimensions that should be considered as important in motor speech treatment include preparing for movement initiation; postural pretuning of the speech mechanism; production of volitional, fractionated speech movements; scaling of motor output; establishing appropriate degrees of freedom for speech movements; encouraging kinetic melody; and establishing control over production of speech motor sequences.

Speech Errors in Aphasia

A great deal of research over the last half-century regarding speech production deficits in aphasia has sought to establish whether a phonological or phonetic disorder accounts for deviant speech production. A phonological impairment would reflect an inability to appropriately access and/or select a phonological representation of a particular lexical item or utterance. In contrast, a phonetic disorder would reflect an inability to appropriately translate or execute the phonological representation into its correct articulatory realization because of defective motor operations.

Blumstein (1998) concluded, from a review of literature, that aphasic patients make both phonological and phonetic speech errors. There is, however, a prevalence of phonetic errors of speech production among many aphasic individuals, especially those classified with Broca's aphasia. Methodologies to study aphasic speech production have included perceptual error analysis (Odell et al., 1991) and acoustic analysis (Kent & Rosenbek, 1983). Both methodologies have resulted in inference of the articulatory states giving rise to the acoustic patterns. More direct methods of articulatory movement have used fiberoptics (Itoh & Sasanuma, 1983), X-ray microbeam tracking (Itoh et al., 1980); strain gauge transducer techniques (McNeil et al., 1989; Forrest, et al., 1991);

TABLE 36–1

Functional Effects on Motor Speech Resulting from Damage to Various Sites in the Dominant Hemisphere

Lesion Site	Suggested Function	Analogous Existing Speech Classification	Speech Symptoms	Perceived Quality
FRONTAL CORTICAL LESION Primary Motor Cortex (Area 4)	■ movement execution ■ activation of distal musculature for fractional movements	■ pseudobulbar palsy ■ upper motoneuron dysarthria	■ slow, effortful speech ■ impaired spatial targeting within vocal tract	■ Dysarthric (Spastic)
Nonprimary Motor Cortex Premotor Area (Areas 6, 44)	■ organization of motor output in relation to sensory information ■ programming of complex, multiple movement sequences "kinetic melody" ■ preparation for movement	■ apraxia of speech, aphemia "small" Broca's aphasia ■ anterior operculum syndrome (with bilateral damage)	■ slow, effortful speech ■ articulatory struggle and groping ■ articulatory distortions ■ dysprosody	■ apraxic ■ dysarthric
Supplementary Motor Area (Area 6)	■ movement initiation ■ scaling of motor output ■ motor sequencing ■ organization and preparation for internally generated motor behaviors	■ akinetic mutism ■ proxysmal speech	■ initiation difficulty ■ dysprosody ■ akinesia ■ dysphonia ■ dysfluency ■ palilalia ■ mutism ■ echolalia	■ dysfluent ■ dysarthric ■ dysphonic ■ initially mute ■ apraxic

Lesion Site	Suggested Function	Analogous Existing Speech Classification	Speech Symptoms	Perceived Quality
FRONTAL SUBCORTICAL LESION Basal Ganglia	■ facilitation or inhibition of cortically initiated movements ■ modulation of frontal lobe functions ■ role in preparation for movement	■ dysarthria, hyperkinetic	■ articulatory inaccuracy ■ prosodic excess ■ prosodic insufficiency ■ reduced volume	■ dysarthric (dystonic)
White Matter Underlying Broca's Area	■ region of afferent and efferent projections with Broca's area	■ dysarthria ■ aphemia	■ slow, effortful speech ■ impaired articulation	■ dysarthric ■ apraxic
Cingulate Cortex	■ role in engaging neocortex for ideational or propositional speech ■ role in learned responses to emotional states	■ possible mutism	????	????
Insula	■ premotor association areas for orofacial behaviors	■ apraxia of speech	■ slow, effortful speech ■ articulatory struggle and groping	■ apraxic
Internal Capsule	■ carries ascending and descending projections from motor cortex	■ dysarthria	■ slow speech ■ impaired articulation	■ dysarthric
PARIETAL CORTICAL LESION Midparietal lobe	■ complex motor sequencing	■ apraxia of speech	■ repetitions, reattempts ■ articulation errors ■ no slowness; word, syllables, and vocalic nuclei of normal duration	■ apraxic

electromyography (Shankweiler & Harris, 1966; Forrest et al., 1991); electropalatography (Hardcastle, 1987), and electromagnetic articulography (Bose et al., 2000; Katz et al., 1990).

In general, the studies of speech production in anterior lesioned patients have shown difficulties in producing phonetic dimensions that require the timing of two independent articulators. Supralaryngeal articulator movement is often mistimed with laryngeal activity, leading to voicing errors. Movement of the velum is mistimed with tongue tip and lip movements, resulting in a blurring of oral and nasal contrast.

The majority of studies that have indicated the phonetic/motoric basis of aphasic speech errors have focused on voice onset time (VOT) (Blumstein et al., 1980; Gandour & Dardarananda, 1984; Shewan et al., 1984; Tuller, 1984), vowel duration (Blumstein & Baum, 1987; Baum et al., 1990; Collins et al., 1983; Duffy & Gawle, 1984; Tuller, 1984), and the duration of frication noise (Code & Ball, 1982; Kent & Rosenbek, 1983; Blumstein & Baum, 1987) for the distinction of voiced and voiceless consonants. Results of such studies have shown that anterior aphasic individuals present significant deficits in voicing, and that these patterns emerge across aphasic speakers in different languages. That is, the errors occur not only in English and Japanese for which VOT distinguishes two categories of voicing, voiced and voiceless, but also in Thai for which VOT distinguishes three categories of voicing in stop consonants, pre-voiced, voiced, and voiceless aspirated (although Ryllas et al., 1995, have found different findings in French-speaking aphasics). Anterior aphasics also have impairment in laryngeal control for voicing for stop consonant (Shinn & Blumstein, 1983) and fricatives (Baum, 1996; Harmes et al., 1984; Kent & Rosenbek, 1983) and for production of intonation contours (Cooper & Sorenson, 1980). Acoustic analysis of formant frequencies of spoken vowel utterances show that anterior aphasics maintain format frequency characteristics of different vowels despite increased variability in their productions (Kent & Rosenbek, 1983; Ryalls, 1981, 1986, 1987). Collectively, the results of such studies confirm the fact that anterior patients have a speech production disorder that affects coordinated timing of particular articulatory maneuvers, i.e., the timing or integration of movements of two independent articulators (Blumstein, 1998). We might also explain these errors as stemming from a decreased ability to produce fractionated movements.

Despite evidence of temporal discoordination between articulators, anterior aphasics do not demonstrate a pervasive timing impairment in speech production. Baum and colleagues (Baum, 1996; Baum et al., 1990) have demonstrated that aphasic patients maintain the intrinsic duration differences characteristic of fricatives varying in place of articulation; for example, /s/ and /ʃ/ are longer in duration than /f/ and /θ/. Although overall vowel duration is longer for anterior aphasics than normals (see Ryalls, 1987, for review), these patients do maintain differences in the intrinsic duration of vowels; for example, tense vowel /i/ is longer than lax vowel /I/.

Studies of coarticulation in anterior aphasia have shown relatively normal anticipatory coarticulation (Katz, 1988; Katz et al., 1990; Sussman et al., 1988). Nonetheless, anticipatory coarticulation may be delayed (Ziegler & von Cramon, 1985, 1986). These results further suggest that phonological planning is relatively intact; but the timing or coordination of the articulatory maneuvers over several subsystems is impaired.

Blumstein (1998) concluded that speech errors in anterior aphasic subjects are not pervasively linguistic in nature. Rather, the majority of errors are phonetic in nature and reflect an inability to implement a particular phonetic feature. The representations for the implementation of phonetic features are not lost as is robustly evidenced in perturbation experiments such as one that demonstrated the preserved ability to compensate for jaw fixation (Baum et al., 1997), and, moreover, the ability to produce coarticulatory effects (Katz et al., 1990). Blumstein, like others, emphasized that "particular maneuvers relating to the timing of articulators seemed to be impaired, ultimately affecting the phonetic realization of some sound segments and of some aspects of speech prosody" (p. 170).

Apraxia of speech (AOS) is often found among the symptom complex of Broca's and conduction aphasia, but at times it is dissociated from aphasia and can be seen (though rarely) in a more or less "pure" form. Thus, it is important to summarize the main characteristics of speech of AOS as they often co-occur or account for Broca's and some conduction aphasic speech errors. These characteristics include inconsistent and variable articulatory movements; increased word or vowel duration patterns; general slowed rate of speaking with resulting prolongations of transitions, segments, and intersyllable pauses; a limited variation in relative peak intensity across syllables resulting in abnormal stress and rhythm patterns; voicing errors; segmental errors; and delayed coarticulation (for review of characteristics of AOS speech see Duffy, 1995; McNeil et al., 1997; and Whiteside & Varely, 1998).

Even though posterior aphasics, e.g., Wernicke's and some conduction, are believed to be unimpaired in their phonetic patterns, there have been reports that demonstrated increased variability in the implementation of a number of phonetic parameters (Kent & McNeil, 1987; Ryalls, 1986). The classification of conduction aphasics is particularly relevant to this discussion. Speech errors of conduction aphasics have been explained by some as having their basis in a deficit in phonological planning (Goodglass, 1992; Kohn, 1984), but McNeil et al. (1997) pointed out that the speech errors of conduction aphasics are very similar to speech errors made by patients with AOS. There may be a physiological explanation for these contradicting views. Metter and colleagues (Kempler et al., 1986) undertook PET studies that demonstrated that there are two subgroups of conduction aphasia as evidenced by brain metabolic patterns: those with hypometabolism to Broca's area and those with only temporoparietal hypometabolism. It might be that at least two subgroups of conduction aphasic individuals exist and that speech errors among conduction aphasics are of varying natures depending on hypometabolic deficits caused by structural lesions.

Studies of posterior aphasics also reveal abnormal patterns in the temporal relations of segmental structure within and between words (Baum, 1992; Baum et al., 1990), and impairments in the production of a number of phonetic dimensions under different speaking rate conditions (Baum, 1993, 1996; Baum & Ryan, 1993; Kent & McNeil, 1987; McNeil et al., 1990). Many phonetic impairments in posterior aphasic patients are subtle and not clinically perceptible but emerge only on acoustic analysis and are, thus, referred to as "subclinical" (Baum et al., 1990; Vijayan & Gandour, 1995). These results lead to the conclusion that speech production involves both anterior and posterior structures of the brain in a complex networking fashion (Blumstein, 1998), a point highlighted in our previous review of neurophysiological mechanisms of the dominant hemisphere that subserve motor speech production.

The preceding review and discussion have provided ample evidence for the probable coexistence of motor speech and language disruptions in many patients who have a verbal production disorder subsequent to dominant hemisphere damage. In the remainder of this chapter, issues regarding the management of neuromotor speech impairments in aphasia will be discussed.

MANAGEMENT OF MOTOR SPEECH DISORDERS ACCOMPANYING APHASIA

The terminological and nosologic confusion that has existed regarding neuromotor speech deficits in aphasia has biased our management of aphasic patients with neuromotor speech impairments. It has been the practice to group patients with motor speech impairments caused by dominant hemisphere damage into the diagnostic category of apraxia of speech (AOS) (Square-Storer, 1989; Wertz et al., 1984). Less frequently, the motor speech disorder has been thought to be dysarthric in nature (Schiff et al., 1983). For those with apraxia of speech, differences among patients have been thought to vary with regard to **severity** rather than combinations of primary and secondary **pathophysiologies**. In accordance, treatment interventions have been advocated for severe, moderate, and mild apraxia of speech, as shown in Table 36–2 (Wertz et al., 1984).

In the last column of Table 36–2, we present a different approach for viewing traditional intervention for AOS. Our analysis presumes three types of deficits and, hence, three

TABLE 36–2

Traditional Approaches for Patients with Apraxia of Speech of Different Degrees of Severity with Speculated Level of Intervention

Severity Level	Recommended Approaches	Level of Intervention
SEVERE	Segmental/syllabic level imitation with • Imitation • Phonetic placement • Phonetic derivation • Derivation + placement • Key word technique Imitation of contrasts Contrastive stress drills	Postural shaping (spatial targeting) and/or production of functional units of speech (coordinative structures) Rate and melodic flow
MODERATE	Intersystemic facilitators • Tapping foot • Tapping leg • Finger counting • Finger tapping Intrasystemic facilitators • Pacing board	Rate and melodic flow
MILD	Expanded contrastive stress drills	Rate and melodic flow

(Wertz et al., 1984)

types of interventions: (1) postural shaping; (2) production of functional units (coordinative structures); and (3) rhythm and pacing. Because we believe that neuromotor speech disruptions in aphasia are not homogeneous, we query whether **severity** is the deciding factor for the appropriate selection of treatment approaches. Perhaps it is the primary pathophysiology that is the determining factor. That is, are the postural shaping methods, especially those that utilize tactile sensation paired with auditory and visual stimulation, more appropriate for patients who cannot volitionally attain appropriate placement of the oral structures to initiate speech? Are methods which focus on coordination of speech subsystems appropriate for patients who cannot produce isolated phonemes and monosyllables? And, are melodic and rate control approaches more appropriate when sequencing disruptions prevail? With regard to the latter, rate and rhythm approaches have been used widely in the treatment of movement disorders, particularly hypokinetic and ataxic dysarthria (Helm, 1979; Beukelman & Yorkston, 1978; Yorkston & Beukelman, 1981; Berry & Goshorn, 1983; Hanson & Metter, 1980, 1983) as well as apraxia of speech (Simmons, 1978; Rubow et al., 1982; Wertz et al., 1984; Square-Storer, 1989). Another important research question is why different treatment approaches are necessary. Are they necessary because some are appropriate for one severity level while others are appropriate for other severity levels? Or, do different treatment approaches target different pathophysiological conditions? (See Kimura, 1982, and Kimura & Watson, 1989; for discussions of oromotor versus sequencing disorders).

Presented in Table 36–3 is a summary of the traditional approaches used for enhancement of speech among dysarthric speakers as derived principally from Yorkston et al. (1988). The similarities and differences between treatment approaches for what we have termed apraxia of speech and dysarthria are easily discerned. First, there is rarely a need to establish physiological support for speech in treatment approaches for the disorder we have termed apraxia of speech; while for dysarthric patients, rehabilitation focused on establishing the physiological support for speech in the respiratory, phonatory, and velopharyngeal systems is typical and often a necessary precursor prior to shifting to methods used for promoting oral spatial and temporal manipulations. Second, for what we have traditionally presumed to be severe and sometimes moderate apraxia of speech, it frequently has been inferred that there may be a need to focus on enhancing spatial and temporal parameters for phonemes and syllable production through tactile techniques such as phonetic placement or kinesthetic techniques such as phonetic derivation. For some dysarthric speakers similar techniques are also required, but generally, once adequate physiological support for speech has been obtained through work on the respiratory, phonatory, and velopharyngeal systems, contrastive articulation drills and intelligibility drills, examples of which are shown in Table 36–3, are the focus of treatment (Yorkston

---

TABLE 36–3

Traditional Speech Treatment Approaches with Acquired Dysarthrias with Speculated Level of Intervention

Establishing Physiological Support for Speech
- Tone, strength
- Coordination of respiratory, phonatory, velopharyngeal

Articulatory Drills
- Vocal tract shaping/production of functional units of speech
  Contrastive stress drills
    pin-bin
    day-may
  Intelligibility drills
    my, hi, buy, dye, sigh
    mail, Mel, mall, meal, mill, mole
    pan, ban, tan, can, ran, man
    lab, lack, lag, lap, laugh

Rate and Stress Drills
- Melodic flow
- Rate control
  Rigid
    Pacing boards (Helm, 1979)
    Alphabet supplementation (Beukelman & Yorkston, 1978)
  Rhythmic cuing
    Computerized (Beukelman, 1983)
    Clinician-controlled reading rule (Yorkston & Beukelman, 1981)
  Other
    Delayed auditory feedback (Hanson & Metter, 1980)
    Oscilloscopic (Berry & Goshorn, 1983)
- Stress
  Natural stress patterning (Yorkston et al., 1988)

(Yorkston et al., 1988)

---

et al., 1988). Thus, it may be inferred that aphasic patients with apraxia of speech are 'more lost' in the oral cavity, or, are more likely to have an impaired guidance system for the coordination of spatial and temporal aspects of correct phoneme production. Furthermore, the adult apraxic speaker usually requires focused attention on the sound, the feel, and the look of speech. Tactile and kinesthetic input paired with auditory and visual stimulation for the placement and movement of the oral structures is generally highlighted more in the treatment of individuals with AOS than those with dysarthria. The differences in treatment approaches for what we have termed apraxia of speech and dysarthria are thus clear.

The similarities in treatment of apraxic and dysarthric speakers are also dramatic as demonstrated by a comparison of the information presented in Tables 36–3 to 36–5. That is, all other traditional therapeutic techniques, whether for AOS or dysarthrias, are those that emphasize postural shaping, the production of functional speech units, melodic flow, and rhythm and rate of speech. Therapies that focus

TABLE 36-4

Most Frequent Speech Symptoms Associated with the Neuromotor Speech Disorders in Aphasia Typically Called "Apraxia of Speech"

Perceived substitutions, distortions
Perceived omissions and additions
Effortful speech
Trial and error grouping
Slow speech
Excess and equal stress
Repetitions
More errors on polysyllabic stimuli
Inconsistent errors
Islands of error-free speech

on rhythm and rate appear to improve prosody and reduce segmental errors. Although the treatment approaches may be summarized in this way, we are not indicating that what we have traditionally termed apraxia of speech is dysarthria or vice-versa. The point we wish to stress is that the neuromotor speech disorder typically observed in aphasic patients is qualitatively different at some levels from those of our traditional dysarthria classifications (Darley et al., 1975); apraxia of speech treatment also has some characteristics that are strikingly similar to some of the those used for the treatment of some of the dysarthrias.

We also are not attempting to diminish the fact that different treatment approaches are required for patients who are principally dysarthric or principally apraxic. However, it is our view that similarities exist when apraxic and dysarthric speakers have impairments to similar basic mechanisms that control motor speech production. The similarities result in large part due to the intimacy of the interconnections of systems and the fact that the motor control mechanisms operate dynamically and influence one another. These points were highlighted in the preceding review of the neurophysiological mechanisms of movement control.

Because we believe that the neuromotor speech disorder syndrome that accompanies aphasia is most likely variable across patients with regard to pathophysiology and symptomatology, we also believe that it is necessary for treatment approaches to be guided more by the nature of the symptomatology and the correlative underlying pathophysiologies and their interactions rather than by the name of the disorder. Traditionally, treatment has been targeted toward the underlying pathophysiology for dysarthric speakers (Rosenbek & LaPointe, 1978, 1985; Yorkston et al., 1988), rather than specifying treatments based upon classification or type of dysarthria, e.g., hypokinetic, hyperkinetic, spastic. Instead, assessments for dysarthria determine (1) what aspects of physiological support require modifications with regard to tone, strength; (2) how maximal physiological support for speech may be attained through coordination of speech subsystems, respiration, phonation, resonance, articulation; (3) whether and when articulation drills need to be included; and (4) whether and when prosody and rate should be worked upon. For patients with neuromotor speech disorders and aphasia, a similar approach may be advantageous.

A Framework for Establishing Treatment Goals for Neuromotor Speech Disorders Associated with Aphasia

A possible alternative method to severity level of "apraxia of speech" for establishing treatment goals may be one that is based upon the observable deviant speech and orofacial

TABLE 36-5

Possible Pathophysiological Processes Underlying the Clinical Symptoms of Apraxia of Speech and Speculated Therapeutic Facilitators

Possible Pathophysiological Process	Probable Primary Facilitators
Spatial targeting deficit Use of too many or too few degrees of freedom Inability to set parameters of movement Reduced ability to produce fractionated movements Abnormal tone and strength	Therapy approaches for postural shaping and production of functional units of speech
Reduced ability to scale range, rate, and timing of movements Dysfluency and/or compensation Reduced ability to coordinate speech systems Reduced ability to sequence complex volitional movements	Therapy approaches for rate and melodic flow

control behaviors of the patient elicited under a variety of conditions. Deviant speech motor control characteristics must be considered in the context of aphasic impairments to verbal expression, as well. The assessment batteries for motor speech proposed by Wertz et al. (1984), Yorkston et al. (1988), Wertz (1985), and Darley et al. (1975) may form the basis for observing the predominant deficits of speech and orofacial motor control. Spontaneous propositional verbal output, when obtainable, should also be analyzed with regard to speech "movement control"and should be used to supplement the results of standard assessment batteries. That is, no one speech sample or motor speech battery should be used in isolation when developing a patient's treatment program.

Typical qualities of speech output of aphasic patients with motor speech dysfunction are summarized in Table 36–4. Table 36–5 includes hypothetical information about the possible pathophysiology, all of which requires further empirical validation; nonetheless, based upon the current state of knowledge, the information presented in Table 36–5 is inferentially logical. The table represents a preliminary attempt to provide for clinicians a framework for deciding what motor treatment approach(es) may be most facilitative. It becomes immediately clear that a variety of deviant processes may underlie disordered speech output. These may include **spatial targeting deficits; abnormal tone and strength; reduced ability to produce fractionated movements (e.g., tongue movements independent of jaw); reduced ability to sequence complex volitional movements; reduced ability to coordinate speech subsystems, i.e., to produce functional units of speech behavior; reduced ability to scale movements with regard to range, rate, and timing; use of too many or too few degrees of freedom of movement; and/or inability to set the boundaries of movement (movement parameters) of one or several speech subsystems.** The second column of Table 36–5 provides a summary of the treatment approaches that most logically would influence the symptoms. The key concept here is that treatment aimed at one or several of **three** levels may be appropriate for the aphasic patient with neuromotor speech impairment. Again, those levels are **postural shaping of the vocal tract; production of functional units of speech (coordinative structures); and rhythm and pacing.**

There are few formalized guidelines for selection of the most efficacious approach to treatment correlative to the constellation of symptoms observed and abilities preserved and lost. As shown in Table 36–2, an attempt was made by Wertz et al. (1984) to provide guidelines based upon presumed severity level, and, as shown in Table 36–5, by us based upon predominance of speech symptoms. Nonetheless, there exist no empirical data to substantiate the validity of either approach for establishing treatment goals. We, like Wertz et al. (1984), advocate that a sufficient period of diagnostic treatment is useful in order to determine the most facilitative treatment approaches.

Therapeutic Techniques Viewed from Motor Speech Control Perspective

The current literature concerning speech motor control has provided us with several constructs. These include the role of sensory input; establishing parameters of vocal tract movement from existing multiple degrees of freedom; developing functional coordinative units of action; developing the ability for online shaping; and utilizing an internal oscillatory mechanism as a macrostructural organizer of speech. Excellent discussions of these concepts are presented by Abbs (1989) and Gracco (1990). These constructs may explain the usefulness of many of the facilitative techniques used in aiding aphasic individuals to regain control over their speech output. Brief discussions of motor speech control constructs as they may relate to treatment approaches are presented in the following sections.

Enhancing Postural Shaping and Re-establishing Functional Units of Speech

Traditional Techniques

For the patient who requires re-acquisition of small units of speech, i.e., segments and syllables, a variety of approaches that facilitate the re-establishment of accurate spatial targeting and production of functional units have been reported (Wertz et al., 1984; Square-Storer, 1989). These have been written about extensively in the speech literature since the 1930s (Van Riper, 1939) and include, among others, phonetic placement and phonetic derivation. Explanations of these facilitative techniques used with aphasic-apraxic patients are presented in detail by Wertz et al. (1984) and Square-Storer (1989). Phonetic placement techniques involve the use of descriptions of where (place) and how (manner, voice) sounds are made, the use of figures and models, imagery such as hissing for /s/, and/or manipulation of the orofacial musculature by the clinician. Phonetic derivation techniques are those that build upon an orofacial skill already in the patient's repertoire. For instance, if the patient can produce nonspeech lip popping, this action may serve as the basis for providing both place and manner of production for /p/ and /b/. Or, using speech, a patient may be able to produce /s/ but not /ʃ/; /ʃ/ may be derived from /s/ by having the patient slowly draw his or he tongue posteriorly along the palate. Such methods bring to a conscious level of awareness kinesthetic cues for correct spatial and temporal aspects of production of the speech movement.

The **key word** technique may also be used. In this approach, a word that the patient can produce acceptably and which contains the target sound being worked upon is produced by the patient while the clinician calls to his/her attention the feel (tactile and kinesthetic) of the sound. For instance, if the goal is volitional control over the production of /s/, and the patient can produce her husband's name, 'Sam,' the name would be used to enhance the feel of /s/ so that this movement can be produced volitionally in other words.

We speculate that the use of phonetic placement, derivation techniques, and key words aid aphasic patients with neuromotor speech disorders to re-establish a corpus of **functional units** of (speech) action, i.e., coordinative structures. As explained by Gracco (1990), even the production of an isolated vowel requires a functional unit of behavior in that adjustment of respiratory muscles, tension in the vocal folds, adjustments in the compliance of the oropharyngeal walls, shaping of the tongue, positioning of the jaw, elevation of the velum, and some lip shaping all contribute in a coordinated fashion. Indeed, it is the coordination of multiple actions in the vocal tract that has been viewed by some as the primary deficit underlying apraxia (Itoh et al., 1980; Itoh & Sasanuma, 1983), and aphasia (Baum et al., 1990; Blumstein, 1998; Blumstein & Baum, 1987). Another way to view neuromotor speech pathologies is in terms of the number of degrees of freedom available to the impaired system. For example, in hyperkinesia extraneous involuntary movements occur. Such pathological movements may increase the degrees of freedom with which the system must contend to produce a given trajectory. However, in some cases of hypokinesia, the system may have far fewer degrees of freedom of movement. As Gracco (1990) points out, the degrees of freedom available to the normal speaker are naturally limited by the fact that functional units of behavior have been firmly established. A possible positive symptom of neurologic damage cortically and/or subcortically to the dominant frontal lobe is the alteration of functional units. Indeed, it has been our clinical observation that many aphasic patients with neuromotor speech impairments utilize excessive and erroneous degrees of freedom for jaw, lip, and tongue speech movements (see, for example, Square-Storer et al., 1989).

Whiteside and Varley (1998) also concluded that individuals with apraxia of speech use excessive degrees of freedom. Examples that we have observed frequently include jaw opening with too great amplitude or with lateral or anterior jaw sliding. These are examples of degrees of freedom of movement NOT normally used in speech. Similarly, we have frequently observed aberrant degrees of freedom of lip movement. Examples include visible contraction of only one-half of the upper lip, and bottom lip protrusion accompanying bilabial closure. These movements are not common in the speech of individuals without brain damage. As another example, aberrant tongue movements not common to those used for speech production, such as lateral curling of the tongue margin, may occur but, of course, these are far less visible. What is known, however, is that aberrant movements in one speech oral subsystem (jaw, lips, and/or tongue) most likely have the effect of creating aberrations of movements in articulators throughout the netted vocal tract (Munhall et al., 1994). Thus, impairments to only one subsystem (jaw, lips, or tongue) probably have widespread effects throughout the speech system.

Imitation of contrasts is a traditional therapeutic technique that seems to be useful once some functional units of speech at the phoneme level have been re-established. This method is described comprehensively by Wertz et al. (1984). Advocated by Rosenbek and LaPointe (1978, 1985), the technique relies on integral stimulation ('Watch me. Listen to me.') for input, thus bringing to a conscious level of awareness the 'look' and 'sound' of the movement pattern. Wertz et al.(1984) stress that work should usually begin on a single target such as /s/ embedded in a variable CV or VC environment or minimally different 'functional' units (e.g., say, sigh, so, see). The clinician stresses to the patient the slowing in the production of the syllables while feeling the movement patterns.

An investigation using minimal contrasts, integral stimulation, phonetic placement, and other traditional techniques on the acquisition, generalization, and maintenance effects of treatment for speech sound errors in three speakers with chronic apraxia of speech and aphasia was undertaken by Wambaugh and colleagues (Wambaugh et al., 1998). Using a multiple baseline design across speakers and behaviors, it was demonstrated that the aphasic-apractic speakers improved in correct production of sounds for both trained and untrained words. Varied response generalization and some positive maintenance effects were also noted in the subjects.

Imitation of contrast such as see-tea, toe-sew, is also advised by Wertz et al. (1984) for aphasic patients with neuromotor speech deficits, as well as by Yorkston et al. (1988) for dysarthric individuals. Both indicate the usefulness of producing numerous consonantal targets in a list in which the vowel nucleus remains stable, e.g., pie-die-I-sigh-rye-tie-lie-my. Such drills, when used with aphasic individuals with neuromotor speech deficits, may highlight for the patient a kinesthetic (conscious) awareness for movement units. As such, this type of motor speech practice may promote the re-establishment of sensorimotor contingencies of functional units. For example, in the CV sequence /s/ + vowel, the production of /s/ varies in relation to vowel context, i.e., high-low-front-back. The sensorimotor specifications for /s/ in these various environments is different. Imitation of these contrasts may provide the opportunity for the system to experience the various sensorimotor specifications related to such functional units of speech.

Parameter and Complex PROMPTs

Another method of improving motor speech control in cases of neuromotor speech disorders of aphasia is to provide enhanced sensory feedback through the **pairing of dynamic tactile-kinesthetic input with auditory and visual stimulation.** Aspects of dynamic movement relate to information regarding onset and offset, velocity, and the newly achieved positions of the system (McCloskey, 1978; Ro & Capra, 1995; Burgess et al., 1982; Gordon & Ghez, 1991). The unconscious information is referred to as *kinesthesia*. Cerebral integration of kinesthetic information allows for motor learning and production of goal-coordinated movements.

PROMPT (Prompts for Restructuring Oral Muscular Phonetic Targets) was developed by Chumpelik (Hayden) (1984) and is a dynamic, tactile-kinesthetic treatment approach. It may be used to stabilize degrees of freedom and to re-establish parameterization for speech movements within the articulatory subsystems—i.e., jaw, lips, tongue—by bringing to a level of conscious awareness the feel of speech movements. When PROMPTs are used to normalize parameters of action and degrees of freedom, they are referred to as **Parameter PROMPTs** (see Appendix 36–1 for definitions from Hayden, 1999). For instance, if labial control is principally disturbed, tactile kinesthetic input that moves the lips symmetrically for speech units involving lip retraction or lip rounding are targeted in functional words such as 'no', 'shoe', 'more', 'go'. Labial movements are guided by the clinician in functional words until normal **parameters** of movement and **appropriate degrees of freedom** for labial speech movements are re-established, i.e., produced semi-consistently with volitional control. Thus, re-establishment of functional speech units with precise movement control with regard to **parameter estimation** and **appropriate degrees of freedom of movement for speech** is achieved through passive movement applied by the clinician to guide the patients' speech movements. It may be that work at the segmental and syllable level (VC or CV) using techniques such as phonetic placement and phonetic derivation aid the aphasic patient with neuromotor speech disorders to also achieve these goals. However, we believe that the application of tactile-kinesthetic PROMPTing is more direct and efficient for relearning the appropriate degrees of freedom and parameterization of speech movements.

We prefer to pair the three sensory modalities: auditory, visual, and tactile-kinesthetic, when treating aphasic individuals with neuromotor speech impairments. Special emphasis is given to dynamic tactile-kinesthetic cues to guide the oral mechanism through movement sequences. Others have found, however, that enhancing visual feedback may be sufficient to effect speech changes. Howard and Varley (1995) reported that the use of visual biofeedback using electropalatography (EPG) with one severe apraxic speaker was successful in ameliorating certain articulatory errors. They speculated that EPG visual biofeedback clarified aspects of oral movements for speech that were not salient to their patient when auditory stimulation alone was used.

Another fundamental underlying deficit of motor speech control thought to be deviant in apraxia of speech is the loss or degradation of speech motor programs (Darley et al., 1975). Gracco (1990) describes motor programs as the assembly of functional units of action organized into larger systems. He stresses that based upon results of previous studies (Abbs et al., 1984; Gracco, 1987), ". . .a motor program is not a process but a set of *sensorimotor specifications identifying* the relative contribution of the vocal tract *structures* to the overall vocal tract configuration" (Gracco, 1990, p. 10). For this reason, we believe that speech movements rather than speech sounds should be the focus of the treatment. For example, if the jaw is a deviant subsystem, we may contrast words with low vowels (e.g., hot, map, hat, Bob) versus high vowels (e.g., heat, me, shoe, Lee) to first establish the jaw parameterization for speech, i.e., greatest degree of mandibular opening versus least degree of mandibular opening in functional speech. Our clinical observations have led us to conclude that parameterization of speech movement is disordered in some patients diagnosed with apraxia of speech. Clinical observation has recently received some support from a physiological study undertaken by Clarke and Robin (1998) that concluded that speech parameterization is aberrant in apraxic speakers. Once maximal and minimal parameters of jaw opening for speech are established, the PROMPT method focuses on words with mid vowels (sit, up, luck). The PROMPT method would then work on functional words to encourage control over dynamic jaw gradations, such as focusing on words with diphthongs (I, boy, why, Roy, Hi). In order to maximize the sensorimotor specifications, tactile-kinesthetic PROMPTing would be paired with auditory and visual input and gradually sensory support would be faded as the patient (re)gains refined volitional control of speech movements in useful words of personal relevance. In this example, the emphasis of the PROMPT method is not on phoneme contrasts, but instead is on subsystem control, in this case mandibular parameterization. First, the maximal limits of jaw movements in speech are established. Control of gradation of movement is then introduced using tactile-kinesthetic guidance.

PROMPT treatment focuses on contrastive speech *movements*, rather than contrasting minimal pairs of phonemes. The importance of sensory enhancement and pairing all sensory inputs maximally in a coordinated manner (visual, auditory, and tactile-kinesthetic), is fundamental. Using PROMPT, it is not at all unusual for a patient to be able to produce up to five new functionally relevant words with good motor control within one session of treatment. For generalization, however, the patients' caretakers are asked to ensure that the patient uses the acquired PROMPTed words in daily activities without PROMPT assistance. This method helps to "hardwire" the newly (re) acquired parameters for functional, highly used, relevant words. On a regular basis, the clinician sees the patient for PROMPT treatment that focuses on re-orienting the supraglottal articulators to the appropriate parameters for speech subsystem and **degrees of freedom of movement for each subsystem.**

PROMPT may also be used to re-establish efficient production of "phonemes." Hayden (1999) refers to such PROMPTs as **complex PROMPTS** (see Appendix 36–1). Complex PROMPTs focus on re-establishment of "coordinative structures." That is, tactile kinesthetic feedback is given for phonemes that indicate a constellation of actions throughout the speech system for production of an individual sound. Phoneme or **complex PROMPTs** cue place, duration of contraction, muscle tension, manner, and voicing. Although PROMPT treatment usually focuses on classes of *speech movements*, treatment that focuses on sound groups has been the traditional approach and is used occasionally in PROMPT treatment. Indeed, evidence for the effectiveness of treatment based on speech sound groups comes from a recent study by Wambaugh et al. (1998). Using a multiple baseline design with a severe aphasic-apractic speaker, it was demonstrated that combined treatment resulted in improved production for trained sound groups, with response generalization closely following acquisition effects. Generalization across sound groups, however, was negligible for the subject studied.

Enhancing the Rhythmic Substrate and Slowing Motor Speech Production

Other therapeutic techniques that focus on slowing speech production and/or enhancing speech rhythm have been used successfully with aphasic patients with neuromotor speech disorders. Most of these techniques are summarized in Table 36–6. Six of them will be discussed briefly in this section as facilitation techniques: Singing (Keith & Aronson, 1975); vibrotactile stimulation (Rubow et al., 1982); metronomic pacing (Shane & Darley, 1978; Dworkin et al., 1988); prolonged speech (Southwood, 1987); use of the pacing board (Helm, 1979); and surface PROMPTing (Hayden, 1999). In a subsequent section of this chapter, those rhythmic and pacing methods which constitute more

---

TABLE 36–6

Pacing and Rhythmic Approaches for the Treatment of Neuromotor Speech Deficits in Aphasia

- Metronomic pacing (Dworkin et al., 1988; Shane & Darley, 1978)
- Prolonged speech (Southwood, 1987)
- Finger counting (Simmons, 1978)
- Vibrotactile stimulation (Rubow et al., 1982)
- Singing (Keith & Aronson, 1975)
- Melodic Intonation Therapy (Sparks & Deck, 1986)
- Surface PROMPT (Square et al., 1985; Square et al., 1986)

---

formalized treatment programs, including finger counting (Simmons, 1978), Melodic Intonation Therapy (Sparks & Deck, 1986) and surface PROMPT (Hayden, 1999), will be discussed.

Although rhythmic and pacing facilitators are common in the treatment of speech disorders in patients with aphasia accompanied by neuromotor speech deficits, it appears that the various methods may be tapping different processes. That is, some of these techniques are rigid pacing techniques while others exaggerate the natural rhythm and stress patterns of the language. The rigid **pacing techniques** include the **metronome, prolonged speech,** and **pacing boards.** Those facilitators that enhance natural **rhythm** and **stress** include **contrastive stress drills, vibrotactile stimulation, singing,** and **surface PROMPT.** All of these methods also slow the rate of speech production. Unfortunately, the clinical literature does not include research that has attempted to determine whether it is the slowed rate or enhanced rhythm that positively affects speech production. In addition, there is no research that has compared the relative effectiveness of these techniques, nor are there indications of patient types for whom each is appropriate. Clinical research addressing these issues is greatly needed.

Singing

The use of singing as a facilitator for motor speech production in nonfluent aphasic individuals has long been recognised (Head, 1926 [1963]). It is the opinion of Lebrun (1989), however, that singing is helpful for Broca's aphasic patients and not for patients designated as having apraxia of speech and minimal or no clinically discernible aphasia. Indeed, the one contemporary published case study documenting the facilitative effect of singing was of a patient with moderate to severe aphasia as measured by the PICA (Porch, 1967) who also had a significant coexisting neuromotor speech disorder (Keith & Aronson, 1975). Singing therapy began after 3 weeks of traditional therapy in which limited gains were made. A close procedure was used whereby the patient completed a phrase by singing the final word. That is, the clinician would sing, 'This is my_____.', while pointing to his hand and the patient would name the body part (or object), thus completing the sentence by singing, 'hand.' The patient was also encouraged to sing functional phrases such as, 'I want coffee.', 'How are you?' etc. The patient transferred the facilitative technique to her environment with rhythm and pitch patterns that had a definite musical quality. In less than a month, her PICA overall score improved by three points (from 7.93 to 10.99) and her verbal subtest score by seven points (from 3.55 to 10.55). A month later the patient was doing well in speaking situations at home although word finding and grammatical errors were noticeable. She had completely given up singing as a facilitative approach but was using an enhanced melodic structure and slower rate in the natural context. Her verbal subtests on the PICA were almost two points higher (from 10.55 to 12.50) and her overall score, almost one point higher (from 10.99 to 11.93). Keith and Aronson (1975) acknowledged that the "...patient might have improved to a similar extent had conventional therapy been continued or no therapy instituted at all" (p. 488), but, given their clinical acumen, they felt the case to be sufficiently noteworthy to report in the literature.

Vibrotactile Stimulation

Another preliminary yet promising study of the effectiveness of rhythm, stress, and pacing to promote articulatory accuracy in aphasic subjects with apraxia of speech was one which used **vibrotactile stimulation** (Rubow et al., 1982). A 50-Hz vibration was applied to the velar surface of the index finger and vibratory tactile stimulation was delivered for every syllable in three-syllable words. Because the clinician could control the timing, duration, and intensity (high or low) of the signal, the stimulation could indicate primary, secondary, and tertiary stress in three-syllable words such as 'sensation.' One subject was exposed to two alternating treatments, imitation treatment for a list of plosive-laden polysyllabic words (e.g., tobacco) and vibrotactile stimulation for a list of fricative-laden words (e.g., sensation). A 16-point multidimensional scoring system for the evaluation of apraxia of speech errors (Collins et al., 1980) was used to determine mean performance on both word lists pre- and post-therapy. At the beginning of treatment, the mean score for both word lists was 5. After 14 sessions of treatment over 7 days, post-therapy scores indicated that the words trained using imitation improved only 1.9 points, whereas the word-list trained using vibrotactile stimulation improved 5.8 points.

Metronomic Pacing

Other attempts have been made to use rhythm and pacing as facilitators of motor speech. Shane and Darley (1978) utilized a **metronome** paired with the reading of passages and set for three rates: normal speaking rate, a slower rate, and a faster rate. The external source of rhythm actually had a deleterious effect on accuracy of connected speech production compared with a control condition in which the metronome was not used. Further, there were no significant differences in articulation accuracy over the three rates of paced speaking. Despite these findings, Dworkin et al. (1988) utilized a metronome set at various speeds when treating a patient on the following and more finite tasks: a nonverbal neuromotor control task; alternate motion rates; word production; and sentence production in which sentences consisted of five words. Although no conjecture can be made about the facilitative effects of the metronome, it is interesting that Dworkin and colleagues, clinicians with exceptional backgrounds in the treatment of apraxia of speech, utilized the approach

when working on shorter units of movement. Their patient improved on all tasks, but she may have also demonstrated such improvement without the metronome.

Prolonged Speech

A study by Southwood (1987) of two patients who were considered to be principally apraxic, one mild and one moderate, provided quantifiable evidence of the facilitative effects of pacing. Southwood used the technique of **prolonged speech** in which speech rates were systematically reduced through conscious prolongation of vocalic nuclei. Systematic decreases in speech rate accompanied by visual guidance from a computer screen display resulted in substantially reduced speech errors. In a reversal phase, systematic increases in speaking rate resulted in an increase in errors. The prolonged speech technique, however, did not generalize, possibly because of its 'bizarre' quality. Southwood recommended that, as in the prolonged speech program formulated for stutterers by Ingam (1983), generalization might be achieved if therapy directed at 'naturalness' training is used as a supplement to the prolonged speech technique. It may be that the metronome and prolonged speech, like speech supplemented by gestures, "...do nothing as grand as reorganizing neuromotor control, (but) they do slow the patient down, heighten rhythm and stress profiles, and they serve to remind the patient that he must attend to each syllable of an utterance" (Rosenbek, 1983, p. 53).

Pacing Board

A similar facilitative effect may be derived with use of the **pacing board** (Helm, 1979). Such a board is approximately 13″ long and is divided horizontally every 2″ by a divider. Patients are trained to touch each consecutive square on the board for each unit of speech. Although we have no experimental data regarding the use of the pacing board with aphasic individuals with neuromotor speech disorders, the method is commonly suggested (e.g., Wertz et al., 1984).

Surface PROMPTs

PROMPT may also be used as a rhythmic and pacing approach. Hayden (1999), in addition to describing complex PROMPTs and parameter PROMPTs, also describes **surface PROMPTs** (see Appendix 36–1). Surface PROMPTs are those which deliver tactile-kinesthetic information about salient aspects of motor production of syllables and which highlight tempo and stress patterns. Square and Chumpelik (Hayden) (1989) described subjects' acquisition of PROMPTed and unPROMPTed trisyllabic words such as "sensation" and "tobacco" in which surface PROMPTs were used to indicate oral spatial parameters of the coda of each syllable as well as rate, meter, and syllabic stress. Rate and meter were indicated by the speed at which PROMPTs were delivered. Syllabic stress was indicated by the pressure and timing of PROMPTs. Surface PROMPTing can thus be thought of as a rhythmic and pacing approach to treatment. For the patients studied, learning curves were both rapid and accelerated when polysyllabic works and functional phrases were treated with surface PROMPT.

Contrastive Stress Drills

The use of **contrastive stress drills** is advocated by many as a potent type of treatment (e.g., Rosenbek, 1983). Such drills can be thought of more as an approach to treatment rather than a facilitative technique but are discussed here because of their hypothesized underlying speech control mechanism, as an enhancement of an underlying **rhythmic** or **oscillatory mechanism.** Contrastive stress drills were first proposed by Fairbanks (1960) and popularized by Rosenbek (1976, 1983) for the treatment of acquired apraxia of speech. Question and answer dialogues which consist of short phrases centered on one or two phonemes are used. Thus, previously practiced functional units are embedded in connected interactive speech. Primary and secondary stress are the factors which are thought to promote improved speech movement. A typical dialogue may be:

Cl: What did you do?
Pt: I *ate* one.
Cl: You ate three?
Pt: No, I ate *one*.
Cl: Tom ate one.
Pt: No, *I* ate one.
Cl: You drank one?
Pt: No, I *ate* one.
Cl: You ate one!
Pt: Yes, *I* ate one.

A hierarchy for helping to ensure success for the patient is described fully by Wertz et al. (1984) and the reader is urged to consult that text.

The possible speech control mechanisms that may be affected using this method are enhancement of an underlying speech rhythm and, possibly, online shaping of speech movements. That is, contrastive stress drills utilize a limited set of phonemes and the segments are fitted into phrasal structures while speaking rate is reduced and sentential stress patterns are maximized. With regard to the rhythm and stress aspects of such drills, Gracco (1990) notes that numerous aspects of motor behavior seem to be guided by an underlying internal oscillatory mechanism and that speech may be no exception. He reported that, in normal speakers, there is an undeniable consistency in repetition suggesting " . . . an underlying periodicity indicative of a rhythmic process" (p. 18). We propose that contrastive stress drills may enhance the production of functional units in the context of enhanced rhythm

and reduced rate that capitalize upon a repeated and heightened speech periodicity. Further, it is speculated that the instances of changing patterns of sentential stress in these drills may enhance flexibility in the motor programs. Wertz et al. (1984) state that, "The contrastive stress drill may be one of the most potent techniques for stabilizing apraxic articulation and improving prosodic profiles (p. 260)." We speculate that this is so because a guiding rhythm is brought to consciousness and the system is required to make specific stress changes within a relatively constant phonetic (movement) environment.

Formalized Treatment Programs

Several formalized treatment approaches for neuromotor speech disorders in aphasia have appeared in the literature. These approaches have been of two types: **microstructural bottom-up approaches** and **macrostructural top-down approaches.** An issue of primary importance is whether a patient requires either a micro- or macrostructural approach or both approaches to treatment in order to improve his/her motor speech control. That is, does first oral speech posturing and then functional units of speech, i.e., phonemes and syllables, or *movement constellations*, need to be re-established and built upon in order to improve functional verbal communication? Or, are macrostructural approaches that enhance suprasegmentals and which are applied at the phrase and sentence levels most facilitative? The unresolved issues are how to determine whether to use bottom-up microstructure versus top-down macrostructure methods, and for what types of patients each is appropriate. The bottom-up microstructure approaches include those methods which begin at either the nonverbal oromotor movement level or segment level. The most notable are those that have been advocated by Dabul and Bollier (1976), Rosenbek (1983), Wertz et al. (1984), and Dworkin et al. (1988). As suggested above, we speculate that these bottom-up approaches aid the impaired system to (1) select the specific spatial parameters to manipulate from the multiple degrees of freedom available to the pathological speech system; (2) establish and refine functional units of action; and (3) ready the system to superimpose these functional units onto a melodic line. The best-known top-down or macrostructure approaches for the treatment of neuromotor speech disorders in aphasia are: Melodic Intonation Therapy (Naeser & Helm-Estabrooks, 1985); surface PROMPT (Freed et al., 1997; Square et al., 1985; Square-Storer & Hayden, 1989); and the eight-step task continuum as applied to functional sentences and phrases (Rosenbek et al., 1973). We speculate that these approaches help re-establish an underlying melody and rate for speech production. The macro-approach of finger counting is less well known. It provides for the patient a rigid pacing for slowing speech production. Each approach will be discussed in the next section.

Microstructural Approaches

Dabul and Bollier (1976) based their approach on the premise that the patient with apraxia of speech must first re-establish the ability to accurately attain articulatory postures at the phone level. Once the posturing for a particular 'phone' is stabilized, reduplication of the consonant in the rapid reproduction of the 'consonant + /a/' is prescribed. A criterion level of rapid accurate reduplication (60 syllables per 15 seconds) is set, and once attained, production of the phone in monosyllable CVC or CVCV nonword combinations is advocated to establish volitional control of nonmeaningful syllable combinations. Finally, word attack skills are recommended in that it is assumed that the patient has acquired, through the previous exercises, a solid basic 'vocabulary' of articulatory skills. Each sound in a word is attacked in isolation and then the patient is encouraged to blend phonemes together.

Rosenbek (1983) and Wertz et al. (1984) do not present such a rigid approach to bottom-up treatment for patients with apraxia of speech but do advocate an approach in which sounds are turned into syllables, and syllables into words. The strength of their belief in this sort of building block approach, is highlighted in the following quote from Rosenbek (1983): "Once the apraxic talker has begun to recall how sounds are made, to contrast those sounds with others, and to combine them into words and short phrases, traditional methods like imitation, placement and derivation can be replaced by methods that slow connected speech and heighten rhythm and stress profiles (p. 52)."

Dworkin and colleagues (1988) reported on treatment of one patient with apraxia of speech. A multiple probe design was applied to a therapeutic regime which consisted of four levels of oromotor complexity including nonverbal tongue tip raising and lowering with a bite block; performance of alternate motion rates on the syllables /pʌtʌkʌ/ and /kʌpʌtʌ/; isolated word training; and sentence training under two conditions, a stressed and unstressed one. The patient's performances improved on all tasks but, "these findings produced no evidence to suggest that successful performance at an earlier step in the treatment regime generalized to later, ostensibly more complex, speech control activities" (p. 287). Although we cannot infer that similar results would be found across subjects, this finding indicates that further research is warranted regarding the validity of and criteria for beginning treatment at the micro-level of speech for aphasic individuals with neuromotor speech disorders.

Macrostructural Approaches

Melodic Intonation Therapy

There is evidence in the literature as well that certain top-down approaches may be effective for establishing functional speech in aphasic individuals with neuromotor speech disorders. That is, the results of these approaches have demonstrated that a 'building-block' approach to treatment is not always necessary. The most notable of these macrostructure techniques is **Melodic Intonation Therapy.** The method of Melodic Intonation Therapy is fully described by Sparks (1981). Elements of inter- and intrasystemic organization (Luria, 1970; Rosenbek & LaPointe, 1978, 1985; Rosenbek et al., 1976) are incorporated into the intoning technique for phrase and sentence production. The intersystemic component consists of hand gestures coupled with word production, while the intrasystemic aspect is reflected in the production of 'intoned' rather than spoken speech. Meaningful phrases such as 'I want coffee' and 'Go to bed' are often produced fluently once a patient has worked through the various steps of the program, and in our experience, performance is usually quite good throughout the program, but few empirical data exist regarding generalization. The startling aspect of this method is that even patients who appear to be totally 'lost' in their vocal tracts and who have extreme difficulty initiating speech are greatly facilitated by this top-down approach. That is, there would appear to be little advantage for working on functional units of speech and building upon those units for phrase production if, in fact, it could be empirically shown that MIT promotes generalization to novel productions. It appears that the macrostructure of the prosody enhanced by the intersystemic hand movement aid the patient in producing intelligible functional phrases. We must also consider whether the linguistic structures of target phrases contribute to the facilitatory aspect of aphasic patients. It has been our observation as well as that of many others that even severe Broca's patients who demonstrate some agrammatism and anomia produce fully syntactic utterances when facilitated by MIT if the syntactic structure of those utterances is simplistic. That is, active declarative sentences, the copula, articles, and verb inflections are usually produced when sentences are facilitated by MIT. The question then becomes one of what aspect of this top-down approach accounts for the facilitative effect—intersystemic hand tapping, intrasystemic melodic speech production, the linguistic template onto which the speech movements are fitted, the rhythmic and melodic template, slowed speech production, or all of the above in varying proportions.

The therapeutic benefits of MIT for chronic nonfluent aphasic patients with good comprehension but minimal speech output were first reported by Albert et al. (1973). In the three cases reported, MIT treatment resulted in increased spontaneous output in the natural environment. One patient required only 2 weeks of treatment to progress from the use of six repetitive phonemes to full responses which were grammatically correct in his natural environment. The other two patients required approximately 1 to 1.5 months of treatment in order to progress from meaningless grunts and stereotyped phonemes to carrying on short but meaningful conversations. Each patient's post-treatment speech, however, was characterized as dysarthric or impaired with regard to articulation and prosody.

Several other reports, however, found that MIT was not effective as measured by improved 'language' test scores for some nonfluent aphasic patients (Sparks et al., 1974; Helm, 1979). In an attempt to provide clearer guidelines for whom MIT was most appropriate, Naeser and Helm-Estabrooks (1985) undertook a study which examined site of lesion correlated with improved 'language' test scores as derived from the Boston Diagnostic Aphasia Examination (BDAE) (Goodglass & Kaplan, 1972) following MIT treatment of eight patients who had also received CT scans. Those patients who responded well to MIT as measured by four subtests of the BDAE had damage to the left frontal motor and premotor areas and adjacent subcortical white matter, in combination with basal ganglia and capsular involvement in one patient. In other words, each of the patients had damage to the left cortical and some damage to the subcortical motor speech control centers *without* involvement of Wernicke's area and/or of the temporal isthmus. Of the four poor responders, three had the above sites of damage *plus* damage to Wernicke's area or the temporal isthmus. The fourth had a patchy frontal Broca's and premotor area lesion, which spared the periventricular white matter and a small lesion deep to the motor cortex face region. Although the later patient was termed a poor responder, it should be noted that this patient, *prior* to treatment, had an articulatory agility score of seven on the BDAE and, as such, was different from the other seven subjects in that he was at ceiling on this measure. These results are impressive, and from them it may be inferred that MIT is an appropriate **motor speech treatment** for nonfluent aphasic subjects with severely restricted verbal output but *without* involvement to the dominant temporal lobe, i.e., without significant aphasic comprehension deficits.

Finger Counting

A macrostructural approach that uses intersystemic reorganization in the form of finger counting to mark the rhythmic flow of speech coupled with a simple linguistic template was reported by Simmons (1978). Although this was a single case study and no known attempt to replicate the findings has been undertaken, this report is of great clinical significance because of the remarkable improvement and description of generalization of verbal expressive output demonstrated by the 'aphasic-apraxic' subject studied. The subject had undergone 9 months of intensive language and speech therapy, showing steady improvement throughout. However, a plateau in performance was subsequently met for 5 months with no discernible improvement as measured by the PICA and by subjective evaluation. During the 5-month period, various approaches to treatment were undertaken including

MIT, imitation, articulatory posturing, contrastive stress drills (Rosenbek et al., 1976), Amerind (Skelly et al., 1974), and language master programming for production of utterances. Subsequent treatment was directed at the production of utterances of the linguistic form, 'Pronoun + Verb + Preposition + Article + Noun.' The patient was trained to hold up one finger for each word (finger counting), thus producing one syllable for each finger raised. The training consisted of the five-task continuum shown in Appendix 36–2. Therapy was administered for 4-months with marked improvement in production of treated utterances. Generalization was demonstrated by the patient's outstanding improvement on the PICA verbal subtests of 21 percentile points. The patient was observed to transfer the finger counting approach to her natural environment, and significant others commented upon her increased sentence length and fluency.

Finger counting, like MIT, is an approach that couples intersystemic re-organization with a linguistic template. The coupling of a language template with intersystemic reorganization could have an interactive facilitative effect on the accuracy of verbal output in aphasic individuals with neuromotor speech disorders. Another additional possible explanation for the dramatic improvement demonstrated by this patient is that the rhythmic finger counting provides the patient with an internal tempo and, possibly, a rhythmic oscillation upon which the speech stream may be superimposed. It might also be that the limb movement helps to re-establish a paced oscillatory rhythm onto which the functional units of speech may be mapped. Further research is needed.

Surface PROMPTs

The application of PROMPT (Chumpelik [Hayden], 1984) produces similar successful results for the acquisition of a limited set of functional phrases and sentences (Freed et al., 1997; Square et al., 1985; Square et al., 1986; Square-Storer & Hayden, 1989). **Surface PROMPTs** (see Appendix 36–1) focus on temporal flow. Rate of speech production is regulated by the timing of delivery of spatial and trajectory cues, and the pressure and duration of the cues. As temporal flow is regulated, the patient becomes consciously aware of the feel of dynamic speech movements (articulatory kinesthesia) as the clinician guides both the spatial and temporal parameters of speech production. Surface PROMPTs are delivered to the orofacial structures by the clinician while the patient produces a target utterance. They are gradually withdrawn until the patient can produce the utterance with less support.

Surface PROMPT therapy programs focus on the motor speech aspects of verbal production while also taking into consideration the patient's social, emotional, cognitive, and language status. Hayden (1999) has put forward the USE Model (see Appendix 36–1) to aid clinicians in determining the types of language utterances to train using surface PROMPTing. The USE Model stresses that surface PROMPTing will be successful only if the patient's linguistic, social, behavioral, cognitive, and pragmatic attributes are also considered. Phrases to be used for PROMPTing must be chosen so as to be personally relevant and environmentally useful. The language construction should be within the language formulation competence of the aphasic patient. Finally, the patient's environment should be assessed with regard to support for carryover and generalization of use of the phrases to contexts in which the patient naturally interacts.

Using single-case study designs and replication on four chronic severe Broca's patients with limited propositional output and severe neuromotor speech involvement, it was demonstrated that phrases can be 'programmed in' for functional communication using this top-down macro-structure approach (Square et al., 1985, 1986; Square-Storer & Hayden, 1989). According to reports from spouses, two patients reported on by Square et al. (1986) generalized treated phrases (e.g., 'Stop it.'; 'I want more'; etc.) to daily life. One patient was re-evaluated 2 months after termination of treatment and was found to have retained trained functional phrases with the same level of perceived efficiency as attained in treatment (Square-Storer & Hayden, 1989). Freed et al. (1997) studied the effect of PROMPT on acquisition and long-term maintenance of functional vocabulary items and some phrases for one severe apractic-aphasic individual. With application of PROMPT the subject acquired 30 target words and phrases which were maintained following the termination of treatment. We speculate that surface PROMPTing, like MIT and finger-tapping strategies, provides patients with a macrostructural linguistic template coupled with a paced rhythmic template and possibly facilitation of a rhythmic oscillatory template for production of phrases.

In the application of PROMPT, not all possible cues for every speech sound and its coarticulation in context are delivered to the patient for every macrostructure. Instead, the master clinician constantly monitors performance and delivers only those surface PROMPTs necessary to improve speech accuracy. What PROMPT appears to achieve in a short time is the hardwiring of programs of several functional phrases in Broca's aphasic patients. The rapidity with which the phrases become hardwired is demonstrated by the accelerated learning curves for phrase production included in clinical research reports (Freed et al., 1997; Square et al., 1985; Square et al., 1986; Square-Storer & Hayden, 1989). Future PROMPT research must address generalization of the approach to novel phrases. Another issue that needs to be addressed is if, in fact, generalization occurs with PROMPT, is it of a sufficient quantity and quality to justify the costliness of one-to-one treatment for the aphasic patient with neuromotor speech impairments? A recent study has demonstrated that significant verbal and nonverbal functional communication gains in 'information transfer' can be made

by chronic Broca's aphasic patients using generic aphasia and speech treatments concentrated over short periods of several months (Brindley et al., 1989). Is it the case that PROMPT effects even greater changes? Further clinical research is needed.

Integral Stimulation and the Rosenbek Continuum

The final macrostructure approach to treatment to be discussed is one of the first approaches reported in the contemporary literature for apraxia of speech. Rosenbek et al. (1973), when first reporting on the efficacy of their integral stimulation approach (i.e., 'Watch me', 'Listen to me') within the context of their eight-step continuum of treatment for apraxia of speech, trained 'functional phrases' in two of three aphasic patients with moderate to severe language and speech disturbance of not longer than 1-year duration. (The eight-step continuum prescribed by Rosenbek et al. is presented in Appendix 36–3). Five phrases for training were individually selected for each patient based upon their personal circumstances. No attempt was made to control for linguistic or phonetic complexity or for length. Both subjects acquired all five sentences within treatment. Carryover was informally assessed for one subject at 3-months post-treatment. At that time, carryover was evident for three of the five phrases. For both subjects, the most time-consuming step in therapy was Step 1, 'Watch me. Listen to me' with simultaneous production with the clinician.

Deal and Florence (1978) essentially replicated the findings of Rosenbek et al. (1973) in their application of the eight-step continuum to four patients, three of whom were more than 1-year post-onset. Two of the patients had essentially no functional speech at the beginning of treatment. Although a different learning criterion was used in the study of Deal and Florence, they too found Step 1 to be the most laborious. Nonetheless, once the criterion was achieved on the initial step, patients progressed rapidly. Further, Steps 1 through 4 seemed to constitute a unit, but not every patient needed all four of the steps. Level 8 was found useful for home programming.

The conclusion of Rosenbek and colleagues (1973) as well as Deal and Florence (1978) was that the eight-step continuum could help restore some communicative ability to *some* severely apraxic patients. Selection criteria for the most appropriate patients were not specified. A general description was that each was severely limited in speech output.

Choosing a Macrostructural Versus a Microstructural Approach

There are no empirical reports nor scholarly discussions that exist in the literature regarding the selection of micro- versus macrostructural methods of treatment for neuromotor speech disorders in aphasia. In fact, to our knowledge, we were the first to have presented therapeutic approaches within the microstructural versus macrostructural framework (Square & Martin, 1994). While guidelines for selecting micro- versus macrostructural treatment are lacking, it would seem logical to start with a macrostructural approach when initiating treatment with the aphasic patient with significant speech involvement. First, we agree with Wertz et al. (1984) that it is extremely important to begin treatment on a positive note and that several of the macrostructural approaches such as surface PROMPTing and MIT appear to have the power to rapidly facilitate the production of functional phrases in aphasic patients with neuromotor speech deficits. Second, there are indications in the literature that not all patients require a bottom-up approach. There have been several clinical reports which have indicated that some aphasic patients with neuromotor speech deficits can transfer strategies from macrostructural approaches to control their speech in their natural environments (Albert et al., 1973; Rosenbek et al., 1973; Deal & Florence, 1978). Finally, bottom-up approaches require a time-consuming hierarchical process in which there is a time delay before functionality or patient self-control of speech emerges. It appears prudent to provide the patient with control over several functional phrases of personal value as early as possible, especially in the United States where there is a $1500 Medicare cap on rehabilitation.

For some patients, it may be that progress is significant with macrostructural approaches. In these cases, there are no logical reasons to incorporate microstructural regimes, although microstructural facilitative techniques may be applied liberally within the frameworks of macrostructural approaches. For other patients, especially those who appear to have the potential to achieve motor control over self-formulated discourse, it is our belief that microstructural approaches may be of great value. These approaches may be especially useful for patients with minimal aphasia and with keen insight about speech production and good self-evaluative skills.

A final issue which requires consideration is treating patients whose language remains relatively intact but who have neuromotor speech deficits because of dominant hemisphere damage versus treating the aphasic individual with neuromotor speech deficits. Square-Storer et al. (1988) demonstrated empirically that apraxia of speech and aphasia were distinct disorders. It would thus seem logical that left-hemisphere–lesioned subjects with significant speech impairment and *no* or *relatively little* aphasia would require treatment approaches different from those applied to subjects with aphasia complicated by significant motor speech disruption. One conclusion which resonates in the clinical treatment literature is that macro-structural treatment approaches that provide for patients not only the rhythmic and rate structure but also a linguistic substrate are successful. The efficacy studies of PROMPT were undertaken with patients classified as Broca's (Square et al., 1985) on the

Western Aphasia Battery (Kertesz, 1982). The Melodic Intonation Therapy reports of effectiveness were based upon the performances of patients with aphasia and limited verbal output (Albert et al., 1973). The eight-step continuum was shown by Rosenbek et al. (1973) to be effective for patients with moderate aphasia and apraxia of speech, some of whom also demonstrated mild dysarthria. And, Simmons's finger-counting program with a linguistic template was successful with an aphasic patient with apraxia of speech. To date, none has been reported to be successful with relatively pure neuromotor speech disorder following left hemisphere lesion.

Again, common to each of the successful macrostructural techniques for aphasic-apraxic patients are three elements: rhythm, pacing, and linguistic templates. Extensive research is much needed regarding the basis of success of the macrostructural approaches as well as for what type of patient each is most effective.

For patients with little or no aphasia but a significant motor speech impairment following left-hemisphere damage, it would appear that microstructural approaches which emphasize the establishment of functional units, parameter estimation, online shaping, and re-establishment of an underlying oscillatory mechanism may be most appropriate. Careful study of the writings of the pre-eminent clinicians in this area by Wertz et al. (1984) indicates that this building block approach is prescribed for the patient with minimal aphasia and a significant neuromotor speech disorder—what they term the *mild* and *moderate apraxic patient*.

Thus, some guideposts have been established for the clinician with regard to selecting the most appropriate approaches to treatment for left-hemisphere–lesioned patients with neuromotor speech involvement both with and without aphasia. However, no empirically validated principles for selection have been reported (see Wambaugh & Doyle, 1994, for a review). Criteria for selection of therapy methods is a fertile area for further research in our discipline.

A final word relates to treatment efficacy for chronic Broca's aphasic patients. Many of the above studies have demonstrated that such individual progress in treatment occurs even after many years post-onset. One research report confirms this point (Brindley et al., 1989). More importantly, however, was the finding that of the five parameters measured using the Functional Communication Profile (Sarno, 1965)—movement, speech, understanding, reading, and other—it was the speech ratings followed by movement which improved most significantly following 3-months of traditional intensive therapy of various generic types. The results of this report are most convincing regarding the efficacy of treatment for aphasic patients who also have significant neuromotor speech involvement.

The tenet of this chapter has been that many verbal production disorders in aphasia are both linguistic and motoric in nature. Clinicians must be trained and encouraged to manage both the language and motor dimensions of verbal production disorders caused by left-hemisphere brain damage. Studies such as the one by Brindley and colleagues (1989) as well as many treatment reports (e.g., Keith & Aronson, 1975; Freed et al., 1997; Rubow et al., 1982; Simmons, 1978; Square-Storer & Hayden, 1989) provide ample evidence for the power of effecting change in the motor speech control abilities of patients with dominant-hemisphere brain damage. It is our hope that our readers have been convinced of the dual nature—linguistic and motor—of verbal production disorders associated with many types of aphasia.

FUTURE TRENDS

This chapter has raised more questions than answers. One central issue which has been clarified, however, is that dominant-hemisphere perisylvian lesions, both cortical and subcortical, most likely result in significant neuromotor deficits for speech production. Well-controlled research studies that correlate both site of structural damage and abnormal patterns of brain metabolism with motor speech performances are needed to determine whether different lesion sites induce functionally different patterns of brain metabolism and whether different pathometabolic states are associated with different constellations of deviant speech and oral movement characteristics.

Answers to the following questions are also crucial to improve our clinical management of aphasic patients. Is there but one aphasia caused by damage to the temporal lobe? Are nonfluent aphasias simply aphasia complicated by motor speech impairment? What are the specific natures of the motor speech impairments accompanying frontal cortical and subcortical lesions to the dominant hemisphere—apraxic, dystonic, ataxic, paretic? When and for whom should microstructural versus macrostructural approaches to treatment be used? Is it true that the macrostructural approaches are successful for nonfluent aphasic patients for two reasons, motoric in that oscillatory and rate mechanisms are re-established and linguistic in that a template of semantic and syntactic structure is provided? How efficacious is each approach when studied with regard to increased verbal communication in the natural environment as well as changes in speech and nonspeech kinematics and coordination? When measures of social validation and consumer satisfaction are used in conjunction with measures of speech intelligibility and speech kinematics/coordination as well as standardized tests, are the treatments we administer efficacious and economically sound?

Even though many unanswered questions remain, some issues regarding speech disorders that accompany language disorders in patients with dominant-hemisphere damage have been amplified via inductive and deductive reasoning. We therefore, albeit tentatively, put forward the following key points.

KEY POINTS

1. Lesions of the perisylvian zone of the dominant hemisphere, both cortical and/or subcortical, most likely result in either subclinical or clinically significant motor deficits, particularly motor speech control deficits, as well as aphasia.
2. "Apraxia of speech" and/or various forms of dysarthria often occur with aphasia and in many instances compound the devastating effects of aphasia, particularly in the modality of verbal expression. That is, the verbal production deficits in aphasia, while always linguistic in nature, are frequently compounded by motor speech control impairments.
3. The interaction of both linguistic and motor control impairments likely exacerbates the severity of verbal production disorders in aphasic patients.
4. Clinicians must be cognizant of the significance of both the language and motor dimensions of verbal production disorders associated with left-hemisphere brain damage.
5. Clinicians should assess and treat the motor speech disorder accompanying aphasia based upon the constellation of predominant characteristics of deviant motor speech control demonstrated by each patient.
6. Motor speech control is likely to be better for aphasic patients when language formulation demands are minimized.

From the standpoint of issues regarding neuroanatomy and neurophysiology, we as a behavioral neuroscience, must utilize more extensively the body of knowledge from the basic neurosciences to better understand the natures of neurologic communication disorders. We must be much less influenced by structural lesions correlated with symptomatology and endeavor to gain an appreciation of the dynamic aspects of brain, functioning. Unfortunately, like our predecessors, we have matched symptoms to static lesion sites, sometimes clouding, our understanding of aphasia and related disorders, more than clarifying them. Finally, research partnerships must be forged which explore the integration of the basic motor neurophysiology and the clinical science of communication disorders for the sake of advancement of both sciences. This chapter has been one attempt to interrelate these areas with the objective of enhancing our level of understanding regarding neuromotor speech disorders in aphasia.

References

Abbs, J.H., Gracco, V.L., & Cole, K.J. (1984). Control of multi-movement coordination: Sensorimotor mechanisms in speech motor programming. *Journal of Motor Behaviour, 16(2),* 195–232.

Abbs, J.H. & Welt, C. (1985). Lateral precentral cortex in speech motor control. In R.G. Daniloff (ed.), *Recent advances in speech science*. San Diego, CA: College Hill Press.

Abbs, J.H. (1989). Neurophysiologic processes of speech movement control. In Lass (ed.), *Handbook of speech-language pathology and audiology* (pp. 154–170). Toronto: BC Decker.

Alajouanine, T., Ombredane, A., & Durand, M. (1939). *Le syndrome de désintégration phonetique dans l'aphasie*. Paris: Masson.

Alajouanine, T., Castaigne, P., Sabouraud, O., & Contamin, F. (1959). Palilalie paraxystique et vocalizations iteratives au cours de crises epileptiques par lesion interessant l'aire motrice supplementaire. *Revue Neurologique, 101*, 186–202.

Albert, M.L., Spades, R.W., & Helm, N.A. (1973). Melodic intonation therapy for aphasia. *Archives of Neurology, 29*, 130–131.

Alexander, M.P., Benson, D.F., & Stuss, D.T. (1989). Frontal lobes and language. *Brain and Language, 37*, 656–691.

Alexander, G.E. & Crutcher, M.D. (1990). Functional architecture of basal ganglia circuits: Neural substrates of parallel processing. *Trends in Neuroscience, 13*, 266–271.

Alexander, G.E., Delong, M.R., & Strick, P.L. (1986). Parallel organization of functionally segregated circuits linking basal ganglia and cortex. *Annual Review of Neuroscience, 9*, 357–381.

Ardila, A., Benson, F.D., & Flynn, F.G. (1997). Participation of the insula in language. *Aphasiology, 11*, 1159–1169.

Asanuma, H. (1989). *The motor cortex*. New York: Raven Press.

Asanuma, H. & Arissian, K. (1984). Experiments in functional role of peripheral input to motor cortex during voluntary movements in the monkey. *Journal of Neurophysiology, 52*, 212–227.

Asanuma, H., Thach, W.T., & Jones, E.G. (1983). Distribution of cerebellar terminations in the ventral lateral thalamic region in the monkey. *Brain Research Review, 5*, 219–235.

Augustine, J.R. (1985). The insular lobe in primates including humans. *Neurological Research, 7*, 2–10.

Barbas, H. & Pandya, D.N. (1987). Architecture and frontal cortical connections of the premotor cortex (area 6) in the rhesus monkey. *Journal of Comparative Neurology, 256*, 211–228.

Baum, S.R. (1992). The influence of word length on syllable duration in aphasia: Acoustic analyses. *Aphasiology, 6*, 501–513.

Baum, S.R. (1993). An acoustic analysis of rate of speech effects on vowel production in aphasia. *Brain and Language, 44*, 414–430.

Baum, S.R. (1996). Fricative production in aphasia: Effects of speaking rate. *Brain and Language, 52*, 328–341.

Baum, S.R., Blumstein, S.E., Naeser, M.A., & Palumbo, C.L. (1990). Temporal dimensions of consonant and vowel production: An acoustic and CT scan analysis of aphasic speech. *Brain and Language, 39*, 33–56.

Baum, S.R., Kim, J.A., & Katz, W.F. (1997). Compensation for jaw fixation by aphasic patients. *Brain and Language, 56*, 354–376.

Baum, S.R. & Ryan, L.R. (1993). Rate of speech effects in aphasia. *Brain and Language, 44*, 431–445.

Bay, E. (1962). Aphasia and non-verbal disorders of language. *Brain, 85*, 412–426.

Bennett, S. & Netsell, R. (1999). Possible roles of the insula in speech and language processing: Directions for research. *Journal of Medical Speech-Language Pathology, 7*, 253–270.

Berry, W.R. & Goshorn, E.L. (1983). Immediate visual feedback in the treatment of ataxic dysarthria: A case study. In W.R. Berry (ed.), *Clinical dysarthria*. San Diego, CA: College Hill Press.

Beukelman, D.R. (1983). Treatment of hyperkinetic dysarthria. In W.H. Perkins (ed.), *Dysarthia and apraxia*. New York: Thieme-Stratton.

Beukelman, D.R. & Yorkston, K.M. (1978). Communication options for patient with brain stem lesions. *Archives of Physical Medicine and Rehabilitation, 59*, 337–340.

Blumstein (1998). Phonological aspects of aphasia. In M. Sarno (ed.), *Acquired aphasia* (3rd ed.) (pp. 157–185). New York: Academic Press.

Blumstein, S.E., Baker, E., & Goodglass, H. (1977). Phonological factors in auditory comprehension in aphasia. *Neuropsychologia, 15*, 19–30.

Blumstein, S.E. & Baum, S.R. (1987). Consonant production deficits in aphasia. In J. Ryalls (ed.), *Phonetic approaches to speech production in aphasia and related disorders* (pp. 3–22). Boston: College-Hill Press.

Blumstein, S.E., Cooper, W.E., Goodglass, H., Statlender, S., & Gottlieb, J. (1980). Production deficits in aphasia: A voice onset time analysis. *Brain and Language, 9*, 153–170.

Bose, A., van Lieshout, P., & Square, P.A. (2000). *Speech-motor coordination in aphasia with apraxia*. Paper presented to the Motor Speech Conference, San Antonio, TX.

Bouillaud, J. (1825). Recherches cliniques propres a domontrer que la perte de la parole correspond à la lesion des lobules anterieurs du cerveau, a confirmer l'opinion de M. Gall sur le siège de l'organe du langage articule. *Archives Generales de Médecine, 8*, 25–45.

Brindley, P., Copeland, M., DeMain, C., & Martyn, P. (1989). A comparison of the speech of 10 chronic Broca's aphasics. *Aphasiology, 3*, 695–707.

Broca, P. (1861). Remarques sur le siège de la faculté de langage suivies d'une observation d'aphémie. *Bulletin de la Societe d'Anatomie, 6*, 330–357.

Buckingham, H. (1979). Explanations in apraxia with consequences for the concept of apraxia of speech. *Brain and Language, 8*, 202–226.

Buckingham, H. (1983). Apraxia of language vs. apraxia of speech. In R.A. Magill (ed.), *Memory and control of action*. Amsterdam: North-Holland.

Buckingham, H. (1998). Explanations for the concept of apraxia of speech. In M. Sarno (ed.), *Acquired aphasia* (3rd ed.) (pp. 269–307). New York: Academic Press.

Burgess, P.R., Wei, J.Y., Clark, F.J., & Simon, J. (1982). Signaling of kinesthetic information by peripheral sensory recpetors. *Annual Reviews of Neuroscience, 5*, 171–187.

Chauvel, P., Bancaud, J., & Buser, P. (1985). Participation of the supplementary motor area in speech. *Experimental Brain Research, 58*, A14–A15.

Chen, D.F., Hyland, B., Maier, V., Palmeri, A., & Wiesendanger, M. (1991). Comparison of neural activity in the supplementary motor area and in the primary motor cortex in monkeys. *Somatosensory and Motor Research, 8*, 27–44.

Chumpelik (Hayden), D. (1984). The PROMPT system of therapy. *Seminars in Speech and Language, 5*, 139–156.

Clark, H.M. & Robin, D.A. (1998). Generalized motor programme and parameterization accuracy in apraxia of speech and conduction aphasia. *Aphasiology, 12,* 699–713.

Code, C. & Ball, M. (1982). Fricative production in Broca's aphasia: A spectographic analysis. *Journal of Phonetics, 10,* 325–331.

Collins, M., Cariski, D., Longstreath, D., & Rosenbek, J.C. (1980). Patterns of articulatory behaviour in selected motor speech programming disorders. In R.H. Brookshire (ed.), *Clinical aphasiology: Conference proceedings* (pp. 196–208). Minneapolis, MN: BRK.

Collins, M., Rosenbek, J.C., & Wertz, R.T. (1983). Spectographic analysis of vowel and word duration in apraxia of speech. *Journal of Speech and Hearing Research, 26,* 224–230.

Cooper, W.E. & Sorenson, J.M. (1980). *Fundamental frequency in sentence production.* New York: Springer.

Critchley, M. (1952). Articulatory defects in aphasia. *Journal of Laryngology and Otology, 66,* 1–17.

Dabul, B. & Bollier, B. (1976). Therapeutic approaches to apraxia. *Journal of Speech and Hearing Disorders, 41,* 268–276.

Damasio, A.R. (1991). Aphasia. *The New England Journal of Medicine, 326,* 531–539.

Damasio, H. & Damasio, A.R.(1980). The anatomical basis of conduction aphasia. *Brain, 103,* 337–350.

Damasio, A.R., Damasio, H., Rizzo, M., Varney, N., & Gersh, F. (1982). Aphasia with nonhemorrhagic lesions in the basal ganglia and internal capsule. *Archives of Neurology, 39,* 15–24.

Damasio, A.R. & Geschwind, N. (1984). The neural basis of language. *Annual Review of Neuroscience, 7,* 127–147.

Damasio, A.R. & Van Hoesen, G.W. (1980). Structure and function of the supplementary motor area. *Neurology, 30,* 359.

Darley, F.L. (1968). Apraxia of speech: 107 Years of terminological confusion. Paper presented to the American Speech and Hearing Association, Denver, CO.

Darley, F.L. (1975). Treatment of acquired aphasia. In W. Friedlander (ed.), *Advances in neurology* (pp. 112–145). New York: Raven Press.

Darley, F.L., Aronson, A.E., & Brown, J. (1975). *Motor speech disorders.* Philadelphia: WB Saunders.

Darley, F.L. (1977). A retrospective review of aphasia. *Journal of Speech and Hearing Disorders, 42,* 161–169.

Deal, J. & Florence, C. (1978). Modification of the eight-step continuum for treatment of apraxia of speech in adults. *Journal of Speech and Hearing Disorders, 43,* 89–95.

Déjèrine, J. (1901). Semiologie du systéme nerveux. *Traite de Pathologie Generale, 5,* 391–471.

Delong, M.R. (1990). Primate models of movement disorders of basal ganglia origin. *Trends in Neuroscience, 13,* 281–285.

Denny-Brown, D. (1965). Physiological aspects of disturbances of speech. *Australian Journal of Experimental Biological Medicine and Science, 43,* 455–474.

Deutsch, S.E. (1984). Prediction of site of lesion from speech apraxic error patterns. In J.C. Rosenbek, M.R. McNeil, & A.E. Aronson (eds.), *Apraxia of speech: Physiology, acoustics, linguistics and management* (pp. 113–134). San Diego, CA: College Hill Press.

Devinsky, O., Morrell, M.J., & Vogt, B.A. (1995). Contributions of anterior cingulate cortex to behaviour. *Brain, 118,* 279–306.

Dronkers, N.F. (1996). A new brain region for coordinating speech articulation. *Nature, 384,* 159–161.

Dronkers, N.F., Shapiro, J.K., Redfern, B.B., & Knight, J. K.

(1992). The role of Broca's area in Broca's aphasia. *Journal of Clinical and Experimental Neuropsychology, 14,* 52–53.

Duffy, J.R. (1995). *Motor speech disorders: Substrates, differential diagnosis, and management.* St Louis: Mosby.

Duffy, J.R. & Folger, W.N. (1986). Dysarthria in unilateral central nervous system lesion: A retrospective study. Paper presented at the Annual Convention of the American Speech, Language, and Hearing Association, Detroit, MI.

Duffy, J.R. & Gawle, C.A. (1984). Apraxic speakers' vowel duration in consonant-vowel-consonant syllables. In J.C. Rosenbek, M.R. McNeil, & A.E. Aronson (eds.), *Apraxia of speech: Physiology, acoustics, linguistics and management* (pp. 167–196). San Diego, CA: College Hill Press.

Dum, R.P. & Strick, P.L. (1991). The origin of corticospinal projections from the premotor areas in the frontal lobe. *Journal of Neuroscience, 11,* 667–689.

Dum, R.P. & Strick, P.L. (1993). Cingulate motor areas. In B.A. Vogt & M. Graybiel (eds.), *Cingulate cortex and limbic thalamus: A comprehensive handbook* (pp. 415–441). Boston: Birkhauser.

Dworkin, J.P., Abkarian, C.G., & Johns, D.F. (1988). Apraxia of speech: The effectiveness of a treatment regimen. *Journal of Speech and Hearing Disorders, 53,* 280–294.

Evarts, E.V. (1986). Motor cortex outputs in primates. *Cerebral Cortex, 5,* 217–241.

Fairbanks, G. (1960). *Voice and articulation drillbook.* New York: Harper & Row.

Fink, G.R., Frackowiak, R.S.J., Pietrzyk, U., & Passingham, R.E. (1997). Multiple nonprimary motor areas in the human cortex. *Journal of Neurophysiology, 77,* 2164–2174.

Forrest, K., Adams, S.G., McNeil, M.R., & Southwood, H. (1991). Kinematic, electromyographic, and perceptual evaluation of speech apraxia, conduction aphasia, ataxic dysarthria, and normal speech production. In C.A. Moore, K.M. Yorkston, & D.R. Beukelman (eds.), *Dysarthria and apraxia of speech: Perspectives on management* (pp. 145–171). Baltimore, MD: Paul H. Brookes.

Freed, D.B., Marshall, R.C., & Frazier, K.E. (1997). Long term effectiveness of PROMPT treatment in severely apractic-aphasic speakers. *Aphasiology, 11,* 365–372.

Freund, H.J. (1987). Abnormalities of motor behaviour after cortical lesions in humans. In S. Geiger, F. Plum, & V. Mountcastle (eds.), *Handbook of physiology: The nervous system* (pp. 763–810). Bethesda, MD: American Physiological Society.

Freund, H.J. (1990). Premotor area and preparation of movement. *Revue Neurologique, 146,* 543–547.

Fried, I., Katz, A., McCarthy, G., Sass, K., Williamson, R., Spencer, S.S., & Spencer, D.D. (1991). Functional organization of human supplementary motor cortex studied by electrical stimulation. *Journal of Neuroscience, 11,* 3656–3666.

Gandour, J. & Dardarananda, R. (1984). Voice onset time in aphasia: Thai II: Production. *Brain and Language, 18,* 98–114.

Ghez, C. (1991). Voluntary movement. In E.R. Kandel, J.H. Schwartz, & T.M. Jessell, *Principles of neuroscience* (3rd ed.) (pp. 609–625). New York: Elsevier.

Ghika, J., Ghika-Schmid, F., & Bogousslavsky, J. (1998). Parietal motor syndrome: A clinical description in 32 patients in the acute phase of pure parietal strokes studied prospectively. *Clinical Neurology and Neurosurgery, 100,* 271–282.

Godschalk, M., Lemon, R.N., Kuypers, H.G.J. M., & Ronday, H.K. (1984). Cortical afferents and efferents of monkey postarcuate area: An anatomical and electrophysiological study. *Experimental Brain Research, 56,* 410–424.

Goldberg, G. (1985). Supplementary motor area structure and function: Review and hypotheses. *The Behavioral and Brain Sciences, 8,* 567–616.

Goldstein, K. (1948). *Language and language disturbances.* New York: Grune & Stratton.

Goodglass, H. (1992). Diagnosis of conduction aphasia. In S. Kohn (ed.), *Conduction aphasia* (pp. 3–50). Hillsdale NJ: Lawrence & Erlbaum.

Goodglass, H. & Kaplan, E. (1972). *The assessment of aphasia and related disorders.* Philadelphia: Lea Febiger.

Gordon, J. & Ghez, C. (1991). Muscle receptors and spinal reflexes: The stretch reflex. In E.R. Kandel, J.H. Schwartz, & T.M. Jessell, *Principles of neuroscience* (3rd ed.) (pp. 564–580). New York: Elsevier.

Gracco, V.L. (1987). A multi-level control model for speech motor activity. In H. Peters & W. Hulstij (eds.), *Speech motor dynamics in stuttering* (pp. 51–76). Vienna: Springer-Verlag.

Gracco, V.L. & Abbs, J.H. (1987). Programming and execution processes of speech movement control: Potential neural correlates. In L.E. Keller & M. Gopnik (eds.), *Symposium on motor and sensory language processes* (pp. 165–218). Hillsdale NJ: Lawrence Erlbaum.

Gracco, V.L. (1990). Characteristics of speech as a motor control system. In G. Hammond (ed.), *Cerebral control of speech and limb movements: Advances in psychology* (pp. 3–28). Amsterdam: North Holland.

Graybiel, A.M. (1990). Neurotransmitters and neuromodulators in the basal ganglia. *Trends in Neuroscience, 13,* 244–253.

Grillner, S. (1982). Possible analogies in the control of innate motor acts and the production of sound in speech. In S. Grillner, B. Lindblom, J. Labker, & A. Persson (eds.), *Speech motor control* (pp. 217–230). New York: Pergamon Press.

Habib, M., Daquin, G., Milandre, L., Royere, M.L., Rey, M., Lanteri, A., Salamon, G., & Khalil, R. (1995). Mutism and auditory agnosia due to bilateral insular damage—role of the insula in human communication. *Neuropsychologia, 33,* 327–339.

Halsband, U., Ito, N., Tanji, J., & Freund, H.J. (1993). The role of premotor cortex and the supplementary motor area in the temporal control of movement in man. *Brain, 116,* 243–266.

Hanson, W.R. & Metter, E.J. (1980). DAF as instrumental treatment for dysarthria in progressive supranuclear palsy: A case report. *Journal of Speech and Hearing Disorders, 45(2),* 268–276.

Hanson, W.R. & Metter, E.J. (1983). DAF speech rate modification in Parkinson's disease: A case report of two cases. In W. Berry (ed.), *Clinical dysarthria.* San Diego, CA: College Hill Press.

Hardcastle, W.J. (1987). Electropalatographic study of articulation disorders in verbal dyspraxia. In J. Ryalls (ed.), *Phonetic approaches to speech production in aphasia and related disorders* (pp. 113–136). Boston: College-Hill.

Harmes, S., Daniloff, R., Hoffman, P., Lewis, J., Kramer, M., & Absher, R. (1984). Temporal and articulatory control of fricative articulation by speakers with Broca's aphasia. *Journal of Phonetics, 12,* 367–385.

Hartman, D.E. & Abbs, J.H. (1992). Dysarthria associated with focal unilateral upper motor neuron lesion. *European Journal of Disorders of Communication, 27,* 187–196.

Hayden, D. (1999). *PROMPT manual level 1 & 2.* Santa Fe, NM: PROMPT Institute.

Hayden, D.A. (2000). *PROMPT level 11 certification workshop manual.* Santa Fe, NM: PROMPT Institute.

He, S.Q., Dum, R.P., Strick, P.L. (1993). Topographic organization of corticospinal projections from the frontal lobe: Motor areas on the lateral surface of the hemisphere. *Journal of Neuroscience, 13,* 952–980.

He, S.Q., Dum, R.P., & Strick, P.L. (1995). Topographic organization of corticospinal projections from the frontal lobe: Motor areas on the medial surface of the hemisphere. *Journal of Neuroscience, 15,* 3284–3306.

Head, H. (1915). Hughlings Jackson on aphasia and kindred affections of speech. *Brain, 38,* 190.

Head, H. (1926 [1963]). *Aphasia and kindred disorders of speech, Vol. 1 & 2.* New York: Hafner.

Helm, N.A. (1979). Management of palilalia with a pacing board. *Journal of Speech and Hearing Disorders, 44,* 350–353.

Howard, S. & Varley, R. (1995). Using electropalatography to treat severe acquired apraxia of speech. *European Journal of Disorders of Communication, 30,* 246–255.

Huang, C.S., Hiraba, H., Murray, G.M., & Sessle, B.J. (1989). Topographical distribution and functional properties of cortically induced rhythmical jaw movements in the monkey (Macaca fascicularis). *Journal of Neurophysiology, 61,* 635–650.

Huang, C.S., Hiraba, H., & Sessle, B.J. (1989). Input-output relationships of the primary face motor cortex in the monkey. *Journal of Neurophysiology, 61,* 350–362.

Huntley, G.W. & Jones, E.G. (1991). Relationship of intrinsic connections to forelimb movement representations in monkey motor cortex: A correlative anatomic and physiological study. *Journal of Neurophysiology, 66,* 390–401.

Inase, M., Tokuno, H., Nambu, A., Akazawa, T., & Takada, M. (1996). Origin of thalamocortical projections to the presupplementary motor area (pre-SMA) in the macaque monkey. *Neuroscience Research, 25,* 217–227.

Ingham, R.J. (1983). *Stuttering and behaviour therapy: Current status and experimental foundations.* San Diego, CA: College Hill Press.

Itoh, M., Sasanuma, S., Hirose, H., Yoshioka, H., & Yushigima, T. (1980). Abnormal articulatory dynamics in a patient with apraxia of speech: X-ray microbeam observation. *Brain and Language, 11,* 66–75.

Itoh, M. & Sasanuma, S. (1983). Velar movements during speech in two Wernicke aphasic patients. *Brain and Language, 19,* 283–292.

Jonas, E.G. (1981). The supplementary motor region and speech emission. *Journal of Communication Disorders, 14,* 349–373.

Jones, E.G. (1987). Ascending inputs to, and internal organization of, cortical motor areas. In G. Bock, M. O'Connor, & J. Marsh (eds.), *Motor areas of the cerebral cortex: CIBA Foundation symposium* (pp. 21–39). England, Chichester: Wiley.

Jurgens, U. (1985). Efferent connections of the supplementary motor area. *Experimental Brain Research, 58,* A1–A2.

Katz, W. (1988). Anticipatory coarticulation in aphasia: Acoustic and perceptual data. *Brain and Language, 35,* 340–368.

Katz, W., Machetanz, J., Orth, U., & Schonle, P. (1990). A kinematic analysis of anticipatory coarticulation in the speech of anterior aphasic subjects using electromagnetic articulatography. *Brain and Language, 38,* 555–575.

Keith, R.L. & Aronson, A.E. (1975). Singing as therapy for apraxia of speech and aphasia: Report of a case. *Brain and Language, 2,* 483–488.

Kempler, D., Metter, E., Jackson, C., Hanson, W., Reiger, W., Mazziota, J.C., & Phelps, M.A. (1986). Conduction aphasia: Subgroups based on behavior, anatomy and physiology. In R. Brookshire (ed.), *Clinical aphasiology: Conference proceedings, 16,* 105–115. Minneapolis, MN: BRK.

Kent, R.D. (1990). The acoustic and physiologic characteristics of neurologically impaired speech movements. In W. Hardcastle & A. Marchal (eds.), *Speech production and modelling* (pp. 365–401). Dordrecht Netherlands: Kluwer Academic Publishers.

Kent, R.D. & Adams, S.G. (1989). The concept and measurement of coordination in speech disorders. In S.A. Wallace (ed.), *Advances in psychology: Perspectives on the coordination of movement* (pp. 415–450). New York: Elsevier.

Kent, R.D. & McNeil, M.R. (1987). Relative timing of sentence repetition in apraxia of speech and conduction aphasia. In J. Ryalls (ed.), *Phonetic approaches to speech production in aphasia and related disorders* (pp. 181–220). Boston: College-Hill Press.

Kent, R.D., Netsell, R., & Abbs, J.H. (1979). Acoustic characteristics of dysarthria associated with cerebellar disease. *Journal of Speech and Hearing Research, 22,* 627–648.

Kent, R.D. & Rosenbek, J.C. (1983). Acoustic patterns of apraxia of speech. *Journal of Speech and Hearing Research, 26,* 231–249.

Kertesz, A. (1982). *Western Aphasia Battery.* New York: Grune & Stratton.

Kertesz, A., Harlock, W., & Coates, R. (1979). Computer tomographic localization lesion size and prognosis in aphasia and nonverbal impairment. *Brain and Language, 8,* 34–50.

Kimura, D. (1979). Neuromotor mechanisms in the evolution of human communication. In H.D. Steklis & M.J. Raleigh (eds.), *Neurobiology of Social Communication in Primates* (pp. 197–219). New York: Academic Press.

Kimura, D. (1982). Left-hemisphere control of oral and brachial movements and their relation to communication. *Philosophical Transactions of the Royal Society of London, 298,* 135–149.

Kimura, D. & Watson, N. (1989). The relationship between oral movement control and speech. *Brain and Language, 37,* 565–590.

Kohn, S. (1984). The nature of the phonological disorder in conduction aphasia. *Brain and Language, 23,* 97–115.

Kupfermann, I. (1991). Localization of higher cognitive and affective functions: The association cortices. In E.R. Kandel, J.H. Schwartz, & T.M. Jessell, *Principles of neuroscience* (3rd ed.) (pp. 823–838). New York: Elsevier.

Kurata, K. (1992). Somatopy in the human supplementary motor area. *Trends in Neuroscience, 15,* 159–160.

Kuypers, H.G.J.M. (1958a). Corticobulbar connections to the pons and lower brain-stem in man. *Brain, 81,* 364–388.

Kuypers, H.G.J.M. (1958b). Some projections from the peri-central cortex to the pons and lower brain stem in monkey and chimpanzee. *Journal of Comparative Neurology, 1190,* 221–255.

Kwan, H.C., Mackay, W.A., Murphy, J.T., & Wong, Y.C. (1978). Spatial organization of precentral cortex in awake primates: II. Motor outputs. *Journal of Neurophysiology, 41,* 1120–1131.

Larson, C.R., Byrd, K.E., Garthwaite, C.R., & Luschei, E.S. (1980). Alterations in the pattern of mastication after ablations of the lateral precentral cortex in rhesus monkeys. *Experimental Neurology, 70,* 638–651.

Lebrun, Y. (1989). Apraxia of speech: The history of a concept. In P.A. Square-Storer (ed.), *Acquired apraxia of speech in aphasic adults* (pp. 3–19). London: Taylor & Francis.

Lecours, A.R. & Lhermitte, F. (1976). The pure form of the phonetic disintegration syndrome (pure anarthria). *Brain and Language, 3,* 88–113.

Lichtheim, L. (1885). On aphasia. *Brain, 7,* 433–484.

Liepmann, H. (1913). Motorische, aphasie, und apraxie. *Transactions of the 17th International Congress of Medicine, XI,* 97–106.

Lund, J.P. & Lamarre, Y. (1974). Activity of neurons in the lower precentral cortex during voluntary and rhythmical jaw movements in the monkey. *Experimental Brain Research, 19,* 282–299.

Luppino, G., Matelli, M., Camarda, R.M., Gallese, V., & Rizzolatti, G. (1991). Multiple representations of body movements in mesial area 6 and the adjacent cingulate cortex: An intracortical microstimulation study in the macaque monkey. *Journal of Comparative Neurology, 311,* 463–482.

Luria, A.R. (1964). Factors and forms of aphasia. In A.V.S. de Reuck & M. O'Connor (eds.), *Disorders of language.* London: Churchill.

Luria, A.R. (1970). *Traumatic aphasic: Its syndromes, psychology and treatment.* The Hague: Mouton.

Luschei, E.S., Garthwaite, C.R., & Armstrong, M.E. (1971). Relationship of firing patterns of units in face area of monkey precentral cortex to conditioned jaw movements. *Journal of Neurophysiology, 34,* 552–561.

Marie, P. (1906). Révision de la question de l'aphasie: Que fait-il penser des aphasies sous corticales (aphasies pures)? *Semaine Medicale, 26,* 493.

Marie, P., Foix, C., & Bertrand, I. (1917). Topographie cranio-cérébrale. *Annales de Médecine, 55.*

Marsden, C.D., Deecke, L., Freund, H.J., Hallett, M., Passingham, R.E., Shibasaki, H., Tanji, J., & Wiesendanger, M. (1996). The functions of the supplementary motor area: Summary of a workshop. *Advances in Neurology, 70,* 477–487.

Martin, R.E., Murray, G.M., Kemppainen, P., Masuda Y., & Sessle, B.J. (1997). Functional properties of neurons in the primate tongue primary motor cortex during swallowing. *Journal of Neurophysiology, 78,* 1516–1530.

Mateer, C. & Kimura, D. (1977). Impairment of nonverbal oral movements in aphasia. *Brain and Language, 4,* 262–276.

Matelli, M., Camarda, R., Glickstein, M., & Rizzolatti, G. (1986). Afferent and efferent projections of the inferior area 6 in the Macaque monkey. *Journal of Comparative Neurology, 251,* 281–298.

McCloskey, D.I. (1978). Kinesthetic sensibility. *Physiological Reviews, 58,* 763–820.

McLean, M.D., Dostrovsky, J.O., Lee, L., & Tasker, R.R. (1990). Somatosensory neurons in human thalamus respond to speech-induced orofacial movements. *Brain Research, 513,* 343–347.

McNeil, M.R. & Adams, S.G. (1990). A comparison of speech kinematics among apraxic, conduction aphasic, ataxic dysarthric and normal geriatric speakers. In T.E. Prescott (ed.), *Clinical aphasiology* (pp. 279–294). Austin, TX: Pro-Ed.

McNeil, M.R., Caligiuri, M., & Rosenbek, J.C. (1989). A comparison of labiomandibular kinematic durations, displacements, velocities and dysmetrias in apraxic and normal adults. In T.E. Prescott (ed.), *Clinical aphasiology* (pp. 173–179). Boston: College Hill Press.

McNeil, M.R., Robin, D.A., & Schmidt, R.A. (1997). Apraxia of speech: Definition, differentiation, and treatment. In M.R. McNeil (ed.), *Clinical management of sensorimotor speech disorders* (pp. 311–344). New York: Thieme.

McNeil, M.R., Weismer, G., Adams, S.G., & Mulligan, M. (1990). Oral structure non-speech motor control in normal dysarthric, aphasic and apraxic speakers: Isometric force and static fine position control. *Journal of Speech and Hearing Research, 33*, 255–268.

Mesulam, M.M. & Mufson, E.J. (1982). Insula of the old world monkey: I. Architectonics in the insulo-orbito-temporal component of the paralimbic brain. *The Journal of Comparative Neurology, 212*, 1–22.

Mesulam, M.M. & Mufson, E.J. (1985). The insula of Reil in man and monkey. In A. Peters & E. Jones (eds.), *Cerebral cortex* (pp. 179–226). New York: Plenum Press.

Metter, E.J., Hanson, W.R., Jackson, C.A., Kempler, D., & van Lancker, D. (1993). Broca's aphasia: Comparison to metabolically matched aphasic subjects. *Clinical Aphasiology, 21*, 335–341.

Metter, E.J., Kempler, D., Jackson, C.A., Hanson, W.R., Riege, W.H., Camras, L.R., Mazziotta, J.C., & Phelps, M.E. (1989). Cerebral glucose metabolism in Wernicke's, Broca's, and conduction aphasia. *Archives of Neurology, 46*, 27–34.

Metter, E.J., Riege, W.H., Hanson, W.R., Jackson, C.A., Kempler, D., & van Lancker, D. (1988). Subcortical structures in aphasia: Analysis based on FBG, PET and CT. *Archives of Neurology, 45*, 1229–1234.

Metter, E.J., Riege, W.H., Hanson, W.R., Phelps, M.E., & Kuhl, D.E. (1988). Evidence for a caudate role in aphasia from FBG positron computed tomography. *Aphasiology, 2*, 33–43.

Mitz, A.R. & Wise, S.P. (1987). The somatotopic organization of the supplementary motor area: Intracortical microstimulation mapping. *Journal of Neuroscience, 7*, 1010–1021.

Mohr, J.P., Pessin, M.S., Finkelstein, S., Funkenstein, H.H., Duncan, G.W., & Davis, K.R. (1978). Broca's aphasia: Pathologic and clinical. *Neurology, 28*, 311–324.

Mountcastle, V.B., Lynch, J.C., Georgopoulos, A. Sakata, H., & Acuna, C. (1975). Posterior parietal association cortex of the monkey: Command functions for operations within extrapersonal space. *Journal of Neurophysiology, 38*, 871–908.

Morecraft, R.J. & Van Hoesen, G.W. (1998). Convergence of limbic input to the cingulate motor cortex in the rhesus monkey. *Brain Research Bulletin, 45*, 209–232.

Muakkassa, K.F. & Strick, P.L. (1979). Frontal lobe inputs to primate motor cortex: Evidence for four somatotopically organized "premotor" areas. *Brain Research, 177*, 176–182.

Munhall, K.G., Lofqvist, A., & Kelso, J.A.S. (1994). Lip-larynx coordination in speech: Effects of mechanical perturbations to the lower lip. *Journal of Acoustical Society of America, 95*, 3605–3616.

Murphy, K., Corfield, D.R., Guz, A., Fink, G.R., Wise, R.J., Harrison, J., & Adams, L. (1997). Cerebral areas associated with motor control of speech in humans. *Journal of Applied Physiology, 83*, 1438–1447.

Murray, G.M. (1989). An analysis of motor cortex neural activities during trained orofacial motor behaviour in the awake primate (Macaca fascicularis). Unpublished doctoral dissertation, University of Toronto.

Murray, G.M. & Sessle, B.J. (1992a). Functional properties of single neurons in the face primary motor cortex of the primate: III. Relations with different directions of trained tongue protrusion. *Journal of Neurophysiology, 67*, 775–785.

Murray, G.M. & Sessle, B.J. (1992b). Functional properties of single neurons in the face primary motor cortex of the primate: II. Relations with trained orofacial motor behaviour. *Journal of Neurophysiology, 67*, 221–255.

Mushiake, H., Inase, M., & Tanji, J. (1991). Neuronal activity in the primate premotor, supplementary, and precentral motor cortex during visually guided and internally determined sequential movements. *Journal of Neurophysiology, 66*, 705–718.

Naeser, M.A., Alexander, M.P., Helm-Estabrooks, N., Levine, H.L., Laughlin, S.A., & Geschwind, N. (1982). Aphasias with predominantly subcortical lesion sites: Description of three capsular/putaminal aphasia syndromes. *Archives of Neurology, 39*, 2–14.

Naeser, M.A. & Helm-Estabrooks, N. (1985). CT scan lesion localization and response to melodic intonation therapy with nonfluent aphasia cases. *Cortex, 21*, 203–223.

Naeser, M.A., Palumbo, C.L., Helm-Estabrooks, N., Stiassny-Eder, D., & Albert, M.L. (1989). Severe nonfluency in aphasia. *Brain, 112*, 1–38.

Nagafuchi, M., Aoki, Y., Nizuma, H., & Okita, N. (1991). Paroxysmal speech disorder following left-frontal brain damage. *Brain and Language, 40*, 266–273.

Odell, K.H., McNeil, M.R., Rosenbek, J.C., & Hunter, L. (1991). Perceptual characteristics of vowel and prosody production in apraxic, aphasic and dysarthic speakers. *Journal of Speech and Hearing Research, 34*, 67–80.

Okano, K. & Tanji, J. (1987). Neuronal activities in the primate motor fields of the agranular frontal cortex preceding visually triggered and self-paced movement. *Experimental Brain Research, 66*, 155–166.

Ojemann, G. (1988). Effects of cortical and subcortical stimulation on human language and verbal memory. In F. Plum (ed.), *Language, communication and the brain* (pp. 101–115). New York: Raven Press.

Pandya, D.N. & Seltzer, B. (1982). Association areas of the cerebral cortex. *Trends in Neuroscience, 5*, 386–390.

Pandya, D.N. & Barnes, C.L. (1987). Architecture and connections of the frontal lobe. In Anonymous, *Frontal lobes revisited* (pp. 41–72). New York: IRBV Press.

Paus, T., Petrides, M., Evans, A.C., & Meter, E. (1993). Role of the human anterior cingulate cortex in the control of oculomotor, manual and speech responses: A positron emission tomography study. *Journal of Neurophysiology, 70*, 453–459.

Pause, M. & Freund, H.J. (1989). Role of the parietal cortex for sensorimotor transformation: Evidence from clinical observations. *Brain, Behavior & Evolution, 33*, 136–140.

Pause, M., Kunesch, E., Binkofski, F., & Freund, H.J. (1989). Sensorimotor disturbances in patients with lesions of the parietal cortex. *Brain, 112*, 1599–1625.

Pellat, J., Gentil, M., Lyard, G., Vila, A., Tarel, V., Moreau, O., & Benabio, A.L. (1991). Aphemia after a penetrating brain wound: A case study. *Brain and Language, 40*, 459–470.

Penfield, W. & Welch, K. (1951). The supplementary motor area of the cerebral cortex: A clinical and experimental study. *American Medical Association Archives of Neurology and Psychiatry, 66,* 289–317.

Penfield, W. & Roberts, L. (1959). *Speech and brain mechanisms.* Princeton, NJ: Princeton University Press.

Petersen, S.E., Fox, P.T., Posner, M.I., Mintun, M., & Raichle, M.E. (1988). Positron emission tomographic studies of the cortical anatomy of single-word processing. *Nature, 331,* 585–589.

Petrovici, J.N. (1983). Speech disorders in tumors of the supplementary motor area. *Zentralbl fur Neurochirurgie, 44,* 97–104.

Picard, N. & Strick, P.L. (1996). Motor areas of the medial wall: A review of their location and functional activation. *Cerebral Cortex, 6,* 342–353.

Poeck, K., de Blesser, R., & von Keyerlingk, D.G. (1984). Computed tomography localization of standard aphasic syndromes. In F.C. Rose (ed.), *Advances in neurology: Progress in aphasiology, Vol. 22* (pp. 71–89). New York: Raven.

Porch, B.E. (1967). *The Porch Index of Communicative Ability.* Palo Alto, CA: Consulting Psychologists Press.

Rizzolatti, G., Luppino, G., & Matelli, M. (1998). The organization of the cortical motor system: New concepts. *Electroencephalography and Clinical Neurophysiology, 106,* 283–296.

Ro, J.Y. & Capra, N.F. (1995). Encoding of jaw movements by central trigeminal neurons with cutaneous and microneurography. *Experimental Brain Research, 47,* 177–190.

Roland, P.E. (1981). Somatotopic tuning of postcentral gyrus during focal attention in man. *Journal of Neurophysiology, 46,* 744–754.

Rolls, E. & Johnstone, S. (1992). Neurophysiological analysis of striatal function. In G. Vallar, S. Cappa, & C. Wallesch (eds.), *Neurophysiological disorders associated with subcortical disorders* (pp. 61–97). Oxford: Oxford University Press.

Rosenbek, J.C. (1976). Treatment of apraxia of speech: Prevention, facilitation and reorganization. Paper presented to the Annual Meeting of the American Speech and Hearing Association, Houston, TX.

Rosenbek, J.C. (1983). Treatment for apraxia of speech in adults. In W.H. Perkins (ed.), *Dysarthria and apraxia* (pp. 49–57). New York: Thieme-Stratton.

Rosenbek, J.C., Collins, M., & Wertz, R.T. (1976). Intersystemic reorganization for apraxia of speech. In R.H. Brookshire (ed.), *Clinical aphasiology: conference proceedings* (pp. 255–260). Minneapolis, MN: BRK.

Rosenbek, J.C. & LaPointe, L.L. (1978). The dysarthrias: Description, diagnosis and treatment. In D.F. Johns (ed.), *Clinical management of neurogenic communicative disorders* (1st ed.) (pp. 251–311). Boston: Little, Brown.

Rosenbek, J.C. & LaPointe, L.L. (1985). The dysarthrias: Description, diagnosis and treatment. In D.F. Johns (ed.), *Clinical management of neurogenic communicative disorders* (2nd ed.) (pp. 97–152). Boston: Little, Brown.

Rosenbek, J.C., Lemme, M.L., Ahern, M.B., Harris, E.H., & Wertz, R.T. (1973). A treatment for apraxia of speech in adults. *Journal of Speech and Hearing Disorders, 38,* 462–472.

Rosenbek, J.C. & McNeil, M.R. (1991). A discussion of the classification in motor speech disorders: Dysarthria and apraxia of speech. In C.A. Moore, K.M. Yorkston, & D.R. Beukelman (eds.), *Dysarthria and apraxia of speech* (pp. 289–295). Baltimore, MD: Paul H. Brookes.

Rubow, R.T., Rosenbek, J.C., & Collins, M. (1982). Vibrotactile stimulation for intersystemic reorganization in the treatment of apraxia of speech. *Archives of Physical Medicine and Rehabilitation, 63,* 150–153.

Ryalls, J. (1981). Motor aphasia: Acoustic correlates of phonetic disintegration in vowels. *Neuropsychologia, 20,* 355–360.

Ryalls, J. (1986). An acoustic study of vowel production in aphasia. *Brain and Language, 29,* 48–67.

Ryalls, J. (1987). Vowel production in aphasia: Towards an account of the consonant-vowel dissociation. In J. Ryalls (ed.), *Phonetic approaches to speech production in aphasia and related disorders* (pp. 23–44). Boston: College-Hill Press.

Ryalls, J., Provost, H., & Arsenault, N. (1995). Voice onset time production in French speaking aphasics. *Journal of Communication Disorders, 28,* 205–215.

Ryding, E., Bradvik, B., & Ingvar, D.H. (1996). Silent speech activates prefrontal cortical regions asymmetrically, as well as speech-related areas in the dominant hemisphere. *Brain and Language, 52,* 435–451.

Sarno, M.T. (1965). Functional communication profile. *Archives of Physical Medicine and Rehabilitation, 46,* 101–107.

Schell, G.R. & Strick, P.L. (1984). The origin of thalamic inputs to the arcuate premotor and supplementary motor areas. *Journal of Neuroscience, 4,* 539–560.

Schiff, H.B., Alexander, M.P., Naeser, M.A., & Galaburda, A.M. (1983). Aphemia: Clinical-anatomic correlations. *Archives of Neurology, 40,* 720–727.

Schuell, H., Jenkins, J., & Jimenez-Pabon, E. (1964). *Aphasia in adults.* New York: Harper & Row.

Shane, H.C. & Darley, F.L. (1978). The effect of auditory rhythmic stimulation on articulatory accuracy in apraxia of speech. *Cortex, 14,* 444–450.

Shankweiler, D. & Harris, K.S. (1966). An experimental approach to the problem of articulation in aphasia. *Cortex, 2,* 287–292.

Shewan, C.M., Leeper, H., & Booth, J. (1984). An analysis of voice onset time (VOT) in aphasic and normal subjects. In J.C. Rosenbek, M.R. McNeil, & A.E. Aronson (eds.), *Apraxia of speech: Physiology, acoustics, linguistics and management* (pp. 197–220). San Diego, CA: College Hill Press.

Shinn, P. & Blumstein, S.E. (1983). Phonemic disintegration in aphasia: Acoustic analysis of spectral characteristics for place of articulation. *Brain and Language, 20,* 90–114.

Sieron, J., Westphal, K.P., & Johannsen, H.S. (1995). Apraxia of the larynx. *Folia Phoniatrica et Logopedica, 47,* 33–38.

Simmons, N.N. (1978). Finger counting as an intersystemic reorganizer in apraxia of speech. In R.H. Brookshire (ed.), *Clinical aphasiology: Conference proceedings* (pp. 174–179). Minneapolis, MN: BRK.

Sirisko, M.A. & Sessle, B.J. (1983). Corticobulbar profections and orofacial and muscle afferent inputs to neurons in primate sensorimotor cerebral cortex. *Experimental Neurology, 82,* 716–720.

Skelly, M., Schensky, L., Smith, R., & Foust, R. (1974). American Indian Sign (Amerind) as a facilitator of verbalization for the verbal apraxia. *Journal of Speech and Hearing Disorders, 39,* 445–456.

Smith, A. (1992). The control of orofacial movements in speech. *Critical Reviews in Oral Biology and Medicine, 3*, 233–267.

Southwood, H. (1987). The use of prolonged speech in the treatment of apraxia of speech. In R.H. Brookshire (ed.), *Clinical aphasiology: Conference proceedings* (pp. 277–287). Minneapolis, MN: BRK.

Sparks, R.W. (1981). Melodic intonation therapy. In R.H. Chapey (ed.), *Language intervention strategies in adult aphasia* (pp. 265–282). Baltimore, MD: Williams & Wilkins.

Sparks, R.W. & Deck, J.W. (1986). Melodic intonation therapy. In R. Chapey (ed.), *Language intervention strategies in adult aphasia* (1st ed.) (pp. 320–332). Baltimore, MD: Williams & Wilkins.

Sparks, R.W., Helm, N., & Albert, M. (1974). Aphasia rehabilitation resulting from melodic intonation therapy. *Cortex, 10*, 303–316.

Square-Storer, P.A. (1989). Traditional therapies for apraxia of speech—reviewed and rationalized. In P.A. Square-Storer (ed.), *Acquired apraxia of speech in aphasic adults* (pp. 145–161). London: Erlbaum.

Square, P.A. (1995). Apraxia of speech reconsidered. In F. Bell-Berti & L.J. Raphael (eds.), *Producing speech: Contemporary issues* (pp. 375–386). New York: AIP Press.

Square-Storer, P.A. & Apeldoorn, S. (1991). An acoustic study of apraxia of speech in patients with different lesion loci. In C.A. Moore, K.M. Yorkston, & D.R. Beukelman (eds.), *Dysarthria and apraxia of speech: Perspectives on management* (pp. 271–286). Baltimore, MD: Paul H. Brookes.

Square, P.A., Chumpelik (Hayden), D., & Adams, S.G. (1985). Efficacy of the PROMPT system of therapy for the treatment of acquired apraxia of speech. In R.H. Brookshire (ed.), *Clinical aphasiology: Conference proceedings* (pp. 319–320). Minneapolis, MN: BRK.

Square, P.A., Chumpelik (Hayden), D., Morningstar, D., & Adams, S.G. (1986). Efficacy of the PROMPT system of therapy for the treatment of apraxia of speech: A follow-up investigation. In R.H. Brookshire (ed.), *Clinical aphasiology: Conference proceedings* (pp. 221–226). Minneapolis, MN: BRK.

Square, P.A., Darley, F.L., & Sommers, R.K. (1981). Speech perception among patients demonstrating apraxia of speech, aphasia and both disorders. In R.H. Brookshire (ed.), *Clinical aphasiology: Conference proceedings* (pp. 83–88). Minneapolis, MN: BRK.

Square, P.A., Darley, F.L., & Sommers, R.K. (1982). An analysis of the productive errors made by pure apractic speakers with differing loci of lesions. In R.H. Brookshire (ed.), *Clinical aphasiology: Conference proceedings* (pp. 245–250). Minneapolis, MN: BRK.

Square-Storer, P.A., Darley, F.L., & Sommers, R.K. (1988). Speech processing abilities in patients with aphasia and apraxia of speech. *Brain and Language, 33*, 65–85.

Square-Storer, P.A. & Hayden (Chumpelik), D. (1989). PROMPT treatment. In P.A. Square-Storer (ed.), *Acquired apraxia of speech in aphasic adults* (pp. 190–219). London: Taylor & Francis.

Square, P.A. & Martin, R.E. (1994). The nature and treatment of neuromotor speech disorders in aphasia. In R.H. Chapey (ed.), *Language intervention strategies in adult aphasia* (3rd ed.) (pp. 467–499). Baltimore, MD: Williams & Wilkins.

Square, P.A. & Mlcoch, A.G. (1983). The syndrome of subcortical apraxia of speech: An acoustic analysis. In R.H. Brookshire

(ed.), *Clinical aphasiology: Conference proceedings* (pp. 239–243). Minneapolis, MN: BRK.

Square-Storer, P.A., Qualizza, L., & Roy, E.A. (1989). Isolated and sequenced oral motor posture production under different input modalities by left-hemisphere damaged adults. *Cortex, 25*, 371–386.

Square-Storer, P.A., Roy, E.A., & Martin, R.E. (1997). Apraxia of speech: Another form of praxis disruption. In L.J.G. Rothi & K.M. Heilman (eds.), *Apraxia: The neuropsychology of action* (pp. 173–206). UK: Psychology Press, an imprint of Erlbaum (UK) Taylor & Francis.

Sussman, H.M., Marquardt, T.P., MacNeilage, P.F., & Hutchinson, J.A. (1988). Anticipatory coarticulation in aphasia: Some methodological considerations. *Brain and Language, 35*, 369–379.

Tonkonogy, J. & Goodglass, H. (1981). Language function, foot of the third frontal gyrus, and rolandic operculum. *Archives of Neurology, 38*, 486–490.

Tonkovich, J.D. & Peach, R.K. (1989). What to treat: Apraxia of speech, aphasia or both. In P.A. Square-Storer (ed.), *Acquired apraxia of speech in aphasic adults* (pp. 115–144). London: Erlbaum.

Tuller, B. (1984). On categorizing speech errors. *Neuropsychologica, 22*, 547–558.

Van Riper, C. (1939). *Speech correction: Principles and methods.* Englewood Cliffs, NJ: Prentice Hall.

Vijayan, A. & Gandour, J. (1995). On the notion of a 'subtle phonetic deficit' in fluent/posterior aphasia. *Brain and Language, 48*, 106–119.

Wallesch, C.W. (1990). Repetitive verbal behaviour: Functional and neurological considerations. *Aphasiology, 4*, 133–153.

Wambaugh, J.L. & Doyle, P.J. (1994). Treatment for acquired apraxia of speech: A review of efficacy reports. *Clinical Aphasiology, 22*, 231–243.

Wambaugh, J.L., Kalinyak-Fliszar, M.M., West, J.E., & Doyle, P.J. (1998). Effects of treatment for sound errors in apraxia of speech and aphasia. *Journal of Speech, Language, and Hearing Research, 41*, 725–743.

Wernicke, C. (1874). *Der aphasische symptomenkomplex.* Breslau, Germany: Cohn & Weigert.

Wernicke, C. (1885). Die neueren arbeiten uber aphasie. *Fortschritte der Medizin, 3*, 824–830.

Wertz, R.T. (1985). Neuropathologies of speech and language: An introduction to patient management. In D.F. Johns (ed.), *Clinical management of neurogenic communicative disorders.* Boston: Little, Brown.

Wertz, R.T., LaPointe, L.L., & Rosenbek, J.C. (1984). *Apraxia of speech in adults: The disorder and its management.* New York: Grune & Stratton.

Whiteside, S.P. & Varley, R.A. (1998). A reconceptualisation of apraxia of speech: A synthesis of evidence. *Cortex, 34*, 221–231.

Wiesendanger, M. (1986). Resdistributive function of the motor cortex. *Trends in Neuroscience, 93*, 120–125.

Wiesendanger, M. & Wise, S.P. (1992). Current issues concerning the functional organization of motor cortical areas in non-human primates. In P. Chauvel & A.V. Delgado-Escueta (eds.), *Advances in Neurology, 57*, 117–134.

Wiesendanger, R. & Wiesendanger, M. (1985a). Cerebello-cortical linkage in the monkey as revealed by transcellular labeling with the lectin wheat germ agglutinin conjugated to the marker horseradish peroxidase. *Experimental Brain Research, 59,* 105–117.

Wiesendanger, R. & Wiesendanger, M. (1985b). The thalamic connection with medial area 6 (supplementary motor cortex) in the monkey. *Experimental Brain Research, 59,* 91–104.

Wise, S.P. & Strick, P.L. (1984). Anatomical and physiological organization of the non-primary motor cortex. *Trends in Neuroscience, 7,* 442–446.

Wise, S.P. (1985). The primate premotor cortex: Past, present, and preparatory. *Annual Review of Neuroscience, 8,* 1–19.

Yorkston, K.M. & Beukelman, D.R. (1981). Ataxic dysarthria: Treatment sequences based on intelligibility and prosodic considerations. *Journal of Speech and Hearing Disorders, 46,* 398–404.

Yorkston, K.M., Beukelman, D.R., & Bell, K.R. (1988). *Clinical management of dysarthric speakers.* Boston: College Hill Press.

Zeigler, W. & von Cramon, D. (1985). Anticipatory coarticulation in a patient with apraxia of speech. *Brain and Language, 26,* 117–130.

Zeigler, W. & von Cramon, D. (1986). Disturbed coarticulation in apraxia of speech: Acoustic evidence. *Brain and Language, 29,* 34–47.

APPENDIX 36-1

Prompts for Restructuring Oral Muscular Phonetic Targets (PROMPT)

PROMPT is a multidimensional, multisensory, therapeutic philosophy, approach, system, and technique that is holistic and dynamic in nature. PROMPT strives to (re)connect and integrate the motor, sensory, perceptual, cognitive-linguistic, and social-emotional aspects of communication. As a system, PROMPT may be described as one that helps clients gain voluntary control of motor-speech systems and links the necessary motor movements that help create holistic motor-phoneme maps to linguistic (word and phrase) equivalents for use in functional communication.
Hayden, D. (1999). *PROMPT Manual Level 1.* Santa Fe, NM: PROMPT Institute.

Parameter Prompt

These larger, organizing postures or cues focus tactile-kinesthetic-proprioceptive input to the skeletal, muscular, or neurological systems. These supporting, Parameter PROMPTs provide the base support for more complex muscular contractions and intricately timed movements. Parameter PROMPTs provide stability and set the degrees of freedom necessary to allow more complex and overlapping movements. When these are engaged they allow for the involvement of specific, discrete, flexible, and well-balanced muscular contractions needed in speech production.

Complex Prompts

These complex, multidimensional, tactile-kinesthetic-proprioceptive prompts provide input to the neurological, muscular, and sensory systems. They signal the place and dynamic integration needed from phonatory, jaw, labial-facial, and lingual muscles (from broad to narrow contractions), and the length and intensity of contractions. Complex PROMPTing specifies as many components as possible for the holistic construction of a motor-phoneme. Complex PROMPTs, then, provide as much information as possible about what is needed for creating a motor-phoneme map or acoustic production template.

Surface Prompts

Surface PROMPTs are one-dimensional and focus tactile-kinesthetic input to the either the jaw, labial-facial structures, or to the mylohyoid or tongue body. Used in isolation, surface PROMPTS may signal the components of place, timing, and the amount of muscular contraction needed in a target movement. When used in syllables, words, or phrases they act to mainly

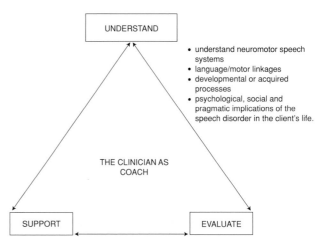

Figure 36A–1. USE Social Application Model. (From Hayden DA [2000]. *PROMPT Level II Certification Workshop Manual.* Santa Fe, NM: PROMPT Institute.)

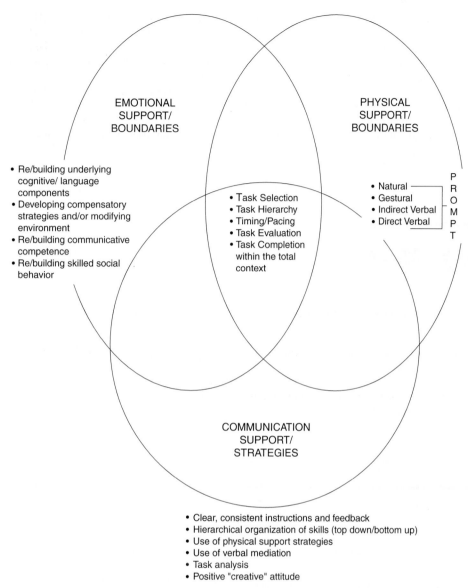

Figure 36A–2. USE Support Function Model. (From Hayden DA [2000]. *PROMPT Level II Certification Workshop Manual.* Santa Fe, NM: PROMPT Institute.)

signal the variables of place, timing, and transition of varying planes of movement. D. Hayden (1999). *PROMPT Manual Level 1* (p. 21). Santa Fe, NM: PROMPT Institute.

The USE Social Application Model

The USE (Understand, Support, and Evaluate) Model was created to provide a social application framework for PROMPT. See Figure 36A–1.

The philosophy of PROMPT stresses the need to thoroughly *evaluate* all areas of client function, to determine the environments in which communication is the "most critical," and to support the client and caregivers by creating a lexicon based on the client's abilities (cognitive, physical, and emotional). The goal of PROMPT is to provide the patient with a lexicon

that is intelligible and useful for interactions with caregivers or peers.

Another part of the framework that is critical to the philosophy of PROMPT is the clinician's ability to *understand* the strengths and weakness in all domains affecting the client's life. This means the clinician must strive to understand how the domains of cognition and social interaction, physical, motor-sensory, and emotional and behavioral conditions impact on the client to produce breakdowns in the acquisition of, or relearning of, information necessary for the formulation of concepts, organization of lexical information and grammatical forms, and the execution and control of motor movements and sequences that result in interactive communication.

The third aspect of the USE model is the *support* that the clinician needs to give to the client in order to create successful communications. This area is often neglected because the goal of therapy is the "production of speech" or the "acquisition of language and form." Support of the client by the clinicians is stressed as the underpinnings of successful communication in PROMPTs.

Other supports such as "boundaries" let the client know when they are correct, incorrect, or may be inappropriate. For example, physically, when they are unable to stop a preservative action or are using too much or too many muscular actions towards a movement, the clinician should direct the patient to stop or produce no movement. If a patient becomes frustrated or angry, the clinician should ask, "Are you mad?" and then help the patient to express his/her feelings

by PROMPTing an appropriate word such as "mad." Boundaries may provide both a safe structure in which to operate as well as a consistent and small-step learning environment. Good boundaries make us feel safe, willing to try, liked whether we fully succeed or not, trust our helpers and caregivers, and most importantly, know that when we are asked to do something we will likely be successful because we have some strategies of how to go about learning. The support functions of PROMPT include physical, emotional, and communication domains. These are depicted and described in Figure 36A–2.

Hayden, D. (1999). *PROMPT Manual Level 2.* Santa Fe, NM: PROMPT Institute.

APPENDIX 36–2

Hierarchy for Finger Tapping Therapy (as specified by Simmons [1978])

1. Patient watches and listens as clinician says each word of sentence, holding one finger up for every word.
2. Unison production.
3. Client production with mimed verbal production by clinician or unison finger counting by clinician.
4. Patient counts off words while choosing written words in proper sequence.
5. Clinician presents a question to which the patient must respond with the practiced sentence using finger counting.

APPENDIX 36–3

Eight-Step Task Continuum with Integral Stimulation (as specified by Rosenbek et al. [1973])

1. Integral stimulation (Watch me, Listen to me) followed by unison production.
2. Integral stimulation. Clinician supports patient's delayed response with mime.
3. Integral stimulation. Patient produces response without support.
4. Integral stimulation followed by successive unsupported productions by patient.
5. Written stimulus with unison production.
6. Written stimulus is provided but is removed before patient responds.
7. Utterance is elicited by a question.
8. Utterance is elicited in role playing.

Subject Index

In this index, *italic* page numbers designate figures; page numbers followed by the letter "t" designate tables; (*see also*) cross-references designate related topics or more detailed subtopic breakdowns.

Author Index

Note: The author index includes only persons whose names appear in the text. Additional co-authors are found following the senior authors' names in the reference list at the end of each chapter.

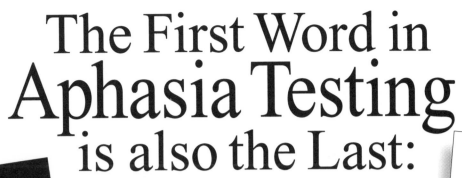
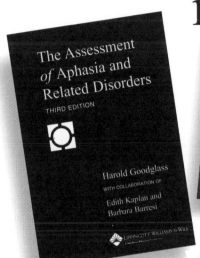
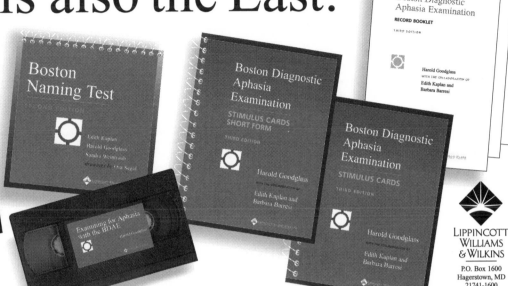